Lecture Notes in Computer Science 9349

More information about this series at http://www.springer.com/series/7412

Nassir Navab · Joachim Hornegger
William M. Wells · Alejandro F. Frangi (Eds.)

Medical Image Computing and Computer-Assisted Intervention – MICCAI 2015

18th International Conference
Munich, Germany, October 5–9, 2015
Proceedings, Part I

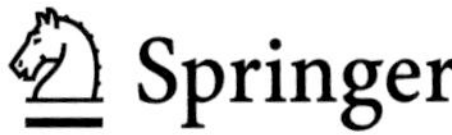

Editors
Nassir Navab
Technische Universität München
Garching
Germany

William M. Wells
Brigham and Women's Hospital
Harvard Medical School
Boston
USA

Joachim Hornegger
Friedrich-Alexander-Universität Erlangen-Nürnberg
Erlangen
Germany

Alejandro F. Frangi
University of Sheffield
Sheffield
UK

ISSN 0302-9743 ISSN 1611-3349 (electronic)
Lecture Notes in Computer Science
ISBN 978-3-319-24552-2 ISBN 978-3-319-24553-9 (eBook)
DOI 10.1007/978-3-319-24553-9

Library of Congress Control Number: 2015949456

LNCS Sublibrary: SL6 – Image Processing, Computer Vision, Pattern Recognition, and Graphics

Springer Cham Heidelberg New York Dordrecht London

Printed on acid-free paper

Springer International Publishing AG Switzerland is part of Springer Science+Business Media
(www.springer.com)

Preface

In 2015, the 18th International Conference on Medical Image Computing and Computer-Assisted Intervention (MICCAI 2015) was held in Munich, Germany. It was organized by the Technical University Munich (TUM) and the Friedrich Alexander University Erlangen-Nuremberg (FAU). The meeting took place in the Philharmonic Hall "Gasteig" during October 6-8, one week after the world-famous Oktoberfest. Satellite events associated with MICCAI 2015 took place on October 5 and October 9 in the Holiday Inn Hotel Munich City Centre and Klinikum rechts der Isar. MICCAI 2015 and its satellite events attracted word-leading scientists, engineers, and clinicians, who presented high-standard papers, aiming at uniting the fields of medical image processing, medical image formation, and medical robotics.

This year the triple anonymous review process was organized in several phases. In total, 810 valid submissions were received. The review process was handled by one primary and two secondary Program Committee members for each paper. It was initiated by the primary Program Committee member, who assigned a minimum of three expert reviewers. Based on these initial reviews, 79 papers were directly accepted and 248 papers were rejected. The remaining papers went to the rebuttal phase, in which the authors had the chance to respond to the concerns raised by reviewers. The reviews and associated rebuttals were subsequently discussed in the next phase among the reviewers leading to the acceptance of another 85 papers and the rejection of 118 papers. Subsequently, secondary Program Committee members issued a recommendation for each paper by weighing both the reviewers' recommendations and the authors' rebuttals. This resulted in "accept" for 67 papers and in "reject" for 120 papers. The remaining 92 papers were discussed at a Program Committee meeting in Garching, Germany, in May 2015, where 36 out of 75 Program Committee members were present. During two days, the 92 papers were examined by experts in the respective fields resulting in another 32 papers being accepted. In total 263 papers of the 810 submitted papers were accepted which corresponds to an acceptance rate of 32.5%.

The frequency of primary and secondary keywords is almost identical in the submitted, the rejected, and the accepted paper pools. The top five keywords of all submissions were machine learning (8.3%), segmentation (7.1%), MRI (6.6%), and CAD (4.9%).

The correlation between the initial keyword counts by category and the accepted papers was 0.98. The correlation with the keyword distribution of the rejected papers was 0.99. The distributions of the intermediate accept and reject phases was also above 0.9 in all cases, i.e., there was a strong relationship between the submitted paper categories and the finally accepted categories. The keyword frequency was essentially not influenced by the review decisions. As a conclusion, we believe the review process was fair and the distribution of topics reflects no favor of any particular topic of the conference.

This year we offered all authors the opportunity of presenting their work in a five-minute talk. These talks were organized in 11 parallel sessions setting the stage for further scientific discussions during the poster sessions of the main single-track conference. Since we consider all of the accepted papers as excellent, the selection of long oral presentations representing different fields in a single track was extremely challenging. Therefore, we decided to organize the papers in these proceedings in a different way than in the conference program. In contrast to the conference program, the proceedings do not differentiate between poster and oral presentations. The proceedings are only organized by conference topics. Only for the sake of the conference program did we decide on oral and poster presentations. In order to help us in the selection process, we asked the authors to submit five-minute short presentations. Based on the five-minute presentations and the recommendations of the reviewers and Program Committee members, we selected 36 papers for oral presentation. We hope these papers to be to some extent representative of the community covering the entire MICCAI spectrum. The difference in raw review score between the poster and oral presentations was not statistically significant ($p > 0.1$). In addition to the oral presentation selection process, all oral presenters were asked to submit their presentations two months prior to the conference for review by the Program Committee who checked the presentations thoroughly and made suggestions for improvement.

Another feature in the conference program is the industry panel that features leading members of the medical software and device companies who gave their opinions and presented their future research directions and their strategies for translating scientific observations and results of the MICCAI community into medical products.

We thank Aslı Okur, who did an excellent job in the preparation of the conference. She took part in every detail of the organization for more than one year. We would also like to thank Andreas Maier, who supported Joachim Hornegger in his editorial tasks following his election as president of the Friedrich Alexander University Erlangen-Nuremberg (FAU) in early 2015. Furthermore, we thank the local Organizing Committee for arranging the wonderful venue and the MICCAI Student Board for organizing the additional student events ranging from a tour to the BMW factory to trips to the world-famous castles of Neuschwanstein and Linderhof. The workshop, challenge, and tutorial chairs did an excellent job in enriching this year's program. In addition, we thank the MICCAI society for provision of support and insightful comments as well as the Program Committee for their support during the review process. Last but not least, we thank our sponsors for the financial support that made the conference possible.

We look forward to seeing you in Istanbul, Turkey in 2016!

October 2015

Nassir Navab
Joachim Hornegger
William M. Wells
Alejandro F. Frangi

Organization

General Chair

Nassir Navab	Technische Universität München, Germany

General Co-chair

Joachim Hornegger	Friedrich-Alexander-Universität Erlangen-Nürnberg, Germany

Program Chairs

Nassir Navab	Technische Universität München, Germany
Joachim Hornegger	Friedrich-Alexander-Universität Erlangen-Nürnberg, Germany
William M. Wells	Harvard Medical School, USA
Alejandro F. Frangi	University of Sheffield, Sheffield, UK

Local Organization Chairs

Ralf Stauder	Technische Universität München, Germany
Aslı Okur	Technische Universität München, Germany
Philipp Matthies	Technische Universität München, Germany
Tobias Zobel	Friedrich-Alexander-Universität Erlangen-Nürnberg, Germany

Publication Chair

Andreas Maier	Friedrich-Alexander-Universität Erlangen-Nürnberg, Germany

Sponsorship and Publicity Chairs

Stefanie Demirci	Technische Universität München, Germany
Su-Lin Lee	Imperial College London, UK

Workshop Chairs

Purang Abolmaesumi	University of British Columbia, Canada
Wolfgang Wein	ImFusion, Germany
Bertrand Thirion	Inria, France
Nicolas Padoy	Université de Strasbourg, France

Challenge Chairs

Björn Menze	Technische Universität München, Germany
Lena Maier-Hein	German Cancer Research Center, Germany
Bram van Ginneken	Radboud University, The Netherlands
Valeria De Luca	ETH Zurich, Switzerland

Tutorial Chairs

Tom Vercauteren	University College London, UK
Tobias Heimann	Siemens Corporate Technology, USA
Sonia Pujol	Harvard Medical School, USA
Carlos Alberola	University of Valladolid, Spain

MICCAI Society Board of Directors

Stephen Aylward	Kitware, Inc., NY, USA
Simon Duchesne	Université Laval, Quebéc, Canada
Gabor Fichtinger (Secretary)	Queen's University, Kingston, ON, Canada
Alejandro F. Frangi	University of Sheffield, Sheffield, UK
Polina Golland	MIT, Cambridge, MA, USA
Pierre Jannin	INSERM/INRIA, Rennes, France
Leo Joskowicz	The Hebrew University of Jerusalem
Wiro Niessen (Executive Director)	Erasmus MC - University Medical Centre, Rotterdam, The Netherlands
Nassir Navab	Technische Universität, München, Germany
Alison Noble (President)	University of Oxford, Oxford, UK
Sebastien Ourselin (Treasurer)	University College, London, UK
Xavier Pennec	INRIA, Sophia Antipolis, France
Josien Pluim	Eindhoven University of Technology, The Netherlands
Dinggang Shen	UNC, Chapel Hill, NC, USA
Li Shen	Indiana University, IN, USA

MICCAI Society Consultants to the Board

Alan Colchester	University of Kent, Canterbury, UK
Terry Peters	University of Western Ontario, London, ON, Canada
Richard Robb	Mayo Clinic College of Medicine, MN, USA

MICCAI Society Staff

Society Secretariat	Janette Wallace, Canada
Recording Secretary	Jackie Williams, Canada
Fellows Nomination Coordinator	Terry Peters, Canada

Program Committee

Acar, Burak
Barbu, Adrian
Ben Ayed, Ismail
Castellani, Umberto
Cattin, Philippe C.
Chung, Albert C.S.
Cootes, Tim
de Bruijne, Marleen
Delingette, Hervé
Fahrig, Rebecca
Falcão, Alexandre
Fichtinger, Gabor
Gerig, Guido
Gholipour, Ali
Glocker, Ben
Greenspan, Hayit
Hager, Gregory D.
Hamarneh, Ghassan
Handels, Heinz
Harders, Matthias
Heinrich, Mattias Paul
Huang, Junzhou
Ionasec, Razvan
Isgum, Ivana
Jannin, Pierre
Joshi, Sarang
Joskowicz, Leo
Kamen, Ali
Kobashi, Syoji
Langs, Georg
Li, Shuo
Linguraru, Marius George
Liu, Huafeng
Lu, Le
Madabhushi, Anant
Maier-Hein, Lena
Martel, Anne
Masamune, Ken
Moradi, Mehdi
Nielsen, Mads
Nielsen, Poul
Niethammer, Marc
Ourselin, Sebastien
Padoy, Nicolas
Papademetris, Xenios
Paragios, Nikos
Pernus, Franjo
Pohl, Kilian
Preim, Bernhard
Prince, Jerry
Radeva, Petia
Rohde, Gustavo
Sabuncu, Mert Rory
Sakuma, Ichiro

Salcudean, Tim
Salvado, Olivier
Sato, Yoshinobu
Schnabel, Julia A.
Shen, Li
Stoyanov, Danail
Studholme, Colin
Syeda-Mahmood, Tanveer
Taylor, Zeike
Unal, Gozde
Van Leemput, Koen
Wassermann, Demian
Weese, Jürgen
Wein, Wolfgang
Wu, Xiaodong
Yang, Guang Zhong
Yap, Pew-Thian
Yin, Zhaozheng
Yuan, Jing
Zheng, Guoyan
Zheng, Yefeng

Additional Reviewers

Abolmaesumi, Purang
Achterberg, Hakim
Acosta-Tamayo, Oscar
Aerts, Hugo
Afacan, Onur
Afsari, Bijan
Aganj, Iman
Ahad, Md. Atiqur Rahman
Ahmidi, Narges
Aichert, André
Akbari, Hamed
Akhondi-Asl, Alireza
Aksoy, Murat
Alam, Saadia
Alberola-López, Carlos
Aljabar, Paul
Allan, Maximilian
Allassonnieres, Stephanie
Antani, Sameer
Antony, Bhavna
Arbel, Tal
Auvray, Vincent
Awate, Suyash
Azzabou, Noura
Bagci, Ulas
Bai, Wenjia
Baka, Nora
Balocco, Simone
Bao, Siqi
Barmpoutis, Angelos
Bartoli, Adrien
Batmanghelich, Kayhan
Baust, Maximilian
Baxter, John
Bazin, Pierre-Louis
Berger, Marie-Odile
Bernal, Jorge
Bernard, Olivier
Bernardis, Elena
Bhatia, Kanwal
Bieth, Marie
Bilgic, Berkin
Birkfellner, Wolfgang
Blaschko, Matthew
Bloch, Isabelle
Boctor, Emad
Bogunovic, Hrvoje
Bouarfa, Loubna
Bouix, Sylvain
Bourgeat, Pierrick
Brady, Michael
Brost, Alexander
Buerger, Christian
Burgert, Oliver
Burschka, Darius
Caan, Matthan
Cahill, Nathan
Cai, Weidong
Carass, Aaron
Cardenes, Ruben

Cardoso, Manuel Jorge
Carmichael, Owen
Caruyer, Emmanuel
Cathier, Pascal
Cerrolaza, Juan
Cetin, Mustafa
Cetingul, Hasan Ertan
Chakravarty, M. Mallar
Chamberland, Maxime
Chapman, Brian E.
Chatelain, Pierre
Chen, Geng
Chen, Shuhang
Chen, Ting
Cheng, Jian
Cheng, Jun
Cheplygina, Veronika
Chicherova, Natalia
Chowdhury, Ananda
Christensen, Gary
Chui, Chee Kong
Cinar Akakin, Hatice
Cinquin, Philippe
Ciompi, Francesco
Clarkson, Matthew
Clarysse, Patrick
Cobzas, Dana
Colliot, Olivier
Commowick, Olivier
Compas, Colin
Corso, Jason
Criminisi, Antonio
Crum, William
Cuingnet, Remi
Daducci, Alessandro
Daga, Pankaj
Dalca, Adrian
Darkner, Sune
Davatzikos, Christos
Dawant, Benoit
Dehghan, Ehsan
Deligianni, Fani
Demirci, Stefanie
Depeursinge, Adrien
Dequidt, Jeremie
Descoteaux, Maxime
Deslauriers-Gauthier, Samuel
DiBella, Edward
Dijkstra, Jouke
Ding, Kai
Ding, Xiaowei
Dojat, Michel
Dong, Xiao
Dowling, Jason
Dowson, Nicholas
Du, Jia
Duchateau, Nicolas
Duchesne, Simon
Duncan, James S.
Dzyubachyk, Oleh
Eavani, Harini
Ebrahimi, Mehran
Ehrhardt, Jan
Eklund, Anders
El-Baz, Ayman
El-Zehiry, Noha
Ellis, Randy
Elson, Daniel
Erdt, Marius
Ernst, Floris
Eslami, Abouzar
Fallavollita, Pascal
Fang, Ruogu
Fenster, Aaron
Feragen, Aasa
Fick, Rutger
Figl, Michael
Fischer, Peter
Fishbaugh, James
Fletcher, P. Thomas
Florack, Luc
Fonov, Vladimir
Forestier, Germain
Fradkin, Maxim
Franz, Alfred
Freiman, Moti
Freysinger, Wolfgang
Fripp, Jurgen
Frisch, Benjamin
Fritscher, Karl

Fundana, Ketut
Gamarnik, Viktor
Gao, Fei
Gao, Mingchen
Gao, Yaozong
Gao, Yue
Gaonkar, Bilwaj
Garvin, Mona
Gaser, Christian
Gass, Tobias
Gatta, Carlo
Georgescu, Bogdan
Gerber, Samuel
Ghesu, Florin-Cristian
Giannarou, Stamatia
Gibaud, Bernard
Gibson, Eli
Gilles, Benjamin
Ginsburg, Shoshana
Girard, Gabriel
Giusti, Alessandro
Goh, Alvina
Goksel, Orcun
Goldberger, Jacob
Golland, Polina
Gooya, Ali
Grady, Leo
Gray, Katherine
Grbic, Sasa
Grisan, Enrico
Grova, Christophe
Gubern-Mérida, Albert
Guevara, Pamela
Guler, Riza Alp
Guo, Peifang B.
Gur, Yaniv
Gutman, Boris
Gómez, Pedro
Hacihaliloglu, Ilker
Haidegger, Tamas
Hajnal, Joseph
Hamamci, Andac
Hammers, Alexander
Han, Dongfeng
Hargreaves, Brian
Hastreiter, Peter
Hatt, Chuck
Hawkes, David
Hayasaka, Satoru
Haynor, David
He, Huiguang
He, Tiancheng
Heckel, Frank
Heckemann, Rolf
Heimann, Tobias
Heng, Pheng Ann
Hennersperger, Christoph
Holden, Matthew
Hong, Byung-Woo
Honnorat, Nicolas
Hoogendoorn, Corné
Hossain, Belayat
Hossain, Shahera
Howe, Robert
Hu, Yipeng
Huang, Heng
Huang, Xiaojie
Huang, Xiaolei
Hutter, Jana
Ibragimov, Bulat
Iglesias, Juan Eugenio
Igual, Laura
Iordachita, Iulian
Irving, Benjamin
Jackowski, Marcel
Jacob, Mathews
Jain, Ameet
Janoos, Firdaus
Janowczyk, Andrew
Jerman, Tim
Ji, Shuiwang
Ji, Songbai
Jiang, Hao
Jiang, Wenchao
Jiang, Xi
Jiao, Fangxiang
Jin, Yan
Jolly, Marie-Pierre
Jomier, Julien
Joshi, Anand

Joshi, Shantanu
Jung, Claudio
K.B., Jayanthi
Kabus, Sven
Kadoury, Samuel
Kahl, Fredrik
Kainmueller, Dagmar
Kainz, Bernhard
Kakadiaris, Ioannis
Kandemir, Melih
Kapoor, Ankur
Kapur, Tina
Katouzian, Amin
Kelm, Michael
Kerrien, Erwan
Kersten-Oertel, Marta
Khan, Ali
Khurd, Parmeshwar
Kiaii, Bob
Kikinis, Ron
Kim, Boklye
Kim, Edward
Kim, Minjeong
Kim, Sungmin
King, Andrew
Klein, Stefan
Klinder, Tobias
Kluckner, Stefan
Kobayahsi, Etsuko
Konukoglu, Ender
Kumar, Puneet
Kunz, Manuela
Köhler, Thomas
Ladikos, Alexander
Landman, Bennett
Lang, Andrew
Lapeer, Rudy
Larrabide, Ignacio
Lasser, Tobias
Lauze, Francois
Lay, Nathan
Le Reste, Pierre-Jean
Lee, Han Sang
Lee, Kangjoo
Lee, Su-Lin
Lefkimmiatis, Stamatis
Lefèvre, Julien
Lekadir, Karim
Lelieveldt, Boudewijn
Lenglet, Christophe
Lepore, Natasha
Lesage, David
Li, Gang
Li, Jiang
Li, Quanzheng
Li, Xiang
Li, Yang
Li, Yeqing
Liang, Liang
Liao, Hongen
Lin, Henry
Lindeman, Robert
Lindner, Claudia
Linte, Cristian
Litjens, Geert
Liu, Feng
Liu, Jiamin
Liu, Jian Fei
Liu, Jundong
Liu, Mingxia
Liu, Sidong
Liu, Tianming
Liu, Ting
Liu, Yinxiao
Lombaert, Herve
Lorenz, Cristian
Lorenzi, Marco
Lou, Xinghua
Lu, Yao
Luo, Xiongbiao
Lv, Jinglei
Lüthi, Marcel
Maass, Nicole
Madooei, Ali
Mahapatra, Dwarikanath
Maier, Andreas
Maier-Hein (né Fritzsche), Klaus Hermann
Majumdar, Angshul
Malandain, Gregoire

Mansi, Tommaso
Mansoor, Awais
Mao, Hongda
Mao, Yunxiang
Marchesseau, Stephanie
Margeta, Jan
Marini Silva, Rafael
Mariottini, Gian Luca
Marsden, Alison
Marsland, Stephen
Martin-Fernandez, Marcos
Martí, Robert
Masutani, Yoshitaka
Mateus, Diana
McClelland, Jamie
McIntosh, Chris
Medrano-Gracia, Pau
Meier, Raphael
Mendizabal-Ruiz, E. Gerardo
Menegaz, Gloria
Menze, Bjoern
Meyer, Chuck
Miga, Michael
Mihalef, Viorel
Miller, James
Miller, Karol
Misaki, Masaya
Modat, Marc
Moghari, Mehdi
Mohamed, Ashraf
Mohareri, Omid
Moore, John
Morales, Hernán G.
Moreno, Rodrigo
Mori, Kensaku
Morimoto, Masakazu
Murphy, Keelin
Müller, Henning
Nabavi, Arya
Nakajima, Yoshikazu
Nakamura, Ryoichi
Napel, Sandy
Nappi, Janne
Nasiriavanaki, Mohammadreza
Nenning, Karl-Heinz
Neumann, Dominik
Neumuth, Thomas
Ng, Bernard
Nguyen Van, Hien
Nicolau, stephane
Ning, Lipeng
Noble, Alison
Noble, Jack
Noblet, Vincent
O'Donnell, Lauren
O'Donnell, Thomas
Oda, Masahiro
Oeltze-Jafra, Steffen
Oh, Junghwan
Oktay, Ayse Betul
Okur, Aslı
Oliver, Arnau
Olivetti, Emanuele
Onofrey, John
Onogi, Shinya
Orihuela-Espina, Felipe
Otake, Yoshito
Ou, Yangming
Ozarslan, Evren
Pace, Danielle
Papa, Joao
Parsopoulos, Konstantinos
Paul, Perrine
Paulsen, Rasmus
Peng, Tingying
Pennec, Xavier
Peruzzo, Denis
Peter, Loic
Peterlik, Igor
Petersen, Jens
Petitjean, Caroline
Peyrat, Jean-Marc
Pham, Dzung
Piella, Gemma
Pitiot, Alain
Pizzolato, Marco
Plenge, Esben
Pluim, Josien
Poline, Jean-Baptiste
Prasad, Gautam

Prastawa, Marcel
Pratt, Philip
Preiswerk, Frank
Preusser, Tobias
Prevost, Raphael
Prieto, Claudia
Punithakumar, Kumaradevan
Putzer, David
Qian, Xiaoning
Qiu, Wu
Quellec, Gwenole
Rafii-Tari, Hedyeh
Rajchl, Martin
Rajpoot, Nasir
Raniga, Parnesh
Rapaka, Saikiran
Rathi, Yogesh
Rathke, Fabian
Rauber, Paulo
Reinertsen, Ingerid
Reinhardt, Joseph
Reiter, Austin
Rekik, Islem
Reyes, Mauricio
Richa, Rogério
Rieke, Nicola
Riess, Christian
Riklin Raviv, Tammy
Risser, Laurent
Rit, Simon
Rivaz, Hassan
Robinson, Emma
Roche, Alexis
Rohling, Robert
Rohr, Karl
Ropinski, Timo
Roth, Holger
Rousseau, François
Rousson, Mikael
Roy, Snehashis
Rueckert, Daniel
Rueda Olarte, Andrea
Ruijters, Daniel
Samaras, Dimitris
Sarry, Laurent
Sato, Joao
Schaap, Michiel
Scheinost, Dustin
Scherrer, Benoit
Schirmer, Markus D.
Schmidt, Frank
Schmidt-Richberg, Alexander
Schneider, Caitlin
Schneider, Matthias
Schultz, Thomas
Schumann, Steffen
Schwartz, Ernst
Sechopoulos, Ioannis
Seiler, Christof
Seitel, Alexander
Sermesant, Maxime
Seshamani, Sharmishtaa
Shahzad, Rahil
Shamir, Reuben R.
Sharma, Puneet
Shen, Xilin
Shi, Feng
Shi, Kuangyu
Shi, Wenzhe
Shi, Yinghuan
Shi, Yonggang
Shin, Hoo-Chang
Simpson, Amber
Singh, Vikas
Sinkus, Ralph
Slabaugh, Greg
Smeets, Dirk
Sona, Diego
Song, Yang
Sotiras, Aristeidis
Speidel, Michael
Speidel, Stefanie
Špiclin, Žiga
Staib, Lawrence
Stamm, Aymeric
Staring, Marius
Stauder, Ralf
Stayman, J. Webster
Steinman, David
Stewart, James

Styles, Iain
Styner, Martin
Su, Hang
Suinesiaputra, Avan
Suk, Heung-Il
Summers, Ronald
Sun, Shanhui
Szekely, Gabor
Sznitman, Raphael
Takeda, Takahiro
Talbot, Hugues
Tam, Roger
Tamura, Manabu
Tang, Lisa
Tao, Lingling
Tasdizen, Tolga
Taylor, Russell
Thirion, Bertrand
Thung, Kim-Han
Tiwari, Pallavi
Toews, Matthew
Toh, Kim-Chuan
Tokuda, Junichi
Tong, Yubing
Tornai, Gábor János
Tosun, Duygu
Totz, Johannes
Tournier, J-Donald
Toussaint, Nicolas
Traub, Joerg
Troccaz, Jocelyne
Tustison, Nicholas
Twinanda, Andru Putra
Twining, Carole
Ukwatta, Eranga
Umadevi Venkataraju, Kannan
Unay, Devrim
Urschler, Martin
Uzunbas, Mustafa
Vaillant, Régis
Vallin Spina, Thiago
Vallotton, Pascal
Van assen, Hans
Van Ginneken, Bram
Van Tulder, Gijs
Van Walsum, Theo
Vandini, Alessandro
Vannier, Michael
Varoquaux, Gael
Vegas-Sánchez-Ferrero, Gonzalo
Venkataraman, Archana
Vercauteren, Tom
Veta, Mtiko
Vignon-Clementel, Irene
Villard, Pierre-Frederic
Visentini-Scarzanella, Marco
Viswanath, Satish
Vitanovski, Dime
Voigt, Ingmar
Von Berg, Jens
Voros, Sandrine
Vrtovec, Tomaz
Wachinger, Christian
Waechter-Stehle, Irina
Wahle, Andreas
Wang, Ancong
Wang, Chaohui
Wang, Haibo
Wang, Hongzhi
Wang, Junchen
Wang, Li
Wang, Liansheng
Wang, Lichao
Wang, Linwei
Wang, Qian
Wang, Qiu
Wang, Song
Wang, Yalin
Wang, Yuanquan
Wee, Chong-Yaw
Wei, Liu
Wels, Michael
Werner, Rene
Wesarg, Stefan
Westin, Carl-Fredrik
Whitaker, Ross
Whitney, Jon
Wiles, Andrew
Wörz, Stefan
Wu, Guorong

Wu, Haiyong
Wu, Yu-Chien
Xie, Yuchen
Xing, Fuyong
Xu, Yanwu
Xu, Ziyue
Xue, Zhong
Yagi, Naomi
Yamazaki, Takaharu
Yan, Pingkun
Yang, Lin
Yang, Ying
Yao, Jianhua
Yaqub, Mohammad
Ye, Dong Hye
Yeo, B.T. Thomas
Ynnermann, Anders
Young, Alistair
Yushkevich, Paul
Zacharaki, Evangelia
Zacur, Ernesto
Zelmann, Rina
Zeng, Wei
Zhan, Liang
Zhan, Yiqiang
Zhang, Daoqiang
Zhang, Hui
Zhang, Ling
Zhang, Miaomiao
Zhang, Pei
Zhang, Shaoting
Zhang, Tianhao
Zhang, Tuo
Zhang, Yong
Zhao, Bo
Zhao, Wei
Zhijun, Zhang
Zhou, jinghao
Zhou, Luping
Zhou, S. Kevin
Zhou, Yan
Zhu, Dajiang
Zhu, Hongtu
Zhu, Yuemin
Zhuang, ling
Zhuang, Xiahai
Zuluaga, Maria A.

Contents – Part I

Advanced MRI: Diffusion, fMRI, DCE

Computer Assisted and Image-Guided Interventions

Computer Aided Diagnosis I: Machine Learning

Contents – Part II

Computer Aided Diagnosis II: Automation

Registration: Method and Advanced Applications

Modeling and Simulation for Diagnosis and Interventional Planning

Reconstruction, Image Formation, Advanced Acquisition - Computational Imaging

Contents – Part III

Quantitative Image Analysis I: Segmentation and Measurement

Quantitative Image Analysis II: Microscopy, Fluorescence and Histological Imagery

Quantitative Image Analysis III: Motion, Deformation, Development and Degeneration

Part I

Advanced MRI: Diffusion, fMRI, DCE

Automatic Segmentation of Renal Compartments in DCE-MRI Images

Xin Yang[1], Hung Le Minh[1], Tim Cheng[2], Kyung Hyun Sung[3], and Wenyu Liu[1]

[1] Huazhong University of Science and Technology, China
[2] University of California, Santa Barbara, USA
[3] University of California, Los Angeles, USA
xinyang2014@hust.edu.cn, leminhhung@hcmutrans.edu.vn,
timcheng@ece.ucsb.edu, ksung@mednet.ucla.edu,
liuwy@mail.hust.edu.cn

Abstract. In this paper, we introduce a method for automatic renal compartment segmentation from Dynamic Contrast-Enhanced MRI (DCE-MRI) images, which is an important problem but existing solutions cannot achieve high accuracy robustly for a wide range of data. The proposed method consists of three main steps. First, the whole kidney is segmented based on the concept of Maximally Stable Temporal Volume (MSTV). The proposed MSTV detects anatomical structures that are stable in both spatial domain and temporal dynamics. MSTV-based kidney segmentation is robust to noises and does not require a training phase. It can well adapt to kidney shape variations caused by renal dysfunction. Second, voxels in the segmented kidney are described by principal components (PCs) to remove temporal redundancy and noises. And then k-means clustering of PCs is applied to separate voxels into cortex, medulla and pelvis. Third, a refinement method is introduced to further remove noises in each segmented compartment. Experimental results on 16 clinical kidney datasets demonstrate that our method reaches a very high level of agreement with manual results and achieves superior performance to three existing baseline methods. The code of the proposed method will be made publicly available with the publication of this paper.

1 Introduction

DCE-MRI has been proved to be the most advantageous imaging modality of the pediatric kidney [1], providing one-stop comprehensive morphological and functional information, without the utilization of ionizing radiation. Accurate segmentation of renal compartments (i.e. cortex, medulla and renal pelvis) from DCE-MRI images is essential for functional kidney evaluation; however, there still lacks of effective and automatic solutions. Several limitations of DCE-MRI images make this task particularly challenging: 1) low spatial resolution, poor signal-to-noise ratio and partial volume effects due to fast and repeated scanning, 2) inhomogeneous intensity changes during perfusion in each compartment, especially for disordered kidneys.

Several papers in the literature tackle the problem of renal compartment segmentation. In [2], authors handled cortex segmentation as a multiple-surface extraction

N. Navab et al. (Eds.): MICCAI 2015, Part I, LNCS 9349, pp. 3–11, 2015.
DOI: 10.1007/978-3-319-24553-9_1

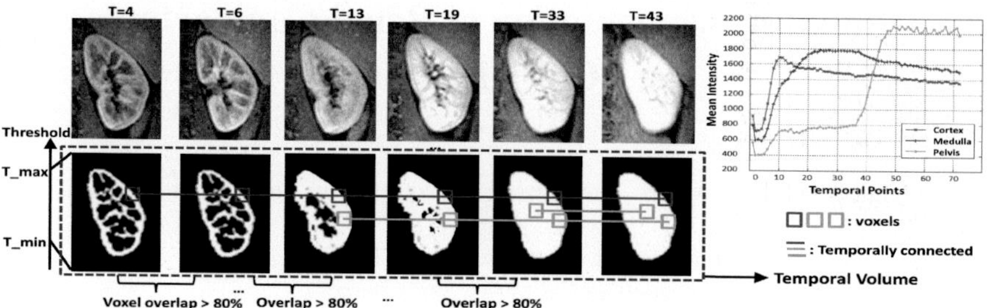

Fig. 1. (1) The top row on the left: a slice of DCE-MRI series taken at 6 temporal points 3, 6, 13, 19, 33 and 43. For this patient, 2448 abdomen images were taken over 72 temporal points. As time increases, the cortex, the medulla and the pelvis are highlighted sequentially. (2) The bottom row on the left: segmentation via thresholding. Red, green and blue rectangles denote voxels at three kidney locations. Voxels connected using solid lines are temporally connected. We define two segmented volumes are temporally connected if they are temporally adjacent and the voxel overlap between them is greater than 80%. A sequence of temporally connected volumes is denoted as a temporal volume (indicated in the purple dashed rectangle). (3) The right figure indicates typical time-intensity curves for compartments of a normal kidney.

problem, which is solved using the optimal surface search method based on a graph construction scheme. This method is primarily designed for 3D CT images and evaluated on CT data, thus valuable temporal information embedded in the intensity time courses of DCE-MRI images is not considered (i.e. the temporal intensity evolution is different for each of the three kidney compartments, as shown in the top row of the left part of Fig. 1 and the chart on the right part of Fig. 1). To address this problem, Sun et al. [3] proposed an energy function that exploits both the spatial correlation among voxels and the intensity change of every voxel across the image sequences. In [4] and [5], the authors employed k-means clustering of temporal intensity evolution to segment the three internal renal structures. However, those methods were evaluated only on normal kidneys; in practice they are sensitive to pathologies. Recently, Khrichenko et al. [1] presented a program, named CHOP-fMRU, for renal compartment segmentation and functional analysis. CHOP-fMRU involves several manual tasks (e.g. manual delineation of a rough kidney contour for initialization) and the quality of the segmentation and analysis results depends heavily on the quality of the manual tasks.

There have been numerous dedicated research efforts [6, 7, 8, 9, 10, 11] for automatic segmentation of whole kidneys. Some of the most popular ones rely on the shape and appearance models learned from a set of previously segmented kidneys. For instance, Spiegel et al. [11] learned the kidney mean shape and principal modes of variation via an Active Shape Model to constrain the segmentation results. Yuksel et al. [10] modeled the kidney shape and intensity distribution using a signed distance map and Gaussian mixture models, respectively. In [8, 9], the authors integrated shape priors into a geometric deformable model to extract the kidney region. Model-based approaches have demonstrated promising results for segmenting an entire healthy kidney. However, the structure of renal compartments is much more challenging to model than a whole kidney due to its high complexity and variability in shape, in particular for those of disordered kidneys. As a result, it's challenging for model-based methods to achieve satisfactory results for dysfunctional kidneys and for inner compartment segmentation.

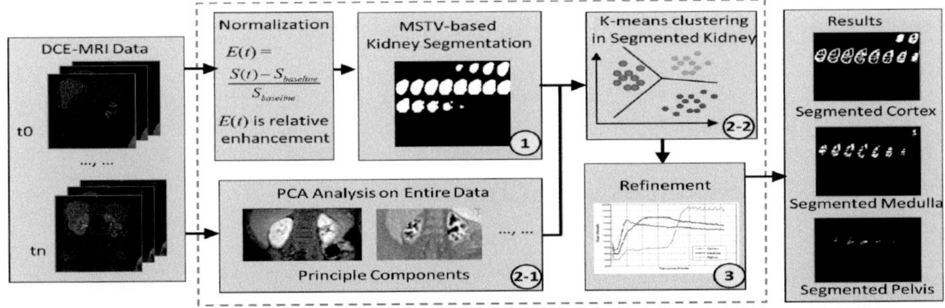

Fig. 2. Illustration of the proposed renal compartment segmentation framework

In this paper, we propose an automatic method which can segment renal compartments for DCE-MRI images from both healthy subjects and patients with kidney problems. The proposed method, which demonstrates excellent agreement with manual segmentation results, consists of three main steps, as illustrated in Fig. 2. First, a whole kidney is automatically segmented from abdominal images based on the detection of *Maximally Stable Temporal Volume* (MSTV). The proposed MSTV exploiting both 3D spatial correlation among voxels and temporal dynamics for each voxel to provide a reliable segmentation robust to noises from surrounding tissues and kidney shape variations. Second, voxels in the segmented kidney are described by N principal components (PCs) where N is an empirical parameter. Our extensive experimental results indicate that for all cases the first 10 PCs capture most information needed for renal compartment segmentation. Thus discarding the rest of the components can effectively remove temporal redundancy and suppress noises with little loss of useful information. K-means clustering of the PCs is then leveraged to cluster voxels into the cortex, the medulla and the pelvis respectively. Third, an effective and fast refinement method is proposed to remove noises in each segmented compartment. The proposed segmentation method has been tested using 16 clinical kidney data and compared with the manual results and the results produced by three baseline methods. The results of the proposed method show excellent agreement with the manual results and superior performance to the baseline methods.

2 Our 3-Step Method

2.1 Step 1 – Initial Segmentation Based on MSTV

As contrast agent perfuses into a kidney, intensity contrast between the kidney and its surrounding tissues are enhanced gradually (as shown in the top row of the left part of Fig. 1). As a result, when binarizing a 3D volume via thresholding after contrast injection, the voxels in the segmented kidney possess three characteristics: 1) they are stable across a wide range of thresholds (as shown in the bottom row of the left part of Fig. 1); 2) most of them are spatially connected (i.e. one voxel is among the other's 26 neighbors of another voxel in the segmented kidney); 3) a large portion of them appear in the temporally adjacent segmented volumes (i.e. having large voxel overlap in their temporal dynamics). In contrast, intensity enhancement of non-kidney tissues is

---

Pseudo Code 1: MSTV-based Whole Kidney Segmentation from a DCE-MRI series

---

Input: DCE-MRI data $\boldsymbol{V} = \{V_1, \dots V_{t-1}, \dots V_T\}$,
All possible thresholds $\boldsymbol{J} = \{1,\dots j,\dots J\}$, j is ranked in an increasing order
Parameters λ , τ and α
Output: Segmentation of a whole kidney
Procedure1: Connected Component Trees Construction
for $V_t = V_1, \dots V_T$
for $j = 1,\dots J$
Binarize V_t using threshold $j \rightarrow$ a list of connected voxels, $\{\dots (v_t^j)_i \dots\}$;
Insert $\{\dots (v_t^j)_i \dots\} \rightarrow$ the jth level of Tree Tr_t ;
Insert Tree $Tr_t \rightarrow$ Connected Component Trees $\boldsymbol{Tr} = \{Tr_1, \dots Tr_t\}$
Procedure2: Maximum Stable Temporal Volumes Detection
for $j = 1,\dots J$
Find temporally connected sequence $\vartheta_j^k = \{\dots, v_{t-1}^j, \dots\}_k$ $(1 \le k \le K)$
K is the total number of temporal volumes in level j
Transverse $\boldsymbol{Tr}$ from root to the level J to detect M sequences of nested temporal volume $\{\vartheta_1, \dots, \vartheta_{j-1}, \vartheta_j \dots\}_m$ $(1 \le m \le M)$
Calculate $S_m(j*)$ for each $\{\vartheta_1, \dots, \vartheta_{j-1}, \vartheta_j \dots\}_m$
Search $m*$ which achieves maximum $S_m(j*)$,and sequence is $\{\vartheta_{j*-\beta_{j*}}, \dots, \vartheta_{j*}\}_{m*}$
Procedure3: MSTV-based Whole Kidney Segmentation
Construct histogram $\boldsymbol{H}=\{h_1,\dots,h_N\}$ for voxels in $\{\vartheta_{j*-\beta_{j*}}, \dots, \vartheta_{j*}\}_{m*}$, $N = |\vartheta_{j*}|$
for $\vartheta_k = \{\vartheta_{j*-\beta_{j*}}, \dots, \vartheta_{j*}\}_{m*}$
Update corresponding items of $\boldsymbol{H}$ for voxels appear in ϑ_k
Select voxels whose votes in $\boldsymbol{H}$ is greater than $\alpha \rightarrow$ whole kidney segmentation

---

rare and random; therefore, segmented non-kidney voxels are sensitive to thresholds, usually are not spatially connected and have small overlap in temporal domain. Based on the characteristics described above, in the following we describe a concept of *Maximally Stable Temporal Volume* (MSTV) and propose its application to whole kidney segmentation. Formal definitions *Temporal Volume* and MSTV are as follows:

1) **Temporal Volume.** We denote v_t $(1 \le t \le T)$ as a set of spatially connected voxels segmented from original 3D volume at temporal point t by thresholding. T is the total number of temporal points in a DCE-MRI series. We define v_{t-1}, v_t $(1 \le t-1 < t \le T)$ are *temporally connected* if v_{t-1}, v_t have greater than λ (λ is 80% in this study) segmented voxels in common (i.e. voxel overlap between them > λ). If a sequence $\vartheta = \{v_1, \dots, v_{t-1}, v_t\}$ $(t \ge 2)$ that any two temporally consecutive voxel sets in the sequence are *temporally connected*, we denote the sequence ϑ as a temporal volume. The cardinality of ϑ is defined as $|\vartheta| = \sum_1^t |v_i|$

2) **Maximally Stable Temporal Volume.** If ϑ_{j-1}, ϑ_j are two temporal volumes obtained using threshold j-1 and j respectively, and $v_1^{j-1} \subseteq v_1^j, \dots, v_{t-1}^{j-1} \subseteq v_{t-1}^j$, $v_t^{j-1} \subseteq v_t^j$, then ϑ_{j-1} is a subset of ϑ_j i.e. $\vartheta_{j-1} \subseteq \vartheta_j$. Let $\{\vartheta_1, \dots, \vartheta_{j-1}, \vartheta_j \dots\}_m$ $(1 \le m \le M)$

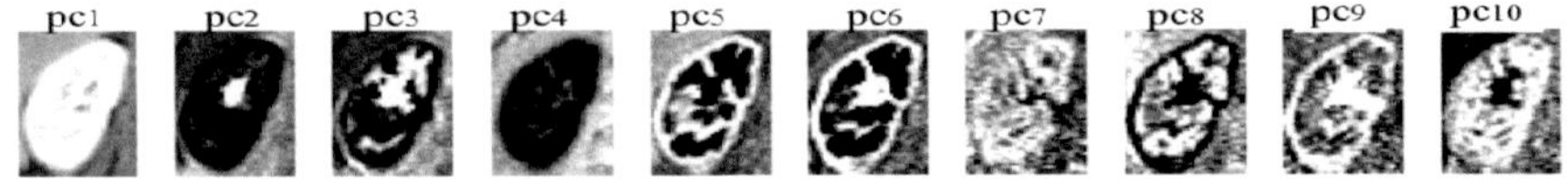

Fig. 3. First 10 PCs of a dynamic DCE-MRI data

be a sequence of nested temporal volumes, M is the total number of nested sequences detected in DCE-MRI data, the stability of the sequence is defined as:

$$S(j) = \beta_j \times |\vartheta_j| \tag{1}$$

Eq.(1) evaluates the stability of a segmentation, where β_j and $|\vartheta_j|$iindicate across how many consecutive thresholds and how many temporally adjacent trees the segmentation could remain stable respectively. We search $j*$ which provides maximum $S_m(j*)$ for $\{\vartheta_1, ..., \vartheta_{j-1}, \vartheta_j ...\}_m$. For all M sequences of nested temporal volumes, we select $m*$ which achieves a maximum $S_{m*}(j*)$ which implies a combination of both large cardinality of ϑ_{j*} and stability of ϑ_{j*} across a wide range of parameters.

The detection process of MSTV is illustrated in Pseudo Code 1. First, for every volumetric data at time t ($1 \le t \le T$), a *connected component tree* Tr_t is constructed by binarizing the volume v_t using all possible thresholds j's ($1 \le j \le J$,). A node at level j of tree Tr_t consists of a group of spatially connected voxels. Second, for every threshold i (i.e. level j of the trees), we transverse trees $\boldsymbol{Tr} = \{Tr_1, ... Tr_T\}$ along temporal axis to search for all temporal volumes. Then we transverse trees $\boldsymbol{Tr}$ vertically from roots to the last level J to detect MSTV. Third, we select voxels which appear in most temporal volumes in MSTV to form initial whole kidney segmentation. A dilation operation is also applied to fill holes inside the kidney segmentation.

Our MSTV can be considered as an extension of *Maximally Stable Extremal Region* (MSER) [13], one of the best interest point detectors in computer vision, from 2D to 4D. Meanwhile, we propose a MSTV detection method based on connected component trees and apply it for kidney segmentation. Our MSTV does not impose any shape constraints on the segmentation results, thus it can adapt to kidney shape variations caused by renal dysfunction.

2.2 Step 2 – PCA-kmeans Clustering for Renal Compartment Segmentation

Time intensity curves associated with the cortex, the medulla and the pelvis voxels are distinguishable from each other (as shown in the right chart of Fig.1). Therefore, they could be separated by unsupervised clustering of time intensity curves. However, the raw temporal data often has a high dimension, which increases the computation cost and induces numerical problems. Moreover, not all voxels of the same tissue are highlighted at the same moment, leading to misalignment of curves which belong to the same tissue and in turn resulting in mis-classification. In addition, most dimensions in the raw temporal data are redundant; the redundancy would dilute the useful information and disturb the true distribution.

To address these problems, we employ Principal Component Analysis (PCA) to reduce the dimension of the temporal data. Voxel features in the temporal dimension are then described by a set of principal components (PCs). PCA transforms the raw data into a new coordinate space, such that the greatest variance lies along the first coordinate (denoted as 1st PC), the second greatest variance along the second coordinate, and so on. By discarding the less significant components, PCA can reduce the dimension of dynamic data and suppress noises. In addition, by linearly combining several temporal dimensions to form a new feature dimension, misalignment can be avoided. Thorough analysis of our experimental results show that, for all cases we experimented with, greater than 99.4% of the total information is included in the first 10 PCs. As illustrated in Fig. 3, the 1st principal component captures most global information of a kidney, and the 2nd to the 10th components encode detailed information of inner structures. For the later PCs, the variances tend to be more dominantly affected by noise. Based on our experiment study, we choose 10 PCs for further analysis.

Once voxels in the segmented kidney are described by the first 10 PCs, unsupervised clustering is applied to separate voxels into three groups: the cortex, the medulla and the pelvis. Among a number of suitable clustering methods, we choose k-means clustering in this study due to its simplicity, efficiency and effectiveness.

2.3 Step 3 – Refinement

We propose a refinement method for removing noise induced in Step 1 and for recovering mis-classification due to ambiguous boundaries between clusters in the principal component space. The refinement method starts from the segmented cortex, to the medulla and then to the pelvis. First, for each candidate cortex voxel obtained in Step 2 we calculate its *maximum intensity enhancement* (MIE) by subtracting its pre-contrast intensity from its maximum intensity. Based on the fact that cortex voxels are mostly highlighted at similar moments, we compute the average intensity of all cortex voxels at each temporal point and select a point t_{max} whose average intensity reaches the maximum. We consider t_{max} and its neighboring temporal points $t_{max\text{-}1}$ and t_{max+1} as the candidate moments at which the cortex tissues are maximally highlighted. Accordingly, MIE for cortex voxel i is calculated based on Eq. (2):

$$MIE_{cortex}(i) = \max\left\{\left(S_{t_{max-1}}(i) - S_b(i)\right),\ \left(S_{t_{max}}(i) - S_b(i)\right),\ \left(S_{t_{max+1}}(i) - S_b(i)\right)\right\}\quad i \subset \{\text{candidate cortex voxels}\} \tag{2}$$

At $t_{max\text{-}1}$, t_{max} and t_{max+1}, the intensities of medulla and non-kidney tissues do not change too much from their pre-contrast intensities. Thus, at those moments, the MIE of voxels should be much smaller than the cortex voxels and hence can be easily excluded by thresholding. The threshold is automatically selected via the Otsu method [15]. Second, we attempt to recover the mis-detection of true cortex voxels. For every non-cortex voxel within the segmented kidney, we examine its spatially adjacent voxels. If all of them are labeled as cortex voxels after the noise removal step described above, we re-label it from a non-cortex to a cortex voxel. Similarly, this refinement method is also applied to the segmented medulla and pelvis.

3 Experimental Results

This study, approved by the local institutional review board, consists of evaluation of 16 kidney cases: 7 normal cases, 7 disordered cases, and 2 cases with operations where the medulla and the pelvis were removed. The MRI data acquisition was

Table 1. Comparison of Segmentation Methods

	Compartment	Our method	w/o MSTV	w/o PCA	Region Completion
Disordered Kidneys	Cortex	0.86	0.72	0.54	0.59
	Medulla	0.95	0.65	0.51	0.52
	Pelvis	0.69	0.54	0.56	0.60
Kidneys with Op.	Cortex	0.92	0.39	0.47	0.45
Healthy Kidneys	Cortex	0.97	0.74	0.58	0.49
	Medulla	0.98	0.74	0.51	0.52
	Pelvis	0.95	0.79	0.74	0.60

performed using a 3.0T GE MR 750 system. To minimize the risk of gadolinium in patients with impaired kidney function, a low dose at 1/5 of Gadovist was used as the contrast agent with the injection rate of 0.3 mL/s, followed by 10mL saline chaser at the same rate. The DCE-MRI data sets were acquired by ventilator controlled breath-hold and have sufficient temporal alignment in most cases. Bellows respiratory triggering was implemented resulting in a temporal phase every two respiratory cycles. A 3D T1-weighted gradient echo sequence with a dual-echo bipolar readout was used for data acquisition, and we used an in-house variable density Cartesian undersampling scheme called DISCO to perform high spatiotemporal resolution dynamic MRU [14]. A two-point Dixon reconstruction was used for robust fat–water separation. Imaging parameters were: flip angle is 15°, TR=3.56ms, matrix size=256×256, FOV= 340×340 mm^2, the total number of slices is 34, and slice thickness is 4 mm.

We evaluated the segmentation accuracy using the Dice Similarity Coefficient (DSC), a widely used metric to evaluate segmentation algorithms for different medical image modalities. The DSC is defined as:

$$DSC(S,G)=\frac{2\times|S\cap G|}{|S|+|G|} \tag{3}$$

where S and G represent the sets of automatically segmented voxels and manually segmented voxels respectively; $|\cdot|$ denotes the set cardinality. The DSC ranges from 0, if S and G do not overlap at all, to 1, if S and G are identical.

We compare our method with three baseline methods: Region Competition [12], a popular active contour method for segmentation, our method without MSTV-based kidney segmentation (denoted as w/o MSTV) and our method without PCA dimension reduction (denoted as w/o PCA). We used the implementation in ITK-SNAP for Region Competition. Since Region Competition is originally designed for 2D or 3D, but not 4D, data, we manually selected 3D volumes at those temporal points when the cortex, the parenchyma (i.e. the cortex and the medulla) and a whole kidney respectively seem maximally highlighted. Region Competition is applied to each 3D volume to segment the cortex, the parenchyma and a whole kidney; the medulla and the pelvis were obtained by subtracting the cortex from the segmented parenchyma, and by subtracting the parenchyma from the whole kidney, respectively.

Table 1 summarizes the average DSC for all four methods. Three observations can be made from Table 1. First, the DSC achieved by our method is over 0.9 for most cases except for the cortex (0.86) and the pelvis (0.69) of disordered kidneys. This might be because part of the cortex and pelvis tissues were not highlighted due to the

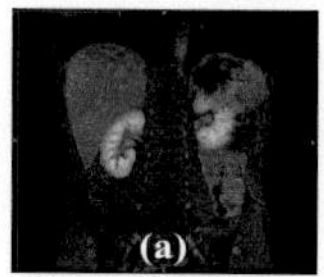

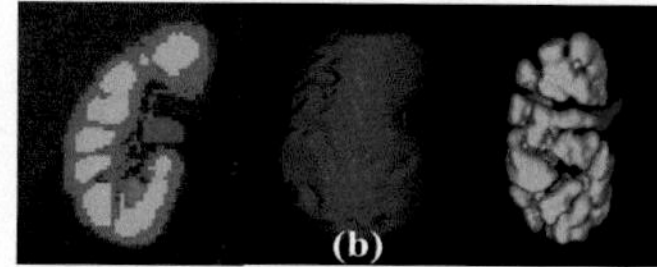

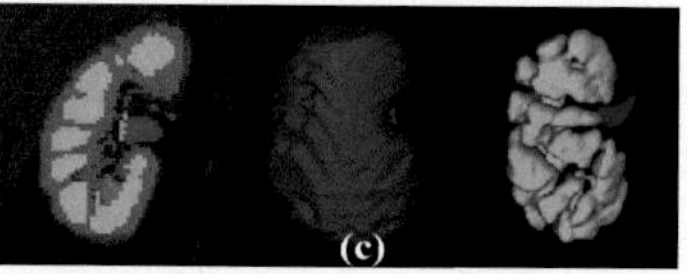

Fig. 4. (a) An exemplar abdominal image from DCE-MRI data. 2D and 3D segmentation of inner compartments based on (b) manual label and (c) our method.

renal disease, causing disconnection among voxels in the spatial and temporal domains. Second, MSTV and PCA dimension reduction are essential and complementary to accurate segmentation results, i.e. 14%~59% and 13%~48% improvements are achieved by using the MSTV-based whole kidney segmentation and by PCA dimension reduction, respectively. Third, the average DSC of our method is 9%~51% higher than those of Region Competition. We believe Region Competition's poor performance is mainly due to the highly varying contrast during perfusion. Although we manually selected the most relevant volumes in different phases of perfusion, it remains challenging to distinguish internal renal structures from a single image sequence. Fig. 4 illustrates an image from a DCE-MRI sequence and the corresponding segmentation results based on manual labeling (b) and our automatic method (c).

4 Conclusion and Future Work

We present a method for automatic renal compartment segmentation from DCE-MRI. The proposed method first segments a whole kidney based on the detection of MSTV. MSTV is a collection of spatially and temporally connected voxels that can be robustly segmented across a wide range of thresholds and temporal dynamics. Voxels in an MSTV well represents characteristics of kidney voxels and hence is applicable to whole kidney segmentation. MSTV-based kidney segmentation is robust to noises and can adapt to kidney shape variations due to renal dysfunction. With a whole kidney segmented, the proposed method clusters the segmented kidney voxels into three groups: the cortex, the medulla and the pelvis, via PCA and k-means clustering. Experimental results show that PCA plays an essential role for high segmentation accuracy. Finally, a refinement method based on maximum intensity enhancement is employed for removing noise and for recovering mis-detected kidney voxels. Our future work includes further acceleration of the current method, further accuracy improvement through renal compartment recognition, and proper motion correction via image registration.

References

1. Khrichenko, D., Darge, K.: Functional Analysis in MR Urography – Made Simple. Pediatr. Radiol. 40, 182–199 (2010)
2. Li, X., Chen, X., Yao, J., Zhang, X., Tian, J.: Renal cortex segmentation using optimal surface search with novel graph construction. In: Fichtinger, G., Martel, A., Peters, T. (eds.) MICCAI 2011, Part III. LNCS, vol. 6893, pp. 387–394. Springer, Heidelberg (2011)

3. Sun, Y., Moura, M.F., Yang, D., Ye, Q., Ho, C.: Kidney Segmentation in MRI Sequences using Temproal Dynamics. In: Proc. of IEEE ISBI, pp. 98–101 (2002)
4. Zollner, F.G., Sance, R., Rogelj, P., Ledesma-Carbayo, M.J., Rorvik, J., Santos, A., Lundervold, A.: Assessment of 3D DCE-MRI of the Kidneys using Non-rigid Image Registration and Segmentation of Voxel Time Courses. Comput. Med. Imag. and Gra., 171–181 (2009)
5. Chevaillier, B., Ponvianne, Y., Collette, J.L., Mandry, D., Claudon, M., Pietquin, O.: Functional Semi-automated Segmentation of Renal DCE-MRI Sequences. In: Proc. of ICASSP (2008)
6. Goceri, E.: Automatic Kidney Segmentation Using Gaussian Mixture Model on MRI Sequences. In: Electrical Power System and Computers, vol. 99, pp. 23–29 (2009)
7. Cuingnet, R., Prevost, R., Lesage, D., Cohen, L.D., Mory, B., Ardon, R.: Automatic detection and segmentation of kidneys in 3D CT images using random forests. In: Ayache, N., Delingette, H., Golland, P., Mori, K. (eds.) MICCAI 2012, Part III. LNCS, vol. 7512, pp. 66–74. Springer, Heidelberg (2012)
8. Mory, B., Somphone, O., Prevost, R., Ardon, R.: Real-Time 3D Image Segmentation by User-Constrained Template Deformation. In: Ayache, N., Delingette, H., Golland, P., Mori, K. (eds.) MICCAI 2012, Part I. LNCS, vol. 7510, pp. 561–568. Springer, Heidelberg (2012)
9. Khalifa, F., Elnakib, A., Beache, G.M., Gimel'farb, G., El-Ghar, M.A., Ouseph, R., Sokhadze, G., Manning, S., McClure, P., El-Baz, A.: 3D Kidney Segmentation from CT Images Using a Level Set Approach Guided by a Novel Stochastic Speed Function. In: Fichtinger, G., Martel, A., Peters, T. (eds.) MICCAI 2011, Part III. LNCS, vol. 6893, pp. 587–594. Springer, Heidelberg (2011)
10. Yuksel, S.E., El-Baz, A., Farag, A.A.: A Kidney Segmentation Framework for Dynamic Contrast Enhanced Magnetic Resonance Imaging. J. of Vibr. and Con. 12(9-10), 1505–1516 (2007)
11. Spiegel, M., Hahn, D., Daum, V., Wasza, J., Hornegger, J.: Segmentation of Kidneys using A New Active Shape Model Generation Technique based on Non-Rigid Image Registration. In: Comput. Med. Imaging Graph, vol. 33(1), pp. 29–39 (2009)
12. Zhu, S.C., Yullie, A.: Region Competition: Unifying Snakes, Region Growing, and Bayes/MDL for Multiband Image Segmentation. IEEE Trans. on PAMI, 884–900 (1996)
13. Matas, J., Chum, O., Urban, M., Pajdla, T.: Robust Wide Baseline Stereo from Maximally Stable Extremal Regions. In: Proc. of BMVC, pp. 384–396 (2002)
14. Saranathan, M., Rettmann, D.W., Hargreaves, B.A., Clarke, S.E., Vasanawala, S.S.: Differential Subsampling with Cartesian Ordering (DISCO): A High Spatio-Temporal Resolution Dixon Imaging Sequence for Multiphasic Contrast Enhanced Abdominal Imaging. J. Magn. Reson. Imaging 35(6), 1484–1492 (2012)
15. Otsu, N.: A Threshold Selection Method from Gray-Level Histograms. IEEE Trans. Sys. Man. Cyber 9(1), 62–66 (1979)

Harmonizing Diffusion MRI Data Across Multiple Sites and Scanners

Hengameh Mirzaalian, Amicie de Pierrefeu, Peter Savadjiev, Ofer Pasternak, Sylvain Bouix, Marek Kubicki, Carl-Fredrik Westin, Martha E. Shenton, and Yogesh Rathi

Harvard Medical School and Brigham and Women's Hospital, Boston, USA

Abstract. Harmonizing diffusion MRI (dMRI) images across multiple sites is imperative for joint analysis of the data to significantly increase the sample size and statistical power of neuroimaging studies. In this work, we develop a method to harmonize diffusion MRI data across multiple sites and scanners that incorporates two main novelties: i) we take into account the spatial variability of the signal (for different sites) in different parts of the brain as opposed to existing methods, which consider one linear statistical covariate for the entire brain; ii) our method is model-free, in that no *a-priori* model of diffusion (e.g., tensor, compartmental models, etc.) is assumed and the signal itself is corrected for scanner related differences. We use spherical harmonic basis functions to represent the signal and compute several rotation invariant features, which are used to estimate a regionally specific linear mapping between signal from different sites (and scanners). We validate our method on diffusion data acquired from four different sites (including two GE and two Siemens scanners) on a group of healthy subjects. Diffusion measures such fractional anisotropy, mean diffusivity and generalized fractional anisotropy are compared across multiple sites before and after the mapping. Our experimental results demonstrate that, for identical acquisition protocol across sites, scanner-specific differences can be accurately removed using the proposed method.

1 Introduction

Multi-site diffusion imaging studies are increasingly being used to study several disorders such, Alzheimer's disease, Huntington's disease, schizophrenia etc. However, intra-site variability in the acquired data sets poses a potential problem for joint analysis of diffusion MRI data [1,2]. Thus, aggregating data sets from different sites is challenging due to the inherent differences in the acquired images from different scanners. Although the inter-site variability of neuroanatomical measurements can be minimized by acquiring images using similar type of scanners (same vendor and version) with similar pulse sequence parameters and same field strength [3], many recent studies have shown that there still exist large differences between diffusion measurements from different sites [4]. This inter-site variability in the measurements can come from several sources, e.g., subject physiological motion, number of head coils used for

N. Navab et al. (Eds.): MICCAI 2015, Part I, LNCS 9349, pp. 12–19, 2015.
DOI: 10.1007/978-3-319-24553-9_2

measurement (16 or 32 channel head coil), imaging gradient non-linearity as well as scanner related factors [5]. This can cause non-linear changes in the images acquired as well as the estimated diffusion measures such as fractional anisotropy (FA) and mean diffusivity (MD). Inter-site variability in FA can be upto 5% in major white matter tracts and between 10-15% in gray matter areas [1]. On the other hand, FA differences in diseases such as schizophrenia are often of the order of 5%. Thus, harmonizing data across sites is imperative for joint analysis of the data.

Broadly, there are two approaches used to combine data sets from multiple sites. One approach is to perform the analysis at each site separately, followed by a meta-analysis as in [6]. Another standard practice is to use a statistical covariate to account for signal changes that are scanner-specific [7]. The first approach (meta-analysis) does not allow for a "true" joint analysis of the data, while the second method requires the use of a statistical covariate for each diffusion measure analyzed. Further, the latter method is inadequate to analyze results from tractography where tracts travel between distant regions. For example, in the cortico-spinal tract, scanner related differences in the brain stem might be quite different from those in the cortical motor region. Thus, using a single statistical covariate for the entire tract may produce false positive or false negative results. Consequently, region-specific scanner differences should be taken into account for such type of analyses. Another alternative is to add a statistical covariate at each voxel in a voxel based analysis method, however, such methods are susceptible to registration errors.

2 Our Contributions

In this work, we propose a novel scheme to harmonize diffusion MRI data from multiple scanners, taking into account the brain region-specific difference in the acquired signal from different scanners. Our method harmonizes the acquired signal at each site compared to a reference site using several rotation invariant spherical harmonic (RISH) features. A region specific linear mapping is proposed between the rotation invariant features to remove scanner specific differences in the white matter between a group of age-matched subjects at each site. The method uses model-free SH features[1] and thus is independent of any modeling assumptions, making it useful to be used for any type of future analysis (e.g., using single or multi-compartment models). To the best of our knowledge, this is a first work that has explicitly addressed the issue of dMRI data harmonization without the use of statistical covariates. Since the mapping is obtained from a set of healthy controls, it will not alter the signal due to disease or pathology, while ensuring that we do not directly modify model-based diffusion features such as FA, which are used in population studies [6].

[1]Note that spherical harmonics is a non-parametric basis and does not assume any particular *model* of diffusion as in the case of single tensor, or multi-compartment models (nothing a-priori is assumed about the diffusion process in terms of the compartments or number of fiber bundles).

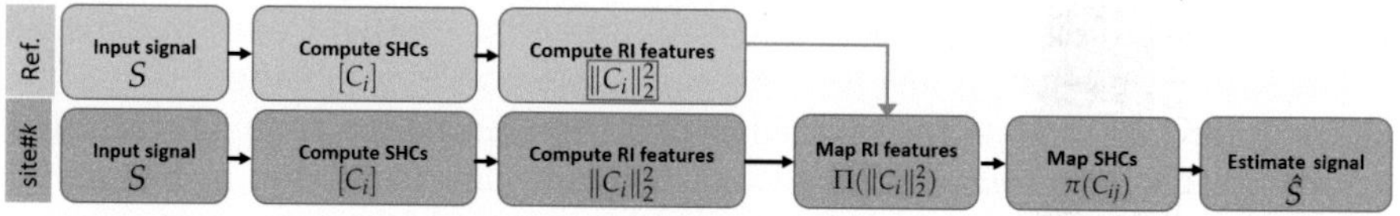

Fig. 1. Outline of the proposed method for inter-site dMRI data harmonization

3 Method

Figure 1 shows an outline of the proposed dMRI data harmonization method. Our goal is to map the dMRI data from a target site to an arbitrarily chosen reference site. We start by computing a set of rotation invariant spherical harmonic (RISH) features from the estimated SH coefficients. A region-specific linear mapping between the RISH features is then computed to map the dMRI data from target site to the reference site. Next, a secondary mapping is computed that appropriately updates each of the SH coefficients at each voxel in the brain. From the mapped SH coefficients, the mapped diffusion signal is computed at the desired set of gradient directions for each subject in the target site.

3.1 Diffusion MRI and RISH Features

Let $S = [s_1 ... s_G]^{\mathrm{T}}$ represent the dMRI signal along G unique gradient directions. In the spherical harmonic (SH) basis, the signal S can be written as [8]: $S \approx \sum_i \sum_j C_{ij} Y_{ij}$, where Y_{ij} is a SH basis function of order i and phase j and C_{ij} are the corresponding SH coefficients. It is well-known that the "energy" or $\mathbb{L}_2$ norm of the SH coefficients for each order forms a set of rotation invariant (RISH) features [9]:

$$\|C_i\|^2 = \sum_{j=1}^{2i+1} (C_{ij})^2. \tag{1}$$

One can think of the RISH features $\|C_i\|^2$ as being the total energy at a particular frequency (order) in the SH space. Given the RISH features for N_k subjects for the kth site (the target site), we compute the expected value as the sample mean:

$$\mathbb{E}_k([\|C_i\|^2]) = \sum_{n=1}^{N_k} [\|C_i(n)\|^2] / N_k. \tag{2}$$

In this work, we computed the RISH features for order $\{0, 2, 4, 6\}$ and ignored the higher order terms as they are the high frequency terms primarily capturing noise in the data. However, if required, the proposed methodology is quite general and can be extended to SH of any order.

3.2 Mapping RISH Features Between Sites

Figure 2 shows the RISH features of different orders computed for each site as well as for different anatomical regions of the brain. In particular, we used

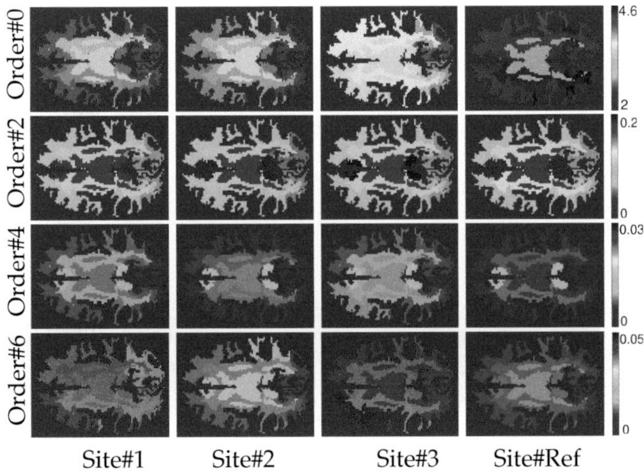

Fig. 2. RISH features in the white matter for different SH orders and sites.

Freesurfer [10] software to parcellate the brain into different regions and subsequently grouped them into the following anatomical regions for each hemisphere: frontal, parietal, temporal, occipital, brain stem, cerebellum, the cingulate-corpus-callosum complex and centrumsemiovale-insula. For each of these white matter regions and for each site, we computed the sample average $\mathbb{E}_k(\cdot)$ (Eq. 2) of the RISH features shown in Figure 2. Clearly, these features vary significantly between sites as well as for different regions, showing that a regionally specific mapping is required to ensure proper harmonization of the diffusion data.

Given two groups of subjects that are matched for age, gender, handedness and socio-economic status, we expect that at a group level, they will have similar diffusion profiles and hence none of the RISH features should be statistically different between any two sites (or scanners). In other words, the diffusion measures between two groups of matched subjects (healthy) are statistically different only due to scanner differences. Thus, our aim is to find a proper mapping $\Pi(\cdot)$ for the RISH features such that all scanner related group differences between two sites are removed, i.e.,

$$\mathbb{E}_k(\Pi(\|C_i\|^2)) = \mathbb{E}_r(\|C_i\|^2), \tag{3}$$

where r is the reference site and k is the target site. Any difference in the sample mean for the two sites (or scanners) k and r can be computed as the difference $\Delta\mathbb{E} = \mathbb{E}_r - \mathbb{E}_k$. By linearity of the expectation operator, the mapping for each subject n is given by:

$$\Pi(\|C_i(n)\|^2) = \|C_i(n)\|^2 + \mathbb{E}_r - \mathbb{E}_k. \tag{4}$$

Note that, this mapping $\Pi(\cdot)$ only gives the amount of shift required to remove any scanner specific "group" differences. Thus, this mapping is only at the population level and a separate mapping is required that will change the individual SH coefficient at each voxel such that equation Eq. 4 is satisfied . We should also note that the mapping $\Pi(\cdot)$ is different for different RISH features even for the same ROI. For a subject n, we have the following map:

$$\Pi(\|C_i(n)\|^2) = \sum_{j=1}^{2i+1} \pi(C_{ij}(n)^2) = \|C_i(n)\|^2 + \Delta\mathbb{E} = \sum_{j=1}^{2i+1} C_{ij}(n)^2 + \Delta\mathbb{E}. \quad (5)$$

We extend this mapping to each voxel in an ROI, by uniformly changing the SH coefficients at each voxel v (we do not include the voxel indexing in our equations to keep the notation simple). There are two possible ways to obtain a mapping $\pi(\cdot)$ for each SH coefficient C_{ij}. One possibility is to use $\pi(C_{ij}) = C_{ij} + \delta$ (for all j) such that Eq. 5 is satisfied. However, this would entail adding a positive or negative constant δ to all coefficients (i.e. shifting the coefficients), which could potentially lead to a change in sign for coefficients that are smaller than δ. The effect of such a "shifting" operation is shown in Figure 3 (b), where the sign of some of the coefficients was changed by adding a small constant δ. This leads to a change in orientation and shape of the signal, which is erroneous and undesirable.

A better mapping $\pi(\cdot)$ is to uniformly scale all the SH coefficients (belonging to a given SH order) so that Eq. 5 is satisfied. Such a mapping is given by:

$$\pi(C_{ij}) = \ell C_{ij}, \quad \text{where:} \quad \ell = \sqrt{\frac{\Pi(\|C_i(n)\|^2)}{\|C_i(n)\|^2}}. \quad (6)$$

Such scaling only changes the "size" of the signal and not its orientation, as seen in Figure 3 and as shown via experiments in the results section. The harmonized diffusion signal at each voxel v of a given ROI (for each subject n) is then computed using the mapped coefficients using $\hat{S}(v,n) = \sum_i \sum_j \pi(C_{ij}(v,n))Y_{ij}$. Such a unique mapping is computed for each ROI and each subject in the target site.

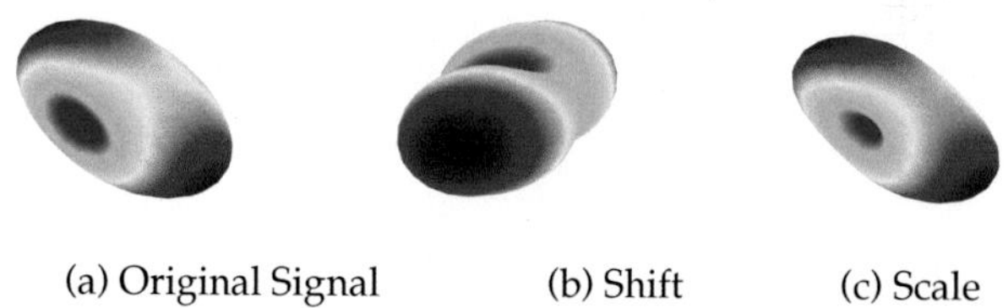

(a) Original Signal (b) Shift (c) Scale

Fig. 3. Effect of using different mapping functions π - shift vs scale. (a) Original dMRI signal. (b) π used as a shift map, (c) Estimated signal with π as a scaling map (Eq. 6).

4 Results

We used our method on data set acquired from 4 different sites and scanners; see Table 1 for details about each scanner as well as the number of subjects from each site. Nearly identical dMRI scan protocol was used at each site with the following acquisition parameters: spatial resolution of $2 \times 2 \times 2\text{mm}^3$, maximum b-value of $b = 900s/\text{mm}^2$ and $TE/TR = 87/10000$ ms. For the GE sites, the data was acquired with a 5/8 partial Fourier encoding, while the Siemens used 6/8 partial Fourier acquisition. Subjects at each site were age-matched to the group at the reference site.

Table 1. Scanner details and subject numbers for each site.

Site#	Manufacturer	Field strength	Model	Software version	# of channels	# of subjects	# of directions
1	GE	3T	MR750	20xM4	8	10	86
2	GE	3T	MR750	M4	8	6	86
3	Siemens	3T	Tim Trio (102x32)	vb17	12	14	87
Ref.	Siemens	3T	Tim Trio (102x18)	VB15	12	10	87

An appropriate mapping was computed for each of the ROIs (obtained from Freesurfer) in each hemisphere of the brain as defined earlier. We tested our method by computing the p-value for the RISH features as well as standard diffusion measures. For each ROI, we computed if the RISH features were statistically different between the reference site and each of the target sites (site #1, #2, #3) and then used the algorithm described above to obtain the mapped signal. Due to space limitations, we have not provided the p-values for the RISH features in this paper, but all statistical differences were removed after the mapping. We also extensively tested our method on diffusion features that were not explicitly used in the mapping procedure, such as MD, FA, GFA and tensor orientation.

Table 2. P-values before and after mapping for MD, FA, GFA for different sites and ROIs.

	MD						FA						GFA					
	Site#1		Site#2		Site#3		Site#1		Site#2		Site#3		Site#1		Site#2		Site#3	
	Before	After	Before	After	Before	After	Before	After	Before	After	Before	After	Before	After	Before	After	Before	After
lFrontal	**2.4e-06**	1	**1.7e-08**	1	**1.6e-07**	1	0.45	0.54	**2.8e-02**	0.43	0.21	0.93	**6.0e-16**	0.4	**6.9e-03**	0.62	**2.6e-08**	0.49
lParietal	**6.5e-08**	1	**2.5e-07**	1	**1.1e-07**	1	**1.0e-04**	0.25	**7.8e-04**	0.27	**1.5e-03**	0.41	**1.5e-08**	0.77	6.3e-02	0.53	**1.1e-09**	0.66
lTemporal	**5.4e-09**	1	**3.3e-08**	1	**5.4e-08**	1	0.18	0.47	**3.9e-02**	0.95	**6.4e-02**	0.71	**3.8e-09**	0.75	5.6e-02	0.84	**4.2e-08**	0.73
lOccipital	**7.1e-06**	1	**2.2e-02**	1	**8.7e-07**	1	6.4e-02	0.81	**2.7e-02**	0.76	**3.3e-02**	0.81	**2.8e-08**	0.93	0.82	0.85	**1.6e-06**	0.97
lCentrumSemi.	**1.5e-10**	1	**8.9e-08**	1	**2.0e-08**	1	**4.7e-03**	0.62	**1.3e-05**	0.90	**1.3e-02**	0.93	**2.2e-12**	0.93	0.42	0.7	**7.8e-09**	0.74
lCerebellum	**5.6e-07**	1	**8.6e-05**	1	**1.7e-07**	1	0.79	0.34	0.77	0.72	**3.3e-02**	0.73	**7.5e-09**	0.86	6.4e-02	0.86	**1.1e-07**	0.92
rFrontal	**4.8e-06**	1	**1.7e-08**	1	**5.8e-10**	1	0.19	0.61	8.6e-02	0.39	0.13	0.18	**4.0e-09**	0.89	**1.4e-03**	0.71	**1.0e-09**	0.23
rParietal	**1.6e-06**	1	**2.1e-06**	1	**1.8e-07**	1	**2.8e-02**	0.51	**1.4e-03**	0.84	7.7e-02	0.54	**1.8e-07**	0.91	0.2	0.94	**4.5e-09**	0.62
rTemporal	**1.4e-06**	1	**7.4e-05**	1	**1.6e-06**	1	0.55	0.39	**9.6e-03**	0.77	0.63	0.65	**4.4e-08**	0.86	7.5e-02	0.96	**5.9e-08**	0.62
rOccipital	**5.5e-05**	1	**1.3e-02**	1	**3.0e-02**	1	9.6e-02	0.91	1.2e-02	0.83	0.38	0.81	**5.0e-07**	0.89	7.4e-02	0.75	**4.2e-09**	0.71
rCentrumSemi.	**8.7e-13**	1	**7.0e-09**	1	**3.7e-10**	1	**8.5e-04**	0.98	**8.8e-04**	0.83	**2.2e-03**	0.78	**6.4e-10**	0.68	0.25	0.61	**5.5e-06**	0.50
rCerebellum	**1.3e-06**	1	**4.9e-04**	1	0.11	1	0.27	0.59	0.79	0.87	**8.5e-04**	0.95	**5.1e-08**	0.98	0.10	0.91	**1.8e-08**	0.90
BrainStem	**5.6e-10**	1	**7.4e-06**	1	**1.2e-05**	1	**2.4e-04**	0.67	**7.6e-04**	0.99	0.49	0.80	**2.2e-06**	0.65	0.22	0.88	**4.0e-08**	0.64

Table 2 gives the p-values for each of the ROIs (nomenclature – lFrontal is left-frontal and rFrontal is right-frontal lobe) before and after the harmonization of the data. Notice that MD was statistically different for almost all regions and sites as compared to the reference site, but these differences were completely removed. The p-value after mapping is almost 1 in this case following Eq. 6 and the fact that MD is directly proportional to the $\mathbb{L}_2$ norm of the SH coefficients. All statistical group differences between FA and GFA are also removed for each of the sites.

We also ran a TBSS study [11] for the FA values for each of the sites. Figure 4 shows widespread group differences between the subjects from the reference

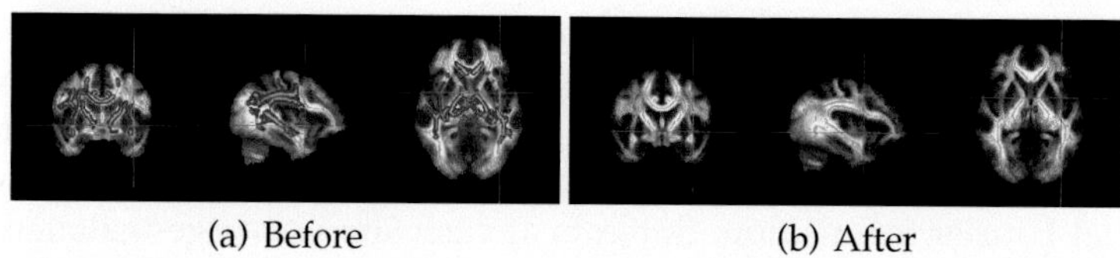

(a) Before (b) After

Fig. 4. TBSS results for site #1 before (a) and after (b) applying our method. The yellow-red colormap displays p-values less than 0.05. Only white matter regions were used in this work, and sub-cortical gray matter regions were not harmonized resulting in a statistical group difference in that region in (b).

site (Siemens scanner) and site #1 (GE scanner). After data harmonization, most white matter group differences were removed confirming the results seen in Table 2. However, group differences in the sub-cortical regions are still seen, as that region was not "harmonized" or mapped for scanner differences. Extending the current methodology to gray matter and sub-cortical region is part of our future work.

We also compared the average error in degrees in the orientation of the fibers (estimated using the single tensor model and SH-based orientation distribution function (ODF)) at each voxel, before and after the mapping. For the tensor based model, the average change in orientation at each voxel was always less that 1° resulting in the following average whole brain change in orientation for each site $0.7606 \pm 0.1250^\circ$, $0.1400 \pm 0.0830^\circ$ and $0.7259 \pm 0.2180^\circ$, respectively. Change in orientations estimated from the discretized ODF's were 0.24e-5°, 0.17e-5° and 0.26e-5°, respectively for each site. We also computed the coefficient of variation (CV) in FA [1] for each site before and after the harmonization procedure (CV, before: $0.0321 \pm 0.0121, 0.0285 \pm 0.0137, 0.0579 \pm 0.0097$ and after 0.0315 ± 0.0114, 0.0272 ± 0.0142, 0.0595 ± 0.0128 respectively). Thus the within site CV did not change much after the mapping.

5 Conclusion and Limitations

In this work, we proposed a novel method that allows to harmonize the dMRI signal from different sites in a region-specific, subject-dependent manner, while maintaining the inter-subject variability at each site but removing scanner specific differences in the signal. Once such a mapping is computed from healthy subjects, it can then be used to map another cohort of diseased subjects without altering the signal due to disease or pathology. The proposed method is model independent and directly maps the signal to the reference site. The method can be of great use to aggregate data from multiple sites and making it feasible to do joint analysis of a large sample of data. We should note that, to the best of our knowledge, this is a first work that has explicitly addressed the issue of dMRI data harmonization without the use of statistical covariates.

Nevertheless, the proposed method has some limitations that we note: 1). It is dependent on the accuracy of Freesurfer segmentations, 2). It is possible that the

ROIs used in this work are too large to remove local scanner-specific differences. One way to address this concern is to test if any sub-region within an ROI is still statistically different between two sites and subsequently obtain a separate mapping for such "smaller ROIs". In this work, we did not harmonize gray matter and sub-cortical structures, however, the proposed method is general enough to be applied to these areas of the brain as well. Our future work will involve ways to address all these limitations. Further, the proposed method can be used to separately harmonize each b-value shell for multi-shell diffusion data.

References

1. Vollmar, C., Muircheartaigh, J., Barker, G., Symms, M., Thompson, P., Kumari, V., Duncan, J., Richardson, M., Koepp, M.: Identical, but not the same: Intra-site and inter-site reproducibility of fractional anisotropy measures on two 3.0 T scanners. NeuroImage, 1384–1394 (2010)
2. Matsui, J.: Development of image processing tools and procedures for analyzing multi-site longitudinal diffusion-weighted imaging studies. Phd Thesis, University of IowaFollow (2014)
3. Cannon, T., McEwen, F.S.S., Abd, G., He, X.P., Erp, T., Jacobson, A., Beardon, C., Walker, E.: Reliability of neuroanatomical measurements in a multi-site longitudinal study of youth at risk for psychosis. Human Brain Mapping 35, 2424–2434 (2014) (in press)
4. Foxa, R., Sakaieb, K., Leec, J., Debbinse, J., Liuf, Y., Arnoldg, D., Melhem, E., Smithh, C., Philipsb, M., Loweb, M., Fisherd, E.: A validation study of multicenter diffusion tensor imaging: Reliability of fractional anisotropy and diffusivity values. AJNR Am. J. Neuroradiol. 33, 695–700 (2012)
5. Zhu, T., Hu, R., Qiu, X., Taylor, M., Tso, Y., Yiannoutsos, C., Navia, B., Mori, S., Ekholm, S., Schifitto, G., Zhong, J.: Quantification of accuracy and precision of multicenter dti measurements: a diffusion phantom and human brain study. Neuroimage 56, 1398–1411 (2011)
6. Salimi-Khorshidi, G., Smith, S., Keltner, J., Wager, T., Nichols, T.: Meta-analysis of neuroimaging data: a comparison of image-based and coordinate-based pooling of studies. Neuroimage 25, 810–823 (2009)
7. Forsyth, J., Cannon, T., et al.: Reliability of functional magnetic resonance imaging activation during working memory in a multi-site study: analysis from the north american prodrome longitudinal study. Neuroimage 97, 41–52 (2014)
8. Descoteaux, M., Angelino, E., Fitzgibbons, S., Deriche, R.: Regularized, fast, and robust analytical q-ball imaging. MRM 58, 497–510 (2007)
9. Kazhdan, M., Funkhouser, T., Rusinkiewicz, S.: Rotation invariant spherical harmonic representation of 3D shape descriptors. In: Symposium on Geometry Processing (2003)
10. Fischl, B., Liu, A., Dale, A.: Automated manifold surgery: Constructing geometrically accurate and topologically correct models of the human cerebral cortex. IEEE TMI 20, 70–80 (2001)
11. Smitha, S., Jenkinsona, M., Johansen-Berga, H., Rueckertb, D., Nicholsc, T., Mackaya, C., Watkinsa, K., Ciccarellid, O., Cadera, Z., Matthewsa, P., Behrensa, T.: Tract-based spatial statistics: Voxelwise analysis of multi-subject diffusion data. NeuroImage 31, 1487–1505 (2006)

Track Filtering via Iterative Correction of TDI Topology

Dogu Baran Aydogan and Yonggang Shi

Laboratory of Neuro Imaging, USC Stevens Neuroimaging and Informatics Institute, Keck School of Medicine, University of Southern California, Los Angeles, USA

Abstract. We propose a new technique to clean outlier tracks from fiber bundles reconstructed by tractography. Previous techniques were mainly based on computing pair-wise distances and clustering methods to identify unwanted tracks, which relied heavy upon user inputs for parameter tuning. In this work, we propose the use of topological information in track density images (TDI) to achieve a more robust filtering of tracks. There are two main steps of our iterative algorithm. Given a fiber bundle, we first convert it to a TDI, then extract and score its critical points. After that, tracks that contribute to high scoring loops are identified and removed using the Reeb graph of the level set surface of the TDI. Our approach is geometrically intuitive and relies only on a single parameter that enables the user to decide on the length of insignificant loops. In our experiments, we use our method to reconstruct the optic radiation in human brain using the multi-shell HARDI data from the human connectome project (HCP). We compare our results against spectral filtering and show that our approach can achieve cleaner reconstructions. We also apply our method to 215 HCP subjects to test for asymmetry of the optic radiation and obtain statistically significant results that are consistent with post-mortem studies.

Keywords: Computational topology, Tractography, Topological filtering.

1 Introduction

Tractography has become a widely used technique to study neurological and neurosurgical pathologies. However its anatomical accuracy is known to be limited [1], its reproducibility has not been throughly studied [2], and obtaining quantitative measures is still a big challenge [3]. The accuracy and reliability are continuously improved by means of devising better tractography techniques [4,5] and validating tracks against the diffusion signal [6,7,8]. In addition to these efforts, there have been numerous studies made to improve and utilize the already available tractography information. So far this problem has been addressed mainly from three different angles: (i) restricting and identifying tracks using anatomical region of interest (ROIs) [9,10]; (ii) defining pairwise similarity measures between tracks and clustering [11,12,13]; (iii) hybrid use of (i) and (ii) [14]. In addition, there have also been approaches proposed in the literature using Dirichlet processes [15].

N. Navab et al. (Eds.): MICCAI 2015, Part I, LNCS 9349, pp. 20–27, 2015.
DOI: 10.1007/978-3-319-24553-9_3

We propose in this work a new technique that uses tools from computational topology to detect and remove outlier tracks. One key property of our method is the incorporation of track density imaging (TDI) [16] for topological analysis. To the best of our knowledge, there has not been any study in the literature that uses the topological information obtained from TDI for the analysis of fiber tracks. Our technique identifies and preserves relevant and coherent bundles without the use of a track similarity measure nor anatomical ROIs. By identifying and iteratively correcting the topology of TDI, we show that competitive and promising results are obtained with a single user defined parameter.

2 Methods

Overview of the Approach: Fig. 1 shows the flowchart for the whole process to remove unwanted tracks. Starting from a set of tracks and a user defined threshold for the maximum allowed loop length, the method iteratively cleans the tracks until no more track can be removed. The process starts with the computation of TDI, then the critical points of TDI are computed. Local maxima and minima correspond to points where densest and least dense tracks exist. Whereas saddles correspond to points where loops are completed. For each loop, we compute a geodesic distance as a score. If there is no loop with a larger score than the threshold, the iteration is stopped; otherwise we compute a Reeb graph to identify the points on the loop and get a list of tracks to remove. After cleaning these tracks, we repeat the same process until no more removal is possible.

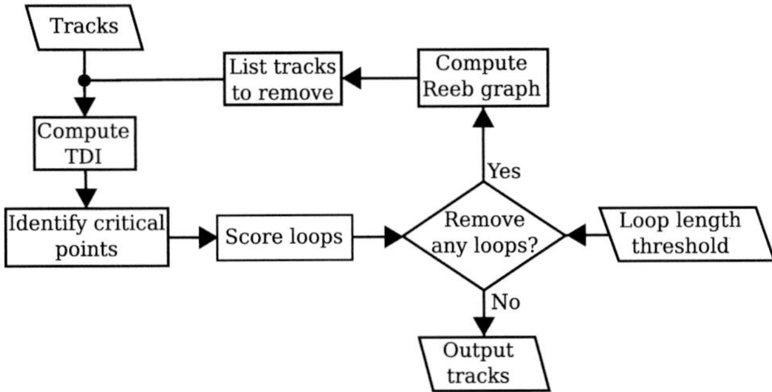

Fig. 1. The process iteratively computes TDI, removes loops larger than the threshold and updates TDI for new iteration until no more removal is possible.

Track Density Imaging (TDI): TDI is a technique to acquire super-resolution images from diffusion MRI [16]. Because TDI boosts anatomical contrast, it is mainly used to perform virtual histologies [17]. Another aspect of TDI is that, it is a representation of track densities on rectangular lattice, thus a conversion from tractography domain to a scalar field on regular image domain. To obtain TDI, we used MRTrix's `tracks2prob` command with `-template` argument [18].

Topology of Scalar Fields: If M is an n-manifold and $f\colon M \to \mathbb{R}$ is a smooth mapping then a point $p \in M$ is called a *critical point* if all the partial derivatives of f at p are 0. A mapping $f\colon M \to \mathbb{R}$ is a *Morse function* if all its critical points are *nondegenerate*, that is $\det H_f(p) \neq 0$ where $H_f(p)$ is the Hessian matrix. A Morse function can be obtained by perturbation in which a very small number is added to each data point according to its location. Morse lemma states that nondegenerate critical points are isolated; thus Morse functions have finitely many critical points which can be computed to fully learn the topological properties of such scalar fields [19]. Fig. 2 shows all possible nondegenerate critical points on a 3-manifold. For each critical point, the *index*, $\gamma(p)$, that is the number of the negative eigenvalues of $H_f(p)$, is written on top.

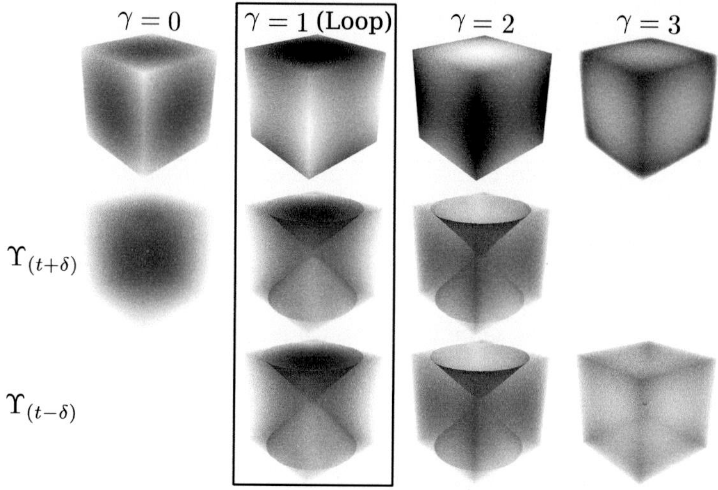

Fig. 2. For a Morse function f, all possible critical points, p, are shown on the first row with their indices on top. Upper ($\Upsilon_{(t+\delta)}$) and lower ($\Upsilon_{(t-\delta)}$) level sets are shown on the second and third rows (for $t = f(p)$ and δ being a small positive number). The case where a loop forms by tracks in TDI is shown in the box.

Localization of Loops: The indices of critical points outline the topology of a scalar field. $\gamma = 0$ and $\gamma = 3$ are local minima and maxima where level sets vanish and appear. These points correspond to least dense and densest points in TDI. $\gamma = 1$ and $\gamma = 2$ are saddles where level sets split and merge. In a TDI, these points correspond to loops generated by tracks ($\gamma = 1$) and empty space ($\gamma = 2$), thus our focus are the critical points with $\gamma = 1$. Fig. 2 shows this case in a box. To find all the critical points, two sweeps are needed, one from top to bottom and another from bottom to top. However, because we are only interested in the critical points with $\gamma = 1$, a single sweep from top to bottom is sufficient. Algorithm 1 shows how to identify critical points for detecting loops.

Computation of Loop Lengths and Scoring: We continue by computing loop lengths. In order to do this, we reconstruct a surface mesh for the upper

Algorithm 1. Identification of critical points for loop detection

Input : I: track density image
Output: $\mathcal{L}_{ind}$, $\mathcal{L}^{\rightarrow}_{ind}$, $\mathcal{L}^{\leftarrow}_{ind}$: Indices of critical points with $\gamma = 1$ ($\mathcal{L}_{ind}$) and indices of two voxels ($\mathcal{L}^{\rightarrow}_{ind}$, $\mathcal{L}^{\leftarrow}_{ind}$) that are joined together

Set $\mathcal{L}_{ind} = \mathcal{L}^{\rightarrow}_{ind} = \mathcal{L}^{\leftarrow}_{ind} = \{\}$;
Perturb and sort the elements of I in descending order to form the index list I_d;
Initialize an empty union-find data structure, UF;
for $i = I_d(first) \rightarrow I_d(last)$ **do**
    Set $Region = \{\}$;
    for $n =$ *neighbors of* i **do**
        Add $UF_{\text{Find}}(n)$ to $Region$;
    if $Region = \{\}$ **then** // the case for $\gamma = 0$
        Add i to UF;
    else if *Region has 1 element* **then** // the case for a regular point
        $UF_{\text{Union}}(i, Region)$;
    else // the case for $\gamma = 1$
        Add i to $\mathcal{L}_{ind}$;
        Add different *Region* elements to $\mathcal{L}^{\rightarrow}_{ind}$ and $\mathcal{L}^{\leftarrow}_{ind}$;
        $UF_{\text{Union}}(i, Region)$;

level set (Fig. 2 for $\gamma = 1$ and $\Upsilon_{(t+\delta)}$). Knowing the two end points of the loop, $\mathcal{L}^{\rightarrow}_{ind}$, $\mathcal{L}^{\leftarrow}_{ind}$ from Algorithm 1, we compute the geodesic distance, thus the length of the loop which is used for scoring.

Reeb Graphs: To obtain the points on the loop, we compute the Reeb graph of the lower level set (Fig. 2 for $\gamma = 1$ and $\Upsilon_{(t-\delta)}$). A Reeb graph is an intuitive graph representation of the topological properties of a manifold, M [19]. For a Morse function $f\colon M \rightarrow \mathbb{R}$, the Reeb graph, is defined as the quotient space with its topology defined through the equivalent relation $x \simeq y$ if $f(x) = f(y)$ for $\forall x, y \in M$. Here we used the Laplace-Beltrami (LB) eigenfunctions as the Morse function, f. We used the algorithms proposed in [20] for accurate reconstruction the surfaces, computation of LB and the Reeb graph.

3 Test Subjects and Data Preparation

We used the multi-shell HARDI data provided by the human connectome project (HCP) between Q1-Q3 [21] to test our method. This release includes 225 subjects, however, only 215 subjects completed both T1 and dMRI scans. We used these 215 subjects' dMRI data for fiber bundle reconstruction. In order to fully utilize the multi-shell HARDI data and obtain very sharp fiber orientation distributions (FODs), we used the recently proposed algorithm in [22]. This method represents FODs by spherical harmonics (SPHARM) and is fully compatible with existing tools developed for tractography.

We focused on the reconstruction of clean fiber bundles that represent the optic radiation in human brains. To obtain the tracks, we used the probabilistic tractography tool in MRTrix [18] between two automatically generated ROIs:

lateral geniculate nucleus (LGN) and primary visual cortex (V1) [23]. One salient feature of the optic radiation is that its fibers are organized retinotopically as they travel from the LGN to the visual cortex. The optic radiation is often considered as composed of three sub-bundles: superior, central, and inferior bundles that correspond to the inferior, foveal, and superior part of the visual field. Most notably the Meyer's loop of the inferior bundle first courses anteriorly before it runs posteriorly toward the visual cortex. This unconventional trajectory is especially challenging for tracking algorithms. To capture the Meyer's loop, it is necessary to lower the curvature threshold in tractography, but this also increases the chance of getting outliers in the result. Thus it is critical to filter out these outliers without sacrificing the ability of capturing the Meyer's loop.

4 Results and Discussions

Demonstrative Study: Fig. 3 shows an example to demonstrate how our method works. We used fiber bundles from the optical radiation, to be precise, bundles from LGN to V1. We chose these fiber bundles because of their inherent challenge due to Meyer's loop. Because our method is based on removing loops, we aimed to show that our approach is stable, not very sensitive to changes in input parameters and can easily be tuned to preserve important features while removing others. Starting with input tracks, the process in the box (Fig. 3) is iterated until no more removal is possible. The final output is clear of loops that are larger than the threshold provided by the user (14mm in this case). The input tracks shown on the left and the final output on the right are a part of the actual study. The upper ($\Upsilon_{(t+\delta)}$) and lower ($\Upsilon_{(t-\delta)}$) level sets shown in Fig. 2 are also indicated on top of corresponding surfaces for clarity in Fig. 3.

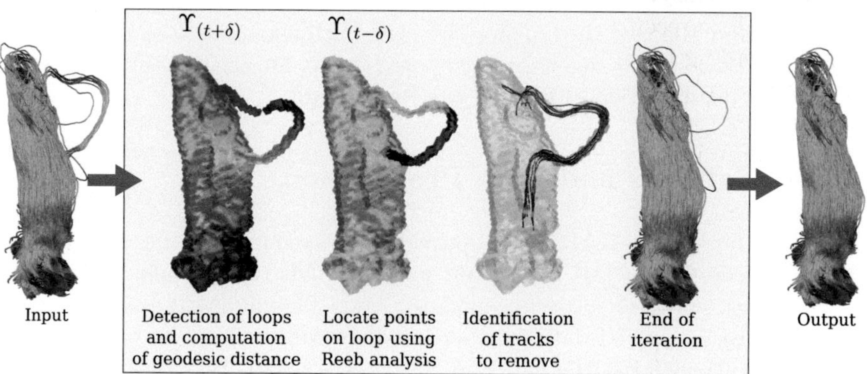

Fig. 3. Demonstrative example. Given input tracks, an iterative process shown in the box is run until no more tracks can be removed.

Comparative Study Against Spectral Filtering: We compared the results of our method against spectral filtering. For that, we used a similar algorithm to [10]. Fig. 4 shows two different subjects used in our study. Red arrows indicate tracks that should have been removed, green circles indicate tracks that are correctly preserved, i.e: those which project to the primary visual cortex. For our method, we used threshold levels of 12mm and 14mm for the subjects on the left and right respectively. Compared to spectral filtering, our method successfully detects and removes outliers while keeping relevant tracks. Although spectral filtering can be fine tuned for a single subject, this process is complicated, time consuming and not practical for studying populations. On the other hand, our method can easily be tuned with a single geometrically intuitive parameter.

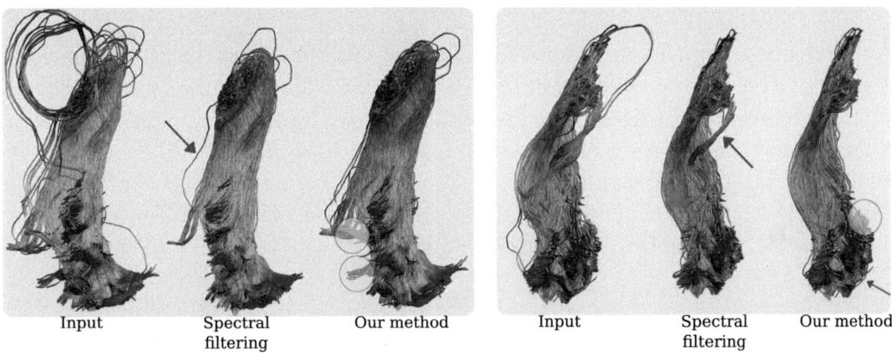

Fig. 4. Visual comparison of our method against spectral filtering on two subjects shown in different boxes. Our method keeps some important tracks shown in green circles. Red arrows indicate tracks that should have been removed.

Population Study: We applied our method to all the 215 subjects from HCP to obtain a clean reconstruction of the optic radiation using a threshold value of 14mm. According to the post-mortem study in [24], there is a left-ward asymmetry of the optic radiation in human brains. To test this asymmetry in our in-vivo reconstructions, we converted each reconstructed optic radiation into a TDI with 1mm isotropic resolution and counted the number of non-zero voxels as its volume. A two-tailed t-test was then applied to test for differences between left and right hemispheres. Table 1 shows the volumes and the p-value.

Table 1. Asymmetry of the optic radiation.

	Left hemisphere	**Right hemisphere**	**P-value**
Vol (mm^3)	$1.36E4 \pm 2.29E3$	$1.27E4 \pm 1.98E3$	$9.1E - 11$

Earlier research as outlined in section 1 mainly focused on using tractography and anatomical information for categorizing tracks. In contrast, we make use of the track density information with tractography. Therefore we take advantage of the familiar image domain which not only enables us to develop mathematically sound and clear methods but also technically unambiguous and easy to use tools.

To validate the accuracy of our track filtering method, we made a large scale study using 215 subjects from HCP. The results in Table 1 show that, our method produced tracks that show highly significant differences between left and right which is consistent with earlier post-mortem studies [24].

Our current code is in MATLAB® and C++. Using an Intel® Core™i7-4700MQ (2.40GHz×8), each block of our method (Fig. 1) is computed in a few seconds. The complete filtering of a single subject takes however ~5min which is similar to the speed of spectral filtering.

5 Conclusion

We developed a novel technique for filtering out unwanted tracks from tractography. The main contribution of this work is the use of topological analysis for the processing of tracks. Our method provides a geometrically intuitive way of controlling the filtering of outliers. In our experiments, we demonstrated its ability in obtaining cleaner tracks than spectral filtering. We also performed a population study on HCP data and obtained statistically significant results on the left-ward asymmetry of the optic radiation.

Acknowledgements. This work was in part supported by the National Institute of Health (NIH) under Grant K01EB013633, P41EB015922, P50AG005142.

References

1. Thomas, C., Ye, F.Q., Irfanoglu, M.O., Modi, P., Saleem, K.S., Leopold, D.A., Pierpaoli, C.: Anatomical accuracy of brain connections derived from diffusion MRI tractography is inherently limited. PNAS 111(46), 16574–16579 (2014)
2. Besseling, R., Jansen, J., Overvliet, G., Vaessen, M., Braakman, H., Hofman, P., Aldenkamp, A., Backes, W.: Tract specific reproducibility of tractography based morphology and diffusion metrics. PLoS ONE 7(4) (2012)
3. Girard, G., Whittingstall, K., Deriche, R., Descoteaux, M.: Towards quantitative connectivity analysis: reducing tractography biases. NeuroImage 98, 266–278 (2014)
4. Fillard, P., Descoteaux, M., Goh, A., Gouttard, S., Jeurissen, B., Malcolm, J., Ramirez-Manzanares, A., Reisert, M., Sakaie, K., Tensaouti, F., Yo, T., Mangin, J.F., Poupon, C.: Quantitative evaluation of 10 tractography algorithms on a realistic diffusion MR phantom. NeuroImage 56(1), 220–234 (2011)
5. Mangin, J.F., Fillard, P., Cointepas, Y., Le Bihan, D., Frouin, V., Poupon, C.: Toward global tractography. NeuroImage 80, 290–296 (2013)
6. Daducci, A., Dal Palu, A., Lemkaddem, A., Thiran, J.P.: COMMIT: Convex Optimization Modeling for Microstructure Informed Tractography. IEEE Transactions on Medical Imaging 34(1), 246–257 (2015)
7. Pestilli, F., Yeatman, J., Rokem, A., Kay, K., Wandell, B.: Evaluation and statistical inference for living connectomes. Nature Methods 11(10), 1058–1063 (2014)
8. Smith, R.E., Tournier, J.D., Calamante, F., Connelly, A.: SIFT: Spherical-deconvolution informed filtering of tractograms. NeuroImage 67, 298–312 (2013)

9. Xia, Y., Turken, A.U., Whitfield-Gabrieli, S.L., Gabrieli, J.D.: Knowledge-Based Classification of Neuronal Fibers in Entire Brain. In: Duncan, J.S., Gerig, G. (eds.) MICCAI 2005. LNCS, vol. 3749, pp. 205–212. Springer, Heidelberg (2005)
10. O'Donnell, L., Westin, C.F.: Automatic Tractography Segmentation Using a High-Dimensional White Matter Atlas. IEEE Trans. Med. Img. 26(11), 1562–1575 (2007)
11. Brun, A., Knutsson, H., Park, H.-J., Shenton, M.E., Westin, C.-F.: Clustering Fiber Traces Using Normalized Cuts. In: Barillot, C., Haynor, D.R., Hellier, P. (eds.) MICCAI 2004. LNCS, vol. 3216, pp. 368–375. Springer, Heidelberg (2004)
12. Tsai, A., Westin, C.F., Hero, A., Willsky, A.: Fiber Tract Clustering on Manifolds With Dual Rooted-Graphs. In: Proc. CVPR, pp. 1–6 (2007)
13. Wassermann, D., Bloy, L., Kanterakis, E., Verma, R., Deriche, R.: Unsupervised white matter fiber clustering and tract probability map generation: Applications of a Gaussian process framework for white matter fibers. NeuroImage 51(1), 228–241 (2010)
14. Li, H., Xue, Z., Guo, L., Liu, T., Hunter, J., Wong, S.T.C.: A hybrid approach to automatic clustering of white matter fibers. NeuroImage 49(2), 1249–1258 (2010)
15. Wang, X., Grimson, W.E.L., Westin, C.F.: Tractography segmentation using a hierarchical Dirichlet processes mixture model. NeuroImage 54(1), 290–302 (2011)
16. Calamante, F., Tournier, J.D., Jackson, G.D., Connelly, A.: Track-density imaging (TDI): Super-resolution white matter imaging using whole-brain track-density mapping. NeuroImage 53(4), 1233–1243 (2010)
17. Calamante, F., Tournier, J.D., Kurniawan, N.D., Yang, Z., Gyengesi, E., Galloway, G.J., Reutens, D.C., Connelly, A.: Super-resolution track-density imaging studies of mouse brain: Comparison to histology. NeuroImage 59(1), 286–296 (2012)
18. Tournier, J.D., Calamante, F., Connelly, A.: MRtrix: Diffusion tractography in crossing fiber regions. Int. J. of Imag. Syst. Tech. 22(1), 53–66 (2012)
19. Edelsbrunner, H., Harer, J.: Computational Topology: An Introduction. American Mathematical Soc. (2010)
20. Shi, Y., Lai, R., Toga, A.W.: Alzheimer's Disease Neuroimaging Initiative: Cortical surface reconstruction via unified Reeb analysis of geometric and topological outliers in magnetic resonance images. IEEE Trans. Med. Img. 32(3), 511–530 (2013)
21. Essen, D.V., Ugurbil, K., Auerbach, E., Barch, D., Behrens, T., Bucholz, R., Chang, A., Chen, L., Corbetta, M., Curtiss, S., Penna, S.D., Feinberg, D., Glasser, M., Harel, N., Heath, A., Larson-Prior, L., Marcus, D., Michalareas, G., Moeller, S., Oostenveld, R., Petersen, S., Prior, F., Schlaggar, B., Smith, S., Snyder, A., Xu, J., Yacoub, E.: The human connectome project: A data acquisition perspective. NeuroImage 62(4), 2222–2231 (2012)
22. Tran, G., Shi, Y.: Fiber Orientation and Compartment Parameter Estimation from Multi-Shell Diffusion Imaging. IEEE Transactions on Medical Imaging (in press, 2015)
23. Benson, N.C., Butt, O.H., Datta, R., Radoeva, P.D., Brainard, D.H., Aguirre, G.K.: The retinotopic organization of striate cortex is well predicted by surface topology. Current Biology 22(21), 2081–2085 (2012)
24. Burgel, U., Schormann, T., Schleicher, A., Zilles, K.: Mapping of histologically identified long fiber tracts in human cerebral hemispheres to the MRI volume of a reference brain: Position and spatial variability of the optic radiation. NeuroImage 10(5), 489–499 (1999)

Novel Single and Multiple Shell Uniform Sampling Schemes for Diffusion MRI Using Spherical Codes

Jian Cheng[1], Dinggang Shen[2], Pew-Thian Yap[2], and Peter J. Basser[1]

[1] Section on Tissue Biophysics and Biomimetics (STBB), PPITS, NICHD, NIBIB
[2] Department of Radiology and BRIC, University of North Carolina at Chapel Hill, USA
jian.cheng@nih.gov

Abstract. A good data sampling scheme is important for diffusion MRI acquisition and reconstruction. Diffusion Weighted Imaging (DWI) data is normally acquired on single or multiple shells in $\mathbf{q}$-space. The samples in different shells are typically distributed uniformly, because they should be invariant to the orientation of structures within tissue, or the laboratory coordinate frame. The Electrostatic Energy Minimization (EEM) method, originally proposed for single shell sampling scheme in dMRI by Jones et al., was recently generalized to the multi-shell case, called generalized EEM (GEEM). GEEM has been successfully used in the Human Connectome Project (HCP). Recently, the Spherical Code (SC) concept was proposed to maximize the minimal angle between different samples in single or multiple shells, producing a larger angular separation and better rotational invariance than the GEEM method. In this paper, we propose two novel algorithms based on the SC concept: 1) an efficient incremental constructive method, called Iterative Maximum Overlap Construction (IMOC), to generate a sampling scheme on a discretized sphere; 2) a constrained non-linear optimization (CNLO) method to update a given initial scheme on the continuous sphere. Compared to existing incremental estimation methods, IMOC obtains schemes with much larger separation angles between samples, which are very close to the best known solutions in single shell case. Compared to the existing Riemannian gradient descent method, CNLO is more robust and stable. Experiments demonstrated that the two proposed methods provide larger separation angles and better rotational invariance than the state-of-the-art GEEM and methods based on the SC concept.

1 Introduction

Diffusion MRI (dMRI) is a unique imaging technique to explore microstructure properties of white matter in the human brain by mapping local diffusion of water molecules. In dMRI, one obtains a limited number of samples of the 3D diffusion signal attenuation $E(\mathbf{q})$ in $\mathbf{q}$-space. Reconstruction in dMRI is to recover the continuous $E(\mathbf{q})$ from these scanned measurements and to estimate some meaningful quantities including the diffusion tensor, the Ensemble Average Propagator (EAP), etc. An appropriate sampling scheme in $\mathbf{q}$-space is important for all dMRI acquisition and reconstruction applications in order to recover as much information as possible using a minimal number of measurements. It is infeasible to develop a general optimal sampling scheme that works best for all signal types and all reconstruction methods. However, a necessary property for an optimal sampling scheme is that the samples should be spherically uniformly

N. Navab et al. (Eds.): MICCAI 2015, Part I, LNCS 9349, pp. 28–36, 2015.
DOI: 10.1007/978-3-319-24553-9_4

distributed with no directional preference, such that the sampling scheme is invariant to the orientation of tissue structures, or the laboratory coordinate frame of scanner.

Uniform single shell sampling schemes are widely used in dMRI, where samples in $\mathbf{q}$-space are uniformly distributed in a sphere with a fixed b-value. The Electrostatic Energy Minimization (EEM) method proposed in dMRI by Jones et al., [1] is the most popular way to generate a general single shell sampling scheme with an arbitrary number of samples. EEM considers the samples as electrons in sphere, and estimates the sample configuration by minimizing the electrostatic repulsive force based on the Coulomb's law, i.e., $\min_{\{\mathbf{u}_i\}_{i=1}^K} \sum_{j<i} \frac{1}{\|\mathbf{u}_i - \mathbf{u}_j\|_2^2} + \frac{1}{\|\mathbf{u}_i + \mathbf{u}_j\|_2^2}$, where antipodal symmetry is considered because antipodal symmetric samples have the same role in dMRI data reconstruction. Some solutions to the EEM problem with different number K have been collected in CAMINO [2]. Recently [4] generalized EEM from single shell to multiple shell, called generalized EEM (GEEM), by considering the electrostatic energies both in each individual shell and in the combined shell with all samples. The obtained multi-shell schemes have been successfully used in the Human Connectome Project (HCP). Although EEM and GEEM are widely used, the electrostatic energy formulation does not directly maximize the angular separation between measurements. There is no study to validate how the electrostatic energy is related with dMRI data reconstruction.

The Spherical Code (SC)[1] was recently proposed to design single and multiple shell sampling schemes [5]. The SC formulation directly maximizes the separation angles between samples in each shell and in the combined shell for all samples, which is more natural than the electrostatic energy formulation. In [5] three algorithms were proposed based on the SC formulation. Although these three methods have larger separation angles compared to GEEM, they have limitations which will be discussed later.

In this paper, we propose two novel methods based on the SC concept to design single and multi-shell schemes. We propose a very efficient method, called Iterative Maximum Overlap Construction (IMOC), to incrementally generate samples from a given fine uniform sampling scheme. Although IMOC is a greedy method, it obtains globally optimal solutions in $\mathbb{S}^1$ for the 2D case and approximately globally optimal solutions in $\mathbb{S}^2$ for single shell scheme design in dMRI. The separation angles by IMOC are much larger than EEM, GEEM and the incremental SC (ISC) in [5]. We also propose Constrained Non-Linear Optimization (CNLO) to produce a local optimal solution from a given initialization. CNLO is more stable and generates larger separation angles than Riemannian gradient descent (RGD) in [5]. Experimental results demonstrate that the proposed methods yield larger separation angles and better rotational invariance than the state-of-the-art GEEM used in the HCP [4], and existing methods based on SC [5].

2 Methods

2.1 Spherical Code (SC) Formulation: Maximize the Minimal Separation Angle

The *covering radius* of a given sampling scheme $\{\mathbf{u}_i\}_{i=1}^K$ is the minimal angular distance between samples, i.e.,

$$d(\{\mathbf{u}_i\}_{i=1}^K) = \min_{i \neq j} \arccos |\mathbf{u}_i^T \mathbf{u}_j|, \tag{1}$$

[1] http://mathworld.wolfram.com/SphericalCode.html

where the absolute value operator is used because the antipodal symmetric samples have the same role in dMRI data reconstruction. The SC formulation on a single shell is to find K samples $\{\mathbf{u}_i\}_{i=1}^K$ such that the covering radius is maximized [5], i.e.,

$$\max_{\{\mathbf{u}_i \in \mathbb{S}^2\}_{i=1}^K} d(\{\mathbf{u}_i\}_{i=1}^K) \tag{2}$$

The SC formulation is also called as Tammes problem[2], which is well studied in the mathematics literature. [6] proposed to iteratively optimize a continuous cost function that approximates the original discontinuous cost function in Eq. (2), and the authors also released a collection of best known solutions to the SC problem in $\mathbb{S}^2$ [6][3].

[5] generalized SC problem from single shell case in mathematics to multiple shell case in dMRI field by solving

$$\max_{\{\mathbf{u}_{s,i} \in \mathbb{S}^2\}} wS^{-1} \sum_{s=1}^{S} d(\{\mathbf{u}_{s,i}\}_{i=1}^{K_s}) + (1-w) d(\{\mathbf{u}_{s,i}\}_{i=1,\ldots,K_s; s=1,\ldots,S}), \tag{3}$$

where S is the number of shells, K_s is the number of points on the s-th shell, $\mathbf{u}_{s,i}$ is the i-th point on the s-th shell, and w is a weighting factor between the mean covering radius of the S shells and the covering radius of the combined shell containing all points from the S shells. It is normally set as 0.5. [5] proposed three algorithms to solve the SC problem in Eq. (2) and Eq. (3), i.e., a greedy method called Incremental SC (ISC), a Mixed Integer Linear Programming (MILP) method, a Riemannian Gradient Descent (RGD) method. MILP selects globally optimal one or multiple subsets of points from a given full set of points. However, MILP is known to be NP hard, thus it is impractical to select samples from a very fine uniform sample set, and [5] obtains an acceptable scheme by MILP within 10 minutes from 321 uniform samples generated by sphere tessellation. RGD updates a given sampling scheme to a better local optimal solution. However the cost functions in Eq. (2) and Eq. (3) are not continuous, and the gradients of the cost functions which are determined by the sample pairs that have the minimal separation angle are not continuous neither. Moreover, the implementation of RGD needs a threshold to determine the sample pairs that can be considered to be equal to the minimal separation angle, and a little change of the threshold can significantly change the final results, which makes RGD unstable.

2.2 Constrained Non-Linear Optimization (CNLO)

Since RGD is not stable due to the reasons we discussed above, we propose a stable method, called Constrained Non-Linear Optimization (CNLO), to obtain a local minimum. SC problem in Eq. (2) can be solved using CNLO in Eq. (4a), where Eq. (4b) means all separation angles are larger than θ.

$$\max_{\theta, \{\mathbf{u}_i\}_{i=1}^K} \theta \tag{4a}$$

$$\text{s.t. } |\mathbf{u}_i^T \mathbf{u}_j| \leq \cos\theta, \ \ \forall i < j \leq K; \tag{4b}$$

$$\mathbf{u}_i^T \mathbf{u}_i = 1, \ \forall i; \tag{4c}$$

[2] http://en.wikipedia.org/wiki/Tammes_problem

[3] http://neilsloane.com/grass/dim3/

Note that both cost function and constraints are continuous, considering $|\mathbf{u}_i^T \mathbf{u}_j| \leq \cos\theta$ means $-\cos\theta \leq \mathbf{u}_i^T \mathbf{u}_j \leq \cos\theta$. CNLO does not need to determine the sample sets with the minimal separation angle, which is more robust and avoids the threshold in RGD.

Multi-shell SC problem in Eq. (3) can be solved using CNLO in Eq. (5a):

$$\max_{\{\theta_s\},\theta_0,\{\mathbf{u}_{s,i}\}} \quad w\frac{1}{S}\sum_{i=1}^{S}\theta_s + (1-w)\theta_0 \tag{5a}$$

$$\text{s.t. } |\mathbf{u}_{s,i}^T \mathbf{u}_{s,j}| \leq \cos\theta_s, \quad \forall s,\ \forall i < j \leq K_s; \tag{5b}$$

$$|\mathbf{u}_{s,i}^T \mathbf{u}_{s',j}| \leq \cos\theta_0, \quad \forall s < s',\ \forall i \leq K_s,\ \forall j \leq K_{s'}; \tag{5c}$$

$$\theta_s \geq \theta_0, \quad \forall s; \tag{5d}$$

$$\mathbf{u}_{s,i}^T \mathbf{u}_{s,i} = 1, \ \forall s, i; \tag{5e}$$

Eq. (5b) means that the separation angles of samples in the s-th shell are larger than its corresponding covering radius θ_s. Eq. (5c) means that the separation angles of samples in two different shells are larger than the covering radius θ_0 for the combined shell with all samples. Eq. (5d) means that the covering radii for all single shells are always larger than the covering radius for the combined shell. In other words, Eq. (5d) means that the separation angles of samples in the same shell are larger than θ_0, because of Eq. (5b).

CNLO in Eq. (4a) and Eq. (5a) are continuous non-convex constrained optimization problems. We use sequential quadratic programming (SQP) to solve them. In each step, SQP solves a quadratic programming problem which locally approximates the original optimization problem. In practice, we use the SQP solver in NLOPT library [7]. CNLO obtains a locally optimal solution with a given initialization. The initialization can be set as a set of random samples, or the schemes provided by other methods.

2.3 Iterative Maximum Overlap Construction (IMOC)

Incremental sampling scheme design methods, i.e., incremental EEM [3], incremental GEEM (IGEEM) [4], and incremental SC (ISC) [5], were proposed to obtain reasonable uniform coverage when the acquisition is terminated and only a subset of the first several samples is used. These incremental scheme design methods are all greedy methods. In each step, they select the best sample from a fine uniform sample set based on the chosen samples in previous steps. They have the same limitations. 1) Since they are devised to work reasonably well for any subset with first several samples, the electrostatic energy or covering radius of the full sample set is not good, compared to optimization based methods. 2) If a finer uniform sample set is used, the electrostatic energy or covering radius of the obtained sampling scheme may not improve, which is beyond our expectation.

Here we propose Iterative Maximum Overlap Construction (IMOC) to overcome the above two limitations. See the IMOC algorithm in Alg. 1 for designing multi-shell schemes, whose simplified version with $S = 1$ is for single shell case. IMOC uses MOC in Alg. 2 to verify whether a candidate covering radius set $(\theta_0, \theta_1, \dots, \theta_S)$ is able to construct an acceptable scheme with $(K_1, \dots, K_s)$ samples for S shells. We define the coverage set of a point $\boldsymbol{x}$ as $C(\boldsymbol{x}, \theta) = \{\boldsymbol{y} \mid \arccos(|\boldsymbol{y}^T \boldsymbol{x}|) < \theta\}$. With a given candidate $(\theta_0, \theta_1, \dots, \theta_S)$, MOC constructs samples one by one. In the i-th step,

Algorithm 1. IMOC for Multiple shell Scheme Design:

Input: number of samples for S shells: $\{K_s\}_{s=1}^S$
Output: $\{\mathbf{u}_{s,i}\}_{i=1}^{K_s}$.
// binary search $\{\theta_s\}$ from $\{(0, \theta_s^{\text{ub}})\}$. $\{\theta_s^{\text{ub}}\}_{s=0}^S$ are the upper bounds of the covering radii;
$\theta_s^0 = 0$, $\theta_s^1 = \theta_s^{\text{ub}}$, $\forall s = 0, 1, \ldots, S$;
repeat
  $\theta_s = (\theta_s^0 + \theta_s^1)/2$, $\forall s = 0, 1, \ldots, S$;
  [IsSatisfied, $\{\mathbf{u}_{s,i}\}$] = **MOC**($\{\theta_s\}_{s=0}^S$, $\{K_s\}_{s=1}^S$);
  if *IsSatisfied* **then** $\theta_s^0 = \theta_s$, $\forall s = 0, 1, \ldots, S$;
  else $\theta_s^1 = \theta_s$, $\forall s = 0, 1, \ldots, S$;
until θ_s *does not change*, $\forall s = 0, 1, \ldots, S$;

Algorithm 2. MOC for Multiple shell Scheme Design:

Input: $\{\theta_s\}_{s=0}^S$, $\{K_s\}_{s=1}^S$
Output: IsSatisfied, $\{\mathbf{u}_{s,i}\}_{i=1}^{K_s}$.
Initialize coverage sets $\{\text{CS}_s\}_{s=0}^S$ as $S+1$ empty sets, and initialize $N_s = 0, \forall s \in [1, S]$;
for $n = 1$ **to** $\sum_{s=1}^S K_s$ **do**
  if $n == 1$ **then** choose any point as $\mathbf{u}_{1,1}$, $s \leftarrow 1$, $i \leftarrow 1$;
  if $1 < n \leq S$ **then** $s \leftarrow n$, $i \leftarrow 1$, choose $\mathbf{u}_{s,i}$ in $(\mathbb{S}^2 - \text{CS}_0)$ such that the set $C(\mathbf{u}_{s,i}, \theta_0) \cap \text{CS}_0$ has the largest area ;
  if $n > S$ **then**
    Set V as an empty set;
    for $s' = 1$ **to** S **do**
      if $N_{s'} < K_{s'}$ ***and*** $(\mathbb{S}^2 - (CS_{s'} \cup CS_0))$ *is not empty* **then**
        choose $\boldsymbol{v}_{s'}$ in $(\mathbb{S}^2 - (\text{CS}_{s'} \cup \text{CS}_0))$ such that the overlap set $C(\boldsymbol{v}_{s'}, \theta_{s'}) \cap (\text{CS}_{s'} \cup \text{CS}_0)$ has the largest area denoted as $A_{s'}$;
        $V \leftarrow V \cup \{\boldsymbol{v}_{s'}\}$;
      end
    end
    if V *is empty* **then**
      IsSatisfied = **False**; **return**
    else
      choose s and $\boldsymbol{v}_s \in V$ such that their corresponding area A_s is the largest one among $\{A_{s'}\}_{s'=1}^S$;
      $i \leftarrow N_s + 1$, $\mathbf{u}_{s,i} \leftarrow \boldsymbol{v}_s$;
    end
  end
  $\text{CS}_s \leftarrow \text{CS}_s \cup C(\mathbf{u}_{s,i}, \theta_s)$; $\text{CS}_0 \leftarrow \text{CS}_0 \cup C(\mathbf{u}_{s,i}, \theta_0)$; $N_s \leftarrow N_s + 1$;
end
IsSatisfied=**True**; **return**;

MOC searches the best point $\mathbf{u}_{s,i}$ for the s-th shell such that its coverage $C(\mathbf{u}_{s,i}, \theta_s)$ has the largest overlap with the existing total coverage set $\text{CS}_s \cup \text{CS}_0$ among all possible samples and possible shells, and then adds $C(\mathbf{u}_{i,s}, \theta_s)$ into CS_s, $C(\mathbf{u}_{i,s}, \theta_0)$ into CS_0. IMOC performs a binary search of the covering radii $\{\theta_s\}_{s=0}^S$ along the line segment determined by $\{\theta_s^{\text{ub}}\}_{s=0}^S$, where $\theta_s^{\text{ub}} = \arccos\sqrt{4 - \csc^2\left(\frac{\pi K_s}{6(K_s-1)}\right)}$ is a upper bound of the covering radius with K_s symmetric points [5,8]. The one dimension search provides good results in compromise for both individual shells and the combined shell.

Note that for single shell case, it is easy to see that IMOC yields the *globally optimal solution* for K samples in $\mathbb{S}^1$ in the 2D case, while ISC and IGEEM cannot. Similarly with ISC, IMOC can analytically select the best point in each iteration in 2D case from all points in $\mathbb{S}^1$. However for $\mathbb{S}^2$ IMOC requires a fine uniform discretization of the sphere to find the best point in each step with the largest overlap area by counting the number of points in overlap sets. We consider several issues for efficient implementation of IMOC. 1) KD-tree is used for efficient nearest neighbor search. 2) In the $(i+1)$-th step, the overlap area $A_s(\boldsymbol{x})$ is different from the i-th step and needs to be re-calculated only if the determined point $\mathbf{u}_{s',i}$ in the i-th step satisfies $\arccos(|\boldsymbol{x}^T\mathbf{u}_{s',i}|) < \theta_0$, if $s \neq s'$, or $\arccos(|\boldsymbol{x}^T\mathbf{u}_{s',i}|) < \theta_s$, if $s = s'$. 3) In MOC, the candidate points can be selected from a small "outside surface" of CS, i.e., $\{\boldsymbol{x} \mid \boldsymbol{x} \notin \text{CS}, \exists \boldsymbol{y} \in \text{CS}, \text{s.t.} \arccos(|\boldsymbol{x}^T\boldsymbol{y}|) \leq \delta\}$, instead of the whole complementary set $(\mathbb{S}^2 - \text{CS})$. δ is set as twice of the covering radius of the fine uniform sampling set used in IMOC. This modification does not change the results by IMOC in our experiments, although we currently have no proof for this phenomenon. These three issues significantly speed up MOC, because they reduce the time for each neighborhood search, and reduce the number of neighborhood search. In our implementation, IMOC only requires a few seconds on an ordinary laptop.

3 Experiments

Effect of Discretization in Incremental Methods. These incremental methods, i.e., Incremental EEM (IEEM) [3], IGEEM [4], ISC [5], and IMOC, all require a uniform sample set as a discretization of $\mathbb{S}^2$ to determine the best sample in each step. We would like to test whether a finer discretization in $\mathbb{S}^2$ can obtain better schemes with larger separation angles. Two uniform sample sets respectively with 81 samples and 20482 samples from sphere tessellation were used for comparison. With these two uniform sets, IEEM, ISC, and IMOC were performed to generate single shell schemes with $K \in [5, 80]$. The left subfigure of Fig. 1 shows the covering radii of schemes obtained by different methods using two uniform discretization. It also shows the best known single shell schemes using EEM in CAMINO [2]. Note that when $K \in [50, 80]$ is close to 81, covering radii by IEEM and ISC using finer discretization are actually smaller than using coarse discretization, and only when $K < 50$ is far from 81, IEEM and ISC obtain larger covering radii using finer discretization. When using finer discretization, covering radii by IMOC are always improved, and are even larger than the well optimized schemes by EEM in CAMINO. ISC and IMOC were performed to generate schemes with 3 shells, $K \in [5, 25]$ per shell. The right subfigure of Fig. 1 shows mean of covering radii of three shells (θ_s) and the covering radii of the combined shell (θ_0). It also demonstrates that when $K \times 3$ is close to 81, covering radius of the combined shell by ISC is not improved using the finer discretization, while IMOC has no such issue.

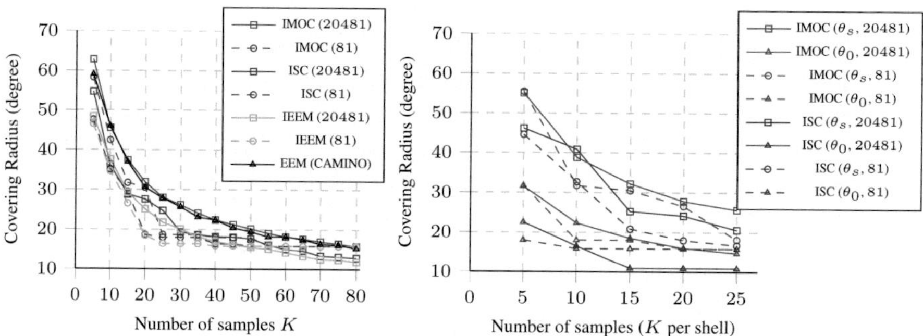

Fig. 1. Effect of discretization. Covering radii of sampling schemes (K in left side, $K \times 3$ in right side) by different methods with two uniform discretization (81 samples and 20481 samples).

Table 1. Covering radii of multi-shell sampling schemes with 28×3 samples generated by various methods. The best known schemes by EEM are individually for each single shell.

	Shell 1 (28)	Shell 2 (28)	Shell 3 (28)	Combined (28×3)
GEEM [4]	$22.2°$	$22.2°$	$22.0°$	$13.2°$
IGEEM [4]	$19.2°$	$19.7°$	$19.3°$	$4.7°$
ISC ($N = 20481$) [5]	$21.3°$	$19.3°$	$21.1°$	$10.5°$
MILP ($N = 321$) [5]	$23.8°$	$23.8°$	$24.3°$	$13.3°$
MILP + RGD [5]	$25.7°$	$25.7°$	$25.4°$	$13.6°$
IMOC ($N = 20481$)	$24.3°$	$24.3°$	$24.3°$	$14.0°$
IMOC + CNLO	**26.3°**	**25.9°**	**26.6°**	**14.6°**
EEM (CAMINO) [1,2]	$25.7°$	$25.7°$	$25.7°$	$15.6°$

Covering Radii in Sampling Schemes. We evaluated the proposed method by generating a multi-shell scheme with 28×3 samples, which was also used for evaluation in [5] and [4]. Table 1 shows the covering radii of the schemes obtained by different methods, where MILP+RGD means RGD using the result by MILP as the initialization, IMOC+CNLO means CNLO using the result by IMOC as the initialization. The results by GEEM, IGEEM in [4], and ISC, MILP, MILP+RGD in [5] were directly extracted from the papers. The single shell schemes with 28 and 28×3 samples using EEM from CAMINO [2] were also listed as references. IMOC obtains better covering radii than existing incremental methods, and even better than MILP. IMOC+CNLO obtains largest covering radii in both 3 individual shells and the combined shell, and the covering radii by IMOC+CNLO in these 3 shells are even better than best known scheme collected in CAMINO using EEM [1,2], similarly with Fig. 1.

Rotational Invariance in Reconstruction. We would like to test rotational invariance of the schemes with 28×3 samples by different methods in Table 1. We generated synthetic diffusion signals from a mixture tensor model $E(q\mathbf{u}) = 0.5\exp(-q^2\mathbf{u}^T\mathbf{D}_1\mathbf{u}) + 0.5\exp(-q^2\mathbf{u}^T\mathbf{D}_2\mathbf{u})$, where $b = q^2 = 1000, 2000, 3000\,\mathrm{s/mm}^2$, and these two tensors have the same eigenvalues $[1.7, 0.2, 0.2] \times 10^{-3}\,\mathrm{mm}^2/\mathrm{s}$ with a crossing angle of $55°$. With each tested scheme, we rotated the model and generated signals 20481 times with the rotation angles determined by the uniform sample set with 20481 samples. Then we performed Spherical Polar Fourier Imaging with spherical order 6 and radial order

Table 2. Angular differences between estimated directions and ground-truth fiber directions using different schemes by various methods.

	IGEEM [4]	ISC [5]	MILP [5]	MILP + RGD [5]	IMOC	IMOC+CNLO
Angular Difference (55° crossing)	$3.56^\circ \pm 1.36^\circ$	$2.72^\circ \pm 1.11^\circ$	$2.46^\circ \pm 1.04^\circ$	$2.45^\circ \pm 1.01^\circ$	$2.43^\circ \pm 1.04^\circ$	$\mathbf{2.37}^\circ \pm \mathbf{0.93}^\circ$

2 [9] to estimate the EAP profiles with radius of 15μm, detected the peaks of the EAP profiles, and calculated the mean angular differences by comparing the detected peaks with the ground-truth fiber directions in these 20481 tests. Table 2 lists the mean and standard deviation of angular differences obtained by different schemes. IMOC+CNLO yields the significantly lowest angular differences (paired t-test, $p < 0.001$) with the lowest deviation, and IMOC has the lower mean and deviation than other incremental methods.

4 Conclusion

We propose IMOC and CNLO based on the SC concept to design single and multiple shell uniform sampling schemes. IMOC is a very efficient incremental method which obtains globally optimal solutions in the 2D case. For the 3D case in dMRI, covering radii of IMOC schemes are even larger than EEM in CAMINO. IMOC obtains better schemes when using a finer discretization, while existing incremental methods (IEEM [3], IGEEM [4], ISC [5]) may have a worse result when using finer discretization. CNLO is a local optimization method which has better theoretical properties than RGD in [5]. The multi-shell scheme by CNLO using IMOC as initialization obtains larger covering radii and better rotational invariance than existing methods [4,5] based on electrostatic energy and the SC formulation. The codes and best known schemes will be released in DMRITool package (https://github.com/DiffusionMRITool).

Acknowledgement. This work is supported in part by NICHD and NIBIB Intramural Research Programs, a UNC BRIC-Radiology start-up fund, and NIH grants (EB006733, EB009634, AG041721, MH100217, and 1UL1TR001111).

References

1. Jones, D.K., Horsfield, M.A., Simmons, A.: Optimal strategies for measuring diffusion in anisotropic systems by magnetic resonance imaging. Magnetic Resonance in Medicine (1999)
2. Cook, P., Bai, Y., Nedjati-Gilani, S., Seunarine, K., Hall, M., Parker, G., Alexander, D.: Camino: Open-source diffusion-MRI reconstruction and processing. In: ISMRM (2006)
3. Deriche, R., Calder, J., Descoteaux, M.: Optimal real-time q-ball imaging using regularized kalman filtering with incremental orientation sets. Medical Image Analysis 13(4) (2009)
4. Caruyer, E., Lenglet, C., Sapiro, G., Deriche, R.: Design of multishell sampling schemes with uniform coverage in diffusion MRI. Magnetic Resonance in Medicine (2013)
5. Cheng, J., Shen, D., Yap, P.-T.: Designing single- and multiple-shell sampling schemes for diffusion MRI using spherical code. In: Golland, P., Hata, N., Barillot, C., Hornegger, J., Howe, R. (eds.) MICCAI 2014, Part III. LNCS, vol. 8675, pp. 281–288. Springer, Heidelberg (2014)

6. Conway, J.H., Hardin, R.H., Sloane, N.J.: Packing lines, planes, etc.: Packings in Grassmannian spaces. Experimental Mathematics 5(2), 139–159 (1996)
7. Johnson, S.G.: The nlopt nonlinear-optimization package, `http://ab-initio.mit.edu/nlopt`
8. Tóth, L.F.: On the densest packing of spherical caps. The American Mathematical Monthly 56(5), 330–331 (1949)
9. Cheng, J., Ghosh, A., Jiang, T., Deriche, R.: Model-Free and Analytical EAP Reconstruction via Spherical Polar Fourier Diffusion MRI. In: Jiang, T., Navab, N., Pluim, J.P.W., Viergever, M.A. (eds.) MICCAI 2010, Part I. LNCS, vol. 6361, pp. 590–597. Springer, Heidelberg (2010)

q-Space Deep Learning for Twelve-Fold Shorter and Model-Free Diffusion MRI Scans

Vladimir Golkov[1], Alexey Dosovitskiy[2], Philipp Sämann[3], Jonathan I. Sperl[4], Tim Sprenger[1,4], Michael Czisch[3], Marion I. Menzel[4], Pedro A. Gómez[1,4], Axel Haase[1], Thomas Brox[2], and Daniel Cremers[1]

[1] Technische Universität München, Garching, Germany
[2] University of Freiburg, Freiburg, Germany
[3] Max Planck Institute of Psychiatry, Munich, Germany
[4] GE Global Research, Garching, Germany
golkov@cs.tum.edu

Abstract. Diffusion MRI uses a multi-step data processing pipeline. With certain steps being prone to instabilities, the pipeline relies on considerable amounts of partly redundant input data, which requires long acquisition time. This leads to high scan costs and makes advanced diffusion models such as diffusion kurtosis imaging (DKI) and neurite orientation dispersion and density imaging (NODDI) inapplicable for children and adults who are uncooperative, uncomfortable or unwell. We demonstrate how deep learning, a group of algorithms in the field of artificial neural networks, can be applied to reduce diffusion MRI data processing to a single optimized step. This method allows obtaining scalar measures from advanced models at twelve-fold reduced scan time and detecting abnormalities without using diffusion models.

1 Introduction

Advanced diffusion MRI models such as DKI [1] and NODDI [2] are preferable over traditional diffusion MRI models because they provide more accurate characterization of tissue microstructure. However, they require long acquisition times. This can be problematic in clinical applications due to high scan costs or if the patient is uncooperative, uncomfortable or unwell.

In diffusion MRI, a number of diffusion-weighted images (DWIs) for different diffusion weightings and directions (constituting the so-called three-dimensional q-space) are acquired. The task in quantitative diffusion MRI is to find a mapping from a limited number of noisy signal samples to rotationally invariant scalar measures that quantify microstructural tissue properties. This inverse problem is solved in each image voxel. The classical approach consists of fitting [3] a diffusion model and calculating rotationally invariant measures from the fitted model parameters. Another approach to calculate scalar measures is approximation, particularly machine learning. Simulations of simplified tissue models with extensive sets of diffusion weightings [4, 5] indicate that standard model fitting procedures can be replaced by approximation methods. On the basis of

N. Navab et al. (Eds.): MICCAI 2015, Part I, LNCS 9349, pp. 37–44, 2015.
DOI: 10.1007/978-3-319-24553-9_5

these observations, we apply deep learning [6–9] for accurate approximation and present a deep learning framework for different inputs (full and subsampled sets of regular DWIs, non-diffusion contrasts) and outputs (denoising, missing DWI reconstruction, scalar measure estimation, tissue segmentation). We term this framework *q-space deep learning* (q-DL). Scalar measure estimation from twelve-fold shortened acquisition is demonstrated on two advanced models: DKI and NODDI. By shortening the acquisition duration of advanced models by an order of magnitude, we strongly improve their potential for clinical use.

Recent applications of machine learning in diffusion MRI [10–12] use fitted model parameters as learning inputs, whereas we omit model fitting altogether by using the DWIs themselves, which allows the use of unprecedented subsampling factors that model fitting (Fig. 1a–d) cannot handle.

Besides, our framework allows tissue segmentation and lesion detection in diffusion MRI without using diffusion models.

2 Methods

Deep learning [6–9] is a set of algorithms for learning of input-output-mappings. It can outperform other machine learning methods and has recently been successfully applied in a variety of fields such as computer vision, natural language processing and drug discovery. It is based on artificial neural networks, where input data is propagated through several layers of hidden units (artificial neurons). Each layer is a data transformation step. The classical diffusion MRI pipeline also consists of several steps: in DKI, approximately 150 measurements are reduced to 22 model parameters, then to a few rotationally invariant measures, and finally (implicitly or explicitly) to the tissue property of interest. In every step, information is partly lost by reducing the degrees of freedom. However, the classical pipeline does not provide feedback to the earlier steps with regard to what part of the information should be retained or discarded and which transformations should be applied. Thus, the pipeline relies on handcrafting and fixing each step. Deep learning takes a more holistic approach: all layers are optimized jointly in terms of the final objective, namely minimizing the output error. This prevents the loss of information at intermediate steps.

In an artificial neural network with L layers (particularly in a so-called multilayer perceptron), the data transformation in layer $i \in \{1, \ldots, L\}$ depends on the weight matrix $\boldsymbol{W}^{(i)}$ and bias term $\boldsymbol{b}^{(i)}$ according to the rule $\boldsymbol{a}_j^{(i)} = s_i(\boldsymbol{W}^{(i)}\boldsymbol{a}_j^{(i-1)} + \boldsymbol{b}^{(i)})$, where $\boldsymbol{a}_j^{(i)}$ are the output vectors of layer i for data sample j, the $\boldsymbol{a}_j^{(0)}$ are the input *vectors* of the network, and s_i are nonlinearities (see below). During training, all weight matrices and bias terms are jointly adjusted such that the output vectors $\boldsymbol{a}_j^{(L)}$ for each training sample j (in our case: each image voxel j) well approximate the target output vectors $\boldsymbol{y}_j$. This adjustment is achieved by using the backpropagation algorithm (implementation [13]) to solve $\arg\min_{\boldsymbol{W},\boldsymbol{b}} \sum_j \left\| \boldsymbol{a}_j^{(L)} - \boldsymbol{y}_j \right\|^2$, where the sum of errors is taken over all training samples j, and outputs $\boldsymbol{a}_j^{(i)}$ recursively depend on $\boldsymbol{W}, \boldsymbol{b}$. In all experiments, training data originate from different human subjects than test data. The network thus does not "know" the true output vectors of the test data but rather estimates them based on the input-output-mapping learned from training data. Each voxel j is treated individually as a data sample. The algorithm does not know its location in the image. We introduce several input-output-mapping tasks. Different deep networks are trained for different tasks:

Denoising. For denoising, the signal $\boldsymbol{S}_j$ from all DWIs in voxel j is used as both the input $\boldsymbol{a}_j^{(0)}$ and target $\boldsymbol{y}_j$ of the neural network. The number of network inputs is the number n of used DWIs, i.e. each input vector $\boldsymbol{a}_j^{(0)} = \boldsymbol{S}_j$ has length n (for every j). The length of the output vector $\boldsymbol{a}_j^{(L)}$ is also n. A network trained to reconstruct its own inputs is known as an autoencoder [7]. Its approximate nature and dropout-based training [8] prevent overfitting and reduce noise.

Reconstruction of Missing DWIs. For q-DL-based Reconstruction of missing DWIs (q-DL-R), a neural network is trained to predict the signal $\boldsymbol{S}_j$ in all DWIs (voxel j) from a reduced subset $\boldsymbol{S}_{j,\alpha}$ where α is a pseudorandom subsampling multi-index (such that the q-space sampling is consistent across training and test data). The length of the input vector $\boldsymbol{a}_j^{(0)} = \boldsymbol{S}_{j,\alpha}$ is $|\alpha|$. Due to partial data redundancy in q-space, missing DWIs can be reconstructed from a reduced subset.

Estimation of Scalar Measures. A network is trained to predict microstructure-characterizing scalar measures $\boldsymbol{m}_j$ directly from the (reduced set of) DWIs $\boldsymbol{S}_{j,\alpha}$. In other words, inputs are $\boldsymbol{a}_j^{(0)} = \boldsymbol{S}_{j,\alpha}$ and targets are $\boldsymbol{y}_j = \boldsymbol{m}_j$. The length of the output vector is the number of considered scalar measures. Training targets $\boldsymbol{y}_j = \boldsymbol{m}_j$ are obtained from a fully sampled training dataset by model fitting.

Model-Free Segmentation. Tissue segmentation is achieved by training a neural network to discriminate between several tissue types. We propose modifying the approach [14] of multi-parametric MRI tissue characterization by artificial neural networks such that the DWIs are directly used as inputs rather than using scalar measures obtained from model fitting. State-of-the-art automatic segmentation [15, 16] (based on non-diffusion images with spatial priors) into healthy white matter (WM), grey matter (GM), cerebrospinal fluid (CSF) and multiple sclerosis lesions was used as ground truth for our proof-of-concept model-free segmentation (based on diffusion images without spatial priors). The q-DL framework allows incorporating additional contrasts other than DWIs as inputs to the learning algorithm. We used fluid-attenuated inversion recovery (FLAIR) signal as an additional input. The length of the output vector is the number of tissue classes (with each output representing a relative class membership "likeliness" using softmax, see below).

Additional Remarks. The trained network with optimized $\boldsymbol{W}^{(i)}$ and $\boldsymbol{b}^{(i)}$ is then applied to other datasets using the recursive formula for $\boldsymbol{a}_j^{(i)}$. In the case of

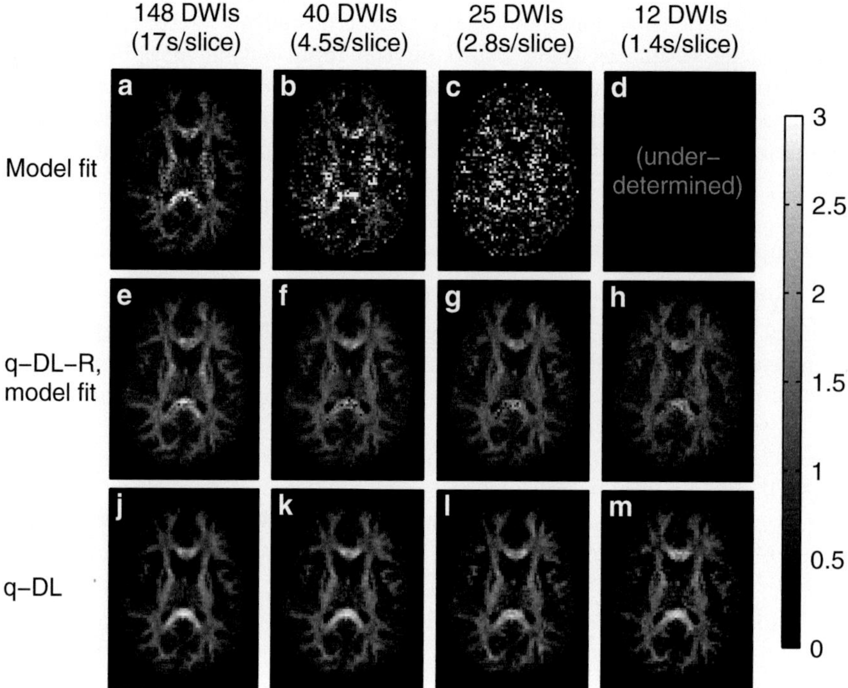

Fig. 1. Maps of radial kurtosis in the human brain for various methods and MRI scan acceleration factors. 148, 40, 25 and 12 randomly selected DWIs are used; required scan time for each scheme is shown in seconds per slice. (a–d) Standard processing (model fitting followed by radial kurtosis calculation). (e–h) q-DL-R, followed by model fitting and radial kurtosis calculation. (j–m) q-DL.

α-subsampling, a large number of DWIs is required only once (for the training dataset) in order to estimate target scalar measures $\boldsymbol{m}$ using model fitting. Subsequently, training is performed using few DWIs as inputs, and the trained network can be applied to any number of previously unseen test datasets which have only few DWIs (same subsampling scheme).

The deep learning toolbox [13] was used for experiments. In each of the described tasks, the neural network architecture used is a multilayer perceptron with three fully connected hidden layers, each consisting of 150 rectified linear units [6], i.e. $s_i(\boldsymbol{z}) = \max(\boldsymbol{0}, \boldsymbol{z})$. Linear units $s_L(\boldsymbol{z}) = \boldsymbol{z}$ are used in the output layer L for fitting tasks and softmax outputs $s_L(\boldsymbol{z}) = \exp(\boldsymbol{z})/\|\exp(\boldsymbol{z})\|_1$ for classification tasks. Each input and output of the neural network is scaled to the interval $[0, 1]$ during training, and the same linear transformation is applied to test data. We found that results improve if the network is pre-trained [7] using training data or initialized with orthogonal random weights [9]. We use

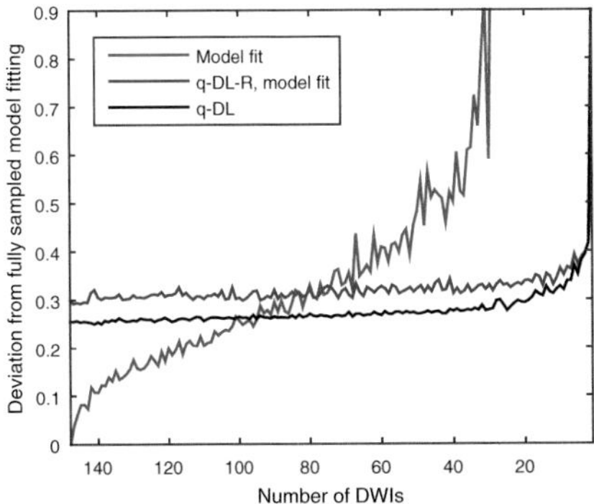

Fig. 2. Error evaluation of different methods at different acceleration factors. Root-mean-square deviation from the radial kurtosis estimated by the standard pipeline (fully sampled model fitting) is used as error metric. Model fitting is outperformed by the proposed methods when less than 70 DWIs are used.

a dropout [8] fraction of 0.1, stochastic gradient descent with momentum 0.9, batch size 128, learning rate 0.01, warm-up learning rate 0.001 for first 10 epochs.

Datasets. The *in vivo* protocols were approved by our institutional review board and prior informed consent was obtained. Two data sets of healthy volunteers were acquired using a scheme optimized [17, 18] for DKI and suitable for NODDI: three shells ($b = 750, 1070, 3000\,\mathrm{s/mm^2}$) with 25, 40, 75 directions, respectively, and eight $b = 0$ images. This is a non-radial multi-shell q-space acquisition scheme for which no missing data reconstruction algorithm exists to the best of our knowledge. Echo-planar imaging was performed using a 3T GE MR750 MR scanner (GE Healthcare, Waukesha, WI, USA) equipped with a 32-channel head coil ($T_E = 80.7\,\mathrm{ms}, T_R = 2\,\mathrm{s}$, FOV $= 24 \times 24 \times 4\,\mathrm{cm}$, isotropic voxel size 2.5 mm, ASSET factor 2). All data underwent FSL topup distortion correction [19]. For the tissue segmentation experiments, six multiple sclerosis patients were scanned using a diffusion spectrum uniform sampling pattern [20] with 167 DWIs ($b_{\max} = 3000\,\mathrm{s/mm^2}$, $T_E = 80.3\,\mathrm{ms}$, $T_R = 5.4\,\mathrm{s}$, FOV $= 24 \times 24 \times 12\,\mathrm{cm}$, isotropic voxel size 2.5 mm, ASSET factor 2).

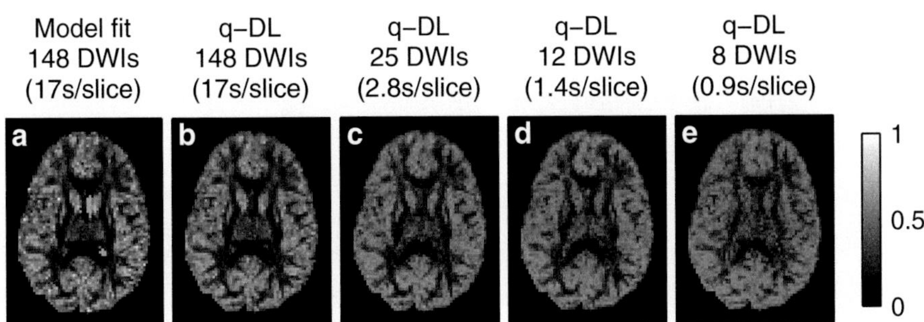

Fig. 3. Comparison of (a) model fitting and (b–e) q-DL for neurite orientation dispersion index based on NODDI. q-DL allows strong scan time reduction with moderate contrast loss.

3 Results

In Fig. 1, we show the radial kurtosis [21] measure based on DKI because of its particular susceptibility to noise and because no analytical solutions are known. In the case of denoising and q-DL-R, model parameters are estimated from the reconstructed DWIs by standard model fitting [3] for comparison.

DKI results of denoising for fully sampled data (Fig. 1e) exhibit slightly less noise than the standard pipeline (Fig. 1a) without sacrificing spatial resolution. Moreover, compared with the standard pipeline (Fig. 1a–d), results of q-DL-R (Fig. 1e–h) and of q-DL (Fig. 1j–m) exhibit feasibility of scan time reduction by a factor of twelve. Fig. 2 compares the methods in terms of root-mean-square deviation from model-fitting results of fully sampled data. Despite their approximate nature leading to disparity with model fitting, the proposed methods outperform model fitting when less than 70 DWIs are used. NODDI results (Fig. 3) demonstrate strong scan time reduction with moderate contrast loss when using q-DL. Segmentation results are shown in Fig. 4. The area under the curve (AUC) of the receiver operating characteristic (ROC) for lesions ranged between 0.869 and 0.934 for six different patients. AUC for WM, GM and CSF was consistently above 0.894 for all patients. Thus, q-space data can be used for segmentation directly without a diffusion model, i.e. without the intermediate information loss detailed above. Results were slightly worse when not using FLAIR (between 0.859 and 0.934 for lesions; above 0.892 for WM, GM, CSF). Tailoring the protocol to optimal results in specific applications is subject of future research.

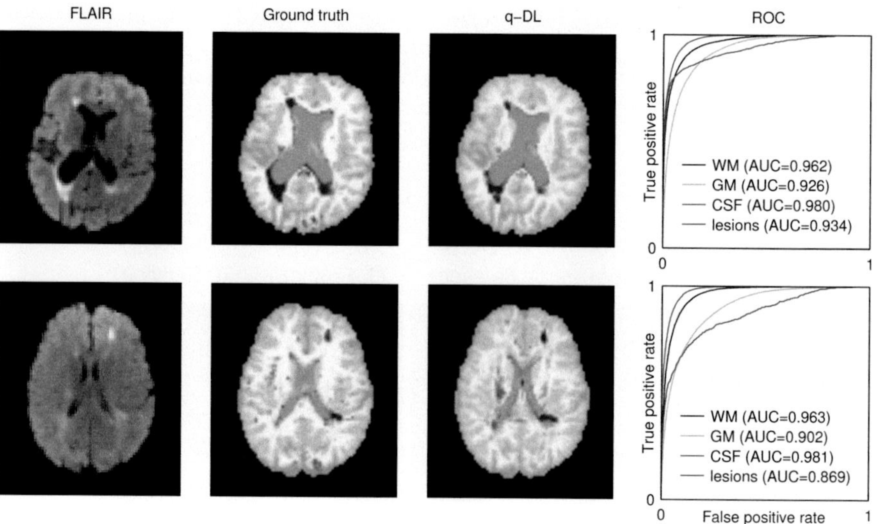

Fig. 4. Direct model-free segmentation. Slices from datasets with the best (upper row, 0.934) and worst lesion AUC (lower row, 0.869) are shown.

4 Discussion

The presented short-scan and model-free protocols open interesting research directions. While state-of-the-art methods [12, 22] require 30 DWIs for NODDI and 64 for radial kurtosis, we require only 8 and 12, respectively. Our results indicate that a considerable amount of information is contained in a limited number of DWIs, and that this information can be better retrieved by deep learning than by model fitting. The network architecture is quite simple compared to other works in deep learning, and yet it works surprisingly well for diffusion MRI. In all presented applications, neural network training takes about one minute on a desktop computer. The network needs to be trained only once and can be applied to any number of datasets, taking 0.03 seconds per dataset, as opposed to several minutes per dataset required by most model fitting methods. Analytical solutions of scalar measure estimation [23] provide reduction of scan time and processing time comparable to q-DL, but are limited to specific scalar measures and acquisition schemes, as opposed to q-DL. A combination with multi-slice imaging is straightforward, yielding additional scan time reduction. Benefits of using spatial neighborhoods [12] for q-DL and (Rician-)noise-robust training [7] can be explored in the future. Our methods require full sampling of the training data only; subsequently, the network can be applied to new subsampled data.

Acknowledgments. We are grateful to S. Pölsterl and B. Menze (TU München) for discussions. V. Golkov is supported by the Deutsche Telekom Foundation.

References

1. Jensen, J.H., Helpern, J.A., Ramani, A., Lu, H., Kaczynski, K.: Diffusional kurtosis imaging: the quantification of non-Gaussian water diffusion by means of magnetic resonance imaging. Magnetic Resonance in Medicine 53(6), 1432–1440 (2005)
2. Zhang, H., Schneider, T., Wheeler-Kingshott, C.A., Alexander, D.C.: NODDI: practical in vivo neurite orientation dispersion and density imaging of the human brain. NeuroImage 61(4), 1000–1016 (2012)
3. Veraart, J., Sijbers, J., Sunaert, S., Leemans, A., Jeurissen, B.: Weighted linear least squares estimation of diffusion MRI parameters: strengths, limitations, and pitfalls. NeuroImage 81, 335–346 (2013)
4. Nilsson, M., Alerstam, E., Wirestam, R., Ståhlberg, F., Brockstedt, S., Lätt, J.: Evaluating the accuracy and precision of a two-compartment Kärger model using Monte Carlo simulations. Journal of Magnetic Resonance 206, 59–67 (2010)
5. Nedjati-Gilani, G., Hall, M.G., Wheeler-Kingshott, C.A.M., Alexander, D.C.: Learning microstructure parameters from diffusion-weighted MRI using random forests. Joint Annual Meeting ISMRM-ESMRMB, 2626 (2014)
6. Jarrett, K., Kavukcuoglu, K., Ranzato, M.A., LeCun, Y.: What is the best multi-stage architecture for object recognition? In: IEEE 12th International Conference on Computer Vision, pp. 2146–2153 (2009)
7. Vincent, P., Larochelle, H., Lajoie, I., Bengio, Y., Manzagol, P.A.: Stacked denoising autoencoders: learning useful representations in a deep network with a local denoising criterion. Journal of Machine Learning Research 11, 3371–3408 (2010)

8. Hinton, G.E., Srivastava, N., Krizhevsky, A., Sutskever, I., Salakhutdinov, R.R.: Improving neural networks by preventing co-adaptation of feature detectors. arXiv:1207.0580 (2012)
9. Saxe, A.M., McClelland, J.L., Ganguli, S.: Exact solutions to the nonlinear dynamics of learning in deep linear neural networks. In: International Conference on Learning Representations, Banff, Canada (2014)
10. Schultz, T.: Learning a reliable estimate of the number of fiber directions in diffusion MRI. In: Ayache, N., Delingette, H., Golland, P., Mori, K. (eds.) MICCAI 2012, Part III. LNCS, vol. 7512, pp. 493–500. Springer, Heidelberg (2012)
11. Nedjati-Gilani, G.L., Schneider, T., Hall, M.G., Wheeler-Kingshott, C.A.M., Alexander, D.C.: Machine learning based compartment models with permeability for white matter microstructure imaging. In: Golland, P., Hata, N., Barillot, C., Hornegger, J., Howe, R. (eds.) MICCAI 2014, Part III. LNCS, vol. 8675, pp. 257–264. Springer, Heidelberg (2014)
12. Alexander, D.C., Zikic, D., Zhang, J., Zhang, H., Criminisi, A.: Image quality transfer via random forest regression: applications in diffusion MRI. In: Golland, P., Hata, N., Barillot, C., Hornegger, J., Howe, R. (eds.) MICCAI 2014, Part III. LNCS, vol. 8675, pp. 225–232. Springer, Heidelberg (2014)
13. Palm, R.B.: Prediction as a candidate for learning deep hierarchical models of data. Master's thesis, Technical University of Denmark (2012)
14. Bagher-Ebadian, H., Jafari-Khouzani, K., Mitsias, P.D., Lu, M., Soltanian-Zadeh, H., Chopp, M., Ewing, J.R.: Predicting final extent of ischemic infarction using artificial neural network analysis of multi-parametric MRI in patients with stroke. PLoS ONE 6(8) (2011)
15. Ashburner, J., Friston, K.J.: Unified segmentation. NeuroImage 26, 839–851 (2005)
16. Van Leemput, K., Maes, F., Vandermeulen, D., Colchester, A., Suetens, P.: Automated segmentation of multiple sclerosis lesions by model outlier detection. IEEE Transactions on Medical Imaging 20, 677–688 (2001)
17. Poot, D.H.J., den Dekker, A.J., Achten, E., Verhoye, M., Sijbers, J.: Optimal experimental design for diffusion kurtosis imaging. IEEE Transactions on Medical Imaging 29(3), 819–829 (2010)
18. Veraart, J., Van Hecke, W., Sijbers, J.: Constrained maximum likelihood estimation of the diffusion kurtosis tensor using a Rician noise model. Magnetic Resonance in Medicine 66(3), 678–686 (2011)
19. Andersson, J.L.R., Skare, S., Ashburner, J.: How to correct susceptibility distortions in spin-echo echo-planar images: application to diffusion tensor imaging. NeuroImage 20(2), 870–888 (2003)
20. Menzel, M.I., Tan, E.T., Khare, K., Sperl, J.I., King, K.F., Tao, X., Hardy, C.J., Marinelli, L.: Accelerated diffusion spectrum imaging in the human brain using compressed sensing. Magnetic Resonance in Medicine 66(5), 1226–1233 (2011)
21. Hui, E.S., Cheung, M.M., Qi, L., Wu, E.X.: Towards better MR characterization of neural tissues using directional diffusion kurtosis analysis. NeuroImage 42(1), 122–134 (2008)
22. Paquette, M., Merlet, S., Gilbert, G., Deriche, R., Descoteaux, M.: Comparison of sampling strategies and sparsifying transforms to improve compressed sensing diffusion spectrum imaging. Magnetic Resonance in Medicine 73, 401–416 (2015)
23. Hansen, B., Lund, T.E., Sangill, R., Jespersen, S.N.: Experimentally and computationally fast method for estimation of a mean kurtosis. Magnetic Resonance in Medicine 69(6), 1754–1760 (2013)

A Machine Learning Based Approach to Fiber Tractography Using Classifier Voting

Peter F. Neher, Michael Götz, Tobias Norajitra, Christian Weber, and Klaus H. Maier-Hein*

Medical Image Computing, German Cancer Research Center (DKFZ)
k.maier-hein@dkfz.de

Abstract. Current tractography pipelines incorporate several modelling assumptions about the nature of the diffusion-weighted signal. We present an approach that tracks fiber pathways based on a random forest classification and voting process, guiding each step of the streamline progression by directly processing raw signal intensities. We evaluated our approach quantitatively and qualitatively using phantom and *in vivo* data. The presented machine learning based approach to fiber tractography is the first of its kind and our experiments showed auspicious performance compared to 12 established state of the art tractography pipelines. Due to its distinctly increased sensitivity and specificity regarding tract connectivity and morphology, the presented approach is a valuable addition to the repertoire of currently available tractography methods and promises to be beneficial for all applications that build upon tractography results.

1 Introduction

Fiber tractography on the basis of diffusion-weighted magnetic resonance imaging (DW-MRI) enables the spatial reconstruction of white matter pathways connecting the different regions of the brain. Despite the efforts invested into developing novel diffusion modeling and fiber tractography methods, ranging from local deterministic approaches through probabilistic methods to global tractography, several studies have shown that the task of fiber tractography is far from being solved. Current tractography algorithms still struggle with simultaneously achieving a high sensitivity and specificity regarding inter-regional connectivity as well as tract morphology [1,2]. This directly impacts processing and analysis steps, such as cortical connectivity analysis, that build upon the tractography result.

Initial studies have successfully shown the potential of machine learning techniques in the context of DW-MRI analysis, e.g. for the tasks of image quality transfer and tissue micro-structure analysis [3] and to estimate the number of distinct fiber clusters per voxel [4]. In this work we present a purely data-driven and thus fundamentally new approach to reconstruct fiber pathways by directly processing raw signal intensities using machine learning methods. In contrast

* Corresponding author.

N. Navab et al. (Eds.): MICCAI 2015, Part I, LNCS 9349, pp. 45–52, 2015.
DOI: 10.1007/978-3-319-24553-9_6

to other current tractography pipelines that incorporate several modelling assumptions about the nature of the underlying diffusion-weighted signal, this model-free approach has several advantages:

1. No simplifying and possibly inaccurate assumptions about the diffusion propagator are made (e.g. Gaussianity). Subsequently, the subtleties of the signal are not blurred by an abstracting modeling approach.
2. Artifacts are directly learned from data. Simplified noise models that are inadequate for modern coil configurations and acquisition methods become obsolete (e.g. Ricianity).
3. Tissue probabilities are learned from the data. Model derived thresholds, such as on the FA, are obsolete.

The presented method is based on random-forest classification applied to signal samples from the local neighborhood guiding each step of the streamline progression. This is based on the hypothesis that sensitivity and specificity of the tractography process can be increased by exploiting the richness of the diffusion-weighted signal not only at the current streamline position but also in its vicinity.

2 Materials and Methods

Standard streamline tractography approaches reconstruct a fiber by iteratively extending the fiber in a direction depending on the current position. The directional information is usually inferred from a signal model at the respective location, such as the diffusion tensor (DT), fiber orientation distribution functions (fODF) or diffusion orientation distribution functions (dODF). The method presented in this work also iteratively extends the current fiber but in contrast to standard streamline approaches, the determination of the next progression direction relies on a completely different concept:

1. Instead of mathematically modeling the signal the presented method employs a random forest classifier working on the raw diffusion-weighted image values in order to obtain information about local tissue properties, such as tissue type (white matter or not white-matter) and fiber direction (cf. sec. 2.1).
2. To progress or possibly terminate a streamline, not only the image information at the current location but also at several sampling points distributed in the neighborhood are taken into account. The final decision on the next action is then based on a voting process among the individual classification results at these sampling points (cf. sec. 2.2).

2.1 Classifier Training

Classification Features: To become independent of the gradient scheme, the signal is resampled to 100 directions equally distributed over the hemisphere using spherical harmonics. These values are directly used as input features for the classifier. Additionally, the normalized previous streamline direction is added to the list of classification features, thus enabling the method to better overcome ambiguous situations. In total, this results in 103 feature values.

Reference Directions: To train the classifier, reference fiber tracts corresponding to the respective diffusion-weighted image are necessary. For the initial experiments presented in this work, we use a previously performed standard tractography to obtain these tracts. The impact of the tractography algorithm choice on the presented approach was systematically evaluated in our experiments. While this approach introduces an indirect dependence of the training step on the modelling and quality of the training tractograms, our plans to overcome this issue are outlined in section 4.

Classifier Output: The classifier produces a probability $P(v_i)$ for each of 100 different possible fiber directions v_i $(1 \leq i \leq 100)$ corresponding to the 100 signal directions used during training as well as a non-fiber probability P_{nofib}.

2.2 Streamline Propagation

At each step of the streamline progression the signal is sampled at N random positions p^j $(1 \leq j \leq N)$ within a distance r of the current streamline position p. Classification is performed at each p^j to infer the local direction proposal v^j. The subsequent streamline direction v is determined by voting of the weighted proposals: $v = \sum_j v^j$. Each v^j is determined based on the normalized previous streamline direction v_{old} and the probabilities $P^j(v_i)$ of each possible direction: $v^j = \sum_i w_i v_i$, with $w_i = P^j(v_i) \cdot \langle v_i, v_{old} \rangle$. The dot product is a directional prior that promotes straight fibers. An additional hard curvature threshold is employed that, when exceeded, sets $w_i = 0$.

If the non-fiber probability of sample j exceeds the cumulated weighted probabilities of all possible directions ($P^j_{nofib} > \sum_i w_i$), a potential tract boundary is identified and a vote for termination of sample j is considered. Now, the position vector $d = p^j - p$ is related to the previous direction v_{old} in order to decide whether termination is preferable or should be avoided. A termination is considered more likely if non-fiber regions lie straight ahead (i.e. in the current direction of streamline progression v_{old}). If the streamline progresses relatively parallel to the detected fiber bundle margin, a premature termination is rather avoided. To this end an auxiliary sample position $\hat{p}^j$ is evaluated that is determined by a 180° rotation of d around v_{old}:

$$\hat{p}^j = p - d + 2 \cdot \langle v_{old}, \bar{d} \rangle \cdot v_{old}$$

with $\bar{d} = \frac{d}{\|d\|}$. If P_{nofib} at the new position $\hat{p}^j$ is $> \sum_i w_i$ as well, v^j is set to $(0,0,0)$ (vote for termination, cf. Fig. 1a), otherwise v^j is set to $\hat{d} = \hat{p}^j - p$ to deflect the streamline from the detected fiber margin (cf. Fig. 1b). A streamline terminates if all sampling positions vote for termination. To avoid backward orientations of v^j (with respect to v_{old}), positions that are located behind the current sampling position, i.e. behind the plane with origin p and normal v_{old}, are mirrored on the plane before the alternative sampling point $\hat{p}^j$ is determined. After this additional step, the process is the same for all points p^j.

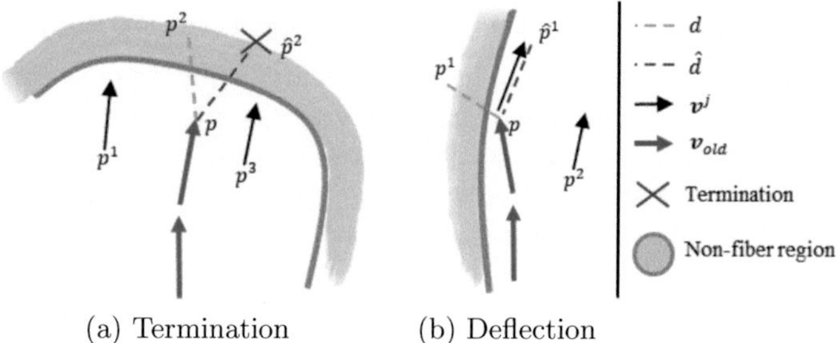

(a) Termination (b) Deflection

Fig. 1. Illustration of the voting process leading to a termination after the next one or two steps (a) and a streamline deflection (b).

2.3 Experiments

The approach was evaluated in comparison to 12 state of the art tractography pipelines using a simulated replication of the *FiberCup* phantom (cf. Fig. 2) (30 gradient directions, b-value $1000\,\mathrm{s\,mm}^{-2}$, 3 mm isotropic voxels, signal-to-noise ratio ~ 40) generated with the *Fiberfox* simulation tool [5] and an *in vivo* dataset (81 gradient directions, b-value $3000\,\mathrm{s\,mm}^{-2}$, 2.5 mm isotropic voxels). Both datasets are available for download at `nitrc.org/projects/diffusion-data/`. All possible configurations of the following openly available and widely known tractography algorithms and local modeling techniques were used as benchmark for the presented approach (cf. Fig. 3 for corresponding toolkits):

- Tractography algorithms:
  - Deterministic streamline tractography (DET)
  - Fiber assignment by continuous tracking (FACT)
  - Tensor deflection tractography (TEND)
  - Probabilistic streamline tractography (PROB)
  - Global Gibbs tractography
- Local modeling techniques:
  - Single-Tensor model (DT)
  - Two-Tensor model (DT-2)
  - Constrained spherical deconvolution (CSD)
  - Constant solid angle Q-ball (CSA)

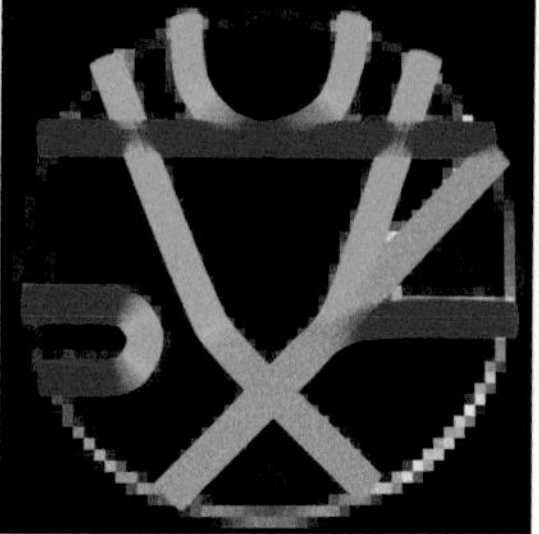

Fig. 2. Structure of the *FiberCup* phantom.

Seeding was performed homogeneously within the brain mask. All tractography algorithms were run with their default parametrization. Only when tracking the simulated phantom image, the stopping criteria (FA and ODF peak thresholds) were manually adjusted to obtain plausible results (FA threshold 0.15, peak threshold for CSA 0.085 and peak threshold for CSD 0.15).

The presented method uses $N = 50$ sampling points, a step size of $0.5 \cdot f$ (f is the minimal voxel size), $r = 0.25 \cdot f$, and a hard curvature threshold at a

Model	Type	No	Valid Connection	Invalid	Bundle Coverage	Angular Error
DT[1]	DET[1]	60%	25%	15%	21%	5°
DT[1]	FACT[1]	62%	23%	14%	24%	6°
DT[1]	TEND[1]	84%	8%	8%	21%	10°
DT[2]	PROB[2]	57%	23%	20%	27%	8°
DT[1]	Global[1]	82%	10%	8%	42%	12°
CSA[1]	DET[3]	24%	67%	9%	70%	8°
CSA[1]	PROB[3]	91%	5%	4%	83%	18°
CSA[1]	Global[1]	81%	14%	5%	74%	13°
DT-2[2]	DET[2]	60%	37%	3%	58%	6°
CSD[3]	DET[3]	21%	78%	1%	86%	4°
CSD[3]	PROB[3]	66%	28%	7%	93%	4°
CSD[3]	Global[1]	81%	17%	2%	72%	12°
-	Proposed	3%	93%	4%	94%	4°

[1]MITK Diffusion (mitk.org/wiki/DiffusionImaging) [2]Camino (cmic.cs.ucl.ac.uk/camino/) [3]MRtrix (brain.org.au/software/mrtrix/)

Fig. 3. Quantitative results on the software phantom. The cells are colored relative to the best (green) and worst (red) result per metric.

maximum angle of 45° between two steps or a maximum directional standard deviation of 30° over the last centimeter by default. The classifier was trained using 30 trees, a maximum tree depth of 50 and a Gini splitting criterion. The training data was sampled equidistantly $(0.5 \cdot f)$ along the input tractogram fibers as well as on 50 randomly placed points in each non-fiber voxel. The defaults for step size and angular thresholds were chosen based on previous experiments with standard streamline approaches. The number of sampling points and the forest parameters yielded stable results in a broad range and increasing them further would mainly impact the computational cost of the proposed approach. Depending on the size of the datasets and the parametrization used for training and tractography the corresponding computation times varied between about 15 minutes (phantom dataset) and 4 hours (*in vivo* dataset) (3.20 GHz Intel® Core^{TM} i7).

To quantitatively assess the impact of the choice of tractography method used for training the classifier, the presented approach was trained individually with each of the benchmark tractograms obtained from the phantom image using the twelve methods described above. Based on the results of this analysis, the most promising algorithm was chosen to obtain the training tractogram for the *in vivo* experiment. To evaluate the presented approach quantitatively, the following metrics from the Tractometer evaluation protocol [1] were analyzed for the phantom-based tractography: the fraction of *no connections*, *valid connections*, *invalid connections* and *bundle coverage*, as well as an additional measure for the local angular error. The *in vivo* tractograms were qualitatively evaluated on basis of reconstructions of the corticospinal tract (CST) and by an analysis of the spatial distribution of fiber end points.

3 Results

The best results on the phantom image were obtained using the CSD DET tractography [6] for training our approach. With this configuration, the presented approach outperformed all benchmark methods in four out of the five metrics

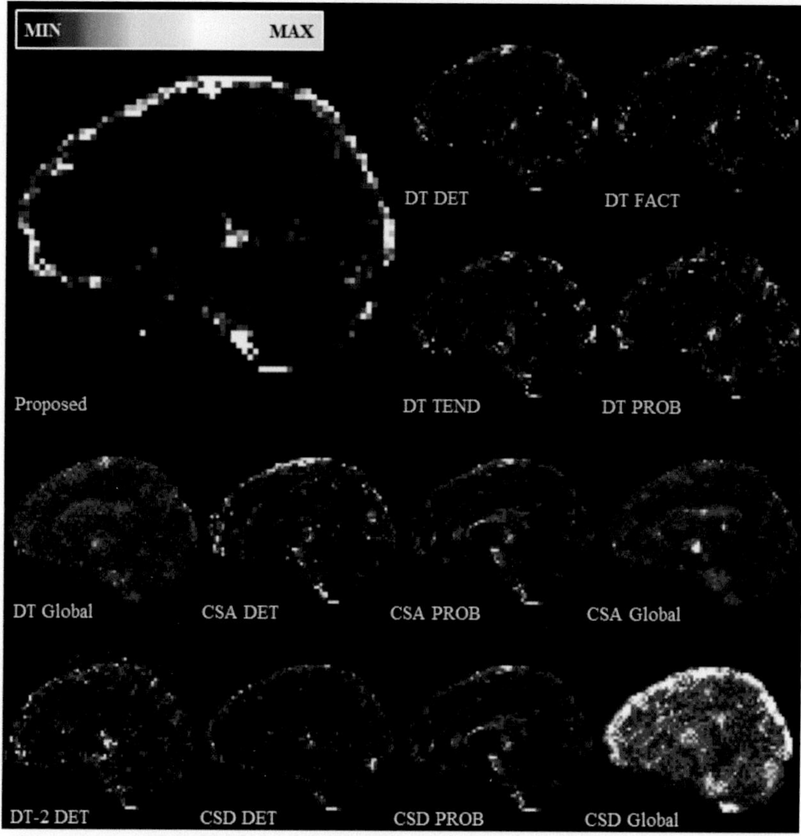

(a) Fiber end-point distributions

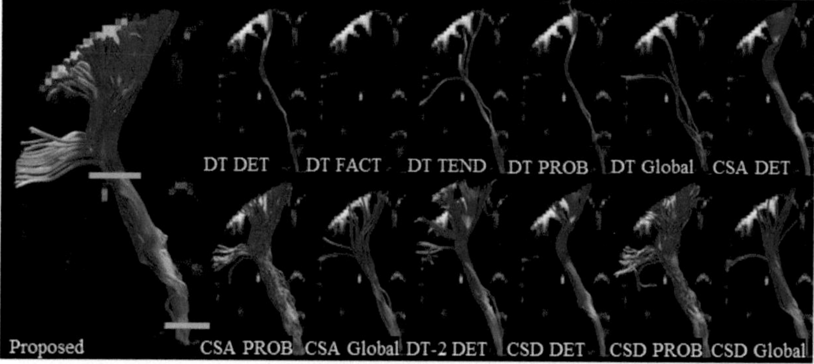

(b) Corticospinal tracts

Fig. 4. Results on the *in vivo* dataset. (a) shows the max-normalized voxel-wise number of fiber endpoints, maximum intensity projected over 20 sagittal slices. (b) shows the corticospinal tracts obtained with all 13 algorithms. The green bars schematically depict the inclusion regions used for all whole brain tractograms to extract the respective CST.

(cf. Fig. 3). Only 3% of the tracts terminated prematurely. Furthermore, the proposed approach yielded the highest percentage of valid connections (93%), the highest bundle coverage rate (94%) and the lowest local angular error (4%). All 7 valid bundles in the phantom were reconstructed successfully. Also, the percentage of invalid connections (4%) is rather low compared to the majority of benchmark algorithms (rank 4 out of 13). When varying the method that was used for training, the percentage of prematurely ending fibers and valid connections yielded by the presented approach improved on average by 56% and 36% respectively as compared to the benchmark tractograms. The average percentage of invalid connections, however, was increased by 21%.

Based on these results, the CSD DET tractography was used to train the classifier for the *in vivo* experiments. *In vivo*, our approach successfully reconstructed a whole brain tractogram including challenging regions such as the crossing between the corpus callosum, the CST and the superior longitudinal fasciculus. Our method was furthermore able to reconstruct parts of the CST that other approaches often missed (cf. lateral projections of the CST in Fig. 4b). In comparison to the benchmark algorithms, most of the fibers reconstructed by the presented approach correctly terminated in the cortex (cf. Fig. 4b).

4 Discussion and Conclusion

The methodological contribution of this work is a random-forest classification-based approach to fiber tractography using neighborhood information that guides each step of the streamline progression. The presented machine learning-based approach is the first of its kind and quantitative as well as qualitative phantom and *in vivo* experiments show promising performance compared to 12 established state-of-the-art tractography pipelines. The quantitative results on the phantom dataset showed a distinctly improved sensitivity and specificity of our method. Especially the number of prematurely ending fibers was strongly reduced as compared to the other methods while also yielding very good results with respect to all other metrics. These results were confirmed by the *in vivo* experiments where our approach yielded very good results in reconstructing difficult tracts (e.g. the lateral projections of the CST) and a much lower number of fibers ending prematurely inside the brain. As expected, tensor based approaches had difficulties in detecting the lateral projections of the CST. However, even the benchmark method that performed best in the phantom experiments (CSD DET) was unable to detect these projection fibers. The benchmark methods that showed a relatively high sensitivity in this region (CSA+CSD PROB and DT-2 DET) displayed a very low specificity in the phantom experiments as well as with respect to the *in vivo* end-point distribution. In contrast, the proposed algorithm showed a constantly high sensitivity and specificity.

The parameters of the proposed method (step size, curvature threshold, number and placement of neighborhood sampling points) have not been optimized explicitly. Previous studies showed that such an optimization has a strong effect on the quality of the resulting tractograms [1] and might improve the results yielded by the presented approach even further. While the parameters of the reference methods have not been optimized either, we used their respective default parametrizations which have already been field-tested.

Future efforts will be undertaken to assess how the machine learning-based approach to process raw signal intensities can be exploited further. An extension of the method to directly include a distinction between different non-white matter tissue types, such as gray matter and corticospinal fluid, seems promising to further improve the decision on terminating the fiber progression. To this end additional contrasts, such as T1-weighted imaging, could be directly included in the presented machine learning-based approach. Another area of interest for further improvements of the method is the training procedure, which is currently based on a previously obtained tractogram. While the choice of this algorithm has been systematically evaluated and the approach already yielded promising results it introduces an indirect dependence on the limitations of the chosen tractography method. To overcome this issue we are investigating the potential of realistically simulated training datasets with known ground truth [5].

The source-code of all methods presented in this work is available open-source and integrated into the Medical Imaging Interaction Toolkit (MITK) [7]. Binaries for all standard platforms (Windows, Linux and Mac) will be published online as free download in one of the next releases.

References

1. Cote, M.A., Girard, G., Bore, A., Garyfallidis, E., Houde, J.C., Descoteaux, M.: Tractometer: Towards validation of tractography pipelines. Med. Image Anal. 17, 844–857 (2013)
2. Fillard, P., Descoteaux, M., Goh, A., Gouttard, S., Jeurissen, B., Malcolm, J., Ramirez-Manzanares, A., Reisert, M., Sakaie, K., Tensaouti, F., Yo, T., Mangin, J.F., Poupon, C.: Quantitative evaluation of 10 tractography algorithms on a realistic diffusion MR phantom. Neuroimage 56, 220–234 (2011)
3. Alexander, D.C., Zikic, D., Zhang, J., Zhang, H.,, C.: Image quality transfer via random forest regression: applications in diffusion MRI. Med. Image Comput. Comput. Assist. Interv. 17(Pt 3), 225–232 (2014)
4. Schultz, T.: Learning a reliable estimate of the number of fiber directions in diffusion MRI. Med. Image Comput. Comput. Assist. Interv. 15(Pt 3), 493–500 (2012)
5. Neher, P.F., Laun, F.B., Stieltjes, B., Maier-Hein, K.H.: Fiberfox: facilitating the creation of realistic white matter software phantoms. Magn. Reson. Med. 72(5), 1460–1470 (2014)
6. Tournier, J.D., Calamante, F., Connelly, A.: MRtrix: Diffusion tractography in crossing fiber regions. International Journal of Imaging Systems and Technology 22, 53–66 (2012)
7. Maier-Hein (ne Fritzsche), K., Neher, P., Reicht, I., van Bruggen, T., Goch, C., Reisert, M., Nolden, M., Zelzer, S., Meinzer, H.P., Stieltjes, B.: MITK diffusion imaging. Method. Inform. Med. 51, 441–448 (2012)

Symmetric Wiener Processes for Probabilistic Tractography and Connectivity Estimation

M. Reisert[1], B. Dihtal[1], E. Kellner[1], H. Skibbe[3], and C. Kaller[2]

[1] Medical Physics, University Medical Center Freiburg, Germany
[2] Freiburg Brain Imaging Center, University Medical Center Freiburg, Germany
[3] Graduate School of Informatics, Kyoto University, Japan

Abstract. Probabilistic tractography based on diffusion weighted MRI has become a powerful approach for quantifying structural brain connectivities. In several works the similarity of probabilistic tractography and path integrals was already pointed out. This work investigates this connection more deeply. For the so called Wiener process, a Gaussian random walker, the equivalence is worked out. We identify the source of the asymmetry of usual random walker approaches and show that there is a proper symmetrization, which leads to a new symmetric connectivity measure. To compute this measure we will use the Fokker-Planck equation, which is an equivalent representation of a Wiener process in terms of a partial differential equation. In experiments we show that the proposed approach leads to a symmetric and robust connectivity measure.

1 Introduction

Diffusion MRI has become a very important tool for understanding the living brain tissue. It can reveal both macro- and microstructural features of the neuronal network of the human brain. Tractography tries to characterize the structural connectome to understand the details of the interregional relationships of the human brain. Tractography algorithms may be divided in deterministic, streamline-based methods, probabilistic approaches and global approaches. In probabilistic tractography one basically draws samples from a distribution over paths and computes some statistics over these paths, for example, recording their endpoints. In some works, the similarity to the notion of path integrals appearing in quantum mechanics [2] and statistical physics [5] was already pointed out [3,1]. Rigorous mathematical investigations show that the basic stochastic process behind path integrals is a so called Wiener process, a continuous Gaussian random walker [10]. In this work we will recap the foundations of the theory of Wiener processes and path integrals. Based on this we build a path integral that leads to a symmetric brain connectivity measure. Besides the walker perspective and path integrals, there is a third, equivalent approach, which describes expectation values of Wiener walkers by partial differential equations (PDE). This equivalence will be used to give an algorithm for the computation of the connectivity measure. It will be based on solving a large linear system, describing a mixed diffusion/convection process.

N. Navab et al. (Eds.): MICCAI 2015, Part I, LNCS 9349, pp. 53–60, 2015.
DOI: 10.1007/978-3-319-24553-9_7

2 Method

Apart from a few examples most methods to estimate brain connectivity are based on the walker principle. Fiber tracts are initiated from certain seed points and are iteratively built by following locally defined directions. While the deterministic tracking approaches are more used for illustrative purposes, the probabilistic ones are more related to quantitative connectivity analysis. In this work we will describe probabilistic tracking in terms of so called Wiener processes. Probabilistic tractography can be described as follows: if we call $\mathbf{s}(t)$ the current state of the tracker at step t, then the next state $\mathbf{s}(t+1)$ is drawn from some transition probability density $W(\mathbf{s}(t+1)|\mathbf{s}(t))$, which depends in some way on the DW-measurement. If W is Gaussian, it is possible to formulate the limit for very small time steps, which results in a Wiener process. In literature [10] these Wiener processes can be described by Langevin equations. To give an example (actually this example already covers everything we need later) we want to consider a simple diffusion process with some additional drift. Let the state of the 'tracker' be $\mathbf{s} \in \mathbb{R}^3$ and $\mathbf{v}$ a vector field causing the drift. Then, the corresponding Langevin equation is $\dot{\mathbf{s}}(t) = \mathbf{v}(\mathbf{s}(t)) + \eta(t)$, where η stands for mean free white noise with variance σ^2 per unit time. It is uncorrelated in time, meaning $\langle \eta(t)\eta(t')\rangle = \sigma^2\delta(t-t')$. The dot in $\dot{\mathbf{s}}$ means time differentiation. An approximative numerical integration gives rise to the propagation scheme: $\mathbf{s}(t+\Delta t) = \mathbf{s}(t) + \mathbf{v}(\mathbf{s}(t))\Delta t + \mathbf{u}(t)\sqrt{\Delta t}$. The first term $\mathbf{v}(\mathbf{s}(t))\Delta t$ looks like ordinary Euler integration. The second, stochastic term $\mathbf{u}(t)$ is drawn independently for each time step from $\mathcal{N}(0, \sigma^2)$. There is a second perspective of this process in terms of its expectation values. Let $\mathcal{S}$ be an ensemble of random walkers described by the above random process. Then, the density of such walkers follows the Fokker-Planck equation (FPE), in this case $\dot{p_t} = -\nabla \cdot (\mathbf{v}p_t) + \frac{\sigma^2}{2}\Delta p_t = \mathcal{H}p_t$ where ∇ is the usual gradient operator in $\mathbb{R}^3$ and Δ the Laplacian. From the form of $\mathcal{H}$ we can already guess that there is an asymmetry: suppose we initiate some walkers at some location $\mathbf{x}_0$, i.e. $p_0(\mathbf{x}) = \delta(\mathbf{x} - \mathbf{x}_0)$ and let the system evolve for some time T and look at the density p_T at some point $\mathbf{x}_1$. We call this number $p_T(\mathbf{x}|\mathbf{x}_0)$. Or, contrarily, we flip the velocity $\mathbf{v}$ to $-\mathbf{v}$, seed the walkers at $\mathbf{x}_1$ and wait for some T and look at $\mathbf{x}_0$. If $\mathbf{v}$ is not divergence free, both processes will lead to different results, i.e. $p_T(\mathbf{x}_1|\mathbf{x}_0) \neq p_T^-(\mathbf{x}_0|\mathbf{x}_1)$, where p^- refers to the $(-\mathbf{v})$ process (for details see our companion report [4]). To symmetrize the process to get a symmetric connectivity measure we use the third perspective: the path integral concept. From the viewpoint of a brain connectivity, the theory of path integrals is probably the most appealing one. The idea is that the connection probability is the sum over all paths weighted by their probability:

$$p_T(\mathbf{x}|\mathbf{x}_0) = \frac{1}{Z}\int_{\{\mathbf{s}\}\in\mathcal{P}_T^{(\mathbf{x}|\mathbf{x}_0)}} \exp\left(-\int_0^T L(\mathbf{s}, \dot{\mathbf{s}})dt\right) \tag{1}$$

where $\mathcal{P}_T^{(\mathbf{x}|\mathbf{x}_0)}$ denotes the set of all paths of length T starting in $\mathbf{x}_0$ and terminating at $\mathbf{x}$. The function L is the Lagrangian, or Osager-Machlup functional [10], describing the cost of the path. For our example it is $L(\mathbf{s}, \dot{\mathbf{s}}) = \frac{1}{2\sigma^2}(\dot{\mathbf{s}} - \mathbf{v}(\mathbf{s}))^2 + \frac{1}{2}(\nabla \cdot \mathbf{v})(\mathbf{s})$, which shows more clearly the above mentioned asymmetry, which is caused by the second term reflecting the divergence of $\mathbf{v}$. If $\mathbf{v}$ and $\dot{\mathbf{s}}$ flip their signs, the value of L changes. A much more reasonable choice is $L_{\mathrm{sym}}(\mathbf{s}, \dot{\mathbf{s}}) = \frac{1}{2\sigma^2}(\dot{\mathbf{s}} - \mathbf{v}(\mathbf{s}))^2$, which is symmetric and results in the following Fokker Planck equation (see [4]):

$$\dot{p}_t = \frac{\sigma^2}{2}\Delta p - \frac{1}{2}(\mathbf{v} \cdot \nabla p_t + \nabla \cdot (\mathbf{v} p_t)) = \mathcal{H} p_t \tag{2}$$

This equation describes paths of a certain length t, however, we are actually interested in *all* paths without any length restriction. That is, we want to sum over all paths of arbitrary length connecting $\mathbf{x}_0$ and $\mathbf{x}$ to get a density $p(\mathbf{x}|\mathbf{x}_0)$ which is independent of T, i.e. $p(\mathbf{x}|\mathbf{x}_0) = \int_0^\infty dT\ p_T(\mathbf{x}|\mathbf{x}_0)$. With the assumption $\lim_{T\to\infty} p_T(\mathbf{x}|\mathbf{x}_0) = 0$, i.e. all walkers eventually die, the function $p(\mathbf{x}|\mathbf{x}_0)$ is the steady state solution of the corresponding FPE, i.e. $p(\mathbf{x}|\mathbf{x}_0)$ is the solution of the equation $-\mathcal{H}p(\mathbf{x}|\mathbf{x}_0) = \delta(\mathbf{x} - \mathbf{x}_0)$. This is the basic type of equation we will solve to estimate brain connectivities. To use the above concepts for DWI connectivity analysis we have to understand that usual probabilistic tractography is markovian with respect to the position $\mathbf{r} \in \mathbb{R}^3$ *and* orientation $\mathbf{n} \in S_2$. So, the state space of the tracker is the joint space of position and orientation $\mathbf{s} = (\mathbf{r}, \mathbf{n})$, where $\mathbf{r} \in \mathbb{R}^3$ and $\mathbf{n} \in S_2$. Also, the data we get from the diffusion measurement is basically a fiber orientation distribution $f(\mathbf{r}, \mathbf{n})$ defined on this joint position/orientation space. We propose to use the following Lagrangian

$$L(\mathbf{r}, \dot{\mathbf{r}}, \mathbf{n}, \dot{\mathbf{n}}) = \frac{1}{2\sigma_r^2}(\dot{\mathbf{r}} - \mathbf{n} f(\mathbf{r}, \mathbf{n}))^2 + \frac{1}{2\sigma_n^2}\dot{\mathbf{n}}^2 \tag{3}$$

as path-costs. Paths with $\dot{\mathbf{s}} \sim \mathbf{n}f$ and small changes in $\mathbf{n}$ are assigned with small costs, and hence, with high probability. From the walker perspective, there is a convective force which drives a walker with internal state $\mathbf{n}$ into direction $\mathbf{n}$, while the speed is proportional to the data term f. Additionally there is diffusion on the orientation variable, enabling the walker to change its directions, or conversely, penalizes too strong bending. The FPE operator looks like

$$\mathcal{H} = \frac{1}{2}(\sigma_r^2 \Delta_{\mathbf{r}} + \sigma_n^2 \Delta_{\mathbf{n}}) - \frac{1}{2}(\mathbf{v} \cdot \nabla_{\mathbf{r}} + \nabla_{\mathbf{r}} \cdot \mathbf{v}) \tag{4}$$

where the velocity is defined by $\mathbf{v}(\mathbf{r}, \mathbf{n}) = \mathbf{n} f(\mathbf{r}, \mathbf{n})$. If we now think of some function $a(\mathbf{r}, \mathbf{n})$ describing a seed point density, and $b(\mathbf{r}, \mathbf{n})$ a terminal density, both may be interpreted as indicator functions describing some cortical region of interests. Then, we can define the symmetric connectivity measure $c(a, b)$ to be $c(a, b) := -\langle a|\mathcal{Z}\mathcal{H}^{-1}b\rangle$, where the operator $\mathcal{Z}$ does a point reflection by $(\mathcal{Z}a)(\mathbf{r}, \mathbf{n}) := a(\mathbf{r}, -\mathbf{n})$. The bra-ket $\langle a|b\rangle$ notation refers to to the standard L_2- inner product. To understand the symmetry properties of the operator $\mathcal{H}$ (and why we get a symmetric connectivity measure) we just have to note that $\mathcal{H}\mathcal{Z} = \mathcal{Z}\mathcal{H}^+$ holds, because the data f is symmetric $\mathcal{Z}f = f$ (here $\mathcal{H}^+$ denotes the adjoint operator of $\mathcal{H}$). In other words, the operator $\mathcal{H}\mathcal{Z}$ is selfadjoint and hence the connectivity amplitudes are symmetric. The interpretation of $c(a, b)$

is straight-forward, it is the sum over all paths connecting region a with region b weighted by their probability according to L in equation (3). Usually the seed functions a and b do not depend on $\mathbf{n}$ because we do not have any preference for the starting orientation, so $\mathcal{Z}a = a$ and $\mathcal{Z}b = b$, so $c(a,b) = \langle a|\mathcal{H}^{-1}|b\rangle$. In all experiments below we will report the normalized connectivity amplitudes $c_n(a,b) = \frac{c(a,b)}{\sqrt{c(a,a)c(b,b)}}$.

2.1 Angular Constraint and Implementation

The Lagrangian (3) penalizes bending, which is a good prior for straight fibers, but underestimates curved fibers. In [1] this problem does not appear, because the walker is always back projected onto the nearest fiber direction in a voxel. Such a behavior cannot be realized by a Wiener process. However, we can mimic such a behavior by an angular constraint such that the walkers do not deviate too strong from the main fiber directions. That is, we only simulate paths where $\mathbf{n}$ is not too far away from the main fiber directions, which is similar to the maximum angle thresholds known from ordinary streamline algorithms, but not so rigorous (it is still possible to find paths where the spatial tangent $\dot{\mathbf{r}}$ to the path is not perfectly $\mathbf{n}$).

The diffusion parameters σ_n and σ_r (see equation (3)) are free parameters of the approach and control the trade-off between angular and spatial uncertainty. Due to implementational reasons (see the companion report [4]) they are linked by $\sigma_r = 5/\pi\sigma_n$, so there is just one parameter left, which we will analyze in the experiments. The speed function f, which represents the DW-data, is constructed from the N local maxima $\mathbf{d}_i$ of a L1-constrained spherical deconvolution result [7]. Specifically, we use $f(\mathbf{n}) = \sum_{i=1}^{N}(\mathbf{n}\cdot\mathbf{d}_i)^{2n}$ with $n = 10$. The simulation domain is defined by thresholding this speed function, i.e. we only consider regions with $f > \epsilon$. In the experiments we used $\epsilon = 0.02$. To solve the FPE we have to set some boundary conditions. It is natural to let the walkers die once they touch the boundary of the domain, which is equivalent to a zero Dirichlet conditions at the boundary. So the complete problem we want to solve is $-\mathcal{H}p = a$ with $p(\partial\Omega) = 0$, where $\partial\Omega$ denotes the boundary of the simulation domain, p the unknown steady state solution and a the seed region where the walkers are emitted. In order to solve this equation we have to discretize the operator $\mathcal{H}$. Details of the discretization scheme can be found in the companion report [4]. The sphere is discretized by 128 directions. The whole matrix is scattered with MATLAB's sparse matrix capabilities. We found the GMRES linear solver the most stable and efficient [8] solver, we just used the MATLAB's `gmres` command. As number of restarts we used 5. The tolerance value is set to 10^{-6} in all experiments. The running time depends on the size of the problem. If we use the setting as described above we get a system with about $2-3\cdot10^6$ variables, which is scattered in $1-2$ minutes on a common Desktop PC (Intel I7, 16GB). Solving the equation also takes about one minute.

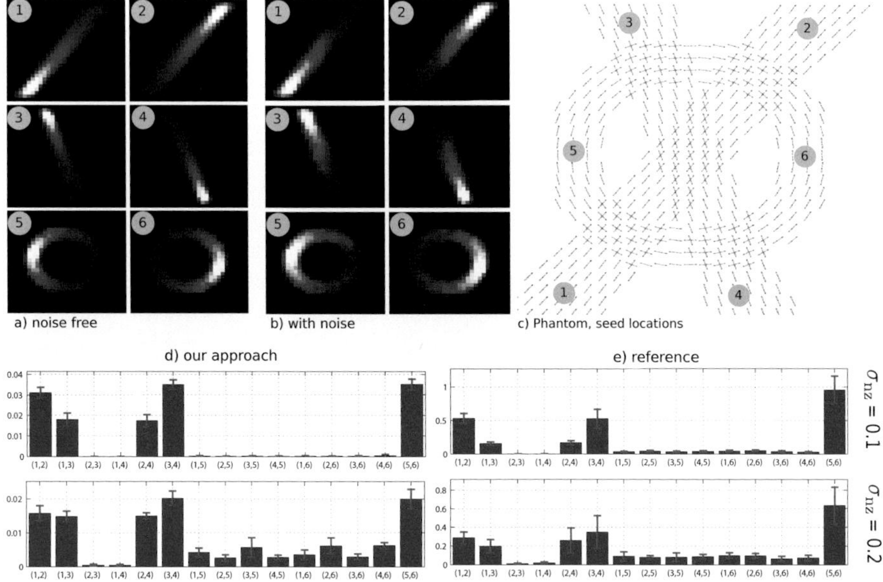

Fig. 1. In (a-b) connectivity amplitudes for two different settings are shown, the color scaling is fixed and the same for both settings. In (c) the FOD of the phantom together with the seed locations is given. The barplots (d,e) show the quantitative analysis of connectivity values (c-values) over 50 trials. The plots show mean c-values together with standard deviations. The x-axis indicates all possible seed pairs (i, j) for $i, j = 1, \ldots, 6$ of the numerical phantom.

3 Experiments

To demonstrate our approach we constructed a numerical phantom consisting of crossing and bending configurations (see Figure 1c)). Six seed locations $\mathbf{r}_1, \ldots, \mathbf{r}_6$ were selected such that they are pairwise connected as (1-2), (3-4) and (5-6). We did not simulate the MR-signal, but created the underlying directions directly. The directions $\mathbf{d}_i$ are created continuously (not aligned with the discretized sphere directions), and a pseudo FOD is generated using $\sum_i \exp(\alpha((\mathbf{d}_i\mathbf{n})^2 - 1)$ woth $\alpha = 10$, which is shown in Figure 1c). For robustness analysis we distorted the directions by Gaussian noise. Figure 1a-b) gives results of our approach for angular diffusion $\sigma_n = 0.2$. The connectivity amplitudes $c(\mathbf{r}, \mathbf{r}_i)$ are displayed as probability maps, where $\mathbf{r}_i$ is one of the fixed seed point. Figure 1a) shows c without noise and b) with noise ($\sigma_{\text{nz}} = 0.1$). To get a quantitative picture we repeated the above experiment for different noise levels $\sigma_{\text{nz}} = 0.1, 0.2$. As reference approach we followed [1], with a stepwidth of $\Delta s = 1$ without revisits and with length bias correction. To keep the approaches comparable, we used exactly the same directions as for the proposed approach and used a backprojected Gaussian distribution for generation of the direction samples with $\sigma = 0.2$ (which we found to work optimal for the phantom). Figure 1d,e) shows barplots of the normalized connectivity amplitudes $c_n(\mathbf{r}_i, \mathbf{r}_j)$ for all pairs of seeds averaged over 50 runs together with its standard deviation.

3.1 In-Vivo Human Brain

For investigations on real DWI data we considered 28 scans of healthy volunteers at a b-value of $1\text{ms}/\mu m^2$ with 61 diffusion directions and an isotropic resolution of $2mm$. A white matter probability map was generated with SPM (Version 8, *http://www.fil.ion.ucl.ac.uk/spm/*) on a T1-weighted scan, which was co-registered to the b_0-scan of the diffusion sequence. For each subject the scans were repeated two times (in two different sessions) to allow to investigate the robustness of the approach. To estimate the fiber orientation distribution we used L1-constrained spherical deconvolution [7]. The fiber response function (FRF) was chosen as $FRF(\mathbf{n}) = \exp(-bD_1(n_i^{\text{fib}} n_i)^2)$ with $D_1 = 1\mu m^2/ms$ for all subjects. The FRF was fixed for all subjects, because in this way also changes of the microstructural parameters are reflected by the FOD. Spurious local maximas were filtered out by neglecting all maximas smaller than 20% of the global one. The speed function is constructed in the same way as for the numerical phantom. The probabilistic white matter segmentation of SPM was thresholded at 0.5 and used as white matter mask. To compare and analyze the group, the AAL atlas [9] was registered to the subjects' native space, normalization was done with SPM 8. The first 90 ROIs (distributed over the cerebral cortex) of the AAL atlas were used to compute connectivity matrices. Figure 2a-c) show examples of the mean connectivity matrices (CM) over the whole group. The first 45 ROIs belong to the right hemisphere, the last 45 to the left hemisphere. The CMs are shown in logarithmic scaling. To get a comparable contrast we used the following formula $c_{\log}(a,b) = \log(t + c_n(a,b))$ where t is the 20% quantile of c_n over all regions. The CMs obtained by our approach for different settings of σ_n are compared to the reference approach [1] (Figure 2d)). As performance measure the intraclass correlation coefficient (ICC)[1] for each connectivity value (c-value) in the CM is used. We also varied the σ parameter $(0.2, 0.5)$ of the reference approach [1] and tried it with and without revisits. It is common to put thresholds to get a binary decision of connectivity. To see how robust the approaches are with respect to such a thresholding operation an agreement measure is calculated as follows: let t be some threshold, then $a = |c_1 < t \wedge c_2 < t|$ denotes the number of regions that are not connected in scan 1 and in scan 2, where the number is counted over all possible ROI pairs and subjects. The agreement value a is normalized by the total number of non-connected regions $s = |c_1 < t| + |c_2 < t|$, and hence, a/s is a number between 0 and 1. If we now vary over all thresholds t and plot a/s as a function of s we get plots displayed in Figure 2e).

[1] If c_1 and c_2 are c-values in the CM for scan 1 and scan 2, respectively, then the ICC is $ICC(c) = \langle (c_1 - \bar{c})(c_2 - \bar{c}) \rangle / \langle (c - \bar{c})^2 \rangle)$, where $\langle\rangle$ denotes the expectation over the whole group and $\bar{c} = \langle (c_1 + c_2)/2 \rangle$. The ICC is 1 if all the variance of the c-value can be explained by differences amongst the subjects.

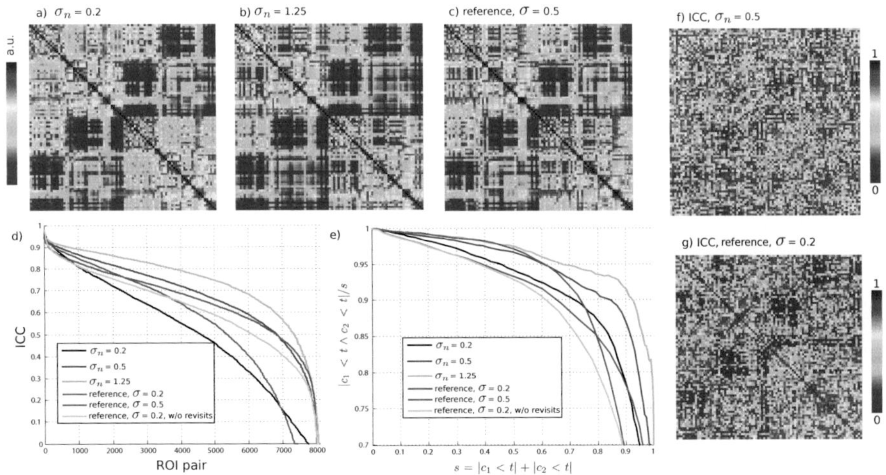

Fig. 2. In (a-c) average connectivty matrices (CM) for different approaches are shown. The matrices in (f,g) show ICC values for individual c-values. Plot (d) displays the ICC for all c-values (all ROI pairs) in the CM sorted by magnitude. Plot (e) shows agreement values.

4 Discussion

We proposed to use a Wiener process for the estimation of structural brain connectivities. The path integral perspective gave us the insight why the usual random walker principle leads to asymmetric connectivities. To symmetrize the solution, the divergence term was omitted, which symmetrized the path integral and the convection part of the Fokker Planck equation. Quantitative experiments show that it leads to a robust connectivity measure. Compared to [1] the new approach shows smaller connectivity values for bending configurations, which is due to the bending penalty inherent to the new approach (see Figure 1). The increased robustness compared to [1] is mainly bought by an increase in σ_n which increases spatial and angular smearing and decreases the bending penalty. The higher σ_n, the more brain anatomy and morphology comes into the play. However, high σ_n emphasizes the length bias, i.e. underestimates long range connections, which is a inherent problem with probabilistic approaches [6]. This is also the main difference to [1], where the curvature is controlled differently. If we want our approach to have a higher connectivity for bending fibers (ROIs (5,6)), then we also get higher c-values for (1,3) and (2,4). For [1] it is different, the step directions are always back projected onto the nearest most likely fiber direction, which results in higher c-values for the bending (5,6). To investigate the new approach in-vivo, we considered a group of volunteers which were all scanned twice. We did a ROI-based approach based on the AAL-atlas. Overall, the CMs obtained from our approach and the reference are similar. As one might expect, with our approach strong bending fibers (like the connection between

'Occipital Sup L' to 'Occipital Sup R') are assigned smaller connectivity values. Analysis of the intraclass correlations of c-values shows that the new approach is quite robust. Higher angular diffusion σ_n gives more robust c-values. Compared to [1] our approach shows higher robustness, however this is mainly caused by the high σ_n values. One can see that in regions with low connectivity [1] has problems (see Figure 2f,g)). We found [1] to work best for $\Delta s = 1$, $\sigma = 0.2$, revisits are allowed and with length bias correction (see [4] for details). In this setting the median ICC is 0.68 which is acceptable, 50% of the c-values have a ICC higher than 0.68. The highest value we can achieve with our approach is a median of 0.78. The agreement scores obtained from thresholded c-values show a similar but more pronounced picture (see Figure 2e)).

Acknowledgement. MR is supported by the DFG, grant RE 3286/2-1 and thanks J. Solera for fruitful discussions. HS is supported by 'Bioinformatics for Brain Sciences', by the MEXT (Japan). CK is partly supported by the BLBT Cluster of Excellence funded by the DFG, grant EXC1086

References

1. Behrens, T.E.J., Berg, H.J., Jbabdi, S., Rushworth, M.F.S., Woolrich, M.W.: Probabilistic diffusion tractography with multiple fibre orientations: What can we gain? Neuroimage 34(1), 1053–8119 (2007); English Article 1053-8119
2. Feynman, R.P., Hibbs, A.R.: Quantum mechanics and path integrals: Emended edition. Courier Dover Publications (2012)
3. Friman, O., Farneback, G.: A bayesian approach for stochastic white matter tractography. IEEE Transactions on Medical Imaging 25(8), 965–978 (2006)
4. Marco Reisert Probabilistic tractography, Path Integrals and the Fokker Planck equation arXiv preprint arXiv:1502.06793 (2015)
5. Kleinert, H.: Path integrals in quantum mechanics, statistics, polymer physics, and financial markets. World Scientific (2009)
6. Jones, D.: Challenges and limitations of quantifying brain connectivity in vivo with diffusion MRI. Future Medicine 2(3), 341–355 (2010)
7. Michailovich, O.: Spatially regularized compressed sensing for high angular resolution diffusion imaging. IEEE Transactions on Medical Imaging 30, 1100–1115 (2011)
8. Saad, Y., Schultz, M.H.: Gmres: A generalized minimal residual algorithm for solving nonsymmetric linear systems. SIAM Journal on Scientific and Statistical Computing 7(3), 856–869 (1986)
9. Tzourio-Mazoyer, N., Landeau, B., Papathanassiou, D., Crivello, F., Etard, O., Delcroix, N., Mazoyer, B., Joliot, M.: Automated anatomical labeling of activations in spm using a macroscopic anatomical parcellation of the mni mri single-subject brain. Neuroimage 15(1), 273–289 (2002)
10. Van Kampen, N.G.: Stochastic processes in physics and chemistry, vol. 1. Elsevier (1992)

An Iterated Complex Matrix Approach for Simulation and Analysis of Diffusion MRI Processes

Hans Knutsson, Magnus Herberthson, and Carl-Fredrik Westin

[1] Biomedical Engineering, CMIV, Linköping University, Sweden
[2] Brigham and Women's Hospital Harvard Medical School, USA
hans.knutsson@liu.se, westin@bwh.harvard.edu

Abstract. We present a novel approach to investigate the properties of diffusion weighted magnetic resonance imaging (dMRI). The process of restricted diffusion of spin particles in the presence of a magnetic field is simulated by an iterated complex matrix multiplication approach. The approach is based on first principles and provides a flexible, transparent and fast simulation tool. The experiments carried out reveals fundamental features of the dMRI process. A particularly interesting observation is that the induced speed of the local spatial spin angle rate of change is highly shift variant. Hence, the encoding basis functions are not the complex exponentials associated with the Fourier transform as commonly assumed. Thus, reconstructing the signal using the inverse Fourier transform leads to large compartment estimation errors, which is demonstrated in a number of 1D and 2D examples. In accordance with previous investigations the compartment size is under-estimated. More interestingly, however, we show that the estimated shape is likely to be far from the true shape using state of the art clinical MRI scanners.

1 Introduction

The field of diffusion weighted magnetic resonance imaging (dMRI) has developed rapidly over recent years and continues to attract a lot of attention. The dMRI observables can be taken as rough measures of tissue micro-structure, cell shape and general directions of the nerve fiber bundles. To move towards more precise measurements require a thorough understanding the process of restricted diffusion in the presence of a magnetic field gradient. To be able to correctly interpret the measurements attained by any given diffusion MR scan is of crucial importance. The commonly used q-space concept is equivalent to assuming a constant rate of spin angle phase change, i.e. constant local spatial frequency, across the compartment. A number of results exist showing that this concept holds an oversimplification of the process [1,2,3,4,5,6]. We present a novel simulation approach enabling a local spatial frequency analysis of the process which demonstrates that this is indeed the case. This fact and the intractability of analytic solutions have prompted a number of researcher to develop dMRI simulator tools [7,8,9,10,11]. Many simulators, however, invoke a boundary condition

N. Navab et al. (Eds.): MICCAI 2015, Part I, LNCS 9349, pp. 61–68, 2015.
DOI: 10.1007/978-3-319-24553-9_8

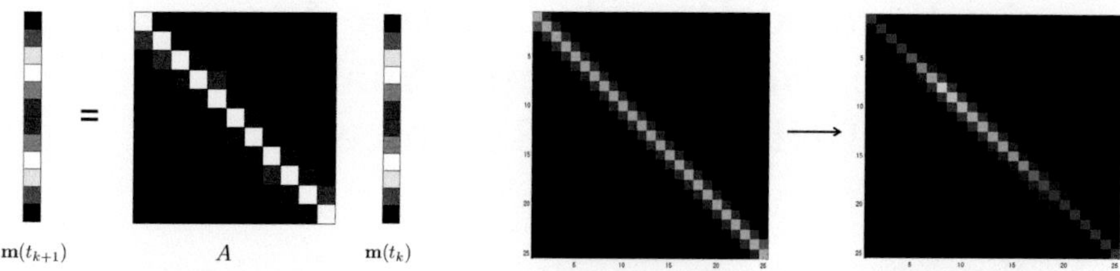

Fig. 1. Left - The process of diffusion can be formulated as an iterative matrix multiplication. **Right** - Color coded simulation matrices: A pure diffusion matrix is shown to the left. The matrix to the right shows how the strength of the local magnetic field increments the phase of the proton spins at each location. Zero phase is coded green, a phase of π is coded red. Blue and yellow codes for $\pi/2$ and $-\pi/2$ respectively. The same color code is used in figures 2 and 4.

motivated, demodulation type, variable change, which is directly linked to the concept of q-space. Our approach is free from this type of *a-priori* modeling.

We believe the main advantages of our iterated complex matrix approach to be: **First principles** – Directly models local diffusion and spin phase change at all points, no additional boundary conditions needed. **Flexibility** – Any compartment shape can be easily specified as a function on a discrete grid and the gradient can be individually specified for each time step. **Transparency** – The development of the local magnetization can be monitored at all points and all times. **Speed** – A matlab simulation providing 10.000 measurements can typically be performed in less than a minute on a modern laptop computer.

We have taken advantage of features listed above and continue to discuss some important consequences of the analysis carried out.

2 Theory and Method

Our method simulates the process of restricted diffusion of spin particles in the presence of a magnetic field by iterated matrix multiplications. To design the simulation matrix and carry out the experiments we used a nearest neighbor approach. The assumption made is that a quantized space-time can provide a good approximation of the continuous process. As illustrated in figure 1, the quantized diffusion process can be expressed as:

$$\mathbf{m}(t_{k+1}) = A\,\mathbf{m}(t_k). \tag{1}$$

Here $\mathbf{m}$ is a complex vector of length N holding the magnetization vectors for each unit. The simulation matrix, A, is an $N \times N$ complex matrix and k is an integer indicating the diffusion time step number. This time step can be large, but initially A is constructed for small time steps (see section 2.1) where A then factors into two matrices: One matrix, D simulating the diffusion process and one matrix, G, simulating the effect on the particle spin angles due to the applied magnetic field. Symmetrizing the process yields:

$$A = G^{1/2} D\, G^{1/2} \tag{2}$$

The diffusion matrix, D, is a real-valued matrix simulating only nearest neighbour interactions thus making it tri-diagonal in the 1-dimensional case. The construction is done in two steps: First the off-diagonal terms are set to specify the amount of particles that flow from the center unit to the neighbouring units. Conservation of mass requires that the columns of the resulting matrix are normalized to unity, i.e. D is a left stochastic matrix. This implies that the columns will hold the probabilities for the new locations of the center unit particles after one time step. The rows specify the relative amount of particles in the adjacent units that move to the center unit. Thus, in general, D will not be symmetric. The spin matrix, G, specifying the spin phase increment occurring during one time step, is a complex diagonal matrix: $G = \text{diag}[\exp((i\gamma g x \Delta t))]$, where γ is the gyromagnetic ratio, g is the applied magnetic gradient strength and x is the spatial position of the corresponding unit.

2.1 The Short Time Limit, $\Delta t \to 0$

Letting the time step become infinitely small by introducing a variable $n \to \infty$ we can express A for finite times as:

$$A = A_0^n = (G_0^{1/2} D_0 \, G_0^{1/2})^n \qquad \text{where } D_0 = I + B \, \tfrac{\Delta t}{n} \quad \text{and} \quad G_0 = I + i \, \underbrace{\gamma \, g \, \text{diag}\, [x_1, ..., x_n]}_{C} \, \tfrac{\Delta t}{n} \tag{3}$$

Here B is tri-diagonal, and C is diagonal. Note that the diffusion mass conservation requirement of D implies that the column sums of B equal zero. Examining A_0, which depends on n, leads to:

$$\begin{aligned} A_0 &= G_0^{1/2} D_0 \, G_0^{1/2} \approx (I + \tfrac{iC\Delta t}{2n})(I + \tfrac{B\Delta t}{n})(I + \tfrac{iC\Delta t}{2n}) \\ &\approx I + (B + iC)\tfrac{\Delta t}{n} \end{aligned} \tag{4}$$

In the limit $\Delta t \to 0$ equation 4 can analytically be shown to be equivalent to the left equation below. Further, by combining equations 1 and 4 in the limit $\Delta t \to 0$, the process can be expressed as the differential equation to the right below.

$$A = e^{(B+iC)\Delta t} \qquad \longleftrightarrow \qquad \frac{\partial \mathbf{m}}{\partial t} = (B + iC)\, \mathbf{m} \tag{5}$$

This highlights the fundamental structure of the process of diffusing spin particles in the presence of a magnetic field gradient. The differential equation above can, in fact, be seen as equivalent to the Bloch-Torre equation, [1], on a discrete grid, which is an indication of the soundness of our matrix simulation approach.

2.2 From Compartment Shape to Simulation Matrix

A major advantage over traditional simulation approaches is that our simulation matrix approach allows compartments of any shape to be specified. The compartment is specified as a function on a grid in any dimension and the matrix components can then be directly found. Work aiming in a similar direction can

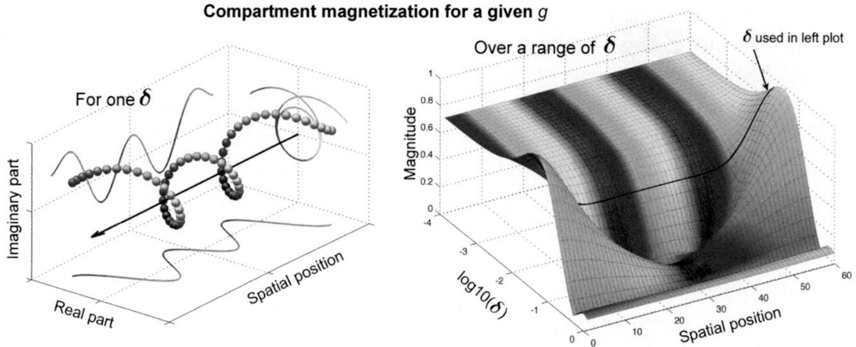

Fig. 2. Left - Positions in the complex plane of 60 magnetization vectors across the compartment for one gradient strength and $\delta = 0.05\ \Delta$. Colors indicate phase angle. The real part is plotted on the back plane and the imaginary part on the bottom plane. The same color code as in figure 1 is used for both plots. **Right** - Magnetization across the compartment (positions 1 to 60) for δ from $10^{-4}\ \Delta$ to $1.0\ \Delta$ (log10 scale). Z-axis shows magnitude and color shows phase. The black line marks $\delta = 0.05\ \Delta$.

be found in [7,10,11]. In the 1D experiments presented here the compartment was quantized to consist of 60 adjacent units. The compartment sizes were found by equidistant sampling of a specified continuous compartment function. The interface sizes were found as the harmonic mean of the flanking compartment sizes. The off diagonal terms in D were set to be proportional to the interface size.

The principles behind the simulation matrix design are readily generalized to higher dimensions. In 2 dimensions we use 4-connectivity and both the diffusion matrix, D, and the spin matrix, G, become block matrices. As before D hold the probabilities of a particle moving from the center unit to an adjacent unit but is now a block tri-diagonal matrix. Further, the gradient, g, and the spatial position, x, become vectors, $\mathbf{g}$ and $\mathbf{x}$. Thus, in 2D, the components of the spin matrix will be given by:

$$G = \text{blockdiag}\left[e^{i\,\gamma\,\mathbf{g}^T\mathbf{x}\,\Delta t} \right] \tag{6}$$

3 Results

The results presented below are from simulations in one and two dimension. The method is, however, equally applicable in three (and higher) dimensions. Results on local frequency are for visualization purposes shown using 1-dimensional compartments. The simulations studying compartment estimation are carried out for 2-dimensional compartments.

Simulated Sequences – The sequences simulated in the experiments were the standard single PFG sequences with encoding parameters δ and Δ and gradient strength g. The length of δ was varied logarithmically from $10^{-4}\Delta$ to $1\ \Delta$, corresponding to the number of time steps, K, ranging from 50 to 500 000. The simulation time for 2000 instances (40 δ, 50 g) was 13 seconds running matlab on a mac book pro.

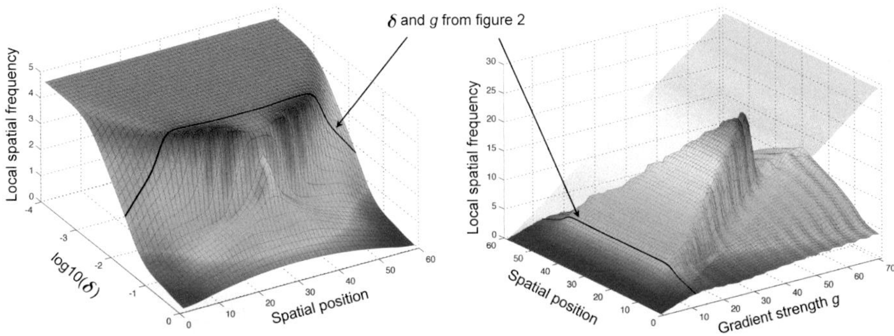

Fig. 3. Left - Color and height shows the local spatial frequency of the magnetization for a given gradient strength. x- and y-axis same as in figure 2 right. The black line marks $\delta = 0.05\ \Delta$. **Right** - Color and height shows the local frequency for different positions across the compartment for $\delta = 0.05\ \Delta$. Spatial position (1-60) is indicated on the x-axis. The y- axis indicates the applied gradient strength. The black lines mark the δ and g used in figure 2.

Local Spatial Frequency – To analyze the diffusion process, the local spatial frequency of the magnetization $\omega(x)$ was computed. The standard definition of local frequency, i.e. the rate of change of the magnetization spin angle, is:

$$\omega(x) = \frac{\partial \arg(\mathbf{m})}{\partial(x)} \tag{7}$$

Figure 2 (left) visualizes compartment magnetization for g corresponding to 2.60 cycles across the compartment using the short pulse approximation (SPA). SPA predicts a complex exponential magnetization across the compartment, i.e. constant local spatial frequency. Even though δ is very short the simulated magnetization clearly deviates from the perfect spiral of a complex exponential and the total number of cycles is only 2.20. Figure 2 (right) shows the compartment magnetization when varying δ. The well known edge effects [2,3,4,5] are noticeable already for $\delta = 10^{-3}\ \Delta$ and increase to be extreme roughly at $\delta = 0.1\ \Delta$. For longer δ the averaging effect of the diffusion effectively prevents a build up of a strong local magnetization. The black line indicates the location of $\delta = 0.05\ \Delta$, the value used to render the left plot.

Figure 3 (left) shows the local frequency dependency on δ for the same g as in figure 2. For lengths up to $\delta = 10^{-3}\ \Delta$ the SPA is valid and the local frequency constant across the compartment. For longer δ the local frequency consistently decreases as the position approaches the compartment edges. The distance from the edge at which the decrease begins increases with increasing δ and at $\delta = 0.1\ \Delta$ this edge effect reaches all the way to the center of the compartment. For longer δ the local frequency is everywhere much lower than predicted by the SPA. Figure 3 (right) shows the local frequency dependence on g for $\delta = 0.05\ \Delta$. For reference the transparent plane shows the SPA prediction. As g increases the local frequency drop gets more pronounced and the effect spreads toward the compartment center. At a g corresponding to 7 cycles across the compartment the edge effect reaches all the way to the center. The black lines in figure 3 indicate the location of $\delta = 0.05\ \Delta$, thus showing the same function but in different contexts.

Simplistically summarized – High b-values do not necessarily lead to high q-values.

Magnetization and Geometry – To illustrate the generality of our approach and the interplay between geometry and local magnetization during a dMRI scan a more elaborate 2-dimensional compartment was designed. Figure 4 shows the local magnetization for a spiral compartment at one measurement point in q-space. The lower plot clearly demonstrates that the encoding basis functions are far from the top plot complex exponentials commonly assumed. It is clear that the basis created will be dependent on the geometry of each individual compartment present in one voxel. Thus, to quote a giant in the field, '...the concept of q-space no longer has any meaning...' [1] p356.

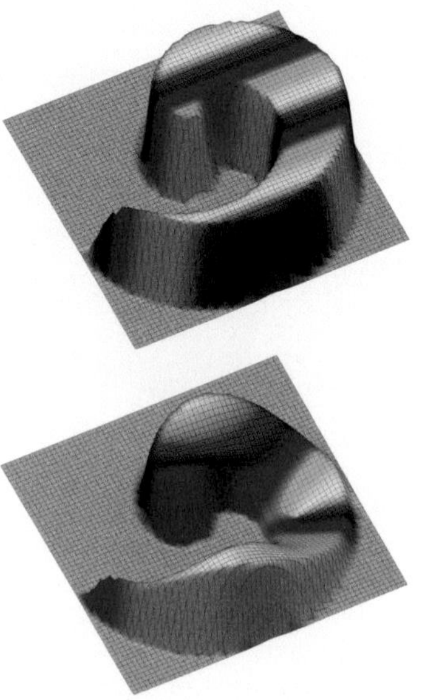

Fig. 4. A spiral compartment demonstrating the effect of geometry on local magnetization for one measurement point in q-space. The magnetization magnitude is given by the height and color indicates phase (the same color code as in figures 1 and 2). The ideal case is shown on top, the lower plot shows a realistic case.

3.1 Compartment Estimation

In this section we present results showing how a Fourier transform based estimation of the spatial compartment shape will appear for in a number of different situations. The results presented correspond to the use of a sPFG sequence consisting of a first gradient, $\mathbf{g}$, applied during a time δ followed by a very weak gradient, $\mathbf{g}_l$, of the opposite sign during a long time, δ_l, where $\mathbf{g}_l\delta_l = -\mathbf{g}\delta$. This type of 'short-long' sPFG pulses will lead to that the measurement attained give the Fourier transform of the compartment [6]. Hence deviations can be studied by making 'reconstructions' using an inverse Fourier transform.

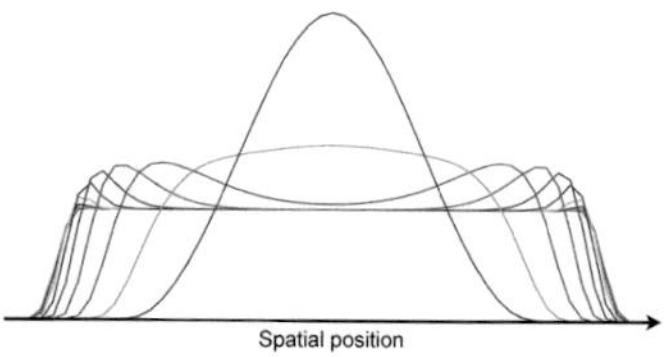

Fig. 5. Reconstructions in 1-dimension using the 'short-long' single PFG sequence: The different curves represent reconstructions when δ is varied logarithmically over a range of 10^5 keeping the product $g\delta$ constant.

Compartment Estimation in one Dimension – To show the general features of the dMRI measurement protocol 1D simulations followed by an inverse Fourier transform were performed. Figure 5 shows the reults when varying δ logarithmically over

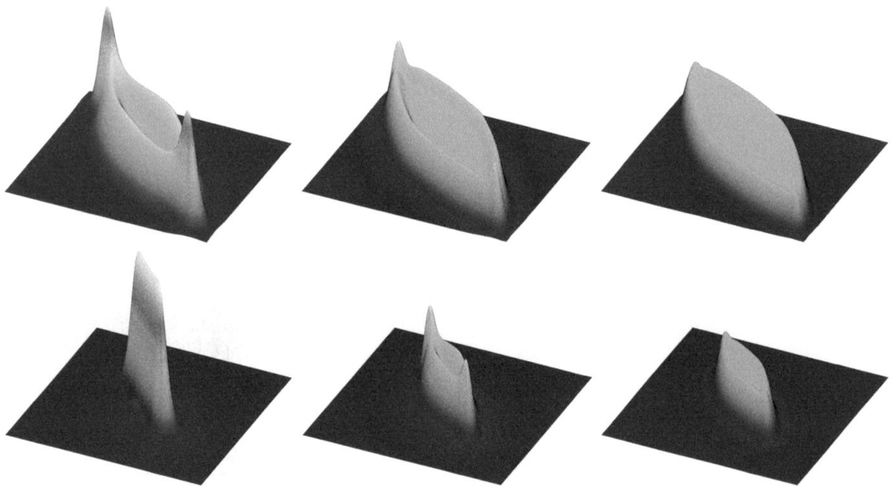

Fig. 6. 2D reconstruction results for two different compartment sizes and three different scanner settings. Top row compartment size = $14 \times 40\,\mu m$. Bottom row compartment size = $7 \times 20\,\mu m$. Parameters from left to wright: **(1)** $\delta_{Max} = 80\,mS$, $g = 150\,mT/m$, **(2)** $\delta_{Max} = 8\,mS$, $g = 1500\,mT/m$, **(3)** $\delta_{Max} = 0.8\,mS$, $g = 15\,T/m$.

a range of 10^5 keeping the q-values, i.e the products $g\delta$, identical. The results are consistent with the findings studying local frequency and show that very short delta, $\delta = 10^{-3}\Delta$ or shorter, are needed for a good reconstruction. At $\delta = 5\ 10^{-3}\ \Delta$ (the black curve) the edge effect is clearly visible and at $\delta = 0.3\ \Delta$ (the cyan curve) the reconstruction distortion is severe.

Compartment Estimation in Two Dimensions – Results from different 2D reconstructions of two compartments having the same shape, a super-quadric with exponent 1.5, but different sizes are shown in figure 6. The leftmost plots show results using parameters corresponding to a good MR scanner. The middle and right plots show the results if 10 (middle) or 100 (right) times higher gradients were available. It is clear that the distorting 'edge effects' seen in 1D become much more complex in 2D and here also radically changes the apparent shape of the compartment. Only at the unrealistic g-value of 15 T/m are the compartment reconstructions good replicas of the true shapes. Interestingly, the distortions clearly increases compartment anisotropy.

4 Conclusion and Discussion

We have presented a novel simulation tool to study diffusion weighted magnetic resonance imaging (dMRI). The flexibility, transparency and speed of our iterated matrix approach has allowed us to investigate a number of important properties of dMRI. We have shown that there is a significant decrease of the local spatial frequency of the magnetization at the compartment at clinical values of δ and that this will have a major impact on compartment size and shape estimates using traditional modeling. However, diffusion MRI scans will continue to hold a lot of information and following the leads presented above we feel confident that better models for extracting micro structure properties will be put forward. The power of these models can then be tested using simulations and, when found to be improvements on state of the art, find their way into clinical practise.

Acknowledgement. The authors wish to thank Jens Sjölund and Mats Andersson for valuable comments on the manuscript. The authors acknowledge the VR grants 2011-5176, 2012-3682, SSF AM13-0090, CADICS Linneaus research environment and NIH grants R01MH074794 and P41EB015902.

References

1. Callaghan, P.T.: Principles of nuclear magnetic resonance microscopy, vol. 3. Clarendon Press, Oxford (1991)
2. Mitra, P., Halperin, B.: Effects of finite gradient-pulse widths in pulsed-field-gradient diffusion measurements. JMR, Series A 113(1), 94–101 (1995)
3. Stepisnik, J., Duh, A., Mohoric, A., Sersa, I.: MRI edge enhancement as a diffusive discord of spin phase structure. JMR (San Diego, Calif: 1997) 137(1), 154–160 (1999)
4. Åslund, I., Cabaleiro-Lago, C., Söderman, O., Topgaard, D.: Diffusion NMR for determining the homogeneous length-scale in lamellar phases. The Journal of Physical Chemistry. B 112(10), 2782–2794 (2008)
5. Åslund, I., Topgaard, D.: Determination of the self-diffusion coefficient of intracellular water using PGSE NMR with variable gradient pulse length. JMR (San Diego, Calif: 1997) 201(2), 250–254 (2009)
6. Laun, F.B., Kuder, T.A., Wetscherek, A., Stieltjes, B., Semmler, W.: NMR-based diffusion pore imaging. Physical Review E 86(2), 021906 (2012)
7. Hwang, S.N., Chin, C.L., Wehrli, F.W., Hackney, D.B.: An image-based finite difference model for simulating restricted diffusion. Magnetic Resonance in Medicine 50(2), 373–382 (2003)
8. Drobnjak, I., Siow, B., Alexander, D.C.: Optimizing gradient waveforms for microstructure sensitivity in diffusion-weighted MR. Journal of Magnetic Resonance 206(1), 41–51 (2010)
9. Russell, G., Harkins, K.D., Secomb, T.W., Galons, J.P., Trouard, T.P.: A finite difference method with periodic boundary conditions for simulations of diffusion-weighted magnetic resonance experiments in tissue. Physics in Medicine and Biology 57(4), N35 (2012)
10. Nguyen, D.V., Li, J.R., Grebenkov, D., Bihan, D.L.: A finite elements method to solve the Bloch-Torrey equation applied to diffusion magnetic resonance imaging. Journal of Computational Physics 263(0), 283–302 (2014)
11. Li, J.R., Calhoun, D., Poupon, C., Le Bihan, D.: Numerical simulation of diffusion MRI signals using an adaptive time-stepping method. Physics in Medicine and Biology 59(2), 441 (2014)

Prediction of Motor Function in Very Preterm Infants Using Connectome Features and Local Synthetic Instances

Colin J. Brown[1], Steven P. Miller[2], Brian G. Booth[1], Kenneth J. Poskitt[3], Vann Chau[2], Anne R. Synnes[3], Jill G. Zwicker[3], Ruth E. Grunau[3], and Ghassan Hamarneh[1]

[1] Simon Fraser University, BC, Canada
[2] The Hospital for Sick Children and The University of Toronto, ON, Canada
[3] University of British Columbia and Child and Family Research Institute, BC, Canada

Abstract. We propose a method to identify preterm infants at highest risk of adverse motor function (identified at 18 months of age) using connectome features from a diffusion tensor image (DTI) acquired shortly after birth. For each full-brain DTI, a connectome is constructed and network features are extracted. After further reducing the dimensionality of the feature vector via PCA, SVM is used to discriminate between normal and abnormal motor scores. We further introduce a novel method to produce realistic synthetic training data in order to reduce the effects of class imbalance. Our method is tested on a dataset of 168 DTIs of 115 very preterm infants, scanned between 27 and 45 weeks post-menstrual age. We show that using our synthesized training data can consistently improve classification accuracy while setting a baseline for this challenging prediction problem. This work presents the first image analysis approach to predicting impairment in motor function in preterm-born infants.

1 Introduction

Every year, an estimated 2.2 million babies worldwide are born very preterm (born at 32 weeks gestation or younger) [6]. Very preterm birth puts newborns at a high risk of long-term motor dysfunction (e.g. cerebral palsy), which places significant burdens on the child, the family and the community [2,12]. Early detection of motor dysfunction could enable more rapid identification of infants who would benefit from rehabilitative interventions. While motor outcomes can be assessed in preterm-born infants at 18 months of age using the Bayley Scales of Infant and Toddler Development, Third Edition (Bayley-III) [4], we desire earlier identification of infants at risk in order to inform care and ongoing monitoring.

Certain brain pathologies, such as white matter injury (WMI) and intraventricular hemorrhaging (IVH) are detectable in a structural MRI scan of an infant's brain. It is also known that some of these pathologies, as well as findings from more advanced MR methods such as diffusion tensor imaging (DTI), are associated with later neurodevelopmental outcomes [3,8]. However, most studies to date have

N. Navab et al. (Eds.): MICCAI 2015, Part I, LNCS 9349, pp. 69–76, 2015.
DOI: 10.1007/978-3-319-24553-9_9

focused on group differences or correlations between specific DTI measures and motor outcomes. For example, Chau et al. recently reported that the trajectory of brain maturation from early in life to term-equivalent age, using region-of-interest-based DTI measures, was associated with neurodevelopmental outcomes [8]. Ball et al. examined the relationship between connectivity in the thalamo-cortical connectome in preterm infants and Bayley-III scores [3]. They found that the strength of certain connections were significantly correlated with outcomes.

In comparison to finding correlations, prediction is a harder problem. In order to predict accurately, the complete set of factors contributing to outcome must be modelled. Prediction of motor function from brain structure at birth is thus very challenging due to the large number of confounding factors affecting brain development, including potentially unknown genetic and environmental factors. It is especially difficult in young infants due to the combination of limited image resolution and small brain sizes, artifacts due to motion and rapid structural change across a small temporal window [5]. Furthermore, datasets are often class-imbalanced, containing fewer abnormal cases. This last issue is of particular importance to prediction since many prediction models are highly sensitive to imbalanced training data [10].

Strategies exist in the literature to alleviate this class imbalance problem by augmenting the training set. For example, the synthetic minority over-sampling technique (SMOTE) finds K nearest neighbours to each training instance and interpolates new instances randomly along lines connecting neighbours [9]. Another method is to sample synthetic instances from an approximate distribution of positive instances, learned using kernel density estimation (KDE). Alternatively, the dominant modes of variation for positive training instances can be learned using principal component analysis (PCA), then sampled to generate new instances. The method that generates the most realistic synthetic instances (i.e., those which improve prediction accuracy the most) is likely application dependent, making class imbalance challenging for prediction problems.

Despite the challenges, prediction of long-term motor dysfunction within the first few weeks of birth remains a desirable goal as it would enable better treatment planning and a more informed assessment of patient outcome. Recently, Ziv et al. used connectome based features from term infants scanned at 6 months of age to predict general neurological outcome at 12 months [18]. Here we set the goal of predicting motor outcome at 18 months from scans taken within the first weeks after birth. In our study, the earlier post-menstrual age (PMA) at scan and the larger temporal gap between scan and outcome makes our task even more challenging. Similar to Ziv et al. we use dimensionality-reduced connectome features and a support vector machine (SVM) classifier to achieve this goal. However, we also introduce a novel method for generating synthetic training samples designed to tackle the specific challenges in our data. Our training data contains only a small number of positive instances existing in a high-dimensional space, likely constrained to a complex manifold. In order to only generate realistic data, we propose a data interpolation technique that generates synthetic instances which are restricted to be more similar to individual known instances.

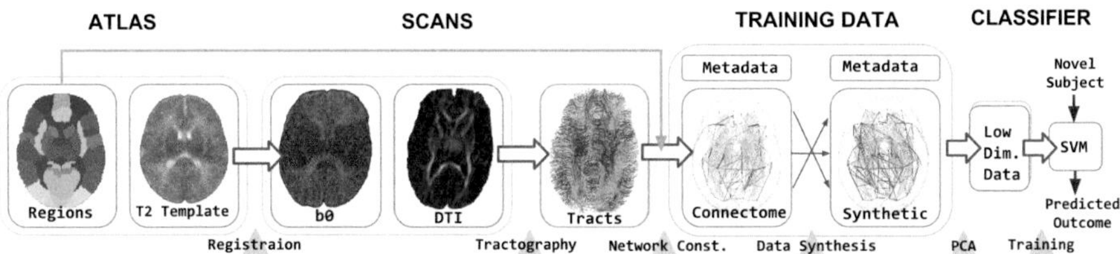

Fig. 1. High level schematic representation of connectome and training pipeline.

In this paper, we show for the first time that 18-month motor outcomes, assessed with the Bayley-III, can be predicted from an MRI taken in the first weeks of a preterm neonate's life. Our method achieves an accuracy of > 70%, which establishes a baseline level of accuracy for this important yet very challenging task. Further, we demonstrate that data augmentation can reliably improve prediction scores and that our novel method for generating local synthetic instances outperforms competing methods.

2 Methods

In Fig. 1, we present a schematic diagram of our supervised learning framework for predicting motor function at 18 months from DTI scans acquired in the first weeks of life. Details for this pipeline are presented below.

Dataset: The cohort used in this study was a group of 115 preterm infants born between 24 and 32 weeks PMA. Neonates underwent a brain MRI between 27 and 45 weeks PMA on a Siemens (Erlangen, Germany) 1.5T Avanto using VB 13A software. Each scan was a multi-slice 2D axial EPI diffusion MR acquisition (TR 4900 ms; TE 104 ms; FOV 160 mm; slice thickness 3 mm; no gap) with 3 averages of 12 non-colinear gradient directions, with an isotropic in-plane resolution of 0.625 mm. Two such acquisitions were performed: one at $b = 600$ s/mm^2 and one at $b = 700$ s/mm^2. The combined diffusion weighted image set was preprocessed using the FSL Diffusion Toolbox (FDT) pipeline[1] and tensors were fit using RESTORE [7]. Nearly half of the subjects (53) were scanned twice for a total of 168 diffusion tensor images.

At 18 months, each subject was evaluated using the Bayley-III test which produces three composite scores of cognitive, language and motor skills [4]. The scores are normalized with mean of 100 and standard deviation of 15; we considered adverse motor outcomes as scores below 85 (i.e., −1 std.). In our cohort, 146 scans were of infants with normal motor function at 18 months, and 22 scans were of infants with abnormal motor function.

Connectome Construction and Analysis: Each DTI was segmented using a neonatal atlas of 90 brain regions from the IDEA group at University of North Carolina (UNC) School of Medicine, Chapel Hill [15]. The atlas' associated T2 template was aligned to the b0 image of each DTI scan in order to segment each brain. Alignment was performed as a rigid registration using FMRIB's

[1] http://fsl.fmrib.ox.ac.uk/fsl/fslwiki/FDT

Linear Image Registration Tool (FLIRT) [11] followed by a deformable registration using the MATLAB Image Registration Toolbox (MIRT)[2]. Full-brain tractography was performed on each scan using TrackVis [16]. Each connectome was constructed by grouping tracts according to their endpoint regions. Following [5], we constructed three connectome types for each scan, including a mean-FA weighted connectome, a tract-count connectome and a normalized tract-count connectome. Network measures summarizing the connectome's topological properties were computed for each connectome type. Ten individual network measures were extracted: 1) mean nodal degree, 2) transitivity, 3) global efficiency, 4,5) raw and normalized modularity, 6,7) raw and normalized clustering coefficient, 8,9) raw and normalized characteristic path length and 10) small-worldness. Each measure was computed for mean-FA, tract-count and normalized tract-count connectomes giving a total of $30 = 10 \times 3$ measures. For a comprehensive summary of network measures and their meanings, see [13].

Classification: For each DTI scan, metadata and connectome features were extracted. See Table 1 for a full list of feature types. Metadata features included gender, age-at-scan and age-at-birth. Age-at-scan is included because we expect it to be an important co-variate given the rapid development of the brain across the age range of our cohort. Connectome features included mean FA across each of the $4005 = 90 \times 89/2$ edges and other high-level network features as described above. WMI severity (graded $[0,3]$) and IVH severity (graded $[0,4]$), assessed from a T1 MRI by an experienced neuroradiologist (KJP), were included as additional features. All features were concatenated into one feature vector.

Feature vectors from the training set were processed using PCA to extract, at most, the top m modes of variation. At test time, instances were projected into this PCA space. A linear dimensionality reduction method was used instead of, for instance, a kernel based method in order to prevent over-fitting to our sparsely sampled, high-dimensional training set. An SVM classifier was then trained on the instances in this reduced space.

Local Synthetic Instances (LSI): Due to the limited number of cases in our cohort that show motor dysfunction (22 out of 168), our training set has a severe class imbalance ($>$ 6:1). We compensate for this by both replicating existing positive instances, $\mathbf{t}_i$ (i.e., feature vectors), and by generating new synthetic positive instances, $\mathbf{s}_j$. New instances are generated by interpolating instance feature vectors within the training set of N positive instances.

We do not know the true distribution of positive instances but we assume that it is locally smooth. Under this assumption, we can generate reasonable synthetic instances as long as they are near existing positive training instances. To this end, we seek an interpolant that satisfies two conditions: (i) gives the majority of weight to one training instance and (ii) gives some non-zero weight to other instances to ensure some variation. We achieve this by randomly assigning elements from a normalized p-series as weights to each instance. Let P^j be a random $N \times N$ permutation matrix and $\mathbf{r}^j = P^j[1, 2, ..., N]^T$. Then, the elements,

[2] https://sites.google.com/site/myronenko/research/mirt

r_i^j, of $\mathbf{r}^j$ are numbers from 1 to N and the vector $\mathbf{r}^j$ is randomly ordered and,

$$\mathbf{s}_j = \sum_{i=1}^{N} w(r_i^j)\mathbf{t}_i \qquad \text{where} \qquad w(i) = \frac{i^{-p}}{\sum_{n=1}^{N} n^{-p}}. \tag{1}$$

Thus, for the jth synthetic instance, $\mathbf{s}_j$, $\mathbf{r}^j$ randomly assigns weights to training instances without replacement. Note that $\sum_{i=1}^{N} w(i) = 1$. Also, note that $\forall i > 1, w(1) \geq 2^p w(i)$ and for $p = 2$ (and in fact, any $p >$ 1.7287), $w(1) > \sum_{i=2}^{N} w(i)$ for any N. In other words, the weight on one instance dominates the others and each synthetic instance will be generated local to one training instance as desired. Fig. 2a is a schematic example of synthetic instances generated from three real instances.

The proposed LSI method has desirable properties compared to other existing methods in the case of high-dimensional data and small number of training instances, as we have here. For instance, while samples from a KDE-estimated distribution are likely to be near training instances, a fixed kernel is used, resulting in new instances that may not vary away from training instances in a realistic way. Instead, LSI encourages new instances to be near training instances but requires variation to be towards known training data. Furthermore, unlike KDE, LSI does not allow extrapolation. This is adventageous since, given a small training size, extrapolation is unlikely to yield realistic samples (Fig. 2b(i)). SMOTE generates instances local to a subset of known instances but fails where the manifold of positive instances is too sparsely sampled to be approximated using nearest neighbours (Fig. 2b(ii)). Sampling from PCA modes ensures that new instances only vary along primary modes of variation but may generate samples that are anatomically implausible since they may not be near any training instance (Fig. 2b(iii)). In comparison, the proposed method offers a balance between trusting local instances and using global information.

3 Results

We evaluated our method using a variety of feature subsets and instance synthesis methods. We assessed classification accuracy for different sets of feature types (Table 1) via 1000 rounds of cross-validation. In each round, one positive and one negative instance were left out for testing. Test subjects were omitted from training data and, since some subjects were scanned twice, the total training set varied between 164 and 166 scans. For these tests, we set $m = 20$, which explains $> 99\%$ of the variance and set $p = 2$. SVM misclassification penalty was set empirically to $C = 2^{-7}$ but test accuracy was relatively insensitive to this value, varying only about 1% for $2^{-8} < C < 2^{-6}$. Classes were balanced by weighting positive instances via replication. Table 2 shows prediction results for different sets of features and compares those tests run with synthetic training data versus those without. In the tests with synthetic data, the training set was first doubled by generating synthetic instances, then real positive training instances were replicated until the classes were balanced.

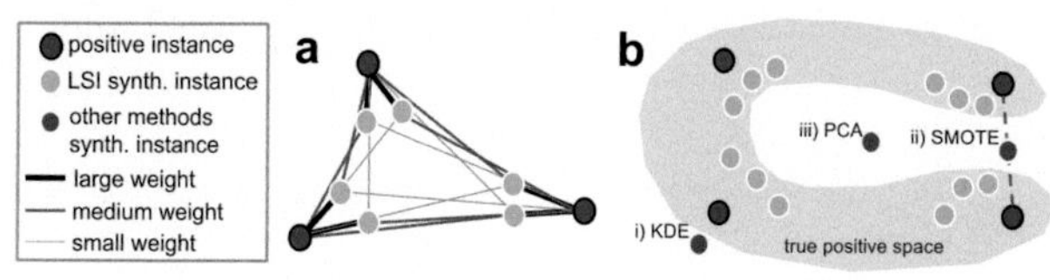

Fig. 2. a) Schematic representation of LSI weights for 6 synthesized instances. b) Possible failure cases for other data augmentation methods.

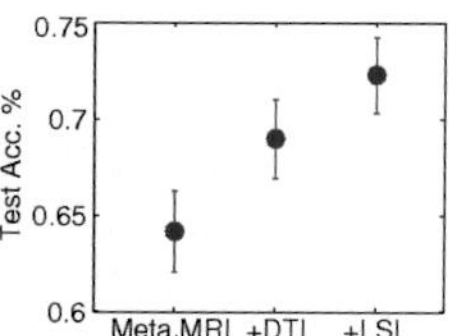

Fig. 3. Test accuracy and 95% CIs for select tests from Table 2.

Table 1. Name and description of each feature type.

Name	Description (# features)	Name	Description (# features)
Meta	Birth age, scan age and gender (3)	MRI	WMI and IVH scores at birth (2)
Edge	Connectome edge FA values (4005)	Network	High-level network measures (30)

Table 2. Mean training (Tr) and test accuracy, sensitivity (Sn) and specificity (Sp) for 1000 rounds of leave-2-out cross validation. Tests marked * are plotted in Fig 3. Best test accuracy is in **bold**.

	No Synth. Data				With Synth. Data			
Feature Types Used	Tr	Test	Sn	Sp	Tr	Test	Sn	Sp
Meta, MRI	69.0	64.2*	0.46	0.83	69.9	64.4	0.47	0.82
Meta, Edge	85.0	58.5	0.33	0.84	86.1	58.5	0.34	0.83
Meta, Edge, Network	85.5	61.2	0.34	0.82	85.7	62.8	0.43	0.83
Meta, Edge, Network, MRI	84.4	64.7	0.51	0.79	85.0	64.7	0.49	0.81
Meta, Network, MRI	77.5	69.0*	0.56	0.82	79.3	**72.3***	0.66	0.79

Note that the addition of synthetically-generated instances improved our highest test accuracy by 3%. Furthermore, as expected, the inclusion of high-level connectome features and MRI-based gradings (i.e. WMI & IVH grades) consistently boosted accuracy on average by about 3% each. Interestingly, *excluding* edge FA features causes the classification accuracy to *improve* when network measures and MRI-based scores are included. This is likely because the edge features are noisy and that much of the relevant structural information from the edge features is captured more succinctly in the network measures, WMI grade, and IVH grade. It may also suggest that no single white-matter fibre bundle is strongly tied to motor-outcome and instead that more widespread factors are at work. This finding is consistent with recent work in [2] which showed that the causes of poor motor outcome are multi-faceted. Note also that while metadata and MRI based information alone provides reasonable predictive power, it is clearly advantageous to include connectome information derived from DTI. This is shown in Fig. 3 with 95% confidence intervals (CI) for each result.

For the test using the subset of features that gave the highest test accuracy (Meta, Network, MRI), test accuracy was 69% across an infant's first scans and 74% across their second scans. This suggests that the later scans may be at some advantage in their ability to predict outcome. This is not surprising since the temporal gap between scan-time and assessment for these scans is smaller.

Again using the same features and ratio of synthetic to training instances that achieved the highest accuracy in the above experiment, we tested four different instance synthesis methods (Table 3). For KDE, a Gaussian kernel was used and, after checking a range of scales, a standard deviation equal to the mean distance between samples was found to give the highest accuracy. SMOTE with different costs (SDC) is a variant of SMOTE, improved to better handle imbalanced classes [1]. For SDC, we set $K = 1$ as it was found to give highest accuracy over range $[1, 5]$. For PCA, once the variation modes were learned, new instances were generated by sampling the Gaussian distribution defined by the variation modes. To be consistent with the PCA step used for classification, again the top $m = 20$ modes of variation were used. We also compared these synthesis methods against subset sampling optimization (SSO) [17], a state-of-the-art undersampling method, and weighted Lagrangian twin SVM (WLT), a classifier designed to natively deal with class imbalance [14]. No replicated or synthetic instances were used with these methods. Note that since we use non-image data in our feature vector, data augmentation methods which modify the images directly are not applicable here, and so were not tested. Table 3 shows that our proposed method outperforms the competing methods. These findings agree with our hypothesis at the end of Section 2, that LSI is well suited to a small sample size from a complex manifold in high-dimensional space.

Table 3. Comparison between class balancing methods. Test accuracies with 95% CIs plotted on right.

Method	Tr	Test	Sn	Sp	Method	Tr	Test	Sn	Sp
WLT	74.2	54.3	0.23	0.85	PCA	79.0	68.5	0.57	0.80
SSO	88.8	62.1	0.56	0.68	KDE	79.7	68.9	0.57	0.81
SDC	78.3	67.6	0.56	0.80	LSI	79.3	**72.3**	0.66	0.79

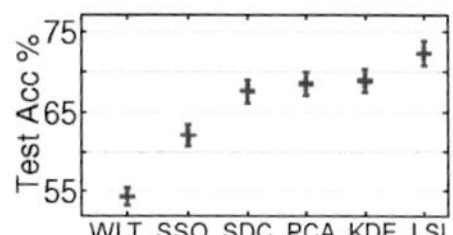

4 Conclusions

In this paper, we predicted preterm infant motor outcomes at 18 months using structural connectome features from DTI scans taken at birth. In doing so, we established a baseline accuracy of over 70% for this challenging but important task. We also proposed a novel method to mitigate the effects of small positive sample sizes common to normal/abnormal datasets. Our approach improved prediction accuracy and outperformed a variety of other methods for this application. In future works, we plan to more thoroughly explore the characteristics of our LSI method and find ways (e.g. via other engineered or learned features and different machine learning techniques) of improving prediction accuracy even further.

Acknowledgements. We thank NSERC, CIHR, NeuroDevNet and the Michael Smith Foundation for Health Research for their financial support.

References

1. Akbani, R., Kwek, S., Japkowicz, N.: Applying support vector machines to imbalanced datasets. In: Boulicaut, J.-F., Esposito, F., Giannotti, F., Pedreschi, D. (eds.) ECML 2004. LNCS (LNAI), vol. 3201, pp. 39–50. Springer, Heidelberg (2004)
2. Back, S.A., Miller, S.P.: Brain injury in premature neonates: A primary cerebral dysmaturation disorder? Annals of Neurology 75(4), 469–486 (2014)
3. Ball, G., Pazderova, L., Chew, A., Tusor, N., Merchant, N., Arichi, T., Allsop, J.M., Cowan, F.M., Edwards, A.D., Counsell, S.J.: Thalamocortical connectivity predicts cognition in children born preterm. Cerebral Cortex p. bhu 331 (2015)
4. Bayley, N.: Manual for the Bayley Scales of Infant Development, 3rd edn. Harcourt, San Antonio (2006)
5. Brown, C.J., Miller, S.P., Booth, B.G., Andrews, S., Chau, V., Poskitt, K.J., Hamarneh, G.: Structural network analysis of brain development in young preterm neonates. NeuroImage 101, 667–680 (2014)
6. Howson, C.P., Kinney, M.V., Lawn, J.L.: Born too soon: The global action report on preterm birth. World Health Organization, Geneva (2012)
7. Chang, L.C., Jones, D.K., Pierpaoli, C.: RESTORE: Robust estimation of tensors by outlier rejection. Magnetic Resonance in Medicine 53, 1088–1095 (2005)
8. Chau, V., Synnes, A., Grunau, R.E., Poskitt, K.J., Brant, R., Miller, S.P.: Abnormal brain maturation in preterm neonates associated with adverse developmental outcomes. Neurology 81(24), 2082–2089 (2013)
9. Chawla, N.V., Bowyer, K.W., Hall, L.O., Kegelmeyer, W.P.: Smote: synthetic minority over-sampling technique. Journal of AI Research 16(1), 321–357 (2002)
10. Japkowicz, N., Stephen, S.: The class imbalance problem: A systematic study. Intelligent Data Analysis 6(5), 429–449 (2002)
11. Jenkinson, M., Bannister, P., Brady, M., Smith, S.: Improved optimization for the robust and accurate linear registration and motion correction of brain images. Neuroimage 17(2), 825–841 (2002)
12. Miller, S.P., Ferriero, D.M., Leonard, C., Piecuch, R., Glidden, D.V., Partridge, J.C., Perez, M., Mukherjee, P., Vigneron, D.B., Barkovich, A.J.: Early brain injury in premature newborns detected with mri is associated with adverse early neurodevelopmental outcome. The Journal of Pediatrics 147(5), 609–616 (2005)
13. Rubinov, M., Sporns, O.: Complex network measures of brain connectivity: Uses and interpretations. NeuroImage 52(3), 1059–1069 (2010)
14. Shao, Y.H., Chen, W.J., Zhang, J.J., Wang, Z., Deng, N.Y.: An efficient weighted lagrangian twin support vector machine for imbalanced data classification. Pattern Recognition 47(9), 3158–3167 (2014)
15. Shi, F., Yap, P.T., Wu, G., Jia, H., Gilmore, J.H., Lin, W., Shen, D.: Infant brain atlases from neonates to 1-and 2-year-olds. PLoS One 6(4), e18746 (2011)
16. Wang, R., Benner, T., Sorensen, A.G., Wedeen, V.J.: Diffusion toolkit: a software package for diffusion imaging data processing and tractography. Proc. Intl. Soc. Mag. Reson. Med. 15, 3720 (2007)
17. Yang, P., Zhang, Z., Zhou, B.B., Zomaya, A.Y.: Sample subset optimization for classifying imbalanced biological data. In: Huang, J.Z., Cao, L., Srivastava, J. (eds.) PAKDD 2011, Part II. LNCS, vol. 6635, pp. 333–344. Springer, Heidelberg (2011)
18. Ziv, E., Tymofiyeva, O., Ferriero, D.M., Barkovich, A.J., Hess, C.P., Xu, D.: A machine learning approach to automated structural network analysis: application to neonatal encephalopathy. PloS One 8(11), e78824 (2013)

Segmenting Kidney DCE-MRI Using 1st-Order Shape and 5th-Order Appearance Priors

Ni Liu*, Ahmed Soliman*, Georgy Gimel'farb[1], and Ayman El-Baz[2]**

[1] Department of Computer Science, University of Auckland, Auckland, New Zealand
aselba01@louisville.edu
[2] Bioengineering Department, University of Louisville, Louisville, KY, USA

Abstract. Kidney segmentation from dynamic contrast enhanced magnetic resonance images (DCE-MRI) is vital for computer-aided early assessment of kidney functions. To accurately extract kidneys in the presence of inherently inhomogeneous contrast deviations, we control an evolving geometric deformable boundary using specific prior models of kidney shape and visual appearance. Due to analytical estimates from the training data, these priors make the kidney segmentation fast and accurate, offering the prospect of clinical applications. Experiments with 50 DCE-MRI *in-vivo* data sets confirmed that the proposed approach outperforms three more conventional counterparts.

1 Introduction

Accurate delineation of kidney borders in dynamic perfusion images is essential for their automated analysis. However, it meets with challenges due to the need to maintain adequate spatial resolution while acquiring images very quickly to capture the transient first-pass transit event; varying signal intensities (gray levels) over the time course of agent transit; and motion-induced artefacts related to intrinsic pulsate effects, breathing, or transmitted effects from adjacent structures, such as the bowel. To address these challenges, De Priester et al. [1] obtained a kidney mask by thresholding the difference between averaged pre-contrast and early-enhanced images, removing objects smaller than a certain size, and smoothing the remaining object by morphological closing and manual processing. This approach was further expanded by Giele [2], obtaining the kidney contour as the morphological inner gradient, or difference between the initial and eroded mask. Koh et al. [3] segmented kidneys with a morphological 3D H-maxima transform, using rectangular masks and edge information to avoid prior knowledge or training. Nonetheless, similar intensities in the kidney and surrounding background tissues make segmentation by straightforward signal thresholding mostly inaccurate. To circumvent these drawbacks, the kidney and its internal structures were segmented by Chevaillier et al. [4] by using a semi-automated k-means clustering of pixel-wise temporal intensity curves to

* Shared first authorship (equal contribution)
** Corresponding author.

N. Navab et al. (Eds.): MICCAI 2015, Part I, LNCS 9349, pp. 77–84, 2015.
DOI: 10.1007/978-3-319-24553-9_10

classify the pixels. An automated wavelet-based k-means partitioning was applied also by Li et al. [5] for segmenting the kidneys and tested successfully on a small number of subjects (four volunteers and three patients).

However, the most accurate kidney segmentation is obtained by evolving a deformable boundary with due account of visual appearance and shape of the kidney or its element of interest. Sun et al. [6] guided the evolution in a DCE-MRI towards the kidney borders with a variational level set integrating a temporal smoothness constraint and spatial inter-pixel correlations and employed the Chan-Vese's level set framework [7] for segmenting the cortex and medulla. Later on, the accuracy of kidney segmentation using a variational level set was improved by incorporating statistical image data [8], or prior knowledge about the kidney's visual appearance (texture) and shape [9]. A level set-based guidance by Gloger et al. [10] also used the shape prior and Bayesian statistical inference for generating the shape probability maps. But the existing techniques usually take no account of inter-pixel dependencies governing visual appearance and shape of the kidney and its structural elements. As a result, even most efficient today's deformable boundaries remain too sensitive to fuzzy kidney borders and image noise, involving spatially variant contrast and offset deviations.

To partially overcome these limitations and handle spatial inhomogeneities and contrast variations in the DCE-MRI, a probabilistic shape prior is appended below with a new visual appearance prior based on a 5th-order translation and contrast/offset invariant MGRF. In addition to the latter prior with analytical parameter estimation, we integrate the appearance and shape priors into a novel energy function resulting in a more effective stochastic guiding force for a level-set-based evolution of a deformable boundary.

2 Shape-Appearance Guided Deformable Boundary

Geometric (level-set based) deformable object-background boundaries are popular and powerful tools in segmenting medical images due to their flexible and parameter-independent evolving on the (x, y)-plane [7]. At each moment t the boundary is represented by a zero level $\phi_t(x, y) = 0$ of an implicit level-set function – a distance map $\phi_t(x, y)$ of the signed minimum Euclidean distances from every point (x, y) to the boundary. The distance is negative for the interior and positive for the exterior points, and the distance map evolves iteratively [7]: $\phi_{n+1}(x, y) = \phi_n(x, y) - \tau\nu_n(x, y)|\nabla\phi_n(x, y)|$ where n is an integer instant of time $t = n\tau$ measured with a step $\tau > 0$; $\nu_n(x, y)$ is a speed function guiding the evolution, and $\nabla\phi_n = \left[\frac{\partial\phi_n}{\partial x}, \frac{\partial\phi_n}{\partial y}\right]$ denotes the spatial gradient of the distance map. Conventional speed functions accounting for image intensities, object edges, gradient vector flow, *etc.*, are unsuccessful on noisy images with low object-background intensity gradients, such as kidney DCE-MRI. Since kidneys have well-defined shapes and distinct visual appearances, our stochastic speed function combines both the kidney's shape and appearance priors to increase the segmentation accuracy.

Adaptive 1st*-order Kidney Shape Prior.* Let $\mathbb{R} = \{(x, y) : x = 0, \ldots, X - 1; y = 0, \ldots, Y - 1\}$ be a finite 2D lattice supporting greyscale kidney images and their region maps. Our shape prior is modeled with a spatially variant independent random field (IRF) of binary region labels ($\mathbb{L} = \{1(\text{kidney}), 0(\text{background})\}$), such that maps $\mathbf{m} : \mathbb{R} \to \mathbb{L}$ of regions in the DCE-MRI with labels $\mathbf{m} = [m(x, y) : (x, y) \in \mathbb{R}; m(x, y) \in \mathbb{L}]$ are sampled from. To learn the model from a set of training DCE-MRI, $\mathbf{m}_n^\circ$; $n = 1, \ldots, N$, from different subjects, geometric deviations between their kidney shapes are reduced by mutual alignment using non-rigid B-spline-based deformations [11]. After a medical expert delineates kidneys borders in the training images, the shape prior is specified by an empirical joint probability disturbution, $P_{\text{sh}}(\mathbf{m}) = \prod_{(x,y) \in \mathrm{R}} p_{\text{sh}:x,y}(m(x, y))$. Here, each label $m(x, y) = 1$ or 0, and $p_{\text{sh}:x,y}(1) = \frac{1}{n} \sum_{n=1}^{N} m_n^\circ(x, y)$ is the empirical pixel-wise kidney probability for a stack of the co-aligned training images $\mathbf{m}_n^\circ$.

Learnable 5th*-order MGRF Appearance Prior.* Let $\mathbb{Q} = \{0, \ldots, Q - 1\}$ denote a finite set of signals (intensities, or grey levels), in the DCE-MRI, $g : \mathbb{R} \to \mathbb{Q}$, with signals $\mathbf{g} = [g(x, y) : (x, y) \in \mathbb{R}]$. Probabilistic signal dependencies in the images are quantified with an interaction graph, $\Gamma = (\mathbb{R}, \mathbb{A})$, with nodes at the lattice sites (pixels or voxels), $(x, y) \in \mathbb{R}$, and edges, or arcs $((x, y), (x', y')) \in \mathbb{A} \subseteq \mathbb{R}^2$ connecting interdependent, or interacting pairs of the nodes, called neighbours. An MGRF of images is defined by a Gibbs probability distribution (GPD), $\mathbf{P} = \left[P(\mathbf{g}) : \mathbf{g} \in \mathbb{Q}^{|\mathbb{R}|}; \sum_{\mathbf{g} \in \mathbb{Q}^{|\mathbb{R}|}} P(\mathbf{g}) = 1\right]$, factored over a set $\mathbb{C}$ of cliques in Γ supporting non-constant factors, logarithms of which are Gibbs potentials (functions of clique-wise signals) [12].

Let a translation-invariant K-order interaction structure on $\mathbb{R}$ be represented by A, $A \geq 1$, families, $\mathbb{C}_a$; $a = 1, \ldots, A$, of K-order cliques, $\mathbf{c}_{a:x,y} \in \mathbb{C}_a$, of the same shape and size. Every clique is associated with a certain pixel, $(x, y) \in \mathbb{R}$, acting as the origin, and supports the same K-variate scalar potential function, $V_a : \mathbb{Q}^K \to (-\infty, \infty)$, depending only on specific ordinal relations between the clique-wise signals. The GPD for this translation- and contrast/offset-invariant MGRF is $P_K(\mathbf{g}) = \frac{1}{Z} \psi(\mathbf{g}) \exp(-E_K(\mathbf{g}))$ where $E_K(\mathbf{g}) = \sum_{a=1}^{A} E_{K:a}(\mathbf{g})$ and $E_{K:a}(\mathbf{g}) = \sum_{\mathbf{c}_{a:x,y} \in \mathbb{C}_a} V_{K:a}(g(x', y') : (x', y') \in \mathbf{c}_{a:x,y})$ denote the Gibbs energy for all the clique families and for each individual family, respectively; $\psi(\mathbf{g})$ is a core distribution (if all the Gibbs potentials are equal to zero), and the partition function Z normalizes the GPD over the parent population of images.

Because kidneys appearance in the DCE-MRI is mostly the same under locally varying contrast, ordinal image descriptors, such as, e.g., local binary (LBP) or ternary patterns (LTP) [13] are more reasonable, than signal co-occurrences. Below, a motivated by the LBP/LTPs new class of high-order MGRFs, introduced in [14,15], is applied to model the kidney appearance priors. Its learning framework generalizes the analytical 2nd-order one in [16].

Given a training image $\mathbf{g}^\circ$, the maximum likelihood estimates (MLE) of the Gibbs potentials for the above generic K-order MGRF model with the simplest core, being an independent random field (IRF) of signals, can be approximated

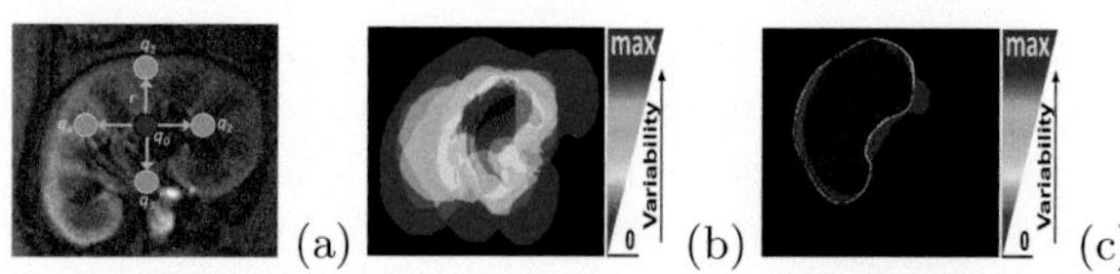

(a) (b) (c)

Fig. 1. The 5th-order clique (a): signals $q_0, q_1, \ldots, q_4$ are at the central pixel and its four central-symmetric neighbours at the radial distance r, respectively, and the color-coded shape prior before (b) and after (c) the nonrigid registration.

by generalizing the analytical approximation in [16] of the MLEs of potentials for a generic 2nd-order MGRF:

$$V_{K:a}(\beta) = \frac{F_{K:a:\text{core}}(\beta) - F_{K:a}(\beta|\mathbf{g}^\circ)}{F_{K:a:\text{core}}(\beta)(1 - F_{K:a:\text{core}}(\beta))};\ a = 1, \ldots, A;\ \beta \in \mathbb{B}_K$$

where β denotes a numerical code (value) of a particular K-order relation between the K signals on the clique; $\mathbb{B}_K$ is a set of these codes for all K-order signal co-occurrences; $F_{K:a}(\mathbf{g}^\circ)$ is an empirical marginal probability of the relation β; $\beta \in \mathbb{B}_K$, over the K-order clique family $\mathbb{C}_{K:a}$ for the training image $\mathbf{g}^\circ$, and $F_{K:a:\text{core}}(\beta)$ is the like probability for the core distribution.

Algorithm 1. Learning the 5th-order MGRF appearance models.

1. Given a training DCE-MRI $\mathbf{g}^\circ$, find the empirical kidney ($l = 1$) and background ($l = 0$) probability distributions, $\mathbf{F}_{l:5:r}(\mathbf{g}^\circ) = [F_{l:5:r}(\beta|\mathbf{g}^\circ) : \beta \in \mathbb{B}]$ of the LBP-based descriptors for different clique sizes $r \in \{1, \ldots, r_{\max}\}$ where the top size $r_{\max} = 10$ in our experiments below.
2. Find the empirical distributions $\mathbf{F}_{5:r:\text{core}} = [F_{5:r:\text{core}}(\beta) : \beta \in \mathbb{B}]$ of the same descriptors for the core IRF $\psi(\mathbf{g})$, e.g., for an image, sampled from the core.
3. Find the approximate potentials' MLE $V_{l:5:r}(\beta) = \frac{F_{5:r:\text{core}}(\beta) - F_{l:5:r}(\beta|\mathbf{g}^\circ)}{F_{5:r:\text{core}}(\beta) \cdot (1 - F_{5:r:\text{core}}(\beta))}$.
4. Compute partial Gibbs energies of the descriptors for equal and all other clique-wise signals over the training image for the clique sizes $r = 1, 2, \ldots, 10$ to choose the size ρ_l, making both the energies the closest one to another.

To demonstrate advantages of capturing constrained high-order signal relations, the kidney and background appearances are quantified below, for simplicity, by pixel-wise Gibbs energies for two 5th-order translation- and contrast/offset-invariant MGRFs, each with a single family of fixed-shape central-symmetric cliques $\mathbf{c}_{x,y} = \{(x, y), (x \pm r, y), (x, y \pm r)\}$, shown in Fig. 1. Their potentials and radial distances, r, between the peripheral and central lattice cites are learned from the training image. Each LBP-based clique descriptor accounts for binary ordinal relations between grey values in the central, q_0, and four peripheral pixels, $q_1, \ldots, q_4$, i.e., $b(q_i, q_0) = 0$ if $q_i = q_0$ and 1 otherwise; $i = 1, \ldots, 4$, giving 16 codes per clique. To further detail the clique-wise signal relations, our descriptor accounts also for the number τ; $\tau = 1, \ldots, 5$, of signals, being equal to or greater than their mean, $\widehat{q} = \frac{1}{5}(q_0 + q_1 + \ldots + q_4)$, making in total up to 80 distinct codes β; $\beta \in \mathbb{B} = \{0, \ldots, 79\}$, per clique.

Algorithm 2. Kidney segmentation with a geometric deformable boundary.

1. Equalize a DCE-MRI $\mathbf{g}$ using its cumulative probability distribution of signals.
2. Select among the training images a reference image, $\mathbf{g}_{\mathrm{ref}}$, having the minimum Kullback-Leibler divergence from the equalized DCE-MRI $\mathbf{g}$.
3. Align $\mathbf{g}$ with $\mathbf{g}_{\mathrm{ref}}$ using the non-rigid deformations [11].
4. Evolve a deformable boundary with the speed function depending on the appearance and shape priors: $\nu(x, y) = \kappa\theta(x, y)$ where κ is the mean curvature and $\theta(x, y)$ defines the pixel-wise evolution magnitude and direction: $\theta(x, y) = -P_{1:x,y}$ if $P_{1:x,y} > P_{0:x,y}$ and $\theta(x, y) = P_{0:x,y}$ otherwise where $P_{l:x,y} = \left(\frac{E_{l:5:\rho_l:x,y}(\mathbf{g})}{E_{0:5:\rho_0:x,y}(\mathbf{g})+E_{1:5:\rho_1:x,y}(\mathbf{g})}\right) p_{\mathrm{sh}:l}(x, y);\ l \in \mathbb{L} = \{1, 0\}$.
5. Transfer the final boundary to the initial (non-aligned) DCE-MRI by reversing the non-rigid deformations, which have been estimated for the alignment.

Algorithms 1 and 2 outline learning the kidney and background appearance priors and basic steps of segmenting the kidney DCE-MRI with these and shape priors, respectively. The pixel-wise energies, $E_{l:5:\rho_l:x,y}(\mathbf{g});\ l \in \mathbb{L}$, summing the learned potentials for the five cliques, containing the pixel (x, y), characterize in Algorithm 2 to what extent that pixel of the image $\mathbf{g}$ can be assigned to the background or kidney in accord with their appearance priors.

3 Experimental Validation and Conclusions

The proposed approach has been tested on the 3D (2D + time) DCE-MRI data sets collected from 50 subjects (35 men and 15 women from 10 to 56 years old (the mean age of $31_{\pm 11}$ years). The temporal sampling was adequate to characterize the transit of the clinical gadoteric acid contrast agent (Dotarem 0.5 *mmol/mL*; Guerbet, France), injected at the rate of 3-4 *ml/sec*, at the dose of 0.2 *ml/kgBW*. The gradient-echo T1 imaging employed a 1.5 T MRI scanner Signa Horizon LX Echo speed (GE Medical Systems, USA) with a phased-array torso surface coil; slice thickness: 5 *mm*; TR = 30-40 *msec*; TE = 2-3 *msec*; flip angle 70°; FOV = $38{\times}38\ cm^2$, and matrix size = $256{\times}160$. To obtain representative sampling to characterize perfusion for each patient, a single coronal image section was used at the level of the renal hilum of the transplanted kidney. Approximately 80 repeated temporal frames were obtained at 3 *sec* intervals.

Basic steps of the proposed level set-based segmentation are shown in Fig. 2, which also compares, together with Table 1 and Figs. 3 and 4, our segmentation accuracy with the vector level set (VLS) algorithm by Abdelmunim and Farag [9] and the parametric kernel graph cut (PKGC) with morphological and connectivity post-analysis by Salah et al. [17]. Differences between the mean Dice similarity coefficients (DSC) for our and other algorithms in Table 1 are statistically significant by the paired t-test. In total, embedding the proposed simple 5th-order MGRF appearance model, together with our earlier shape prior, into

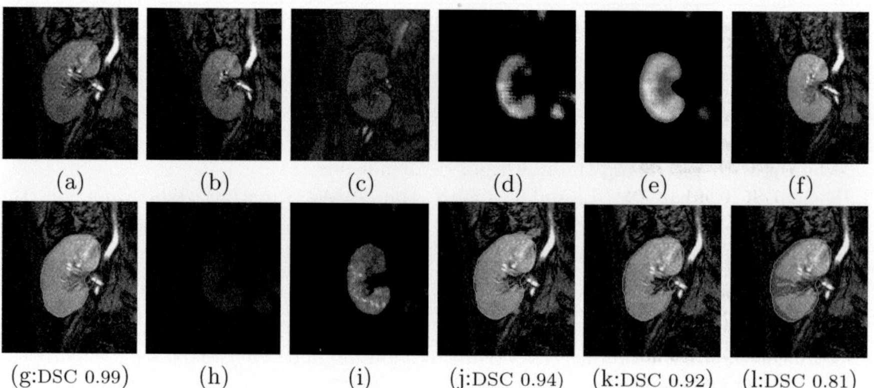

Fig. 2. The image (a) to be segmented; its alignment (b) [11] to a selected training reference image (c); the pixel-wise Gibbs energy (d) of our 5th-order MGRF model; the total energy (e) after fusing that energy with the shape prior; the segmented aligned kidney (f); the final segmentation (g) after reversing to the original image (a); the pixel-wise Gibbs energy (h) for the 2nd-order MGRF appearance model [16]; the total energy (i) after fusing with the shape prior; the PKGC segmentation (j) [17]; the segmentation (k) with the 2nd-order MGRF prior; and the VLS segmentation (l) [9]. The ground truth is in green.

Table 1. Accuracy of our level-set based kidney segmentation with the 5th- or only 2nd-order appearance prior w.r.t. the vector level set (VLS) [9] and parametric kernel graph cut (PKGC) [17] algorithms on the 50 data sets.

	5th-order prior	2nd-order prior	VLS	PKGC
DSC: mean$_{\pm \text{st.dev.}}$	$0.99_{\pm 0.02}$	$0.91_{\pm 0.03}$	$0.90_{\pm 0.08}$	$0.82_{\pm 0.18}$
p-value		$\leq 10^{-4}$	$\leq 10^{-4}$	$\leq 10^{-4}$

the speed function of the level-set-guided boundary evolution results in more accurate segmentation of complex 3D (2D + time) kidney DCE-MRI.

These qualitative and quantitative comparisons use the ground truth obtained manually by an MRI expert. To highlight advantages of the proposed 5th-order MGRF priors, the pixel-wise Gibbs energies were compared in Fig. 2,h–k, and Table 1 with the like energies for the 2nd-order priors [16]. Obviously, the latter priors describe the object appearance less accurately. The considerably more distinct 5th-order pixel-wise Gibbs energies for the kidney and background (see Figs. 2,d,e,h,i) ensure better guidance of the evolving level-sets-based boundary.

Our present mixed-code implementation (Matlab and C++) on a T7500 workstation (Intel quad-core processor; 3.33 GHz each with 48 GB of memory) takes about 125 ± 10 *sec* for segmenting 79 DCE-MRI time series images, each of size 256×256 pixels.

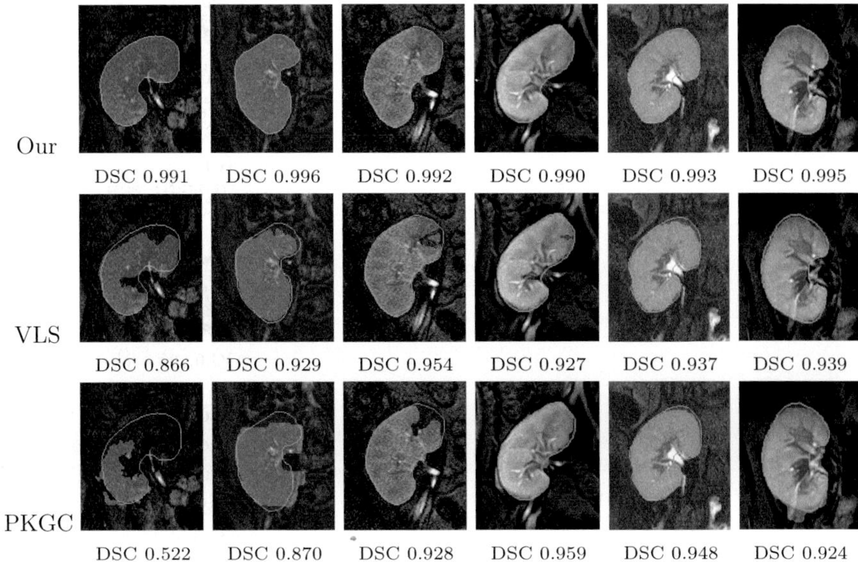

Fig. 3. Comparison to the VLS [9] and PKGC [17] (green – the ground truth).

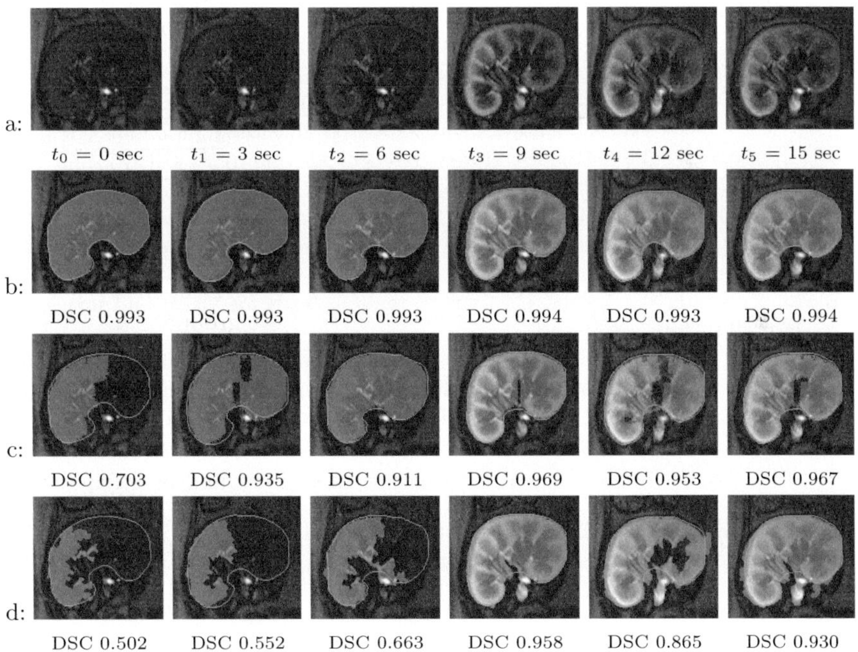

Fig. 4. Original first 6 images (a) of one of the DCE-MRI sequences and our segmentation (b) w.r.t. the VLS [9] (c) and PKGC [17] (d).

References

1. de Priester, J., Kessels, A., Giele, E., den Boer, J., Christiaans, M., Hasman, A., van Engelshoven, J.: MR renography by semiautomated image analysis: Performance in renal transplant recipients. J. M.R.I. 14(2), 134–140 (2001)
2. Giele, E., De Priester, J., Blom, J., den Boer, J., Van Engelshoven, J., Hasman, A., Geerlings, M.: Movement correction of the kidney in dynamic MRI scans using FFT phase difference movement detection. J. M.R.I. 14(6), 741–749 (2001)
3. Koh, H., Shen, W., Shuter, B., Kassim, A.A.: Segmentation of kidney cortex in MRI studies using a constrained morphological 3D H-maxima transform. In: Proc. ICARCV, pp. 1–5 (2006)
4. Chevaillier, B., Ponvianne, Y., Collette, J.L., Mandry, D., Claudon, M., Pietquin, O.: Functional semi-automated segmentation of renal DCE-MRI sequences. In: Proc. ICASSP, pp. 525–528 (2008)
5. Li, S., Zöllner, F.G., Merrem, A.D., Peng, Y., Roervik, J., Lundervold, A., Schad, L.R.: Wavelet-based segmentation of renal compartments in DCE-MRI of human kidney: initial results in patients and healthy volunteers. Comput. Med. Imaging Graph. 36(2), 108–118 (2012)
6. Sun, Y., Moura, J., Yang, D., Ye, Q., Ho, C.: Kidney segmentation in MRI sequences using temporal dynamics. In: Proc. ISBI, pp. 98–101 (2002)
7. Chan, T.F., Vese, L.A.: Active contours without edges. IEEE Trans. Image Process. 10(2), 266–277 (2001)
8. Wu, C.H., Sun, Y.N.: Segmentation of kidney from ultrasound B-mode images with texture-based classification. Comput. Meth. Prog. Biomed. 84(2), 114–123 (2006)
9. El Munim, H.E.A., Farag, A.A.: Curve/surface representation and evolution using vector level sets with application to the shape-based segmentation problem. IEEE Trans. Pattern Anal. Mach. Intell. 29(6), 945–958 (2007)
10. Gloger, O., Tonnies, K.D., Liebscher, V., Kugelmann, B., Laqua, R., Volzke, H.: Prior shape level set segmentation on multistep generated probability maps of MR datasets for fully automatic kidney parenchyma volumetry. IEEE Trans. Med. Imaging 31(2), 312–325 (2012)
11. Rueckert, D., Sonoda, L.I., Hayes, C., Hill, D.L., Leach, M.O., Hawkes, D.J.: Non-rigid registration using free-form deformations: application to breast MR images. IEEE Trans. Med. Imaging 18(8), 712–721 (1999)
12. Blake, A., Kohli, P., Rother, C.: Markov random fields for vision and image processing. MIT Press (2011)
13. Ojala, T., Pietikainen, M., Maenpaa, T.: Multiresolution gray-scale and rotation invariant texture classification with local binary patterns. IEEE Trans. Pattern Anal. Mach. Intell. 24(7), 971–987 (2002)
14. Liu, N., Gimel'farb, G., Delmas, P., Chan, Y.H.: Contrast/offset-invariant generic low-order MGRF models of uniform textures. In: AIP Conf. Proc., vol. 1559(1), pp. 145–154 (2013)
15. Liu, N., Gimel'farb, G., Delmas, P.: High-order MGRF models for contrast/offset invariant texture retrieval. In: Proc. Int. Conf. Image Vision Computing, pp. 96–101. ACM, New Zealand (2014)
16. Gimel'farb, G., Zhou, D.: Texture analysis by accurate identification of a generic Markov–Gibbs model. In: Gimel'farb, G., Zhou, D. (eds.) Applied Pattern Recognition. SCI, vol. 91, pp. 221–245. Springer, Heidelberg (2008)
17. Salah, M.B., Mitiche, A., Ayed, I.B.: Multiregion image segmentation by parametric kernel graph cuts. IEEE Trans. Image Process. 20(2), 545–557 (2011)

Comparison of Stochastic and Variational Solutions to ASL fMRI Data Analysis

Aina Frau-Pascual[1,3], Florence Forbes[1], and Philippe Ciuciu[2,3]

[1] INRIA, Univ. Grenoble Alpes, LJK, Grenoble, France
[2] CEA/DSV/I^{2}BM/NeuroSpin, Bât. 145, F-91191 Gif-sur-Yvette, France
[3] INRIA/CEA Parietal team, NeuroSpin, Bât. 145, F-91191 Gif-sur-Yvette, France

Abstract. Functional Arterial Spin Labeling (fASL) MRI can provide a quantitative measurement of changes of cerebral blood flow induced by stimulation or task performance. fASL data is commonly analysed using a general linear model (GLM) with regressors based on the canonical hemodynamic response function. In this work, we consider instead a joint detection-estimation (JDE) framework which has the advantage of allowing the extraction of both task-related perfusion and hemodynamic responses not restricted to canonical shapes. Previous JDE attempts for ASL have been based on computer intensive sampling (MCMC) methods. Our contribution is to provide a comparison with an alternative variational expectation-maximization (VEM) algorithm on synthetic and real data.

1 Introduction

Arterial Spin Labeling (ASL) [1] is a MRI modality that is able to provide a quantitative measurement of cerebral blood flow (CBF). ASL data consists of alternating pairs of control and magnetically tagged ("tag") images. Local CBF or perfusion changes can be measured by considering the "control-tag" difference. Many control-tag pairs (> 50) need to be acquired to compensate for the low Signal-to-Noise Ratio (SNR) of this difference ($\simeq$1-2%). Aside from its main use in static measurements, ASL has also been used in functional MRI (functional ASL or fASL) as an alternative quantitative imaging technique to the standard blood-oxygen-level-dependent (BOLD) [2] contrast imaging modality. fASL can provide more specific information about brain function but its lower SNR and temporal resolution make its analysis more challenging. The standard approach for fASL data analysis is the general linear model (GLM) [3,4]. It relies on the canonical hemodynamic response function (HRF) for defining the hemodynamic and perfusion-related regressors, although the HRF has been calibrated in BOLD experiments only. Moreover, there has been strong evidence in the literature for space-varying and subject-specific HRF shape [5,6]. To deal with this issue, a joint detection-estimation (JDE) framework, originally developed for BOLD data analysis [7,8], has been extended in [9] to allow for the extraction of both task-related perfusion and hemodynamic responses while recovering perfusion-related and BOLD-related maps of evoked activity. Previous JDE implementations for ASL have been based on Markov Chain Monte Carlo (MCMC) techniques. In this

N. Navab et al. (Eds.): MICCAI 2015, Part I, LNCS 9349, pp. 85–92, 2015.
DOI: 10.1007/978-3-319-24553-9_11

work, following the spirit of [8], we provide an alternative solution based on the variational expectation-maximization (VEM) algorithm and compare its performance to its MCMC alternative. In both solutions, prior knowledge is introduced on the relationship between perfusion and hemodynamic responses (resp. PRF and HRF) derived from physiological models [10]. This prior allows us to benefit from a better estimation of the HRF due to higher SNR of the BOLD component in the ASL signal to inform the PRF estimation. As already observed in [8] for the BOLD case, JDE-VEM provides comparable results to JDE-MCMC for a lower computational load. On top of that, JDE-VEM is more convenient to handle identifiability constraints (eg, unit norm or positivity constraint of the response shapes for solving the scale ambiguity issue in Eq. (1)).

2 Joint Detection Estimation Model for fASL Data

The JDE formalism is a region-based approach that considers hemodynamically homogeneous regions. In a region $\mathcal{P}$ comprising J voxels, the ASL JDE model [9,11] defines voxel-specific ASL time series as the linear superposition of the M task-induced (or stimulus-specific) responses:

$$\forall j \in \mathcal{P}, \;\; \boldsymbol{y}_j = \sum_{m=1}^{M} \big[\underbrace{a_j^m \boldsymbol{X}^m \boldsymbol{h}}_{(a)} + \underbrace{c_j^m \boldsymbol{W} \boldsymbol{X}^m \boldsymbol{g}}_{(b)}\big] + \underbrace{\alpha_j \boldsymbol{w}}_{(c)} + \underbrace{\boldsymbol{P}\boldsymbol{\ell}_j}_{(d)} + \underbrace{\boldsymbol{b}_j}_{(e)} \qquad (1)$$

Each time series $\boldsymbol{y}_j \in \mathbb{R}^N$ is decomposed into (a) task-related hemodynamic and (b) perfusion components, (c) a perfusion baseline term $\alpha_j \boldsymbol{w}^1$ which completes the modelling of the perfusion component, (d) a drift component $\boldsymbol{P}\boldsymbol{\ell}_j$ and (e) a noise term, assumed white Gaussian with variance σ_j^2. The control/tag effect is modelled in Eq. (1) by making use of $\boldsymbol{w}$ and $\boldsymbol{W} = \mathrm{diag}(\boldsymbol{w})$. Vectors $\boldsymbol{h}$ and $\boldsymbol{g}$ represent the D-dimensional ($D < N$) unknown HRF and PRF shapes, constant within $\mathcal{P}$. The magnitudes of activation or response levels for hemodynamic and perfusion components are $\boldsymbol{a} = \{a_j^m\}$ and $\boldsymbol{c} = \{c_j^m\}$ and referred to as HRLs and PRLs (hemodynamic and perfusion response levels) hereafter. $\boldsymbol{X} \in \mathbb{R}^{N \times D}$ is a binary matrix that encodes the lagged onset stimuli. The response levels are assumed to follow different Gaussian mixture models but governed by M common binary hidden Markov random fields $\boldsymbol{q}^m$ with $\boldsymbol{q}^m = \{q_j^m, j \in \mathcal{P}\}$ encoding voxels activation states for each experimental condition m. HRLs and PRLs are assumed independent conditionally to these activation labels $\boldsymbol{q} = \{\boldsymbol{q}^m, m = 1 : M\}$. For further details, please refer to [9].

As already mentioned, the perfusion component in the ASL signal has a very low SNR owing to its small size captured by the "control-tag" subtraction. To address this issue, we make use of a link derived in [10] from physiological models between the two responses $\boldsymbol{g} = \boldsymbol{\Omega}\boldsymbol{h}$. As a difference with [9], we then consider that HRF and PRF shapes follow prior Gaussian distributions $\boldsymbol{h} \sim \mathcal{N}(\boldsymbol{0}, v_{\boldsymbol{h}}\boldsymbol{\Sigma}_{\boldsymbol{h}})$

[1] Vector $\boldsymbol{w}$ is N-dimensional such that $w_{t_n} = 1/2$ if t_n is even (control) and $w_{t_n} = -1/2$ otherwise (tagged).

and $\boldsymbol{g}|\boldsymbol{h} \sim \mathcal{N}(\boldsymbol{\Omega h}, v_g \boldsymbol{\Sigma}_g)$, with covariance matrices $\boldsymbol{\Sigma}_h$ and $\boldsymbol{\Sigma}_g$ encoding a constraint on the second order derivatives so as to account for temporal smoothness of $\boldsymbol{h}$ and $\boldsymbol{g}$, respectively. We also consider constraints on the response functions to enforce their L_2-norm to be unitary.

3 Variational EM Estimation

In a first attempt to estimate the ASL JDE model, an intensive sampling MCMC procedure has been used in a Bayesian setting [10]. This provides an elegant way to estimate the missing model variables $\boldsymbol{a} \in \mathcal{A}$, $\boldsymbol{h} \in \mathcal{H}$, $\boldsymbol{c} \in \mathcal{C}$, $\boldsymbol{g} \in \mathcal{G}$, $\boldsymbol{q} \in \mathcal{Q}$ via the sampling of the posterior distribution $p(\boldsymbol{a}, \boldsymbol{h}, \boldsymbol{c}, \boldsymbol{g}, \boldsymbol{q}|\boldsymbol{y})$ whose direct computation or maximization is intractable. When the model involves a lot of missing variables, such an approach is not easy to monitor and not that flexible. Additional information or constraints on the response function shapes (*i.e.*, unit L_2-norm) cannot be easily integrated. Following the lead of [8], we propose an alternative Expectation-Maximization (EM) framework. Let $\mathcal{D}$ be the set of all probability distributions on $\mathcal{A} \times \mathcal{H} \times \mathcal{C} \times \mathcal{G} \times \mathcal{Q}$. EM can be viewed as an alternating maximization procedure of a function F such that for any $\tilde{p} \in \mathcal{D}$, $F(\tilde{p}, \boldsymbol{\theta}) = \mathrm{E}_{\tilde{p}}\big[\log p(\boldsymbol{y}, \boldsymbol{a}, \boldsymbol{h}, \boldsymbol{c}, \boldsymbol{g}, \boldsymbol{q}\ ;\ \boldsymbol{\theta})\big] + I[\tilde{p}]$ where $I[\tilde{p}] = -\mathrm{E}_{\tilde{p}}\big[\log \tilde{p}(\boldsymbol{a}, \boldsymbol{h}, \boldsymbol{c}, \boldsymbol{g}, \boldsymbol{q})\big]$ is the entropy of $\tilde{p}$, $\mathrm{E}_{\tilde{p}}[]$ denotes the expectation with respect to $\tilde{p}$ and $\boldsymbol{\theta}$ is the set of parameters. Maximizing function F is equivalent to minimizing the Kullback-Leibler divergence between $\tilde{p}$ and the true posterior of interest $p(\boldsymbol{a}, \boldsymbol{h}, \boldsymbol{c}, \boldsymbol{g}, \boldsymbol{q}|\boldsymbol{y})$. This view of EM has led to a number of variants in which the E-step is solved over a restricted class of probability distributions, $\tilde{\mathcal{D}}$. The variational approach corresponds to choosing $\tilde{\mathcal{D}}$ as the set of distributions that factorize over the set of missing variables: $\tilde{p}(\boldsymbol{a}, \boldsymbol{h}, \boldsymbol{c}, \boldsymbol{g}, \boldsymbol{q}) = \tilde{p}_a(\boldsymbol{a})\ \tilde{p}_h(\boldsymbol{h})\ \tilde{p}_c(\boldsymbol{c})\ \tilde{p}_g(\boldsymbol{g})\ \tilde{p}_q(\boldsymbol{q})$ where $\tilde{p}_a \in \mathcal{D}_A$, $\tilde{p}_h \in \mathcal{D}_H$, $\tilde{p}_c \in \mathcal{D}_C$, $\tilde{p}_g \in \mathcal{D}_G$ and $\tilde{p}_q \in \mathcal{D}_Q$, the sets of probability distributions on $\mathcal{A}, \mathcal{H}, \mathcal{C}, \mathcal{G}, \mathcal{Q}$ respectively. The E-step becomes an approximate E-step that can be further decomposed into five stages updating the different variables in turn. At iteration (r), with current estimates denoted by $\tilde{p}_a^{(r-1)}, \tilde{p}_h^{(r-1)}, \tilde{p}_c^{(r-1)}, \tilde{p}_g^{(r-1)}, \tilde{p}_q^{(r-1)}$ and $\boldsymbol{\theta}^{(r-1)}$, where $\boldsymbol{\theta} = \big\{\boldsymbol{\alpha}, \boldsymbol{\ell}, \boldsymbol{\sigma}^2, \boldsymbol{\mu}_{a,c}, \boldsymbol{\sigma}_{a,c}, v_h, v_g, \boldsymbol{\beta}\big\}$, the updating formulae are of the form:

$$\textbf{E-H-step:}\ \ \tilde{p}_h^{(r)} = \arg\max_{\tilde{p}_h \in \mathcal{D}_H} F(\tilde{p}_a^{(r-1)}\ \tilde{p}_h\ \tilde{p}_c^{(r-1)}\ \tilde{p}_g^{(r-1)}\ \tilde{p}_q^{(r-1)}; \boldsymbol{\theta}^{(r-1)}) \quad (2)$$

$$\textbf{E-G-step:}\ \ \tilde{p}_g^{(r)} = \arg\max_{\tilde{p}_g \in \mathcal{D}_G} F(\tilde{p}_a^{(r-1)}\ \tilde{p}_h^{(r)}\ \tilde{p}_c^{(r-1)}\ \tilde{p}_g\ \tilde{p}_q^{(r-1)}; \boldsymbol{\theta}^{(r-1)}) \quad (3)$$

with similar expressions for the other steps obtained by permuting the roles of the variables. Hereafter, for the ease of presentation, the (r) and $(r-1)$ superscripts are omitted. In contrast to the standard setting, to introduce normalisation constraints on $\boldsymbol{h}$ and $\boldsymbol{g}$, we modify the sought variational approximation into $\tilde{p} = \tilde{p}_a\ \delta_{\tilde{\boldsymbol{h}}}\ \tilde{p}_c\ \delta_{\tilde{\boldsymbol{g}}}\ \tilde{p}_q$, where the distributions on $\boldsymbol{h}$ and $\boldsymbol{g}$ are replaced by Dirac functions. This reduces the search to pointwise estimates $\tilde{\boldsymbol{h}}$ and $\tilde{\boldsymbol{g}}$. The E-H and E-G steps in Eqs. (2)-(3) then yield maximization problems which are easily constrained to account for normalisation:

$$\textbf{E-H:}\ \tilde{\boldsymbol{h}} = \arg\max_{\boldsymbol{h}} \mathrm{E}_{\tilde{p}_a\tilde{p}_c\tilde{p}_q}\big[\log p(\boldsymbol{h} \mid \boldsymbol{y}, \boldsymbol{a}, \boldsymbol{c}, \tilde{\boldsymbol{g}}, \boldsymbol{q}; \boldsymbol{\theta})\big] \tag{4}$$

$$\textbf{E-G:}\ \tilde{\boldsymbol{g}} = \arg\max_{\boldsymbol{g}} \mathrm{E}_{\tilde{p}_a\tilde{p}_c\tilde{p}_q}\big[\log p(\boldsymbol{g} \mid \boldsymbol{y}, \boldsymbol{a}, \tilde{\boldsymbol{h}}, \boldsymbol{c}, \boldsymbol{q}; \boldsymbol{\theta})\big] \tag{5}$$

Solving Eqs. (4)-(5) amounts to minimizing a quadratic function under a quadratic constraint, namely $\|\boldsymbol{h}\|_2^2 = 1$ and $\|\boldsymbol{g}\|_2^2 = 1$ respectively. The other E-steps can be derived from standard expressions in [8] replacing expectations over $\boldsymbol{h}$ and $\boldsymbol{g}$ by $\tilde{\boldsymbol{h}}$ and $\tilde{\boldsymbol{g}}$, *e.g.*

$$\textbf{E-Q:}\ \tilde{p}_q(\boldsymbol{q}) \propto \exp\left(\mathrm{E}_{\tilde{p}_a\tilde{p}_c}\big[\log p(\boldsymbol{q} \mid \boldsymbol{y}, \boldsymbol{a}, \tilde{\boldsymbol{h}}, \boldsymbol{c}, \tilde{\boldsymbol{g}}; \boldsymbol{\theta})\big]\right), \tag{6}$$

with similar expressions for the E-A and E-C steps. The corresponding **M-step** for the update of $\boldsymbol{\theta}$ can be divided into separate M-substeps, as in [8]:

$$\begin{aligned}\boldsymbol{\theta} = \arg\max_{\boldsymbol{\theta}\in\boldsymbol{\Theta}} \Big[&\mathrm{E}_{\tilde{p}_a\tilde{p}_c}\big[\log p(\boldsymbol{y} \mid \boldsymbol{a}, \tilde{\boldsymbol{h}}, \boldsymbol{c}, \tilde{\boldsymbol{g}}; \boldsymbol{\alpha}, \boldsymbol{\ell}, \boldsymbol{\sigma}^2)\big] + \mathrm{E}_{\tilde{p}_a\tilde{p}_q}\big[\log p(\boldsymbol{a} \mid \boldsymbol{q}; \boldsymbol{\mu}_a, \boldsymbol{\sigma}_a)\big] \\ &+ \log p(\tilde{\boldsymbol{h}}; v_h) + \mathrm{E}_{\tilde{p}_c\tilde{p}_q}\big[\log p(\boldsymbol{c} \mid \boldsymbol{q}; \boldsymbol{\mu}_c, \boldsymbol{\sigma}_c)\big] + \log p(\tilde{\boldsymbol{g}}; v_g) + \mathrm{E}_{\tilde{p}_q}\big[\log p(\boldsymbol{q}; \boldsymbol{\beta})\big]\Big].\end{aligned}$$

It follows a VEM procedure in which missing quantities are updated in turn. Compare to an MCMC solution, the variational approach is based on an approximation of the full posterior distribution. The dependencies between te random variables in the JDE model are reduced to dependencies between their moments that appear in the successive E-steps. No theoretical results exist that would guarantee the quality of such an approximation but the performance comparison provided in the next section suggests that VEM is still able to capture enough information amongst the original dependencies.

4 Results

Different data sets have been analysed to assess the performance of the VEM and MCMC approaches: first, artificial data synthesized with the generative model (1), and second real data acquired on different individuals from the AINSI initiative (`http://thalie.ujf-grenoble.fr/ainsi`).

4.1 Artificial Data

$N = 292$ ASL artificial images (i.e., 146 control/tag pairs) have been simulated using a realistic SNR ($\simeq 3$ dB) according to Eq. (1) considering $\boldsymbol{h}$ and $\boldsymbol{g}$ as depicted in Fig.1(a)-(b) by dashed lines. To emulate the slow sampling rate of ASL images, Eq. (1) was synthesized at $\Delta t = 1$ sec and then undersampled at $TR = 3$ sec. Here, we considered a fast event-related paradigm comprising two conditions ($M = 2$). Drift coefficients and noise realizations were drawn according to $\boldsymbol{\ell}_j \sim \mathcal{N}(0, 10\boldsymbol{I}_O)$ and $\boldsymbol{b}_j \sim \mathcal{N}(0, 2\boldsymbol{I}_N)$, respectively. HRLs were generated with $(a_j^m | q_j^m = 1) \sim \mathcal{N}(2.2, 0.3)$ for active voxels and $(a_j^m | q_j^m = 0) \sim \mathcal{N}(0, 0.3)$ for inactive ones. To make this synthetic setting realistic, PRLs were generated with a lower contrast than HRLs: $(c_j^m|q_j^m = 1) \sim \mathcal{N}(1.6, 0.3)$ and $(c_j^m|q_j^m = 0) \sim \mathcal{N}(0, 0.3)$. Activation states (assignment variables $\boldsymbol{q}$) are set by a hand-drawn map, as illustrated on the first column maps of Fig. 2.

Fig. 1(a-d) shows the HRF and PRF estimates obtained for two different noise levels. Both response functions were well recovered with MCMC and VEM at 3 dB SNR with an acceptable degradation at lower SNR (i.e. 0.5 dB). In the latter case, MCMC recovers slightly better the peak. The labels (activated/non-activated) in Fig. 2 are well recovered with both MCMC and VEM at the higher SNR. At the lower one, both solutions fail to recover accurate label maps. As typical of VEM, labels maps are more *contrasted* than with MCMC which is likely to better estimate variability. Fig. 3 shows the root mean squared errors (RMSE) for a range of SNR levels. Response functions are well recovered with small RMSE in all cases (Fig. 3(a)) but with better estimations with MCMC. In contrast, response levels are better recovered with VEM (Fig. 3(b)). This is consistent with previous comparisons between VEM and MCMC on BOLD signals [8].

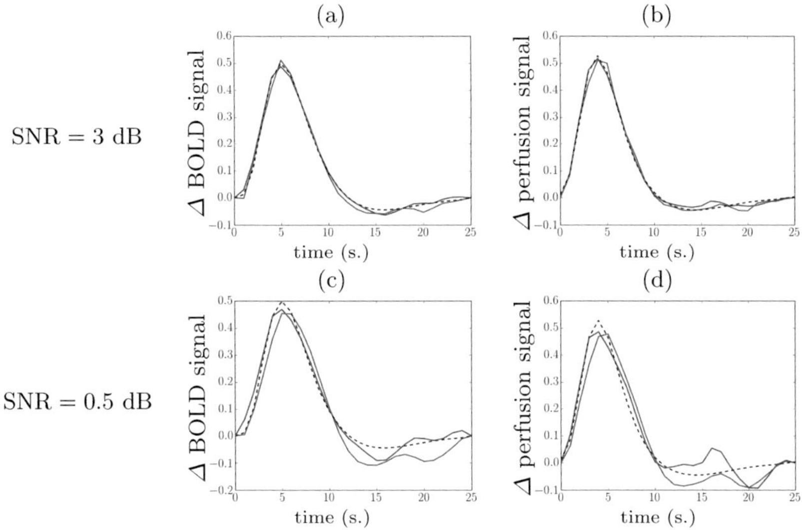

Fig. 1. Artificial data with 2 noise settings: (a, b) SNR = 3 dB, (c, d) SNR = 0.5 dB. Ground-truth response curves (black dashed lines) and estimated hemodynamic (a, c) and perfusion (b, d) response functions with MCMC in blue and VEM in red.

4.2 Real Data

Real ASL data were recorded during an experiment designed to map auditory and visual brain functions, which consisted of $N = 291$ scans lasting TR = 3000 ms, with TE = 18 ms, FoV 192 mm, each yielding a 3-D volume composed of $64 \times 64 \times 22$ voxels (spatial resolution of $3 \times 3 \times 7$ mm^3). The tagging scheme used was PICORE Q2T, with $(\mathrm{TI}_1, \mathrm{TI}_2) = (700, 1700)$ ms. A fast event-related

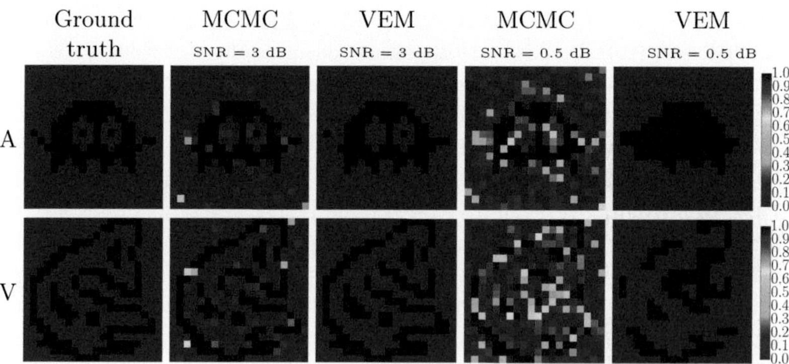

Fig. 2. Results on artificial data for labels $\boldsymbol{q}$. The probability to be activated is shown for each voxel, for 2 experimental conditions, namely auditory (A) and visual (V) stimuli. The ground truth as well as the MCMC and VEM activation probability estimates are shown in two different SNR scenarios.

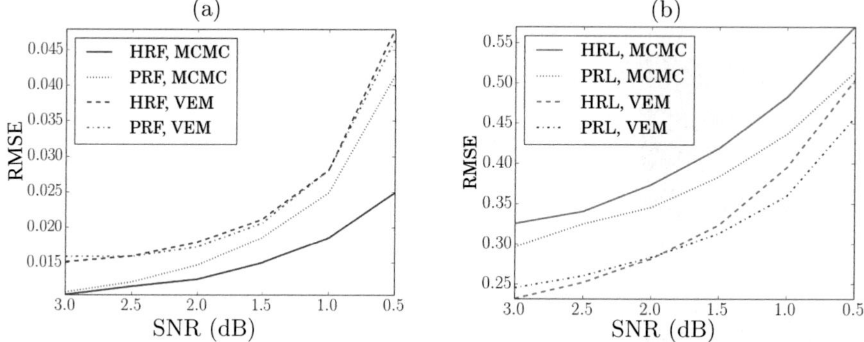

Fig. 3. RMSE comparison between MCMC and VEM approaches. (a) Response functions HRF and PRF. (b) Mean over conditions of the RMSE of the response levels HRL and PRL.

paradigm comprising sixty auditory and visual stimuli, randomly distributed according to a mean inter-stimulus interval of 5.1 sec, was run during acquisition.

In Fig. 4, the MCMC and VEM results are shown in the left and right visual and auditory cortices. The HRL maps in Fig. 4(a) are very similar for the two approaches and for A and V conditions in contrast to the larger variability reported in the PRL maps owing to the lower effect size. Interestingly, the PRL maps yielded by the two algorithms are consistent for the V condition in contrast to what we observed for the A condition. The regions of interest (ROI) in Fig. 4(b) correspond to the parcels with stronger mean HRL and PRL values for each condition respectively. The HRF and PRF estimates in these ROIs have plausible shapes and both approaches recover similar profiles. For both conditions, the PRF peaks before the HRF, as enforced by the physiological prior.

Regarding computational times, a substantial decrease was observed for VEM as compared to the MCMC solution, which is consistent with previous reports [8].

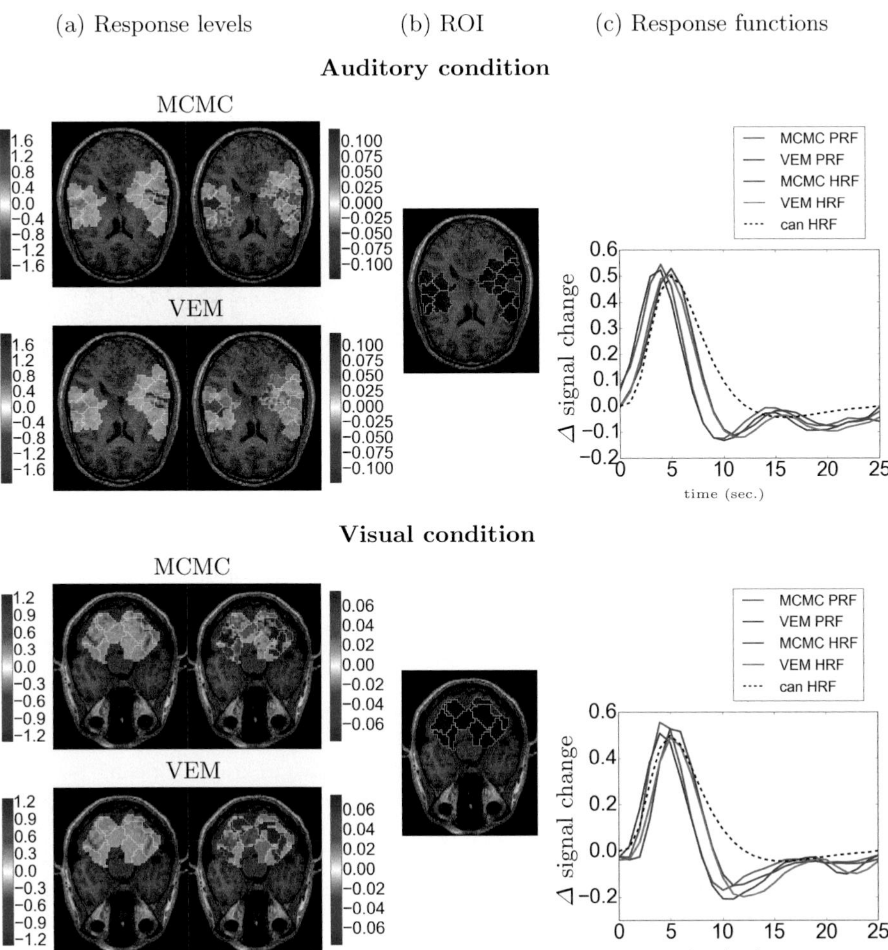

Fig. 4. Results on real fASL data for a single subject of the AINSI database for both conditions: Auditory (top) and Visual (bottom). (a) HRL on the left and PRL on the right; (b) region of interest (ROI) where the response functions in (c) are estimated. In (c) and as indicated in the legend, the red and blue curves represent the PRF and HRF respectively for the MCMC approach, and the magenta and green curves represent the PRF and HRF respectively for the VEM approach. As a reference, we depicted the canonical HRF with a black dashed line.

5 Conclusion

A VEM algorithm has been proposed to address the issue of jointly detecting evoked activity and estimating the associated hemodynamic and perfusion responses from functional ASL data. Compared to MCMC, VEM delivers estimations in analytic form for each latent variable. Although the VEM setting remains an approximation, it facilitates the inclusion of additional information such as constraints. Our results demonstrate a good performance of VEM when compared to MCMC at a significantly lower computation time. This suggests VEM as a fast and valid alternative for functional ASL data analysis.

References

1. Williams, D., Detre, J., Leigh, J., Koretsky, A.: Magnetic resonance imaging of perfusion using spin inversion of arterial water. Proceedings of the National Academy of Sciences 89(1), 212–216 (1992)
2. Ogawa, S., Tank, D.W., Menon, R., Ellermann, J.M., Kim, S.-G., Merkle, H., Ugurbil, K.: Intrinsic signal changes accompanying sensory stimulation: functional brain mapping with magnetic resonance imaging. Proceedings of the National Academy of Sciences 89, 5951–5955 (1992)
3. Hernandez-Garcia, L., Jahanian, H., Rowe, D.B.: Quantitative analysis of arterial spin labeling fMRI data using a general linear model. Magnetic Resonance Imaging 28(7), 919–927 (2010)
4. Mumford, J.A., Hernandez-Garcia, L., Lee, G.R., Nichols, T.E.: Estimation efficiency and statistical power in arterial spin labeling fMRI. Neuroimage 33(1), 103–114 (2006)
5. Handwerker, D.A., Ollinger, J.M., Mark, D.: Variation of BOLD hemodynamic responses across subjects and brain regions and their effects on statistical analyses. Neuroimage 21, 1639–1651 (2004)
6. Badillo, S., Vincent, T., Ciuciu, P.: Group-level impacts of within- and between-subject hemodynamic variability in fMRI. Neuroimage 82, 433–448 (2013)
7. Vincent, T., Risser, L., Ciuciu, P.: Spatially adaptive mixture modeling for analysis of within-subject fMRI time series. IEEE Trans. on Medical Imaging 29(4), 1059–1074 (2010)
8. Chaari, L., Vincent, T., Forbes, F., Dojat, M., Ciuciu, P.: Fast joint detection-estimation of evoked brain activity in event-related fMRI using a variational approach. IEEE Trans. on Medical Imaging 32(5), 821–837 (2013)
9. Vincent, T., Warnking, J., Villien, M., Krainik, A., Ciuciu, P., Forbes, F.: Bayesian Joint Detection-Estimation of Cerebral Vasoreactivity from ASL fMRI Data. In: Mori, K., Sakuma, I., Sato, Y., Barillot, C., Navab, N. (eds.) MICCAI 2013, Part II. LNCS, vol. 8150, pp. 616–624. Springer, Heidelberg (2013)
10. Frau-Pascual, A., Vincent, T., Sloboda, J., Ciuciu, P., Forbes, F.: Physiologically Informed Bayesian Analysis of ASL fMRI Data. In: Cardoso, M.J., Simpson, I., Arbel, T., Precup, D., Ribbens, A. (eds.) BAMBI 2014. LNCS, vol. 8677, pp. 37–48. Springer, Heidelberg (2014)
11. Vincent, T., Forbes, F., Ciuciu, P.: Bayesian BOLD and perfusion source separation and deconvolution from functional ASL imaging. In: 38th Proc. IEEE ICASSP, Vancouver, Canada, pp. 1003–1007 (May 2013)

Prediction of CT Substitutes from MR Images Based on Local Sparse Correspondence Combination

Yao Wu, Wei Yang, Lijun Lu, Zhentai Lu, Liming Zhong, Ru Yang, Meiyan Huang, Yanqiu Feng, Wufan Chen, and Qianjin Feng*

School of Biomedical Engineering, Southern Medical University, Guangdong, China

Abstract. Prediction of CT substitutes from MR images are clinically desired for dose planning in MR-based radiation therapy and attenuation correction in PET/MR. Considering that there is no global relation between intensities in MR and CT images, we propose local sparse correspondence combination (LSCC) for the prediction of CT substitutes from MR images. In LSCC, we assume that MR and CT patches are located on two nonlinear manifolds and the mapping from the MR manifold to the CT manifold approximates a diffeomorphism under a local constraint. Several techniques are used to constrain locality: 1) for each patch in the testing MR image, a local search window is used to extract patches from the training MR/CT pairs to construct MR and CT dictionaries; 2) *k*-Nearest Neighbors is used to constrain locality in the MR dictionary; 3) outlier detection is performed to constrain locality in the CT dictionary; 4) Local Anchor Embedding is used to solve the MR dictionary coefficients when representing the MR testing sample. Under these local constraints, the coefficient weights are linearly transferred from MR to CT, and used to combine the samples in the CT dictionary to generate CT predictions. The proposed method has been evaluated for brain images on a dataset of 13 subjects. Each subject has T1- and T2-weighted MR images, as well as a CT image with a total of 39 images. Results show the effectiveness of the proposed method which provides CT predictions with a mean absolute error of 113.8 HU compared with real CTs.

Keywords: CT Prediction, Outlier Detection, Local Anchor Embedding.

1 Introduction

Prediction of CT substitutes from MR images is important for dose planning in MR-based radiation therapy [1] and attenuation correction in PET/MR [2, 3]. MR images have shown many advantages compared to CT for radiation treatment planning, such as reducing X ray irradiation and improving target delineation. However, MR images do not contain electron density information which is needed for dose calculations in radiotherapy. In addition, PET/MR has shown its advantages and been used in many applications. To accurately quantify the radionuclide uptake, PET images need to be corrected for photon attenuation. However, the signals in MR images are not directly

* Corresponding author.

N. Navab et al. (Eds.): MICCAI 2015, Part I, LNCS 9349, pp. 93–100, 2015.
DOI: 10.1007/978-3-319-24553-9_12

related to the attenuation coefficients of radiation. Given that CT intensity is directly related to electron density, CT images are usually used for MR-based dose planning and attenuation correction for PET imaging. Therefore, accurate prediction of CT images from MR images is highly desired for clinical applications.

Recently, various methods for prediction of CT substitutes from MR data have been proposed. These methods mainly belong to two categories: segmentation-based and atlas-based methods. Segmentation-based methods [4, 5] usually classify voxels in MR images into different tissues, and assign linear attenuation coefficients or CT values. However, accurate segmentation is hard to obtain in some complicated regions such as the sinuses [3]. Atlas-based methods [1-3] usually use deformable image registration between training MR/CT pairs and the testing MR image to help CT predictions. These methods highly depend on the accuracy of the deformable registration results. In addition, many atlas-based methods [2, 3, 6] learn a regression from MR intensities to CT values, where a one-to-one correspondence between MR and CT intensities should be assumed. However, the relationship between MR and CT without any constraint is not a bijection, since materials such as air and cerebrospinal fluid have similar intensities in T1-weighted MR images but different CT values. Patch matching has shown its advantages on image synthesis and been applied in CT predictions [7].

In this study, a patch-based method for predicting CT substitutes from MR images is developed. Considering that the relationship between MR and CT intensities is not a bijection, we assume that MR patches and CT patches are located on two different nonlinear manifolds and the mapping from the MR manifold to the CT manifold approximates a diffeomorphism under a local constraint. In our study, we emphasize the locality on each manifold and propose local sparse correspondence combination (LSCC) to predict CT substitutes. The proposed method is evaluated on brain data for 13 subjects using a leave-one-subject-out cross-validation. Results show that our method can generate promising CT predictions.

2 CT Prediction by LSCC

2.1 Basic Idea of LSCC

Assumption I: Samples from different modalities are located on different nonlinear manifolds, and a sample can be approximately represented as a linear combination of several nearest neighbors from its manifold.

Assumption II: Under a local constraint, the mapping from the MR manifold to the CT manifold $\boldsymbol{f}: \mathbf{M} \rightarrow \mathbf{N}$ approximates a diffeomorphism.

Assumption I has been applied in many studies [8, 9], where an MR testing sample x can be linearly represented by its neighbors on the MR manifold:

$$x = \boldsymbol{D}\vec{w} + \boldsymbol{\varepsilon} = \sum_{i=1}^{\eta} d_i w_i + \boldsymbol{\varepsilon} \tag{1}$$

$$s.t. \|\boldsymbol{\varepsilon}\| < \tau;\ \forall d_i \notin O_x(L), w_i = 0;$$

$$\sum_{i=1}^{\eta} w_i = 1, w_i \geq 0.$$

where $\boldsymbol{D} = [d_1, d_2, \dots, d_\eta]$ is a dictionary which contains η MR training samples. $\vec{w}$ is a coefficient vector. $O_x(L)$ is a set of L nearest neighbors of x in $\boldsymbol{D}$. $\boldsymbol{\varepsilon}$ is the reconstruction error. The sum to one and non-negative constraints of coefficients ensure x is located in a small convex region on a hyperplane spanned by the closest neighbors [10], which ensures the locality of the linear representation.

Based on assumption II, the mapping from MR to CT approximates a diffeomorphism under a local constraint (i.e., $\boldsymbol{f}(\boldsymbol{D}) = \boldsymbol{C}$). $\boldsymbol{C}$ is a dictionary which contains CT training samples with the same locations as samples in $\boldsymbol{D}$. Given that Eq. (1) constrains the linear representation in a local space, $\boldsymbol{f}$ is linear in this local region. Therefore, $\vec{w}$ can be written out of $\boldsymbol{f}$ and transferred from MR to CT:

$$\boldsymbol{f}(x) \approx \boldsymbol{f}(\boldsymbol{D}\vec{w}) = \boldsymbol{f}(\boldsymbol{D})\vec{w} = \boldsymbol{C}\vec{w} \tag{2}$$

Combining $\boldsymbol{C}$ with $\vec{w}$ is used to predict the CT intensity at point x (Section 2.4).

Assumption II is crucial in LSCC. Given that the mapping from MR to CT is a diffeomorphism, $\vec{w}$ can be transferred from MR to CT. Given two manifolds **M** and **N**, the mapping $\boldsymbol{f}$: **M**→**N** is called a diffeomorphism if it is differentiable and bijective, and its inverse $\boldsymbol{f}^{-1}$: **N**→**M** is also differentiable. Based on assumption II, a local region on manifold **M** can be mapped onto a local region on manifold **N** by $\boldsymbol{f}$, wherein $\boldsymbol{f}$ is approximately linear. However, the relationship between the MR manifold and the CT manifold is not a bijection, since several materials have similar intensities in MR images but different CT values and vice versa.

To support assumption II, four steps are used to emphasize the local constraint: **1)** for each patch in the testing MR image, use a local search window to extract MR and CT training samples; **2)** use *k*NN to constrain the MR dictionary in a local space; **3)** delete outliers in the CT dictionary to ensure the locality; **4)** use Local Anchor Embedding (LAE), which emphasizes the locality of the representation, to solve MR dictionary coefficients in representing the MR testing sample. Detailed steps of LSCC are shown in Fig. 1. There are three main parts in LSCC: **local dictionary construction, local linear representation,** and **prediction.**

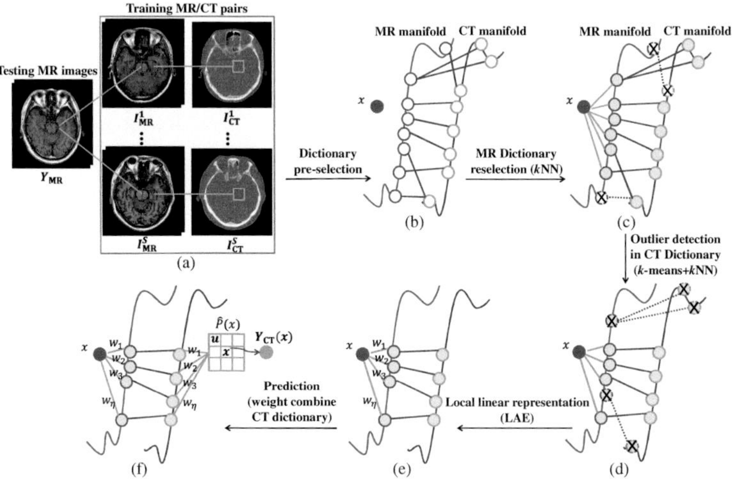

Fig. 1. Detailed steps of LSCC.

2.2 Local Dictionary Construction

We use $\boldsymbol{I} = \{I_t^s | s = 1, \dots, S; t = \text{T1}, \text{T2}, \text{CT}\}$ to denote the training dataset, where S denotes the number of training subjects and t denotes the image modality. For a new subject Y, we denote its T1- and T2-weighted MR images as Y_t $(t = \text{T1}, \text{T2})$. This step aims to construct MR and CT local dictionaries for each point in Y_t. Detailed procedures are described below:

Dictionary Pre-selection: First, we rigidly align Y_t $(t = \text{T1}, \text{T2})$ to the space in training MR/CT pairs by using FLIRT in FSL package[1]. Then, we extract patch-based features $\overrightarrow{f_x^1} \in R^{m\times 1}$ and $\overrightarrow{f_x^2} \in R^{m\times 1}$ centered at point x in Y_{T1} and Y_{T2}, where m denotes the number of points in the MR image patch. The patch-based feature is obtained by vectorizing the intensities of the image patch centered at x. Feature vector $\overrightarrow{f_x^1}$ and $\overrightarrow{f_x^2}$ are combined to represent the final feature of x, denoted as $\overrightarrow{f_x} = [\overrightarrow{f_x^1}; \overrightarrow{f_x^2}] \in R^{2m\times 1}$. For point x, we collect a set of patches within a local search window centered at x (i.e., red and green boxes in Fig. 1(a)) across all training images to generate an MR dictionary $\boldsymbol{D}(x)$ and a CT dictionary $\boldsymbol{C}(x)$.

Dictionary Reselection: Assumption II requires a local constraint. This step aims to constrain the MR dictionary in a local space, where we use *k*NN to find k nearest vectors of $\overrightarrow{f_x}$ from $\boldsymbol{D}(x)$, thus generating a new dictionary $\boldsymbol{D}_k(x) = [\vec{d}_1, \vec{d}_2, \dots, \vec{d}_k] \in R^{2m\times k}$. Based on the k samples in $\boldsymbol{D}_k(x)$, k CT correspondences can be obtained in $\boldsymbol{C}(x)$ through the MR/CT image patch pairs, thereby generating CT dictionary $\boldsymbol{C}_k(x) = [\vec{c}_1, \vec{c}_2, \dots, \vec{c}_k] \in R^{l\times k}$, where l denotes the number of points in the CT image patch.

Outlier Detection: In dictionary reselection, *k*NN is used to constrain the MR dictionary in a local space. To guarantee the locality in the CT dictionary, the outlier detection is performed to constrain CT training samples in a local space.

Various outlier detection methods are available, such as *k*NN, local outlier factor [11], one class support vector machines [12], and cluster-based method [13]. After comparing different outlier detection methods, we choose *k*-means clustering combined with *k*NN to detect outliers in $\boldsymbol{C}_k(x)$. We first use *k*-means to get a clustering center in $\boldsymbol{C}_k(x)$ and further use *k*NN to find ç nearest samples of the clustering center, constructing a new CT dictionary $\boldsymbol{C}_ç(x) = [\vec{c}_1, \vec{c}_2, \dots, \vec{c}_ç] \in R^{l\times ç}$. Accordingly, we delete the samples in $\boldsymbol{D}_k(x)$ with the same locations as the outliers in $\boldsymbol{C}_k(x)$, obtaining MR dictionary $\boldsymbol{D}_ç(x) = [\vec{d}_1, \vec{d}_2, \dots, \vec{d}_ç] \in R^{2m\times ç}$.

[1] http://fsl.fmrib.ox.ac.uk/fsl/fslwiki/

2.3 Local Linear Representation

Based on assumption I, we use the MR dictionary to linearly represent the MR testing sample. Various techniques are available to solve the dictionary coefficients. Sparse coding with L_1 LASSO constraint [14] emphasizes the sparsity of the representation and uses training samples with non-zero coefficients to linearly represent the testing sample. Locality-constrained linear coding (LLC) [15] focuses on locality by limiting linear coding within a local space. Compared to LLC, LAE [10] adds a nonnegative constraint to the coefficients. In LAE (Eq. (1)), the reconstructed sample is located in a convex region on a hyperplane spanned by its closest neighbors. Given that locality is important in this study, LAE is used to ensure the locality of the representation in solving the dictionary coefficients.

2.4 Prediction

For point x, we have an MR dictionary $\boldsymbol{D}_{ç}(x)$ and a CT dictionary $\boldsymbol{C}_{ç}(x)$. Both $\boldsymbol{D}_{ç}(x)$ and $\boldsymbol{C}_{ç}(x)$ are constrained to a local space, and they are assumed to be diffeomorphic (i.e., $\boldsymbol{f}(\boldsymbol{D}_{ç}) = \boldsymbol{C}_{ç}$). After using LAE to solve the MR dictionary coefficients, $\vec{w}$ can be transferred to the CT manifold based on Eq. (2). A vector $\vec{b}$ can be obtained: $\vec{b} \leftarrow \boldsymbol{C}_{ç}\vec{w}$, $\vec{b} \in R^{l}$. Vector $\vec{b}$ is reshaped to an image patch $\widehat{P}(x)$ (i.e., green grid in Fig. 1(f)) centered at x in the CT substitute Y_{CT}. After predicting an image patch for each point, we weighted average the overlapped patches to obtain the CT prediction. The weight of point u in patch $\widehat{P}(x)$ is defined as:

$$\omega_x^u = a^{D(u,x)}, \; 0 < a < 1 \tag{3}$$

where $D(u,x)$ is the Euclidean distance between u and x. As u gets away from x, the weight at u decreases, which means that the image patch makes a greater contribution in predicting the central points than the peripheral points. Finally, the predicted CT intensity at x in Y_{CT} is calculated as:

$$Y_{\text{CT}}(x) = \frac{\sum_{u \in \widehat{P}(x)} \omega_u^x \hat{I}_u^x}{\sum_{u \in \widehat{P}(x)} \omega_u^x} \tag{4}$$

where u is a point in patch $\widehat{P}(x)$. $\hat{I}_u^x$ is the intensity at point x in patch $\widehat{P}(u)$.

3 Experimental Results

We applied the proposed method to 13 subjects. Each subject has T1- and T2-weighted MR images and a CT image. Necessary pre-processing was applied to all images in the dataset. The N3 package[2] was used to remove bias field artifacts from the MR images. Intensity normalization of the MR images was performed to reduce the variance across images from different subjects. The head in each CT image was

[2] http://en.wikibooks.org/wiki/MINC/Tools/N3

separated from the bed using a thresholding technique as used in [3]. Our method was evaluated in a leave-one-subject-out cross-validation, where the CT substitute was compared to the real CT by calculating the mean absolute error (MAE) in Hounsfield units (HU) for all voxels in the brain volume.

3.1 Performance of Using Multimodality MR Images

To evaluate the impact of using different modalities, the performance is evaluated using only T1 or T2, and T1+T2. Statistical results are shown in Fig. 2. Mean $\pm$ standard deviation MAEs obtained using T1, T2, and T1+T2 are 124.6 $\pm$ 14.2 HU, 123.9 $\pm$ 17.1 HU, 113.8 $\pm$ 16.8 HU, respectively. The mean MAE using T1 and T2 images is 10.8 HU/10.1 HU lower than that of using a single T1/T2 image (paired t-test; $p < 0.001$). Using a single T1 or T2, there is no statistically significant difference between the results (paired t-test; $p > 0.05$).

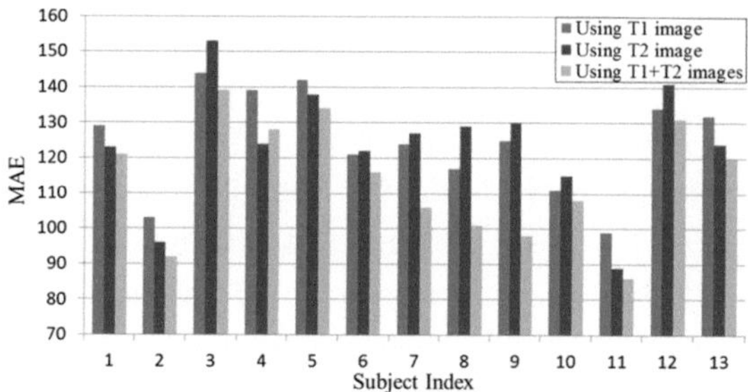

Fig. 2. MAEs of all 13 subjects obtained by using T1, T2, and T1+T2 images.

Fig. 3 shows the results of one slice obtained using T1, T2, and T1+T2. The first row shows the real CT image, CT substitutes obtained by using T1, T2, and T1+T2, respectively. The second row shows T1, T2, and difference images by using T1, T2, and T1+T2, respectively. The left scale bar shows the intensity distribution of real and substitute CT images and the right scale bar shows the values in difference images. Red in the right bar means a higher intensity in the real CT image and blue indicates a higher intensity in the CT substitute.

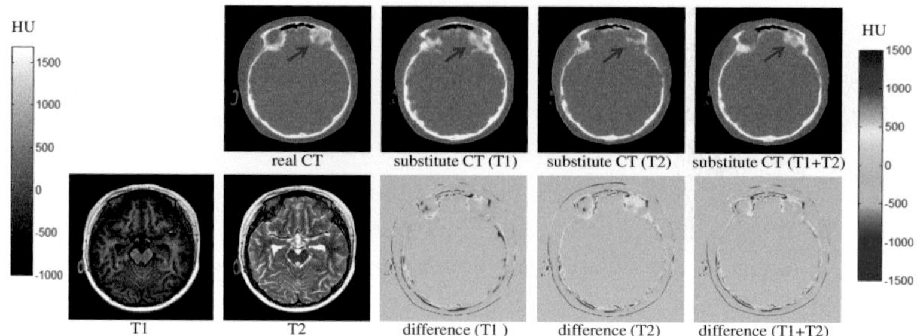

Fig. 3. Results of one slice generated by using T1, T2, and T1+T2 images. MAEs obtained by using T1, T2, T1+T2 are 95 HU, 89 HU, 83 HU, respectively.

3.2 Comparison with the Relevant Methods

The proposed LSCC is compared with Burgos *et al.*[3] [3] and Ta *et al.*[16]. Burgos *et al.* [3] also considered the local information and used the local image similarity measure to match between a given MR image and each of the MR/CT pairs in CT prediction. Ta *et al.* [16] combined patch matching with label fusion, which can be used in CT prediction by replacing label fusion with CT intensity fusion. Since the testing image is a single MR image in Burgos *et al.* [3], we compare these three methods using a single T1 or T2 image. Results obtained by Burgos *et al.* [3], Ta *et al.*[16] and LSCC based on T1 and T2 are shown in Fig. 4 (a) and (b), respectively. The mean ± standard deviation MAEs of all subjects using T1 by Burgos *et al.* [3], Ta *et al.*[16] and LSCC are 146.5 ± 25.6 HU, 134.8±14.4 HU and 124.6 ± 14.2 HU, respectively. When using T2, the mean ± standard deviation MAEs obtained by Burgos *et al.* [3], Ta *et al.*[16] and LSCC are 140.2 ± 26.0 HU, 133.2 ± 18.2 HU and 123.9 ± 17.1 HU, respectively. LSCC achieves significantly lower MAEs than the other two methods, which would bring an improvement in PET reconstruction and radiation dose planning.

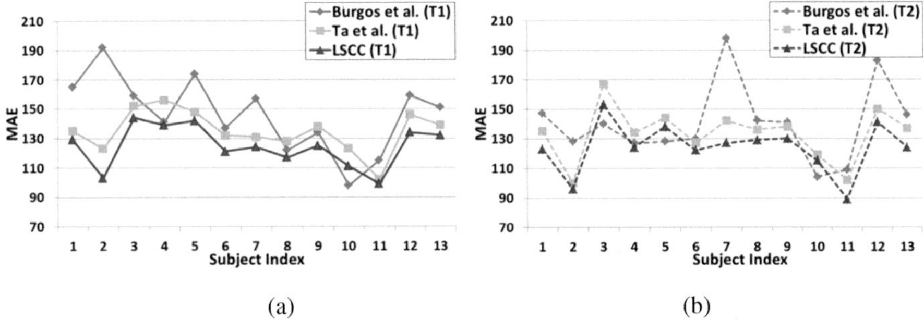

Fig. 4. MAEs of all 13 subjects obtained by Burgos *et al.* [3] (blue), Ta *et al.*[16] (green) and LSCC (red) using the T1 image (a) and T2 image (b) as the testing MR image, respectively.

Fig. 5 shows the results by Burgos *et al.* [3], Ta *et al.*[16] and LSCC. The first/second row shows the results using the T1/T2 image. Columns (a) to (h) are real CT, T1 or T2, CT substitutes and difference images by Burgos *et al.* [3], Ta *et al.*[16], and LSCC, respectively. Improvements by LSCC are shown in red arrows.

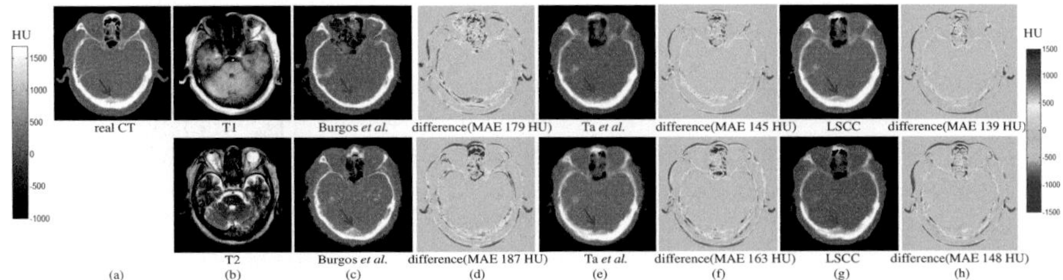

Fig. 5. Results by Burgos *et al.* [3], Ta *et al.* [16] and LSCC based on the T1 or T2 image.

---

[3] http://cmictig.cs.ucl.ac.uk/niftyweb/program.php?p=PCT

4 Conclusion

This study presents a novel method for the prediction of CT substitutes from MR images. In the proposed LSCC, we assume that MR patches and CT patches are located on two nonlinear manifolds, and the mapping from the MR manifold to the CT manifold approximates a diffeomorphism under a local constraint. Several techniques are used to constrain locality in both MR and CT dictionaries. The testing sample is locally represented by its MR dictionary. The coefficients are transferred from the MR manifold to the CT manifold and are further used to combine samples in the CT dictionary to generate CT predictions. Our method is evaluated for brain images on a dataset of 13 MR/CT pairs, and demonstrates superior performance compared to the competing CT prediction methods.

References

1. Uh, J., et al.: MRI-based treatment planning with pseudo CT generated through atlas registration. Med. Phys. 41, 051711 (2014)
2. Hofmann, M., et al.: "MRI-based attenuation correction for PET/MRI: a novel approach combining pattern recognition and atlas registration. J. Nucl. Med. 49, 1875–1883 (2008)
3. Burgos, N., et al.: Attenuation Correction Synthesis for Hybrid PET-MR Scanners: Application to Brain Studies. IEEE Trans. Med. Imaging 33, 2332–2341 (2014)
4. Keereman, V.: MRI-based attenuation correction for PET/MRI using ultrashort echo time sequences. Journal of Nuclear Medicine 51, 812–818 (2010)
5. Catana, C.: Toward implementing an MRI-based PET attenuation-correction method for neurologic studies on the MR-PET brain prototype. Journal of Nuclear Medicine (2010)
6. Hofmann, M., et al.: MRI-based attenuation correction for whole-body PET/MRI: quantitative evaluation of segmentation- and atlas-based methods. Journal of Nuclear Medicine 52, 1392–1399 (2011)
7. Roy, S., et al.: PET attenuation correction using synthetic CT from ultrashort echo-time MR imaging. Journal of Nuclear Medicine 55 (2014)
8. Roweis, S.T., Saul, L.K.: Nonlinear dimensionality reduction by locally linear embedding. Science 290, 2323–2326 (2000)
9. Wu, Y., et al.: Prostate segmentation based on variant scale patch and local independent projection. IEEE Trans. Med. Imaging 33, 1290–1303 (2014)
10. Liu, W., et al.: Large graph construction for scalable semi-supervised learning. In: Proceedings of the 27th International Conference on Machine Learning, pp. 679–686 (2010)
11. Breunig, M.M.: LOF: identifying density-based local outliers. ACM Sigmod Record, 93–104 (2000)
12. Mourao-Miranda, J., et al.: Patient classification as an outlier detection problem: an application of the One-Class Support Vector Machine. Neuroimage 58, 793–804 (2011)
13. He, Z., et al.: Discovering cluster-based local outliers. Pattern Recognition Letters (2003)
14. Tibshirani, R.: Regression shrinkage and selection via the lasso. Journal of the Royal Statistical Society. Series B (Methodological), 267–288 (1996)
15. Wang, J., et al.: Locality-constrained linear coding for image classification. In: IEEE Conference on Computer Vision and Pattern Recognition, pp. 3360–3367 (2010)
16. Ta, V.-T., Giraud, R., Collins, D.L., Coupé, P.: Optimized PatchMatch for Near Real Time and Accurate Label Fusion. In: Golland, P., Hata, N., Barillot, C., Hornegger, J., Howe, R. (eds.) MICCAI 2014, Part III. LNCS, vol. 8675, pp. 105–112. Springer, Heidelberg (2014)

Robust Automated White Matter Pathway Reconstruction for Large Studies

Jalmar Teeuw, Matthan W.A. Caan, and Silvia D. Olabarriaga*

Academic Medical Center Amsterdam, Amsterdam, The Netherlands
jalmar@me.com

Abstract. Automated probabilistic reconstruction of white matter pathways facilitates tractography in large studies. TRACULA (TRActs Constrained by UnderLying Anatomy) follows a Markov-chain Monte Carlo (MCMC) approach that is compute-intensive. TRACULA is available on our Neuroscience Gateway (NSG), a user-friendly environment for fully automated data processing on grid computing resources. Despite the robustness of TRACULA, our users and others have reported incidents of partially reconstructed tracts. Investigation revealed that in these situations the MCMC algorithm is caught in local minima. We developed a method that detects unsuccessful tract reconstructions and iteratively repeats the sampling procedure while maintaining the anatomical priors to reduce computation time. The anatomical priors are recomputed only after several unsuccessful iterations. Our method detects affected tract reconstructions by analyzing the dependency between samples produced by the MCMC algorithm. We extensively validated the original and the modified methods by performing five repeated reconstructions on a dataset of 74 HIV-positive patients and 47 healthy controls. Our method increased the rate of successful reconstruction in the two most prominently affected tracts (forceps major and minor) on average from 74% to 99%. In these tracts, no group difference in FA and MD was found, while a significant association with age could be confirmed.

1 Introduction

White matter bundles are known to degenerate with aging [5] and may also be affected by neurodegenerative diseases. They are therefore extensively studied in population imaging and comparative studies. Different approaches exist to reconstruct pathways in Diffusion Weighted Images (DWI) [4]. Deterministic streamline tractography models a path as a one-dimensional curve, rendering it sensitive to noise. Probabilistic tractography takes the uncertainty in the principal diffusion orientation into account but might miss a sparse pathway that is dominated by another denser pathway. Global tractography defines the tract end-points and searches the space for all possible connections.

* The AGEhIV Study Group and Co-morbidity in Relation to AIDS (COBRA) Study Group.

N. Navab et al. (Eds.): MICCAI 2015, Part I, LNCS 9349, pp. 101–108, 2015.
DOI: 10.1007/978-3-319-24553-9_13

Tractography relies on anatomical landmarks that define the pathway. Conventionally, these landmarks are manually annotated by an operator, which is a time-consuming and subjective procedure. This may be overcome by adopting a white matter parcellation atlas, built by populating tract probability maps of a cohort of healthy subjects [6]. Such an atlas averages out inter-subject morphological variation. Instead, landmarks may be retrieved from an atlas, transformed to subject space and used to obtain subject-specific tractography [10]. Additional subject-specific prior information may be obtained from an automated segmentation and parcellation of a high-resolution structural scan. This allows automatic delineation of 18 tracts constrained by underlying anatomy, in a method coined TRACULA (TRActs Constrained by UnderLying Anatomy) [9], which alleviates the need of manual tracing. TRACULA is one of the few methods providing an automated probabilistic method to segment individual pathways.

The adoption of TRACULA in practice imposes two challenges. First, it needs to be robust to be adopted in large imaging studies. For example, Figure 1 shows partial reconstruction in a subset of tracts [2] requiring manual intervention, which would not be feasible for large studies. Second, processing the data is compute-intensive, estimated to one CPU-year for a study of 100 subjects. To facilitate the adoption of such methods in clinical research, in our hospital we offer them as service available on our Neuroscience Gateway (NSG, https://neuro.ebioscience.amc.nl) [7]. From a web interface, the user browses the scans based on metadata, and runs applications such as TRACULA on the selected scans. The computations are performed seamlessly on a grid infrastructure, including the transport of data from the data server to the grid storage, and of results back to the data server. In the case of TRACULA, however, we

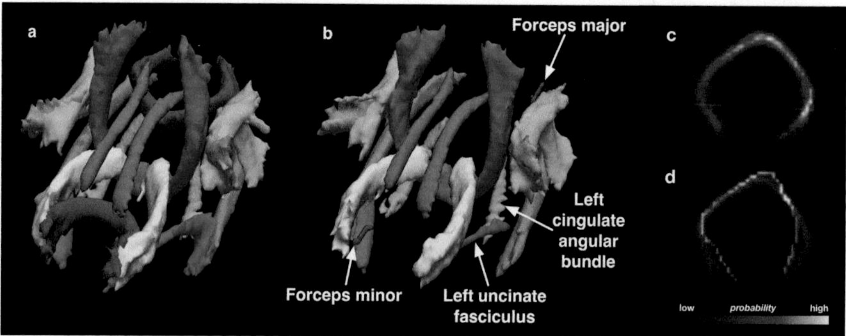

Fig. 1. Example 3D models (isosurface at 20% of maximum probability) of all tracts and maximum intensity projection along the inferior-superior axis of the probability density (PD) maps of forceps major for two repeated runs of TRACULA on the same subject scan. (***a***) successful reconstruction of all 18 tracts. (***b***) partial reconstruction of forceps major, forceps minor, left uncinate fasciculus, and left cingulate angular bundle. (***c***) PD map of successful reconstruction of forceps major. (***d***) PD map of partial reconstruction of forceps major showing artificially high probability for the track sample where the MCMC algorithm is caught in a local minimum.

observed that human interaction would be necessary in a large number of cases to deliver a complete reconstruction of all tracts; therefore we tried to find a solution to reduce this manual intervention.

In this paper we propose a robust and automated white matter pathway reconstruction method that detects unsuccessful tract reconstructions. It iteratively repeats the sampling procedure of TRACULA and updates anatomical priors only if needed. The method is implemented on the NSG, enabling it to be run by clinical researchers on their data.

2 Method

Automated Tract Reconstruction. TRACULA builds upon a Bayesian framework for global tractography [3] in which a pathway $\mathcal{F}$ is estimated from DWIs $\mathbf{Y}$ via the posterior distribution $p(\mathcal{F} \mid \mathbf{Y}) \propto p(\mathbf{Y} \mid \mathcal{F}) p(\mathcal{F})$. The likelihood $p(\mathbf{Y} \mid \mathcal{F})$ encapsulates the variability in the measured data given the pathway, assuming a "ball-and-stick" diffusion model [8]. The prior $p(\mathcal{F})$ is informed by an anatomical segmentation map of a structural scan [1], providing information of intersecting and adjacent structures along the pathway. The posterior distribution $p(\mathcal{F} \mid \mathbf{Y})$ is estimated via the Markov Chain Monte Carlo (MCMC) algorithm, which after a burn-in period runs a set of sampling iterations. A sample produced by the MCMC algorithm consists of perturbed spatial coordinates (x, y, z) for a set of control points that define a path through the tract by spline interpolation. The perturbation can be accepted or rejected, and in the latter case the perturbation is undone before the next iteration. Practically, separate steps can be run in TRACULA as follows: *a*) preparation (`trac-all -prep`), includes computing anatomical priors; *b*) reconstruction (`trac-all -path`), this runs the MCMC algorithm and produces statistics on the reconstructed tracts; and *c*) preparation step *a* with reinitialization of initial control points (`set reinit = 1` option).

Detecting Local Minima. By default the MCMC algorithm is run for 7500 iterations, but only every 5th iteration produces a sample in order to reduce the dependency between samples, resulting in 1500 samples. We observed that in partially reconstructed tracts a high number of duplicate samples were produced. We suspect that this occurs for example near the edge of a tract, where a random perturbation of control points likely leads to a rejected state outside the white matter. In such cases, $p(\mathcal{F} \mid \mathbf{Y})$ will then be biased to the edge of the tract, resulting in a 'narrow' pathway $\mathcal{F}$. We therefore try to detect when the MCMC algorithm was caught in such local minima by analyzing the presence of duplicate samples in the logs of TRACULA. We consider two samples duplicate when all x, y, z values of corresponding control points are identical. A sample is considered unique when it occurs only once in the set of 1500 samples. A local minimum can then be detected when *a*) there are less than A unique samples in the set; or *b*) the most frequently occurring duplicate has more than B samples in the set.

Robust Pathway Reconstruction. We propose an augmented sampling strategy that aims to automatically recover partially reconstructed tracts. The proposed method consist of three stages. In the first stage we obtain an initial reconstruction of the tracts by running step a followed by step b. In the second stage, partially reconstructed tracts are detected as described above. For these tracts, we attempt to increase the likelihood of obtaining a fully sampled tract by repeating step b maximally k times. In the third stage, if necessary, the anatomical priors $p(\mathcal{F})$ are recomputed and a different set of initial control points is chosen than in previous runs. This is done by running step c followed by step b a maximum of m times. This three-stage approach minimizes computing time by only recalculating partially reconstructed tracts and recomputing anatomical priors only when necessary.

3 Experiments

We performed four experiments to analyze the performance of our method using a large dataset of 121 subjects from the AGEhIV Cohort Study, consisting of 74 HIV positive patients and 47 healthy controls. Subjects were scanned on a 3.0 Tesla Philips Intera system. T1-weighted structural scans were acquired at a resolution of 1mm^3 and DWIs at 2mm^3 along 64 gradient directions with $b = 1000 s/mm^2$ and 6 non-diffusion weighted images ($b = 0 s/mm^2$). The structural MRI scans are processed with Freesurfer v5.3 [1] to obtain brain segmentations that are used to compute the anatomical priors in TRACULA. The DWI scans are preprocessed with an in-house developed pipeline. The preprocessed DWI scans are then processed with FSL BedpostX [8] v5.0.5 to obtain probabilistic diffusion parameters using a two-compartment model. The output of all three applications is merged and used as input for TRACULA. Default parameters are used for all three software packages. All the experiments were performed using the NSG within one week and consumed an estimated amount of 8228 computing hours (almost a full year) and 726 GB of data.

The *first experiment* assesses reproducibility of the problem of partial reconstructed tracts and validates our approach to detect the occurrence of this problem. We applied the original TRACULA implementation five times to reconstruct all 18 tracts in all 121 subjects. The detection method described in Section 2 was applied off-line to determine the number of unsuccessful reconstructions per scan and individually for each of the tracts in all 605 subject reconstructions. The results of the reconstructions for the first 55 subjects were verified by visual inspection. All 18 tracts were checked to determine if the result of the detection method is a true positive (TP), i.e. correctly detected unsuccessful reconstructions; false positive (FP), i.e. incorrectly detected successful reconstructions which our method superfluously recomputes; false negative (FN), i.e. incorrectly detected unsuccessful reconstructions representing missed cases of partial reconstruction; or true negative (TN), i.e. correctly detected successful reconstructions.

The *second experiment* investigates the behavior of the parameters A and B used by the proposed method. The parameters were varied within plausible

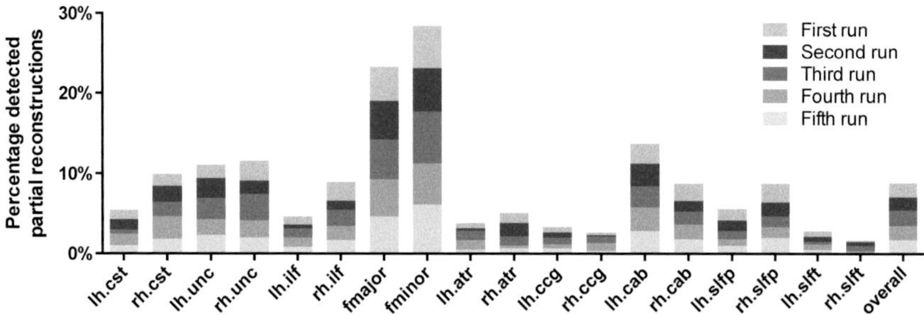

Fig. 2. Detected partial reconstructions of Tracula for five runs (different shadings).

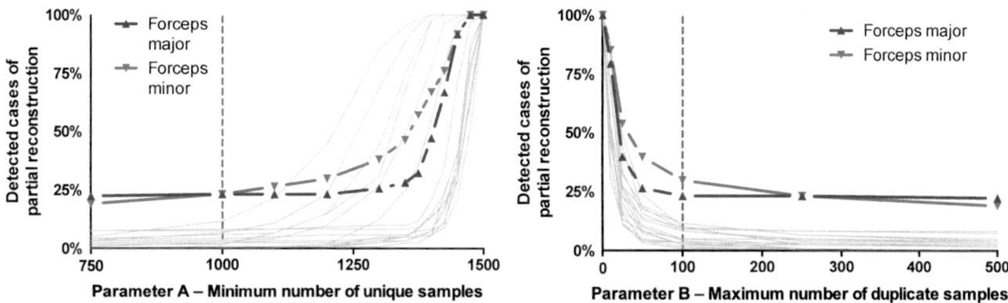

Fig. 3. Response curves per tract as percentage of detected cases for values of parameters A (left) and B (right). Dashed lines indicate values chosen for experiments.

range and the method was repetitively applied to a single run of TRACULA on all 121 subjects. We again applied the detection method from Section 2 and determined the number of failed reconstructions individually for each tract.

The *third experiment* aims at assessing the performance of the proposed method. Thresholds $A = 1000$ and $B = 100$ were set based on results from the second experiment. The other parameters were set empirically to $k = 7$ and $m = 3$, for a maximum of $n = k + m = 10$ iterations. Based on the results of the 605 subject reconstructions with our method we quantified the incidence rate of partially reconstructed tracts. We also assessed the behavior of our method by analyzing the number of iterations necessary to generate a successful reconstruction. We compared the reported volume and the weighted average fractional anisotropy (FA) of the tracts to the results obtained in the first experiment.

Finally, in the *fourth experiment*, a general linear model was fitted to the weighted average FA in the forceps major with age, group and reconstruction method as predictors.

4 Results

Figure 2 illustrates the number of unsuccessful reconstructions for each tract in all the five runs of Tracula from the first experiment. Note that there are variations between the runs, and that some tracts (e.g. the forceps major and

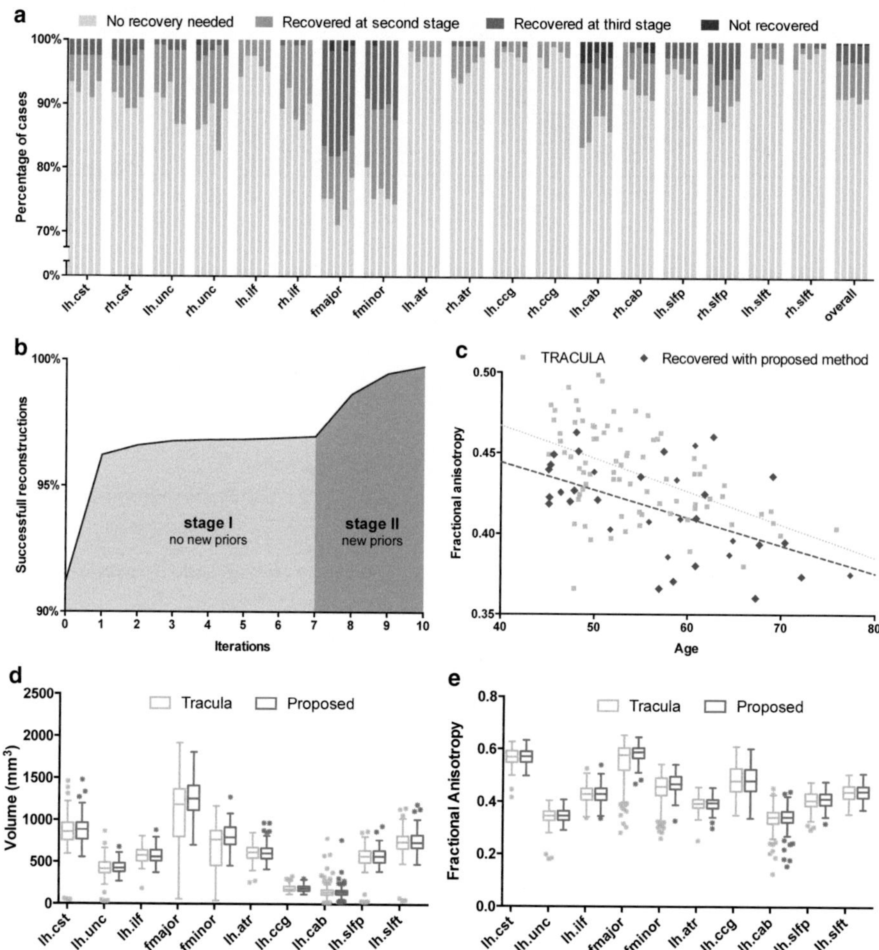

Fig. 4. (***a***) Percentage of successfully reconstructed tracts in each stage of our method (light blue=first, medium blue=second, dark blue=third). In darkest blue are tracts that failed after the maximum number of iterations. The overall (average of all tracts) is shown in the last column. (***b***) Percentage of successfully reconstructed tracts at each iteration of our method. (***c***) Scatter plot of FA as a function of age for TRACULA and proposed method, with trend lines for each group. There is a significant effect of age ($p = 0.015$) and reconstruction method (TRACULA versus proposed method, $p = 0.0002$). (***d***) Box plot of the segmented volumes per tract for TRACULA and the proposed method. Right hemisphere tracts show comparable results to the left hemisphere and are omitted. (***e***) Box plot of the weighted average FA per tract for TRACULA and the proposed method.

minor) are more prone to failure than others. The results of the second experiment are presented in Figure 3. When parameters A, B are too strict, too many reconstructions are detected as partial reconstruction. We chose $A = 1000$ and $B = 100$ as optimal values to be used in the remaining experiments.

Figure 4a synthesizes the results obtained for the original method and the proposed robust method. On overall, 8.8% of the tracts were identified by our method as partial reconstruction. The variability in success rate between repeated runs of the initial reconstruction is low at $\leq 5\%$. Differences between hemispheres are negligible. Figure 4b reveals that 65% of the detected cases were successfully reconstructed during stage two of our method, and another 32% during stage three, i.e. after recomputing anatomical priors. The overall success rate increases from 91.2% to 99.7%. The few failed cases were detected in the forceps major and minor and cingulum angular bundles. From this experiment we can optimize the number of iterations for stage 2 and set $k = 2$ in the future.

Visual inspection of the first 55 subject reconstructions, for a total of 990 tract reconstructions, produced by the first run of TRACULA produced the following results: 5.86% of the detected cases were true positive, 2.63% false positive, 0.71% false negative, and 90.81% true negatives. The cingulum angular bundle and cingulumcingulate gyrus, both thin elongated tracts, are most often wrongly detected as partial reconstruction (i.e. detected as FP).

The effect of the recovery strategy is most prominently seen in the volume measures of the tracts (Figure 4d). The partially reconstructed tracts no longer appear as outliers with small volume when using the proposed method. The 25-75 percentile volume range of the forceps major and minor are reduced by approximately a factor of two and the median volume is marginally increased. Similar effects can be witnessed for the weighted average FA of the tracts (Figure 4e). This supports our suspicion that partially reconstructed tracts are biased toward the edge of the tract, resulting in a lower average FA.

Comparing FA values in the forceps major, no group difference was found, while a significantly association with age could be confirmed ($p = 0.015$, Figure 4c). FA was significantly lower among the subgroup recovered using the proposed method compared to the set reconstructed with TRACULA ($p = 0.0002$).

5 Discussion and Conclusions

The high curvature of the forceps major and forceps minor could have caused a lower success rate compared to the other tracts. Future work may consider increasing the number of control points for these highly curved tracts. In general, optimizing the parameter settings per tract individually, including the number of control points and number of samples, would be recommended.

When applying the method to a dataset of HIV positive patients and healthy controls, the weighted average FA in the successfully reconstructed forceps major using the proposed method was significantly lower than those obtained using TRACULA. The uncertainty in the principal diffusion orientation is known to be inversely related to FA. This makes tractography more challenging in subjects with low FA and may explain the higher failure rate. Failing to include these subjects in the analysis may bias the statistical comparison between patients and controls, illustrating the importance of robust pathway reconstruction in comparative studies.

We presented a method for robust and automated white matter pathway segmentation. The proposed method provides efficient recovery of partially reconstructed tracts by repeated MCMC sampling, and only having to recompute the anatomical priors when necessary. The method is effective in improving the success rate for the two most prominently affected tracts (i.e. the forceps major and minor) from 74% to 99%, and on overall from 91.2% to 99.7%.

References

1. Fischl, B.: FreeSurfer. NeuroImage 62(2), 774–781 (2012)
2. Hatton, S.N., Lagopoulos, J., Hermens, D.F., Hickie, I.B., Scott, E., Bennett, M.R.: White matter tractography in early psychosis: clinical and neurocognitive associations. Journal of Psychiatry & Neuroscience: JPN 39(6), 417–427 (2014)
3. Jbabdi, S., Woolrich, M.W., Andersson, J.L.R., Behrens, T.E.J.: A Bayesian framework for global tractography. NeuroImage 37(1), 116–129 (2007)
4. Lazar, M.: Mapping brain anatomical connectivity using white matter tractography. NMR in Biomedicine 23(7), 821–835 (2010)
5. Lebel, C., Gee, M., Camicioli, R., Wieler, M., Martin, W., Beaulieu, C.: Diffusion tensor imaging of white matter tract evolution over the lifespan. NeuroImage 60(1), 340–352 (2012)
6. Mori, S., Oishi, K., Jiang, H., Jiang, L., Li, X., Akhter, K., Hua, K., Faria, A.V., Mahmood, A., Woods, R., Toga, A., Pike, G., Neto, P., Evans, A., Zhang, J., Huang, H., Miller, M., van Zijl, P., Mazziotta, J.: Stereotaxic white matter atlas based on diffusion tensor imaging in an ICBM template. NeuroImage 40(2), 570–582 (2008)
7. Shahand, S., Benabdelkader, A., Jaghoori, M.M., al Mourabit, M., Huguet, J., Caan, M.W.A., van Kampen, A.H.C., Olabarriaga, S.D.: A Data-Centric Neuroscience Gateway: Design, Implementation, and Experiences. Concurrency and Computation: Practice and Experience 27(2), 489–506 (2015)
8. Woolrich, M.W., Jbabdi, S., Patenaude, B., Chappell, M., Makni, S., Behrens, T., Beckmann, C., Jenkinson, M., Smith, S.M.: Bayesian analysis of neuroimaging data in FSL. NeuroImage 45(1), S173–S186 (2009)
9. Yendiki, A., Panneck, P., Srinivasan, P., Stevens, A., Zöllei, L., Augustinack, J., Wang, R., Salat, D., Ehrlich, S., Behrens, T., Jbabdi, S., Gollub, R., Fischl, B.: Automated probabilistic reconstruction of white-matter pathways in health and disease using an atlas of the underlying anatomy. Frontiers in Neuroinformatics 5(23), 1–12 (2011)
10. Zhang, W., Olivi, A., Hertig, S., Zijl, P.V., Mori, S.: Automated fiber tracking of human brain white matter using diffusion tensor imaging. Neuroimage 42(2), 771–777 (2008)

Exploiting the Phase in Diffusion MRI for Microstructure Recovery: Towards Axonal Tortuosity via Asymmetric Diffusion Processes

Marco Pizzolato[1,⋆,⋆⋆], Demian Wassermann[1,⋆], Timothé Boutelier[2], and Rachid Deriche[1]

[1] Athena, Inria Sophia Antipolis - Méditerranée, France
{marco.pizzolato,demian.wassermann,rachid.deriche}@inria.fr
[2] Olea Medical, La Ciotat, France
timothe.boutelier@olea-medical.com

Abstract. Microstructure recovery procedures via Diffusion-Weighted Magnetic Resonance Imaging (DW-MRI) usually discard the signal's phase, assuming symmetry in the underlying diffusion process. We propose to recover the Ensemble Average Propagator (EAP) directly from the complex DW signal in order to describe also eventual diffusional asymmetry, thus obtaining an asymmetric EAP. The asymmetry of the EAP is then related to tortuosity of undulated white matter axons, which are found in pathological scenarios associated with axonal elongation or compression. We derive a model of the EAP for this geometry and quantify its asymmetry. Results show that the EAP obtained when accounting for the DW signal's phase provides useful microstructural information in such pathological scenarios. Furthermore, we validate these results in-silico through 3D Monte-Carlo simulations of white matter tissue that has experienced different degrees of elongation/compression.

Keywords: Diffusion MRI, Phase, EAP, Asymmetry, Tortuosity, Axon.

1 Introduction

A rather unexplored field in Diffusion-Weighted Magnetic Resonance Imaging (DW-MRI) is the use of the phase component of the signal to quantify white matter microstructural characteristics. Despite the DW signal's complex nature, current approaches discard the phase and characterize microstructure using just the signal's magnitude [1,2,3]. In this paper, we show that the signal's phase component plays an important role in microstructure characterization. It provides a novel approach towards the quantification of diffusion properties. Particularly, we exploit the signal's phase to quantify different levels of tortuosity in undulated axons within a voxel, which can be associated with pathology through, for instance, axonal compression.

⋆ Marco Pizzolato and Demian Wassermann contributed equally to this work.

⋆⋆ The author expresses his thanks to Olea Medical and the Provence-Alpes-Côte d'Azur (PACA) Regional Council for providing grant and support for this work.

N. Navab et al. (Eds.): MICCAI 2015, Part I, LNCS 9349, pp. 109–116, 2015.
DOI: 10.1007/978-3-319-24553-9_14

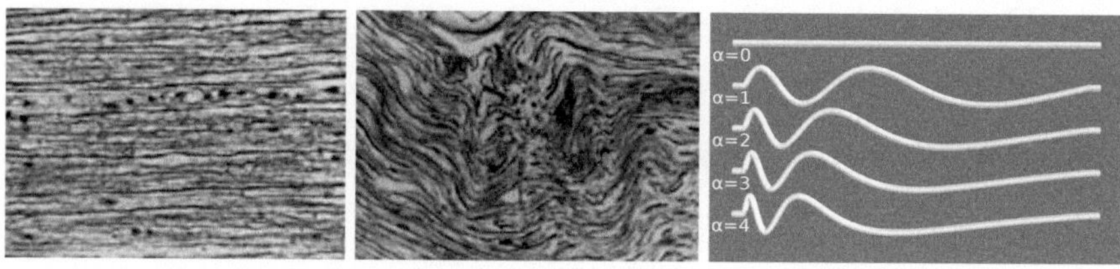

Fig. 1. From left to right: elongated and compressed WM tissue, reproduced with permission from [5]; straight/undulated axonal models for different tortuosity rates α.

White matter (WM) tissue may present different microstructural organizations depending on its nature and pathological condition. For instance, axons composing the tissue can be straight as shown in fig. 1 left. However axons may appear sinusoidal, and pathological conditions such as those caused by cervical cord injury can result in changes of undulation amplitude and tortuosity due to longitudinal elongation or compression [4,5], as shown in central fig. 1. The movement of spins within the WM tissue is influenced by the type of organization. Thus, a profound knowledge of the diffusion process can give insights into its microstructural properties.

DW-MRI allows to probe diffusion in a tissue sample by measuring a complex-valued signal related to the displacement probability of spins. The average displacement probability of the ensemble of spins contained within a voxel is known as Ensemble Average Propagator (EAP), and is related to the signal attenuation via an inverse Fourier transform [6]. Tissue microstructure influences spins displacements. Hence, EAP and DW signal can be exploited to measure microstructural properties. Recent work [4] proves that undulated axons, modeled as sinusoids, are a confound on axonal diameter estimation from DW images.

We show that by exploiting the DW signal's phase it is possible to characterize axonal tortuosity, which can be linked to elongation/compression phenomena in pathological scenarios. Compressed axons are partially convoluted and show irregular undulation with a non-uniform tortuosity along the longitudinal direction (see fig. 1 right). Hence, we model the compressed axon as a sinusoid with varying tortuosity, inducing asymmetry in its shape. Moreover, as the degree of compression increases, the tortuosity variation rate along the axon also increases. Spins diffusing within these axons undergo an asymmetric diffusion process resulting in an informative DW signal's phase, sensible to increasing tortuosity rates. The amount of diffusion asymmetry thus gives important insights into the underlying degree of compression.

Diffusion process asymmetries have already been investigated [7]. However, current approaches to obtain the EAP only use the DW magnitude signal and assume axial symmetry along each diffusion direction. We show that, by exploiting the DW signal's phase component, we recover an EAP describing also asymmetric diffusion which asymmetry is linked to the axonal tortuosity rate, and thus compression. To prove this, we first derive an analytic model of the EAP corresponding to the proposed axonal geometry, and obtain the correspondent DW complex signal. Using the complex signal we recompute the EAPs for increasing tortuosity rates, corresponding to scenarios of increasing axonal compression. We propose to quantify asymmetry as the Hellinger distance [8] between each EAP and its axially reflected version. We finally present experiments elucidating the link between EAP asymmetry and axonal tortuosity rates, thus compression degrees. Results are shown for EAPs generated analytically in 2D and validated by means of 3D Monte-Carlo simulations performed with Camino [9].

2 Theory and Methods

In this section, we introduce a model describing the undulated axon geometry with varying tortuosity. We derive the corresponding equations for the 2D Ensemble Average Propagator (EAP) and discuss its relation with the magnitude and phase of the DW-MRI signal.

2.1 Tortuous Axon Model

To analyze the DW signal in axonal compression cases, we model straight axons, in agreement with the usual hypothesis in the area, and undulated axons showing tortuosity. Our model for undulated axons is an extension of that proposed in [4]. We consider a sinusoidal axon that lies in the xz-plane and evolves along z with oscillations along x. Our axon model has infinitesimal thickness and goes through two full periods within the interval $[-Z, Z]$ with $Z > 0$:

$$x = f(z) = A \sin\left(\frac{2\pi(z - Z)}{L(z, \alpha)}\right) \tag{1}$$

where A and $L(z, \alpha)$ are respectively the amplitude and the wavelength of the sinusoid, with $0 < A \leq X$ and $L(z, \alpha) > 0$. We model the varying wavelength as

$$L(z, \alpha) = \alpha(z + Z) + l, \; for \, \alpha > 0 \tag{2}$$

where α is the spatial rate regulating the wavelength increment along the z-axis. The wavelength increases progressively along the z-axis starting from a minimum value l in $z = -Z$. The spatial rate α is related to the degree of intrinsic asymmetry induced in the undulated shape along the z-axis. We consider the case where $\alpha = 0$ as the straight axon, that is when $A = 0$, as shown in fig. 1 right. To derive the EAP in the following section it is useful to define the curve length for eq. (1). In particular the length between z and $z + \Delta z$ is given by

$$s(\Delta z; z) = \int_{z}^{z+\Delta z} \sqrt{1 + \left[A \cos\left(\frac{2\pi(\zeta - Z)}{L(\zeta, \alpha)}\right) \frac{2\pi(l + 2\alpha Z)}{L(\zeta, \alpha)^2}\right]^2} \, d\zeta \tag{3}$$

where Δz is a displacement along the z-axis with respect to the coordinate z.

2.2 Ensemble Average Propagator for Tortuous Axons

To obtain the complex DW signal in the case of tortuous axons model in section 2.1, we derive the correspondent Ensemble Average Propagator (EAP). The EAP for a spin displacement $(\Delta x, \Delta z)$ subject to a diffusion time t_d is [6]

$$\begin{aligned} \mathrm{EAP}(\Delta x, \Delta z; t_d) &= \iint_{-\infty}^{\infty} \rho_0(x,z) P(\Delta x, \Delta z | x, z, t_d)\, dxdz \\ &= \int_{-\infty}^{\infty} \rho_0(z) P(\Delta x, \Delta z | z, t_d)\, dz \end{aligned} \tag{4}$$

where ρ_0 is the initial spin density and P is the displacement pdf. The second equality in eq. (4) is due to our model parametrization in eq. (1). We compute ρ_0 by assuming an initial uniform spin density along our axon model

$$\rho_0(z) = \cos\left(\arctan\left[f'(z)\right]\right)^{-1} \tag{5}$$

where $f'(z)$ is the derivative of f in eq. (1). To produce an approximation for the displacement probability P in eq. (4), we decompose it using:

$$P(\Delta x, \Delta z | z, t_d) = P(\Delta x | \Delta z, z) P(\Delta z | z, t_d). \tag{6}$$

Using this decomposition, we assume that spins diffuse freely along the curve, i.e. they follow a normal distribution with variance $2Dt_d$ where D is the self-diffusion coefficient of water. Then, the probability of a spin experiencing a net displacement along the z-axis Δz can be approximated by [4]

$$P(\Delta z | z, t_d) = \frac{1}{\sqrt{4\pi D t_d}} e^{-\frac{s(\Delta z; z)^2}{4Dt_d}} \tag{7}$$

where s, the arc length of the axon between z and $z + \Delta_z$, is in eq. (3). As the coordinate x on the axon is univocally determined by z, as specified in eq. (1), the displacement density along x provided that we know Δz and z is [4]

$$P(\Delta x | \Delta z, z) = \delta_D\left(f(z) + \Delta x - f(z + \Delta z)\right) \tag{8}$$

where δ_D is the Dirac delta function. Given eqs. (5) to (8), the EAP of a tortuous axon, according to our model in section 2.1, can be obtained by simple numerical integration of eq. (4).

We proceed to express the relationship between EAP and signal, then we quintify EAP asymmetry by exploiting the phase information.

2.3 Diffusion Signal and EAP Asymmetry

The signal acquired in DW-MRI can be represented as function of the diffusion time t_d and frequency vector $\mathbf{q} = \gamma\delta\mathbf{G}/2\pi$ where γ is the gyromagnetic ratio, δ is the diffusion pulse duration and $\mathbf{G}$ is the diffusion gradient vector.

The measured **q**-dependent signal $S(\mathbf{q})$ has a complex nature and its attenuation $E(\mathbf{q}) = S(\mathbf{q})/S(0)$ is related to the EAP via a Fourier relationship [6]:

$$E(q_x, q_z; t_d) = \iint_{-\infty}^{\infty} \mathrm{EAP}(\Delta x, \Delta z | t_d) e^{-j2\pi(q_x \Delta x + q_z \Delta z)}\, d\Delta z\, d\Delta x \qquad (9)$$

which is valid under narrow pulse approximation and where q_x and q_z are the components of the frequency vector **q**. The EAP usually calculated from the magnitude attenuation $|E|$ via inverse Fourier transform is symmetric due to the zero phase assumption [10]. We consider instead the complex attenuation and characterize the asymmetry of the diffusion process by measuring the distance between the corresponding EAP and its axially reflected version. Despite different measures are possible, after defining the displacement vector $\mathbf{r} = (\Delta x, \Delta z)$, we adopt the Hellinger distance [8] because it constitutes a proper metric between probability measures

$$H^2 = \frac{1}{2} \int \left(\sqrt{\mathrm{EAP}(\mathbf{r}|t_d)} - \sqrt{\mathrm{EAP}(-\mathbf{r}|t_d)} \right)^2 d\mathbf{r} \qquad (10)$$

where $0 \leq H \leq 1$, 0 corresponding to equality and 1 to maximum inequality.

2.4 Monte-Carlo Simulation of DW-MRI in Tortuous Axons

To validate analytic results, we generate the DW complex signal by performing 3D Monte-Carlo simulations using an in-house customized version of Camino [9] that allows to obtain both Magnitude and Phase. This is done by considering both real and imaginary parts of the signal, thus replacing eq. (7) in [9] with

$$S(\mathbf{G}, \Delta, \delta) = S(0, \Delta, \delta) \int_{-\infty}^{\infty} P(\phi) \left(\cos(\phi) + j \sin(\phi)\right) d\phi \qquad (11)$$

where ϕ is the phase accumulation, $P(\phi)$ the spin phase distribution and Δ the time separation between diffusion gradients.

3 Experiments

In this section we present experiments showing the relationship between EAP asymmetry and axonal tortuosity for the EAP obtained as described in section 2.2 and with 3D Monte-Carlo simulations.

In the first case we compute the EAP of straight and undulated axons via eq. (4) for increasing tortuosity rates $\alpha \in [1, 8]$. Axons present undulation amplitude $A = 4\,\mu m$ with a basal wavelength $l = 50\,\mu m$ [4]. We set $D = 2 \times 10^{-9}\, m^2 s^{-1}$ [9] and $t_d = 28.6\, ms$ according to a realistic scenario. We fix the maximum observable displacement in both directions to $X = Z = 50\,\mu m$ and we define the observation frame as the xz-plane limited to the interval $[-X, X]$ along x and $[-Z, Z]$ along z. As α increases along the z-axis, eq. (2), the undulated axonal trajectory becomes compressed towards the frame's negative bound $-Z$

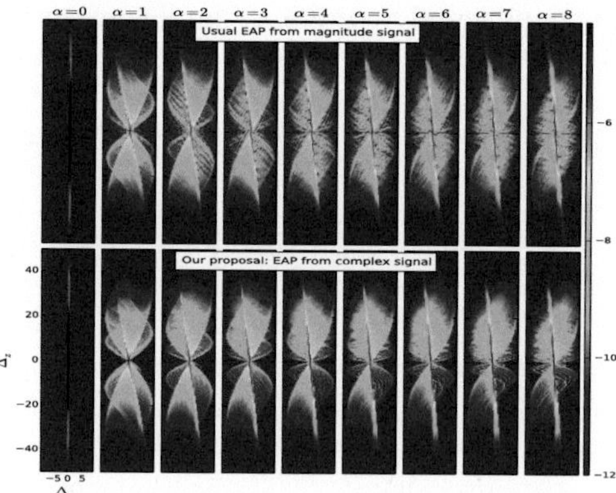

Fig. 2. Log-scaled EAPs obtained for straight and undulated axons with different tortuosity rates α. The first row shows EAPs obtained via inverse Fourier transform of the magnitude signal attenuation: EAPs show axial symmetry with respect to the axis passing through the origin. The second row shows EAPs obtained from the complex signal: axial asymmetry is present and increases with the tortuosity rate α.

(see fig. 1 right). The observation frame is discretized over a 257×257 displacement grid, and the EAP is calculated for each sample via numerical evaluation of eq. (4). The complex signal attenuation is obtained, for each considered α, as the Fourier transform of the EAP over the displacement grid according to eq. (9). The EAPs are then calculated as the inverse Fourier transform of both the complex and magnitude signal attenuations.

Images in fig. 2 show the log-transformed EAPs calculated for the straight axon ($\alpha = 0$) and for different degrees of axonal compression ($\alpha > 0$). The first row contains the EAPs as usually calculated from the magnitude signal. The second row shows the EAPs obtained from the complex signal. We note that no differences exist for the straight axon $\alpha = 0$. Despite the shape of the magnitude-derived EAP changes as α increases, we note that it always shows axial symmetry. On the other end, evident asymmetry is present in the case of the complex-derived EAPs for $\alpha > 0$. When looking at the EAPs in the second row of fig. 2, the difference between the upper and lower lobes of each EAP clearly appears. We further note that the degree of asymmetry between the lobes is more marked at high α, for instance the difference between the lower and upper lobes for $\alpha = 8$ is more accentuated than in the case of $\alpha = 1$.

We quantify asymmetry in the EAPs by computing the proposed Hellinger distance, eq. (10), as function of α (fig. 3 left). We note the incremental trend between the complex-derived EAP asymmetry and the tortuosity rate, in agreement with images in the second row of fig. 2. To validate the results for the more realistic case in which axons have finite diameter, we reproduce experiments using 3D Monte-Carlo simulations. Complex signals are obtained via PGSE sequences with $\Delta = 24.3\,ms$, $\delta = 12.9\,ms$ and maximum gradient strength $|\mathbf{G}_{max}| = 0.8\,Tm^{-1}$. Gradient directions are selected over the undersampled 29×29 displacement grid. Simulations are carried out considering 10^5 spins diffusing within the axon [9]. We generate meshes for axons with $\alpha = 0, 1, 2, 3, 4$

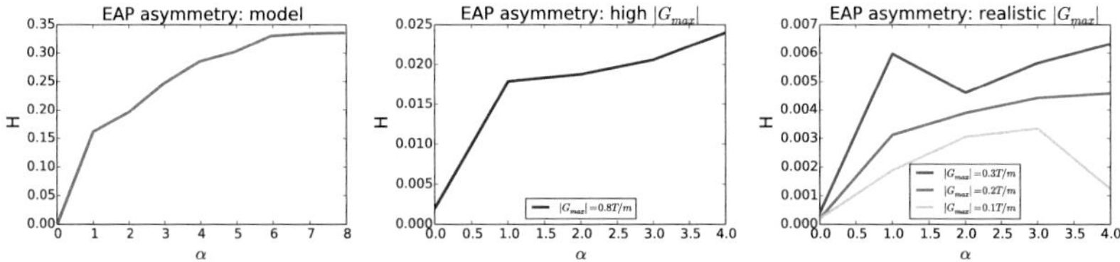

Fig. 3. Hellinger distances as function of tortuosity rate α obtained for the analytic model (left) and via Monte-Carlo simulation (central, right). Right figure shows the behaviour for state-of-the-art human MRI scanners such as the HCP one.

considering a diameter $d = 1\,\mu m$ [4], as shown in fig. 1 right. Meshes have impermeable walls with zero thickness. As for the analytic case we obtain the complex-derived EAPs for increasing α and compute the Hellinger distance to measure the asymmetry, as shown in central fig. 3. To assess the feasibility of the technique in state-of-the-art human settings, such as in the Human Connectome Project, we explore the behavior of the Hellinger distance at different gradient strengths $|\mathbf{G}_{max}| = 0.1, 0.2, 0.3\,Tm^{-1}$, as shown in fig. 3 right.

4 Discussion and Conclusion

The overall objective of this work is to assess the use of the DW signal's phase as microstructural marker. We show that the phase becomes informative whenever the underlying diffusion process manifests asymmetry along specific directions as a consequence of, for instance, a variation in the axonal tortuosity.

EAP asymmetry Increases with Larger Tortuosity Rates in our 2D Model. This is observable in fig. 3 left and fig. 2 (second row), where values along radial lines passing through the origin are asymmetric for $\alpha > 0$. The explanation of this phenomenon lies in the spin displacements asymmetry along the axes. Indeed the maximum distance a spin can travel along an axon evolving along the z-axis is defined by the diffusion coefficient and time. This distance is fixed irrespective of the fact that the spin displaces, along the axon, towards the positive or the negative values of the z-axis. This is the case of the straight axon ($\alpha = 0$) where diffusion occurs equally in each direction (fig. 2). With undulation the maximum displacement along z, resulting from a movement along the axon, depends on the movement direction of the spin, and precisely on the average tortuosity the axon shows in each direction: the ratio between the length of the trajectory and the corresponding length along the z-axis. If the tortuosity in the two directions is different ($\alpha > 0$), then the displacement probability of the spin along the z-axis, thus the x-axis, is asymmetric with respect to the origin. Since the EAP accounts for all of the contributions of the spin displacement probabilities along the axon, the EAP is symmetric when axonal tortuosity is constant ($\alpha = 0$), and is asymmetric otherwise ($\alpha > 0$).

EAP Asymmetry is Sensible to Axonal Tortuosity in Realistic Scenarios. In 3D experiments spins diffuse transversely to the axon as well as along it.

Hence, the trajectory a spin performs is convoluted and leads to smaller displacements along the axon, causing the asymmetry to have a milder effect on the overall EAP. This directly implies that a good characterization of the EAP asymmetry may be better achieved at very high $|\mathbf{q}|$ values as shown in fig. 3 central and right. Lower gradient strengths, hence displacement resolutions, affect the measured asymmetry at very short wavelengths as for the case of $\alpha = 4$ and $|\mathbf{G}_{max}| = 0.1\,Tm^{-1}$. However, our proposed measure of asymmetry using the complex signal combined with the Hellinger distance, *eq.* (10), as microstructure marker for axonal tortuosity/compression, remains effective. As a future work we suggest to explore higher diffusion times, and thus Δ. While a very high $|\mathbf{q}|$ is hard to achieve, longer diffusion times allow spins to diffuse more thus sensing the asymmetry at greater displacements, which are observable also at lower $|\mathbf{q}|$.

Real data acquisition for this scenario is challenging, specially due to technical difficulties such as the extreme sensibility of phase to noise. However, although other techniques assume straight axons, simulations show that undulation combined with tortuosity significantly affect the DW signal and can be detected through diffusion asymmetry by exploiting the phase. We strongly believe that this pioneering work opens new roads and perspectives towards measuring WM tissue properties via DW-MRI.

References

1. Assaf, Y., Blumenfeld-Katzir, T., Yovel, Y., Basser, P.J.: AxCaliber: a method for measuring axon diameter distribution from diffusion MRI. MRM 59(6), 1347–1354 (2008)
2. Zhang, H., Schneider, T., Wheeler-Kingshott, C.A., Alexander, D.C.: NODDI: practical in vivo neurite orientation dispersion and density imaging of the human brain. Neuroimage 61(4), 1000–1016 (2012)
3. Alexander, D.C.: A general framework for experiment design in diffusion MRI and its application in measuring direct tissue-microstructure features. MRN 60(2), 439–448 (2008)
4. Nilsson, M., Lätt, J., Stahlberg, F., Westen, D., Hagsltt, H.: The importance of axonal undulation in diffusion MR measurements: a Monte Carlo simulation study. NMR in Biomedicine 25(5), 795 (2012)
5. Shacklock, M.: Biomechanics of the Nervous System: Breig Revisited. Neurodynamics Solutions, Adelaide (2007)
6. Tanner, J.E., Stejskal, E.: Restricted Self-Diffusion of Protons in Colloidal Systems by the Pulsed-Gradient, Spin-Echo Method. JCP 49(4), 1768–1777 (1968)
7. Özarslan, E., Koay, C.G., Basser, P.J.: Remarks on q-space MR propagator in partially restricted, axially-symmetric, and isotropic environments. MRI 27(6), 834–844 (2009)
8. Hellinger, E.: Neue Begründung der Theorie quadratischer Formen von unendlichvielen Veränderlichen. Journal für die reine und angewandte Mathematik (1909)
9. Hall, M.G., Alexander, D.C.: Convergence and parameter choice for Monte-Carlo simulations of diffusion MRI. IEEE TMI 28, 1354–1364 (2009)
10. Bracewell, R.: The Fourier transform and its applications, New York (2000)

Sparse Bayesian Inference of White Matter Fiber Orientations from Compressed Multi-resolution Diffusion MRI

Pramod Kumar Pisharady[1], Julio M. Duarte-Carvajalino[1], Stamatios N. Sotiropoulos[2], Guillermo Sapiro[3,4], and Christophe Lenglet[1]

[1] CMRR, Radiology, University of Minnesota, Minneapolis, Minnesota, USA
pramodkp@umn.edu
[2] FMRIB, John Radcliffe Hospital, University of Oxford, Headington, UK
[3] Electrical and Computer Engineering, Duke University, Durham, USA
[4] Biomedical Engineering and Computer Science, Duke University, Durham, USA

Abstract. The RubiX [1] algorithm combines high SNR characteristics of low resolution data with high spacial specificity of high resolution data, to extract microstructural tissue parameters from diffusion MRI. In this paper we focus on estimating crossing fiber orientations and introduce sparsity to the RubiX algorithm, making it suitable for reconstruction from compressed (under-sampled) data. We propose a sparse Bayesian algorithm for estimation of fiber orientations and volume fractions from compressed diffusion MRI. The data at high resolution is modeled using a parametric spherical deconvolution approach and represented using a dictionary created with the exponential decay components along different possible directions. Volume fractions of fibers along these orientations define the dictionary weights. The data at low resolution is modeled using a spatial partial volume representation. The proposed dictionary representation and sparsity priors consider the dependence between fiber orientations and the spatial redundancy in data representation. Our method exploits the sparsity of fiber orientations, therefore facilitating inference from under-sampled data. Experimental results show improved accuracy and decreased uncertainty in fiber orientation estimates. For under-sampled data, the proposed method is also shown to produce more robust estimates of fiber orientations.

Keywords: Sparse Bayesian inference, Compressive sensing, Linear un-mixing, Diffusion MRI, Fiber orientation, Brain imaging.

1 Introduction

Multi-compartment models [2,3] are used to represent the diffusion MR signal from the brain white matter and to estimate microstructure features of the imaged tissue. Estimation of orientations and volume fractions of anisotropic compartments in these models helps infer the white matter fiber anatomy [4]. However accurate estimation of these parameters is challenged by the relatively

N. Navab et al. (Eds.): MICCAI 2015, Part I, LNCS 9349, pp. 117–124, 2015.
DOI: 10.1007/978-3-319-24553-9_15

limited spatial resolution of acquired diffusion MRI (dMRI) data. Advances in magnetic field strength has significantly improved spatial resolution [5,6], although it may lead to increased noise and scanning time. Computational approach to improve the scan resolution includes the super resolution reconstruction proposed by Scherrer *et al.* [7]. One effective way to mitigate the effects of noise is the multi-resolution data fusion approach introduced in RubiX [1], which combines high SNR characteristics of low resolution (LR) data with high spatial specificity of high resolution (HR) data. This further allows combining images with different diffusion contrast at different spatial resolutions without reducing the SNR. Compressed sensing approaches [8,9,10,11] are effective ways to deal with increased scan time, which result in less measurements (diffusion directions) within a voxel.

Considering the limited number of crossing fiber bundles within a voxel, sparsity can be introduced for better and faster inference on the anisotropic compartments. In this paper, we introduce sparsity based representation and inference into the data fusion approach of RubiX, combining the benefits of regularized noise and reduced scan time. Finding volume fractions and fiber directions with a large number of possible fiber orientations is computationally expensive. We demonstrate that sparsity based approaches are useful in addressing this issue.

Without loss of generality, we represent the HR data using the ball & stick model [2,3], in a convenient dictionary form. The volume fractions of compartments, which form the dictionary weights, are all positive and those sum to one [3]. The positivity and sum-to-one constraints, the natural constraints for fiber volume fraction estimation, make the sparse representation and inference especially challenging. We formulate the estimation of volume fractions as a linear un-mixing inference problem [12]. The volume fractions and fiber directions are estimated using a semi-supervised hierarchical Bayesian linear un-mixing approach, which is an extension of sparse Bayesian inference dealing with constraints [13,8].

2 Methods

2.1 Dictionary Representation of High Resolution Data

The HR data is represented using a dictionary containing exponential decay component vectors in the compartment model. The measured dMRI signal at each HR voxel is first modeled using the ball & stick (1) model [2,3].

$$S_{HR}^k = S_{HR}^0 \left[\left(1 - \sum_{n=1}^{N} f_n\right) e^{-b_k d} + \sum_{n=1}^{N} f_n e^{-b_k d (g_k^T v_n)^2} \right] \tag{1}$$

where,

S_{HR}^k the signal at HR voxel after application of kth diffusion-sensitizing gradient with direction g_k and b-value b_k,

S_{HR}^0 the HR signal without diffusion gradient applied,

f_n the volume fraction of anisotropic compartment with orientation v_n, and

d the apparent diffusivity.

The measured signal at an HR voxel is the sum of the attenuation signal and measurement noise (2).

$$y^k_{HR} = \frac{S^k_{HR}}{S^0_{HR}} + \eta^k_{HR} \tag{2}$$

Based on (1) and (2), the measured signal along all K diffusion-sensitizing directions can be written in a *dictionary* form (3) as follows:

$$\mathbf{y_{HR}} = \begin{pmatrix} e^{-b_1 d} & e^{-b_1 d(g_1^T v_1)^2} & \ldots & e^{-b_1 d(g_1^T v_N)^2} \\ \vdots & \vdots & \ddots & \vdots \\ e^{-b_K d} & e^{-b_K d(g_K^T v_1)^2} & \ldots & e^{-b_K d(g_K^T v_N)^2} \end{pmatrix} \begin{pmatrix} f_0 \\ f_1 \\ \vdots \\ f_N \end{pmatrix} + \boldsymbol{\eta_{HR}} \tag{3}$$

where,

$$f_0 = \left(1 - \sum_{n=1}^{N} f_n\right), f_n \geq 0.$$

Hence,

$$\mathbf{y_{HR}} = \mathbf{Ef} + \eta_{\mathbf{HR}} \tag{4}$$

In equation (4), $\mathbf{E}$ represents the local dictionary for the HR diffusion data and $\mathbf{f}$ is the sparse representation of the HR data in this dictionary $\mathbf{E}$. The non-zero entries in $\mathbf{f}$ define the number and orientation of fibers (*sticks*) in a voxel. The possible orientations of anisotropic components in the dictionary (second column onwards) are pre-specified and formed using a 5th order icosahedral tessellation of the sphere with 10242 points.

2.2 Partial Volume Representation of Low Resolution Data

In the RubiX framework, the LR data and HR data are collected from the same subject through two scans at different spatial resolutions (voxel sizes). The two datasets are aligned (if necessary) using rigid body transformations. Once the data is aligned, the LR data can be represented using corresponding HR data (data that correspond to the same physical location, but at a different spatial resolution grid), with a partial volume model [1]. The model calculates attenuation signal at an LR voxel as a linear combination of the signals at overlapping M HR voxels.

$$\frac{S^k_{LR}}{S^0_{LR}} = \sum_{m=1}^{M} \alpha_m \frac{S^{km}_{HR}}{S^{0m}_{HR}}, \qquad \alpha_m = e^{-\frac{\|r_m - r_0\|^2}{\gamma^2}} \tag{5}$$

The HR signal contributes to the LR signal via a discretized Gaussian point spread function (PSF) with weights α_m given by the normalized Euclidean distance between the PSF center r_0 at LR voxel and the spatial position of each HR voxel r_m, and the unknown standard deviation of the PSF, γ.

2.3 Bayesian Linear Un-mixing Inference

Finding the volume fractions **f** in (4) with a large number (N) of possible fiber orientations is an ill-posed problem. We introduce sparsity in the dictionary and estimation process to propose an efficient algorithm for volume fraction and fiber orientation estimation. The positivity and sum-to-one constraints of volume fractions make the sparse representation and inference especially difficult. We fix the sparsity level (maximum number of fiber orientations to be considered) to a small number ($n_0, n_0 << N$). The problem is then formulated as a linear un-mixing inference where the diffusion signals correspond to a mixture of the dictionary components with positive weights **f**. We follow a semi-supervised hierarchical Bayesian linear un-mixing approach [12] for sparsity-based inference of fibers. The method is semi-supervised because the dictionary is known for a given diffusivity, gradient directions, b-values, and possible orientations, but we do not know either the fiber orientations or the volume fractions within each compartment.

The likelihood function of the HR data can be expressed by (6)

$$p\left(y_{HR}|f,\sigma^2\right) = \left(\frac{1}{2\pi\sigma^2}\right)^{\frac{K}{2}} e^{-\frac{\|y_{HR}-Ef\|_2^2}{2\sigma^2}} \tag{6}$$

where σ^2 corresponds to the variance of the error in representation of y_{HR} by using dictionary **E** and volume fractions **f**. Let $f^+ = [f_1, \ldots, f_N]^T$ be the volume fractions of the anisotropic compartments, then f^+ belongs to a simplex S (7).

$$S = \left\{ f^+|f_n \geq 0, \forall n = 1, \ldots, N, \sum_{n=1}^{N} f_n \leq 1 \right\} \tag{7}$$

A sparsity-promoting prior (section 2.4) is used for the anisotropic volume fractions. The volume fractions posterior is given by (8) [8,12].

$$p\left(f^+|y_{HR},\sigma^2\right) \sim e^{-\left(f^+-\mu_f\right)^T \Lambda_f^{-1}\left(f^+-\mu_f\right)} 1_S(f^+) \tag{8}$$

where

$$\Lambda_f = \left[\sigma^{-2}\left(E_{n0}^+ - e_0 u^T\right)^T \left(E_{n0}^+ - e_0 u^T\right)\right]^{-1}, \tag{9}$$

$$\mu_f = \sigma^{-2}\Lambda_f\left(E_{n0}^+ - e_0 u^T\right)^T\left(y_{HR} - e_0\right), \tag{10}$$

with $u = [1, \ldots, 1]^T$. E_{n0}^+ contains the columns of E that correspond to the $n0$ non-zero coefficients in f^+ (effective dictionary) and e_0 is the column corresponding to the isotropic compartment (*ball*). $1_S(f^+)$ is one if $f^+ \in S$ and zero otherwise.

The posterior of σ^2 given the data and sparse representation is given by the inverse Gamma (IG) distribution (11) [12]

$$p(\sigma^2|y_{HR}, f) \sim IG(K/2, \|y_{HR} - Ef\|^2/2). \tag{11}$$

The generation of samples according to (8-10) is accomplished using a Gibbs sampler, where a column in the effective dictionary E_{n0}^+ can be switched at random with another to test a different fiber orientation.

2.4 Priors

We utilized a sparsity promoting prior for the volume fractions estimation. The prior utilized is a dirichlet prior (12) [13] which depends on the data.

$$p\left(f_n\right) = \prod_{n=1}^{N} f_n^{\phi-1}, \phi < 1 \tag{12}$$

When the hyper-parameter ϕ is small ($\phi < 1$), the prior takes a larger value as the number of volume fractions whose values are close to zero increases, which is desirable for enforcing sparsity.

We followed the rest of the parameter priors and inference procedure as in RubiX [1]. The priors used for S^0 and σ are unconditional and non-informative (uniform). Conditional priors are used for orientation and diffusivity and are defined as a mixture of Watson distributions with non-informative hyper-parameter for orientation and normal distribution with informative hyper-parameter for diffusivity.

3 Experiments and Results

3.1 Simulated Data

Synthetic data is simulated using Camino [14] (Diffusion Tensor-Cylinder-Sphere model) to have the ground truth for comparison of estimated fiber orientations. Single and crossing fiber structures (with 2 and 3 fibers) with image size 10x10x2 (LR) and 20x20x4 (HR) are simulated. The orientations of fibers at each LR voxel are randomly selected. Diffusion signals are simulated along 133 uniformly distributed directions. The noise free HR signal is created by expanding the LR image size to HR image size along all three coordinates without partial voluming. Rician noise is added to both LR and HR images by adding zero-mean Gaussian signal in quadrature. A factor of $8/\sqrt{2}$ is maintained [1] in the ratio of SNR of LR to that of HR signal (lesser noise in LR data). Data with two SNRs, 15 and 25, are simulated. Under-sampling of diffusion directions is done by a factor of up to 4 to simulate acceleration in image acquisition.

The algorithm performance is compared with the ball & stick model applied to the HR dataset (using *bedpostX* tool [4] in FSL) and RubiX [1] applied to HR and LR datasets. Both RubiX and the proposed method are applied to HR and LR datasets, with the first 67 measurements forming the *no-acceleration* data. This is done in order to match the acquisition time, making the comparisons fair. The 67 measurements are under-sampled again up to a factor of 4 to simulate accelerations. For under-sampling we used the protocol proposed by Caruyer *et al.* [15], which makes any first N samples isotropic. Fig. 1 shows the error in orientation estimation and its variation with acceleration. On comparison, the proposed sparse approach provided better accuracy in estimation. The variation in accuracy with acceleration is less in the proposed approach. Fig. 2 (a) shows mean span of the 95% cones of orientational uncertainty, which is a measure of the width of estimated distribution, representing the uncertainty in estimation. On comparison, the proposed method yielded lower estimation uncertainty.

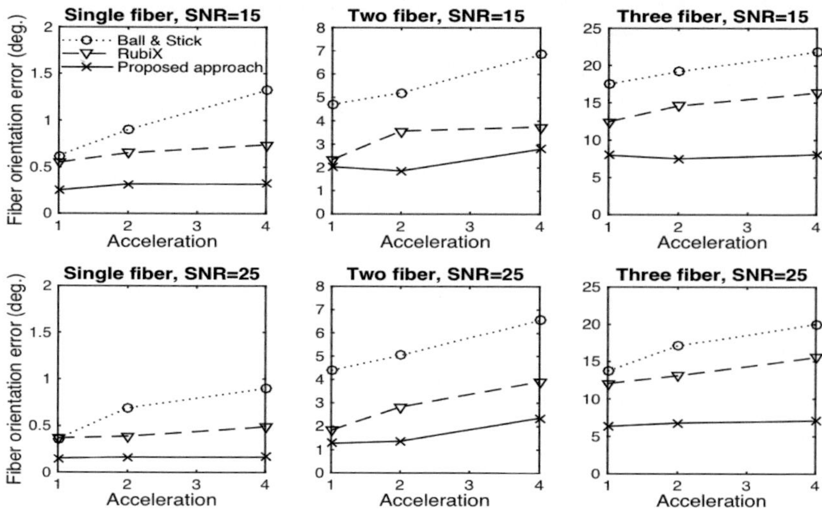

Fig. 1. Comparison of fiber orientation estimation error and its variation with acceleration. Acceleration of 1, 2 and 4 represent the cases of no-acceleration, acceleration by a factor of 50% and that by a factor of 75% respectively. Y-axis represents mean error in 2 and 3 fiber cases.

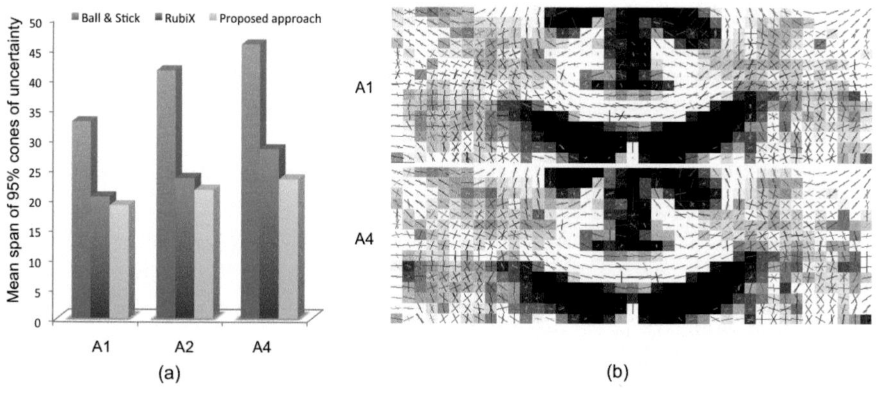

Fig. 2. (a) Mean span of 95% cones of uncertainty (representative simulation case, 2 fiber, SNR 15), (b) Comparison showing the stability of fiber orientation estimates with acceleration (in-vivo data, overlapped on sum of anisotropic volume fractions). A1-A4 represent accelerations up to 4.

3.2 In-Vivo MRI Data

We acquired in-vivo dMRI data from a healthy subject using a 3T Siemens Prisma scanner. For HR acquisitions the acquisition matrix was 140x140x92 voxels with a resolution of 1.5x1.5x1.5 mm^3. For LR acquisitions the resolution was reduced to 3x3x3 mm^3 for an acquisition matrix size 70x70x46 voxels. Diffusion weighting was applied in 200 evenly spaced directions with a b-value of 1500 s/mm^2. Twenty one volumes without diffusion weighting are equally interleaved in the dataset.

Fig. 2 (b) shows a representative comparison of fiber orientation estimates from Corpus Callosum area, demonstrating the invariance in estimates with acceleration. In addition we analyzed several regions of interest (ROIs) in the brain and found that the proposed method resolved more number of fiber crossings at a lesser uncertainty. Included result (Fig. 3) is the number of two and three fiber crossings from left/right superior longitudinal fasciculus (SLF) and left/right posterior corona radiata (PCR). It can be noticed that, while RubiX tends to recover fewer second and third fiber crossings as under-sampling factor increases, the proposed method performs equally well even with only a quarter of the original diffusion gradients.

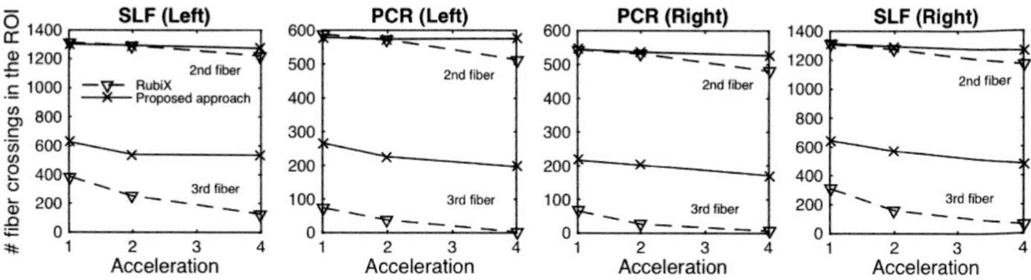

Fig. 3. Variation in number of second and third fiber crossings (with volume fraction greater than 5%) in four ROIs, left/right superior longitudinal fasciculus (SLF) and left/right posterior corona radiata (PCR).

4 Conclusions

Reducing acquisition time and maintaining SNR are two challenging goals in dMRI acquisition. We proposed a processing method to achieve these goals simultaneously, extending and improving an existing multi-resolution approach (RubiX) by introducing sparsity. The proposed sparse Bayesian algorithm is useful in reconstructing fiber orientations from accelerated (under-sampled) dMRI data. The algorithm provided better estimation accuracy at lower uncertainty. The near linear behavior of the estimation error and the number of detected fiber crossings with acceleration shows the utility of the proposed approach.

Acknowledgements. This work was partly supported by NIH grants P41 EB015894, P30 NS076408, R01 EB008432, and the Human Connectome Project (U54 MH091657).

References

1. Sotiropoulos, S.N., Jbabdi, S., Andersson, J.L., Woolrich, M.W., Ugurbil, K., Behrens, T.E.J.: Rubix: Combining spatial resolutions for bayesian inference of crossing fibers in diffusion mri. IEEE Trans. Med. Imag. 32, 969–982 (2013)
2. Behrens, T.E., Woolrich, M.W., Jenkinson, M., Johansen-Berg, H., Nunes, R.G., Clare, S., Matthews, P.M., et al.: Characterization and propagation of uncertainty in diffusion-weighted mr imaging. Magn. Reson. Med. 50, 1077–1088 (2003)
3. Panagiotaki, E., Schneider, T., Siow, B., Hall, M.G., Lythgoe, M.F., Alexander, D.C.: Compartment models of the diffusion mr signal in brain white matter: A taxonomy and comparison. NeuroImage 59, 2241–2254 (2012)
4. Behrens, T.E., Berg, H.J., Jbabdi, S., et al.: Probabilistic diffusion tractography with multiple fibre orientations: What can we gain? Neuroimage 34, 144–155 (2007)
5. Ugurbil, K., et al.: Pushing spatial and temporal resolution for functional and diffusion mri in the human connectome project. Neuroimage 80, 80–104 (2013)
6. Sotiropoulos, S.N., Jbabdi, S., Xu, J., Andersson, J.L., Moeller, S., et al.: Advances in diffusion mri acquisition and processing in the human connectome project. Neuroimage 80, 125–143 (2013)
7. Scherrer, B., Gholipour, A., Warfield, S.K.: Super-resolution reconstruction to increase the spatial resolution of diffusion weighted images from orthogonal anisotropic acquisitions. Medical Image Analysis 16, 1465–1476 (2012)
8. Tipping, M.E.: Sparse bayesian learning and the relevance vector machine. Journal of Machine Learning Research 1, 211–244 (2001)
9. Ji, S., Dunson, D., Carin, L.: Multitask compressive sensing. IEEE Transactions on Signal Processing 57, 92–106 (2009)
10. Otazo, R., Cande‘s, E., Sodickson, D.K.: Low-rank plus sparse matrix decomposition for accelerated dynamic mri with separation of background and dynamic components. Magnetic Resonance in Medicine 73, 1125–1136 (2015)
11. Paquette, M., Merlet, S., Gilbert, G., Deriche, R., Descoteaux, M.: Comparison of sampling strategies and sparsifying transforms to improve compressed sensing diffusion spectrum imaging. Magnetic Resonance in Medicine 73, 401–416 (2015)
12. Dobigeon, N., Tourneret, J.Y., Chang, C.I.: Semi-supervised linear spectral unmixing using a hierarchical bayesian model for hyperspectral imagery. IEEE Transactions on Signal Processing 56, 2684–2695 (2008)
13. Araki, S., Nakatani, T., Sawada, H., Makino, S.: Ieee: Blind sparse source separation for unknown number of sources using gaussian mixture model fitting with dirichlet prior. In: IEEE ICASSP Proceedings, pp. 33–36 (2009)
14. Cook, P.A., Bai, Y., Nedjati-Gilani, S., Seunarine, K.K., Hall, M.G., Parker, G., Alexander, D.C.: Camino: Open-source diffusion-mri reconstruction and processing. In: Scientific Meeting of ISMRM, Seattle, WA, USA (2006)
15. Caruyer, E., Cheng, J., Lenglet, C., Sapiro, G., Jiang, T., Deriche, R.: Optimal design of multiple q-shells experiments for diffusion mri. In: MICCAI Workshop Comput. Diffusion MRI (CDMRI) (2011)

Classification of MRI under the Presence of Disease Heterogeneity using Multi-Task Learning: Application to Bipolar Disorder

Xiangyang Wang[1,2], Tianhao Zhang[1,⋆], Tiffany M. Chaim[3], Marcus V. Zanetti[3], and Christos Davatzikos[1]

[1] Center for Biomedical Image Computing and Analytics, and Department of Radiology, University of Pennsylvania, Philadelphia PA 19104, United States
[2] School of Communication and Information Engineering, Shanghai University, 200444, Shanghai, China
[3] Laboratory of Psychiatric Neuroimaging (LIM-21), Department and Institute of Psychiatry, Faculty of Medicine, University of São Paulo, São Paulo, Brazil
tianhao.zhang@uphs.upenn.edu

Abstract. Heterogeneity in psychiatric and neurological disorders has undermined our ability to understand the pathophysiology underlying their clinical manifestations. In an effort to better distinguish clinical subtypes, many disorders, such as Bipolar Disorder, have been further sub-categorized into subgroups, albeit with criteria that are not very clear, reproducible and objective. Imaging, along with pattern analysis and classification methods, offers promise for developing objective and quantitative ways for disease subtype categorization. Herein, we develop such a method using learning multiple tasks, assuming that each task corresponds to a disease subtype but that subtypes share some common imaging characteristics, along with having distinct features. In particular, we extend the original SVM method by incorporating the sparsity and the group sparsity techniques to allow simultaneous joint learning for all diagnostic tasks. Experiments on Multi-Task Bipolar Disorder classification demonstrate the advantages of our proposed methods compared to other state-of-art pattern analysis approaches.

1 Introduction

Most neurodegenerative and neuropsychiatric disorders are very heterogeneous, both from an imaging and from a clinical perspective, likely reflecting underlying complex genetic and environmental factors. Heterogeneity is further complicated by the fact that oftentimes different pathologies co-exist in the same individual, thereby confounding the structural and the clinical phenotypes. In the past decade, we have witnessed a great deal of progress in the use of advanced pattern analysis and machine learning methods for the classification of individuals, which is important for diagnostic and predictive purposes, and ultimately

⋆ Corresponding author.

N. Navab et al. (Eds.): MICCAI 2015, Part I, LNCS 9349, pp. 125–132, 2015.
DOI: 10.1007/978-3-319-24553-9_16

for individualized medicine. To date, however, most attempts for multivariate pattern analysis (MVPA) methods, such as Support Vector Machines (SVM), especially linear formulations, are primarily focused on the problem of finding a single direction separating two groups, and not on capturing multiple directions in heterogeneous populations.

For example, Bipolar Disorder (BD) mainly consists of BD type I and type II [1]. Multiple tasks of classifications including the whole patients (BD) vs normal controls (NC), each subtype of BD vs NC (i.e., BD I vs NC and BD II vs NC), and the distinguishing between different subtypes of BD (BD I vs BD II), are thereby more necessarily implemented rather than simple binary categorization of BD vs NC for computerized MRI diagnosis.

Multi-task learning [2] is a relatively recent development in the field of machine learning, and might be better suited for classification under phenotypic heterogeneity, as it simultaneously solves multiple classification tasks. Herein, we develop a novel multi-task SVM method, named Multi-Task $l_{2,1} + l_1$-norm SVM (mtSVM$L21L1$), which can work in the context of multiple classification tasks, by solving the multi-task hinge loss with sparsity [3] and group sparsity [4] regularization minimization problem. The learned weight coefficients W which defining the hyperplane are endowed with group sparsity property across multiple tasks while allow different patterns between tasks. This, therefore, can facilitate us to select a subset of features from the original input variables, which are meaningful for all the tasks. Our method is different from the multi-task feature learning methods [5][6][7][8][9][10][11] which are based on the least square (LS) loss technique. Actually, hinge loss based SVM (adopted in our method) has been validated [12][13] to have better performance than LS based methods for feature selection and classification. To the best of our knowledge, this is the first multi-task pattern classification method invented to identify the individual-level biomarkers for diagnosis of the heterogeneous neuropsychiatric data.

2 Multi-Task $l_{2,1} + l_1$-norm Support Vector Machine

2.1 Formulation

Assuming that we have t supervised learning tasks, let $X_i = [x_1, x_2, \cdots, x_n] \in \mathbb{R}^{d\times n}$ as the training data matrix on i^{th} task, $i = 1, \cdots, t$, where d is the feature dimension, n is the number of input data samples, and let $Y_i = [y_1, y_2, \cdots, y_n] \in \mathbb{R}^n$ is the corresponding labels from these training samples for task i, where $y_j \in \{+1, -1\}$ is the binary label for each task. Let $W = [w_1, w_2, \cdots, w_t] \in \mathbb{R}^{d\times t}$ be the weight coefficient matrix for all t tasks, whose column $w_i \in \mathbb{R}^d$ parameteries the linear discriminant function and whose row $w^k \in \mathbb{R}^t$ is the vector of coefficients associated with the kth feature across different tasks. Then the hinge loss based multi-task model, i.e., Multi-Task $l_{2,1}+l_1$-norm SVM (mtSVM$L21L1$) can be defined by the following minimization problem:

$$\min_W \sum_{i=1}^{t} f(w_i^T X_i, Y_i) + \alpha\|W\|_{2,1} + \beta\|W\|_1 \quad (1)$$

where f is the hinge loss function as used in standard SVM [14] and defined as:

$$f(w_i^T X_i, Y_i) = \sum_{i=1}^{n} (1 - y_{ji}(w_i^T x_{ji} + b_i))_+ \tag{2}$$

where $(a)_+$ =max$(0, a)$, b is the bias term. In the second term of (1), $\|W\|_{2,1} = \sum_{k=1}^{d} \|w^k\|_2$ is the structural sparsity, i.e., $l_{2,1}$-norm regularization [4], which encourages the weight coefficient matrix with many near-zero rows, while endows the coefficients that are significant to all the tasks to have larger weights. It will make sense if all classification tasks more or less share some common features. This may be true in our BD problem, because some brain regions might be abnormal in all subgroups (BD I, BD II) here. However, on the other hand, each task may have its specific features that are important for this task while unimportant for some others. So the l_1-norm regularization term $\|W\|_1$ is included in (1) in order to induce sparsity among tasks. This idea can be illustrated by Fig. 1: Fig. 1A is the standard sparsity pattern, and the models for different tasks are built independently; Fig. 1B is the pattern learned by the model with only $l_{2,1}$-norm, which enforces all models from different tasks to select a common set of features; Fig. 1C shows the learned pattern with $l_{2,1} + l_1$-norm, which makes sparsity weight coefficients that are similar, but not identical, across tasks.

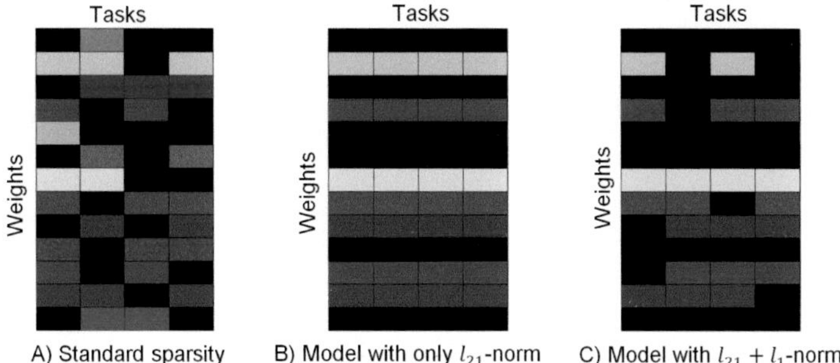

Fig. 1. Illustrations of sparsity effects. Different colors indicate different weight coefficients. A) Standard sparsity; B) Model with only $l_{2,1}$-norm; C)Model with $l_{2,1}$+l_1-norm.

2.2 Solution

We use the Optimal Stochastic Alternating Direction Method of Multipliers (SADMM) method [15] to solve our $l_{2,1}$+l_1-norm SVM problem. We first convert (1) to the following equivalent problem:

$$\min_{W} \sum_{i=1}^{t} \sum_{j=1}^{n} \max(0, 1 - y_{ji} w_i^T x_{ji}) + \alpha \|Z\|_{2,1} + \beta \|Z\|_1 \quad \text{s.t. } Z = W \tag{3}$$

This is a non-smooth but strongly convex problem. Let $f(w,\xi) = \max(0, 1 - yw^T x)$, where $\xi = \{x, y\}$ is a feature-label pair, and $h(Z) = \alpha\|Z\|_{2,1} + \beta\|Z\|_1$, the augmented Lagrangian will be:

$$\begin{aligned} L_\mu^k(W,Z,\lambda) = f(W_k) + < g_k, W > + \tfrac{1}{2\eta_k}\|W - W_k\|_2^2 + h(Z) \\ - < \lambda, Z - W > + \tfrac{\mu}{2}\|Z - W\|_2^2 \end{aligned} \tag{4}$$

where $g_k = f'(W_k, \xi_{k+1})$ is a stochastic sub-gradient of $f(W_k)$ at the current search point W_k of the kth iteration, λ is the Lagrangian multipliers, $\mu > 0$ is a penalty parameter, $< A, B >= \text{trace}(A^T B)$, η_k is the step size and is set as $\eta_k = 2/\gamma(k+2)$ as well as in [15]. Applying SADMM to problem (4) produces closed-form updating rules as follows:

$$\begin{aligned} W_{k+1} &= \arg\min_W W^T f'(W_k, \xi_{k+1}) + \tfrac{\mu}{2}\|Z_k - W - \tfrac{\lambda_k}{\mu}\|_2^2 + \tfrac{1}{2\eta_k}\|W - W_k\|_2^2 \\ Z_{k+1} &= \arg\min_Z \alpha\|Z\|_{2,1} + \beta\|Z\|_1 + \tfrac{\mu}{2}\|Z - W_{k+1} - \tfrac{\lambda_k}{\mu}\|_2^2 \\ \lambda_{k+1} &= \lambda_k - \mu(Z_{k+1} - W_{k+1}) \end{aligned} \tag{5}$$

Let $L_\mu^k(W) = W^T f'(W_k, \xi_{k+1}) + \frac{\mu}{2}\|Z_k - W - \frac{\lambda_k}{\mu}\|_2^2 + \frac{1}{2\eta_k}\|W - W_k\|_2^2$, have $\partial L_\mu^k(W)/\partial W = 0$, and then we get the updating rule:

$$W_{k+1} = (\frac{1}{\eta_k} + \mu)^{-1}\left[\mu Z_k - \lambda_k + \frac{1}{\eta_k}W_k - f'(W_k, \xi_{k+1})\right] \tag{6}$$

where $f'(w,\xi) = -yx$, if $yw^T x < 1$; otherwise 0.

The implementation of the method can be summarized in **Algorithm 1**. Note that the Step 4 is solved by utilizing the decomposition property [7]. For further details see **Supplementary Material**[1], in which we also provided the proof on the convergence property of the algorithm.

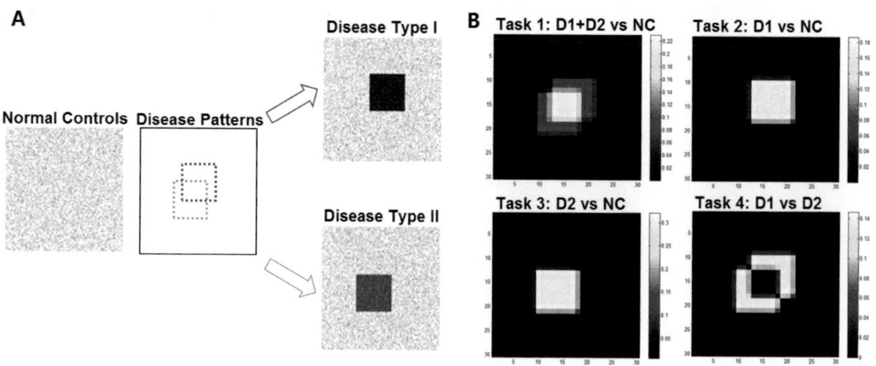

Fig. 2. Simulated data and results. A) Data generation; B) Learned weight coefficients.

[1] www.cbica.upenn.edu/sbia/Tianhao.Zhang/MICCAI2015.html

Algorithm 1. Multi-Task $l_{2,1} + l_1$-norm SVM (mtSVM$L21L1$)

Input: data matrix X, labels Y, and parameters α, β
Initialize: $W_0 = Z_0 = \lambda_0 = 0$, $\mu = 10^{-6}$, $\mu_{max} = 10^{10}$, $\rho_0 = 1.1$, $\epsilon = 10^{-8}$, $\gamma = 2$, maxIter$= 10^3$, $k = 0$.
Output: W
while not converge, $k <$maxIter, **do**
  $\eta_k = 2/\gamma(k+2)$
  Obtain stochastic gradient g_k; build L_μ^k via (4)
  Fix the others and update W by (6)
  Fix the others and update Z by:
    $Z_{k+1} = \arg\min_Z \alpha\|Z\|_{2,1} + \beta\|Z\|_1 + \frac{\mu}{2}\|Z - W_{k+1} - \frac{\lambda_k}{\mu}\|_2^2$
  Update the multiplier λ by: $\lambda_{k+1} = \lambda_k - \mu\,(Z_{k+1} - W_{k+1})$
  Update the parameter μ by: $\mu = \min(\rho_0\mu, \mu_{max})$
  Check the convergence conditions: $\|Z_{k+1} - W_{k+1}\|_\infty < \epsilon$
  $k = k+1$
end while

3 Results

3.1 Multi-Task Feature Learning on the Simulated Data

The Data: We generated three groups of images: 1) disease type I (D1) data, 2) disease type II (D2) data, and 3) normal control data (NC). Each group had 30 samples, resulting in a total of 90 samples. All images are of size 100×100. The data are generated as follows. For each of the normal data, the mean is in [0.8, 0.95] with some Gaussian noise. In D1 and D2 images, there is an area of size 30×30, in which the values are decreased to [0.1, 0.6] with some Gaussian noise. The locations of such patches in D1 and D2 are not identical, but they have an overlapping area of size 20×20. The generation is illustrated in Fig. 2A.

The Results: The results obtained by mtSVM$L21L1$ are shown in Fig. 2B. Both disease patterns are identified in the comparison of D1+D2 vs NC (Task 1), with their overlapping area being more highlighted. In Task 2, it's shown that the abnormal patch in D1 is identified, while in Task 3, the abnormal patch in D2 is well marked. In Task 4, we can see that only the differences between D1 and D2 are highlighted. Taken together, the simulation results show our proposed method works effectively and correctly for multi-task feature learning.

3.2 Multi-Task Classification on the Bipolar Disorder Data

The Data: We evaluated the proposed methods using the structural brain MRIs on Bipolar Disorder (BD), a typical heterogeneous neuropsychiatric illness. From the total of 71 subjects, 44 were treatment-naive patients of BD and 27 were age and gender matched normal controls (NC). According to the DSM-IV criteria, each patient was assigned into BD I (22 subjects) or BD II (22 subjects) subgroups. Details on demographic characteristics, and image acquisition and preprocessing can be found in [16]. T1-weighted images were preprocessed according to a number of steps [16], including 1) AC-PC plane alignment; 2) Skull removal; 3) Tissue segmentation into gray matter (GM), white matter (WM), and cerebrospinal fluid (CSF); and 4) High-dimensional image warping to a standard MNI space, resulting in the mass-preserved tissue density maps.

Experimental Design: Based on the voxel-wise tissue density values of GM, we performed the multiple classification tasks, including 1) Task 1: BD vs NC, 2) Task 2: BD I vs NC, 3) Task 3: BD II vs NC, and 4) Task 4: BD I vs BD II. According to the absolute values of weight coefficients W, we select the respective K top-ranked features [6][12] for each task, with which the linear SVM is used in the final step for the binary classification for each task. Other than the proposed mtSVM$L21L1$ method, some comparative methods are also carried out as below: 1) stLS$L1$: Single Task l_1-norm Least Square (LS) loss function feature selection; 2) stSVM$L1$: Single Task l_1-norm SVM feature selection; 3) mtLS$L21$: Multi-Task $l_{2,1}$-norm LS loss function feature selection [6][7]; 4) mtSVM$L21$: Multi-Task $l_{2,1}$-norm SVM, i.e., the case that only $l_{2,1}$-norm term is included in Equation (1); 5) mtLS$L21L1$: Multi-Task $l_{2,1} + l_1$-norm LS loss function [17] feature selection. mtLS$L21L1$ is built upon mtLS$L21$ by adding the l_1-norm, and solved by using the Accelerated Proximal Gradient (APG) [7] method. To compare all methods, we used 5-fold cross-validation: four random subsets for training and the remaining one subset for testing.

Parameters Tuning: The above methods can be classified into three groups according to regularization terms: 1)l_1-norm: stLS$L1$ and stSVM$L1$; 2)$l_{2,1}$-norm: mtLS$L21$ and mtSVM$L21$; 3)$l_{2,1} + l_1$-norm: mtLS$L21L1$ and mtSVM$L21L1$. They are related with two parameters, α or/and β which regulate the effects of the $l_{2,1}$ or/and l_1 terms respectively. We searched them in the range of $\alpha, \beta \in \left[10^{-5}, \cdots, 10^{-1}, 0.5, 1, 10^1, \cdots, 10^5\right]$. Another important parameter is K, i.e., the number of features which are selected from tasks. In our experiments, this number is in the area of [5, 5500].

Table 1. The ACCs (%) and the AUCs of the competing methods, calculated from four different tasks, respectively. The right columns list the average values.

Methods	Task 1		Task 2		Task 3		Task 4		ACC (avg)	AUC (avg)
	ACC	AUC	ACC	AUC	ACC	AUC	ACC	AUC		
stLS$L1$	59.23	0.49	51.78	0.54	48.79	0.44	46.80	0.42	51.65	0.47
stSVM$L1$	56.48	0.47	51.79	0.54	53.52	0.43	50.81	0.45	53.15	0.48
mtLS$L21$	67.52	0.61	66.75	0.62	58.52	0.56	68.52	0.61	65.33	0.60
mtSVM$L21$	70.38	0.66	74.78	0.73	72.43	0.73	71.42	0.61	72.25	0.68
mtLS$L21L1$	76.00	0.64	74.83	0.64	74.28	0.61	72.34	0.63	74.36	0.63
mtSVM$L21L1$	**78.95**	**0.67**	**84.23**	**0.76**	**84.18**	**0.77**	**78.35**	**0.71**	**81.42**	**0.72**

Classification Results: The optimal classification accuracy (ACC) and the area under curve (AUC) measures of all methods are listed in Table 1. As shown, Multi-Task methods performed better than Single Task ones. Among all the methods, mtSVM$L21L1$ has the best performances. The fact that mtSVM$L21L1$ outperformed mtSVM$L21$ reveals the benefit of characterizing specific patterns related to different tasks. The heterogeneity in the BD group resulted in inferior performance of BD vs NC than BD I/II vs NC. In addition, we find that BD I vs BD II is the most difficult task, and likely requires a much larger training set.

Feature Interpretations: We overlaid the output weight coefficients obtained by mtSVM$L21L1$ onto the standard template for visual inspection. The representative sections are displayed in Fig. 3. We can see that BD I and BD II share similar patterns of GM abnormalities around the Frontal Pole (Fig. 3A) and the Precuneus (Fig. 3B) which are present in the results of Tasks 1, 2, and 3 (namely, BD vs NC, BD I vs NC, BD II vs NC), but not in Task 4 (BD I vs BD II). Relative to BD I vs NC (Task 2), BD II vs NC (Task 3) demonstrated more widely spread patterns including not only the Frontal Pole and the Precuneus but also more signals around the Cerebellum (Fig. 3C), and the Middle Frontal Gyrus (Fig. 3D) which were further confirmed by the direct comparison between BD I and BD II, that is, Task 4.

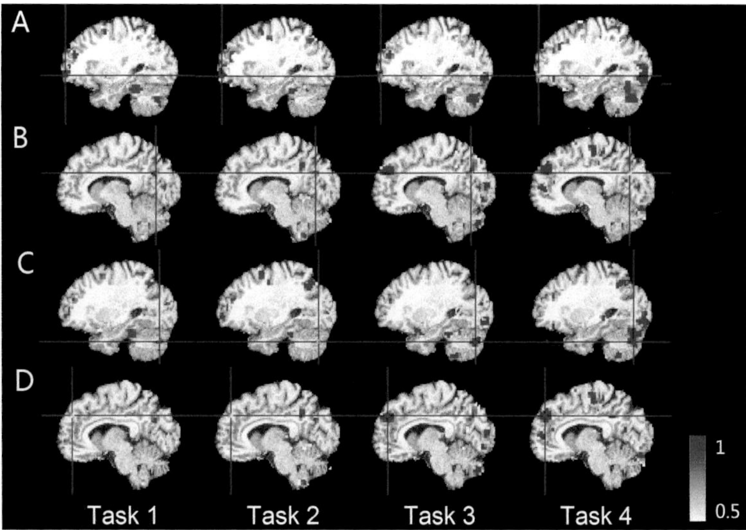

Fig. 3. Representative slices of regions, including A) Frontal Pole, B) Precuneus, C) Cerebellum, and D) Middle Frontal Gyrus, obtained from all four tasks. The scale indicates the absolute values of weights.

4 Conclusions

In this paper, we propose a novel method named Multi-Task $l_{2,1} + l_1$-norm Support Vector Machine (mtSVM$L21L1$) for classifying Bipolar Disorder (BD) disease under the presence of phenotypic heterogeneity. We adopt the framework of multi-task hinge loss with sparsity regularization terms to jointly learn features that are commonly shared among all the tasks and which are characterized with specific patterns in each task. Experimental results have shown that, compared with other state-of-the-art methods, our proposed method can achieve the best performances for multi-tasks, also yielding better results than previous works on MRI-based classification in BD [16]. Furthermore, the features learned by the proposed method reveals the heterogeneous patterns of structural abnormalities from different tasks. Taken together, the proposed methods have deepened our insight into the neurobiological basis of the disorder's clinical heterogeneity and helped us make progress on individual-level patient stratification.

Acknowledgement. This was supported in part by NIH R01AG14971, CNPq-Brazil & NARSAD (for clinical data), and FAPESP 13/03905-4 (to M.V.Z).

References

1. Dunner, D.L., Gershon, E.S., Goodwin, F.K.: Heritable factors in the severity of affective illness. Biological Psychiatry 11(1), 31–42 (1976)
2. Caruana, R.: Multitask learning. Machine Learning 28(1), 41–75 (1997)
3. Tibshirani, R.: Regression shrinkage and selection via the lasso. Journal of the Royal Statistical Society: Series B 58(1), 267–288 (1996)
4. Yuan, M., Lin, Y.: Model selection and estimation in regression with grouped variables. Journal of the Royal Statistical Society: Series B 68(1), 49–67 (2006)
5. Evgeniou, A., Pontil, M.: Multi-task feature learning. In: NIPS, pp. 41–48 (2007)
6. Wang, H., Nie, F., Huang, H., Risacher, S., et al.: Sparse multi-task regression and feature selection to identify brain imaging predictors for memory performance. In: ICCV, pp. 557–562 (2011)
7. Zhou, J., Liu, J., Narayan, V.A., Ye, J.: Modeling disease progression via multi-task learning. NeuroImage 78, 233–248 (2013)
8. Rao, N., Cox, C., Nowak, R., Rogers, T.T.: Sparse overlapping sets lasso for multi-task learning and its application to fmri analysis. In: NIPS, pp. 2202–2210 (2013)
9. Jie, B., Zhang, D., Cheng, B., Shen, D.: Manifold regularized multitask feature learning for multimodality disease classification. Human Brain Mapping 36(2), 489–507 (2015)
10. Metsis, V., Makedon, F., Shen, D., Huang, H.: DNA copy number selection using robust structured sparsity-inducing norms. IEEE/ACM Transactions on Computational Biology and Bioinformatics 11(1), 168–181 (2014)
11. Nie, F., Huang, H., Cai, X., Ding, C.H.: Efficient and robust feature selection via joint $l2$, 1-norms minimization. In: NIPS, pp. 1813–1821 (2010)
12. Cai, X., Nie, F., Huang, H., Ding, C.: Multi-class l2, 1-norm support vector machine. In: ICDM, pp. 91–100 (2011)
13. Chang, C.C., Lin, C.J.: LIBSVM: a library for support vector machines. ACM Transactions on Intelligent Systems and Technology 2(3), 28–55 (2011)
14. Scholkopf, B., Smola, A.J.: Learning with kernels: Support vector machines, regularization, optimization, and beyond. MIT Press (2002)
15. Azadi, S., Sra, S.: Towards an optimal stochastic alternating direction method of multipliers. In: ICML, pp. 620–628 (2014)
16. Serpa, M.H., Ou, Y., Schaufelberger, M.S., Doshi, J., et al.: Neuroanatomical classification in a population-based sample of psychotic major depression and bipolar I disorder with 1 year of diagnostic stability. BioMed Research International (2014)
17. Simon, N., Friedman, J., Hastie, T., Tibshirani, R.: A sparse-group lasso. Journal of Computational and Graphical Statistics 22(2), 231–245 (2013)

Fiber Connection Pattern-Guided Structured Sparse Representation of Whole-Brain fMRI Signals for Functional Network Inference

Xi Jiang[1], Tuo Zhang[2,1], Qinghua Zhao[3], Jianfeng Lu[3], Lei Guo[2], and Tianming Liu[1]

[1] Cortical Architecture Imaging and Discovery Laboratory, Department of Computer Science and Bioimaging Research Center, The University of Georgia, Athens, GA, USA
superjx2318@gmail.com

[2] School of Automation, Northwestern Polytechnical University, Xi'an, P. R. China

[3] School of Computer Science and Engineering, Nanjing University of Science and Technology, Nanjing, P. R. China

Abstract. A variety of studies in the brain mapping field have reported that the dictionary learning and sparse representation framework is efficient and effective in reconstructing concurrent functional brain networks based on the functional magnetic resonance imaging (fMRI) signals. However, previous approaches are pure data-driven and do not integrate brain science domain knowledge when reconstructing functional networks. The group-wise correspondence of the reconstructed functional networks across individual subjects is thus not well guaranteed. Moreover, the fiber connection pattern consistency of those functional networks across subjects is largely unknown. To tackle these challenges, in this paper, we propose a novel fiber connection pattern-guided structured sparse representation of whole-brain resting state fMRI (rsfMRI) signals to infer functional networks. In particular, the fiber connection patterns derived from diffusion tensor imaging (DTI) data are adopted as the connectional features to perform consistent cortical parcellation across subjects. Those consistent parcellated regions with similar fiber connection patterns are then employed as the group structured constraint to guide group-wise multi-task sparse representation of whole-brain rsfMRI signals to reconstruct functional networks. Using the recently publicly released high quality Human Connectome Project (HCP) rsfMRI and DTI data, our experimental results demonstrate that the identified functional networks via the proposed approach have both reasonable spatial pattern correspondence and fiber connection pattern consistency across individual subjects.

Keywords: Structured sparse representation, functional network, fiber connection pattern, resting state functional MRI, diffusion tensor imaging.

1 Introduction

Sparse representation has received increasing interests in the brain mapping field for functional magnetic resonance imaging (fMRI) signal analysis and functional brain network inference based on the assumption that each brain fMRI signal can be

N. Navab et al. (Eds.): MICCAI 2015, Part I, LNCS 9349, pp. 133–141, 2015.
DOI: 10.1007/978-3-319-24553-9_17

represented as sparse linear combination of a set of signal basis [1-3]. Recent studies have widely reported that the dictionary learning and sparse representation framework is efficient and effective in reconstructing concurrent functional brain networks based on either task-based or resting state fMRI (rsfMRI) data [1-3]. One possible limitation of previous approaches, however, is that it is a pure data-driven regression procedure and does not integrate brain science domain knowledge when reconstructing functional networks. The group-wise correspondence of the functional networks across subjects is thus not well guaranteed. Moreover, the fiber connection pattern consistency of the reconstructed functional networks across subjects is largely unknown. In the neuroscience field, it is widely believed that the fiber connections are the substrates of brain functions [4].

To tackle the above-mentioned two challenges, in this paper, we propose a novel fiber connection pattern-guided structured sparse representation of whole-brain rsfMRI signals to infer functional networks. Note that previous efforts have been devoted to fiber connectivity-constrained conventional functional network (node and connectivity) analysis (e.g., [5]), while we focus on fiber connection pattern-constrained identification of functionally consistent brain regions, which are simply called 'functional network' in this paper. In particular, the fiber connection patterns derived from diffusion tensor imaging (DTI) data are adopted as the connectional features to perform group-wise consistent fine-granularity cortical parcellation across subjects based on our previous methods in [6]. Those consistent parcellated regions are then employed as the group structured constraint to guide group-wise multi-task sparse representation of whole-brain rsfMRI signals to reconstruct functional networks. Theoretically, structured multi-task sparse representation [7] defines a specific structure (e.g., groups, trees, or graphs) on the multi-tasks, and achieves both intra-group homogeneity and intra/inter-group sparsity via combined ℓ_1 and ℓ_2 -norms [7]. Our premise is that cortical vertices within the same parcellated cortical region which have similar fiber connection patterns should potentially play similar roles in brain function. Therefore, integrating those group-wise consistent parcellated regions across subjects as the group structured constraint can effectively handle the above-mentioned two challenges and improve the functional network reconstruction by constraining both intra-group homogeneity and intra/inter-group sparsity.

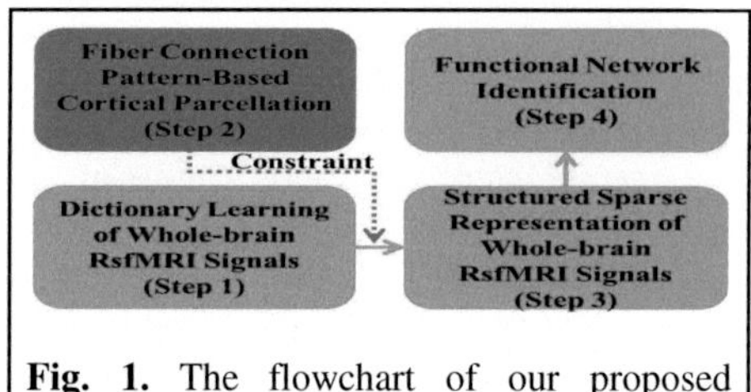

Fig. 1. The flowchart of our proposed framework.

2 Materials and Methods

2.1 Data Acquisition and Pre-processing

We used the high-quality rsfMRI [8] and DTI [9] data in the Human Connectome Project (HCP) (Q1 release) to develop and evaluate the proposed framework (Fig. 1).

Ten subjects were adopted as a test bed in this paper. The major acquisition parameters of rsfMRI data are 220mm/0.72s/33.1ms of FOV/TR/TE, 1200 time points, 90×104×72 dimension, and 2.0mm isotropic voxels. The pre-processing of rsfMRI data is referred to [8]. The major acquisition parameters of DTI data are 210×180/5520ms/89.5ms of FOV/TR/TE, 90 directions, 168×144 matrix, and 1.25mm isotropic voxels. Pre-processing of DTI data is referred to [6].

2.2 Dictionary Learning of Whole-Brain rsfMRI Signals

In our framework (Fig. 1), an over-complete dictionary $\mathbf{D} \epsilon \mathbb{R}^{t \times k}$ (t is the signal time points and k is the dictionary atoms) was firstly learned from the whole-brain rsfMRI signals $\mathbf{X}=[\mathbf{x}_1, \mathbf{x}_2, \ldots, \mathbf{x}_n] \epsilon \mathbb{R}^{t \times n}$ (n is the cortical vertices, $k>t$ and $k<<n$ [10]) of each subject using an effective online dictionary learning algorithm [10] assuming that the rsfMRI signals $\mathbf{X}$ can be represented as sparse linear combination of a set of signal basis (dictionary atoms) [10]. Specifically, for each subject, the whole-brain rsfMRI signals were extracted, normalized to zero mean and standard deviation of 1 [10], and aggregated into a matrix $\mathbf{X} \epsilon \mathbb{R}^{t \times n}$. An empirical cost function considering the average loss of regression to n signal vectors was then defined in Eq. (1):

$$f_n(\mathbf{D}) \triangleq \frac{1}{n} \sum_{i=1}^{n} \ell(\mathbf{x}_i, \mathbf{D}) \tag{1}$$

$$\ell(\mathbf{x}_i, \mathbf{D}) \triangleq \min_{\boldsymbol{\alpha}_i \epsilon \mathbb{R}^k} \frac{1}{2} ||\mathbf{x}_i - \mathbf{D}\boldsymbol{\alpha}_i||_2^2 + \lambda ||\boldsymbol{\alpha}_i||_1 \tag{2}$$

where the ℓ_1 regularization in Eq. (2) was adopted to generate a sparse resolution of $\boldsymbol{\alpha}_i$. $\mathbf{D}$ and $\boldsymbol{\alpha}$ were alternatively updated and learned [10]. The learned $\mathbf{D}$ was adopted as the regressors to perform conventional sparse representation and the proposed structured sparse representation of brain rsfMRI signals as detailed in Section 2.4.

2.3 Fiber Connection Pattern Based Cortical Parcellation for Constraint

We performed fiber connection pattern based cortical parcellation based on DTI data using our methods in [6]. Briefly, for each cortical vertex, we extracted the white matter fiber bundle consisting of fiber tracts emanating from the neighborhood (5 mm sphere) of the cortical vertex. The connection pattern of the extracted fiber bundle was then described as a 144 dimensional connectional descriptor using the trace-map model developed in [11]. Based on the fiber connectional descriptor of each cortical vertex, the cortical parcellation was performed to group-wisely and gradually parcellate cortical surfaces into consistent fine-granularity patches across subjects under a hierarchical scheme. The initial cluster centers and cluster numbers within each hierarchical level were determined via adaptive affinity propagation [6] based on the recently publicly released 358 cortical landmarks [11] which possess consistent white matter fiber connection patterns across subjects. Other cortical vertices were then classified into correspondent clusters based on the similarity of the connectional descriptors to achieve intra-level parcellation using the group-wise implementation of expectation maximization [6] under the spatial constraint of a group of subjects.

The same intra-level parcellation procedure was repeated in the next hierarchical level based on the parcellation results of the previous level. A group-wise hidden Markov random field smoothing approach [6] was also adopted to prevent the potential disconnected clusters. The resulted consistent parcellated cortical regions across subjects were employed as the group structured constraint to guide the sparse representation of rsfMRI signals as illustrated in Fig. 2 and detailed in Section 2.4.

2.4 Structured Sparse Representation of Whole-Brain rsfMRI Signals

The LASSO [12] has been widely used for sparse representation, and is defined as:

$$\hat{\boldsymbol{\alpha}} = argmin \ell(\boldsymbol{\alpha}) + \lambda\phi(\boldsymbol{\alpha}) \tag{3}$$

where $\ell(\boldsymbol{\alpha})$ is the empirical loss function, $\phi(\boldsymbol{\alpha})$ is the penalty term, and $\lambda>0$ is the regularization parameter. As illustrated in Fig. 2a, once we learned dictionary $\mathbf{D}\epsilon\mathbb{R}^{t\times k}$ (Section 2.2), the conventional LASSO to perform regression of rsfMRI signals $\mathbf{X}\epsilon\mathbb{R}^{t\times n}$ to obtain a sparse coefficient matrix $\boldsymbol{\alpha}\epsilon\mathbb{R}^{k\times n}$ was defined as:

$$\hat{\boldsymbol{\alpha}} = argmin \sum_{i=1}^{n} \frac{1}{2}||\mathbf{x}_i - \mathbf{D}\boldsymbol{\alpha}_i||_2^2 + \lambda \sum_{i=1}^{n}\sum_{j=1}^{k} |\boldsymbol{\alpha}_i^j| \tag{4}$$

where $\ell(\boldsymbol{\alpha})$ is defined as the least square loss, and $\phi(\boldsymbol{\alpha})$ is the ℓ_1-norm regularization term to induce sparsity. $\boldsymbol{\alpha}_i^j$ is the coefficient element at the i-th column and j-th row. k and λ were experimentally determined (k=400 and λ=1.5). This conventional LASSO approach in Eq. (4) is pure data-driven.

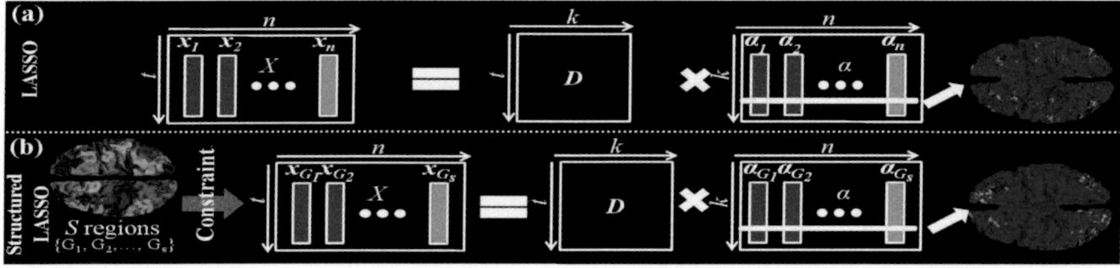

Fig. 2. The illustration of (a) conventional LASSO and (b) the proposed structured LASSO.

In this paper, we proposed a novel structured sparse representation (or structured LASSO) approach. As shown in Fig. 2b, the group-wise consistent parcellated cortical regions (Section 2.3) were adopted as the group structured constraint to guide LASSO. Based on the premise that vertices within the same parcellated cortical region which have similar fiber connection patterns should potentially play similar roles in brain function, the rsfMRI signals of those vertices should share similar regression weights for functional network reconstruction. We aimed to constrain both intra-group homogeneity and intra/inter-group sparsity for LASSO, and defined the structured LASSO as follows:

$$\hat{\boldsymbol{\alpha}} = argmin \sum_{i=1}^{n} \frac{1}{2}||\mathbf{x}_i - \mathbf{D}\boldsymbol{\alpha}_i||_2^2 + \lambda \sum_{i=1}^{n}\sum_{j=1}^{k} |\boldsymbol{\alpha}_i^j| + (1-\lambda)\sum_{j=1}^{k}\sum_{s=1}^{S} \omega_s \left\|\boldsymbol{\alpha}_{G_s}^j\right\|_2 \tag{5}$$

where the rsfMRI signals $\mathbf{X}$ are categorized into S structured groups $\{G_1, G_2, \ldots, G_s\}$ $s = 1, \ldots, S$ based on the S parcellated cortical regions (Fig. 2b). ω_s is the weight coefficient of $\|\boldsymbol{\alpha}_{G_s}^j\|_2$. The conventional LASSO adopted the ℓ_1-norm regularization term to induce sparsity (Eq. (4)), while our proposed structured LASSO introduced a ℓ_2-norm penalty term to improve the intra-group homogeneity, and also kept the ℓ_1-norm penalty to induce both intra- and inter-group sparsity (Eq. (5)). The detailed parameter selection and solution of Eq. (5) was referred to [7]. We adopted the public SLEP software package (http://www.public.asu.edu/~jye02/Software/SLEP/) to solve the problem and to obtain $\boldsymbol{\alpha} \epsilon \mathbb{R}^{k \times n}$. The values of two major parameters k and λ were experimentally determined using cross-validation (k=400 and λ=0.15). From brain science perspective, each learned dictionary can be viewed as the temporal pattern of a functional network, and each row of learned $\boldsymbol{\alpha}$ (non-zeros coefficients) were mapped back to cortical surface (Figs. 2a-2b) to obtain the cortical spatial maps of the network. To identify and quantitatively characterize the meaningful functional networks, we adopted the functional networks templates provided in [13]. The specific row of $\boldsymbol{\alpha}$ with the most spatial pattern similarity (defined as Jaccard similarity coefficient [14] $\mathrm{J(A,T)} = |\mathrm{A} \cap \mathrm{T}|/|\mathrm{A} \cup \mathrm{T}|$, A and T are spatial maps of a specific row of $\boldsymbol{\alpha}$ and a template, respectively) with a specific network template was identified as the corresponding functional network. More details are in [3].

3 Experimental Results

3.1 Comparison of Identified Functional Networks

We compared the identified functional networks via the structured LASSO and conventional LASSO. The widely known 'default mode network' (DMN) [13] was adopted as the example here for demonstration. First, Fig. 3 shows that the spatial patterns of DMN via the structured LASSO (Fig. 3a) have better group-wise correspondence and higher similarity with the DMN template [13] across subjects compared with those via the conventional LASSO (Fig. 3b). Quantitatively, the mean spatial similarity of identified DMNs for each individual subject is 0.31±0.03 via the structured LASSO, which is larger than the conventional LASSO (0.18±0.01). The spatial similarity of group-averaged DMN with the structured LASSO (0.53) is also improved compared with the conventional LASSO.

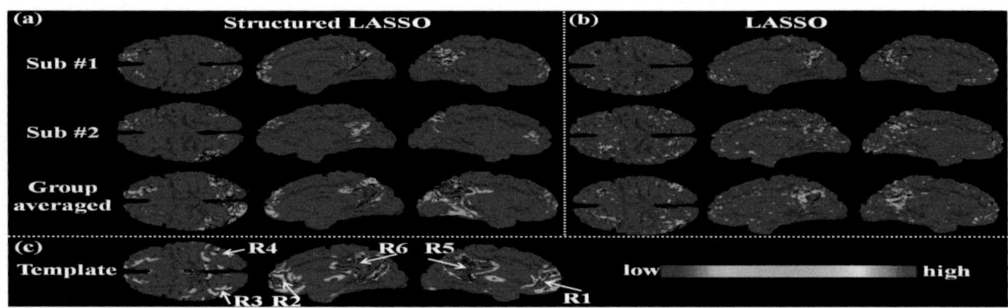

Fig. 3. Spatial patterns of identified DMN via (a) the proposed structured LASSO and (b) conventional LASSO of two example subjects and across all ten subjects. (c) shows the spatial pattern of the DMN template. The six major regions of DMN are labeled as R1 to R6, respectively. The color bar of the spatial patterns is shown in (c).

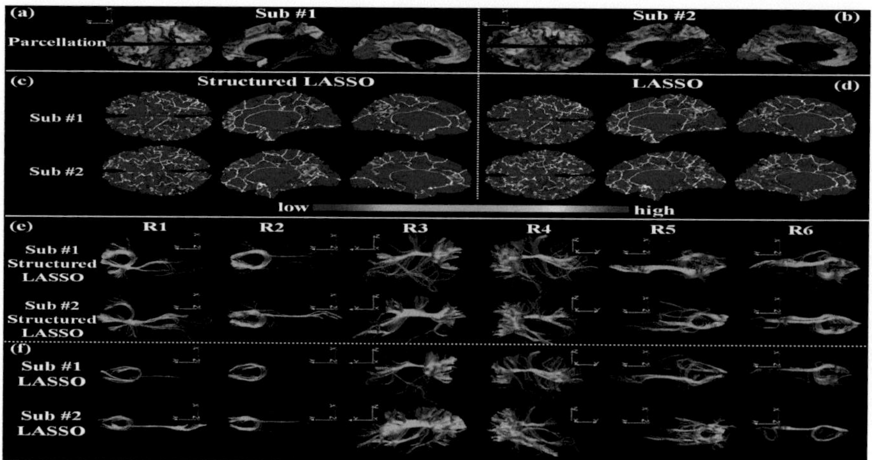

Fig. 4. (a)-(b): Parcellated cortical regions of the two example subjects. The corresponding regions are labeled by the same color. (c)-(d): Co-visualization of the cortical parcellation (white curves delineate the boundaries of regions) and spatial pattern of DMN via the (c) structured LASSO and (d) conventional LASSO of the two subjects. (e)-(f): DTI-derived white matter fiber bundles connecting to the six regions of DMN (R1 to R6 in Fig. 3c) via the (e) structured LASSO and (f) conventional LASSO of the two subjects.

Second, Figs. 4a-4b show that the parcellated cortical regions (65 in total) of the two example subjects have reasonable correspondence as reference. The co-visualization of the cortical parcellation and the spatial pattern of DMN in Figs. 4c-4d shows that all six major regions of DMN (Fig. 3c) have reasonable coincidence with specific parcellated regions via the structured LASSO (Fig. 4c), as expected, while are not well matched with the parcellated regions via the conventional LASSO (Fig. 4d). We further showed the DTI-derived white matter fiber bundles connecting to each of six major regions of DMNs in Figs. 4e-4f. We see that the global fiber shape patterns are reasonably consistent between the two subjects for each of the six regions via the structured LASSO (Fig. 4e), while with considerate variability between those via the conventional LASSO (Fig. 4f). Quantitatively, we represented the connection pattern of a fiber bundle as a 144 dimensional vector descriptor (Section 2.3), and defined the connection pattern consistency of two fiber bundles as the Euclidean distance of the two 144 dimensional vectors. The mean fiber connection pattern consistency across the six regions and across any pair of all subjects is 0.46±0.05 via the structured LASSO and 1.55±0.54 via the conventional LASSO. In conclusion, the identified functional networks via the proposed structured LASSO have both reasonable spatial pattern correspondence and fiber connection pattern consistency across subjects compared with those via the conventional LASSO.

3.2 Functional Networks Guided by Multiple Levels of Cortical Parcellation

We further parcellated the cortical surfaces into finer-granularity group-wise consistent patches under the hierarchical scheme detailed in Section 2.3. Another four levels (159, 222, 243, and 250 regions in total based on [6], respectively) besides the first level (Figs. 4a-4b) were obtained and illustrated in Fig. 5. Here we examined the stability and consistency of reconstructed DMNs via the four different levels of cortical parcellation guided structured LASSO in Figs. 5a-5d. The co-visualization of the cortical parcellation with the spatial pattern of identified DMN at each level (the first row of Figs. 5a-5d, respectively) shows that the major regions of DMNs are reasonably matched with specific parcellated regions at each level. Quantitatively, the mean spatial similarity and fiber connection pattern consistency of DMNs across all ten subjects at each level are shown in Fig. 6. In conclusion, the DMNs based on different hierarchical levels of cortical parcellation guided structured LASSO have both higher spatial pattern similarity with the DMN template and fiber connection pattern consistency across subjects compared with those via the conventional LASSO.

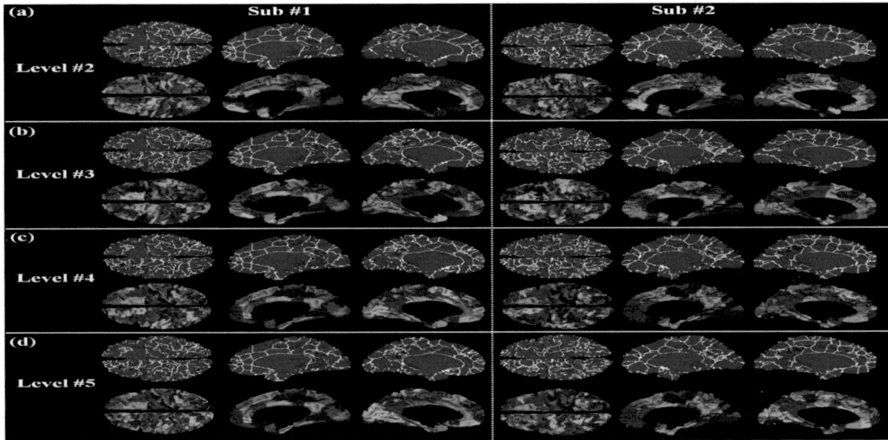

Fig. 5. (a)-(d): Identified DMNs based on another four levels of cortical parcellation guided structured LASSO, respectively. In each sub-figure, the first row shows the co-visualization of the cortical parcellation (white curves delineate the boundaries of regions) and the spatial pattern of DMN, and the second row shows the cortical parcellation at the specific level. The corresponding parcellated regions across subjects are labeled by the same color. Note that there is no correspondence of cortical parcellation color labels across different levels.

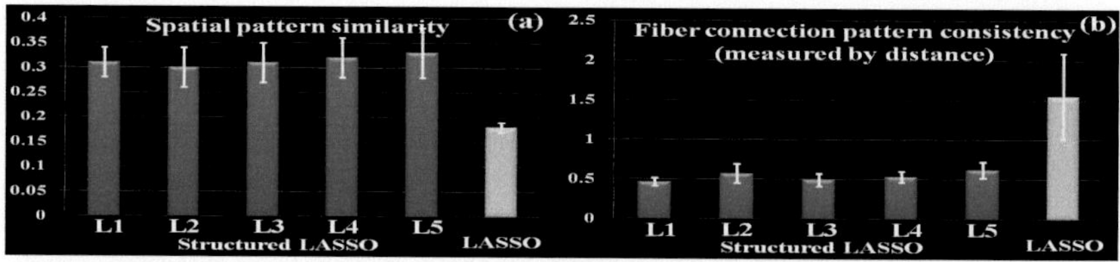

Fig. 6. (a) Mean spatial pattern similarity and (b) fiber connection pattern consistency (defined as the distance in Section 3.1) of DMNs across all ten subjects based on the five levels (indexed by L1 to L5) of cortical parcellation guided structured LASSO and the conventional LASSO.

3.3 Co-visualization of Other Identified Functional Networks

We identified nine functional networks based the network templates in [13]. Note that more networks can be identified if more templates are provided. Fig. 7 co-visualizes the nine functional networks of two example subjects. Specifically, RSNs #1, #2 and #3 are all located at visual cortex. RSNs #4, #5, #6 and #7 are DMN, sensorimotor, auditory, and executive control network, respectively. RSNs #8 and #9 contain middle frontal and superior parietal regions. We see that the major regions of the nine networks have reasonable spatial pattern correspondence and coincidence with specific corresponding parcellated cortical regions across the two example subjects.

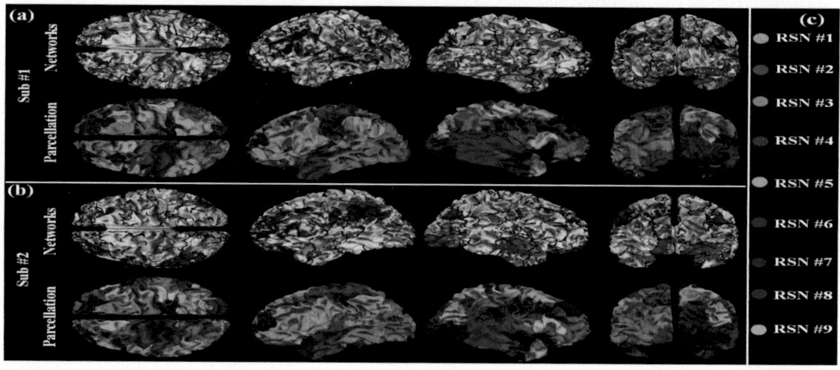

Fig. 7. (a)-(b) Co-visualization of nine functional networks via the structured LASSO of two example subjects. In each sub-figure, the first row co-visualizes the cortical parcellation (black curves delineate the boundaries of regions) and the spatial pattern of nine functional networks. The corresponding functional network is labeled by the same color across subjects as illustrated in (c), and the second row shows the cortical parcellation. The corresponding parcellated regions are labeled by the same color across subjects. Note that there is no correspondence of color labels between functional networks and parcellated regions.

4 Discussion and Conclusion

We proposed a novel fiber connection pattern-guided structured sparse representation of whole-brain rsfMRI signals to infer functionally consistent regions. Experimental results demonstrated that the identified functional networks achieved both reasonable group-wise spatial pattern correspondence and fiber connection pattern consistency across subjects, which were not well addressed in previous functional atlas. Our future work includes adopting our method to identify network nodes based on the orthogonal dictionary atoms and 'network node hubs' based on the non-orthogonal atoms for conventional functional connectivity network analysis.

Acknowledgements. This research was supported in part by the National Institutes of Health (R01DA033393, R01AG042599), by the National Science Foundation Graduate Research Fellowship (NSF CAREER Award IIS-1149260, CBET-1302089, BCS-1439051), by the Jiangsu Natural Science Foundation (Project No. BK20131351), and by the 111 Project (No.B13022).

References

1. Lee, K., et al.: A data-driven sparse GLM for fMRI analysis using sparse dictionary learning with MDL criterion. IEEE Trans. Med. Imaging 30(5), 1076–1089 (2011)
2. Oikonomou, V.P., et al.: A sparse and spatially constrained generative regression model for fMRI data analysis. IEEE Trans. Biomed. Eng. 59(1), 58–67 (2012)
3. Lv, J., et al.: Holistic atlases of functional networks and interactions reveal reciprocal organizational architecture of cortical function. IEEE Trans. Biomed. Eng. (2014). doi: 10.1109/TBME.2014.2369495
4. Passingham, R.E., et al.: The anatomical basis of functional localization in the cortex. Nat. Rev. Neurosci. 3(8), 606–616 (2002)
5. Venkataraman, A., et al.: Joint modeling of anatomical and functional connectivity for population studies. IEEE Trans. Med. Imaging 31(2), 164–182 (2012)
6. Zhang, T., et al.: Group-wise consistent cortical parcellation based on DTI-derived connectional profiles. In: International Symposium on Biomedical Imaging, pp. 826–829 (2014)
7. Liu J., et al.: Multi-task feature learning via efficient $l_{2,1}$-norm minimization. In: Conference on Uncertainty in Artificial Intelligence, pp. 339–348, arXiv:1205.2631 (2009)
8. Smith, S.M., et al.: Resting-state fMRI in the Human Connectome Project. NeuroImage 80, 144–168 (2013)
9. Sotiropoulos, S.N., et al.: Advances in diffusion MRI acquisition and processing in the Human Connectome Project. Neuroimage 80, 125–143 (2013)
10. Mairal, J., et al.: Online learning for matrix factorization and sparse coding. The Journal of Machine Learning Research 11, 19–60 (2010)
11. Zhu, D., et al.: DICCCOL: dense individualized and common connectivity-based cortical landmarks. Cerebral Cortex 23(4), 786–800 (2013)
12. Tibshirani, R.: Regression shrinkage and selection via the LASSO. Journal of the Royal Statistical Society 58, 267–288 (1996)
13. Smith, S.M., et al.: Correspondence of the brain's functional architecture during activation and rest. Proc. Natl. Acad. Sci. U S A 106(31), 13040–13045 (2009)
14. Jaccard, P.: Étude comparative de la distribution florale dans une portion des Alpes et des Jura. Bulletin de la Société Vaudoise des Sciences Naturelles 37, 547–579 (1901)

Joint Estimation of Hemodynamic Response Function and Voxel Activation in Functional MRI Data

Priya Aggarwal, Anubha Gupta, and Ajay Garg

[1] Department of Electronics and Communication Engineering, IIIT-Delhi, India
[2] Department of Neuroradiology, Neurosciences Centre, AIIMS, Delhi, India
{priyaa,anubha}@iiitd.ac.in, drajaygarg@gmail.com

Abstract. This paper proposes a method of voxel-wise hemodynamic response function (HRF) estimation using sparsity and smoothing constraints on the HRF. The slow varying baseline drift at the voxel time-series is initially estimated via empirical mode decomposition (EMD). This estimation is refined by two-stage optimization that estimates HRF and slow-varying noise iteratively. In addition, this paper proposes a novel method of finding voxel activation via projection of voxel time-series on signal subspace constructed using the prior estimates of HRF. The performance of the proposed method is demonstrated on both synthetic and real fMRI data.

Keywords: functional MRI, Hemodynamic Response Function, Activation detection.

1 Introduction

Blood oxygen-level dependent (BOLD) functional magnetic resonance imaging (fMRI) is a non-invasive method to analyze human brain activity under different tasks such as visual, hearing, cognitive, etc [1]. It relates the neural activity with the temporal impulse response which is known as hemodynamic response function (HRF). In this manner, HRF is a proxy measure of underlying neuronal activity in brain. HRF not only varies across multiple subjects, but also in different regions of the brain of a single subject. HRF estimation can play a crucial role in estimating brain voxels activity accurately.

In the literature, HRF estimation has been done by two approaches: via region-based approach and via voxel-based approach [2]. In the region-based approach, regions of interest (ROIs) are extracted by either assuming equally sized regions [3] or via parcellation algorithm [4]. It is assumed that the HRF is same in all the voxels of a region. Hence, the mean of fMRI signal in the ROI is considered for HRF estimation. But, in actual scenario, some voxels may have different HRF within that ROI. Thus, estimated HRF may be suboptimal. In order to overcome the above shortcoming, various methods of voxel-based HRF estimation have been proposed in the literature [5-6]. Here, HRF is assumed to vary across different voxels. However, due to poor signal-to-noise ratio of fMRI time series,

N. Navab et al. (Eds.): MICCAI 2015, Part I, LNCS 9349, pp. 142–149, 2015.
DOI: 10.1007/978-3-319-24553-9_18

HRF estimates may be potentially misleading. Smoothing in the pre-processing stage can overcome this problem.

In addition to the above classification, there are parametric and nonparametric methods of HRF estimation. In the parametric methods, shape of HRF is assumed to be known apriori. However, single nonlinear function is not accurate to model HRFs across the entire brain. Nonparametric methods of HRF estimation do not restrict the shape of HRF and estimate HRF at each time point [5]. In [5], general linear model (GLM) is applied on each voxel to characterize voxel activity via best linear combination of the predictors [5]. The nonparametric method in [6] imposes sparsity constraint on HRF in time-domain. However, sparsity of HRF may be better modeled in the wavelet-domain as compared to the time-domain. In order to account for HRF variability across ROI, this paper considers voxel-based nonparametric approach for HRF estimation. Our method does not require priors on the parameters of HRF. A consistent voxel-wise HRF estimation along with sparsity and smoothing constraint is proposed in this paper. Additionally, estimated HRFs in a region are used to form signal subspace and projection of voxel time-series onto this signal subspace is used for robust detection of active *seed* voxel in the ROI.

This paper is organized as follows. Section 2 describes the fMRI time series model. Section 3 describes the proposed HRF estimation method. This section also presents the proposed method of voxel activation detection via subspace modeling. Simulation results on both simulated and real fMRI data are presented in Section 4. In the end, conclusions are presented in section 5.

Notations: We use lower case bold letters for vectors, upper case bold letters for matrices, and lower case italics letters for scalars.

2 Preliminaries

This section presents a brief background on fMRI signal time series and EMD.

2.1 Cerebral Hemodynamic Response Function

The BOLD fMRI signal is captured via T_2^* weighted imaging via MR scanner. Let us consider that M no. of brain volumes, at time instants t_j where $j = 1, 2, ..., M$ have been captured during an fMRI experiment. The intensity of a particular voxel V_i in the scanned brain volumes can be represented as a time-series $\mathbf{y}_i = [y_{i,1}, y_{i,2}, \cdots, y_{i,M}]$. This signal characterizes the BOLD time-series or signal at a particular voxel in brain.

In general, an fMRI signal is comprised of a) an activity-induced signal modeled as convolution of stimulus function with HRF of that region, b) a slow varying noise component, also called as baseline drift, and c) noise that is generally assumed to be additive white Gaussian noise (AWGN) for the sake of simplicity [6]. In other words, we can write

$$\mathbf{y}_i = \mathbf{S}\mathbf{h}_i + \mathbf{f}_i + \xi_i. \tag{1}$$

where $\mathbf{S}$ is M x L convolution matrix consisting of known lagged stimulus covariates. $\mathbf{S}$ depends on experimental design and is independent of voxel position. $\mathbf{h}_i$

is the amplitude of L-length HRF at voxel V_i, $\mathbf{f}_i$ is the M-time point baseline drift at voxel V_i, and ξ_i is the vector of M-length AWGN with $\xi_i \in N(0, \sigma^2\mathbf{I})$. This model does not assume any apriori shape of HRF. The baseline drift represented by $\mathbf{f}_i = [f_{i,1}, f_{i,2}, \cdots, f_{i,M}]$ is assumed to be independent of the experimental design matrix $\mathbf{S}$. This is to note that, in general, experimental paradigms in fMRI are constructed with single stimulus paradigm as considered in this paper to determine activated regions to build functional connectivity maps. However, the framework can be extended to multiple stimulus (say two) as below:

$$\mathbf{y}_i = \alpha_1\mathbf{S}_1\mathbf{h}_i + \alpha_2\mathbf{S}_2\mathbf{h}_i + \mathbf{f}_i + \xi_i. \tag{2}$$

where $\mathbf{S}_1$ and $\mathbf{S}_1$ are two different stimuli and α_1 and α_2 are the associated constants. However, for this framework, fMRI experiment data has to be captured for two different stimuli one by one in different time slots in the same session.

2.2 Empirical Mode Decomposition

Empirical mode decomposition (EMD) is an adaptive data driven approach that decomposes any nonlinear and non-stationary signal such as biomedical signals into amplitude and frequency modulated (AM-FM) components [7]. These functions are also called as intrinsic mode functions (IMFs) [7]. These IMFs are linearly independent of each other and capture the oscillations (or modes) that are intrinsically part of the given signal [7]. In general, the estimated IMFs are in the order of decreasing frequency. Thus, the first IMF corresponds to the high frequency oscillations, while the last IMF has the slow varying component. In general, signal $f[n]$ can be represented using IMFs as below:

$$f[n] = \sum_{k=1}^{Q} d_k[n] + r_Q[n] \tag{3}$$

where Q = total number of IMFs, $d_k[n]$ for $k = 1, ..., Q$ are the IMFs, $r_Q[n]$ is the last IMF, and stopping criterion defined in the EMD algorithm terminates the iterative procedure providing all IMFs. Currently, this method is being applied in various applications including biomedical, geological time-series analysis, etc. [7, 8].

3 Proposed Estimation of HRF and Voxel Activation

3.1 Proposed HRF Estimation Method

The time-series at a voxel V_i is represented as given in (1). In this equation, there are two unknowns: the HRF $\mathbf{h}_i$ and the slow varying baseline drift $\mathbf{f}_i$. In the literature, the theoretical shape of the HRF is assumed to be the one shown in Fig. 1(a) [3].

From Fig. 1(a), we draw the following assumptions on HRF:

A1) HRF is a smooth function over time. Thus, we can apply the Tikhonov regularisation technique for incorporating a smoothness constraint on the

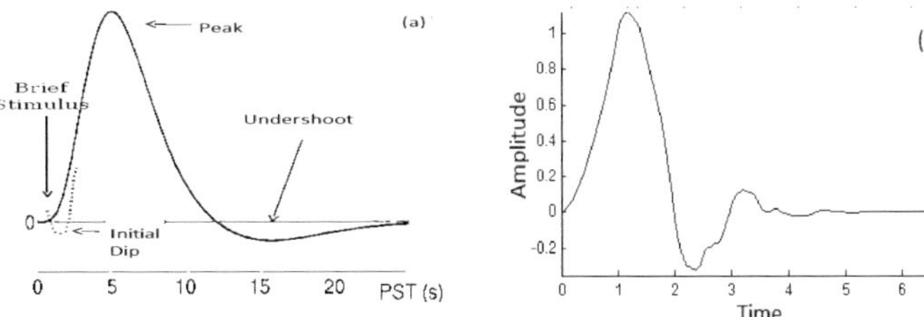

Fig. 1. (*a*):Theoretical shape of HRF; (*b*) Scaling function of *db4*

HRF [4]. This implies that the minimization of l^2 norm of $\mathbf{Dh}_i$ can be used as a constraint, where $\mathbf{D}$ is the second difference matrix operator given as:

$$\mathbf{D} = \begin{array}{ccccccc} 2 & -1 & 0 & . & 0 & 0 & 0 \\ -1 & 2 & -1 & 0 & . & 0 & 0 \\ 0 & -1 & 2 & -1 & 0 & . & . \\ 0 & 0 & . & . & . & . & . \\ . & . & . & . & 2 & -1 & 0 \\ 0 & . & . & . & -1 & 2 & -1 \\ 0 & 0 & . & 0 & 0 & -1 & 2 \end{array}$$

A2) Refer to Fig. 1(b) that shows the shape of the scaling function corresponding to the orthogonal wavelet *Daubechies*-4 (or *db4*). This shape is very similar to the theoretical HRF shape shown in Fig. 1(a). From these two figures, it is obvious that if HRF is analyzed via *db*4, it will be sparse in the wavelet domain. Thus, we assume that $\mathbf{Wh}_i$ is sparse, where $\mathbf{W}$ is the matrix operator corresponding to *db*4.

Using the above assumptions, we formulate the problem of HRF estimation, mathematically, using Lagrangian multiplier method as below:

$$\hat{\mathbf{h}}_i = \underset{h_i}{argmin} \left\|\mathbf{y}_i - \mathbf{Sh}_i - \mathbf{f}_i\right\|_2 + \lambda_1 \left\|\mathbf{Dh}_i\right\|_2 + \lambda_2 \left\|\mathbf{Wh}_i\right\|_1 + \lambda_3 \left\|\mathbf{f}_i\right\|_2 \tag{4}$$

where λ_1, λ_2, and λ_3 are the Lagrangian multipliers or regularization parameters. In (4), baseline drift is also unknown. In order to solve this problem, we carry out optimization in two stages, wherein we solve for $\hat{\mathbf{h}}_i$ and $\hat{\mathbf{f}}_i$ iteratively with the first iteration estimate $\hat{\mathbf{f}}_i^{(1)}$ drawn as the last IMF of EMD decomposition. The pseudo code for the estimation of $\hat{\mathbf{h}}_i$ is provided in Table-1. This is to note that optimization is carried out in CVX, a package for specifying and solving convex programs [8].

3.2 Proposed Voxel Activation Detection via Subspace Modeling

In order to estimate voxel activation, we formulate the following strategy. First, we estimate HRF at N no. of voxels with significant magnitude in the activity sensitive region using *Algorithm*-1. Within a region, the shape of HRF is somewhat similar, hence, we construct the signal subspace using estimated HRFs in that region. To this end, we use the projection operator based approach. First, we convolve each of these N no. of HRFs with the stimulus function $s(n)$ of length M (no. of brain scan volumes) as below:

$$\mathbf{x}_i = x_i[n] = s[n] \otimes h_i[n] = \sum_{k=0}^{L-1} h_i[k]s[n-k] \tag{5}$$

Table-1

Algorithm-1: Pseudo Code for Estimation of $\hat{\mathbf{h}}_i$

Input Parameters

Tikhonov regularisation matrix **D** (size *L* x *L*)
Daubechies-4 matrix **W** (size *L* x *L*)
Stimulus or Design matrix **S** (size *M* x *L*)
Lagrangian multipliers λ_1, λ_2, and λ_3 (scalars)

Input Data

Measured voxel V_i's time series stacked in a column $\mathbf{r}_i$ (size *M* x 1)

Start

Step-1 $\mathbf{y}_i$=detrend($\mathbf{r}_i$)

Step-2 Carry out EMD decomposition of $\mathbf{y}_i$ and initialize $\hat{\mathbf{f}}_i^{(1)} = \text{Last IMF}$.

Step-3 Compute first estimate of HRF $\hat{\mathbf{h}}_i^{(1)}$

$$\hat{\mathbf{h}}_i^{(1)} = \arg\min_{\mathbf{h}_i} \left\| \mathbf{y}_i - \mathbf{S}\mathbf{h}_i - \hat{\mathbf{f}}_i^{(1)} \right\|_2 + \lambda_1 \left\| \mathbf{D}\mathbf{h}_i \right\|_2 + \lambda_2 \left\| \mathbf{W}\mathbf{h}_i \right\|_1$$

Step-4 do

$$\hat{\mathbf{f}}_i^{(k+1)} = \arg\min_{\mathbf{f}_i} \left\| \mathbf{y}_i - \mathbf{S}\hat{\mathbf{h}}_i^{(k)} - \mathbf{f}_i \right\|_2 + \lambda_3 \left\| \mathbf{f}_i \right\|_2$$

$$\hat{\mathbf{h}}_i^{(k+1)} = \arg\min_{\mathbf{h}_i} \left\| \mathbf{y}_i - \mathbf{S}\mathbf{h}_i - \hat{\mathbf{f}}_i^{(k)} \right\|_2 + \lambda_1 \left\| \mathbf{D}\mathbf{h}_i \right\|_2 + \lambda_2 \left\| \mathbf{W}\mathbf{h}_i \right\|_1$$

while $\hat{\mathbf{h}}_i^{(k+1)} \neq \hat{\mathbf{h}}_i^{(k)}$ and $\hat{\mathbf{f}}_i^{(k+1)} \neq \hat{\mathbf{f}}_i^{(k)}$

Output

$\hat{\mathbf{h}}_i^{(k)}$

where $n = 0, 1, \cdots, M-1$ and $i = 0, 1, \cdots, N-1$. Next, we assume that these N no. of vectors $\mathbf{x}_i$ form the basis vectors of signal subspace χ and stack these into the columns of matrix $\mathbf{X}$ of size (M x N). We compute the projection matrix (operator) $\mathbf{P_X}$ corresponding to the signal subspace χ as below [9]:

$$\mathbf{P}_X = \mathbf{X}(\mathbf{X}^T\mathbf{X})^{-1}\mathbf{X}^T \tag{6}$$

where $\mathbf{P_X}$ is a symmetric and idempotent projection matrix. Since this signal subspace has been constructed from the estimated HRFs of the voxels with significant magnitude, this space will not be influenced largely with AWGN noise and the baseline drift. Now, this projection matrix $\mathbf{P_X}$ is used to project a detrended voxel time series $\mathbf{y}_k$ onto signal subspace χ as below:

$$\mathbf{w}_k = \mathbf{P_X}\mathbf{y}_k \tag{7}$$

for $k = 0, 1, \cdots, p-1$ where p corresponds to the no. of voxels in the activity-sensitive region of the brain. The norm of vectors $\mathbf{w}_k$ are computed for all p voxels. The voxel with the highest norm is labeled as the *seed* voxel of this region. This approach will take care of any inhomogeneity left in the neighborhood even after motion correction, removal of drift noise, etc. that might confound seed voxel. Voxels with norm greater than the threshold γ are declared as active voxels, i.e.,

$$\text{Declare } V_k = \text{active} \quad if\ norm(\mathbf{w}_k) > \gamma \tag{8}$$

4 Validation of the Proposed Method

In this section, we test the proposed joint method of HRF estimation and activation detection on the synthetic and real fMRI data.

4.1 Results on Synthetic fMRI Data

We generated a synthetic fMRI time series by convolving the stimulus function with the canonical HRF. Our canonical HRF of length L=20 is constructed using the difference of two gamma functions [4]. The plot of HRF $h[n]$ is shown in Fig. 2(a). We generated 200 time points of the synthetic BOLD fMRI signal as below:

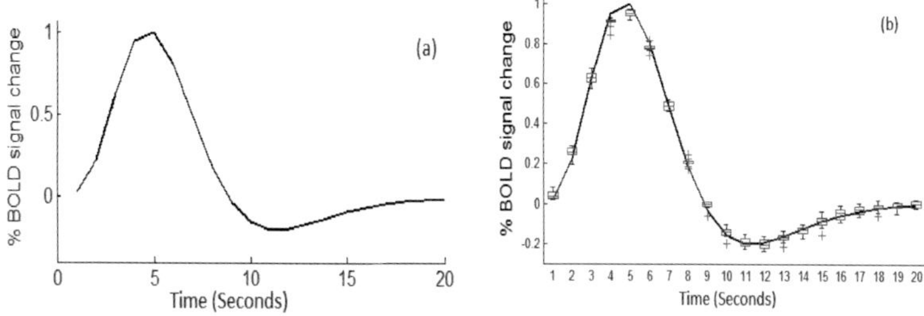

Fig. 2. (a): Synthetic HRF $h[n]$; (b) Estimated HRF $\hat{\mathbf{h}}_i$ using *Algorithm*-1

$$\mathbf{y} \equiv y[n] = s[n] \otimes h[n] + \xi[n] \tag{9}$$

Since we used real data with block-stimulus experiment design, we generated synthetic data with the same experimental paradigm. In the block experiment, block of 60s is generated with 30s on and 30s off time. Additive white Gaussion noise is generated with variances 0.75, 0.5, 0.25, 0.1, and 0.05. For computing the mean square error (MSE), 500 Monte Carlo cycles have been performed over voxel time-series (i.e., considering 500 different realizations of noise time-series). MSE between the canonical and estimated HRF is calculated as below:

$$MSE = \frac{1}{500} \sum_{k=1}^{500} \left[\frac{1}{L} \sum_{n=0}^{L-1} (\hat{h}_k[n] - h_k[n])^2 \right] \tag{10}$$

Since we did not corrupt the synthetic data with the slow varying baseline drift, only HRF was required to be estimated using *Algorithm*-1. The estimated HRF for noise variance $\sigma^2 = 0.1$ and with regularization parameters of $\lambda_1 = 1$ and $\lambda_2 = 0.2$ (determined empirically) is shown in Fig. 2(b).

The results of proposed algorithm are compared with the method of [6] and tabulated in Table-2. In [6], sparsity on HRF is imposed in the time-domain, while based on the shape and our discussion in Section 3.1, we find it more

Table-2: MSE calculated between estimated and canonical (assumed) HRF

	Noise Variance σ^2				
	0.05	0.1	0.25	0.5	0.75
Method of [6]	0.0522	0.0839	0.1689	0.3405	0.6474
Proposed	0.0153	0.0186	0.0374	0.0744	0.1012
Proposed without smoothing	0.0179	0.0361	0.0697	0.1253	0.2406

appropriate to consider sparsity of HRF in the wavelet-domain. In addition, we have imposed smoothness constraint on HRF that was not imposed in [6]. From Table-2, we observe that the proposed method with both smoothing and wavelet-domain sparsity constraint outperforms [6].

4.2 Results on Real fMRI Data

For testing the proposed framework on real fMRI data, we utilized the block design paradigm based auditory fMRI dataset available at SPM website [10]. This auditory dataset consists of acquisitions of 64 contiguous slices with 64x64x64 voxels of voxel size 3x3x3 mm^3. It contains 96 time points (or 96 acquisitions) with repetition time of 7s. Pre-processing of this data has been carried out using SPM8 toolbox with the procedure as outlined specifically for this dataset in Chapter 28 of SPM8 manual [10]. Pre-processing steps include realignment (with the first scan for removal of motion artefact), co-registration (with the mean fMRI scan generated in the step of realignment), normalisation (with the MNI atlas), and smoothing (using a 6mm full width at half maximum (FWHM) Gaussian kernel). These steps provided 96 brain volumes of 79x95x68 voxels each. First 12 scans were discarded, resulting in 84 brain volumes. Subject was given stimulus starting with the condition of rest, auditory, rest, and so on.

In general, Brodmann regions 22, 40, 41 are found to be associated with the auditory stimulus. We have tested the proposed methodology on Brodmann region 22. We extracted this ROI (Z) using *WFU Pickatlas Tool* [11]. Total 1720 voxels were extracted from this ROI. Next, we estimated HRF at 10 voxels with the highest norm, out of which 2 HRFs are shown in Fig. 3(a). The regularization parameters of $\lambda_1 = 1$, $\lambda_2 = 0.2$ (same as used for synthetic data) and $\lambda_3 = 0.1$ were used in the optimization routine for HRF estimation.

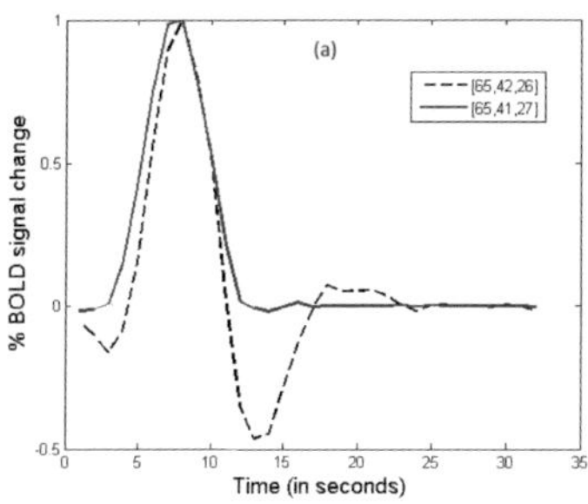

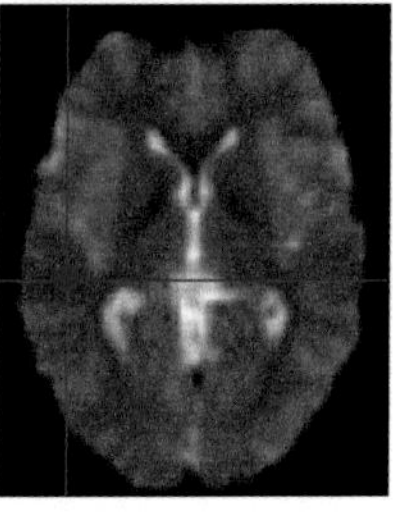

Fig. 3. (a): Estimated HRF estimated using *Algorithm*-1 on voxel positions ([65,41,27]-solid line;[65,42,26]-dotted line); (b) Active Seed Voxel [65,42,25]

Next, we constructed the projection operator using the estimated HRFs at 30 highest norm voxels as discussed in Section 3.2, projected the de-trended time-series $\mathbf{y}_k$ of all the voxels p of region Z using (7). Thereafter, we computed norm of vectors $\mathbf{w}_k$ of all p voxels. In the end, we declare the voxel with the highest norm as the seed voxel of activity-specific region Z. The coordinates of *seed* voxel on MNI frame of reference are found to be [65,42,25], and is shown on a 10mm diameter in Fig. 3(b). The position of seed voxel was validated by the radiologist.

5 Conclusion

In this paper, we have presented a joint method of voxel-wise hemodynamic response function (HRF) estimation and voxel activation detection. We removed the slow varying baseline drift using EMD along with the constraint optimization using sparsity on HRF in the wavelet-domain and smoothness of HRF in time-domain. This estimation is refined by two-stage optimization that estimates HRF and slow-varying noise iteratively. In addition, we propose a novel method of finding active seed voxel via projection of voxels time series on signal subspace constructed using the estimates of HRF. Since the proposed framework estimates HRF voxel-wise instead of region-wise, the determination of seed voxel in a region will be more accurate.

References

1. Ogawa, S., et al.: Brain magnetic resonance imaging with contrast dependent on blood oxygenation. In: PNAS, USA, vol. 87(24), pp. 9868–9872 (1990)
2. Glover, G.: Deconvolution of impulse response in event related BOLD fMRI. Neuroimage 9, 416–429 (1999)
3. Makni, S., et al.: A fully Bayesian approach to the parcel-based detection-estimation of brain activity in fMRI. NeuroImage 41, 941–969 (2008)
4. Bezargani, N., Nostratinia, A.: Joint maximum likelihood estimation of activation and Hemodynamic Response Function for fMRI. Elsevier Medical Image Analysis 18, 711–724 (2014)
5. Sole, A.F., et al.: Anisotropic 2-D and 3-D averaging of fMRI signals. IEEE Trans. Med. Imag. 20, 86–93 (2001)
6. Seghouane, A.K., Johnston, L.A.: Consistent hemodynamic response estimation function in fMRI using sparse prior information. In: IEEE ISBI, pp. 596–599, May 2014
7. Huang, N.E., et al.: The empirical mode decomposition and hilbert spectrum for nonlinear and nonstationary time series analysis. Proc. Roy. Soc. London, 454–460 (1998)
8. Grant, M., Boyd, S.: CVX: Matlab software for disciplined convex programming, version 2.0 beta (September 2013). `http://cvxr.com/cvx`
9. Agarwal, S., Gupta, A.: Fractal and EMD based Removal of Baseline Wander and Powerline Interference from ECG Signals. Computers in Biology and Medicine 43(11), 1889–1899 (2013)
10. `http://www.fil.ion.ucl.ac.uk/spm/data/`
11. Maldjian, J.A., et al.: An automated method for neuroanatomic and cytoarchitectonic atlas-based interrogation of fmri data sets (WFU Pickatlas, version 3.05). NeuroImage 19, 1233–1239

Quantifying Microstructure in Fiber Crossings with Diffusional Kurtosis

Michael Ankele and Thomas Schultz

University of Bonn, Germany*

Abstract. Diffusional Kurtosis Imaging (DKI) is able to capture non-Gaussian diffusion and has become a popular complement to the more traditional Diffusion Tensor Imaging (DTI). In this paper, we demonstrate how strongly the presence of fiber crossings and the exact crossing angle affect measures from diffusional kurtosis, limiting their interpretability as indicators of tissue microstructure. We alleviate this limitation by modeling fiber crossings with a mixture of cylindrically symmetric kurtosis models. Based on results on simulated and on real-world data, we conclude that explicitly including crossing geometry in kurtosis models leads to parameters that are more specific to other aspects of tissue microstructure, such as scale and homogeneity.

1 Introduction

Diffusional Kurtosis Imaging (DKI) is a natural and popular extension of Diffusion Tensor Imaging (DTI) that accounts for the empirically observed non-Gaussianity of diffusion in biological tissue. Measures of diffusional kurtosis are known to be affected by factors such as the scale and homogeneity of obstacles to the molecular motion [4], and therefore provide useful information on tissue microstructure, complementing the information captured in the diffusion tensor.

Many studies of white matter are motivated by an interest in structural parameters, such as nerve fiber density or myelination. They use diffusion MRI because it provides quantities that are affected by such factors, and that are easy and safe to obtain *in vivo*. A known limitation of diffusion tensor imaging is the fact that measures such as fractional anisotropy are sensitive, but not specific to those parameters of interest: The effect of confounding factors, such as the presence of orientational dispersion or fiber crossings, can be substantial.

In Section 3 of this paper, we discuss an analogous limitation in DKI: We show that common measures of diffusional kurtosis are not specific to microstructural parameters of individual fibers, but are heavily affected by the presence, and the exact angle, of fiber crossings. This motivates development of a novel computational method in Section 4, in which the impact of those nuisance parameters is

* This work was supported by the DFG under grant SCHU 3040/1-1. Data were provided by the Human Connectome Project, WU-Minn Consortium (Principal Investigators: David Van Essen and Kamil Ugurbil; 1U54MH091657) funded by the 16 NIH Institutes and Centers that support the NIH Blueprint for Neuroscience Research; and by the McDonnell Center for Systems Neuroscience at Washington University.

N. Navab et al. (Eds.): MICCAI 2015, Part I, LNCS 9349, pp. 150–157, 2015.
DOI: 10.1007/978-3-319-24553-9_19

greatly reduced. Its building block is a cylindrically symmetric kurtosis model. In Section 5, we present results on simulated data, confirming that our newly derived kurtosis measures are affected far less by the crossing angle than results of traditional DKI. We also show parameter maps that demonstrate the effectiveness of our method on real data.

2 Related Work

Several recent works have aimed to reduce the effects of fiber crossings and orientational dispersion on quantitative markers from diffusion MRI. NODDI disentangles the effects of neurite orientation dispersion and density, but does not model fiber crossings [16]. Spherical deconvolution can be used to quantify fiber properties in a way that is robust to fiber crossings, either by analyzing the fiber orientation distribution function after using a fixed deconvolution kernel [8,2], or by calibrating the kernel itself [10]. Finally, estimation of per-compartment diffusion parameters can be integrated into crossing-fiber tractography [6,9].

Our work is most closely related to a series of approaches that have fitted multiple diffusion tensors [15,5,13]. However, none of them model diffusional kurtosis. We demonstrate how fiber crossings affect kurtosis measures and propose novel kurtosis measures whose sensitivity to crossings is greatly reduced.

3 How Fiber Crossings Affect Diffusional Kurtosis

It is well-known that fiber crossings strongly affect measures derived from the diffusion tensor model, such as Fractional Anisotropy (FA). It is unsurprising that the same is true for measures of diffusional kurtosis. Our first goal is to systematically demonstrate the exact extent of this dependence.

We have synthesized crossings with varying crossing angles between 0 and 90 degrees, and created plots of how diffusional kurtosis depends on it. Signal synthesis was performed in a data-driven manner from a subject from the Human Connectome Project (288 DWIs on shells at $b \approx \{5, 1000, 2000, 3000\}\,\mathrm{s/mm^2}$). It is based on 300 voxels thought to contain a single dominant fiber compartment, given as the voxels with highest FA within a white matter mask. The DKI model was fit to the data, and model parameters were analytically rotated by the desired crossing angle. Diffusion-weighted signals were computed from the original and rotated model, and averaged. This simulates two fiber compartments that cross at a known angle, with no significant exchange within the diffusion time. Since we use the full DKI model, it does not impose cylindrical symmetry.

We performed a constrained least squares fit of the diffusional kurtosis model to the simulated data [12]. Fig. 1 plots mean and one standard deviation of the resulting mean, axial, and radial kurtosis, over the 300 voxels used to simulate the crossings. The plots in the top row show that the dependence on the crossing angle is substantial: Compared to the baseline (value for a single fiber compartment, indicated by a green line), the crossing changes radial kurtosis by a factor of up to 4.23, and axial kurtosis up to 5.65. A very similar dependence

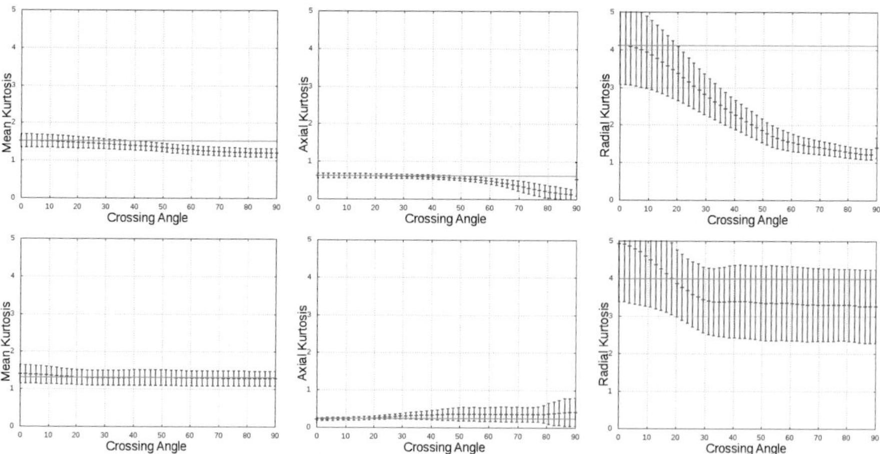

Fig. 1. *Top:* The angle at which fibers cross has a severe impact on the parameters of DKI. *Bottom:* The proposed model reduces effects of crossing geometry, leading to biomarkers that more specifically quantify microstructure properties.

is observed for axial and radial diffusivities (not shown). Studies that aim to use kurtosis to specifically quantify microstructure properties, without confounding effects from crossings, should be aware of this problem. We will now introduce a method to compute novel kurtosis measures, shown in the lower row of Fig. 1, that are less susceptible to the undesired impact of crossing geometry.

4 A Mixture of Kurtosis Models

The general strategy of our method is to fit a mixture of kurtosis models to fiber crossings. In effect, this adds kurtosis to previous methods that have modeled fiber crossings using multiple diffusion tensors.

4.1 A Cylindrically Symmetric Kurtosis Model

The full kurtosis model has six parameters for the diffusion tensor, plus 15 for the kurtosis tensor. This seems prohibitive for fitting a mixture. We thus constrain the kurtosis models that will represent the individual fiber compartments in our mixture to be cylindrically symmetric around the principal diffusion direction.

The same symmetry is frequently assumed in multi-tensor models [15,5]. It reduces the 21 parameters in the full kurtosis model to only 7: Two angles that parameterize a unit vector $\mathbf{v}$ indicating the fiber direction, axial and radial diffusivities ($\lambda_{\|}$, $\lambda_{\perp}$), as well as three kurtosis-related parameters: In addition to $\kappa_{\|}$ and $\kappa_{\perp}$, which are related to axial and radial kurtosis, the fact that kurtosis is a fourth-order quantity introduced a third parameter $\kappa_{\diamond}$. The resulting signal equation as a function of gradient direction $\mathbf{g}$ and b value is

$$\ln \frac{S_{cyl}(\mathbf{g}, b; \mathbf{v})}{S_0} = -b \left[\lambda_\perp + (\lambda_\| - \lambda_\perp)\langle \mathbf{v}, \mathbf{g}\rangle^2\right] + \\ \frac{b^2}{6}\left[\kappa_\perp + (\kappa_\diamond - 2\kappa_\perp)\langle \mathbf{v}, \mathbf{g}\rangle^2 + (\kappa_\| - \kappa_\diamond + \kappa_\perp)\langle \mathbf{v}, \mathbf{g}\rangle^4\right] \quad (1)$$

To simplify Eq. (1), κ_* absorb the square of the mean diffusivity $\bar{\lambda} = (\lambda_\| + 2\lambda_\perp)/3$ that usually occurs as a factor in diffusional kurtosis. This means that axial and radial kurtosis K_* can be computed from our parameters as

$$K_\| = \frac{\kappa_\|}{\lambda_\|^2} \quad \text{and} \quad K_\perp = \frac{\kappa_\perp}{\lambda_\perp^2}. \quad (2)$$

Assuming that the fiber is oriented along the z axis, our model parameters translate to a standard kurtosis tensor via

$$W_{xxxx} = W_{yyyy} = 3W_{xxyy} = \frac{\kappa_\perp}{\bar{\lambda}^2},\ W_{xxzz} = W_{yyzz} = \frac{\kappa_\diamond}{6\,\bar{\lambda}^2},\ W_{zzzz} = \frac{\kappa_\|}{\bar{\lambda}^2}. \quad (3)$$

This allows computation of mean kurtosis MK using the equations given in [12].

We have used the Bayesian Information Criterion (BIC) to compare our cylindrically symmetric model with two variants, one with a ball compartment, the other one with a dot compartment [7], and with the full kurtosis model. Ranking them with respect to their BIC preferred "symmetric+dot" in 96.3% of all cases, "symmetric" in 3.0%, the full kurtosis model in 0.7%, and "symmetric+ball" in 0%. Therefore, we include a dot compartment in all our experiments.

4.2 Strategy for Fitting the Final Mixture

Our final signal equation results from using Eq. (1) to model each of k crossing fiber compartments and adding the dot compartment:

$$S(\mathbf{g}, b) = S_0 \left[f_{dot} + \sum_{i=1}^{k} f_i S_{cyl}(\mathbf{g}, b; \mathbf{v}_i)\right] \quad (4)$$

Volume fractions f_* are constrained to be non-negative, and to add to one. We ensure numerical stability in evaluating Eq. (2), and force $\mathbf{v}_i$ to align with a principal diffusion direction, by constraining $\lambda_\perp \in [0.01\lambda_\|, \lambda_\|]$ and $\lambda_\| > \epsilon$. We also impose the same constraints on our kurtosis parameters as Tabesh et al., $3/(b_{max}\bar{\lambda}) \geq K \geq 0$ [12]. As in the widely used ball-and-stick model [1], the diffusion and kurtosis parameters of all compartments are coupled. Trying to obtain stable estimates without this constraint is a topic for future work.

Even though Eq. (4) is relatively straightforward conceptually, fitting it to a given set of measurements amounts to a difficult non-convex optimization problem. We have developed the following strategy for solving it: A suitable initialization is obtained from a diffusion tensor fit, by setting $\lambda_\|$ to the largest eigenvalue and $\lambda_\perp$ to the mean of the two smaller ones. Fiber volume fractions f_i and directions $\mathbf{v}_i$ are initialized by discretizing an orientation distribution function from spherical deconvolution, as proposed in [11]. The kurtosis parameters and f_{dot} are initialized to zero.

Table 1. Statistics on the difference between kurtosis estimates in simulated crossings and the single fiber voxels from which they were generated quantify the extent to which we reduce the impact of crossings. At low SNR, neither model gives useful results.

	Kurtosis Tensor Model			Our Kurtosis Mixture Model		
SNR	MK	$K_{\parallel}$	$K_{\perp}$	MK	$K_{\parallel}$	$K_{\perp}$
∞	-0.15 ± 0.17	-0.09 ± 0.22	-1.69 ± 1.60	-0.00 ± 0.07	0.02 ± 0.07	-0.20 ± 1.01
40	-0.15 ± 0.28	-0.09 ± 0.21	-1.75 ± 1.76	0.01 ± 0.31	0.02 ± 0.08	-0.14 ± 1.62
30	-0.15 ± 0.28	0.17 ± 0.38	-1.95 ± 1.36	0.16 ± 0.40	0.20 ± 0.50	-0.36 ± 1.48
20	-0.04 ± 0.45	0.35 ± 0.51	-1.89 ± 1.35	0.42 ± 0.84	0.52 ± 1.00	-0.27 ± 1.95
10	0.49 ± 1.18	0.83 ± 0.96	-1.43 ± 2.02	1.79 ± 5.05	1.61 ± 2.52	1.88 ± 14.90

The fitting itself is performed with constrained Levenberg-Marquardt optimization. We found that it can be accelerated greatly by re-parametrizing diffusivity and kurtosis parameters. The actual parameters visible to the optimizer are $\ln(\lambda_{\parallel})$, $\lambda_{\perp}/\lambda_{\parallel}$, $1000\kappa_{\parallel}/\lambda_{\parallel}$, $1000\kappa_{\perp}/\lambda_{\perp}$, $1000\kappa_{\diamond}/\lambda_{\parallel}$. Moreover, we observed that convergence benefits from splitting the parameters into two blocks, and alternating between their optimization. The first block contains the volume fractions and directions, which we parameterize using elevation and azimuth angles. The second block optimizes diffusion and kurtosis. Despite these optimization, processing a slice of 174×145 voxels on 6 cores of a 3.4GHz $i7$ takes 6 minutes.

5 Results

5.1 Simulated Data

As an initial validation of our model and fitting procedure, we applied it to the simulated data that was described in Section 3. The results are shown in the bottom row of Fig. 1. They confirm that our crossing model succeeds in absorbing a significant part of the variation in kurtosis measures which is otherwise caused by crossing geometry. The results remain much closer to the baseline, which is indicated by the green line. Note that differences between the baselines in both rows are due to the presence of the dot compartment.

For a quantitative summary, we have taken the difference of kurtosis parameters estimated in the crossing by the two models, and a baseline, computed by the same method from the single-fiber voxel that was used to simulate the fiber crossing. Table 1 reports the mean and standard deviation of this difference over all 300 voxels and all crossing angles. It confirms that our model greatly reduces the impact of crossings, in particular in case of radial kurtosis. The relatively low standard deviations indicate that fitting works reliably. Table 1 also shows the results of adding Rician noise to the simulation, indicating that our fitting starts to degrade around SNR ≈ 20. At this point, even values from the full model start to exhibit a noticeable bias.

5.2 Real Data

In addition to the quantitative validation on simulated data, we have verified that our model produces plausible results on real human brain scans by fitting

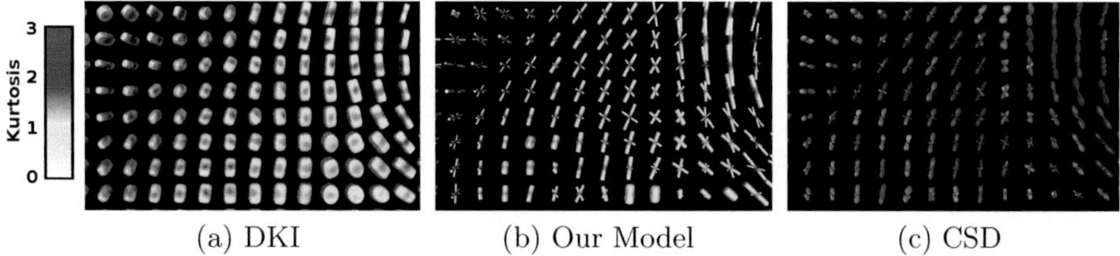

Fig. 2. Our mixture of cylindrically symmetric kurtosis compartments (b) results in principal fiber directions that agree well with constrained spherical deconvolution (c). In contrast to the traditional kurtosis model (a), it leads to measures that disentangle the effects of microstructure and crossing geometry.

it to data from the human connectome project. In each voxel, the BIC has been used to select between models with a single, two, or three cylindrically symmetric kurtosis compartments.

A detail of the result on a coronal slice, in the region where fibers from the corpus callosum, corticospinal tract, and superior longitudinal fasciculus cross, is visualized in Fig. 2 using superquadric glyphs [3] for the diffusion tensor part of the kurtosis model. Glyphs have been scaled with the volume fraction of the respective compartment, and color coded with directional kurtosis. In contrast to the traditional kurtosis model in (a), directions of crossing fibers are immediately apparent from our result (b).

A comparison to the widely used constrained spherical deconvolution model [14], which we fitted to the subset of measurements with $b \approx 3000\,\mathrm{s/mm^2}$, is shown in Fig. 2 (c). The agreement of principal fiber directions and relative volume fractions confirms that the individual kurtosis compartments in our model successfully capture the dominant fiber populations in real crossings.

However, our main interest is in the kurtosis measures themselves, which are mapped in the bottom row of Fig. 3 and compared to the corresponding ones from standard kurtosis imaging in the top row. MK and $K_{\|}$ are mapped with range $[0, 2]$; $K_{\perp}$ is mapped with range $[0, 5]$; FA is shown with range $[0, 1]$.

Within the white matter, our model measures a much lower $K_{\|}$ than the classical DKI model, close to that of free diffusion. In gray matter, our $K_{\|}$ remains high, providing a clear contrast between the two tissue types. This correlates with the volume fraction of the dot compartment; after factoring it out, MK is nearly uniform over the brain tissue (Fig. 3 (e)).

$K_{\perp}$ and FA have been computed from the diffusion tensors of both models. There is a clear visual similarity between structures in Fig. 3 (c) and (d), which is much reduced in the corresponding Fig. 3 (g) and (h): While the FA from our model remains high throughout the white matter (in agreement with the results in [10]), confirming the reduced impact of fiber crossings, our radial kurtosis still shows substantial variation, which reflects more subtle aspects of tissue architecture. We believe that the similarity between Fig. 3 (c) and (d) is caused by the fact that, in standard DKI, FA and $K_{\perp}$ are both reduced in regions of fiber crossings, and that factoring out the effect of crossings emphasizes the information specific to diffusional kurtosis.

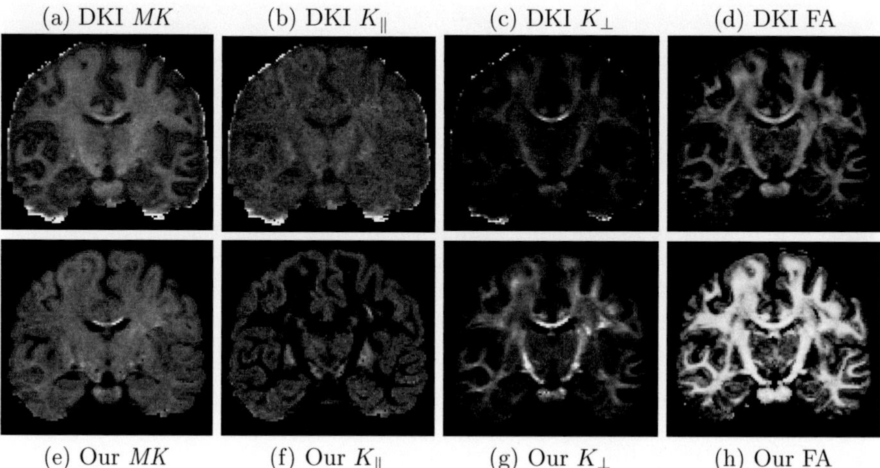

Fig. 3. Differences in MK and $K_{\|}$ between our model and standard DKI appear to be due to including a dot compartment, while those in $K_{\perp}$ and FA are more strongly affected by the reduced impact of fiber crossings.

6 Conclusion

In this work, we have demonstrated how strongly measures from diffusional kurtosis are affected by fiber crossings, which limits their interpretability as indicators of tissue microstructure. To alleviate this, we have explicitly accounted for crossings by adding a cylindrically symmetric kurtosis term to the popular multi-tensor model. Results on simulated data confirm that the resulting model remains tractable, and successfully disentangles the effects of crossings and per-compartment tissue parameters.

In real data, the maps from our model differ significantly from standard diffusional kurtosis imaging; we believe that they more specifically indicate factors such as scale and homogeneity of tissue microstructure. As a next step, we plan to use additional simulations and a systematic comparison to other MR-derived quantities to gain more insight into the exact interpretation of these maps. We also plan to use spatial regularization to achieve stable fitting on noisy data.

References

1. Behrens, T.E.J., Johansen-Berg, H., Jbabdi, S., Rushworth, M.F.S., Woolrich, M.W.: Probabilistic diffusion tractography with multiple fibre orientations: What can we gain? NeuroImage 34, 144–155 (2007)
2. Dell'Acqua, F., Simmons, A., Williams, S.C.R., Catani, M.: Can spherical deconvolution provide more information than fiber orientations? hindrance modulated orientational anisotropy, a true-tract specific index to characterize white matter diffusion. Human Brain Mapping 34(10), 2464–2483 (2013)

3. Ennis, D.B., Kindlmann, G., Rodriguez, I., Helm, P.A., McVeigh, E.R.: Visualization of tensor fields using superquadric glyphs. Magnetic Resonance in Medicine 53(1), 169–176 (2005)
4. Jensen, J.H., Helpern, J.A.: MRI quantification of non-gaussian water diffusion by kurtosis analysis. NMR in Biomedicine 23(7), 698–710 (2010)
5. Kreher, B., Schneider, J., Mader, I., Martin, E., Hennig, J., Il'yasov, K.: Multitensor approach for analysis and tracking of complex fiber configurations. Magnetic Resonance in Medicine 54, 1216–1225 (2005)
6. Malcolm, J.G., Shenton, M.E., Rathi, Y.: Filtered multitensor tractography. IEEE Trans. on Medical Imaging 29(9), 1664–1675 (2010)
7. Panagiotaki, E., Schneider, T., Siow, B., Hall, M.G., Lythgoe, M.F., Alexander, D.C.: Compartment models of the diffusion MR signal in brain white matter: A taxonomy and comparison. NeuroImage 59, 2241–2254 (2012)
8. Raffelt, D., Tournier, J.D., Rose, S., Ridgway, G.R., Henderson, R., Crozier, S., Salvado, O., Connelly, A.: Apparent fibre density: A novel measure for the analysis of diffusion-weighted magnetic resonance images. NeuroImage 59(4), 3976–3994 (2012)
9. Reisert, M., Kiselev, V.G., Dihtal, B., Kellner, E., Novikov, D.S.: MesoFT: unifying diffusion modelling and fiber tracking. In: Golland, P., Hata, N., Barillot, C., Hornegger, J., Howe, R. (eds.) MICCAI 2014, Part III. LNCS, vol. 8675, pp. 201–208. Springer, Heidelberg (2014)
10. Schultz, T., Groeschel, S.: Auto-calibrating spherical deconvolution based on ODF sparsity. In: Mori, K., Sakuma, I., Sato, Y., Barillot, C., Navab, N. (eds.) MICCAI 2013, Part I. LNCS, vol. 8149, pp. 663–670. Springer, Heidelberg (2013)
11. Schultz, T., Westin, C.F., Kindlmann, G.: Multi-diffusion-tensor fitting via spherical deconvolution: A unifying framework. In: Jiang, T., Navab, N., Pluim, J.P.W., Viergever, M.A. (eds.) MICCAI 2010, Part I. LNCS, vol. 6361, pp. 673–680. Springer, Heidelberg (2010)
12. Tabesh, A., Jensen, J.H., Ardekani, B.A., Helpern, J.A.: Estimation of tensors and tensor-derived measures in diffusional kurtosis imaging. Magnetic Resonance in Medicine 65, 823–836 (2011)
13. Taquet, M., Scherrer, B., Boumal, N., Macq, B., Warfield, S.K.: Estimation of a multi-fascicle model from single b-value data with a population-informed prior. In: Mori, K., Sakuma, I., Sato, Y., Barillot, C., Navab, N. (eds.) MICCAI 2013, Part I. LNCS, vol. 8149, pp. 695–702. Springer, Heidelberg (2013)
14. Tournier, J.D., Calamante, F., Connelly, A.: Robust determination of the fibre orientation distribution in diffusion MRI: Non-negativity constrained super-resolved spherical deconvolution. NeuroImage 35, 1459–1472 (2007)
15. Tuch, D.S., Reese, T.G., Wiegell, M.R., Makris, N., Belliveau, J.W., Wedeen, V.J.: High angular resolution diffusion imaging reveals intravoxel white matter fiber heterogeneity. Magnetic Resonance in Medicine 48, 577–582 (2002)
16. Zhang, H., Schneider, T., Wheeler-Kingshott, C.A., Alexander, D.C.: NODDI: practical in vivo neurite orientation dispersion and density imaging of the human brain. NeuroImage 61(4), 1000–1016 (2012)

Which Manifold Should be Used for Group Comparison in Diffusion Tensor Imaging?

A. Bouchon[1], V. Noblet[1], F. Heitz[1],
J. Lamy[1], F. Blanc[1,2], and J.-P. Armspach[1]

[1] ICube, University of Strasbourg, CNRS,
Fédération de Médecine Translationnelle de Strasbourg (FMTS), France
[2] Neuropsychology Service, Department of Neurology,
University Hospital of Strasbourg, France

Abstract. Diffusion Tensor Magnetic Resonance Imaging (DT-MRI) is a modality which allows to investigate the white matter structure by probing water molecule diffusion. A common way to model the diffusion process is to consider a second-order tensor, represented by a symmetric positive-definite matrix. Currently, there is still no consensus on the most appropriate manifold for handling diffusion tensors. We propose to evaluate the influence of considering an Euclidean, a Log-Euclidean or a Riemannian manifold for conducting group comparison in DT-MRI. To this end, we consider a multi-linear regression problem that is solved on each of these manifolds. Statistical analysis is then achieved by computing an F-statistic between two nested (restricted and full) models. Our evaluation on simulated data suggests that the performance of these manifolds varies with the kind of modifications that has to be detected, while the experiments on real data do not exhibit significant difference between the methods.

1 Introduction

Diffusion Tensor Magnetic Resonance Imaging (DT-MRI) is a modality commonly used to investigate the cerebral white matter integrity. There is a great need in the neuroscientific community for efficient tools to compare DT-MRI across cohorts of subjects according to clinical or cognitive data. Most studies focus on the comparison of scalar images derived from DT-MRI such as Fractional Anisotropy (FA) or Mean Diffusivity (MD) using either the voxel-based analysis framework [1] provided in SPM[1] or the tract-based spatial statistics (TBSS) method [2] provided in FSL[2]. However, these methods do not exploit all the information contained in tensor images and thus cannot detect all kind of changes. Different statistical frameworks have been proposed to compare the whole diffusion tensor information [3,4,5,6,7]. Only a few take into account covariates (e.g. age, sex, cognitive scores) [4,6,7]. A convenient way to introduce

[1] http://www.fil.ion.ucl.ac.uk/spm/
[2] http://fsl.fmrib.ox.ac.uk/fsl/

N. Navab et al. (Eds.): MICCAI 2015, Part I, LNCS 9349, pp. 158–165, 2015.
DOI: 10.1007/978-3-319-24553-9_20

these covariates is to consider a linear model [4,6,7]. The regression estimation can be done by considering different metrics to compute the residuals. In this work, we propose to compare the influence of considering either an Euclidean, a Log-Euclidean or a Riemanian metric in the regression problem. A few works have already evaluated the impact of these metrics for various image processing problems [8,9], but there is still no consensus on the most appropriate one, especially in the context of group comparison. To compare the influence of these metrics, a simulation framework has been set up, based on DT-MRI acquisitions of healthy subjects in which different kinds of lesions have been introduced. This study has also been complemented by results on a cohort of patients suffering from neuromyelitis optica (NMO).

2 Methods

2.1 Pre-processing

To conduct group studies at the voxel level, all images should first be registered in a common space. This is done by registering all FA images derived from DT-MRI on a common template using an affine followed by a non-rigid registration method [10]. Spatial transforms estimated from FA images are then applied on tensor images using the Preservation of Principal Direction (PPD) reorientation strategy.

2.2 Multi-linear Regression

Let $\mathcal{M}$ be a manifold and $\{y_i\}_{i\in[1..N]} \in \mathcal{M}$ the observations from N individuals, each individual being characterized by K explanatory variables $\{x_{i,j}\}_{j\in[1..K]}$ such as age, gender or group affiliation. The regression problem consists in estimating a function $f : \mathbb{R}^K \mapsto \mathcal{M}$ that best fits all the couples $(\{x_{i,1} \dots x_{i,K}\}, y_i)$. A simple parametric model is to consider a multi-linear function:

$$y_i = \alpha + \beta_1 x_{i,1} + \beta_2 x_{i,2} + \dots + \beta_K x_{i,K} + \varepsilon_i \tag{1}$$

where α is the intercept, β_i are the regression coefficients and ε_i are the residuals.

Case of Scalar Observations. If y_i are scalar observations (*i.e.*, $\mathcal{M} \subseteq \mathbb{R}$), this regression problem amounts to the general linear model commonly used to perform voxelwise group comparison on scalar images derived from DT-MRI [1]. Let $Y = [y_1 \dots y_i \dots y_N]^t$, $X[i,j] = x_{i,j}$ and $B = [\beta_1 \dots \beta_j \dots \beta_K]^t$. If the residuals ε_i are assumed to be independent and identically distributed according to a normal distribution, then the least squares estimate of B can be obtained analytically:

$$\hat{B} = \arg\min_{B\in\mathbb{R}^K} \|Y - XB\|^2 = (X^t X)^{-1} X^t Y \tag{2}$$

To extend this framework to tensors images, several strategies can be implemented depending on the assumption made on the manifold $\mathcal{M}$.

Euclidean Framework. A diffusion tensor can be represented by $D^i = [D^i_{xx}\ D^i_{xy}\ D^i_{xz}\ D^i_{yy}\ D^i_{yz}\ D^i_{zz}]^t \in \mathbb{R}^6$. The previous regression problem can straightforwardly be extended to the multivariate case by assuming the noise variance on each tensor element to be identical (homoscedasticity assumption) [7]. This method will be referred in the sequel as General Linear Model for Diffusion Tensors (*GLM-DT*).

The basic idea is to concatenate all tensor components of the N individuals in a single vector $Y \in \mathbb{R}^{6N}$. For each explanatory variable, six regressors are estimated, one associated with each tensor component. This is done by constructing a new design matrix $X[i,j] = x_{i,j}$, for $i = 1 \ldots N \times 6$ and $j = 1 \ldots K \times 6$, where each explanatory variable is replicated in six columns: the first column is composed of the values of the explanatory variable for the entries corresponding to the first tensor components D^i_{xx} and of zeros for the others entries, and so on for the five others columns. With that formulation, the least squares estimate of B has also a closed-form solution and leads to the estimation of K regressors of six components [7].

Log-Euclidean Framework. The Euclidean framework does not take into account that diffusion tensors are symetric positive-definite matrices, *i.e.* $\mathcal{M} = \mathrm{Sym}^+(3)$, which is in fact only a subset of $\mathbb{R}^6$. Consequently, the estimated regression can possibly map some sets of explanatory variables to vectors that do not correspond to positive-definite matrices. A way to circumvent this limitation is to conduct the regression on the logarithm of tensors instead on the tensors directly. Indeed, the logarithmic transformation enables to map the space of symmetric positive-definite matrices $\mathrm{Sym}^+(3)$ to the space of symmetric matrices $\mathrm{Sym}(3)$. Thus, the same framework as in [7] can be used for the regression estimation. The corresponding regression model is then given by:

$$Y = \exp(XB + \varepsilon) \tag{3}$$

where $\exp(\cdot)$ stands for the matrix exponential. This method will be referred as General Linear Model for Diffusion Log-Tensors (*GLM-LOG-DT*).

Riemannian Framework. Recently, a multiple geodesic regression model based on Riemannian geometry has been proposed [6]. This framework enables to account for the positive-definite nature of diffusion tensors. The corresponding regression model is given by:

$$y_i = \mathrm{Exp}(\mathrm{Exp}(\alpha, \sum_{j=1}^{N} \beta^j x_{i,j}),\ \varepsilon_i) \tag{4}$$

where Exp refers to the exponential map. The regressors β and the intercept α are simultaneoustly estimated using a gradient descent scheme by minimizing the distance between the data y_i and the estimate $\hat{y}_i = \mathrm{Exp}(\alpha, \sum_{j=1}^{N} \beta^j x_{i,j})$. To this end, the following geodesic distance is used:

$$d(y_i, \hat{y}_i) = \sqrt{\langle \mathrm{Log}(y_i, \hat{y}_i),\ \mathrm{Log}(y_i, \hat{y}_i) \rangle_{y_i}} \tag{5}$$

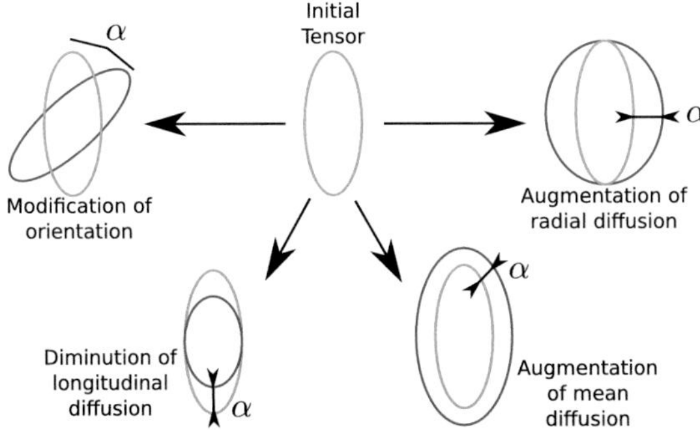

Fig. 1. Representation of the four kinds of lesions. The green and the red tensors represent respectively the initial tensor and the modified tensor.

The implementation of this method has been made available on `https://www.nitrc.org/projects/riem_mglm`. This method will be referred in the sequel as Manifold General Linear Model for Diffusion (*MGLM*).

2.3 Statistical Test

The objective of the statistical test is to evaluate whether a given explanatory variable has a significant contribution in the regression model. To this end, an F-test is used to compare the Residuals Sum of Squares (RSS) of two nested models: a full model taking into account all the covariates (RSS_2) and a restricted model where the covariate of interest is discarded (RSS_1):

$$F = \frac{\frac{RSS_1 - RSS_2}{p_2 - p_1}}{\frac{RSS_2}{N - p_2}} \tag{6}$$

with p_2 and p_1 representing respectively the number of covariates for both models. Assuming that the residuals follow a normal distribution, F follows a Fisher distribution with $p_2 - p_1$ and $N - p_2$ degrees of freedom under the null hypothesis that model 2 does not provide a significantly better fit than model 1. The Gaussianity assumption of the residuals is a reasonable hypothesis for the Euclidean and Log-Euclidean frameworks, but it is no longer valid for the Riemannian framework. Permutations may be used to obtain corresponding p-values in the latter case [6], but it was not done in this work because of prohibitive computational time.

3 Validation Framework

The Euclidean, the Log-Euclidean and the Riemannian frameworks are compared on both simulated and real data. All DT-MRI images were acquired on a 1.5T Siemens scanner with 30 encoding gradients (b-value of 1000 s/mm^2) and two baseline images (*i.e.*, b-value of 0 s/mm^2). The image dimensions are $128 \times 128 \times 41$ and the spatial resolution is $1.8 \times 1.8 \times 3.5\ mm^3$.

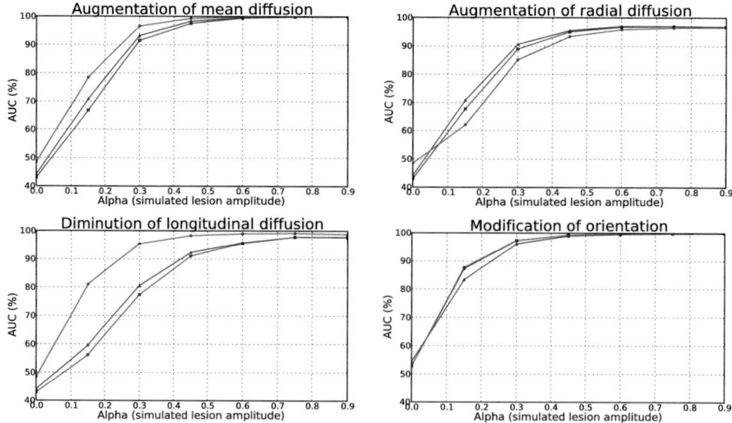

Fig. 2. Area under the ROC curve (AUC) *vs* lesion amplitude (α) (Legend: ● = GLM-DT, ▲ = GLM-LOG-DT, ■ = MGLM)

3.1 Synthetic Data

A set of 11 images with simulated lesions in the corpus callosum (CC) are generated from the DT-MRI acquisitions of 11 healthy subjects. We focused on the CC since it consists of a single direction white matter tract, where the tensor assumption holds. These simulated images, considered in the experiments as the patient group, are compared with the group of 11 images of healthy subjects, introducing age, gender, and group affiliation as covariates. For the statistical test, the group affiliation is discarded in the restricted model. Four kinds of lesions are simulated: mean and radial diffusion augmentation, longitudinal diffusion diminution and diffusion orientation modification. A parameter $\alpha \in [0 : 0.9]$ controls the amplitude of the simulated lesions (Fig.1). An image is generated for each α and each kind of lesions, leading to $4 \times 19 = 76$ groups of 11 patients images. The three first kind of lesion are consistent with real case scenarios [11]. The last one is rather a toy example, since a realistic diffusion orientation modification would imply the deflection of the whole trajectory of a fiber bundle.

Methods are compared using ROC analysis, which allows to compare the statistical maps with the ground truth for various statistical thresholds. The area under the ROC curve (AUC) is computed for each experiment. An AUC of 50% corresponds to a random detection and 100% to a perfect detection. AUCs are plotted with respect to the lesions amplitude α for each kind of simulated lesion (Fig. 2). This way, it is possible to assess the performance of each method for major changes as well as smaller ones and for different types of lesions.

3.2 Neuromyelitis Optica Cohort

The Neuromyelitis Optica (NMO) is an inflammatory disease characterized by alterations of the normal-appearing white matter in relation to several disorders [12]. A group of 34 patients suffering from NMO are compared to a group

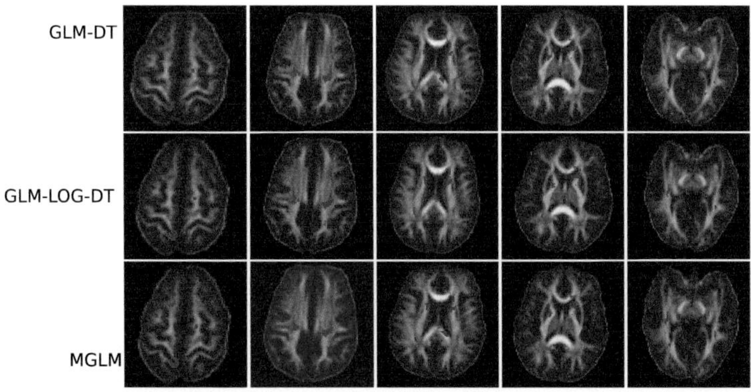

Fig. 3. Results obtained for the three methods on the comparison of NMO patients ($n = 34$) to healthy subjects ($n = 22$). The statistical thresholds have been chosen to detect the 5% most significant voxels within the white matter mask for each method. Clusters of less than 10 voxels are discarded.

of 22 healthy subjects by considering age, gender, and group affiliation as covariates. For the statistical test, the group affiliation is discarded in the restricted model. Since the F-statistic maps may not follow the same distribution for the three methods, they cannot be compared by using the same statistical threshold. To obtain comparable detection maps, the threshold is adjusted for each method to obtain the same number of detected voxels within the white matter mask for each method. To compare the similarity of the detection maps obtained by two methods, the Dice coefficient is computed. This is done for a wide range of thresholds (adjusted for each method) in order to compare the behavior of the three methods for different levels of sensitivity (Fig. 4).

4 Results

4.1 Results on Synthetic Data

The results on simulated data are summed up in Fig. 2. They highlight that the performance of the methods varies with the kind of simulated changes. On one hand, the *GLM-DT* outperforms the two other methods for detecting a mean diffusivity augmentation and a longitudinal diffusion diminution. On the other hand, the *GLM-LOG-DT* and the *MGLM* exhibit better results for detecting an augmentation of the radial diffusion. Notice that all the three methods show similar performance for detecting modifications of orientation. Finally, it has to be pointed out that the Log-Euclidean and Riemannian frameworks lead to very close results.

4.2 Results on NMO Patients

Fig.3 shows the results obtained by the three methods for the comparison of 34 NMO patients to 22 healthy subjects. The statistical thresholds have been

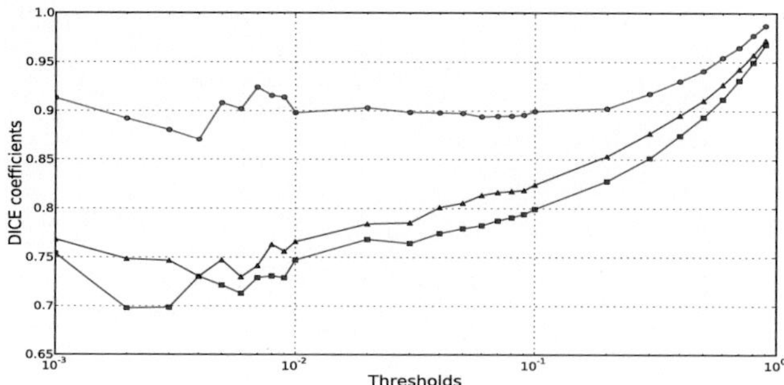

Fig. 4. Dice coefficient *vs* percentage of detected voxels in logarithmic scale (Legend: ● = MGLM / GLM-LOG-DT, ▲ = GLM-DT / GLM-LOG-DT, ■ = MGLM / GLM-DT)

chosen to detect the 5% most significant voxels within the white matter mask for each method. Visually, all three methods lead to very close results, which does not allow us to assert that one method outperforms the others. They succeed to detect the regions involved in the NMO pathology [12]: the visual cortex, the corticospinal tract and the CC that are respectively related to the visual, motor and cognitive disorders induced by the pathology. To strengthen the claim that there is no significant difference between the methods on these data, the Dice coefficient for the three couples are presented in Fig. 4 for several statistical thresholds. It shows a good agreement between the methods, with a Dice coefficient always greater than 70%. The best agreement is obtained between the *GLM-LOG-DT* and *MGLM* frameworks (Dice coefficient greater than 90%), which is in accordance with the conclusion on simulated data.

5 Conclusion and Discussion

In this paper, the Euclidean, the Log-Euclidean and a Riemannian framework have been compared in the context of a DT-MRI group comparison. The experimental results on simulated lesions highlight that all methods can efficiently detect the four kinds of lesions, with performance varying for each framework according to the kind of simulated lesions. The results on the real database confirm the good ability of the three methods to detect the regions affected by the NMO, without exhibiting any significant difference between the detection maps. Typical computation time on a standard workstation is about 2 min for the Euclidean and Log-Euclidean approaches as compared to more than 80 hours for the Riemannian framework on the real database with the provided implemantation. This time gap may probably be reduced by optimizing the implementation of the Riemannian framework, for instance by rewriting the matlab code in C++ language. But in any case, the Riemannian framework would still be much more computationally intensive than the Euclidean and Log-Euclidean approaches. In conclusion, this study suggests that, despite the mathematical elegance offered by the Riemannian framework, its superiority on both simulated and real clinical data could not be demonstrated compared to the Euclidean and Log-Euclidean frameworks. For a similar performance, these two latter methods present the advantage to be easily implementable and computationally effective. Bearing in mind the limitation of tensors to model crossing fibers, we plan to investigate more complex diffusion models.

Acknowledgements. We thank Pr Jérome de Sèze for the recruitment of NMO patients and Pr Stéphane Kremer for image acquisitions.

References

1. Penny, W., Friston, K., Ashburner, J., Kirbel, S., Nichols, T.: Statistical Parametric Mapping: The Analysis of Functional Brain Images. Elsevier LTD, Oxford (2006)
2. Smith, S., Jenkinson, M., Johansen-Berg, H., Rueckert, D., Nichols, T., Mackay, C., Watkins, K., Ciccarelli, O., Cader, M., Matthews, P., Behrens, T.: Tract based spatial statistics: voxelwise analysis of multi-subjects diffusion data. NeuroImage 31(4), 1487–1505 (2006)
3. Whitcher, B., Wisco, J.J., Hadjikhani, N., Tuch, D.S.: Statistical group comparison of diffusion tensors via multivariate hypothesis testing. Magn. Reson. Med. 57(6), 1065–1074 (2007)
4. Zhu, H., Chen, Y., Ibrahim, J., Li, Y., Hall, C., Lin, W.: Intrinsic regression models for positive-definite matrices with applications to Diffusion Tensor Imaging. Journal of the American Statistical Association 104(487), 1203–1212 (2009)
5. Schwartzman, A., Dougherty, R., Taylor, J.: Group comparison of eigenvalues and eigenvectors of diffusion tensors. Journal of the American Statistical Association 105(490), 588–599 (2010)
6. Kim, H., Bendlin, B., Adluru, N., Collins, M., Chung, M., Johnson, S., Davidson, R., Singh, V.: Multivariate General Linear Models (MGLM) on Riemannian Manifolds with Applications to Statistical Analysis of Diffusion Weighted Images. In: 2014 IEEE Conference on Computer Vision and Pattern Recognition (CVPR), pp. 2705–2712 (June 2014)
7. Bouchon, A., Noblet, V., Heitz, F., Lamy, J., Blanc, F., Armspach, J.P.: General linear models for group studies in diffusion tensor imaging. In: Proceedings of International Symposium on Biomedical Imaging: From Nano to Macro, Beijing, China (2014)
8. Arsigny, V., Fillard, P., Pennec, X., Ayache, N.: Log-euclidean metrics for fast and simple calculus on diffusion tensors. In: Magnetic Resonance in Medicine (2006)
9. Pasternak, O., Sochen, N., Basser, P.J.: The effect of metric selection on the analysis of diffusion tensor MRI data. NeuroImage 49(3), 2190–2204 (2010)
10. Noblet, V., Heinrich, C., Heitz, F., Armspach, J.P.: Retrospective evaluation of a topology preserving non-rigid registration method. Medical Image Analysis 10(3), 366–384 (2006)
11. Harsan, L.A., Poulet, P., Guignard, B., Steibel, J., Parizel, N., de Sousa, P., Boehm, N., Grucker, D., Ghandour, M.S.: Brain dysmyelination and recovery assessment by noninvasive in vivo diffusion tensor magnetic resonance imaging. Journal of Neuroscience Research 83(3), 392–402 (2006)
12. Yu, C., Lin, F., Li, K., Jiang, T., Qin, W., Sun, H., Chan, P.: Pathologenesis of normal-appearing white matter damage in neuromyelitis optica: Diffusion-Tensor MR Imaging. Radiology 246(1), 222–228 (2008)

Convex Non-negative Spherical Factorization of Multi-Shell Diffusion-Weighted Images

Daan Christiaens[1,4], Frederik Maes[1,4], Stefan Sunaert[2,4], and Paul Suetens[1,3,4]

[1] KU Leuven, Dept. of Electrical Engineering, ESAT/PSI, Medical Image Computing
[2] KU Leuven, Dept. of Imaging and Pathology, Translational MRI
[3] iMinds, Medical IT Department
[4] UZ Leuven, Medical Imaging Research Center
Herestraat 49 – 7003, 3000 Leuven, Belgium

Abstract. Diffusion-weighted imaging (DWI) allows to probe tissue microstructure non-invasively and study healthy and diseased white matter (WM) in vivo. Yet, less research has focussed on modelling grey matter (GM), cerebrospinal fluid (CSF) and other tissues. Here, we introduce a fully data-driven approach to spherical deconvolution, based on convex non-negative matrix factorization. Our approach decomposes multi-shell DWI data, represented in the basis of spherical harmonics, into tissue-specific orientation distribution functions and corresponding response functions. We evaluate the proposed method in phantom simulations and in vivo brain images, and demonstrate its ability to reconstruct WM, GM and CSF, unsupervised and solely relying on DWI.

1 Introduction

Diffusion-weighted imaging (DWI) is a non-invasive MRI modality that allows to probe tissue microstructure in vivo by measuring its hinderance to the diffusion process of water [1]. DWI has found applications in neuroscientific research into brain organization and disease processes, as well as clinical applications such as diagnosing acute stroke and neurosurgical planning based on tractography.

Since it was recognised that diffusion anisotropy is indicative of axonal structure in the nervous system [2], research has largely focussed on reconstructing fibre orientation and connectivity in white matter (WM). On the one hand, a myriad of biophysical models have been introduced [3], which aim to estimate microstructure parameters such as axon diameter or dispersion. On the other hand, spherical deconvolution (SD) approaches estimate the fibre orientation distribution function (ODF), given a fibre response function (RF) that is typically estimated from and hence adapted to the data at hand [4]. However, this calibration of the RF may severely impact the reconstructed fibre ODF [5, 6]. Additionally, the presence of partial volume effects (PVE), originating from adjacent grey matter (GM) and cerebrospinal fluid (CSF), has been shown to affect SD [7]. Hence, the question arises how to accurately represent both WM and other tissues, as well as pathology.

N. Navab et al. (Eds.): MICCAI 2015, Part I, LNCS 9349, pp. 166–173, 2015.
DOI: 10.1007/978-3-319-24553-9_21

Recent work has extended SD to multiple tissue types [8]. Yet, for calibrating the tissue response functions they rely on a prior tissue segmentation obtained from a T1-weighted MR image, which may not always be available or may not be well aligned to the DWI data, e.g., due to EPI distortion [9]. In this paper, we present a more general take on spherical deconvolution, formulated as convex non-negative matrix factorization (NMF) [10] in the basis of spherical harmonics, in which tissue-specific RFs and ODFs are estimated simultaneously from the DWI data itself, without the need for external input.

NMF has previously been applied to diffusion tensor imaging (DTI) data [11], which we now generalize to (multi-shell) high angular resolution imaging (HARDI). The dictionary learning approach introduced in [12] is also based on NMF but assumes sparsity of the reconstructed ODFs. Here, we do not impose any constraints on the ODFs except for non-negativity. Instead, we constrain the tissue RFs to be convex combinations of the data voxels. As such, physical plausibility of the tissue responses is ensured in a purely data-driven manner.

We evaluate accuracy of the estimated tissue RFs and ODFs in simulations on in silico data, and demonstrate the method on real brain data. In addition, we investigate the required number of NMF sources in healthy subjects and in the presence of pathology, and show that they can be associated to known anatomy.

2 Method

Assuming linear partial volume effect (PVE), the diffusion signal in each voxel, for gradient direction $\boldsymbol{g}$ and given b-value, $S_b(\boldsymbol{g})$, can be decomposed into N tissues, each of which are characterized by an axially symmetric response function $H_{t,b}(\theta)$. Each tissue t then contributes to the signal in a voxel as the spherical convolution of its RF and an orientation distribution $F_t(\theta, \phi)$, i.e.,

$$S_b(\boldsymbol{g}) \approx \sum_{t=1}^{N} (H_{t,b} * F_t)(\boldsymbol{g}) \quad .$$

When S_b and F_t are represented in the basis of real, symmetric spherical harmonics (SH) of maximum order $\ell_{\max}$, and the response functions $H_{t,b}$ are represented as zonal harmonics (phase $m = 0$), the convolution reduces to a multiplication of the coefficients of corresponding order ℓ, i.e., $s_b(\ell, m) = \sum_t \sqrt{\frac{4\pi}{2\ell+1}} h_{t,b}(\ell)\, f_t(\ell, m)$ with $\ell \in \{0, 2, \ldots, \ell_{\max}\}$ and $m \in [-\ell, \ell]$ [4,8]. We then structure the SH coefficients of all voxels v and shells b in the tensor equation

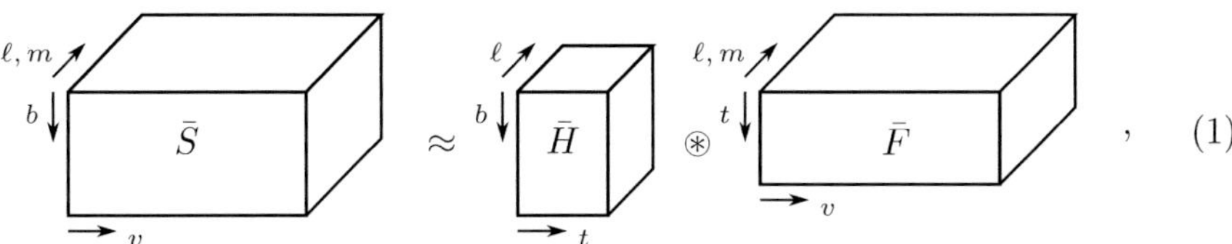

(1)

where $\bar{H}$ contains the RF coefficients and $\bar{F}$ the coefficients of the tissue ODFs. The operator $\circledast$ is used to denote spherical convolution in the SH basis, and corresponds to the matrix product of every slice $F_{\cdot,\cdot,(\ell,m)}$ with slice $H_{\cdot,\cdot,\ell}$ of corresponding order ℓ. For all voxels and tissues, the coefficients $\boldsymbol{f}_{v,t,\cdot}$ are constrained to represent non-negative functions. Note that the $\ell = 0$ coefficients of $\bar{F}$ represent the isotropic volume fraction or density of each tissue.

In this work, we do not assume that the response functions $\bar{H}$ are known a priori. As such, expression (1) becomes a blind source separation problem in the form of non-negative matrix factorization (NMF) [10], in which a data matrix is decomposed as the product of a source matrix and a non-negative weight matrix. In this case, the unknown sources are the tissue-specific response functions, the weights are the tissue ODFs, and we aim to find

$$\bar{H}^{\star}, \bar{F}^{\star} = \arg \min_{(\bar{H},\bar{F})} \|\bar{S} - \bar{H} \circledast \bar{F}\|_F^2, \text{ s.t. } A\,\boldsymbol{f}_{v,t,\cdot} \geq 0 \quad , \tag{2}$$

where A is a matrix that evaluates the SH basis across a dense set of directions and ensures non-negativity of the tissue ODFs. In addition, we impose that all sources H_t are a convex combination of the measured signal after reorientation. To achieve this, we compute an auxiliary tensor $\bar{Z}$ that contains, for each voxel v, the coefficients of the best fitting zonal harmonics to the data S_v across all possible orientations of the symmetry axis. The tissue RFs are then represented as $h_{t,b,\ell} = \boldsymbol{z}_{\cdot,b,\ell} \cdot \boldsymbol{w}_{t,\cdot}$, with voxel weights $W \geq 0$ and $\|\boldsymbol{w}_{t,\cdot}\|_1 = 1$.

The resulting convex non-negative factorization problem is solved by alternatingly solving for $\bar{F}$ and W, starting from an initialization for $\bar{H}$ which we obtain from k-means clustering in the space of best-fitting zonal harmonics $\bar{Z}$. We solve (2) for the ODFs $\bar{F}$ in each voxel by unfolding all tensors along the dimensions of shells and SH coefficients. This results in the constrained least-squares expression identical to multi-shell multi-tissue spherical deconvolution [8], which is solved with quadratic programming (QP) given the non-negativity constraints on $\bar{F}$. Subsequently, (2) can be solved for $\bar{H}$ by unfolding across all voxels and SH coefficients. Imposing the convexity constraint furthermore requires unfolding across shells to solve directly for the weights W in one global QP problem. This procedure is repeated for 10 iterations, which we found to be sufficient for convergence (the relative decrease in residual was consistently $< 1\%$).

We implemented the factorization method in Python, using a custom SH basis implementation and CVXOPT (`cvxopt.org`) for optimizing the QP problems.

3 Experiments and Results

3.1 Monte-Carlo Simulations

We simulated a phantom dataset with the geometry shown in Fig. 1. The phantom contains 3 tissue classes, mimicking WM, GM and CSF regions, each simulated by a ground-truth RF that was originally estimated from in vivo data according to the procedure advised in [8]. The WM ODF is represented at $\ell_{\max} = 10$. GM and CSF are modelled isotropically ($\ell_{\max} = 0$). The original

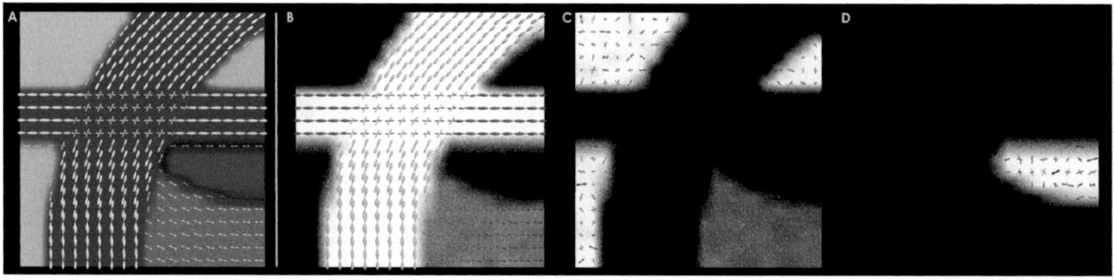

Fig. 1. (A) Ground truth geometry of simulated WM (*blue*), GM (*green*), CSF (*red*), and WM-GM PVE (*cyan*). (B-D) Estimated ODFs of 3 components at SNR 20.

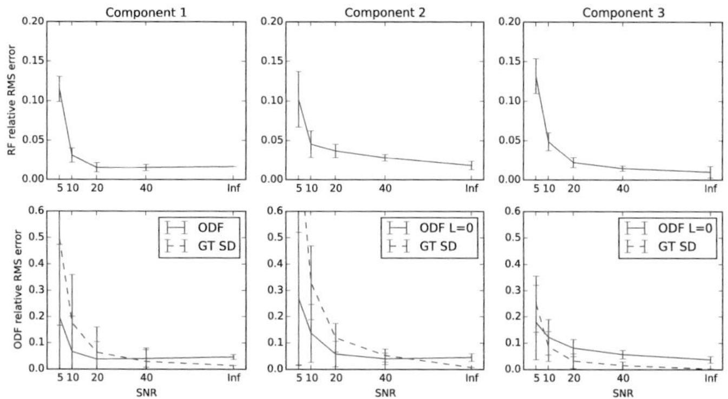

Fig. 2. Measures of accuracy and precision of the proposed method on the simulated phantom. *Top row:* Response function accuracy as a function of signal-to-noise ratio (SNR). *Bottom row:* ODF accuracy as a function of SNR, restricted to the isotropic volume fraction ($\ell_{\max} = 0$) in case of components 2 and 3. The dashed lines represent the ODF accuracy in case of direct deconvolution with the ground truth kernels.

phantom was generated at 100×100 voxels and subsampled to 20×20 voxels to simulate PVE. Finally, we sampled the signal with the gradient scheme of the Human Connectome Project [13], and added Rician noise for signal-to-noise ratios (SNR) ranging from 5 to ∞. At each SNR, 100 noise realizations of the data were generated.

We applied the proposed method to estimate $N = 3$ components in the phantom. Accuracy and precision of the RFs and ODFs are measured by the relative root-mean-square (RMS) error of the amplitude. Results for one noise realization at SNR 20 are shown in Fig. 1. Component 1 corresponds well with WM and the fibre directions are nicely recovered. Components 2 and 3 correspond to GM and CSF. Although the estimated ODFs contain spurious peaks, the isotropic density ($\ell = 0$ coefficient) closely matches the isotropic ground truth. The RF and ODF accuracy and precision are plotted in Fig. 2 and confirm these observations. The accuracy of the estimated RFs is good (error $< 5\%$ for SNR ≥ 10)

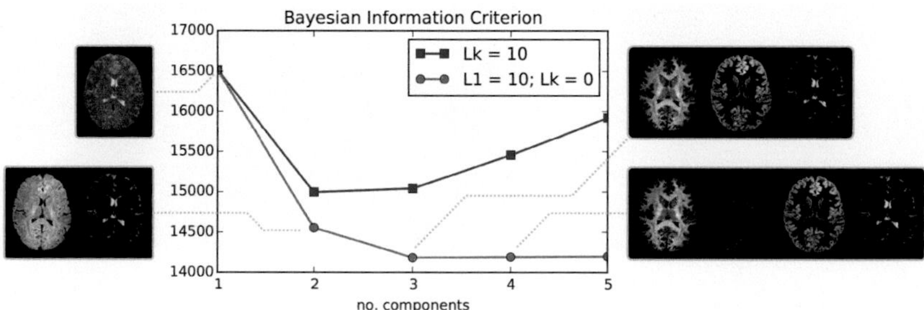

Fig. 3. Model selection for dataset 1. Plot of the Bayesian information criterion for varying no. anisotropic components (blue) and one anisotropic and a range of isotropic components (green), annotated with the volume fractions of the estimated components.

and improves with increasing SNR. The accuracy of the WM ODF and of the density of GM and CSF is in the same range. Notably, our approach outperforms direct SD with the ground-truth RFs in the low SNR range (dashed line). We attribute this to the Rician noise floor, particularly at high *b*-values, which the joint RF estimation may be able to model, whereas direct SD can not.

3.2 Results on Human Brain Data

We evaluate our method in data of two neurologically healthy subjects and in one post-surgery image of a patient who suffered a grade IV glioma in the right temporal lobe. Dataset 1 was provided by the Human Connectome Project [13]. Dataset 2 and 3 were acquired in house on a Philips Achieva 3T system, using an isotropic voxel size of 2.5 mm, and 10, 25, 40, 75 gradients at *b*-values 0, 700, 1000, and 2800 $^{s}/_{mm^2}$ respectively. Dataset 2 was corrected for motion, eddy current, and EPI distortions using reverse-phase encoding in the *b*0 [9].

In order to keep the computational requirements low, we apply our method in a random subset of 1000 voxels, which takes about 8 min. Afterwards, the ODFs of the entire dataset are computed as the deconvolution with the estimated RFs. The estimated RFs were verified to be robust to this subsampling (e.g., the precision of the WM response on 50 runs is $< 5\%$).

First, we investigate the required number of sources and their maximal SH order for the healthy human brain. We vary the number of sources from 1 to 5 and compare two cases, one in which all sources are modelled up to $\ell_{\text{max}} = 10$, and one in which only the first is modelled in this way and all others are modelled isotropically. We use the Bayesian information criterion (BIC) [14] to find the optimal balance between model fit and model complexity. The result is plotted in Fig. 3 and shows that minimal BIC is obtained with one anisotropic and at least two isotropic components. Slices of the corresponding tissue volume fractions are shown as well and allow for a better interpretation of this result. The first 3 components can be associated to WM, GM and CSF. Additional components can not be related to known anatomy. Similar results were obtained in dataset 2.

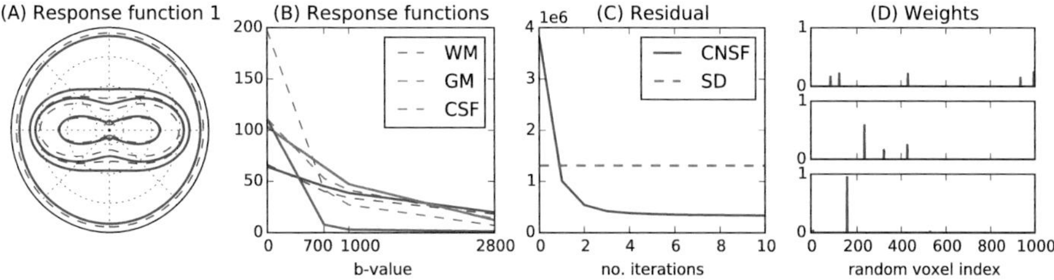

Fig. 4. Estimated response functions for dataset 2. From left to right: (A) anisotropic response function, and (B) radial component of all response functions (full lines), compared to the WM, GM and CSF response estimated as in [8] (dashed lines); (C) residual compared to the supervised method; (D) weights of the response estimation.

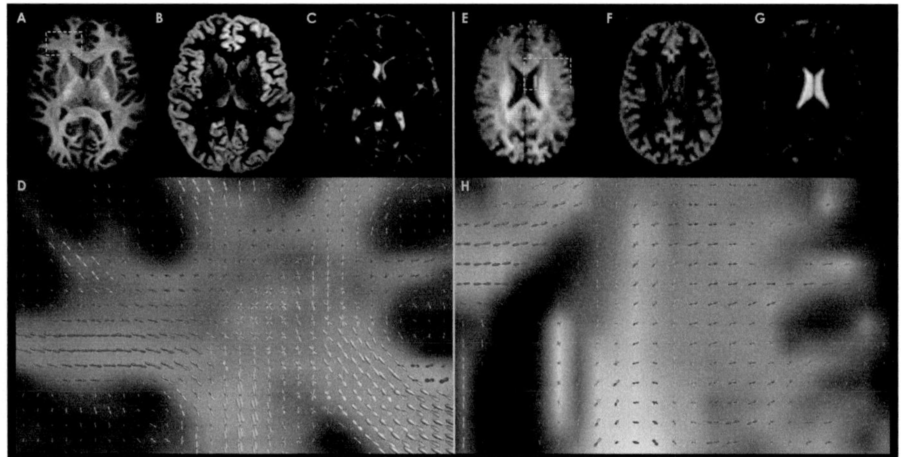

Fig. 5. Estimated tissue ODFs. (A-D) for dataset 1. (E-H) for dataset 2.

Based on the optimal model complexity, we apply the proposed method to decompose both DWI datasets into 3 tissue classes, two of which are modelled isotropically. The response functions of dataset 2 are depicted on the left in Fig. 4, and compared to the response functions of WM, GM, and CSF, estimated as described in [8] based on a prior segmentation of the T1 image (dashed lines). The RFs estimated in our (unsupervised) method qualitatively correspond to those obtained from the supervised method, up to a scaling factor. Moreover, we consistently obtained a smaller residual fitting error given the same model complexity, as shown in Fig. 4. Notice how the algorithm converges after about 5 iterations. The graphs on the right of Fig. 4 show the weights W by which each voxel contributes to the estimated kernels. Interestingly, these are naturally sparse in convex NMF, as pointed out in [10]. In Fig. 5, we show the tissue ODFs for both datasets. The ODF of component 1 closely resembles the fibre ODF in [8] and nicely captures partial voluming at the WM-GM interface.

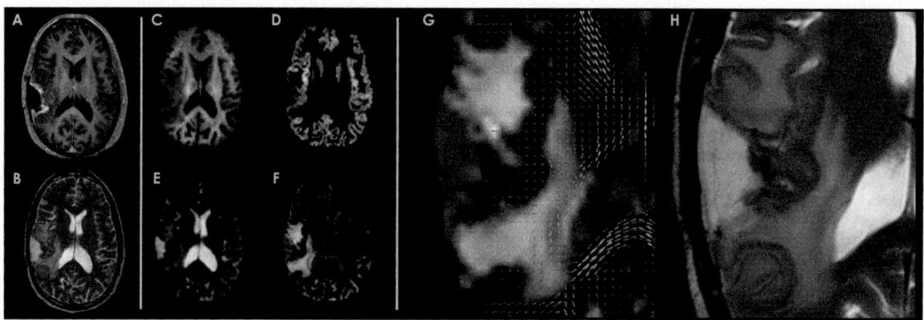

Fig. 6. Results of dataset 3. (A-B) T1 and T2. (C-F) Tissue ODFs of 4 components. (G-H) Close-up of the WM ODF, overlaid onto the estimated edema density, and T2.

For dataset 3, the model selection as described above suggested one anisotropic and 3 isotropic kernels, and the resulting tissue ODFs are shown in Fig. 6. Results indicate that, in addition to WM, GM, and CSF, edema is detected as a 4th component. Notice that CSF is detected in the surgical cavity.

4 Discussion and Conclusion

In this work, we introduced a generalization of multi-tissue SD as a blind source separation problem, formulated as convex NMF in the SH basis. Like SD, our approach assumes non-negativity of the tissue ODFs and spatial invariance of their RFs, but jointly optimizes the RFs instead of assuming them as known.

As such, our method is an unsupervised RF estimation method that, in contrast to [8], does not require (alignment to) a T1-segmentation. Instead, we impose the convexity constraint to ensure that the RF is actually observed in the data, typically in a sparse set of voxels. Not only does this broaden the application of multi-tissue SD to DWI data that could not be corrected for distortions or for which no T1 is available, ultimately a better fit to the data was obtained.

For the normal brain, we found optimal model complexity with one anisotropic and two isotropic RFs, which can be associated to WM, GM, and CSF, and agrees with the model adopted in [8]. Instead of imposing such model explicitly, our method is more flexible in that it allows to estimate the most suitable number of sources and their SH order from the data itself. For instance in brain tumour data, our method detected the need for a 4th component that could be associated to edema. We expect that, by explicitly accounting for edema, the reconstructed WM ODF is less contaminated by the increased diffusion, which may facilitate tracing WM fibre bundles through edema. Possibly, this approach can be extended to characterize tissue heterogeneity within the tumour itself.

In future work, the presented method may be applied to explore tissue microstructure and growth patterns in brain tumours, as well as in other organs. Furthermore, a straightforward extension to multiple subjects can be used for group analyses of patients and controls.

Acknowledgements. D. Christiaens is supported by a Ph.D. grant of the Agency for Innovation by Science and Technology (IWT). Data were provided in part by the Human Connectome Project, WU-Minn Consortium (Principal Investigators: David Van Essen and Kamil Ugurbil; 1U54MH091657) funded by the 16 NIH Institutes and Centers that support the NIH Blueprint for Neuroscience Research; and by the McDonnell Center for Systems Neuroscience at Washington University.

References

1. Le Bihan, D., Breton, E., Lallemand, D., Grenier, P., Cabanis, E., Laval-Jeantet, M.: MR imaging of intravoxel incoherent motions: application to diffusion and perfusion in neurologic disorders. Radiology 161(2), 401–407 (1986)
2. Beaulieu, C.: The basis of anisotropic water diffusion in the nervous system – a technical review. NMR in Biomedicine 15(7-8), 435–455 (2002)
3. Panagiotaki, E., Schneider, T., Siow, B., Hall, M.G., Lythgoe, M.F., Alexander, D.C.: Compartment models of the diffusion MR signal in brain white matter: A taxonomy and comparison. NeuroImage 59(3), 2241–2254 (2012)
4. Tournier, J.-D., Calamante, F., Connelly, A.: Robust determination of the fibre orientation distribution in diffusion MRI: Non-negativity constrained super-resolved spherical deconvolution. NeuroImage 35(4), 1459–1472 (2007)
5. Parker, G.D., Marshall, D., Rosin, P.L., Drage, N., Richmond, S., Jones, D.K.: A pitfall in the reconstruction of fibre ODFs using spherical deconvolution of diffusion MRI data. NeuroImage 65, 433–448 (2013)
6. Schultz, T., Groeschel, S.: Auto-calibrating spherical deconvolution based on ODF sparsity. In: Mori, K., Sakuma, I., Sato, Y., Barillot, C., Navab, N. (eds.) MICCAI 2013, Part I. LNCS, vol. 8149, pp. 663–670. Springer, Heidelberg (2013)
7. Roine, T., Jeurissen, B., Perrone, D., Aelterman, J., Leemans, A., Philips, W., Sijbers, J.: Isotropic non-white matter partial volume effects in constrained spherical deconvolution. Frontiers in Neuroinformatics 8 (2014)
8. Jeurissen, B., Tournier, J.-D., Dhollander, T., Connelly, A., Sijbers, J.: Multi-tissue constrained spherical deconvolution for improved analysis of multi-shell diffusion MRI data. NeuroImage 103, 411–426 (2014)
9. Andersson, J.L.R., Skare, S., Ashburner, J.: How to correct susceptibility distortions in spin-echo echo-planar images: application to diffusion tensor imaging. NeuroImage 20(2), 870–888 (2003)
10. Ding, C.H.Q., Li, T., Jordan, M.I.: Convex and semi-nonnegative matrix factorizations. IEEE Trans. on Pattern Analysis and Machine Intelligence 32(1), 45–55 (2010)
11. Xie, Y., Ho, J., Vemuri, B.: Nonnegative factorization of diffusion tensor images and its applications. In: Szkely, G., Hahn, H. (eds.) Information Processing in Medical Imaging. LNCS, vol. 6801, pp. 550–561. Springer, Heidelberg (2011)
12. Reisert, M., Skibbe, H., Kiselev, V.G.: The diffusion dictionary in the human brain is short: Rotation invariant learning of basis functions. In: Schultz, T., Nedjati-Gilani, G., Venkataraman, A., O'Donnell, L., Panagiotaki, E. (eds.) Computational Diffusion MRI and Brain Connectivity. Mathematics and Visualization, pp. 47–55. Springer, Heidelberg (2014)
13. Van Essen, D., Smith, S., Barch, D., Behrens, T., Yacoub, E., Ugurbil, K.: The WU-Minn human connectome project: An overview. NeuroImage 80, 62–79 (2013)
14. Schwarz, G.: Estimating the dimension of a model. The Annals of Statistics 6(2), 461–464 (1978)

Tensorial Spherical Polar Fourier Diffusion MRI with Optimal Dictionary Learning

Jian Cheng[1], Dinggang Shen[2], Pew-Thian Yap[2], and Peter J. Basser[1]

[1] Section on Tissue Biophysics and Biomimetics (STBB), PPITS, NICHD, NIBIB
[2] Department of Radiology and BRIC, University of North Carolina at Chapel Hill, USA
{jian.cheng,pb12q}@nih.gov

Abstract. High Angular Resolution Diffusion Imaging (HARDI) can characterize complex white matter micro-structure, avoiding the Gaussian diffusion assumption inherent in Diffusion Tensor Imaging (DTI). However, HARDI methods normally require significantly more signal measurements and a longer scan time than DTI, which limits its clinical utility. By considering sparsity of the diffusion signal, Compressed Sensing (CS) allows robust signal reconstruction from relatively fewer samples, reducing the scanning time. A good dictionary that sparsifies the signal is crucial for CS reconstruction. In this paper, we propose a novel method called Tensorial Spherical Polar Fourier Imaging (TSPFI) to recover continuous diffusion signal and diffusion propagator by representing the diffusion signal using an orthonormal TSPF basis. TSPFI is a generalization of the existing model-based method DTI and the model-free method SPFI. We also propose dictionary learning TSPFI (DL-TSPFI) to learn an even sparser dictionary represented as a linear combination of TSPF basis from continuous mixture of Gaussian signals. The learning process is efficiently performed in a small subspace of SPF coefficients, and the learned dictionary is proved to be sparse for all mixture of Gaussian signals by adaptively setting the tensor in TSPF basis. Then the learned DL-TSPF dictionary is optimally and adaptively applied to different voxels using DTI and a weighted LASSO for CS reconstruction. DL-TSPFI is a generalization of DL-SPFI, by considering general adaptive tensor setting instead of a scale value. The experiments demonstrated that the learned DL-TSPF dictionary has a sparser representation and lower reconstruction Root-Mean-Squared-Error (RMSE) than both the original SPF basis and the DL-SPF dictionary.

1 Introduction

Diffusion MRI (dMRI) is a unique non-invasive imaging technique to explore white matter in human brain by measuring the diffusion of water molecules. The diffusion process is fully characterized by the diffusion propagator $P(\mathbf{R})$, called the Ensemble Average Propagator (EAP), in the displacement $\mathbf{R}$-space [1]. With the narrow pulse assumption, the diffusion signal attenuation $E(\mathbf{q})$ is the 3D Fourier transform of $P(\mathbf{R})$, i.e., $P(\mathbf{R}) = \int_{\mathbb{R}^3} E(\mathbf{q}) \exp(-2\pi \mathbf{q}^T \mathbf{R}) d\mathbf{q}$. A hot topic in dMRI is to recover the continuous signal $E(\mathbf{q})$ and the EAP $P(\mathbf{R})$ from a limited number of signal samples with noise.

Diffusion Tensor Imaging (DTI) [2] is the most popular method for diffusion data reconstruction. With the Gaussian diffusion assumption, $E(\mathbf{q}) = \exp(-4\pi^2 \tau \mathbf{q}^T \mathbf{D} \mathbf{q})$ where

N. Navab et al. (Eds.): MICCAI 2015, Part I, LNCS 9349, pp. 174–182, 2015.
DOI: 10.1007/978-3-319-24553-9_22

τ is the diffusion time and $\mathbf{D}$ is the 3×3 diffusion tensor. Many other methods, categorized as High Angular Resolution Diffusion Imaging (HARDI), were proposed to avoid the Gaussian assumption and characterize more general diffusion processes due to complex microstructure. Diffusion spectrum imaging [3] does not impose any assumption on diffusion signal, but it requires a long scan time, and only estimates diffusion signal and propagator in discretized samples, not in a continuous domain. MAP-MRI [4,5] and Spherical Polar Fourier Imaging (SPFI) [6,7] are two state-of-the-art methods, which estimate continuous $E(\mathbf{q})$ and $P(\mathbf{R})$ from arbitrary sampling schemes by representing $E(\mathbf{q})$ using orthonormal basis functions with analytic Fourier transform.

The Compressed Sensing (CS) technique recovers a signal from measurements by considering the sparsity of the signal under a dictionary. CS methods have been proposed in dMRI to recover diffusion signal and propagator using both discretized [8] and continuous bases [7]. The most important advantage of the continuous basis representation is that it allows the analytical Fourier transform without numerical error. In CS reconstruction, a dictionary that yields sparse representation of diffusion signals plays an important role. MAP-MRI was first proposed using an isotropic tensor in its basis [4], then using a general tensor [5]. SPFI first used SPF basis [9,6], then learned an adaptive sparser dictionary based on SPF basis from continuous Gaussian signal space [7]. All those evolutions make the dictionaries in MAP-MRI and SPFI sparser and more suitable for CS reconstruction. However, existing MAP-MRI in [5] still uses manually devised basis without performing dictionary learning, and existing SPFI in [6] and DL-SPFI in [7] use isotropic Gaussian diffusion in its dictionary, which is limited to represent diffusion signals with high anisotropy.

In this paper, we propose Tensorial SPFI which generalizes SPFI [6] by considering a general adaptive tensor setting instead of using just a simple scalar value, and we also propose TSPFI with optimal dictionary learning, called DL-TSPFI, to learn an even sparser dictionary from only a small subspace of SPF coefficients of Gaussian diffusion signals. The learned dictionary is proven to be capable to sparsely represent an arbitrary mixture of Gaussian diffusion signals, by considering an adaptive tensor setting. The learned dictionary is then adaptively applied to all voxels using a weighted LASSO optimization with adaptive tensor setting from DTI for CS reconstruction. Experiments demonstrated that TSPFI and DL-TSPFI provide sparser representation and yield low RMSE in CS reconstruction than the state-of-the-art SPFI [6] and DL-SPFI [7].

2 Tensorial Spherical Polar Fourier Imaging (TSPFI)

The SPF basis is a continuous orthonormal basis that can sparsely represent Gaussian-like 3D signal [9,6]. In SPFI, the diffusion signal is represented by the SPF basis $\{B_{nlm}(\mathbf{q}|\zeta) = G_n(q|\zeta)Y_l^m(\mathbf{u})\}$, i.e.,

$$E(q\mathbf{u}|\zeta) = \sum_{n=0}^{N}\sum_{l=0}^{L}\sum_{m=-l}^{l} a_{nlm} G_n(q|\zeta) Y_l^m(\mathbf{u}),\ G_n(q|\zeta) = \left[\frac{2n!}{\zeta^{3/2}\Gamma(n+3/2)}\right]^{1/2} \exp\left(-\frac{q^2}{2\zeta}\right) L_n^{1/2}\left(\frac{q^2}{\zeta}\right) \tag{1}$$

where $\mathbf{q} = q\mathbf{u}$, $\mathbf{u} \in \mathbb{S}^2$, ζ is the scale parameter and $Y_l^m(\mathbf{u})$ is the real spherical harmonic basis. It was proven that the EAP can be analytically represented by dual SPF basis [6]:

$$P(R\mathbf{r}|\zeta) = \sum_{n=0}^{N}\sum_{l=0}^{L}\sum_{m=-l}^{l} a_{nlm} F_{nl}(R|\zeta) Y_l^m(\mathbf{r}) \qquad B_{nlm}^{\text{dual}}(\mathbf{R}|\zeta) = F_{nl}(R|\zeta) Y_l^m(\mathbf{r}) \tag{2}$$

where $\mathbf{R} = R\mathbf{r}$, $\mathbf{r} \in \mathbb{S}^2$, and the definition of $F_{nl}(R|\zeta)$ can be found in [6]. It can be seen that $B_{000}(\mathbf{q})$ is just an isotropic Gaussian function, which makes the SPF representation sparse for isotropic Gaussian signal $E(\mathbf{q}) = \exp(-4\pi^2\tau\mathbf{q}^T\mathbf{D}\mathbf{q})$. However it requires more basis elements to represent a Gaussian signal with a highly anisotropic tensor. The representation error is actually inevitable for any finite order N and L, although increasing the orders can reduce the representation error. DL-SPFI was proposed in [7] to learn a sparser dictionary from Gaussian diffusion signals with different mean diffusivity and fractional anisotropy (FA), and adaptively set the scale value ζ based on the mean diffusivity. [7] also demonstrated that the DL-SPF dictionary keeps the same level of sparsity for Gaussian diffusion with different FA, while the sparsity in SPF dictionary decreases for signals with higher FA.

Theorem 1 (TSPF Basis and Dual TSPF Basis). *Let* $\mathbf{D}$ *be* 3×3 *positive definite matrix with eigen-decomposition* $\mathbf{D} = Q\Lambda^2 Q^T$, $Q^T Q = I$, *then* $\left\{\sqrt{|\Lambda|} B_{nlm}(\Lambda Q^T \mathbf{q} \mid \zeta)\right\}$ *is an orthonormal basis set, called the Tensorial SPF (TSPF) basis. Its Fourier transform is* $\left\{\frac{1}{\sqrt{|\Lambda|}} B_{nlm}^{dual}(\Lambda^{-1} Q^T \mathbf{R} \mid \zeta)\right\}$ *called the dual TSPF basis, which is also complete and orthonormal in the dual Fourier space.*

We propose Tensorial SPFI (TSPFI) to further sparsely represent Gaussian-like signals. Theorem 1 demonstrates TSPF basis and dual TSPF basis which are the affinely transformed SPF basis and dual SPF basis[1]. TSPFI represents diffusion signal $E(\mathbf{q})$ using TSPF basis in Eq. (3), then the diffusion propagator is analytically represented as dual TSPF basis in Eq. (4), where we set $\zeta_0 = (8\pi^2\tau)^{-1}$ such that $\sqrt{|\Lambda|} B_{000}(\Lambda Q^T \mathbf{q} \mid \zeta_0)$ is proportional to Gaussian function $\exp(-4\pi^2\tau\mathbf{q}^T\mathbf{D}\mathbf{q})$.

$$E(q\mathbf{u} \mid \mathbf{D}) = \sqrt{|\Lambda|} \sum_{n=0}^{N}\sum_{l=0}^{L}\sum_{m=-l}^{l} a_{nlm} G_n\left(q\sqrt{\mathbf{u}^T\mathbf{D}\mathbf{u}} \mid \zeta_0\right) Y_l^m\left(\frac{\Lambda Q^T\mathbf{u}}{\|\Lambda Q^T\mathbf{u}\|}\right) \tag{3}$$

$$P(R\mathbf{r} \mid \mathbf{D}) = \frac{1}{\sqrt{|\Lambda|}} \sum_{nlm} a_{nlm} F_{nl}\left(R\sqrt{\mathbf{r}^T\mathbf{D}^{-1}\mathbf{r}} \mid \zeta_0\right) Y_l^m\left(\frac{\Lambda^{-1}Q^T\mathbf{r}}{\|\Lambda^{-1}Q^T\mathbf{r}\|}\right) \tag{4}$$

The representation using TSPF basis is sparse for Gaussian-like diffusion signals when we set tensor $\mathbf{D}$ appropriately, and the first basis is enough to represent Gaussian diffusion signals. Note that MAP-MRI basis [5] also uses an anisotropic Gaussian function as the zero order basis, while it can be proven that MAP-MRI basis can be linearly represented by the TSPF basis with a finite order, but the opposite is not true, which means TSPF basis is more general than MAP-MRI basis.

Similarly with [7], considering $E(0) = 1$, we have $\sum_0^N a_{nlm} G_n(0) = \sqrt{4\pi}\delta_l^0$, $0 \le l \le L$, $-l \le m \le l$. Then we can separate the coefficient vector $\boldsymbol{a}$ into $\boldsymbol{a} = (\boldsymbol{a}_0^T, \boldsymbol{a}'^T)^T$, where $\boldsymbol{a}_0 = (a_{000}, \ldots, a_{0LL})^T$, $\boldsymbol{a}' = (a_{100}, \ldots, a_{NLL})^T$, and represent $\boldsymbol{a}_0$ using $\boldsymbol{a}'$, i.e.,

$$a_{0lm} = \frac{1}{G_0(0)}\left(\sqrt{4\pi}\delta_l^0 - \sum_{n=1}^{N} a_{nlm} G_n(0)\right), \quad 0 \le l \le L, \quad -l \le m \le l \tag{5}$$

[1] All proofs in this paper are omitted due to space limitation, available upon request.

Then based on Eq. (3), $\boldsymbol{a}'$ can be estimated from measurements of $E(\mathbf{q})$ via weighted LASSO.

$$\min_{\boldsymbol{a}'} \|\mathbf{M}'\boldsymbol{a}' - \boldsymbol{e}'\|_2^2 + \|\mathbf{H}\boldsymbol{a}'\|_1 \tag{6}$$

$$\mathbf{M}' = \begin{bmatrix} \sqrt{|\Lambda|}\Big(B_{100}(\Lambda Q^T\mathbf{q}_1|\zeta_0) - \frac{G_1(0|\zeta_0)}{G_0(0|\zeta_0)} B_{000}(\Lambda Q^T\mathbf{q}_1|\zeta_0)\Big) & \cdots & \sqrt{|\Lambda|}\Big(B_{NLL}(\Lambda Q^T\mathbf{q}_1|\zeta_0) - \frac{G_N(0|\zeta_0)}{G_0(0|\zeta_0)} B_{0LL}(\Lambda Q^T\mathbf{q}_1|\zeta_0)\Big) \\ \vdots & \ddots & \vdots \\ \sqrt{|\Lambda|}\Big(B_{100}(\Lambda Q^T\mathbf{q}_S|\zeta_0) - \frac{G_1(0|\zeta_0)}{G_0(0|\zeta_0)} B_{000}(\Lambda Q^T\mathbf{q}_S|\zeta_0)\Big) & \cdots & \sqrt{|\Lambda|}\Big(B_{NLL}(\Lambda Q^T\mathbf{q}_S|\zeta_0) - \frac{G_N(0|\zeta_0)}{G_0(0|\zeta_0)} B_{0LL}(\Lambda Q^T\mathbf{q}_S|\zeta_0)\Big) \end{bmatrix}, \ \boldsymbol{e}' = \begin{bmatrix} E_1 - \exp(-4\pi^2\tau\mathbf{q}_1^T\mathbf{D}\mathbf{q}_1) \\ \vdots \\ E_S - \exp(-4\pi^2\tau\mathbf{q}_S^T\mathbf{D}\mathbf{q}_S) \end{bmatrix},$$

where $\{E_i\}$ are signal measurements in $\mathbf{q}$-space, $\boldsymbol{e}'$ is the measurement vector removing its Gaussian part, $\mathbf{M}'$ is the basis matrix used for reconstruction, $\mathbf{H}$ is the regularization matrix. After estimating $\boldsymbol{a}'$, $\boldsymbol{a}_0$ can be obtained using Eq. (5), then $E(0) = 1$ is automatically satisfied. For Gaussian diffusion signal, if $\mathbf{D}$ is estimated correctly, then $\boldsymbol{e}' = 0$, $\boldsymbol{a}' = 0$, and only a_{000} is non-zero. Thus Eq. (6) mainly focus on the non-Gaussian fitting.

3 TSPFI with Optimal Dictionary Learning (DL-TSPFI)

Based CS theory [10], a dictionary with sparser representation gives better reconstruction. Following DL-SPFI in [7], we consider a more general formulation:

$$\min_{\boldsymbol{c}} \|\mathbf{M}'\mathbf{W}\boldsymbol{c} - \boldsymbol{e}'\|_2^2 + \|\mathbf{V}\boldsymbol{c}\|_1. \tag{7}$$

Note that Eq. (7) actually considers a general dictionary represented as a linear combination of TSPF basis, i.e., $\mathbf{M}'\mathbf{W}$, where $\mathbf{W}$ is the combination matrix and $\boldsymbol{c}$ is the new coefficient vector under transformed dictionary. When $\mathbf{W}$ is identity, Eq. (7) becomes TSPFI in Eq. (6). As we discussed that MAP-MRI basis can be linearly represented by TSPF basis, $\mathbf{W}$ can be specifically designed such that $\mathbf{M}'\mathbf{W}$ is the MAP-MRI basis removing its Gaussian part, then Eq. (7) becomes MAP-MRI.

Instead of using specific $\mathbf{W}$ in TSPFI and MAP-MRI, we would like performing dictionary learning to learn a good $\mathbf{W}$ as well as a good dictionary $\mathbf{M}'\mathbf{W}$ from a set of given signals $\{\boldsymbol{e}'_i\}$. such that the representation $\{\boldsymbol{c}_i\}$ are all sparse, i.e.

$$\min_{\mathbf{C},\mathbf{W},\mathbf{D}} \sum_i \|\boldsymbol{c}_i\|_1 \quad \text{s.t. } \|\mathbf{M}'\mathbf{W}\boldsymbol{c}_j - \boldsymbol{e}'_j\|_2 \leq \epsilon, \ \forall j. \tag{8}$$

Considering real data always suffers from noise and a limited number of samples, similarly with [7], we perform dictionary learning in synthetic mixture of Gaussian signals. Considering simulated signals can be generated in continuous $\mathbf{q}$-space and TSPF basis is an orthonormal basis showed in Theorem 1, Eq. (8) is equivalent to Eq. (9), where the dictionary learning can be performed in the space of TSPF coefficients with a small dimension, not the space of simulated measurements of $E(\mathbf{q})$ with infinite dimension.

$$\min_{\mathbf{C},\mathbf{W},\mathbf{D}} \sum_i \|\boldsymbol{c}_i\|_1 \quad \text{s.t. } \|\mathbf{W}\boldsymbol{c}_j - \boldsymbol{a}'_j\|_2 \leq \epsilon, \ \forall j, \tag{9}$$

The learned result $(\mathbf{W}^*, \mathbf{D}^*)$ is actually determined by the chosen space of diffusion signals. We have several theoretical results to design a small space for training data to learn a general dictionary. 1) Theorem 2 proved that the single tensor model $\{E(\mathbf{q}) = \exp(-4\pi^2\tau\mathbf{q}^T\mathbf{D}\mathbf{q}) \mid \mathbf{D} \in \mathrm{Sym}_+^3\}$, where Sym_+^3 is the space of 3×3 positive definite matrices, is sufficient to learn a dictionary to sparsely represent signals from mixture of tensor models. The theorem works for both DL-SPFI in [7] and DL-TSPFI. 2) Theorem 3 shows that the dictionary $(\mathbf{W}^*, \mathbf{D}^*)$ can be learned from a small space $S_0 \subset \mathrm{Sym}^3_+$, then the learned dictionary can be affinely transformed to another tensor space. Note that for every single Gaussian signal, the sparsest $\boldsymbol{c}$ is 0 once we set the tensor $\mathbf{D}$ correctly. However this does not help us to handle arbitrary mixture of Gaussian signals with noise where a single tensor $\mathbf{D}$ cannot fully represent all Gaussian components. Thus we have to learn a common dictionary for a subspace of Sym^3_+, such that even when the tensor $\mathbf{D}$ is not correctly set, the learned dictionary still yields a sparse representation. 3) Theorem 4 demonstrated that we can fix a tensor $\mathbf{D}_0$ and learn a sparse dictionary $\mathbf{W}^*$ from Gaussian signals with $\mathbf{D}$ in a geodesic ball $d(\mathbf{D}_0, \mathbf{D}) < \Delta$ [11]. Then the learned dictionary can be adaptively applied to Gaussian signals with $\mathbf{D}$ in another geodesic ball $d(\mathbf{D}_1, \mathbf{D}) < \Delta$ by adaptively setting tensor in TSPF basis as $\mathbf{D}_1$. The geodesic ball actually mimics the difference between the tensor used in TSPF basis and the ground truth tensor in each Gaussian component in the mixture of Gaussian model.

Theorem 2 (Sparsity of Mixture of Tensors [7]). *A dictionary learned from signals generated by single tensor model can sparsely represent signals generated by arbitrary mixture of tensor model.*

Theorem 3 (Optimal Dictionary). *For signals generated from the single tensor model with tensors* $\{\exp(-4\pi^2\tau\mathbf{q}^T\mathbf{D}\mathbf{q}) \mid \mathbf{D} \in S_0\}$, *if the dictionary* $\{\mathbf{W}^*, \mathbf{D}^*\}$ *is the optimal solution for* (9), *then for another space* $\{\exp(-4\pi^2\tau\mathbf{q}^T A\mathbf{D}A^T\mathbf{q}) \mid \mathbf{D} \in S_0\}$ *with non-singular A,* $\{\mathbf{W}^*, A\mathbf{D}^*A^T\}$ *is still the optimal solution.*

Theorem 4 (Traning Space and Adaptive Tensor). *Let* $\mathbf{D}_0$ *be a fixed tensor. If training signals are from* $\{\exp(-4\pi^2\tau\mathbf{q}^T\mathbf{D}\mathbf{q}) \mid d(\mathbf{D}_0, \mathbf{D}) < \Delta\}$, *where* $d(\mathbf{D}_0, \mathbf{D})$ *is the Riemannian distance between* $\mathbf{D}_0$ *and* $\mathbf{D}$ *[11], and if we set* $\mathbf{D}^* = \mathbf{D}_0$ *and estimate* $\mathbf{W}^*$ *in dictionary learning, then* $(\mathbf{W}^*, \mathbf{D}_1)$ *can sparsely represent signals from* $\{\exp(-4\pi^2\tau\mathbf{q}^T\mathbf{D}\mathbf{q}) \mid d(\mathbf{D}_1, \mathbf{D}) < \Delta\}$

Because of Theorem 4, it is possible to choose any $\mathbf{D}_0$ and generate signals from the geodesic ball of $\mathbf{D}_0$. In practice, in order to better mimic the representation error of tensors, we simply set $\mathbf{D}_0 = 0.7 \times 10^{-3}\mathbf{I}$ as a typical isotropic tensor in human brain, and then generated Gaussian signals with mean diffusivity (MD) in range $[0.5, 0.9] \times 10^{-3} mm^2/s$, FA in range $[0, 0.9]$, uniformly orientated in 321 directions from sphere tessellation. Note that we used a relatively small range of MD, while a relatively large range of FA. It is because when using a tensor model to fit a mixture of Gaussian signal, the MD value of the tensor model normally has relatively less error than its FA value compared to the ground truth MD and FA in each Gaussian component. For example, considering a mixture of three Gaussian functions with FA = 0.9 and MD = 0.7×10^{-3} respectively along x, y and z axises, after DTI fitting, the estimated MD is still close to 0.7×10^{-3}, but the estimated FA is close to 0. Note that when choosing isotropic $\mathbf{D}_0$, the TSPF coefficients $\{\boldsymbol{a}_i\}$ become SPF coefficients with the corresponding scale, and the dictionary learning process is the same as the one used in DL-SPFI [7]. The SPF coefficients of the Gaussian signals were calculated via numerical inner product with $N = 4$, $L = 8$. Then we performed an efficient online learning method implemented in the SPAMS toolbox [12] to learn $\mathbf{W}$ with 250 atoms using the initialization of identity matrix. We added the atoms $\{B_{n00}(\mathbf{q})\}_{n=1}^{N}$ back to sparsely represent isotropic signals. Thus we have total 254 columns in the learned $\mathbf{W}$. Then we estimated the energy $\{h_j\}$ of dictionary atoms via the coefficients $\{\boldsymbol{c}_i\}$, and set $\mathbf{V}$ in Eq. (7) as a diagonal matrix with elements $V_j = \frac{S}{h_j}\lambda$, where λ is a tuning regularization parameter, S is the dimension of measurements. This is to penalize the dictionary atom with low energy of coefficients. With the learned $\mathbf{W}$ and $\mathbf{V}$, Eq. (7) first performs DTI to estimate a tensor D for TSPF basis matrix $\mathbf{M}'$, then performs weighted LASSO for CS reconstruction of $\boldsymbol{c}$, then $\boldsymbol{a}' = \mathbf{W}\boldsymbol{c}$, and $\boldsymbol{a}$ can be obtained accordingly based on Eq. (5).

4 Experiments

Signal Sparsity in Miture of Gaussian Model. We would like to demonstrate the importance of adaptive tensor setting and validate the theorems. We generated Gaussian diffusion signals with different FA in range $[0, 0.9]$, along different directions, and with two MD values respectively 0.6×10^{-3} and 1.1×10^{-3}. These signals from single tensor model with the same FA and MD but different orientations were also randomly mixed to obtain mixture of Gaussian signals. Then with $N = 4$, $L = 8$, we performed adaptive scale setting to obtain adaptive SPF basis and DL-SPF basis, and performed adaptive tensor setting to obtain adaptive TSPF basis and DL-TSPF basis. Then for each signal, we calculated the coefficients $\boldsymbol{a}'$ respectively for SPF basis and TSPF basis using numerical inner product, then calculated the coefficients $\boldsymbol{c}$ respectively for DL-SPF and DL-TSPF basis using Eq. (9). For the obtained coefficients under each basis, we calculated the number of non-zero values as the sparsity of the representation. The value in $\boldsymbol{a}'$ or $\boldsymbol{c}$ is considered to be non-zero if its absolute value is larger than $0.01\|\boldsymbol{a}'\|$ or $0.01\|\boldsymbol{c}\|$. The sparsity of signals with two MD values were showed in the top two subfigures of Fig. 1. The top left subfigure showed that although DL-TSPF basis was learned from signal Gaussian diffusion signals, it can sparsely represent signals from mixture of Gaussian functions, which validated Theorem 2 The top right subfigure showed that although the MD value 1.1×10^{-3} is outside of the MD range used in dictionary learning, the sparse representation still holds by adaptively setting diffusion tensor in DL-TSPF basis, which validates Theorem 3 and 4. Both subfigures demonstrated the DL-TSPF basis obtains sparser representation than DL-SPF basis [7], and TSPF basis is sparser than SPF basis.

RMSE in Cylinder Model. We evaluated the different basis using the Söderman cylinder model [13] which is different from the Gaussian signals used in dictionary learning. Using the DSI sampling scheme in [8] with $b_{max} = 8000 s/mm^2$, 514 measurements, we generated ground truth DWI signals from the cylinder model with the default parameters in [13]. Then we estimated the coefficients under different basis from an undersampled dataset with 170 samples and reconstructed the DWI signals in all 514 samples. Root-Mean-Square Error (RMSE), which is defined based on the difference of the estimated signal and ground truth signal in these 514 samples, was used to quantify the reconstruction accuracy. We also added Rician noise with signal-to-noise ratio (SNR) of 20 and performed Monte-Carlo simulation. We set $\lambda = \lambda_l = \lambda_n = 10^{-8}$ for the noise-free dataset and 10^{-5} for the noisy dataset for all methods. The second row of Fig. 1 indicates that DL-TSPFI yields the lowest RMSE than DL-SPFI and L1-SPFI in both noiseless and noisy conditions.

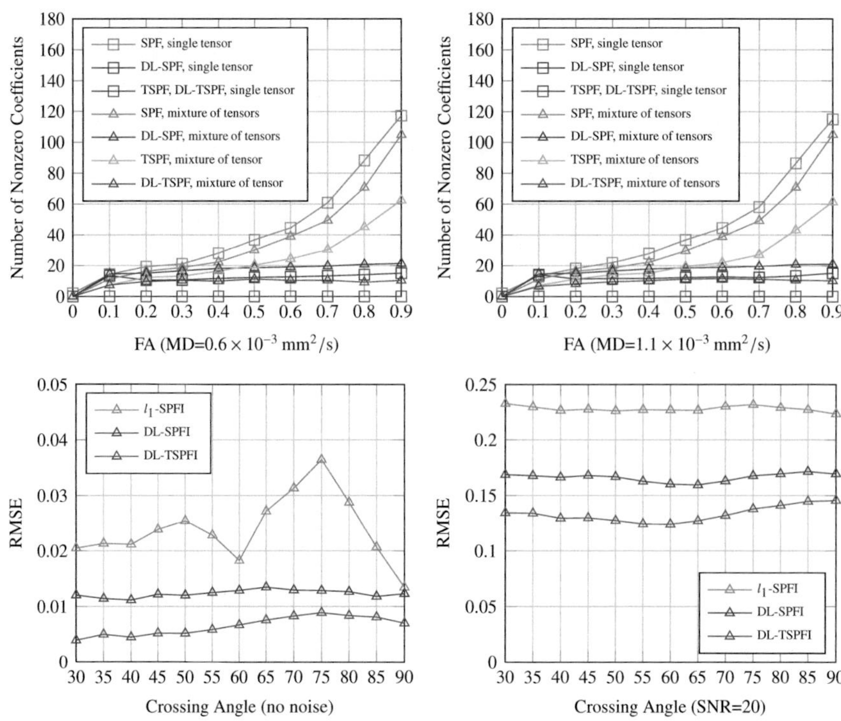

Fig. 1. Synthetic Experiments. First row: the average number of non-zero coefficients for SPF, DL-SPF, TSPF and DL-TSPF basis. Second row: RMSE of different methods using the Söderman cylinder model with and without noise.

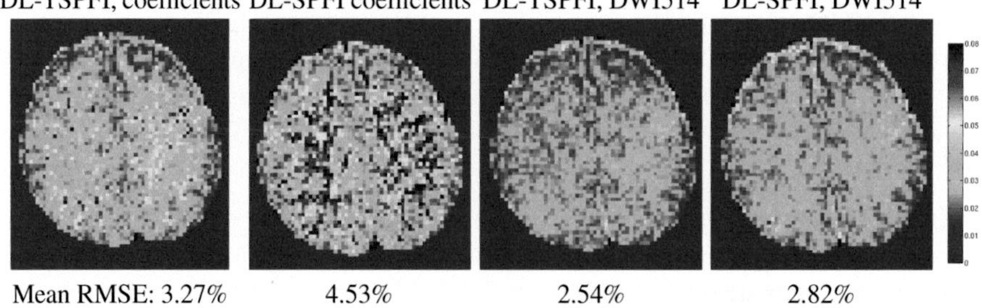

Fig. 2. Real Data Experiment. RMSE calculated from estimated SPF coefficients and recovered 514 DWI samples.

RMSE in Real Data. We also tested CS reconstruction using DL-TSPFI on a real DSI data set released by Bilgic [2], which was also used to validate DL-SPFI [7]. This dataset uses the same DSI sampling scheme as the above cylinder data experiment. With DL-SPFI and DL-TSPFI, we perform CS reconstruction with $\lambda = 10^{-6}$ respectively using full 514 measurements and a subset of 170 samples, then we calculated two RMSEs,

[2] `https://www.martinos.org/~berkin/software.html`

one is based on the difference of coefficients using full measurements and the subset of measurements, and the other one is based on the difference of recovered DWI signals in these 514 points using full samples and subsamples. Fig. 2 showed that DL-TSPFI obtains less RMSE than DL-SPFI, especially for RMSE defined using coefficients in white matter area.

5 Conclusion

In this paper, we propose a novel Tensorial SPFI (TSPFI) which allows a continuous representation for both the diffusion signal and the diffusion propagator. TSPFI is a combination of existing DTI and SPFI. We also propose a dictionary learning strategy, called DL-TSPFI, to learn a sparser dictionary from mixture of Gaussian signals. The learned dictionary can be optimally and adaptively applied to different voxels by adaptive tensor setting. The proposed TSPFI and DL-TSPFI yield a sparser representation with lower CS reconstruction error than existing SPFI and DL-SPFI. The source codes of TSPFI and DL-TSPFI will be available in the DMRITool package [3].

Acknowledgement. This work is supported in part by NICHD and NIBIB Intramural Research Programs, a UNC BRIC-Radiology start-up fund, and NIH grants (EB006733, EB009634, AG041721, MH100217, and 1UL1TR001111).

References

1. Callaghan, P.T.: Principles of nuclear magnetic resonance microscopy. Oxford University Press (1991)
2. Basser, P.J., Mattiello, J., LeBihan, D.: MR diffusion tensor spectroscropy and imaging. Biophysical Journal 66, 259–267 (1994)
3. Wedeen, V.J., Hagmann, P., Tseng, W.Y.I., Reese, T.G., Weisskoff, R.M.: Mapping Complex Tissue Architecture With Diffusion Spectrum Magnetic Resonance Imaging. Magnetic Resonance in Medicine 54, 1377–1386 (2005)
4. Özarslan, E., Koay, C., Shepherd, T., Blackband, S., Basser, P.: Simple harmonic oscillator based reconstruction and estimation for three-dimensional q-space MRI. In: ISMRM (2009)
5. Özarslan, E., Koay, C.G., Shepherd, T.M., Komlosh, M.E., İrfanoğlu, M.O., Pierpaoli, C., Basser, P.J.: Mean apparent propagator (map) mri: a novel diffusion imaging method for mapping tissue microstructure. NeuroImage 78, 16–32 (2013)
6. Cheng, J., Ghosh, A., Jiang, T., Deriche, R.: Model-free and Analytical EAP Reconstruction via Spherical Polar Fourier Diffusion MRI. In: Jiang, T., Navab, N., Pluim, J.P.W., Viergever, M.A. (eds.) MICCAI 2010, Part I. LNCS, vol. 6361, pp. 590–597. Springer, Heidelberg (2010)
7. Cheng, J., Jiang, T., Deriche, R., Shen, D., Yap, P.-T.: Regularized Spherical Polar Fourier Diffusion MRI with Optimal Dictionary Learning. In: Mori, K., Sakuma, I., Sato, Y., Barillot, C., Navab, N. (eds.) MICCAI 2013, Part I. LNCS, vol. 8149, pp. 639–646. Springer, Heidelberg (2013)

[3] `https://github.com/DiffusionMRITool`

8. Bilgic, B., Setsompop, K., Cohen-Adad, J., Yendiki, A., Wald, L.L., Adalsteinsson, E.: Accelerated diffusion spectrum imaging with compressed sensing using adaptive dictionaries. Magnetic Resonance in Medicine (2012)
9. Assemlal, H.E., Tschumperlé, D., Brun, L.: Efficient and robust computation of PDF features from diffusion MR signal. Medical Image Analysis 13, 715–729 (2009)
10. Donoho, D.: Compressed sensing. IEEE Transactions on Information Theory 52(4), 1289–1306 (2006)
11. Pennec, X., Fillard, P., Ayache, N.: A Riemannian Framework for Tensor Computing. International Journal of Computer Vision 66, 41–66 (2006)
12. Mairal, J., Bach, F., Ponce, J., Sapiro, G.: Online learning for matrix factorization and sparse coding. The Journal of Machine Learning Research 11, 19–60 (2010)
13. Özarslan, E., Shepherd, T.M., Vemuri, B.C., Blackband, S.J., Mareci, T.H.: Resolution of complex tissue microarchitecture using the diffusion orientation transform (DOT). NeuroImage 31, 1086–1103 (2006)

Diffusion Compartmentalization Using Response Function Groups with Cardinality Penalization*

Pew-Thian Yap[1], Yong Zhang[2], and Dinggang Shen[1]

[1] Department of Radiology and Biomedical Research Imaging Center, The University of North Carolina at Chapel Hill, U.S.A.
[2] Department of Psychiatry and Behavioral Sciences, Stanford University, U.S.A.
ptyap@med.unc.edu

Abstract. Spherical deconvolution (SD) of the white matter (WM) diffusion-attenuated signal with a fiber signal response function has been shown to yield high-quality estimates of fiber orientation distribution functions (FODFs). However, an inherent limitation of this approach is that the response function (RF) is often fixed and assumed to be spatially invariant. This has been reported to result in spurious FODF peaks as the discrepancy of the RF with the data increases. In this paper, we propose to utilize response function groups (RFGs) for robust compartmentalization of diffusion signal and hence improving FODF estimation. Unlike the aforementioned single fixed RF, each RFG consists of a set of RFs that are intentionally varied to capture potential signal variations associated with a fiber bundle. Additional isotropic RFGs are included to account for signal contributions from gray matter (GM) and cerebrospinal fluid (CSF). To estimate the WM FODF and the volume fractions of GM and CSF compartments, the RFGs are fitted to the data in the least-squares sense, penalized by the cardinality of the support of the solution to encourage group sparsity. The volume fractions associated with each compartment are then computed by summing up the volume fractions of the RFs within each RFGs. Experimental results confirm that our method yields estimates of FODFs and volume fractions of diffusion compartments with improved robustness and accuracy.

1 Introduction

Diffusion magnetic resonance imaging (DMRI) is a powerful imaging modality due to its unique ability to extract microstructural information by utilizing restricted diffusion to probe compartments that are much smaller than the voxel size. One important goal of DMRI is to estimate axonal orientations, tracing of which will allow one to gauge connectivity between brain regions. For estimation of axonal orientations, a widely used method, constrained spherical deconvolution (CSD) [1], estimates the fiber orientation distribution function (FODF) by

* This work was supported in part by a UNC BRIC-Radiology start-up fund and NIH grants (EB006733, EB009634, AG041721, MH100217, and 1UL1TR001111).

N. Navab et al. (Eds.): MICCAI 2015, Part I, LNCS 9349, pp. 183–190, 2015.
DOI: 10.1007/978-3-319-24553-9_23

deconvolving the measured diffusion-attenuated signal with a spatially-invariant kernel representing the signal response function (RF) of a single coherent fiber bundle. Unlike the multi-tensor approach, CSD does not require the specification of the number of tensors to fit to the data. However, it has been recently reported that a mismatch between the kernel used in CSD and the actual fiber RF can cause spurious peaks in the estimated FODF [2]. Although CSD has been recently extended to include RFs of not only the white matter (WM), but also the gray matter (GM) and the cerebrospinal fluid (CSF) [3], these RFs remain spatially fixed and similar shortcomings as reported in [2] apply.

In this paper, we propose to estimate the WM FODF and the volume fractions of the GM and CSF compartments by using response function groups (RFGs). Each RFG is a collection of exemplar RFs aimed at capturing the variations of the actual RFs. Unlike the conventional approach of using fixed RFs, the utilization of RFGs will allow tolerance to RF variations and hence minimize estimation error due to RF and data mismatch. Several RFGs are included to cater to the WM, GM, and CSF compartments. The WM is represented by a large number of directional RFGs with orientations distributed uniformly on the unit sphere. Each WM RFG consists of a set of unidirectional axial-symmetric diffusion tensors with a range of typical axial and radial diffusivities. The GM and CSF RFGs consist of isotropic tensors with diffusivities of GM RFs set lower than CSF RFs, consistent with what was reported in [3]. The FODF and compartmental volume fractions for each voxel are estimated by solving a group cardinality (i.e., l_0-"norm") penalized least-squares problem that aims to preserve the group structure of the RPGs while at the same time encourage sparsity. Our work is an integration of concepts presented in [3–5] with a novel estimation framework.

Recently, Daducci et al. [6] linearize the fitting problem of ActiveAx and NODDI to drastically speed up axon diameter and density estimation by a few orders of magnitude. They achieve this by solving an l_1 minimization problem with a design matrix containing instances of the respective biophysical models generated with a discretized range of parameters. The results reported in [6] are supportive of the fact that variation of diffusion signals should be explained not only in terms of varying volume fractions but also in terms of varying model parameters. Similar to [6], we observe that by using RFGs containing RFs of varying parameters, the data can be explained with greater fidelity than by using RFs with a single fixed set of parameters. Dissimilar to [6], our work (i) is not limited to single fiber populations and explicitly considers fiber crossings, (ii) solves a cardinality penalized problem instead of the l_1 problem, and (iii) explicitly considers the natural coupling between RFs via sparse-group estimation, similar but not identical to [7].

We propose here to directly minimize the cardinality penalized problem instead of resorting to reweighted ℓ_1 minimization as performed in [8]. By doing so, we (i) overcome the suboptimality of reweighted minimization, and (ii) improve estimation speed greatly by avoiding having to solve the l_1 minimization problem (especially the sparse-group problem [7]) multiple times to gradually improve sparsity. We will describe in this paper an algorithm based on iterative hard thresholding (IHT) to effectively and efficiently solve the cardinality penalized sparse-group problem.

2 Proposed Approach

2.1 Response Function Groups (RFGs)

At each voxel, the diffusion-attenuated signal $S(b, \hat{\mathbf{g}})$, measured for diffusion weighting b and at direction $\hat{\mathbf{g}}$, can be represented as a mixture of N models: $S(b, \hat{\mathbf{g}}) = \sum_{i=1}^{N} f_i S_i(b, \hat{\mathbf{g}}) + \epsilon(b, \hat{\mathbf{g}})$, where f_i is the volume fraction associated with the i-th model S_i and $\epsilon(b, \hat{\mathbf{g}})$ is the fitting residual. In the current work, we are interested in distinguishing signal contributions from WM, GM, and CSF and choose to use the tensor model $S_i(b, \hat{\mathbf{g}}) = S_0 \exp(-b\hat{\mathbf{g}}^{\mathrm{T}}\mathbf{D}_i\hat{\mathbf{g}})$, where S_0 is the baseline signal with no diffusion weighting and $\mathbf{D}_i$ is a diffusion tensor. This model affords great flexibility in representing different compartments of the diffusion signal. Setting $\mathbf{D} = \lambda\mathbf{I}$, the model represents isotropic diffusion with diffusivity λ. When $\lambda = 0$ and $\lambda > 0$ the model corresponds to the dot model and the ball model, respectively [9]. Setting $\mathbf{D} = (\lambda_{\parallel} - \lambda_{\perp})\hat{\mathbf{v}}\hat{\mathbf{v}}^{\mathrm{T}} + \lambda_{\perp}\mathbf{I}$, $\lambda_{\parallel} > \lambda_{\perp}$, the model represents anisotropic diffusion in principal direction $\hat{\mathbf{v}}$ with diffusivity $\lambda_{\parallel}$ parallel to $\hat{\mathbf{v}}$ and diffusivity $\lambda_{\perp}$ perpendicular to $\hat{\mathbf{v}}$. When $\lambda_{\perp} = 0$ and $\lambda_{\perp} > 0$ the model corresponds to the stick model and the zeppelin model, respectively. In our case, each of these tensor models is a representation of an RF.

The solution to SD [1] can be obtained in discretized form by including in the mixture model a large number of anisotropic tensors uniformly distributed on the unit sphere with fixed $\lambda_{\parallel}$ and $\lambda_{\perp}$ and solving for $\{f_i\}$ by minimizing the error in the least-squares sense with some appropriate regularization, giving us the FODF. In this work, instead of fixing $\lambda_{\parallel}$ and $\lambda_{\perp}$, we allow them to vary across a range of values. Therefore, each principal direction is now represented by a group of RFs, forming a RFG. Additional isotropic RFGs are included to account for signal contributions from GM and CSF. Formally, the representation can be expressed as

$$S(b, \hat{\mathbf{g}}) = \underbrace{\sum_{i=1}^{N_{\mathrm{WM}}} S_i^{\mathrm{WM}}(b, \hat{\mathbf{g}}) + S^{\mathrm{GM}}(b, \hat{\mathbf{g}}) + S^{\mathrm{CSF}}(b, \hat{\mathbf{g}})}_{\hat{S}(b, \hat{\mathbf{g}})} + \epsilon(b, \hat{\mathbf{g}}), \tag{1}$$

where we have N_{WM} WM RFGs, a GM RFG, and a CSF RFG with $S_i^{\mathrm{WM}}(b, \hat{\mathbf{g}}) = \sum_{j=1}^{K_{\mathrm{WM}}} f_{i,j}^{\mathrm{WM}} \exp(-b\hat{\mathbf{g}}^{\mathrm{T}}\mathbf{D}_{i,j}^{\mathrm{WM}}\hat{\mathbf{g}})$, $S^{\mathrm{GM}}(b, \hat{\mathbf{g}}) = \sum_{j=1}^{K_{\mathrm{GM}}} f_j^{\mathrm{GM}} \exp(-b\hat{\mathbf{g}}^{\mathrm{T}}\mathbf{D}_j^{\mathrm{GM}}\hat{\mathbf{g}})$, $S^{\mathrm{CSF}}(b, \hat{\mathbf{g}}) = \sum_{j=1}^{K_{\mathrm{CSF}}} f_j^{\mathrm{CSF}} \exp(-b\hat{\mathbf{g}}^{\mathrm{T}}\mathbf{D}_j^{\mathrm{CSF}}\hat{\mathbf{g}})$, and $\mathbf{D}_{i,j}^{\mathrm{WM}} = (\lambda_{\parallel,j}^{\mathrm{WM}} - \lambda_{\perp,j}^{\mathrm{WM}})\hat{\mathbf{v}}_i\hat{\mathbf{v}}_i^{\mathrm{T}} + \lambda_{\perp,j}^{\mathrm{WM}}\mathbf{I}$, $\mathbf{D}_j^{\mathrm{GM}} = \lambda_j^{\mathrm{GM}}\mathbf{I}$, $\mathbf{D}_j^{\mathrm{CSF}} = \lambda_j^{\mathrm{CSF}}\mathbf{I}$. Given the signal $S(b, \hat{\mathbf{g}})$, we need to estimate the volume fractions $\{f_{i,j}^{\mathrm{WM}}\}$, $\{f_j^{\mathrm{GM}}\}$, and $\{f_j^{\mathrm{CSF}}\}$. Note that we have dropped S_0 here because it can be absorbed into the volume fractions. The normalized volume fractions can be recovered by dividing the unnormalized volume fractions by S_0. It is easy to see that if we take a Fourier transform of (1), these volume fractions are in fact weights that decompose the ensemble average propagator (EAP) of the overall signal as a weighted sum of the EAPs of the individual tensors. The *overall* volume fractions associated with WM, GM, and CSF are $f^{\mathrm{WM}_i} = \sum_{j=1}^{K_{\mathrm{WM}}} f_{i,j}^{\mathrm{WM}}$, $f^{\mathrm{GM}} = \sum_{j=1}^{K_{\mathrm{GM}}} f_j^{\mathrm{GM}}$, $f^{\mathrm{CSF}} = \sum_{j=1}^{K_{\mathrm{CSF}}} f_j^{\mathrm{CSF}}$. The set $\{f^{\mathrm{WM}_i}\}$ over i gives the WM FODF. For notation simplicity, we group the volume fractions into a vector $\mathbf{f} = [\mathbf{f}^{\mathrm{WM}_1}; \ldots; \mathbf{f}^{\mathrm{WM}_{N_{\mathrm{WM}}}}; \mathbf{f}^{\mathrm{GM}}; \mathbf{f}^{\mathrm{CSF}}]$.

2.2 Estimation of Volume Fractions

To obtain an estimate of the volume fractions, we solve the following optimization problem: $\min_{\mathbf{f}\geq 0} \Big\{ \phi(\mathbf{f}) = \|S(b,\mathbf{g}) - \hat{S}(b,\mathbf{g})\|_2^2 + \alpha\gamma\|\mathbf{f}\|_0 + (1-\alpha)\gamma \Big[\sum_{i=1}^{N_{\mathrm{WM}}} \mathcal{I}(\|\mathbf{f}^{\mathrm{WM}_i}\|_2) + \mathcal{I}(\|\mathbf{f}^{\mathrm{GM}}\|_2) + \mathcal{I}(\|\mathbf{f}^{\mathrm{CSF}}\|_2) \Big] \Big\}$, where $\mathcal{I}(z)$ is an indicator function returning 1 if $z \neq 0$ or 0 if otherwise. The l_0-"norm" gives the cardinality of the support, i.e., $\|\mathbf{f}\|_0 = |\mathbf{supp}(\mathbf{f})| = |\{k : f_k \neq 0\}|$. Parameters $\alpha \in [0,1]$ and $\gamma > 0$ are for penalty tuning, analogous to those used in the sparse-group LASSO [7]. Note that $\alpha = 1$ gives the l_0 fit, whereas $\alpha = 0$ gives the group l_0 fit. The problem can be written more succinctly in matrix form: $\min_{\mathbf{f}\geq 0} \Big\{ \phi(\mathbf{f}) = \|\mathbf{Af} - \mathbf{s}\|_2^2 + \alpha\gamma\|\mathbf{f}\|_0 + (1-\alpha)\gamma \sum_{g\in G} \mathcal{I}(\|\mathbf{f}_g\|_2) \Big\}$, where $\mathbf{f}_g$ denotes the subvector containing the elements associated with group $g \in G = \{\mathrm{WM}_1, \ldots, \mathrm{WM}_{N_{\mathrm{WM}}}, \mathrm{GM}, \mathrm{CSF}\}$. If $\mathbf{s}$ is the signal vector acquired at D $(b,\mathbf{g})$-points, $\mathbf{A} = \left[\mathbf{A}^{\mathrm{WM}} | \mathbf{A}^{\mathrm{GM}} | \mathbf{A}^{\mathrm{CSF}}\right]$ is a $D \times N$ matrix ($N = N_{\mathrm{WM}}K_{\mathrm{WM}} + K_{\mathrm{GM}} + K_{\mathrm{CSF}}$) with columns containing all the individual WM, GM, and CSF tensor models sampled at the corresponding D points. To the best of our knowledge, the solution to this problem has not been described elsewhere. We will therefore provide next the details of our algorithm.

2.3 Optimization

The problem we are interested in solving has the following form: $\min_{\mathbf{f}\geq 0}\{\phi(\mathbf{f}) = l(\mathbf{f}) + r(\mathbf{f})\}$, where in our case $l(\mathbf{f}) = \|\mathbf{Af} - \mathbf{s}\|_2^2$ is smooth and convex and $r(\mathbf{f}) = \alpha\gamma\|\mathbf{f}\|_0 + (1-\alpha)\gamma\sum_{g\in G}\mathcal{I}(\|\mathbf{f}_g\|_2)$ is non-convex, non-smooth, and discontinuous. Note that the solution is trivial, i.e., $\mathbf{f}^* = 0$, when $\gamma \geq \|\mathbf{s}\|_2^2$. We will solve this problem using an algorithm called non-monotone iterative hard thresholding (NIHT), as described in the following.

Non-monotone Spectral Projected Gradient: Choose factor $\tau > 1$, step size constants $L_{\min} < L_{\max}$, line search constant $\eta > 0$, stopping tolerance $\epsilon > 0$, and integer-valued non-monotone descent parameter $M > 0$. For iteration $k = 0$, set $L_0^{(0)} = 1$ and initial solution to $\mathbf{f}^{(0)}$. Then proceed with the following steps to obtain the solution:

1) Set $L^{(k)} = L_0^{(k)}$.
   1a) Solve the subproblem

$$\mathbf{f}^{(k+1)} \in \operatorname{Arg}\min_{\mathbf{f}\geq 0} \left\{ l(\mathbf{f}^{(k)}) + \nabla l(\mathbf{f}^{(k)})^{\mathrm{T}}(\mathbf{f}-\mathbf{f}^{(k)}) + \frac{L^{(k)}}{2}\|\mathbf{f}-\mathbf{f}^{(k)}\|_2^2 + r(\mathbf{f}) \right\}.$$

   1b) If $\phi(\mathbf{f}^{(k+1)}) \leq \max_{[k-M]^+ \leq i \leq k} \phi(\mathbf{f}^{(i)}) - \frac{\eta}{2}\|\mathbf{f}^{(k+1)} - \mathbf{f}^{(k)}\|_2^2$ is satisfied, then go to Step 2.
   1c) Set $L^{(k)} \leftarrow \tau L^{(k)}$ and go to Step 1a.
2) If $|\phi(\mathbf{f}^{(k+1)}) - \phi(\mathbf{f}^{(k)})|/\max(\phi(\mathbf{f}^{(k+1)}), 1) < \epsilon$ is satisfied, then return $\mathbf{f}^{(k+1)}$ as a solution. Otherwise, go to Step 3.
3) Set $L_0^{(k+1)} = \max\left\{L_{\min}, \min\left\{L_{\max}, \frac{\Delta l^{\mathrm{T}}\Delta \mathbf{f}}{\|\Delta \mathbf{f}\|_2^2}\right\}\right\}$, where $\Delta \mathbf{f} = \mathbf{f}^{(k+1)} - \mathbf{f}^{(k)}$ and $\Delta l = \nabla l(\mathbf{f}^{(k+1)}) - \nabla l(\mathbf{f}^{(k)})$.
4) Set $k \leftarrow k+1$ and go to Step 1.

The algorithm above seeks the solution via gradient descent using a majorization-minimization (MM) formulation of the problem. Step 1a minimizes the majorization of the objective $\phi(\cdot)$ at $\mathbf{f}^{(k)}$. It can be shown that the minimization involves a gradient descent step with step size $1/L^{(k)}$ (more details in the next section). The parameters $L_{\min}$ and $L_{\max}$ constrain the step size so that it is neither too aggressive nor too conservative (Step 3). We choose the initial step size $1/L_0^{(k)}$ as proposed by Barzilai and Borwein in [10], using a diagonal matrix $1/L_0^{(k)}\mathbf{I}$ to approximate the inverse of the Hessian matrix of $l(\mathbf{f})$ at $\mathbf{f}^{(k)}$ (Step 3). A suitable step size is determined via backtracking line search, where the step size is progressively shrunk by a factor of $1/\tau$ (Step 1c). Parameter η makes sure that the backtracking line search results in a sufficient change of the objective. Since the problem is non-monotone, i.e., the objective function is not guaranteed to decrease at every iteration, we require the objective to be slightly smaller than the largest objective in M previous iterations (Step 1b). For $M > 0$, the algorithm may increase the objective occasionally but will eventually converge faster than the monotone case with $M = 0$. Parameter ϵ controls the stopping condition (Step 2). We divide $|\phi(\mathbf{f}^{(k+1)}) - \phi(\mathbf{f}^{(k)})|$ by $\max(\phi(\mathbf{f}^{(k+1)}), 1)$ to compute the relative change or the absolute change of the objective, whichever is smaller. In this work, the following parameters were used: $L_{\min} = 1 \times 10^{-2}$, $L_{\max} = 1 \times 10^{8}$, $\eta = 1 \times 10^{-4}$, $\tau = 2$, $\epsilon = 1 \times 10^{-3}$, and $M = 10$.

Solution to Subproblem: The subproblem is group separable and can be shown to be equivalent to solving the problem separately for each group $g \in G$. With some algebra, the subproblem associated with group g can be shown to be equivalent to $\mathbf{f}_g^{(k+1)} \in \operatorname{Arg}\min_{\mathbf{f}_g \geq 0} \left\{ \phi_g(\mathbf{f}_g) = \|\mathbf{f}_g - \mathbf{z}_g^{(k)}\|_2^2 + \frac{2}{L^{(k)}} r(\mathbf{f}) \right\}$, where $\mathbf{z}^{(k)} = \mathbf{f}^{(k)} - \nabla l(\mathbf{f}^{(k)})/L^{(k)} = \mathbf{f}^{(k)} - 2\mathbf{A}^{\mathrm{T}}(\mathbf{A}\mathbf{f}^{(k)} - \mathbf{b})/L^{(k)}$ and $\mathbf{z}_g^{(k)}$ is a subvector of $\mathbf{z}^{(k)}$ associated with group g. If we let $\tilde{\gamma}_1^{(k)} = 2\alpha\gamma/L^{(k)}$, and $\tilde{\gamma}_2^{(k)} = 2(1-\alpha)\gamma/L^{(k)}$, the solution to the problem can be obtained by hard thresholding. If $\tilde{\mathbf{z}} = \mathtt{hard}_+(\mathbf{z}_g^{(k)}, \tilde{\gamma}_1^{(k)})$, where $\mathtt{hard}_+(\mathbf{z}, \gamma)_i = z_i$ if if $z_i > \sqrt{\gamma}$ and 0 otherwise,

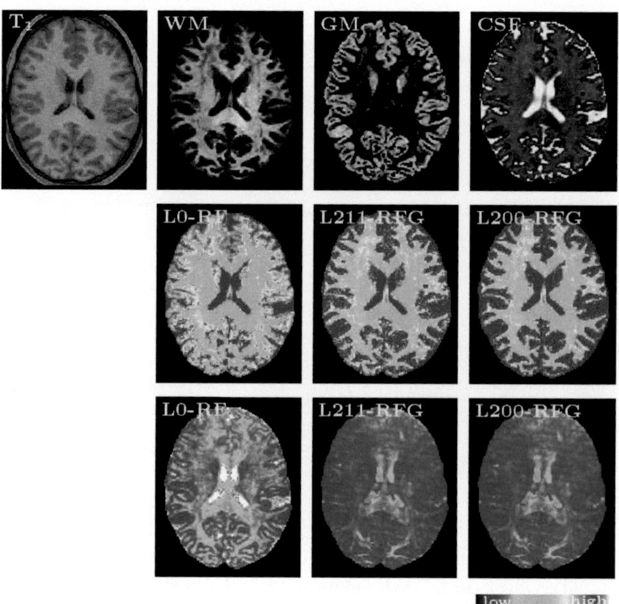

Fig. 1. (Top) Volume fractions of WM, GM, and CSF obtained by the proposed method. The T_1-weighted image is provided for reference. **(Middle)** Color-coded volume fraction images and **(Bottom)** fitting-residual images obtained by the various methods.

the solution to the subproblem is $\mathbf{f}_g^{(k+1)} = \tilde{\mathbf{z}}$ if $\|\tilde{\mathbf{z}}\|_2^2 > \tilde{\gamma}_1^{(k)} \|\tilde{\mathbf{z}}\|_0 + \tilde{\gamma}_2^{(k)}$ and 0 otherwise. Note that the sparse-group LASSO [7] can be implemented in a similar fashion by replacing the above solution with a soft-thresholding version.

3 Experimental Results

3.1 Data

For reproducibility, diffusion weighted (DW) data from the Human Connectome Project (HCP) were used. The $1.25 \times 1.25 \times 1.25\,\text{mm}^3$ data were acquired with diffusion weightings $b = 1000$, 2000, and $3000\,\text{s/mm}^2$ each applied in 90 directions. 18 baseline images with low diffusion weighting $b = 5\,\text{s/mm}^2$ were acquired.

3.2 Diffusion Parameters

The parameters of the RFGs were set to cover the typical values of the diffusivities of the WM, GM, and CSF voxels in the above dataset: $\lambda_{\parallel}^{\text{WM}} = 1 \times 10^{-3}\,\text{mm}^2/s$, $\lambda_{\perp}^{\text{WM}} = [0.1 : 0.1 : 0.3] \times 10^{-3}\,\text{mm}^2/s$, $\lambda^{\text{GM}} = [0.00 : 0.01 : 0.80] \times 10^{-3}\,\text{mm}^2/s$, and $\lambda^{\text{CSF}} = [1.0 : 0.1 : 3.0] \times 10^{-3}\,\text{mm}^2/s$. The notation $[a : s : b]$ denotes values from a to b, inclusive, with step s. Note that in practice, these ranges do not have to be exact but should however cover the range

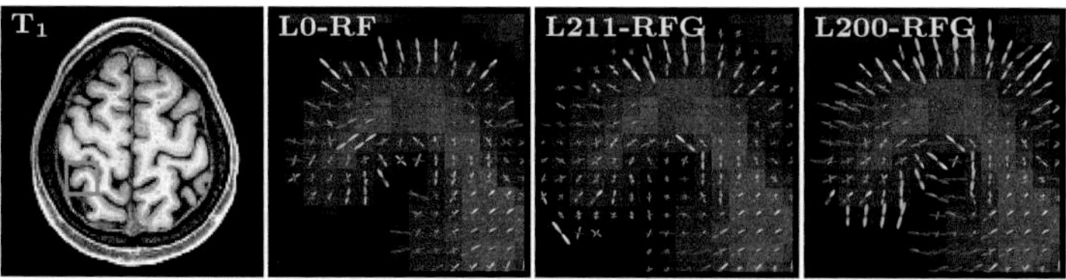

Fig. 2. WM FODFs at WM-GM interface. The glyphs are normalized to have unit integral.

of possible parameter variation. The WM RFGs are distributed evenly on 321 points on a hemisphere, generated by subdivision of the faces of an icosahedron.

3.3 Comparison Methods

We compared the proposed method (**L200-RFG**) with the following methods: **L0-RF**: l_0 minimization using a single RF each for WM, GM, and CSF [3]. Similar to [3], WM-GM-CSF segmentation was used to help determine the parameters for the RFs. The axial and radial diffusivities of the WM RFs were determined based on WM voxels with fractional anisotropy (FA) greater than 0.7. The diffusivity of the isotropic GM/CSF RF was determined based on GM/CSF voxels with FA less than 0.2. **L211-RFG**: Sparse-group LASSO [7] using RFGs identical to the proposed method. Similar to [8], we executed sparse-group LASSO multiple times, each time reweighing the l_{21}-norm and the l_1-norm so that they eventually approximate their l_0 counterparts. The tuning parameter γ was set to 1×10^{-4} for all methods. In addition, we set $\alpha = 0.05$ for the proposed method.

3.4 Results

Volume Fractions: The top row of Fig. 1 shows that the proposed method, even with no spatial regularization, is able to produce WM, GM, CSF volume fraction estimates that match quite well with the anatomy shown by the T_1-weighted image. The second row of the figure shows color-coded volume-fraction images generated by convex combinations of green, blue, and red using the WM, GM, and CSF volume fractions, respectively, as the weights. The results confirm the benefits of using RFGs over just RFs for the WM, GM, and CSF compartments. Compared with l_1 penalization, our method based on cardinality penalization yields cleaner volume fraction estimates especially for cortical GM.

Fitting Residuals: The last row of Fig. 1 indicates that using only a RF for each compartment is inadequate for explaining the data sufficiently, resulting in large fitting errors for some voxels. This also indicates that there is a mismatch between the RFs and the data. By using RFGs, the fitting residuals are smaller and relatively uniform spatially.

FODFs: The FODFs at the WM-GM interface are significantly affected by partial volume effect, with the signal being a mixture of contributions from WM and GM. Fig. 2 shows an example of the WM FODFs estimated at a WM-GM interface. The GM and CSF compartments are discarded and not shown. The proposed method in general yields FODFs that penetrate deeper into the GM when compared with L0-RF and that have a smaller amount of false-positive peaks when compared with L211-RFG. These observations indicate that the proposed method is able to effectively extract directional information that is buried within confounding signals.

4 Conclusion

We have shown that the estimation of the WM FODF and the GM and CSF volume fractions can be improved by using response function groups in a cardinality-penalized estimation framework. Our method provides the flexibility of including different diffusion models in different groupings for robust microstructural estimation. Future work includes incorporating complex diffusion models [9] for estimation of subtle properties such as axonal diameter. We will also apply our method to the investigation of pathological conditions such as edema.

References

1. Tournier, J.-D., Calamante, F., Connelly, A.: Robust determination of the fibre orientation distribution in diffusion MRI: Non-negativity constrained super-resolved spherical deconvolution. NeuroImage 35(4), 1459–1472 (2007)
2. Parker, G.D., Marshall, D., Rosin, P.L., Drage, N., Richmond, S., Jones, D.K.: A pitfall in the reconstruction of fibre ODFs using spherical deconvolution of diffusion MRI data. NeuroImage 65, 433–448 (2013)
3. Jeurissen, B., Tournier, J.D., Dhollander, T., Connelly, A., Sijbers, J.: Multi-tissue constrained spherical deconvolution for improved analysis of multi-shell diffusion MRI data. NeuroImage (2014)
4. Wang, Y., Wang, Q., Haldar, J.P., Yeh, F.C., Xie, M., Sun, P., Tu, T.W., Trinkaus, K., Klein, R.S., Cross, A.H., Song, S.K.: Quantification of increased cellularity during inflammatory demyelination. Brain 134, 3590–3601 (2011)
5. White, N.S., Leergaard, T.B., D'Arceuil, H., Bjaalie, J.G., Dale, A.M.: Probing tissue microstructure with restriction spectrum imaging: Histological and theoretical validation. Human Brain Mapping 34, 327–346 (2013)
6. Daducci, A., Canales-Rodríguez, E.J., Zhang, H., Dyrby, T.B., Alexander, D.C., Thiran, J.-P.: Accelerated microstructure imaging via convex optimization (AMICO) from diffusion MRI data. NeuroImage 105, 32–44 (2015)
7. Simon, N., Friedman, J., Hastie, T., Tibshirani, R.: A sparse-group lasso. Journal of Computational and Graphical Statistics 22(2), 231–245 (2013)
8. Daducci, A., Van De Ville, D., Thiran, J.-P., Wiaux, Y.: Sparse regularization for fiber ODF reconstruction: From the suboptimality of l_2 and l_1 priors to l_0. Medical Image Analysis 18, 820–833 (2014)
9. Panagiotaki, E., Schneider, T., Siow, B., Hall, M.G., Lythgoe, M.F., Alexander, D.C.: Compartment models of the diffusion MR signal in brain white matter: A taxonomy and comparison. NeuroImage 59, 2241–2254 (2012)
10. Barzilai, J., Borwein, J.: Two point step size gradient methods. IMA Journal of Numerical Analysis 8, 141–148 (1988)

V–Bundles: Clustering Fiber Trajectories from Diffusion MRI in Linear Time

Andre Reichenbach[1], Mathias Goldau[1], Christian Heine[2], and Mario Hlawitschka[3]

[1] Image and Signal Processing Group, Computer Sience Institute, Leipzig University, Germany
[reichenbach,math]@informatik.uni-leipzig.de
[2] Visual Computing Group, Department of Computer Science, TU Chemnitz, Germany
christian.heine@informatik.tu-chemnitz.de
[3] Scientific Visualization Group, Computer Sience Institute, Leipzig University, Germany
hlawitschka@informatik.uni-leipzig.de

Abstract. Fiber clustering algorithms are employed to find patterns in the structural connections of the human brain as traced by tractography algorithms. Current clustering algorithms often require the calculation of large similarity matrices and thus do not scale well for datasets beyond 100,000 streamlines. We extended and adapted the 2D vector field k–means algorithm of Ferreira et al. to find bundles in 3D tractography data from diffusion MRI (dMRI) data. The resulting algorithm is linear in the number of line segments in the fiber data and can cluster large datasets without the use of random sampling or complex multipass procedures. It copes with interrupted streamlines and allows multisubject comparisons.

Keywords: diffusion MRI, fiber clustering, vector field.

1 Introduction

Tractography allows estimating the physical paths of neuronal connections in the human brain from diffusion–weighted magnetic resonance imaging (dMRI) data. Existing methods typically generate up to millions of streamlines for a single subject and then group them into bundles. These bundles represent a macro–scale wiring scheme of the brain and thus play a big role in generating atlases of the human white matter. They are also of general interest to neuroscience, in particular the study how structural as well as functional bundle characteristics relate to brain development, aging, and diseases.

To find fiber bundles, many popular methods use similarity measures and employ clustering, e.g., hierarchical clustering [4,9]. This typically requires the computation and storage of pairwise similarities, which grow quadratically in the number of streamlines and thus quickly limit the dataset sizes that can be

N. Navab et al. (Eds.): MICCAI 2015, Part I, LNCS 9349, pp. 191–198, 2015.
DOI: 10.1007/978-3-319-24553-9_24

processed. General strategies to reduce this complexity include random sampling [5,7], culling [10], or preclustering using a faster algorithm. Methods using similarity measures often require the data to be resampled to a fixed number of points or fixed segment length, and thus may loose information. Most similarity measures are not very resistent to interrupted streamlines typically arising from fiber tracers. Among other subquadratic algorithms are greedy approaches (e.g. [3]), procedures based on stochastic processes (e.g. [9,8]), and multiprocedure schemes including voxel–based clustering such as [4]. In contrast to these predominantly data–driven approaches, which are important for inferring structural connectivity without bias, there also are approaches that incorporate anatomical priors, as well as those working directly on the diffusion model omitting the tractography; a thorough review can be found in [6]. Although anatomical priors are designed to help to identify plausible white matter tracts, only little is known on white matter variability, hence essential subject differences may not be regarded.

Determining correspondence between identified clusters among subjects or image acquisitions allows population–averaged atlases or comparing diffusion indices along bundles. In prior work, this has been attempted by means of clustering subjects in unison in a common space [5], by bundle similarity measures [9,10], by using priors learned from training datasets [8,9], or by clustering an inter–subject similarity matrix [1].

In this paper, we adapt the vector field k–means algorithm by Ferreira et al. [2]. It is designed to find movement patterns in 2D directed trajectories by learning "latent" vector fields; we extend it to 3D and undirected streamlines. The result has a runtime complexity linear in the number of input points and naturally copes with interrupted streamlines. The learned vector fields can be used to classify new data or subjects.

2 Methods and Material

We first provide an overview of the vector k–means algorithm by Ferreira et al. [2] and then discuss our changes to make it applicable to streamline data.

2.1 Vector Field k–Means

The input to the algorithm is a set of 2D trajectories, given as lists of points and time stamps. The output is each trajectory's cluster and optionally the regular rectilinear vector fields which serve as cluster descriptors and can be used to classify trajectories not in the training set. The algorithm has three parameters: the vector field resolution R_v, i.e., the number of grid points along each axis, the number of clusters k, and the regularization strength λ to avoid overfitting. The algorithm first splits each trajectory i into a list of line segments $s_1^{(i)}, \ldots, s_{m^i}^{(i)}$, each lying in exactly one grid cell and having its own duration $w_l^{(i)}$.

The algorithm then proceeds iteratively, alternating between assigning the best vector field to each trajectory and fitting each vector field to its currently assigned trajectories. The vector fields $V^{(1)}, \ldots, V^{(k)}$ are represented as $R_v^2 \times 2$ matrices, each line coding the x, y velocity at one grid position. To find the best vector field for a given trajectory the algorithm computes, in terms of squared error, the average match of its line segments with each vector field as follows:

$$e(S^{(i)}, V^{(j)}) = \sum_{l=1}^{m^{(i)}} w_l^{(i)} (C_l^{(i)} V^{(j)} - B_l^{(i)})^2 \ , \tag{1}$$

where $C_l^{(i)}$ and $B_l^{(i)}$ are suitably constructed matrices for each segment that take within–cell interpolation into account. We refer to Ferreira et al. [2] for details.

To fit a vector field $V^{(j)}$ to its currently assigned trajectories, the algorithm computes the coefficients of $V^{(j)}$ that minimize:

$$c(V^{(j)}) = \lambda \|LV\|^2 + \frac{1-\lambda}{W} \sum_{i \in \{i | \phi_i = j\}} e(S^{(i)}, V^{(j)}) \ , \tag{2}$$

where W is the total time length over all line segments and L denotes the Laplacian of the grid. Its purpose is to prefer smooth vector fields. The algorithm is initialized by fitting each cluster to a single trajectory in turn. The first cluster is fitted to a random trajectory and each next cluster is fitted to the trajectory maximizing $e(S^{(i)}, V^{(j)})$ for all clusters already fitted. The algorithm finishes as soon as the assignment of trajectories to clusters no longer changes or a fixed number of iterations is reached. The computational complexity of the algorithm is linear in the total number of line segments, clusters, and grid size.

2.2 V–Bundles

To adapt vector field k–means to streamline data, we first need to extend the algorithm to 3D. Changing the dimension of the matrices suffices, but the size of the grid changes from $O(R_v^2)$ to $O(R_v^3)$, affecting computational complexity. We avoid unnecessary computations due to empty grid cells by initializing the grid using a voxel size parameter r_v instead of the number of points. Second, streamlines lack time information. We therefore replace the time parameter by arc length parameterization in the original trajectory–to–field match cost, implemented by replacing each line segment's duration $w_l^{(i)}$ by its length.

The lack of a direction in streamlines causes a more substantial change. Replacing vector fields by orientation fields is difficult because the latter lack a suitable and fast interpolation scheme. Instead, to determine the match cost between a streamline and a vector field, we treat each streamline as being directed but take the smaller value for both possible directions. The flip is implemented by negating $B_l^{(i)}$ in Equation 1. When fitting the vector field, we originally allowed streamlines to change their direction. Since we observed that only a few, typically outlying, streamlines change their direction and cause only marginal difference in cost, we decided to assign each streamline its direction in each assignment step and keep it fixed during fitting steps. This allows us to use the same technique as Ferreira et al., to stack the matrices $C_l^{(i)}$ and $B_l^{(i)}$ to $C^{(i)}$ and

$B^{(i)}$ in the fitting step and end up with a sparse linear system suitable for efficient solution by conjugate gradient. We also do not use the squared Laplacian, thus we solve the equation system $(L + C^{(i)^T} C^{(i)})V^{(i)} = C^{(i)^T} B^{(i)}$ to compute our vector fields. In order to keep the algorithm deterministic, we use the longest streamline to initialize $V^{(0)}$ instead of a random one.

Finally, we observed that spatially distant bundles were represented by the same vector field due to Laplacian smoothing. To avoid them being added to the same cluster, we employ additional scalar fields $Z^{(i)}$ of voxel size r_z describing the streamline density of each cluster. They are calculated by counting the number of streamlines crossing each cell, normalizing by their total number, smoothing using a Gaussian kernel and then inverting by subtracting each value from 1.0. By changing the assignment cost to $(1-\gamma)e(S^{(i)}, V^{(j)}) + \gamma\|C^{(i)}Z^{(j)}\|^2$, we can choose close by streamlines over distant ones as γ gets larger.

2.3 Material

We tested our algorithm on multiple datasets. To judge the robustness regarding interrupted streamlines, we created two artificial datasets: a crossing with 150 streamlines and a fork with 100 streamlines. In both datasets, runs of successive segments were removed randomly (overall one third of all segments) from the streamlines, breaking them into multiple pieces. We employ the *FiberCup* phantom[1], which is a hardware phantom that was originally developed in order to benchmark tracking algorithms through various types of complex fiber configurations: bundles crossing, forking, and touching. To assess clustering quality on real data, HARDI data of five healthy subjects aged 24 to 31 was acquired using a 3T Siemens Trio MRI scanner, single echo spin echo EPI sequence with GRAPPA on a 32 channel coil, $128 \times 128 \times 72$ image matrix, $1.7 \times 1.7 \times 1.7\,\mathrm{mm}^3$ voxel size, 60 gradient and six non–gradient images at $b = 1000$. The datasets were corrected for motion artifacts and linearly registered to one subject using *FLIRT* (fsl[2]). Registration used fractional anisotropy maps computed from the HARDI data. We traced streamlines using the *tensor toolkit*[3](ttk, version 1.4) and its default parameters (except for $\mathrm{FA}_1 = 0.2$ and $\mathrm{FA}_2 = 0.3$) and its standard interpolation for both the *FiberCup* as well as the human brain data. Furthermore, we created a 500 000–streamline dataset using *mrtrix*[4](version 0.2.11) using its default pipeline, parameters, and interpolation scheme. We resampled this dataset to 1mm segment length (around 28×10^6 segments).

For the purpose of comparison, we implemented four clustering algorithms: Garyfallidis et al. [3] (QuickBundles), a spectral clustering by O'Donnell and Westin [5], a point–based clustering by Zhang et al. [10], and a stochastic–process–based algorithm by Wassermann et al. [9]. The implementations make use of multiple cores where applicable. If not stated otherwise, streamlines were

1 http://www.lnao.fr/spip.php?rubrique79

2 http://fsl.fmrib.ox.ac.uk/fsl/fslwiki/FLIRT/UserGuide

3 https://gforge.inria.fr/projects/ttk/

4 http://www.brain.org.au/software/mrtrix/

resampled to 20 points per streamline in order to save time or because the resampling is required by the algorithm, as in the case of QuickBundles. For V–Bundles, we usually set the maximum number of k–means iterations to 3, $\lambda = 0.1$, $\gamma = 0.6$, $r_v = 15mm$ and $r_z = 9mm$. All algorithms were run on a dual Intel E5-2630v3 CPU, 32GB RAM, NVIDIA GeForce GTX 980, 4GB VRAM.

3 Results

We tested the five clustering algorithms' ability to resolve clusters even in the presence of gaps and short lines using the synthetic datasets. Each parameter was tuned to give a good match with the three, respectively two, contained bundles. The results are shown in Fig. 1. V–Bundles showed the best results, perfectly discerning the bundles in both experiments, but required $\gamma = 0$ to correctly resolve the fork. Spectral clustering came close to resolving the crossing configuration, missing only a few short lines. In all other cases, we did not find parameters that provided reasonable clusters. The similarity-based methods tend to cluster lines by proximity rather than orientation and often put isolated small lines into their own cluster.

We tested the ability to resolve common fiber configurations using the *FiberCup* phantom (Fig. 2). V-Bundles is able to separate lines into meaningful clusters, while QuickBundles easily becomes confused by outliers and interrupted lines. From the dataset we selected only those lines which exactly correspond to the seven known ground truth bundles of the *FiberCup* in order to measure precision and recall (using the clusters that share the largest number of lines with the respective ground truth cluster). V-Bundles shows a perfect recall score of 1 for all ground truth clusters when computing 16 clusters for the dataset using standard parameters. Precision, however, is low due to short fibers getting added to those few clusters. QuickBundles reaches high recall and precision values of 0.97 and 0.75 when creating a large number of clusters (e.g. 73 clusters, $\theta = 230$), but then, most of those fail to capture the patterns inherent to the phantom.

Furthermore, V-Bundles was also able to reliably extract major fiber bundles from a set of full brain tractography data (approx. 88 000 lines). We used the fields output by a run of V-Bundles on a single subject to identify the corresponding clusters in three other subjects. Figure 3 shows clusters located in three well–known fiber bundles in the four subjects.

The computation times for different datasets are shown in Table 1. Note the large influence of the vector grid length r_v, but V-Bundles scales linearly in the number of segments. The scalar grid resolution has little impact on computation time. The algorithms of O'Donnell et al., Zhang et al. and Wassermann et al. fail to cluster moderately large datasets due to resource limitations.

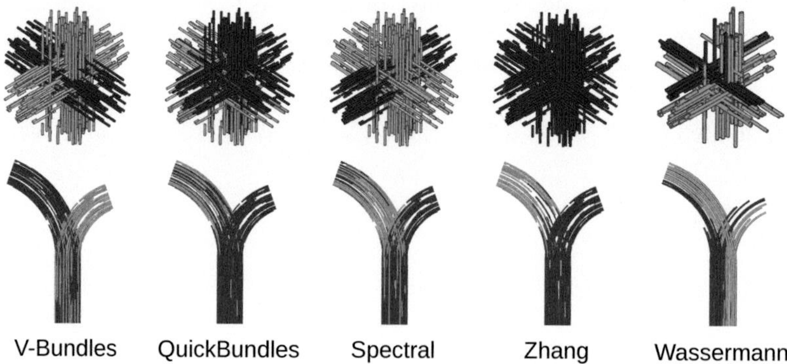

Fig. 1. The best three and two clusters for the crossing and the forking datasets respectively.

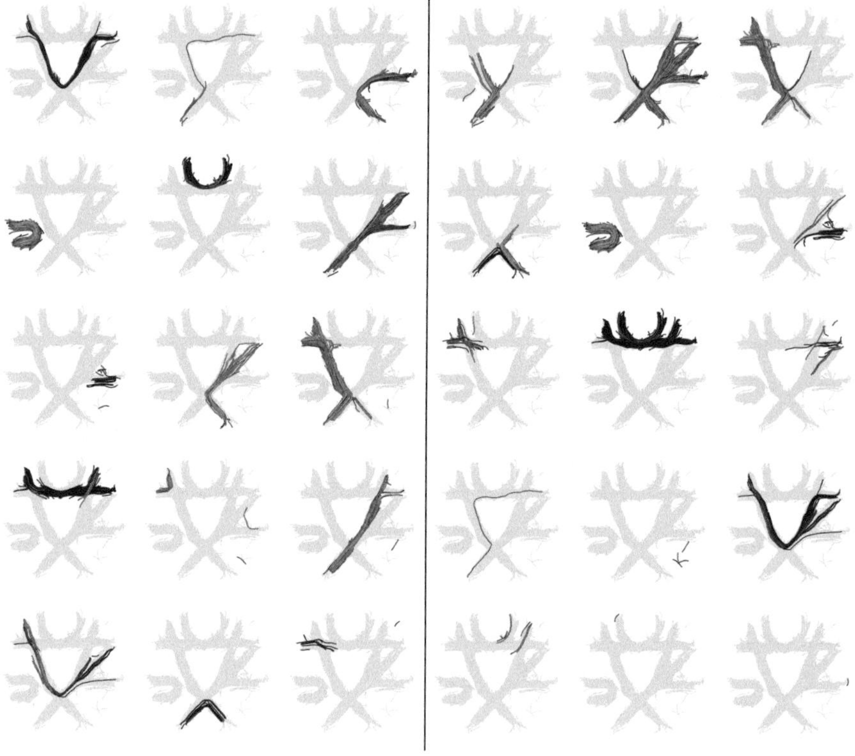

Fig. 2. Partitioning 883 lines tracked on the FiberCup dataset into 15 clusters using V–Bundles (r_v = 15mm, r_z = 9mm, γ = 0.6, λ = 0.001, *left*) and QuickBundles (θ = 620, *right*), respectively. The background shows all lines for context.

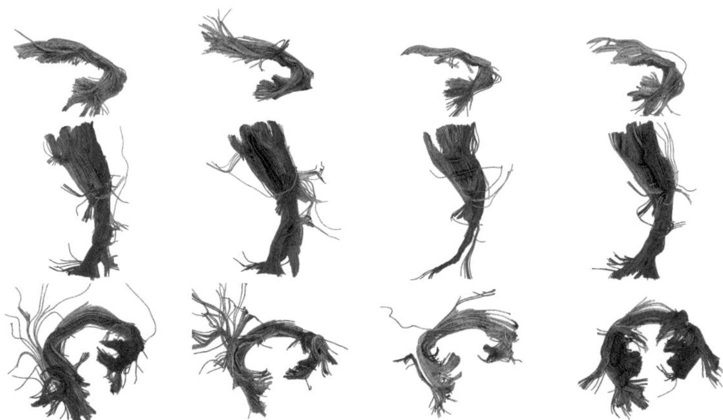

Fig. 3. Corresponding clusters calculated for the uncinate fasciculus (top row), parts of the cortico–spinal tract (mid row), and forceps major over four subjects. Each row has the same camera position. Parameters were $r_v = 15$mm, $r_z = 9$mm, $\lambda = 0.1$, $\gamma = 0.6$, 500 clusters. lines were resampled to 3 mm per segment to improve speed.

Table 1. Computation times, a single run each. The number of lines is denoted in brackets. When an algorithm exceeded 32GB of RAM, it was aborted (marked by –).

	V-Bundles	QuickB.	O'Donnell	Zhang	Wassermann
FiberCup (441)	2.5s	0.025s	0.31s	1.11s	0.67s
FiberCup (883)	3.3s	0.043s	1.08s	1.19s	3.03s
Human Brain (11k)	113s	2.23s	1770s	20.0s	531s
Human Brain (22k)	205s	4.88s	15500s	96.8s	–
Human Brain (44k)	368s	10.8s	108600s	428s	–
Human Brain (88k)	681s	17.0s	–	2260s	–
Human Brain (500k)	2290s	75.3s	–	–	–

4 Discussion and Conclusion

We described an adaption of the vector field k-means algorithm for clustering neuronal pathways. The algorithm handles short and interrupted streamlines, which can make up a significant part of a tractogram, without special treatment. This avoids generating a large number of "outlier"–clusters which need to be removed from the clustering afterwards. However, this property can also lead to bundles that share a common path for a significant part of their lengths to be erroneously clustered into the same cluster. Both increasing the locality parameter γ and reducing the number of clusters aggravates the problem.

As demonstrated, computation time and memory consumption scale linearly in the overall number of streamline segments, whis makes the algorithm applicable to dense sets of 100 000 or more streamlines while keeping computation times reasonably short. It may thus prove to be a useful tool in clinical settings or group studies. Computation time can be significantly reduced by resampling the streamlines to have longer segments. However, the grid resolution currently also has a high impact on performance; thus, in future work, we plan to address this problem by finding a sparser representation of the vector field which could be computed more quickly.

V–Bundles is also capable of finding corresponding clusters in different subjects in a common space, which is done by initializing the algorithm with the output fields of one subject (or possibly the result of combined tractograms of multiple subjects). It would also be conceivable to initialize the algorithm with a clustering created by an expert.

Also, we plan to evaluate different strategies for picking the first streamline in the initialization step. The source code of our reference implementation will be made available at *www.openwalnut.org*.

Acknowledgements. We thank Marcus Stuber for his initial coding effort, Marc Tittgemeyer for providing T1 and HARDI data of human subjects, and the anonymous reviewers for their excellent feedback.

References

1. Dodero, L., Vascon, S., Murino, V., Bifone, A., Gozzi, A., Sona, D.: Automated multi-subject fiber clustering of mouse brain using dominant sets. Frontiers in Neuroinformatics 8, 87 (2015)
2. Ferreira, N., Klosowski, J.T., Scheidegger, C.E., Silva, C.T.: Vector field k–means: Clustering trajectories by fitting multiple vector fields. Computer Graphics Forum 32(3), 201–210 (2013)
3. Garyfallidis, E., Brett, M., Correia, M.M., Williams, G.B., Nimmo-Smith, I.: Quickbundles, a method for tractography simplification. Front. Neurosci. 6 (2012)
4. Guevara, P., Poupon, C.: Inference of a hardi fiber bundle atlas using a two-level clustering strategy. In: Jiang, T., Navab, N., Pluim, J.W., Viergever, M. (eds.) MICCAI 2010. LNCS, vol. 6361, pp. 550–557. Springer, Heidelberg (2010)
5. O'Donnell, L., Westin, C.F.: White matter tract clustering and correspondence in populations. In: Duncan, J., Gerig, G. (eds.) MICCAI 2005. LNCS, vol. 3749, pp. 140–147. Springer, Heidelberg (2005)
6. O'Donnell, L.J., Golby, A.J., Westin, C.F.: Fiber clustering versus the parcellation-based connectome. NeuroImage 80, 283–289 (2013)
7. Visser, E., Nijhuis, E.H., Buitelaar, J.K., Zwiers, M.P.: Partition-based mass clustering of tractography streamlines. NeuroImage 54(1), 303–312 (2011)
8. Wang, X., Grimson, W.E.L., Westin, C.F.: Tractography segmentation using a hierarchical dirichlet processes mixture model. NeuroImage 54(1), 290–302 (2011)
9. Wassermann, D., Bloy, L., Kanterakis, E., Verma, R., Deriche, R.: Unsupervised white matter fiber clustering and tract probability map generation: Applications of a gaussian process framework for white matter fibers. NeuroImage 51(1), 228–241 (2010)
10. Zhang, S., Correia, S., Laidlaw, D.H.: Identifying white-matter fiber bundles in dti data using an automated proximity-based fiber-clustering method. IEEE Transactions on Visualization and Computer Graphics 14(5), 1044–1053 (2008)

Assessment of Mean Apparent Propagator-Based Indices as Biomarkers of Axonal Remodeling after Stroke

Lorenza Brusini[1], Silvia Obertino[1], Mauro Zucchelli[1], Ilaria Boscolo Galazzo[2], Gunnar Krueger[3], Cristina Granziera[4], and Gloria Menegaz[1]

[1] Dept. of Computer Science, University of Verona, Italy
[2] Institute of Nuclear Medicine, University College of London, UK
[3] Siemens Healthcare USA, Boston, USA
[4] Dept. of Clinical Neuroscience, CHUV and University of Lausanne, Switzerland

Abstract. Recently, a robust mathematical formulation has been introduced for the closed-form analytical reconstruction of the signal and the Mean Apparent Propagator (MAP) in diffusion MRI. This is referred to as MAP-MRI or 3D-SHORE depending on the chosen reference frame. From the MAP, microstructural properties can be inferred by the derivation of indices that under certain circumstances allow the estimation of pores' geometry and local diffusivity, holding the potential of becoming the next generation of microstructural numerical biomarkers. In this work, we propose the assessment and validation of a subset of such indices that is RTAP, D, and PA for the quantitative analysis of axonal remodeling in the uninjured motor network after stroke. Diffusion Spectrum Imaging (DSI) was performed on ten patients and ten controls at different time points and the indices were derived and exploited for tract-based quantitative analysis. Our results provide quantitative evidence on the eligibility of the derived indices as microstructural biomarkers.

1 Introduction

Connectivity remodeling after stroke has been reported in both injured [1] and uninjured hemispheres [2,3]. Generalized Fractional Anisotropy (GFA) had previously been successfully exploited to provide evidence of plasticity in the uninjured motor network in stroke patients with motor deficits. Recently, a robust mathematical formulation has been introduced for the closed-form analytical reconstruction of the diffusion signal from which new micro structural indices could be analytically derived. This is referred to as Mean Apparent Propagator (MAP)-MRI and 3D Simple Harmonic Oscillator Based Reconstruction and Estimation (3D-SHORE), respectively, depending on the reference frame. The corresponding MAP, also known in literature as Ensemble Average Propagator (EAP) [4], can then be profitably exploited for deriving information about the ensemble average values of pores' geometry and local diffusivity [4] and hold the potential for eligibility as the next generation of microstructural biomarkers. In particular, an estimation of the axons' cross-sectional area and diameter

N. Navab et al. (Eds.): MICCAI 2015, Part I, LNCS 9349, pp. 199–206, 2015.
DOI: 10.1007/978-3-319-24553-9_25

can be derived analytically in white matter. In this work, we aimed at exploring whether the MAP-derived measures 1) could reveal contralesional structural changes along intracallosal connections after stroke; 2) correlate with the well established GFA index; and 3) jointly with clinical status allow to predict motor outcomes.

2 Materials and Methods

Ten stroke patients [6 males and 4 females (age: 60.3 ± 12.8 years, mean ± SD)] were enrolled in the study; the inclusion criteria, imaging protocol and post-processing were as in [2]. All patients underwent three DSI scans (TR/TE = 6600/138 msec, FOV = 212 × 212 mm, 34 slices, 2.2 × 2.2 × 3 mm resolution, 258 gradient directions, b_{max} = 8000 s/mm^2) within one week (*tp1*), one month (± one week, *tp2*), and six months (± fifteen days, *tp3*) after stroke. Orientation distribution functions were reconstructed using the Diffusion Toolkit (www.trackvis.org/dtk). Fiber-tracking was performed via a streamline algorithm (www.cmtk.org). Patients benefited of clinical assessment (NIHSS: National Institute of Health Stroke Scale), with the motor part (NIHSS motor) derived from items 2 to 7 and 10 (www.nihstrokescale.org/). Ten age and gender matched healthy controls were also included in the study (age: 56.1 ± 17.8 years, mean ± SD). Control group underwent two DSI scans one month apart (*tp1c* and *tp2c*). All subjects provided written informed consent and the Lausanne University Hospital review board approved the study protocol. To the best of our knowledge, this is the first attempt of using MAP-indices in patients, while *in-vivo* acquisition in healthy subjects were reported in [5].

2.1 Analytical Model for Signal Reconstruction

In this work, the orthonormal formulation of the 3D-SHORE model was chosen [6,7]. With respect to MAP, this formulation allows less degrees of freedom in the choice of the scale parameter but there is some evidence for improved capability in resolving complex structural micro-topologies [8]. The diffusion signal is modeled by using the Eigenfunctions of the SHORE as basis. After rotating the reference frame for diagonalizing the stiffness tensor, a separable solution can be obtained [4]

$$\Phi_{N_i}(\mathbf{A}, \mathbf{q}) = \phi_{n_{x(i)}}(u_x, q_x)\phi_{n_{y(i)}}(u_y, q_y)\phi_{n_{z(i)}}(u_z, q_z) \tag{1}$$
$$\text{with} \begin{cases} \phi_n(u, q) = \frac{i^{-n}}{\sqrt{2^n n!}} e^{-2\pi^2 q^2 u^2} H_n(2\pi u q) \\ \mathbf{A} = \mathrm{Diag}(u_x^2, u_y^2, u_z^2) \end{cases}$$

where $N_i = (n_{x(i)}, n_{y(i)}, n_{z(i)})$ is the basis order and H_n a Hermite polynomial. Diagonalization of the stiffness tensor is performed by tensor fitting $\mathbf{A}'$ ($\mathbf{A} = \mathbf{R}\mathbf{A}'\mathbf{R}^T$), where $\mathbf{R}$ consists of the tensor Eigenvectors. Separability enables the anisotropic scaling of the basis functions along the coordinate axes making the 3D basis particularly suited to anisotropic data. The 3D-SHORE model is expressed in spherical coordinates. Separability holds the radial and angular coordinates which prevents the independent scaling of the basis functions along the main coordinate axes. Following the formulation in [9], the basis functions $\Phi_n(q\mathbf{u})$ can be written as

$$\Phi_n(q\mathbf{u}) = R_n(q)Y_n(\mathbf{u}) \tag{2}$$

where $R_n(q)$ models the radial part of the signal and $\{Y_n(\mathbf{u})\}$ are the real spherical harmonics of even order [10]. After a reordering of the terms, the signal model becomes

$$\mathbf{E}(q\mathbf{u}) = \sum_{l=0,even}^{N_{max}} \sum_{n=l}^{(N_{max}+l)/2} \sum_{m=-l}^{l} c_{nlm}\Phi_{nlm}(q\mathbf{u}) \tag{3}$$

$$\Phi_{nlm}(q\mathbf{u}) = \left[\frac{2(n-l)!}{\zeta^{3/2}\Gamma(n+3/2)}\right]^{1/2} \left(\frac{q^2}{\zeta}\right)^{l/2} \exp\left(\frac{-q^2}{2\zeta}\right) L_{n-l}^{l+1/2}\left(\frac{q^2}{\zeta}\right) Y_l^m(\mathbf{u})$$

where N_{max} is the maximal order in the truncated series and $\Phi_{nlm}(\mathbf{q})$ is the orthonormal 3D-SHORE basis, Γ is the Gamma function and ζ is an isotropic scaling parameter. The coefficients are determined by quadratic programming and positivity constraints are imposed to the MAP. The two formulations are equivalent for isotropic scaling.

Under such assumption, in this study we call MAP-based indices the measures derived from 3D-SHORE namely the Return to Axis Probability (RTAP) and Propagator anisotropy (PA). An estimate of the axon diameter (D) was inferred from RTAP as this provides an estimate of the exact statistical average of the cross-sectional area in white matter if some conditions are met [4] as $D = \sqrt{4\pi\ /RTAP}$. The MAP indices were assessed against GFA.

$$\begin{aligned} RTAP &= \sum_{l=0,even}^{N_{max}} \sum_{n=l}^{(N_{max}+l)/2} \sum_{m=-l}^{l} c_{nlm} \left[\frac{\zeta^{1/2}\ 2^{l+3}\pi^2\ \Gamma(l/2+1)^2\ \Gamma(n+3/2)}{(n-l)!\ \Gamma(l+3/2)^2}\right]^{1/2} \times \\ &\quad \times {}_2F_1(l-n, l/2+1, l+3/2, 2)\ P_l(0)\ Y_l^m(\mathbf{u}^*) \\ PA &= \sqrt{1 - \frac{\sum_{l=0}^{N_{max}/2+1} c_{l00}^2}{\sum_{l=0,even}^{N_{max}} \sum_{n=l}^{(N_{max}+l)/2} \sum_{m=-l}^{l} c_{nlm}^2}} \end{aligned} \tag{4}$$

2.2 Tract-Based Quantitative Analysis

The primary motor area (M1), supplementary motor area (SMA), somatosensory cortex (SC) and thalamus (Thl) were considered in the analysis. GFA and MAP-indices were collected along intracallosal fiber bundles connecting those regions to the corpus callosum (CC) in the contralateral (non-lesioned) hemisphere. In particular, GFA, RTAP, D, and PA values were computed for each voxel and then averaged along each tract and among all tracts connecting the regions of interest to the CC.

2.3 Statistical Analysis

Reproducibility of mean GFA, RTAP, D, and PA values along motor tracts was assessed by evaluating statistical differences between *tp1c* and *tp2c* using a paired t-test ($p > 0.05$) after a Kolmogorov-Smirnov normality test. Percentage absolute changes in mean values between time points were evaluated for each index on both groups as

$$\begin{aligned} \Delta_{tp12c}(m) &= |(m_{tp2c} - m_{tp1c})|/m_{tp1c} \\ \Delta_{tp12}(m) &= |(m_{tp2} - m_{tp1})|/m_{tp1} \\ \Delta_{tp23}(m) &= |(m_{tp3} - m_{tp2})|/m_{tp2} \\ \Delta_{tp13}(m) &= |(m_{tp3} - m_{tp1})|/m_{tp1} \end{aligned} \tag{5}$$

where m denotes the mean value of the considered index along the fibers of a given connection, and the subscript c denotes the control group. Normality test (Kolmogorov-Smirnov) revealed that the values were normally distributed enabling the use of parametric statistics. Accordingly, the unpaired t-test with $p < 0.05$ was performed to establish the significant differences between $\Delta_{tp12c}(m)$ and $\Delta_{tp12}(m)$. With the purpose to further characterize the MAP-based indices, Spearman correlation with GFA was performed. In addition, for each patient, the z-score of the mean absolute changes of each index and connection with respect to the same measurement on the control group was calculated in order to highlight and visually render in an intuitive way the distance between each patient and the control group as well as individual changes over time. Finally, the predictive value of each metric was assessed by a linear regression model where the motor outcome at six months after stroke ($tp3$) was the dependent variable and the mean values of each index for all the connections at $tp1$, age, stroke size, and NIHSS motor scores at $tp1$ and $tp2$ were the predictors. A backward selection process was used to select the optimal predictor model with $p = 0.05$ as significance threshold.

3 Results and Discussions

Reproducibility of index values in controls. In controls, reproducibility of the mean GFA, RTAP, D and PA values was observed as confirmed by t-test which showed no statistical significant differences between *tp1c* and *tp2c* ($p > 0.05$). The mean absolute GFA, RTAP, D, and PA changes calculated for all the motor connections between the two time points were: $GFA: 0.0248 \pm 0.0074$, $RTAP: 0.0290 \pm 0.0082$, $D: 0.0205 \pm 0.0047$, $PA: 0.0241 \pm 0.0072$ (mean $\pm$ SEM). Among connections, the largest variability was recorded for SC.

Comparison of absolute GFA, RTAP, D, and PA changes in patients and controls. Figure 1 illustrates the mean absolute percent changes of the different indices for patients and controls. For each index, absolute changes between *tp1* and *tp2* in patients' connections were significantly different from the absolute changes between the same regions in controls between *tp1c* and *tp2c* ($0.01 \leq p \leq 0.05$). However, the thalamic intracallosal connection failed to reach significance in all conditions, and SC-CC did not reach significance for RTAP and D. As it is apparent from Figure 1, PA shows the highest sensitivity in differentiating the patients from the control group, outperforming GFA in the SMA-CC connection and having the same performance for the other considered ones. In particular, both are able to differentiate the groups for the M1 and SC intracallosal connections. RTAP and D also allow differentiating between the two groups for M1 and SMA, while they could not highlight differences for SC. However, RTAP and D provide a richer microstructural information with respect to GFA which only describes the level of anisotropy of restricted diffusion. In connections where RTAP and D are able to split patients and controls, MAP-based indices allow for a more accurate description of the microstructural changes in patients.

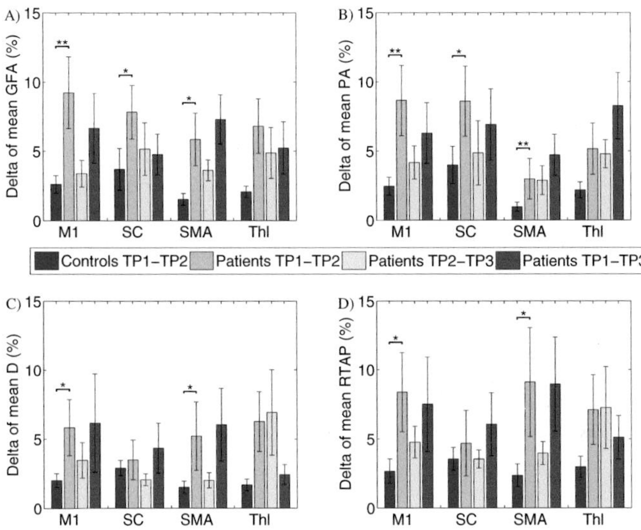

Fig. 1. Longitudinal changes in percent mean absolute values in controls and patients (${}^{*}p < 0.05$, ${}^{**}p < 0.01$). (A) GFA; (B) PA; (C) D; (D) $RTAP$.

Correlations of each absolute descriptor changes with GFA. For both controls and patients, Spearman's correlation ρ showed a significant ($p < 0.05$) monotonic relationship between the mean absolute changes of each MAP-based index and GFA changes. The overall correlation among all the intracallosal connections was assessed, showing the following results: 1) RTAP: $\rho_{tp12c} = 0.48$, $\rho_{tp12} = 0.74$, $\rho_{tp23} = 0.38$, $\rho_{tp13} = 0.65$; 2) D: $\rho_{tp12c} = 0.43$, $\rho_{tp12} = 0.76$, $\rho_{tp23} = 0.37$, $\rho_{tp13} = 0.40$; and 3) PA: $\rho_{tp12c} = 0.51$, $\rho_{tp12} = 0.74$, $\rho_{tp23} = 0.40$, $\rho_{tp13} = 0.64$. In all cases results were significant with $p < 0.05$.

Longitudinal changes in patients. Figure 2 highlights the pattern of the longitudinal changes in the different connections for individual patients with respect to the control group, that appeared to be patient-specific. The largest changes were observed in patients with the more severe motor deficit. The pattern is similar for the different indices providing evidence of the ability to capture the microstructural alterations due to white matter plasticity in the contralesional area. In particular, PA closely reproduces the pattern of GFA, while RTAP and D appear to be less sensitive especially for SC, coherently with the observation that for SC no significant difference between patients and controls could be detected by these two indices (see Figure 1). An increase in axon diameter is seen in patients over time. This could reveal axonal outgrowth and myelin increase due to plasticity as activated in the rehabilitation process [3], [11].

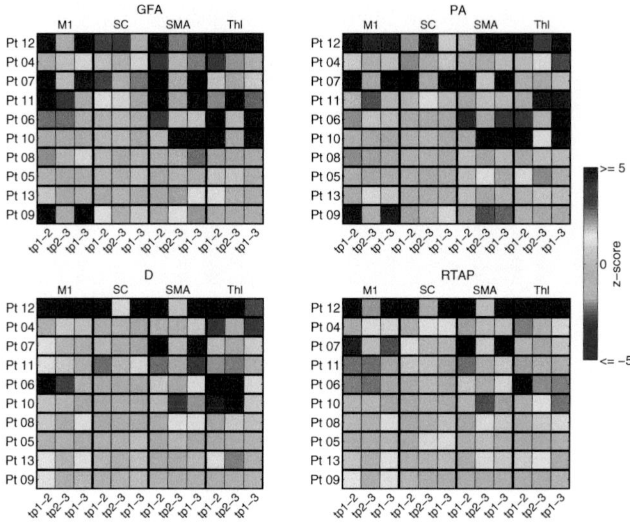

Fig. 2. Patients' individual profiles of mean absolute changes between *tp1* and *tp2* (first column), *tp2* and *tp3* (second column), and *tp1* and *tp3* (third column). Changes were compared to the corresponding controls' mean changes using *z*-scores. Patients are ordered according to the initial NIH Stroke Scale (NIHSS).

Prediction of clinical outcomes in patients for each index. In the patients' group, a linear regression model including only age and NIHSS at *tp1* and *tp2* gave low correlation as well as a model including only NIHSS at *tp1* and *tp2* ($R^2 = 0.691$; adjusted $R^2 = 0.652$). Conversely, for each index, the models including also its mean values across the different connections were able to predict the NIHSS at *tp3* with higher significance (Table 1). In particular, the best prediction model was obtained for D ($R^2 = 0.998$; adjusted $R^2 = 0.990$, $p = 0.008$). The relative importance for each predictor of the different optimal models was evaluated with the Fisher test and reported in Supplementary Materials. However, all models led to high significance, with adjusted $R^2 > 0.8$, confirming the importance of GFA and MAP-based indices for an early prediction of the patient clinical outcome.

Moreover, although GFA and PA are both anisotropy indices, PA has a higher prediction significance pointing at a stronger reliability of this new descriptor.

Table 1. Performance of each prediction model

Index	**Multiple** R^2	**Adjusted** R^2	p
GFA	0.970	0.932	0.004
RTAP	0.919	0.818	0.026
D	0.998	0.990	0.008
PA	0.991	0.973	0.004

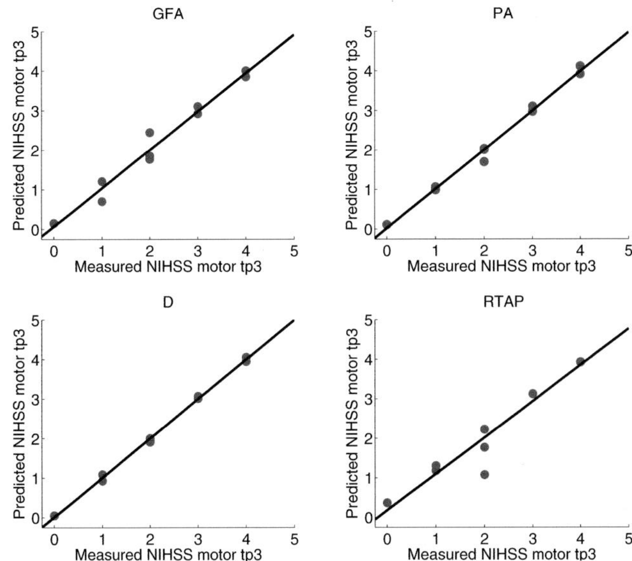

Fig. 3. Representation of the measured and predicted NIHSS at *tp3* using the models described above.

4 Conclusions

In this study, some evidence was provided on the suitability of the MAP-based indices RTAP, D, and PA as numerical biomarkers for stroke. Reproducibility was assessed by the test-retest method on the control group and longitudinal analysis on the patients group highlighted that contralesional structural changes after stroke could be well characterized and monitored by the newly proposed indices. The significant differences between controls and patients over multiple regions of interest lead the way to the application of RTAP, D, and PA as important descriptors for differentiating between the groups. Moreover, the performance of RTAP-, D-, and PA-based clinical regression models emphasized the suitability of these indices as early descriptors of patients' longitudinal changes and predictors of clinical outcomes.

References

1. Sotak, C.: The role of diffusion tensor imaging in the evaluation of ischemic brain injury a review. NMR in Biomedicine 15(7-8), 561–569 (2002)
2. Granziera, C., Daducci, A., Meskaldji, D., Roche, A., Maeder, P., Michel, P., Hadjikhani, N., Sorensen, A., Frackowiak, R., Thiran, J., Meuli, R., Krueger, G.: A new early and automated mri-based predictor of motor improvement after stroke. Neurology 79, 39–46 (2012)
3. Lin, Y., Daducci, A., Meskaldji, D., Thiran, J., Michel, P., Meuli, R., Krueger, G., Menegaz, G., Granziera, C.: Quantitative analysis of myelin and axonal remodeling in the uninjured motor network after stroke. Brain Connectivity (2014)
4. Ozarslan, E., Koay, C., Shepherd, T., Komlosh, M., Irfanoglu, M., Pierpaoli, C., Basser, P.: Mean apparent propagator (map) mri: A novel diffusion imaging method for mapping tissue microstructure. NeuroImage 78, 16–32 (2013)
5. Zucchelli, M., Descoteaux, M., Menegaz, G.: Human brain tissue microstructure characterization using 3D-SHORE on the HCP data. In: ISMRM, Toronto, Ontario, Canada (2015)
6. Ozarslan, E., Koay, C., Shepherd, T., Blackband, S., Basser, P.: Simple harmonic oscillator based reconstruction and estimation for three-dimensional q-space mri. Proc. Intl. Soc. Mag. Reson. Med. 17, 1396 (2009c)
7. Merlet, S., Deriche, R.: Continuous diffusion signal, {EAP} and {ODF} estimation via compressive sensing in diffusion {MRI}. Medical Image Analysis 17(5), 556–572 (2013)
8. Fick, R., Zucchelli, M., Girard, G., Descoteaux, M., Menegaz, G., Deriche, R.: Using 3D-SHORE and MAP-MRI to Obtain Both Tractography and Microstructural Constrast from a Clinical DMRI Acquisition. In: International Symposium on Biomedical Imaging: From Nano to Macro, Brooklyn, New York City, United States (2015)
9. Cheng, J., Jiang, T., Deriche, R.: Theoretical Analysis and Practical Insights on EAP Estimation via a Unified HARDI Framework. In: MICCAI Workshop on Computational Diffusion MRI (CDMRI), Toronto, Canada (2011)
10. Descoteaux, M., Angelino, E., Fitzgibbons, S., Deriche, R.: Regularized, fast, and robust analytical q-ball imaging. Magnetic Resonance in Medicine 58(3), 497–510 (2007)
11. Ueno, Y., Chopp, M., Zhang, L., Buller, B., Liu, Z., Lehman, N., Liu, X., Zhang, Y., Roberts, C., Zhang, Z.: Axonal outgrowth and dendritic plasticity in the cortical peri-infarct area after experimental stroke. Stroke 43(8), 2221–2228 (2012)

Integrating Multimodal Priors in Predictive Models for the Functional Characterization of Alzheimer's Disease

Mehdi Rahim[1,2,3], Bertrand Thirion[1,2], Alexandre Abraham[1,2], Michael Eickenberg[1,2], Elvis Dohmatob[1,2], Claude Comtat[3], and Gael Varoquaux[1,2]

[1] Parietal Team, INRIA Saclay-Île-de-France, Saclay, France
[2] CEA, DSV, I^{2}BM, Neurospin bât 145, 91191 Gif-Sur-Yvette, France
[3] CEA, DSV, I^{2}BM, SHFJ 4, place du Général Leclerc, 91401 Orsay, France
mehdi.rahim@cea.fr

Abstract. Functional brain imaging provides key information to characterize neurodegenerative diseases, such as Alzheimer's disease (AD). Specifically, the metabolic activity measured through fluorodeoxyglucose positron emission tomography (FDG-PET) and the connectivity extracted from resting-state functional magnetic resonance imaging (fMRI), are promising biomarkers that can be used for early assessment and prognosis of the disease and to understand its mechanisms. FDG-PET is the best suited functional marker so far, as it gives a reliable quantitative measure, but is invasive. On the other hand, non-invasive fMRI acquisitions do not provide a straightforward quantification of brain functional activity. To analyze populations solely based on resting-state fMRI, we propose an approach that leverages a metabolic prior learned from FDG-PET. More formally, our classification framework embeds population priors learned from another modality at the voxel-level, which can be seen as a regularization term in the analysis. Experimental results show that our PET-informed approach increases classification accuracy compared to pure fMRI approaches and highlights regions known to be impacted by the disease.

Keywords: Classification, prior, connectivity, metabolism, resting-state fMRI, FDG-PET, Alzheimer's disease.

1 Introduction

Alzheimer's disease (AD) is characterized by a progressive impairment of brain structures and their connections, which leads to a loss of cognitive function. Mild cognitive impairment (MCI) is frequently seen as a prodromal stage of AD. The anatomical and functional changes caused by AD or MCI can be detected via various neuroimaging modalities and machine learning techniques.

Indeed, anatomical measures performed on Magnetic Resonance Images (MRIs) such as hippocampus volume or cortical thickness [8] [6] [5], amyloid-β

N. Navab et al. (Eds.): MICCAI 2015, Part I, LNCS 9349, pp. 207–214, 2015.
DOI: 10.1007/978-3-319-24553-9_26

deposition [12], the quantification of metabolism on fluorodeoxyglucose positron emission tomography (FDG-PET), or cerebrospinal fluid (CSF) measures, can all bring precious biomarkers to help to distinguish AD subjects or MCI subjects who convert later to AD [10].

There is abundant prior art on classification models based on multi-modal images and non-imaging data. For instance [14] used a kernel to combine FDG-PET, anatomical MRI and CSF biomarker measures to obtain a high AD detection accuracy. Here we focus on functional imaging biomarkers involved in AD. Several studies have shown that FDG-PET imaging on MCI and AD subjects reveals significantly reduced metabolic activity. Whether based on brain regions [2] or voxels [9], prediction of AD on FDG-PET yields 90% accuracy. The major drawback of this modality is that it is invasive and involves exposition to gamma-ray radiation. On the other hand, resting-state fMRI captures brain activation via fluctuations of the blood oxygenation level dependent (BOLD) contrast. It is used to estimate functional connectivity, which is measured through the correlation between time courses. As studied in [13] and [4], AD is characterized by widespread decreases in connectivity, especially in the default mode network (DMN). Resting-state fMRI acquisitions are non-invasive and can be easily integrated within a clinical imaging protocol. However, their low signal-to-noise ratio reduces the sensitivity with regards to AD prediction. Also, the selection of prior *seed* regions for connectivity mapping involves a subjective choice which may lead to inaccuracies when analyzing groups of subjects.

Recently, [7] reported a close relationship between the DMN functional connectivity and its metabolic activity at rest, thanks to a study on FDG-PET and resting-state fMRI performed on a PET-MRI scanner. In this paper, we leverage this relationship in a rest-fMRI-based classification framework, constrained by a metabolism-based discriminative pattern learned from a distinct and large FDG-PET dataset. We show that regularization with an FDG-PET prior improves the fMRI classification accuracy and the discriminative pattern identification, compared to various state-of-the-art regularizers applied to the functional connectivity maps. We address the issue of the arbitrary selection of a reference region of interest (ROI) when computing connectivity by using several seed-based correlations of ROIs extracted from a functional atlas, followed by a model that stacks their predictions. The resulting predictor, based on multiple ROIs, gives better accuracy than a single selected ROI. The paper is organized as follows. In section 2, we present our classification framework with the integration of priors. Section 3 presents experiments in which different approaches are compared. Finally section 4 summarizes the results.

2 Multimodal Prior Integration for Model Enhancement

The proposed approach relies on the assumption that information on metabolism alterations measured with FDG-PET images can improve the accuracy of resting-state fMRI-based predictive models. Rather than a multi-modal PET-fMRI prediction in each subject, we derive a population-level PET prior, to avoid as much as possible the recurrent use of PET, since it is invasive. The first step of the proposed framework is to estimate a connectivity-based classification model regularized by a learned metabolic prior, which involves a complementary coupling parameter to adapt this prior. Besides the metabolic prior, we also investigate the usefulness of a spatial prior called the total-variation TV-ℓ_1 prior proposed in [1]. It is composed of a sparse regularization scheme ℓ_1 that displays few salient regions, combined with a TV scheme which promotes spatially grouped regions. The second step combines the predictions computed from the prior-integrated models of all ROIs involved thanks to a stacking model. Typically, a given set of seed-regions are used to compute signal correlations.

Let $\mathbf{X} \in \mathbb{R}^{n \times p}$ denote a voxel-level connectivity matrix relative to a specific ROI, where n and p are respectively the numbers of samples (subjects) and variables (voxels). Let $\mathbf{y} \in \{0,1\}^n$ denote the class (diagnosis) vector of each sample. Our model builds on ridge regression. The classical ridge regression estimates the coefficients $\hat{\mathbf{w}}_{\text{ridge}} \in \mathbb{R}^p$ so that

$$\hat{\mathbf{w}}_{\text{ridge}} = \operatorname{argmin}_{\mathbf{w}} \|\mathbf{X}\mathbf{w} - \mathbf{y}\|_2^2 + \alpha \|\mathbf{w}\|_2^2, \tag{1}$$

where $\alpha > 0$ is a parameter of the coefficient penalization that controls the amount of shrinkage. The proposed model integrates the prior within the penalization term yielding

$$\hat{\mathbf{w}} = \operatorname{argmin}_{\mathbf{w}} \|\mathbf{X}\mathbf{w} - \mathbf{y}\|_2^2 + \alpha \|\mathbf{w} - \lambda \mathbf{w}_{\mathbf{prior}}\|_2^2, \tag{2}$$

where $\mathbf{w}_{\mathbf{prior}}$ is the prior coefficient vector that has already been learned. $\lambda > 0$ is a scaling parameter that adapts the prior to the actual setting. By substituting $\mathbf{b} = \mathbf{w} - \lambda \mathbf{w}_{\mathbf{prior}}$, one falls back to a classical ridge regression formulation. Each of the model parameters λ and α are empirically estimated through a nested cross-validation procedure.

The coefficient vector $\hat{\mathbf{w}}$ of the predictive model is a spatial map that can be regularized with the TV-ℓ_1 spatial prior, in order to obtain more stable discriminative patterns. So the estimation problem is formulated as

$$\hat{\mathbf{w}} = \operatorname{argmin}_{\mathbf{w}} \frac{1}{2} \|\mathbf{X}\mathbf{w} - \mathbf{y}\|_2^2 + \frac{\alpha}{2} \|\mathbf{w} - \lambda \mathbf{w}_{\mathbf{prior}}\|_2^2 + \beta J(\mathbf{w}), \tag{3}$$

where $J(\mathbf{w})$ is the TV-ℓ_1 regularization term expressed as

$$J(\mathbf{w}) = \|\nabla \mathbf{w}\|_{21} + \rho \|\mathbf{w}\|_1. \tag{4}$$

In the stacking stage, the unthresholded prior-model predictions of all ROIs are concatenated, yielding a matrix $\mathbf{S} \in \mathbb{R}^{n \times s}$, where s is the number of ROIs. This summary is used in a logistic regression model to predict the subject class $\mathbf{y}$.

The pipeline corresponding to our model is depicted in Fig. 1. The inputs are the quantitative metabolism on 3D FDG-PET which is used for the prior estimation, the 4D resting-state fMRI and a set of ROIs from which the connectivity is estimated. First, the prior is estimated from FDG-PET thanks to a ridge classifier. Regarding the resting-state fMRI features, ROI-based connectivity maps are computed based on fMRI data as correlations between each voxel

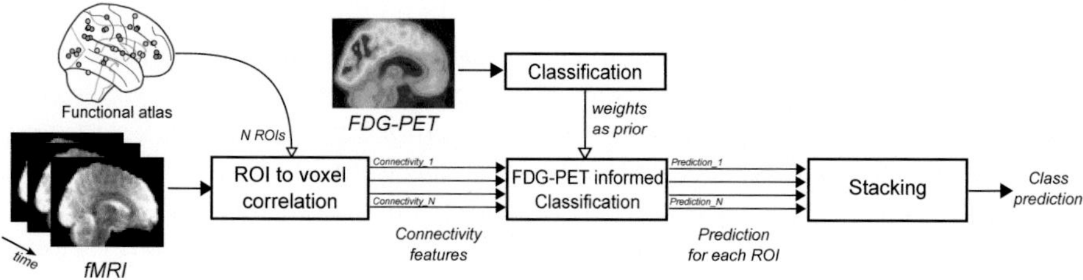

Fig. 1. Overview of the proposed classification pipeline: The inputs are ROI-to-voxel connectivities computed from the rs-fMRI time-series. FDG-PET model weights are integrated as prior for the classification. Then, predictions of all ROIs are the inputs of a stacking model to predict the clinical group.

and signals from the ROI. Unlike what is commonly done, we took as ROIs several regions extracted from a functional brain atlas. Actually, we compared two widely used functional brain atlases. The first atlas (called *Atlas 1* below), comprises 68 seed ROIs extracted from a functional dataset and proposed in [3]. This atlas has been constructed on 892 subjects, and was successfully used to characterize differences between AD subjects and cognitively normal ones. The second functional atlas (*Atlas 2*) has been proposed in [11], it contains 39 ROIs learned from resting-state fMRI data. Then, the regression model informed by the FDG-PET prior is estimated. This yields one model per ROI. Finally, the global classification on fMRI is performed via a logistic regression which estimates the target from the stacked predictions of each ROI-based model.

3 Experiments

Datasets. Data used in this study are taken from the Alzheimer's Disease Neuroimaging Initiative (ADNI) database (`adni.loni.ucla.edu`). In this work, two subject-distinct subsets were extracted for each modality (FDG-PET and fMRI) at baseline. We wish to study and predict conversion of MCI subjects to AD. However, the resting-state fMRI protocol has been integrated only recently in the ADNI study (from ADNI-GO phase), and we have merely 5 MCI converters that have fMRI acquisitions, which is not sufficient for estimation. We thus consider a proxy, namely the classification between MCI and AD subjects.

We applied a preprocessing pipeline which is composed of the following steps: removing the three first frames, motion correction, normalization to the MNI template, spatial smoothing (Gaussian, FWHM 5mm) and temporal detrending. After a quality check, we selected 94 subjects (21 AD and 73 MCI) out of 110 from ADNI-GO and ADNI-2 phases. Regarding the FDG-PET acquisitions, the downloaded data had already been preprocessed and quality-checked. The FDG-PET data used are 3D averaged images which have undergone co-registration, intensity standardization and a spatial normalization. Overall, we have images from 627 subjects (147 AD and 480 MCI) acquired mainly during ADNI-1 phase.

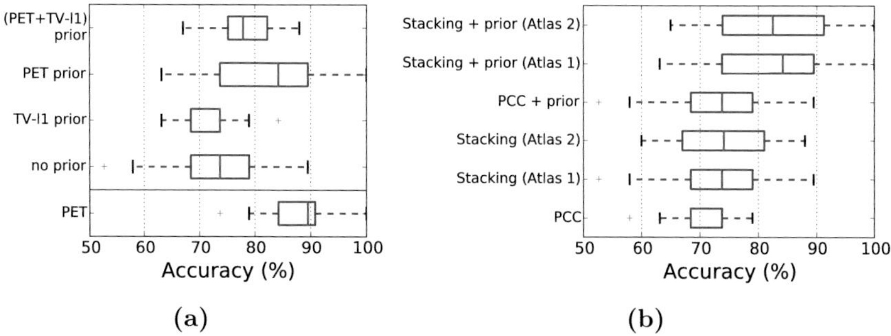

Fig. 2. Classification accuracies of : (a) PET prior and TV-ℓ_1 prior classifiers compared to pure connectivity classifier (no prior). (b) Atlas based stacking approach compared to a single ROI connectivity.

Note that the datasets of the two modalities are from two completely distinct groups of subjects.

Experiment settings. We evaluate the impact of : *i)* The regularization (metabolic, spatial, both, none). *ii)* The selection of the ROIs (*Atlas 1*, *Atlas 2*, posterior cingulate cortex region) on the connectivity-based classification. The model without regularization relies on a ridge regression on each ROI stacked under a logistic regression classifier. The evaluation of the two models is done by cross-validation, which consists of a stratified-shuffle split loop with 100 iterations and a test fold size of 20% of the whole dataset. The classification hyper-parameters (α, λ, β, ρ) are estimated by a nested 4-fold cross-validation. Moreover, the accuracy differences between test folds across iterations are measured through a two-sided Wilcoxon test.

4 Results and Discussion

Classification accuracy. Fig. 2a shows the accuracy of the cross-validated classification for the classical connectivity, the TV-ℓ_1 prior and the proposed metabolic prior. These results show that the proposed prior method outperformed the pure functional connectivity method. Indeed, the mean gain is relatively substantial (around 8%), as reported in Table 1, which summarizes the mean differences and the p-values calculated from the two-sided Wilcoxon test between each pair of models. The spatial TV-ℓ_1 prior does not improve the connectivity classification accuracy, although it produces a more stable model as the cross-validation accuracies have a lower variance. From these results, we conclude that the metabolic prior is more powerful to classify AD subjects than the spatial prior. One could expect that combining both metabolic and spatial priors would increase the connectivity-based prediction. In fact, the spatial penalty limited the metabolic

Table 1. Comparing accuracies on cross-validation folds when including the metabolic and the spatial priors or not. The last three rows report the differences when stacking predictions of ROI set from two functional atlases, and when using a selected ROI (posterior cingulate cortex). P-values from the two-sided Wilcoxon test between each pair of methods are in the last column.

Comparison	Mean difference (%)	p-value
TV-ℓ_1 prior − no prior	-1.9 ± 7.6	6.7×10^{-3}
PET prior − no prior	$+7.9 \pm 9.5$	1.3×10^{-10}
(PET + TV-ℓ_1) prior − no prior	$+4.1 \pm 9.4$	1.8×10^{-4}
PET prior − TV-ℓ_1 prior	$+9.7 \pm 8.8$	1.6×10^{-13}
(PET + TV-ℓ_1) prior − TV-ℓ_1 prior	$+5.9 \pm 7.1$	4.4×10^{-11}
(PET + TV-ℓ_1) prior − PET prior	-3.7 ± 9.6	2.7×10^{-4}
Atlas 1 − PCC	$+9.3 \pm 9.8$	2.6×10^{-12}
Atlas 2 − PCC	$+10.7 \pm 12.2$	6.6×10^{-12}
Atlas 1 − Atlas 2	$+1.4 \pm 9.3$	3.5×10^{-1}

prior influence in terms of accuracy, but decreased the variance. While these results should be interpreted with caution, given the size of the dataset, the overall accuracy increase is significant. It suggests that the metabolic prior estimated from FDG-PET data (whose consistency has been validated) permits the highlighting of biomarkers that the small fMRI dataset alone fails to bring. Spatial regularization does not enhance the scarce information provided by fMRI maps.

Regarding the stacking approach, Fig. 2b represents the accuracy distribution when stacking ROIs-based connectivity estimates compared to single-ROI connectivity. We note that, despite a higher variance introduced, calculating the connectivity from various ROIs and combining them allows a significant prediction accuracy enhancement: in Table 1, the accuracies are 10% higher than the PCC connectivity usually used in the analysis of resting-state fMRI connectivity. The comparison between the two atlases reveals that the models produced by each of them are quite similar in terms of accuracy. This shows that, in order to set up more robust connectivity-based models that classify AD, it is important not to restrict the analysis to a single region, but to extend it to several functional regions that bring complementary information.

Discriminative spatial patterns. Since we perform a voxel-level brain analysis, it is easy to visualize discriminant patterns between AD subjects and MCI subjects to interpret the estimated classification model coefficients. Learned brain spatial models, which consist of averaged classifier weights across cross-validation folds, are shown in Fig. 3.

Fig. 3a shows the spatial distribution map of the learned FDG-PET prior model, the map values are the coefficients of a cross-validated ridge classifier, with an overall accuracy of $88.0 \pm 5.7\%$. This difference map clearly outlines some cerebral regions, such as the posterior cingulate cortex (PCC), the precuneus, and parts of the parietal lobe. These structures, which are part of the DMN, are known to characterize AD with a decreased metabolism.

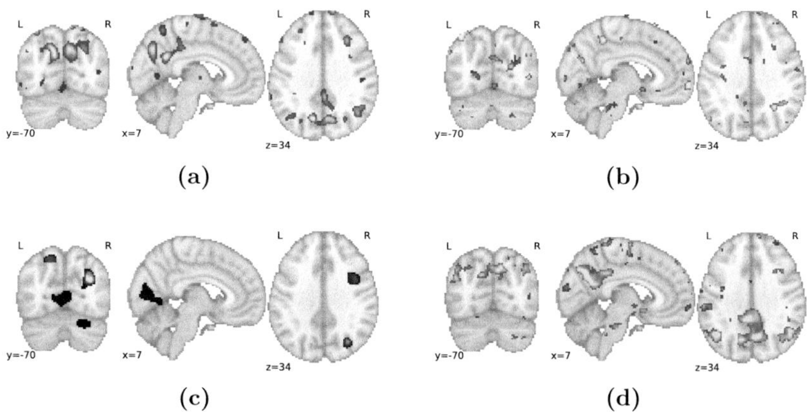

Fig. 3. Maps of AD discriminative spatial patterns extracted from : (a) the FDG-PET model used as prior. (b) the fMRI seed-to-voxel connectivity. (c) the fMRI with the spatial prior. (d) the fMRI with the metabolic prior.

The regions formed by the weights of the classification model estimated from PCC functional connectivity are plotted in Fig. 3b. Although the patterns are quite noisy, these regions describe some meaningful functional structures such as the default mode network, and parts of the parietal lobe.

The spatial TV-ℓ_1 prior in Fig. 3c did not bring supplementary information, but as expected, the sparse ℓ_1 constraint yielded less noisy patterns and the total-variation constraint produced more focused regions.

The impact of the FDG-PET prior is shown in Fig. 3d, where we see that the metabolic prior overcame the limitations of the connectivity-based discriminant patterns. We observe in particular patterns that are smoother than fMRI only, e.g. the clearly outstanding default mode network. This finding is in agreement with AD studies that showed the functional connectivity differences observed on resting-state fMRI, but it is hard to obtain from functional connectivity only.

5 Conclusion

We introduced in this paper a learning framework that integrates multi-modal prior knowledge from a distinct cohort. We addressed the ROI selection issue when computing the functional connectivity by proposing a stacking model that couples a set of ROIs. Experimental results confirm that the metabolism activity of brain structures measured on the FDG-PET images is linked to the connectivity measured by resting-state fMRI. In our experiments on the ADNI fMRI dataset, within the context of AD/MCI prediction, we validated the proposed method, since it improved the accuracy of the classification of AD subjects better than a spatial prior, and highlighted meaningful functional regions related to state-of-the-art studies on AD. It overcomes the limitations of fMRI data (small dataset, noisy data) with a pre-established model validated on a consistent fold of subjects. We showed that the stacking approach has a significant impact on the prediction accuracy, and using a validated functional atlas allowed us to be insensitive to the ROI selection. Moreover, our experiments showed that existing datasets are a very useful resource to investigate more difficult questions such as the prognosis of conversions from MCI to AD.

Acknowledgements. This work is supported by the Lidex PIM project funded by the IDEX Paris-Saclay, ANR-11-IDEX-003-02. We also acknowledge funding from the NiConnect project (ANR-11-BINF-0004_NiConnect).

References

1. Gramfort, A., Thirion, B., Varoquaux, G.: Identifying predictive regions from fMRI with TV-L1 prior. In: Pattern Recognition in Neuroimaging (PRNI), p. 17 (2013)
2. Gray, K.R., Wolz, R., Heckemann, R.A., Aljabar, P., Hammers, A., Rueckert, D.: Multi-region analysis of longitudinal FDG-PET for the classification of Alzheimer's disease. NeuroImage 60(1), 221–229 (2012)
3. Jones, D.T., Vemuri, P., Murphy, M.C., et al.: Non-stationarity in the "resting brain's" modular architecture. PloS One 7(6), e39731 (2012)
4. Koch, W., Teipel, S., Mueller, S., Benninghoff, J., Wagner, M., et al.: Diagnostic power of default mode network resting state fMRI in the detection of Alzheimer's disease. Neurobiology of Aging 33(3), 466–478 (2012)
5. Lillemark, L., Sørensen, L., et al.: Brain region's relative proximity as marker for Alzheimer's disease based on structural MRI. BMC Med. Imag. 14(1), 21 (2014)
6. Prados, F., Cardoso, M.J., et al.: Measuring brain atrophy with a generalized formulation of the boundary shift integral. Neurobiology of Aging 36, 81–90 (2015)
7. Riedl, V., Bienkowska, K., Strobel, C., et al.: Local activity determines functional connectivity in the resting human brain: a simultaneous FDG-PET/fMRI study. Journal of Neuroscience 34(18), 6260–6266 (2014)
8. Sabuncu, M.R., Desikan, R.S., Sepulcre, J., et al.: The dynamics of cortical and hippocampal atrophy in Alzheimer's disease. Archives of Neurology 68, 1040 (2011)
9. Toussaint, P.J., Perlbarg, V., Bellec, P., et al.: Resting state FDG-PET functional connectivity as an early biomarker of Alzheimer's disease using conjoint univariate and independent component analyses. NeuroImage 63(2), 936–946 (2012)
10. Trzepacz, P.T., Yu, P., Sun, J., et al.: Comparison of neuroimaging modalities for the prediction of conversion from mild cognitive impairment to Alzheimer's dementia. Neurobiology of Aging 35(1), 143–151 (2014)
11. Varoquaux, G., Gramfort, A., Pedregosa, F., Michel, V., Thirion, B.: Multi-subject dictionary learning to segment an atlas of brain spontaneous activity. In: Székely, G., Hahn, H.K. (eds.) IPMI 2011. LNCS, vol. 6801, pp. 562–573. Springer, Heidelberg (2011)
12. Villain, N., Chételat, G., et al.: Regional dynamics of amyloid-β deposition in healthy elderly, mild cognitive impairment and Alzheimer's disease: a voxelwise PiB–PET longitudinal study. Brain 135(7), 2126–2139 (2012)
13. Wang, K., Liang, M., Wang, L., Tian, L., Zhang, X., Li, K., Jiang, T.: Altered functional connectivity in early Alzheimer's disease: A resting-state fmri study. Human Brain Mapping 28(10), 967–978 (2007)
14. Zhang, D., Wang, Y., Zhou, L., Yuan, H., Shen, D.: Multimodal classification of Alzheimer's disease and mild cognitive impairment. NeuroImage 55, 856 (2011)

Simultaneous Denoising and Registration for Accurate Cardiac Diffusion Tensor Reconstruction from MRI

Valeriy Vishnevskiy[1], Christian Stoeck[2], Gábor Székely[1], Christine Tanner[1], and Sebastian Kozerke[2]

[1] Computer Vision Laboratory, ETH Zurich, Switzerland
{valeryv,tanner,szekely}@vision.ee.ethz.ch
[2] Institute for Biomedical Engineering, University and ETH Zurich, Switzerland
{stoeck,kozerke}@biomed.ee.ethz.ch

Abstract. Cardiac diffusion tensor MR imaging (DT-MRI) allows to analyze 3D fiber organization of the myocardium which may enhance the understanding of, for example, cardiac remodeling in conditions such as ventricular hypertrophy. Diffusion-weighted MRI (DW-MRI) denoising methods rely on accurate spatial alignment of all acquired DW images. However, due to cardiac and respiratory motion, cardiac DT-MRI suffers from low signal-to-noise ratio (SNR) and large spatial transformations, which result in unusable DT reconstructions. The method proposed in this paper is based on a novel registration-guided denoising algorithm, that explicitly avoids intensity averaging in misaligned regions of the images by imposing a sparsity-inducing norm between corresponding image edges. We compared our method with consecutive registration and denoising of DW images on a high quality *ex vivo* canine dataset. The results show that the proposed method improves DT field reconstruction quality, which yields more accurate measures of fiber helix angle distribution and fractional anisotropy coefficients.

Keywords: denoising, registration, sparsity, primal-dual, DW-MRI.

1 Introduction

Scanning time and subject motion is considered one of the most challenging issues in DW-MRI of the brain [1]. In cardiac *in vivo* DW-MRI breathing and cardiac motion requires shorter acquisition windows which lowers image SNR relative to applications in the brain [2]. Most of DT-MRI denoising algorithms are based on a model of the acquisition process, assuming spatial alignment of the individual DW images. However, image registration is challenging for low SNR. Moreover out-of-plane motion can occur during the acquisition process.

Most of the joint image denoising and registration methods apply explicit or implicit image intensity averaging [3,4,5]. Yet direct averaging can degrade denoising results and is not applicable for DW-MRI data. A novel graph-based approach was proposed by Lombaert and Cheriet in [6], where registration and

N. Navab et al. (Eds.): MICCAI 2015, Part I, LNCS 9349, pp. 215–222, 2015.
DOI: 10.1007/978-3-319-24553-9_27

denoising are combined (via Cartesian product) for a joint label space. The advantage of this method over independent denoising and registration has been shown. Yet its applicability is questionable due to the size of the resulting label space (e.g. 256 "denoising" labels × 1681 displacements $\in \{-20, -19, \ldots, 20\} =$ 4 308 736 labels). Logcut framework [7] might be able to efficiently solve the problem in such a huge label space, but it needs nontrivial tuning for each problem class, which has not been performed to date. Moreover, many image registration regularization measures cannot be expressed with binary energy potentials.

In our simultaneous registration and denoising method we impose the similarity of image gradients instead of intensities using sparsity inducing ℓ_1-norm and linear representation of the image warping operator. Our main motivation is following: (a) gradients are less sensitive to intensity variations and (b) "sparse" constraints automatically "allow" images to be different in some regions, which helps us to correctly treat misalignments and heterogeneities of the images.

2 Methods

2.1 Denoising

The relation of intensity of DW image $\mathbf{y}_i$ at spatial location s with diffusion gradient $\mathbf{g}_i$ and diffusion tensor D_s is given by the following equation:

$$\mathbf{y}_i[s] = \mathbf{y}_0[s] \exp(-b\, \mathbf{g}_i^\top \mathsf{D}_s\, \mathbf{g}_i), \tag{1}$$

where $\mathbf{y}_0$ is the image without diffusion weighting and b is the b-value. Given a sequence of DW images degraded with noise, the set of aligned DW images $\hat{\mathbf{y}}_i$ for N different gradient directions $\mathbf{g}_i$, is obtained using the following MAP estimation formulation [8]:

$$\underset{\mathbf{y}_1,\ldots,\mathbf{y}_N}{\text{minimize}} \; -\sum_{i=1}^{N} \log p(\hat{\mathbf{y}}_i \mid \mathbf{y}_i) + \lambda\, \mathrm{TV}_\phi(\mathbf{y}_1, ..., \mathbf{y}_N), \tag{2}$$

here $p(\hat{\mathbf{y}}_i \mid \mathbf{y}_i)$ is a likelihood function that captures the image noise model, the Rician distribution with parameter σ:

$$p(\hat{\mathbf{y}}_i | \mathbf{y}_i) = \prod_{s \in \text{Pixels}} \frac{\hat{\mathbf{y}}_i[s]}{\sigma^2} \exp\left(-\frac{(\hat{\mathbf{y}}_i[s])^2 + (\mathbf{y}_i[s])^2}{2\sigma^2}\right) \times \mathrm{I}_0\left(\frac{\hat{\mathbf{y}}_i[s]\mathbf{y}_i[s]}{\sigma^2}\right), \tag{3}$$

where I_0 is the zeroth-order-modified Bessel function of the first kind, and σ is the standard deviation of the Gaussian noise in the real and the imaginary images, which is assumed to be equal and spatially invariant. The modified total variation (TV_ϕ) of images is employed as image prior: , i.e. $p(\mathbf{y}_1, \ldots, \mathbf{y}_N) \propto \exp\left(-\lambda\, \mathrm{TV}_\phi(\mathbf{y}_1, \ldots, \mathbf{y}_N)\right)$, with

$$\mathrm{TV}_\phi(\mathbf{y}_1, \ldots, \mathbf{y}_N) = \textstyle\sum_{s \in \text{Pixels}} \phi\left(\sum_{i=1,\ldots,N; k=1,2} (\nabla_k \mathbf{y}_i[s])^2\right), \tag{4}$$

where $\phi(x) = \sqrt{c + x/\tau^2}$, τ scales the gradient magnitude, c controls the smoothness of low contrast regions, $\nabla_k \in \mathbb{R}^{P \times P}$ is the gradient operator in the k-th direction, [.] indexes the vector (s-th element of $\nabla_k \mathbf{y}_i$ in the formula above) and parameter λ controls the amount of regularization.

This denoising formulation is extensively used in image processing, and incorporates the edge information from all components of the image. Rank constraint on matrix $[\mathbf{y}_1, \ldots, \mathbf{y}_N]$ introduced by Lam *et al.* in [9] showed significant improvement compared to other methods, such as non-local means denoising [10], and will be considered in this work as the state-of-the-art for denoising *aligned* DW-MRI data and referred to as rank-edge denoising (RE-denoising).

2.2 Registration-Guided (RG) Denoising

Now consider that DW images $\mathbf{y}_i$ are spatially misaligned and all pairwise mapping estimates are given $\{\mathcal{T}_{ij}\}_{i,j=1}^{N}$, such that $\mathcal{T}_{ij}(\mathbf{y}_i) \approx \mathbf{y}_j$. If all transformations $\{\mathcal{T}_{ij}\}$ were correct, we could use them to warp all images into the common coordinate frame and perform RE-denoising. However, in practice the registrations are not ideal. Moreover, if out-of-plane motion is present, these 2D transformations do not even exist. Ignoring the registration inaccuracies can amplify noise near misaligned edges, decrease denoising quality and create noisy structures. Ideally we want to have a local registration accuracy estimation, that would indicate for every image pixel, if we can use information from the other warped images. Here we propose to enforce *sparse* image edges consistency across the images instead of regularizing them directly. We use a compressed sensing approach to maximize the region of gradient consistency. Here we propose to extend (2), yielding the following registration-guided (RG) denoising model:

$$\min_{\{\mathbf{y}_i\}} -\sum_{i=1}^{N} \log p(\hat{\mathbf{y}}_i|\mathbf{y}_i) + \lambda \sum_{i}^{N} \mathrm{TV}_{\phi}(\mathbf{y}_i) + \beta \sum_{i,j}^{N} \sum_{k=1,2} \underbrace{\|\nabla_k \mathbf{y}_j - \nabla_k \mathsf{R}_{ij} \mathbf{y}_i\|_1}_{\text{sparse gradients consistency}}, \tag{5}$$

where parameter β weights the consistency of the gradients of images i and j. $\mathsf{R}_{ij} = \mathsf{R}(\mathcal{T}_{ij}) \in \mathbb{R}^{P \times P}$ is a sparse matrix which warps an image with a given transformation and depends on the image interpolation scheme $\mathcal{T}_{ij}(\mathbf{y}_i) = \mathsf{R}_{ij}\mathbf{y}_i$. Since the ℓ_1-norm is a convex relaxation of the cardinality measure, this sparsity-inducing term encourages the least number of non-aligned edges.

The problem (5) is not smooth and cannot be solved with ordinary gradient descent methods. We apply the theory of duality, and use the ADMM [11] algorithm. Problem (5) can be transformed to the following equivalent form:

$$\begin{aligned} &\min_{\mathbf{y}_i, \mathbf{f}_i, \mathbf{z}_{ijk}} -\sum_{i}^{N} \log p(\hat{\mathbf{y}}_i|\mathbf{f}_i) + \lambda \sum_{i}^{N} \sum_{s} \phi\left(\sum_{k=1,2} (\mathbf{z}_{iik}[s])^2\right) + \beta \sum_{i,j}^{N} \sum_{k=1}^{2} \|\mathbf{t}_{ijk}\|_1, \\ &\text{s.t.} \quad \mathbf{f}_i = \mathbf{y}_i, \qquad \mathbf{z}_{ijk} = \nabla_k \mathsf{R}_{ij} \mathbf{y}_i, \qquad \mathbf{t}_{ijk} = \nabla_k \mathbf{y}_j - \mathbf{z}_{ijk}, \quad \forall i,j,k \end{aligned} \tag{6}$$

In this form the problem can be solved with an iterative ADMM scheme described in [11].

Algorithm 1. Proposed iterative registration and denoising scheme. The denoising step with the RE-method is performed in the following manner: all images are transformed to the i-th coordinate frame, then the i-th image is denoised with the RE-method and stored as $\mathbf{y}_i^{(k+1)}$. In practice the stopping criteria is reached after 4-10 iterations with $\mathcal{F}_{\text{tol}} = 10^{-2}$.

Initialize $\{\mathbf{y}_i\}^{(1)}$ with single image denoising, $k := 1$
Repeat:
  `for` $i := 1$ to N
    `for` $j := 1$ to N
      $\mathcal{T}_{ij}^{(k+1)} \leftarrow$ `register` $\mathbf{y}_i^{(k)}$ `to` $\mathbf{y}_j^{(k)}$ `with` (7)
    `rof`
  `rof`
  $\{\mathbf{y}_i\}^{(k+1)} \leftarrow$ `denoise images with RG- or RE- method`
  $k \leftarrow k+1$
  $\mathcal{F}^{(k+1)} = \frac{1}{N^2(\#\text{Pixels})} \sum_{ij} \|\mathbf{y}_j^{(k+1)} - \mathcal{T}_{ij}^{(k+1)}(\mathbf{y}_i^{(k+1)})\|_2$
while $\|\mathcal{F}^{(k+1)} - \mathcal{F}^{(k)}\| \geq \mathcal{F}_{\text{tol}}$ and $k \leq k_{\text{max}}$.

2.3 Simultaneous Denoising and Registration

Given two images $\mathbf{y}_i$ and $\mathbf{y}_j$ the registration problem can be modelled as the following optimization task:

$$\underset{\mathcal{T}_{ij} \in \text{Affine}}{\text{minimize}} \ \text{LNCC}(\mathbf{y}_j, \mathcal{T}_{ij}(\mathbf{y}_i)), \tag{7}$$

where LNCC is local normalized cross correlation image metric, a multi-model image similarity metric which is insensitive to local linear contrast changes and can be computed efficiently [12]. Image registration is a highly nonlinear and non-convex problem. To deal with this problems, while aligning low SNR images, we propose to iteratively perform denoising and registration of denoised images. Reducing the image noise should enhance image registration results. The procedure is described in the Algorithm 1.

3 Results

To enable qualitative evaluation, we build on a high-resolution, high-quality, motion-free *ex vivo* canine heart dataset [13] as ground truth and simulate data of *in vivo* quality. The publicly available[1] *ex vivo* data was acquired using a 3D fast spin-echo sequence. Twenty diffusion encoding gradients were used for each imaging slice with in-plane resolutions of $0.31 \times 0.31 \text{mm}^2$ and slice thickness of 0.8 mm. The imaging slices were then stacked and downsampled to $0.6 \times 0.6 \times 1.6 \text{mm}^3$ resolution to produce a plausible *in vivo* gold standard tensor model, to evaluate recovery from simulated noise and spatial transformations as described in the next sections.

[1] `http://cvrgrid.org/data/ex-vivo`

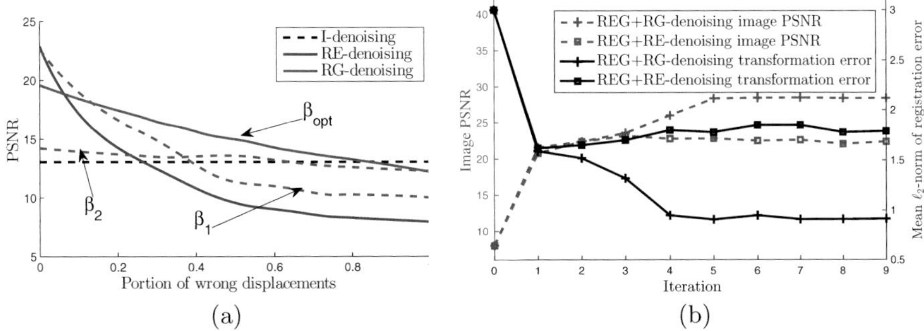

Fig. 1. (a) Dependence between denoising quality (mean image PSNR), registration accuracy and parameter β. The pixel displacement is considered to be wrong, if its length is larger than 1 pixel. $\beta_{\text{opt}} = 0.02, \beta_1 = 0.08, \beta_2 = 0.003$ (b) Mean image denoising and registration performance on the synthetic dataset.

Registration-Guided Denoising. First, we test the ability of the proposed RG-denoising to improve image quality despite inaccurate transformations. For this purpose we fixed a reference imaging slice and created four DW images, deformed with random in-plane ground truth affine transformation M_{ij} such that $|\det(\mathsf{M}_{ij})-1| \leq 0.05$. Random affine transformation matrices with the same properties were then added to produce erroneous transformations $\hat{\mathcal{T}}_{ij}$. Finally, images were degraded with additive Rician noise ($\sigma = 10$). We solve (5) to obtain denoised images and compare the peak SNR (PSNR) of the images.

We compare our RG-denoising with two extreme denoising variants: independent image TV denoising (I-denoising) e.g. solving (2) separately for each image without rank constraint, and RE-denoising. Obviously, if all the transformations are correct, then RE-denoising will give the best possible result for a given edge prior. However, any misalignment will degrade averaging quality. I-denoising does not use any registration information and therefore does not depend on the registration quality. Large (see β in Figure 1a) values of β tend to favor gradients consistency, which results in low restoration quality in cases when there are misaligned images (β_1 Fig. 1a). With small β values, the method ignores gradients consistency and behaves like I-denoising (β_2 Fig. 1a). We could observe that there exist optimal values β_{opt}, such that denoising quality is close to the best when all registrations are correct, and a little worse than single image denoising, when all are wrong (β_{opt} Fig. 1a).

Second, we show that our method is able to improve registration and denoising quality simultaneously. We took the same set of four images and executed Algorithm 1 with RG- and RE- denoising methods. Figure 1(b) shows that our method improves on RE-denoising and registration, which led to more accurate registration estimates as well. Ignoring registration inaccuracies during the denoising step can degrade the estimation results.

DTI Quantitive Assessment. To model the *in vivo* acquisition process accurately, for each axial imaging plane, 10 noncollinear diffusion gradients were

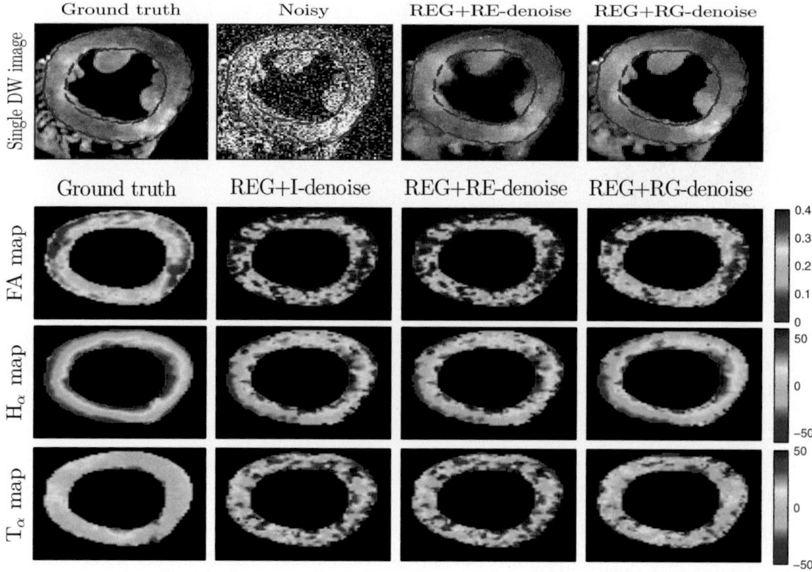

Fig. 2. Comparison of DW intensity, FA, helix and transverse angle maps, from different iterative image registration and denoising schemes. The provided ventricle myocardium segmentation is shown as red lines. Note the edge fuzziness of the RE-denoising based method, caused by misalignments.

chosen. The proposed method was tested for affine transformations, as these capture the components of cardiac deformation due to respiration, e.g. [14], but can also successfully be applied to non-affine deformations (tests not included). For each gradient direction a random affine mapping M_i was applied to the imaging plane, such that the inclination of the mapped plane to the original is less than $10°$ and $|\det(\mathsf{M}) - 1| \leq 0.05$. Corresponding DW images were then computed according to (1) using the finite strain (FS) reorientation strategy described in [15]. After that, Rician noise with $\sigma = 12$ was added to the image, yielding $\hat{\mathbf{y}}_i$. These 10 DW images were denoised and spatially aligned using three methods: (i) registration and I-denoising, (ii) iterative registration and RE-denoising, (iii) iterative registration and RG-denoising. Six iterations of the Algorithm 1 were executed with the following denoising parameters: $\beta = 0.012, \lambda = 0.2, \tau = 3, c = 1$ and a $7 \times 7\text{px}^2$ region was used for the LNCC. A standard least-squares approach together with the FS reorientation strategy was applied to the denoised images using the estimated transformations to produce DT maps of the reference plane. To compare the results of the reconstruction we analyzed the following characteristics of the DT map: (i) fractional anisotropy (FA) RMSE, (ii) mean affine-invariant Riemannian distance [16] between reconstructed and ground truth tensors: $\Delta_{\text{AI}}(\mathsf{D}_1, \mathsf{D}_2) = \| \log(\mathsf{D}_1^{-1/2}\mathsf{D}_2\mathsf{D}_1^{-1/2})\|_F$ and (iii) myocardial fiber helix angle (H_α) and transverse angle (T_α) [17] distributions.

The first row in Figure 2 shows the gold standard DW image together with the denoising results for a single fixed diffusion gradient direction. As can be seen, the

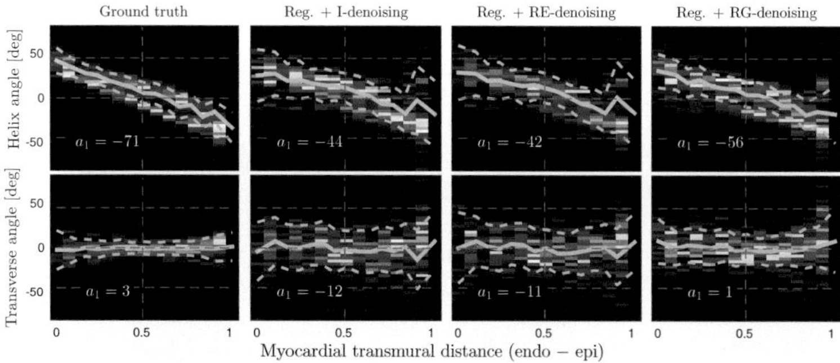

Fig. 3. Myocardial fibers helix and transverse angle distribution with respect to transmural abscissa together with cyan lines showing mean and one standard deviation. a_1 is the regression slope of the linear fit.

Table 1. DTI reconstruction measures computed in the myocardium. Columns H_α-σ and T_α-σ state the standard deviation of the linear model fit for H_α and T_α.

Method	PSNR	FA-RMSE	Δ_{AI}	H_α-RMSE	H_α-σ	T_α-RMSE	T_α-σ
I-denoising	22.8	0.37	0.17	13.7°	28.4°	19.8°	29.1°
RE-denoising	21.4	0.39	0.18	14.0°	28.1°	19.1°	29.8°
RG-denoising	27.6	0.28	0.13	11.5°	20.4°	14.6°	25.8°
No denoising	16.1	0.49	0.70	29.4°	39.1°	31.2°	43.1°

proposed (REG+RG-denoise) noise reduction is more effective, especially at the myocardium edges. Tensor estimate quality and fibre geometry reconstruction also benefit from the proposed method. Illustration of fiber inclination distribution is shown in Figure 3. Studies indicate [18] that there should be linear dependence between helix angle and transmural myocardium distance. The transverse angle is reported to be close to zero inside the myocardium. Standard deviations of these angles from the linear models are reported in the Table 1 together with other performance metrics. We notice that iterative registration with RE-denoising outperforms independent image denoising, which illustrates the danger of ignoring the misalignment errors. The proposed RG-denoising based method showed substantial improvement in denoising and tensor estimation quality.

4 Conclusions

In this paper we have addressed the problem of alignment and denoising of DWI data. Quantitative evaluation, based on simulations from *ex vivo* data, shows that the standard DWI denoising methods can degrade reconstruction results, when either poor alignment or out-of-plane motion occurs. Our proposed method based on a robust groupwise denoising approach, allows to deal with foregoing issues. The method showed qualitative improvement over standard techniques both in the image denoising quality (+21% PSNR) and anatomical characteristics, such as helix (-18% RMSE) and transversal angles of the myocardial fibers.

References

1. Pierpaoli, C.: Artifacts in diffusion MRI. In: Diffusion MRI: Theory, Methods and Applications, pp. 303–318. Oxford University Press, New York (2010)
2. Toussaint, N., Stoeck, C.T., Schaeffter, T., Kozerke, S., Sermesant, M., Batchelor, P.: In vivo human cardiac fibre architecture estimation using shape-based diffusion tensor processing. Medical Image Analysis 17(8), 1243–1255 (2013)
3. Han, J., Berkels, B., Rumpf, M., Hornegger, J., Droske, M., Fried, M., Scorzin, J., Schaller, C.: A variational framework for joint image registration, denoising and edge detection. In: Bildv. Für Die Med. 2006, pp. 246–250. Springer, Heidelberg (2006)
4. Telea, A.C., Preusser, T., Garbe, C.S., Droske, M., Rumpf, M.: A variational approach to joint denoising, edge detection and motion estimation. In: Franke, K., Müller, K.-R., Nickolay, B., Schäfer, R. (eds.) DAGM 2006. LNCS, vol. 4174, pp. 525–535. Springer, Heidelberg (2006)
5. Sanches, J.M., Marques, J.S.: Joint image registration and volume reconstruction for 3D ultrasound. Pattern Recognition Letters 24(4), 791–800 (2003)
6. Lombaert, H., Cheriet, F.: Simultaneous image denoising and registration using graph cuts: Application to corrupted medical images. In: ISSPA, pp. 264–268. IEEE (2012)
7. Lempitsky, V., Rother, C., Blake, A.: Logcut-efficient graph cut optimization for markov random fields. In: ICCV, pp. 1–8. IEEE (2007)
8. Getreuer, P.: Rudin-Osher-Fatemi total variation denoising using split Bregman. IPOL 10 (2012)
9. Lam, F., Babacan, D., Haldar, J., Weiner, M., Schuff, N., Liang, Z.: Denoising diffusion-weighted magnitude MR images using rank and edge constraints. Magnetic Resonance in Medicine 71(3), 1272–1284 (2014)
10. Wiest-Daesslé, N., Prima, S., Coupé, P., Morrissey, S.P., Barillot, C.: Non-local means variants for denoising of diffusion-weighted and diffusion tensor MRI. In: Ayache, N., Ourselin, S., Maeder, A. (eds.) MICCAI 2007, Part II. LNCS, vol. 4792, pp. 344–351. Springer, Heidelberg (2007)
11. Boyd, S., Parikh, N., Chu, E., Peleato, B., Eckstein, J.: Distributed optimization and statistical learning via the alternating direction method of multipliers. Foundations and Trends in ML 3(1), 1–122 (2011)
12. Cachier, P., Bardinet, E., Dormont, D., Pennec, X., Ayache, N.: Iconic feature based nonrigid registration: the PASHA algorithm. Computer Vision and Image Understanding 89(2), 272–298 (2003)
13. Helm, P., Younes, L., Beg, M., Ennis, D., Leclercq, C., Faris, O., McVeigh, E., Kass, D., Miller, M., Winslow, R.: Evidence of structural remodeling in the dyssynchronous failing heart. Circulation Research 98(1), 125–132 (2006)
14. King, A., Rhode, K., Razavi, R., Schaeffter, T.: An adaptive and predictive respiratory motion model for image-guided interventions: theory and first clinical application. T. Med. Imag. 28(12), 2020–2032 (2009)
15. Alexander, D., Pierpaoli, C., Basser, P., Gee, J.: Spatial transformations of diffusion tensor magnetic resonance images. T. Med. Imag. 20(11), 1131–1139 (2001)
16. Fillard, P., Pennec, X., Arsigny, V., Ayache, N.: Clinical DT-MRI estimation, smoothing, and fiber tracking with log-Euclidean metrics. T. Med. Imag. 26(11), 1472–1482 (2007)
17. Scollan, D., Holmes, A., Winslow, R., Forder, J.: Histological validation of myocardial microstructure obtained from diffusion tensor magnetic resonance imaging. Am. J. of Physiology-Heart and Circulatory Phys. 275(6), H2308–H2318 (1998)
18. Lombaert, H., Peyrat, J., Croisille, P., Rapacchi, S., Fanton, L., Clarysse, P., Magnin, I., Delingette, H., Ayache, N.: Human atlas of the cardiac fiber architecture: study on a healthy population. T. Med. Imag. 31(7), 1436–1447 (2012)

Iterative Subspace Screening for Rapid Sparse Estimation of Brain Tissue Microstructural Properties

Pew-Thian Yap[2], Yong Zhang[1], and Dinggang Shen[2]

[1] Department of Radiology and Biomedical Research Imaging Center, The University of North Carolina at Chapel Hill, USA
[2] Department of Psychiatry and Behavioral Sciences, Stanford University, USA
ptyap@med.unc.edu

Abstract. Diffusion magnetic resonance imaging (DMRI) is a powerful imaging modality due to its unique ability to extract microstructural information by utilizing restricted diffusion to probe compartments that are much smaller than the voxel size. Quite commonly, a mixture of models is fitted to the data to infer microstructural properties based on the estimated parameters. The fitting process is often non-linear and computationally very intensive. Recent work by Daducci et al. has shown that speed improvement of several orders of magnitude can be achieved by linearizing and recasting the fitting problem as a linear system, involving the estimation of the volume fractions associated with a set of diffusion basis functions that span the signal space. However, to ensure coverage of the signal space, sufficiently dense sampling of the parameter space is needed. This can be problematic because the number of basis functions increases exponentially with the number of parameters, causing computational intractability. We propose in this paper a method called iterative subspace screening (ISS) for tackling this ultrahigh dimensional problem. ISS requires only solving the problem in a medium-size subspace with a dimension that is much smaller than the original space spanned by all diffusion basis functions but is larger than the expected cardinality of the support of the solution. The solution obtained for this subspace is used to screen the basis functions to identify a new subspace that is pertinent to the target problem. These steps are performed iteratively to seek both the solution subspace and the solution itself. We apply ISS to the estimation of the fiber orientation distribution function (ODF) and demonstrate that it improves estimation robustness and accuracy.

1 Introduction

Microstructural tissue properties can be inferred with the help of diffusion MRI (DMRI) thanks to its sensitivity to the restricted motion of water molecules owing to barriers such as cellular membranes. Microstructural information is typically obtained from diffusion parameters estimated via fitting to the acquired data some biophysical models. Fitting models such as the tensor model [1] is relatively simple and straightforward. But fitting models that are more sophisticated, such as the multi-compartmental models used in AxCaliber [2] and NODDI [3], is much more involved with significantly greater

N. Navab et al. (Eds.): MICCAI 2015, Part I, LNCS 9349, pp. 223–230, 2015.
DOI: 10.1007/978-3-319-24553-9_28

computational load. Computational complexity is further increased when certain structure is imposed on the solution, such as sparsity [4,5].

In a recent work called AMICO [6], the authors show that it is possible to speed up AxCaliber and NODDI estimation several orders of magnitude by re-formulating the fitting problem as a linear system that can be efficiently solved using very fast algorithms. However, this work is limited to a sparse sampling of the parameter space (30 basis functions for AxCaliber and 145 basis functions for NODDI) and is also limited to voxels containing only a single principal diffusion direction. When extending AMICO for the more realistic case of multiple white matter (WM) directions per voxel [7], the number of the basis functions would need to be significantly increased, causing the optimization problem to be very high dimensional and computationally very expensive. A similar situation occurs in the estimation of the fiber orientation distribution function (ODF), as in [5], when one needs to increase the number of angular directions of the basis functions for improving accuracy.

In this paper, we propose a method called iterative subspace screening (ISS) to solve this kind of ultrahigh dimension problem more efficiently. ISS requires only solving the target problem in a medium-size subspace with a dimension that is much smaller than the original space spanned by all the basis functions, but is larger than the expected cardinality of the support of the solution. ISS is a subspace pursuit algorithm [8] involving the following iterative steps:

1. **Subspace Selection:** Select a potential solution subspace by screening out irrelevant basis functions. This is done by element-wise regression of the fitting residual similar to iterative sure independence screening (ISIS) [9] and subspace pursuit (SP) [8].
2. **Subspace Solution:** Solve for the solution, assumed sparse, in the selected subspace and compute the fitting residual. The fitting residual is then used in the subspace selection step above to refine the subspace so that irrelevant basis functions can be discarded and relevant ones can be included.

Such subspace selection approach allows us to remove from consideration many basis functions that might never be active and contribute to the solution. This is motivated by the fact that, in our case, the solution is sparse and hence resides in a small subspace. Since the dimension of the ISS subspace is typically much smaller, the solution can be obtained much faster with potentially lesser local minima that may result from the high dimensionality. We demonstrate the effectiveness of ISS on the problem of fiber ODF estimation and show that significant speed up can be achieved. Extension of ISS for AxCaliber and NODDI, similar to AMICO, should be straightforward.

2 Approach

2.1 Problem Description

The problem we are interested in solving has the following form:

$$\min_{\mathbf{f}\geq 0}\{\phi(\mathbf{f}) = l(\mathbf{f}) + r(\mathbf{f})\}, \tag{1}$$

Algorithm 1. Iterative Subspace Screening

Input : $\mathbf{A}$, s, D

Initialization:

1. $\mathcal{J}^{(0)} = \{D$ indices of the entries with the largest magnitudes in vector $\mathbf{A}^{\mathrm{T}}\mathbf{s}\}$
2. $\mathbf{r}^{(0)} = \mathtt{residual}(\mathbf{s}, \mathbf{A}_{\mathcal{J}^{(0)}})$
3. $\mathbf{f}^{(0)} = \mathbf{0}$

Iteration : At iterations $k = 1, 2, \ldots$, go through the following steps:

1. $\mathcal{J}^{(k)} = \{D$ indices of the non-zeros entries of $\mathbf{f}^{(k-1)}$ and the entries with the largest magnitudes in vector $\mathbf{A}^{\mathrm{T}}\mathbf{r}^{(k-1)}\}$
2. Set $\mathbf{f}^{(k)} = \mathtt{solve}(\mathbf{s}, \mathbf{A}_{\mathcal{J}^{(k)}})$
3. $\mathbf{r}^{(k)} = \mathtt{residual}(\mathbf{s}, \mathbf{A}_{\mathcal{J}^{(k)}})$
4. If $\|\mathbf{r}^{(k)}\| > \|\mathbf{r}^{(k-1)}\|$, quit the iteration.

Output : The solution $\mathbf{f} = \mathbf{f}^{(k-1)}$.

where in our case $l(\mathbf{f}) = \|\mathbf{Af} - \mathbf{s}\|_2^2$ is a smooth and convex data fidelity term with respect to observation vector $\mathbf{s} \in \mathbb{R}^N$ and $r(\mathbf{f})$ is a sparsity-inducing regularization term that is not necessarily smooth or convex. In diffusion MRI, one would typically fill the columns of basis matrix $\mathbf{A} \in \mathbb{R}^{N\times P}$ with the set of basis functions derived from diffusion models with varying parameters, such as orientation and diffusivity. The vector $\mathbf{f} \in \mathbb{R}^P$ consists of the corresponding volume fractions associated with the basis functions. For example, for estimating the fiber ODF as in [5], one would fill the columns of $\mathbf{A}$ with the signal vectors sampled from tensor models oriented uniformly in all directions. For fast AxCaliber [2] and NODDI [3] estimation using a linear system as described in AMICO [6], one would fill the columns of $\mathbf{A}$ with signal vectors from compartment models orientated in a direction estimated via fitting a diffusion tensor. If the parameter space is sampled densely, the above estimation would be computationally very expensive and can be susceptible to local minima due to the high dimensionality and high correlation between the basis functions.

2.2 Iterative Subspace Screening (ISS)

We propose a method called iterative subspace screening (ISS) to tackle this kind of ultrahigh dimension problem more efficiently. ISS requires only solving the target problem (1) in a medium-size subspace with a dimension that is much smaller than the original space spanned by all the basis functions, but is larger than the expected cardinality of the support of the solution. This is based on the observation that the problem (1) can be rewritten as

$$\min_{\mathbf{f}_{\mathcal{J}}\geq\mathbf{0},\mathbf{f}_{\bar{\mathcal{J}}}=\mathbf{0},|\mathcal{J}|=D} \{\phi(\mathbf{f}) = l_{\mathcal{J}}(\mathbf{f}) + r_{\mathcal{J}}(\mathbf{f})\}, \tag{2}$$

subject to $D \ll P$ is larger than the expected cardinality of the support of the solution. Here, $l_{\mathcal{J}}(\mathbf{f}) = \|\mathbf{A}_{\mathcal{J}}\mathbf{f}_{\mathcal{J}} - \mathbf{s}\|_2^2$ with $\mathbf{f}_{\mathcal{J}}$ being the subvector formed by the elements of

$\mathbf{f}$ indexed by set $\mathcal{J} \subseteq \{1, 2, \ldots, P\}$, $\bar{\mathcal{J}} = \{1, 2, \ldots, P\} \setminus \mathcal{J}$, and $\mathbf{A}_{\mathcal{J}}$ being the submatrix formed by the columns of $\mathbf{A}$ indexed by $\mathcal{J}$. The regularization term $r_{\mathcal{J}}(\mathbf{f})$ now penalizes only the elements in $\mathbf{f}$ that are indexed by $\mathcal{J}$. We can think of problem (2) as concurrently solving for the solution subspace and the solution itself. This problem is clearly non-convex, non-smooth, and discontinuous; but decoupling subspace identification from the problem allows us to devise an algorithm that focuses on determining the solution in a subspace that actually contains the solution and not in the original subspace, especially when the original problem (1) is very high dimensional (i.e., P is large). As we shall see later, this subspace can be progressively refined by including basis functions that will contribute to the solution and by discarding those that will not. Since the solution is sparse, most basis functions are irrelevant to the solution and can be removed from consideration, reducing significantly the computation cost. Note that if the solution to (1) resides in the identified subspace, solving for (2) will give the same solution as (1).

Proposed Solution. We propose to solve (2) by alternating between solving for $\mathcal{J}$ and solving for $\mathbf{f}$. At each iteration, one only needs to solve for $\mathbf{f}$ in a medium-size subspace with dimension $D \ll P$. To select the subspace, we perform an element-wise regression of the fitting residual with the basis functions. That is, at the k-th iteration, we first compute the fitting residual $\mathbf{r}^{(k-1)} = \texttt{residual}(\mathbf{s}, \mathbf{A}_{\mathcal{J}^{(k-1)}}) = \mathbf{s} - \mathbf{A}_{\mathcal{J}^{(k-1)}} \mathbf{f}_{\mathcal{J}^{(k-1)}}$ and then use it to determine a subspace of dimension D. This subspace is spanned by the basis functions corresponding to the non-zero elements of $\mathbf{f}^{(k-1)}$ and, in addition, the basis functions corresponding to the largest entries of $\mathbf{A}^{\mathrm{T}}\mathbf{r}^{k-1}$. Based on this new subspace, with the constituent basis functions indexed by $\mathcal{J}^{(k)}$, we solve for $\mathbf{f}^{(k)}$, i.e., $\mathbf{f}^{(k)} = \texttt{solve}(\mathbf{s}, \mathbf{A}_{\mathcal{J}^{(k)}})$, via (2) with $\mathcal{J}^{(k)}$ fixed. This solution can then be used to recompute the residual and refine the subspace. Since at each iteration, the residual vector will be used to screen out a significant number of basis functions, thus removing a big portion of the original subspace, we call our method iterative subspace screening (ISS). See Algorithm 1 for a step-by-step summary of ISS. In addition to reducing significantly the computation time by not having to solve the problem in the original high-dimensional space, ISS can also deal with collinearity between basis functions. By performing subspace screening using the residual vector, some unimportant basis functions that are highly correlated with the important basis functions can be discarded, as observed in [9].

Grouped Variant. We can take advantage of the relationships between basis functions by grouping them [9]. We can divide the pool of P basis functions into disjoint groups, each with a number of basis functions. ISS can then be applied to the selection of basis function groups instead of the individual basis functions. This will reduce the chance of missing important basis functions by taking advantage of the joint information among them, making the estimation more reliable. This can be achieved by modifying Step 1 in the k-loop of Algorithm 1 to select the top D groups of basis functions with the greatest ℓ_2-norm of inner products with the residual vector. We shall show how grouping can be used in ISS to help solve sparse-group approximation problem similar to the one described in [10].

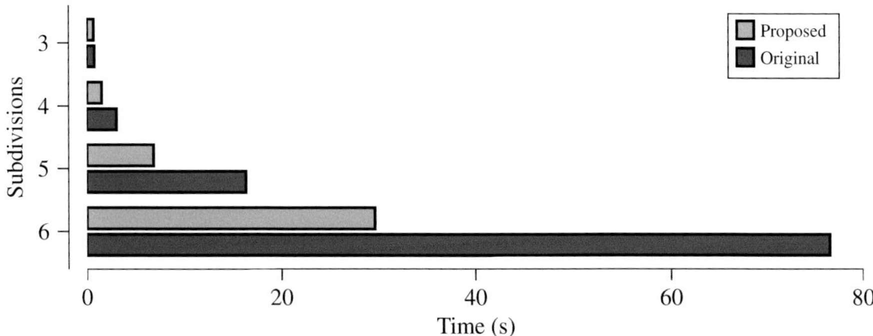

Fig. 1. Computation times.

A Specific Case. To demonstrate the utility of ISS, we select to use the general sparse-group regularization $r(\mathbf{f}) = \gamma \left[\alpha\|\mathbf{f}\|_0 + (1-\alpha)\sum_{g\in G}\mathcal{I}(\|\mathbf{f}_g\|_2)\right]$, where $\mathcal{I}(z)$ is an indicator function returning 1 if $z \neq 0$ or 0 if otherwise. The ℓ_0-"norm" gives the cardinality of the support, i.e., $\|\mathbf{f}\|_0 = |\mathtt{supp}(\mathbf{f})| = |\{k : f_k \neq 0\}|$. Parameters $\alpha \in [0,1]$ and $\gamma > 0$ are for penalty tuning, analogous to those used in the sparse-group LASSO [10]. Note that $\alpha = 1$ gives the ℓ_0 fit, whereas $\alpha = 0$ gives the group ℓ_0 fit. Note that in contrast to the more commonly used ℓ_1-norm penalization, we have chosen here to use ℓ_0-"norm" cardinality-based penalization. As reported in [11], ℓ_1-norm penalization [5] conflicts with the unit sum requirement of the volume fractions and hence results in suboptimal solutions.

3 Experiments

3.1 Data

Synthetic Data: For quantitative evaluation, we generated a synthetic dataset for evaluation of ISS. The dataset was generated using a mixture of four tensor models. Two of which are anisotropic and represent two white matter (WM) compartments that are at an angle of $60°$ with each other. The other two are isotropic and represent the gray matter (GM) and cerebrospinal fluid (CSF) compartments. The generated diffusion-attenuated signals therefore simulate the partial volume effects resulting from these compartments. The volume fractions and the diffusivities of the compartments were allowed to vary in ranges that mimic closely the real data discussed in the next section. Various levels of noise (SNR=10, 20, 30, with respect to the signal value at $b = 0\,\mathrm{s/mm}^2$) was added.

Real Data: Diffusion weighted (DW) data from the Human Connectome Project (HCP) [12] were used. The $1.25 \times 1.25 \times 1.25\,\mathrm{mm}^3$ data were acquired with diffusion weightings $b = 1000, 2000$, and $3000\,\mathrm{s/mm}^2$ each applied in 90 directions. 18 baseline images with low diffusion weighting $b = 5\,\mathrm{s/mm}^2$ were also acquired. All images were acquired with reversed phase encoding for correction of EPI distortion.

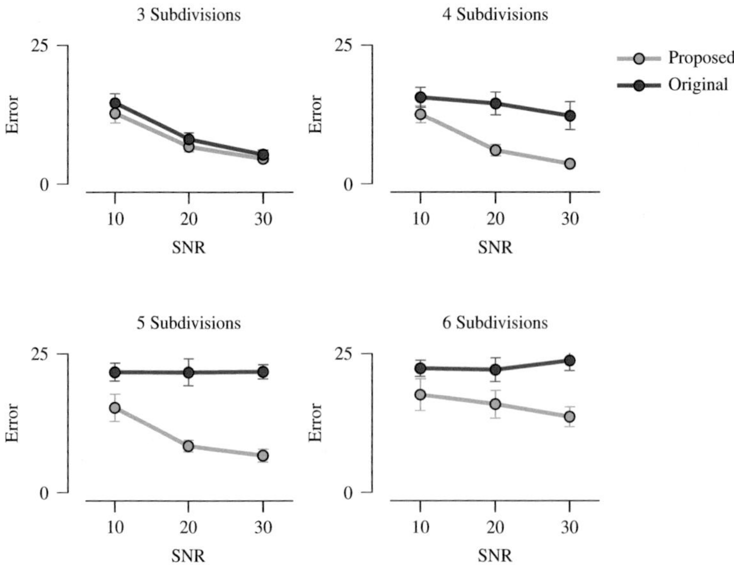

Fig. 2. ODF estimation error measured via orientational discrepancy (OD). The error bars indicate the standard deviations.

3.2 Methods of Evaluation

For the synthetic data, our aim is to estimate the fiber ODFs [13] and evaluate their accuracy by comparing their peaks (local maxima) with respect to the ground truth. The orientational discrepancy (OD) measure defined in [14] was used as a metric for evaluating the accuracy of peak estimation. For the real data, we want to evaluate whether consistent results are given by ISS compared with the original problem (1).

The fiber ODF was estimated by fitting to the data the compartment models for WM, GM, and CSF. Similar to [15], the WM is represented by a large number of anisotropic single-tensor models with orientations distributed evenly on a unit sphere. Dissimilar to [15], however, we allow the axial and radial diffusivities to vary. The GM and CSF are represented using isotropic tensor models with GM having a lower range of diffusivities compared with CSF. Mathematically, this is realized by filling the columns of $\mathbf{A}$ with the above models with different parameters, i.e., orientations and diffusivities, and then solving problem (1) (or (2)) for the corresponding volume fractions $\mathbf{f}$. Structure is imposed on the problem by grouping the WM models for each direction as well as the GM models and the CSF models. The tuning parameters were set as follows: $\gamma = 1 \times 10^{-4}$ and $\alpha = 0.05$. D was set to about 15% of P.

3.3 Results

Synthetic Data: To show that ISS improves the speed of estimation, we evaluated the computation time of ISS in comparison with solving the original problem (1). We perform this for different numbers of subdivisions of the icosahedron, giving different

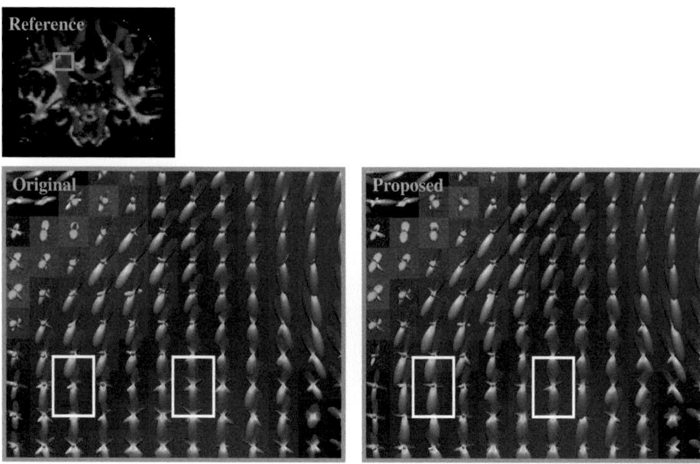

Fig. 3. WM ODF glyphs at the centrum semiovale. White boxes mark examples of improvements given by ISS.

numbers of directions for the WM models and hence different numbers of columns P for $\mathbf{A}$. 3, 4, 5, and 6 subdivisions of the icosahedron give respectively 321, 1281, 5121, and 20481 directions on a hemisphere. Figure 1 shows that ISS improves the speed of convergence remarkably.

Next, we proceeded to evaluate whether such increase in speed implies a decrease in ODF estimation accuracy. Figure 2, perhaps surprisingly, indicate that ISS actually improves ODF estimation accuracy. This can be explained from the fact that solving the problem in a lower-dimensional subspace can help alleviate the problem of local minima, especially when the problem is non-convex as in our case.

Real Data: Figure 3 shows the WM ODF glyphs at a portion of the centrum semiovale. The images show that the centrum semiovale contains elements of the corticospinal tract (blue), corpus callosum (red), and superior longitudinal fasciculus (green), including voxels with two- and three-way intersections of these elements. The images indicate that ISS gives consistent results comparable to the original problem. However, we could observe that ISS in fact improves ODF estimation in some voxels (marked by white boxes) and gives ODF estimates that are more coherent and match better with the underlying anatomy.

4 Conclusion

We have proposed a method for improving the speed and robustness of solving least-squares problems that are regularized by sparse inducing norms. We applied our method called iterative subspace screening (ISS) to ODF estimation and showed that better and faster estimates of the fiber orientations can be obtained. In the future, ISS will be applied to improve the speed and accuracy of estimation techniques for microstructure, such as AxCaliber and NODDI.

Acknowledgment. This work was supported in part by a UNC BRIC-Radiology start-up fund and NIH grants (EB006733, EB009634, AG041721, MH100217, and 1UL1TR001111).

References

1. Basser, P.J., Pierpaoli, C.: Microstructural and physiological features of tissues elucidated by quantitative-diffusion-tensor MRI. Journal of Magnetic Resonance Series B 111(3), 209–219 (1996)
2. Alexander, D.C., Hubbard, P.L., Hall, M.G., Moore, E.A., Ptito, M., Parker, G.J., Dyrby, T.B.: Orientationally invariant indices of axon diameter and density from diffusion MRI. NeuroImage 52, 1374–1389 (2010)
3. Zhang, H., Schneider, T., Wheeler-Kingshott, C.A., Alexander, D.C.: NODDI: Practical in vivo neurite orientation dispersion and density imaging of the human brain. NeuroImage 61, 1000–1016 (2012)
4. Landman, B.A., Bogovic, J.A., Wan, H., ElShahaby, F.E.Z., Bazin, P.L., Prince, J.L.: Resolution of crossing fibers with constrained compressed sensing using diffusion tensor MRI. NeuroImage 59, 2175–2186 (2012)
5. Ramirez-Manzanares, A., Rivera, M., Vemuri, B.C., Carney, P., Mareci, T.: Diffusion basis functions decomposition for estimating white matter intra-voxel fiber geometry. IEEE Transactions on Medical Imaging 26(8), 1091–1102 (2007)
6. Daducci, A., Canales-Rodríguez, E.J., Zhang, H., Dyrby, T.B., Alexander, D.C., Thiran, J.P.: Accelerated microstructure imaging via convex optimization (AMICO) from diffusion MRI data. NeuroImage 105, 32–44 (2015)
7. Zhang, H., Dyrby, T.B., Alexander, D.C.: Axon diameter mapping in crossing fibers with diffusion MRI. In: Fichtinger, G., Martel, A., Peters, T. (eds.) MICCAI 2011, Part II. LNCS, vol. 6892, pp. 82–89. Springer, Heidelberg (2011)
8. Dai, W., Milenkovic, O.: Subspace pursuit for compressive sensing signal reconstruction. IEEE Transactions on Information Theory 55(5), 2230–2249 (2009)
9. Fan, J., Lv, J.: Sure independence screening for ultrahigh dimensional feature space. Journal of the Royal Statistical Society, Series B 70(Part 5), 849–911 (2008)
10. Simon, N., Friedman, J., Hastie, T., Tibshirani, R.: A sparse-group lasso. Journal of Computational and Graphical Statistics 22(2), 231–245 (2013)
11. Daducci, A., Ville, D.V.D., Thiran, J.P., Wiaux, Y.: Sparse regularization for fiber ODF reconstruction: From the suboptimality of ℓ_2 and ℓ_1 priors to ℓ_0. Medical Image Analysis 18, 820–833 (2014)
12. Essen, D.C.V., Smith, S.M., Barch, D.M., Behrens, T.E., Yacoub, E., Ugurbil, K.: The WU-Minn human connectome project: An overview. NeuroImage 80, 62–79 (2013)
13. Tournier, J.D., Calamante, F., Gadian, D.G., Connelly, A.: Direct estimation of the fiber orientation density function from diffusion-weighted MRI data using spherical deconvolution. NeuroImage 23(3), 1176–1185 (2004)
14. Yap, P.T., Chen, Y., An, H., Yang, Y., Gilmore, J.H., Lin, W., Shen, D.: SPHERE: SPherical Harmonic Elastic REgistration of HARDI data. NeuroImage 55(2), 545–556 (2011)
15. Jian, B., Vemuri, B.C.: A unified computational framework for deconvolution to reconstruct multiple fibers from diffusion weighted MRI. IEEE Transactions on Medical Imaging 26(11), 1464–1471 (2007)

Elucidating Intravoxel Geometry in Diffusion-MRI: Asymmetric Orientation Distribution Functions (AODFs) Revealed by a Cone Model

Suheyla Cetin[1], Evren Ozarslan[2], and Gozde Unal[1]

[1] Faculty of Engineering and Natural Sciences, Sabanci University, Turkey
[2] Physics Department, Bogazici University, Turkey
{suheylacetin,gozdeunal}@sabanciuniv.edu, evren.ozarslan@boun.edu.tr

Abstract. A diffusion-MRI processing method is presented for representing the inherent asymmetry of the underlying intravoxel geometry, which emerges in regions with bending, crossing, or sprouting fibers. The orientation distribution functions (ODFs) obtained through conventional approaches such as q-ball imaging and spherical deconvolution result in symmetric ODF profiles at each voxel even when the underlying geometry is asymmetric. To extract such inherent asymmetry, an inter-voxel filtering approach through a cone model is employed. The cone model facilitates a sharpening of the ODFs in some directions while suppressing peaks in other directions, thus yielding an asymmetric ODF (AODF) field. Compared to symmetric ODFs, AODFs reveal more information regarding the cytoarchitectural organization within the voxel. The level of asymmetry is quantified via a new scalar index that could complement standard measures of diffusion anisotropy. Experiments on synthetic geometries of circular, crossing, and kissing fibers show that the estimated AODFs successfully recover the asymmetry of the underlying geometry. The feasibility of the technique is demonstrated on *in vivo* data obtained from the Human Connectome Project.

Keywords: MRI, diffusion, anisotropy, HARDI, ODF, asymmetry.

1 Introduction

Diffusion magnetic resonance imaging (dMRI) provides a powerful means to characterize tissue anisotropy, enabling the computation of neural connections in the nervous system. Diffusion tensor imaging (DTI) based findings have demonstrated the feasibility of such endeavour [1] despite its well-known shortcoming in regions with heterogeneous fiber orientations. In such environments, the unimodal ODF assumed by DTI is incapable of resolving the orientations of distinct fiber bundles within a voxel.

An important advance is the introduction of high angular resolution diffusion imaging (HARDI) acquisitions [2]. Several methods, designed for HARDI data,

N. Navab et al. (Eds.): MICCAI 2015, Part I, LNCS 9349, pp. 231–238, 2015.
DOI: 10.1007/978-3-319-24553-9_29

have managed to overcome DTI's limitation by making it possible to estimate multimodal ODFs.

Although having multimodal distributions is very important for reliably estimating connectivity, the HARDI-based ODFs do not accurately reflect the underlying cellular organization. For example, it has been demonstrated that when the voxel of interest contains Y-shaped crossings [3], or curving fibers [4], the distribution of displacements for water molecules is asymmetric. Due to the Fourier transform relationship between the displacement distribution and the signal, the signal for such regions is predicted to be complex-valued. Consequently, some techniques [3,5,6] have been formulated with the capability of handling complex-valued data to yield asymmetric profiles.

From a practical point-of-view however, obtaining accurate phase information in diffusion-weighted acquisitions is a formidable task particularly in *in vivo* acquisitions. Most important obstacle is the patient motion, which substantially distorts the phase of the signal [7]. Additionally, imperfections in the acquisition (e.g., imperfect B_0 shift compensation), flow, and susceptibility variations within the tissue could all influence the detected signal phase substantially. Thus, attributing the observed phase shifts to diffusion alone would be very problematic. Therefore, current dMRI processing pipelines assume magnitude-valued data. When magnitude-valued data are used, the regions containing Y-shaped crossings or bending fibers might lead to unimodal or star-shaped ODFs.

Several works have been published with varying levels of relevance to our study. In Ref. [8] the authors suggested an ODF field estimation scheme by considering inter-voxel information, which requires a relatively large number of diffusion directions. The high order tensor method and the associated tensor voting scheme introduced in Ref. [9] was shown to provide even-order tensor fields that facilitate fiber reconstruction at crossings, and odd-order fields that differentiate crossings from junctions. In Ref. [10], tracts with high curvature, crossing, branching, bottlenecks and sprouting have been discussed within the context of partial volume averaging of fiber directions and a regularisation technique was introduced. However, there is no mention of AODFs in this work.

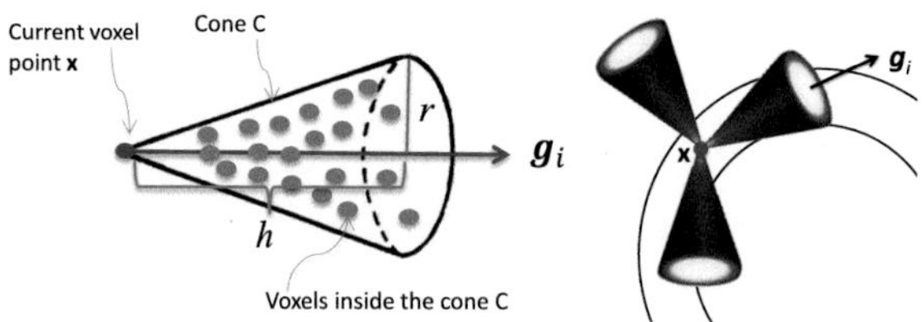

Fig. 1. Left: The cone **C** with a certain height and radius is used in the ODF filtering; Right: An asymmetric ODF is constructed by rotating the cone model along all sampled directions on the unit sphere at each voxel point and performing a weighted averaging using the depicted Gaussian map (shown in hot colours).

In a recent work [11], a regularisation on the ODF field is carried out using a cone model somewhat similar to the one we propose in this work. However, the approach in [11] differs in that ODF regularisation is based on the asymmetric weights assigned to the utilized pair of antipodally-symmetric cones placed at a given voxel. Moreover, neither in the results nor in the discussions is an AODF constructed or depicted.

In this paper, we present a technique for voxel-by-voxel reconstruction of AODFs. To the best of our knowledge this is the first such study.

2 Method

Relying on well-established HARDI techniques[1] that enable estimation of a multi-directional representation of the local fiber orientations, we present a method that exploits voxel-based ODFs in a conic spatial neighborhood to capture underlying asymmetry of the ODF. The ODF is defined at each voxel location $\mathbf{x} = (x, y, z) \in \mathbb{R}^3$ by $\phi_{\mathbf{x}}(\mathbf{g_i})$ for each sampled direction vector $\mathbf{g_i} \in \mathbb{S}^{\mathbf{2}}$. At the given voxel $\mathbf{x}$ and the given direction $\mathbf{g_i}$, a cone $\mathbf{C}$ (Figure 1(a)) is constructed by a certain radius r and height h. Although the directional asymmetry of the fiber pathway cannot be deduced from the ODF of a single voxel, it becomes apparent by considering the information holistically revealed by the ODFs of the voxels in the local volume delimited by the cone $\mathbf{C}$.

2.1 Asymmetric ODFs Based on a Cone Model

We exemplify the idea of a cone-based directional ODF filtering by building a Gaussian function $G(\mathbf{x}, \mathbf{g_i}, \sigma)$ whose center lies on the axis of the cone with a variance parameter σ. At the voxel $\mathbf{x}$, once the cones are constructed along each sampling direction $\mathbf{g}_i$ as in Figure 1(b), the weighted smoothing of the ODFs is carried out. The corresponding Gaussian functions are also visualised in (b) which depicts the nature of the weighting going from highest on the central axis to lowest on the side surface of the cone. This filtering operation is formulated by:

$$f_{\boldsymbol{x}}(\boldsymbol{g}_i) = \sum_{\boldsymbol{v} \in \text{Cone } \boldsymbol{C}} \phi_{\boldsymbol{v}}(\boldsymbol{g}_i) G(\boldsymbol{x}, \boldsymbol{g}_i, \sigma) , \tag{1}$$

where $f_{\boldsymbol{x}}(\cdot)$ is the regularized ODF function at the voxel $\mathbf{x}$. Note that smoothing is performed only along the orientation of the cone $\mathbf{g_i}$, i.e., the ODF values only in the direction corresponding to that of the cone are averaged out over the voxels in the cone. Thus, via the created capability to both seeing further along a given direction in a larger neighbourhood and summing over the corresponding ODF values, the gross orientations are sharpened whereas the less important or less dominant directions are supressed. This leads to extraction of existing local asymmetries in a fiber distribution.

[1] The reconstruction of an ODF is performed by two methods: diffusion orientation transform (DOT) [12] and spherical deconvolution [13] using HARDI tools [14].

2.2 Measuring Asymmetry

Once an AODF field is constructed over the volume of interest, the asymmetry for each voxel can be computed. To this end, we formulate an index based on the angular similarity metric in Ref. [5]. Functions are envisioned to be vectors on an ∞-dimensional Hilbert space, and the cosine of the angle between two functions is a measure of their similarity. When symmetry is concerned, the functions can be taken to be the AODF denoted by $f(\hat{\boldsymbol{u}})$, and its reflection in the origin, $f(-\hat{\boldsymbol{u}})$. Thus, a similarity index is given by

$$\cos\gamma = \frac{\int_S f(\hat{\boldsymbol{u}})f(-\hat{\boldsymbol{u}})d\hat{\boldsymbol{u}}}{\int_S f(\hat{\boldsymbol{u}})^2 d\hat{\boldsymbol{u}}} = \frac{\sum_{l=0}^{l_{\max}}\sum_{m=-l}^{l}(-1)^l\,|a_{lm}|^2}{\sum_{l=0}^{l_{\max}}\sum_{m=-l}^{l}|a_{lm}|^2}\,, \tag{2}$$

where the last expression provides the measure in terms of a_{lm}, which are the coefficients obtained when $f(\hat{\boldsymbol{u}})$ is represented in a series of spherical harmonics. Then an asymmetry index α can be defined simply as

$$\alpha = \sin\gamma. \tag{3}$$

3 Experimental Results

In this section, we will show the results of cone-based directional ODF filtering and asymmetry index maps on synthetic and real data. The parameters cone height h and radius r (defined in § 2.1) are taken to be 2 voxels for synthetic experiments, they are chosen as 4 voxels for real experiments, and σ is taken to be 0.5 for all experiments; these parameters were selected heuristically.

3.1 Synthetic Bending and Crossing Fibers

In Ref. [4], diffusion taking place in a curving fiber within a full circle geometry is considered, and the signal attenuation for each portion of the curving circular fiber is derived. Using this result, we simulated the signal for a set of concentric circularly bending fibers. Then, ODFs that are based on the constructed q-space signals are reconstructed using the DOT approach [12]. One sample simulated data is shown in Figure 2. In (a), the original ODFs are depicted whereas in (b) are the resulting AODFs at each voxel corresponding to those in (a). Clearly, the proposed spatial regularisation of the ODFs resulted in an asymmetric ODF field, which is naturally in line with the underlying curving geometry where the bending structures are now visible at the voxel level. The asymmetry is visibly decreasing for larger circles as expected.

Two more synthetic examples (images are taken from the simulations in [15]) demonstrate the capabilities of the proposed technique. In Figure 3 (a,b), a half circle pattern of fibers meet a straight line of fibers in non-symmetric junctions. The ODF field shown on the left (a) displays the symmetry assumption imposed in conventional HARDI processing as seen from the visualised symmetric ODFs. However, the obtained asymmetric ODF field displayed on the right (b) reveals clearly the bending in the crossing captured at the voxel-level representations of the junction regions.

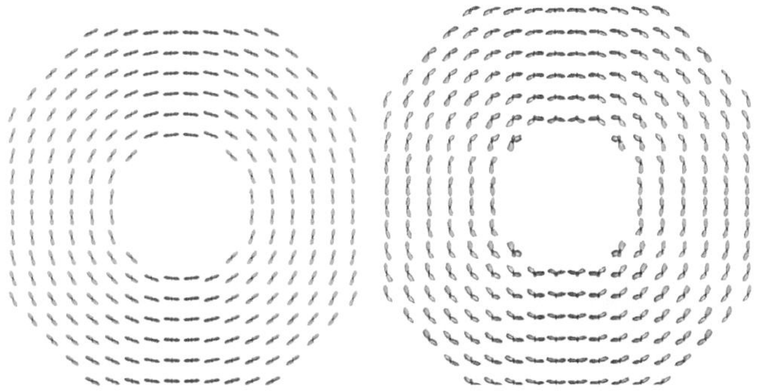

Fig. 2. Circularly bending fibers: ODF field created by the DOT method [12] (Left); asymmetric ODF field created by the proposed technique (Right).

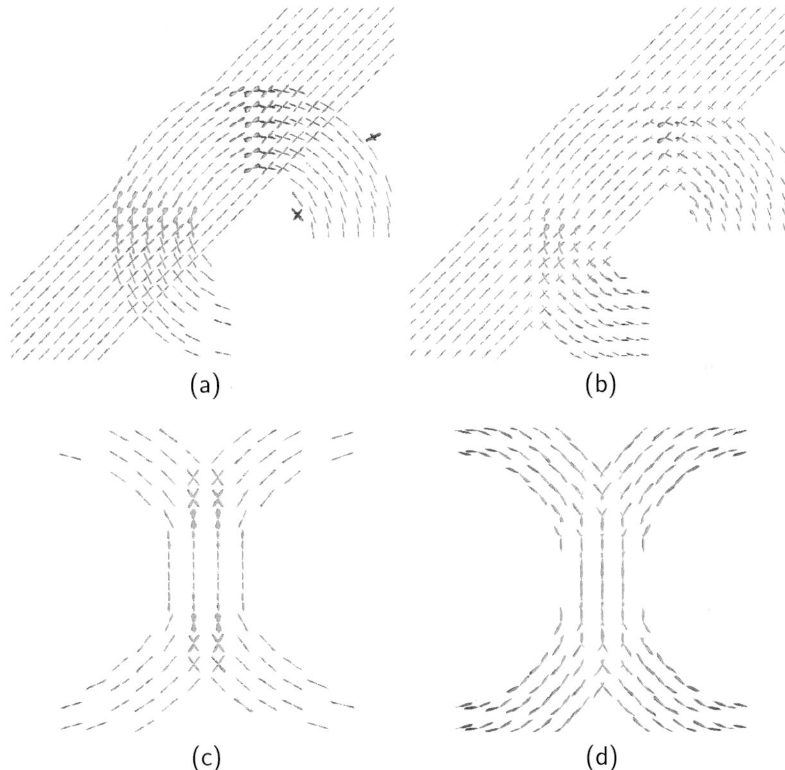

Fig. 3. Simulations for two geometries involving crossing fiber bundles. (a & c): ODFs obtained via the method in Ref. [13]. (b & d) AODF maps obtained by our technique.

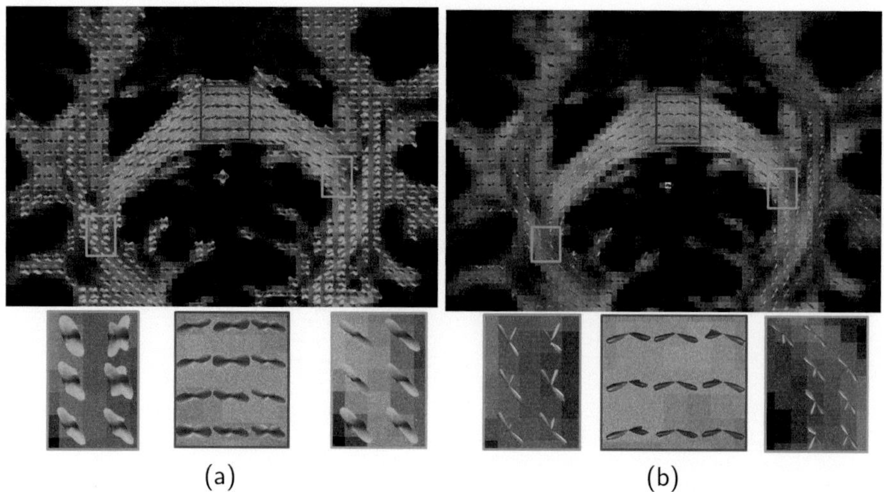

Fig. 4. An axial slice depicting the corpus callosum and Meyer's loop. ODF results obtained by the DOT method (a), and corresponding AODF maps (b) shown on fractional anisotropy maps. Three color-coded regions are magnified in the bottom rows.

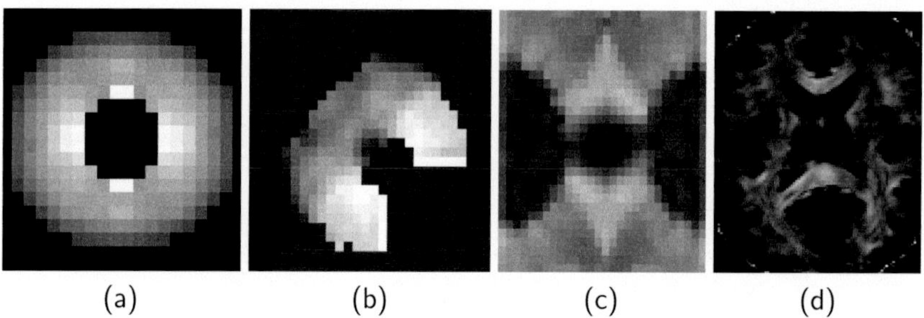

Fig. 5. Asymmetry index (α) maps (bright-to-dark:high-to-low values) calculated for: (a) circular fibers; (b) half circle crossing with a straight bundle; (c) kissing fiber configuration; (d) a slice from the HCP data.

In Figure 3 (c,d), a bottleneck or a kissing fiber geometry is depicted. On the left (c) is the ODF representation of the kissing fibers whereas on the right (d) are the corresponding reconstructed asymmetric ODFs. The resulting representation of the local fiber orientations, particularly in splaying sections of the kissing fibers are clearly observed to exhibit the Y-pattern as desired.

3.2 Results on Real Diffusion MRI Data

HARDI data was obtained from the MGH-USC Human Connectome Project (HCP) database (https://ida.loni.usc.edu/login.jsp), which is acquired from 288 gradient directions with $1.25 \times 1.25 \times 1.25\ mm^3$ voxel size. The ODF field is created by the DOT method [12]. In application of Eq. 1, we inserted a sigmoid function on the ODF to enhance very high components and suppress very low components, which are likely to be due to noise. To focus on fiber pathways that exhibit high curvature, we selected the corpus callosum (CC) and Meyer's Loop (ML) as shown in Figure 4. It is well known that non-invasive extraction of the visual pathways including CC and ML through Diffusion MRI tractography is challenging due to the strong bending, crossing and kissing geometric patterns in the relevant anatomy. The reconstructed asymmetric ODFs clearly display the inherent bending and non-symmetry at the voxel level for those white matter tracts.

3.3 Asymmetry Index Map Results

Figure 5 demonstrates the asymmetry gray scale index maps calculated over a slice of half-circle crossing straight lines, circular fibers, kissing fibers and real white matter fibers. In (a), for the circularly bending fibers, the asymmetry indices are as expected rotationally invariant and decrease from high to low radii. Similarly, the proposed index becomes larger in the asymmetric regions of interest in (b,c): the half circle itself as well as the crossing regions, and in the splaying parts of the kissing fibers, respectively. In both cases, for the fibers lying straight, the asymmetry map values are close to zero as desired. In (d), the asymmetry map for an axial slice is shown. The α values are substantial for regions with fibers featuring relatively high curvature.

4 Discussion and Conclusion

The proposed method provides an alternative representation and visualization of diffusion anisotropy that can overcome the limitations of the conventional symmetric ODF profiles, which are a product of the existing ODF reconstruction techniques. Asymmetry information is captured via an inter-voxel regularisation scheme, which produces asymmetric ODFs, indicative of the intravoxel organization. Based on the latter, an asymmetry index is also introduced.

Our experiments on both synthetic fiber populations and real MRI data demonstrated that the constructed AODFs successfully capture the intra-voxel asymmetry. We expect our method to improve tractography outcomes, where we can simply adjust conventional tractography methods such as [15] and provide faithful extraction of fiber pathways when orientational heterogeneity persists at the voxel level, particularly for fibers that exhibit intravoxel curvature, splaying, or crossings. The generated asymmetry maps were shown to accentuate strongly bending, kissing and crossing regions in fiber pathways. Such maps could be utilised to analyse white matter structures, complementing traditional measures of anisotropy and mean diffusivity in population studies and eventually improve the sensitivity and specificity of diffusion-MRI to different pathologies and processes.

References

1. Basser, P.J., Pajevic, S., Pierpaoli, C., Duda, J., Aldroubi, A.: In vivo fiber tractography using DT-MRI data. Magn. Reson. Med. 44(4), 625–632 (2000)
2. Tuch, D.S., Weisskoff, R.M., Belliveau, J.W., Wedeen, V.J.: High angular resolution diffusion imaging of the human brain. Mag. Reson. Med. 7, 321 (1999)
3. Liu, C., Bammer, R., Acar, B., Moseley, M.E.: Characterizing non-Gaussian diffusion by using generalized diffusion tensors. Magn. Reson. Med. 51(5), 924–937 (2004)
4. Özarslan, E., Koay, C.G., Basser, P.J.: Remarks on q-space MR propagator in partially restricted, axially-symmetric, and isotropic environments. Magn. Reson. Imaging 27(6), 834–844 (2009)
5. Özarslan, E., Koay, C.G., Shepherd, T.M., Komlosh, M.E., İrfanoğlu, M.O., Pierpaoli, C., Basser, P.J.: Mean apparent propagator (MAP) MRI: a novel diffusion imaging method for mapping tissue microstructure. NeuroImage 78, 16–32 (2013)
6. Ozcan, A.: Complete Fourier direct magnetic resonance imaging (CFD-MRI) for diffusion MRI. Front. Integr. Neurosci. 7, 18 (2013)
7. Anderson, A.W., Gore, J.C.: Analysis and correction of motion artifacts in diffusion weighted imaging. Magnetic Resonance in Medicine 32(3), 379–387 (1994)
8. Barmpoutis, A., Vemuri, B.C., Howland, D., Forder, J.R.: Extracting tractosemas from a displacement probability field for tractography in DW-MRI. In: Metaxas, D., Axel, L., Fichtinger, G., Székely, G. (eds.) MICCAI 2008, Part I. LNCS, vol. 5241, pp. 9–16. Springer, Heidelberg (2008)
9. Schultz, T.: Towards resolving fiber crossings with higher order tensor inpainting. In: Laidlaw, D.H., Vilanova, A. (eds.) New Developments in the Visualization and Processing of Tensor Fields, pp. 253–265 (2012)
10. Campbell, J.S.W.: Savadjiev, P., Siddiqi, K., Pike, G.: Validation and Regularization in Diffusion MRI Tractography. In: ISBI, pp. 351–354 (2006)
11. Ehricke, H.H., Otto, K.M., Klose, U.: Regularization of bending and crossing white matter fibers in MRI q-ball fields. Magn. Reson. Imaging 29, 916–926 (2011)
12. Özarslan, E., Shepherd, T.M., Vemuri, B.C., Blackband, S.J., Mareci, T.H.: Resolution of complex tissue microarchitecture using the diffusion orientation transform (DOT). NeuroImage 31(3), 1086–1103 (2006)
13. Dell'Acqua, F., Scifo, P., Rizzo, G., Catani, M., Simmons, A., Scotti, G., Fazio, F.: A modified damped Richardson-Lucy algorithm to reduce isotropic background effects in spherical deconvolution. NeuroImage 49(2), 1446–1458 (2010)
14. Canales-Rodrguez, E.J., Melie-Garca, L., Iturria-Medina, Y., Alemn-Gmez, Y.: High angular resolution diffusion imaging (HARDI) tools. http://neuroimagen.es/webs/hardi_tools/
15. Descoteaux, M., Deriche, R., Knsche, T.R., Anwander, A.: Deterministic and probabilistic tractography based on complex fibre orientation distributions. IEEE Trans. Med. Imaging 28(2), 269–286 (2009)

Modeling Task FMRI Data via Supervised Stochastic Coordinate Coding

Jinglei Lv[1,2], Binbin Lin[3], Wei Zhang[2], Xi Jiang[2], Xintao Hu[1], Junwei Han[1], Lei Guo[1], Jieping Ye[3], and Tianming Liu[2]

[1] School of Automation, Northwestern Polytechnical University, Xi'an, China
[2] Cortical Architecture Imaging and Discovery Lab, Department of Computer Science, The University of Georgia, Athens, GA, USA
[3] Department of Electrical Engineering and Computer Science, University of Michigan, Ann Arbor, MI, USA
lvjinglei@gmail.com

Abstract. Task functional MRI (fMRI) has been widely employed to assess brain activation and networks. Modeling the rich information from the fMRI time series is challenging because of the lack of ground truth and the intrinsic complexity. Model-driven methods such as the general linear model (GLM) regresses exterior task designs from voxel-wise brain functional activity, which is confined because of ignoring the complexity and diversity of concurrent brain networks. Recently, dictionary learning and sparse coding method has attracted increasing attention in the fMRI analysis field. The major advantage of this methodology is its effectiveness in reconstructing concurrent brain networks automatically and systematically. However, the data-driven strategy is, to some extent, arbitrary due to ignoring the prior knowledge of task design and neuroscience knowledge. In this paper, we proposed a novel supervised stochastic coordinate coding (SCC) algorithm for fMRI data analysis, in which certain brain networks are learned with supervised information such as temporal patterns of task designs and spatial patterns of network templates, while other networks are learned automatically from the data. Its application on two independent fMRI datasets has shown the effectiveness of our methods.

Keywords: Task fMRI, Supervised Stochastic Coordinate Coding, Brain network.

1 Introduction

Task-based functional magnetic resonance imaging (fMRI) has been well established for mapping brain activations and networks [1, 2]. How to effectively mine the rich information from fMRI data has been challenging because of the lack of ground truth and the intrinsic complexity of brain function [3]. Among all of state-of-the-art methodologies, the general linear model (GLM) has been the dominant approach in detecting functional networks from task-based fMRI data [2] by regressing the designed task information from fMRI signals. However, the straightforward block-based task designs are limited in inferring concurrent networks that perform diverse activeity [4-6] or recruit various heterogeneous neuroanatomic areas [4-5].

N. Navab et al. (Eds.): MICCAI 2015, Part I, LNCS 9349, pp. 239–246, 2015.
DOI: 10.1007/978-3-319-24553-9_30

Recently, pioneer work that adopted the dictionary learning and sparse representation methods from machine learning field [7] in fMRI data analysis has shown promising performance [3, 8]. The basic idea is to aggregate fMRI signals within the whole-brain of one subject into a sample matrix, based on which an over-complete basis dictionary and sparse code matrix for optimal representation will be learned [3,9]. Particularly, the signal shape of each dictionary atom represents the functional activities of a specific brain network and its corresponding sparse code vector can be reorganized as the spatial distribution of this brain network [3]. An important characteristic of this framework is that concurrent brain networks that are captured by fMRI data can be reconstructed simultaneously in an automatic and optimal way. This novel data-driven strategy naturally accounts for the fact that brain regions might be involved in multiple concurrent functional processes [4-6] and thus their fMRI signals are composed of various heterogeneous components [3,8].

However, the data-driven strategy might be arbitrary due to ignoring the task design and the neuroscience background knowledge [3]. Therefore, adopting the dictionary learning and sparse coding method into neuroscience applications entails a novel, flexible framework that can guide the learning procedure with prior knowledge. Typically, the task design is straightforward information that can be utilized as a reasonable temporal feature, and in the field of neuroscience, a variety of spatial signatures such as network templates or brain mapping atlases are valuable information for brain network inference. If we can adapt such temporal features and spatial signatures into the dictionary learning and model task fMRI data with the prior knowledge, the gap between model-driven method and data-driven method could be significantly bridged and the power of both methods would be boosted at the same time. In this paper, we proposed a novel supervised stochastic coordinate coding (SCC) method that is capable of adopting temporal features such as task designs as part of learned dictionary and supervise the spatial region in which an unknown signal pattern might take major contribution. With our proposed method, meaningful functional networks can be inferred with known temporal and spatial features, and at the same time, other concurrent networks can be learned automatically from the data.

2 Methods

Our supervised stochastic coordinate coding (SCC) framework is summarized in Fig.1. Briefly, fMRI signals extracted from a 3D brain mask are firstly normalized and then organized into a signal matrix S (Fig.1a). The supervised stochastic coordinate coding (SCC) method then decomposes the signal matrix S into a dictionary matrix D and sparse code matrix A (Fig.1b). The learning process will preserve the organization of signals of voxels so that each row in A can be mapped back to brain volume, which we call a brain network [3], as shown in Fig.1c. The SCC can be supervised with fixed temporal features in D and constrained spatial features in A. Specifically, in our supervised SCC, temporal features such as task designs can be fixed in D as $\mathrm{D_C}$ and they keep unchanged during the whole training, while the D_l will be learned automatically. Accordingly, the rows in A_C are the learned spatial distributions of D_C atoms. We can also restrict the spatial patterns of networks in A_R, correspondingly, and in this way we can learn the major signal contribution in D_R of the restricted spatial patterns. More details will be discussed in the following sections.

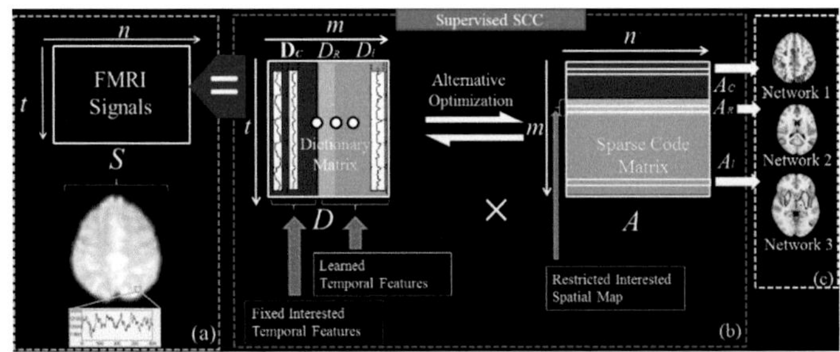

Fig. 1. Illustration of the framework of supervised stochastic coordinate coding (SCC) for fMRI data modeling. (a) FMRI signals from a brain are extracted and organized into a signal matrix *S*. (b) *S* is decomposed into a dictionary matrix *D* and a sparse code matrix *A* by the supervised SCC. (c) Each row of *A* can be mapped back to brain volume as a spatial network.

2.1 Stochastic Coordinate Coding of FMRI Data

Consider signals within the brain is represented as $S = [s_1 \ldots\ldots s_n] \in \mathbb{R}^{t\times n}$, where t is the number of time points in each signal and n is the voxel number in the brain mask. The aim of SCC is to learn a dictionary of signal basis $D \in \mathbb{R}^{t\times m}$, and a sparse code matrix $A \in \mathbb{R}^{m\times n}$, so that each s_i is modeled as a sparse linear combination of learned basis, i.e., $s_i = Da_i$ or written as $S = DA$ [3, 9].

Given the signal s_i, it can be formularized as an optimization problem:

$$\min\ f_i(D, a_i) = \min \frac{1}{2}||s_i - Da_i||^2 + \lambda||a_i||_1, \tag{1}$$

where both *D* and a_i need to be learned and λ is the regularization parameter. Given the whole-brain data set *S*, the minimization function is summarized as follow:

$$\min_{D \in B_m, a_1, \ldots a_n} F(D, a_1, \ldots a_n) \equiv \frac{1}{n}\sum_{i=1}^{n} f_i(D, a_i), \tag{2}$$

where
$$B_m = \left\{D \in \mathbb{R}^{t\times m} : \forall j = 1, \ldots, m, \left\|d_j\right\|_2 \leq 1\right\}. \tag{3}$$

We first define some concepts that will help our method to be illustrated. In our method, each a_i is called *sparse code*. Since a_i is sparse so that there are only a few entries in a_i that are non-zero. We define the non-zero entries as its support, i.e., *support* (a_i) ={ $1, if\ a_{i,j} \neq 0$; $0, if\ a_{i,j} = 0$. } $\in \{0,1\}^{m\times 1}, (j = 1, \ldots, m.)$. The support will be a screen that guides necessary and efficient updating of a_i and *D*. The training process will take a few cycles on the whole data set, and we call each cycle, i.e., each input signal in *S* has been trained once, as an

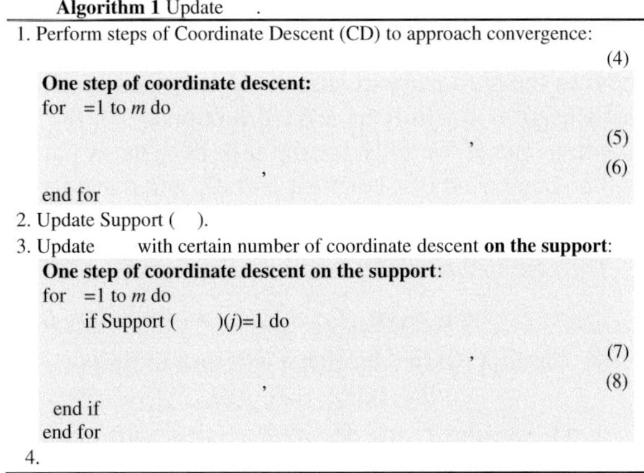
Algorithm 1 Update .

1. Perform steps of Coordinate Descent (CD) to approach convergence: (4)

One step of coordinate descent:
for =1 to *m* do
, (5)
, (6)
end for

2. Update Support ( ).
3. Update with certain number of coordinate descent **on the support**:

One step of coordinate descent on the support:
for =1 to *m* do
if Support ( )(*j*)=1 do
, (7)
, (8)
end if
end for

4.

Algorithm 2 Update *D*

1. Update Support ( ).
2. ,
3. Update the dictionary D by using stochastic gradient descent: (10) (11)

One step of stochastic gradient descent:
for =1 to *m* do
 if Support ( )(j)=1 do
 (12)
 end if
end for

epoch. In the following sections, we will use superscript *k* to represent the number of epochs and we use subscript *i* to represent the index of data samples.

The dictionary is initialized via any initialization method, such as random weights, random patches or k-means [11]. And denote it as D_1^1, Initialize the sparse code a_i^0 =0 ($\mathbb{R}^{m\times 1}$) , for *i*=1,..., *n*, *support*(a_i^0) is all zero. *H* is initialized as 0. Then starting from *k*=1 and *i*=1, we do the following:

1. Get an input sample s_i.
2. Update a_i^k with **Algorithm 1**.
3. Update the dictionary *D* with **Algorithm 2**.
4. $i = i + 1$. If $i > n$, set $D_1^{k+1} = D_{n+1}^k$, $k = k + 1$ and $i = 1$. Go to step 1.

In **Algorithm 1**, updating a_i^k is the classical lasso problem. After a number of Coordinate Decent until approximately convergence, we defined the *support* to accelerate the convergence and for future use. Note that **Support ($\boldsymbol{a_i^{k-1}}$)(j)** denotes the *j*-th value in the vector of **Support ($\boldsymbol{a_i^{k-1}}$).** And while applying the L1 norm, the soft shrinking function is defined as follow:

$$h_\lambda(v) = \begin{cases} v+\lambda, & v < -\lambda \\ 0, & -\lambda \le v \le \lambda \\ v-\lambda, & v > \lambda \end{cases} \tag{9}$$

In **Algorithm 2**, suppose that $a_{i,j}^k = 0$, then $\nabla_{d_{i,j}^k} f_i(D_i^k, a_i^k) = (D_i^k a_i^k - s_i)(a_{i,j}^k)^T = 0$, therefore $d_{i,j}^k$ does not need to be updated. Thus, with the help of the definition of *support,* we can only update the *j*-th column of D_{i+1}^k on which the $a_{i,j}^k$ is non-zero. Note that P_{B_m} in **Algorithm 2** indicates restriction by B_m.

2.2 Fix Temporal Features in Stochastic Coordinate Coding

In our method, we normalize the task designs with the B_m constraint (Eq.(3)) and set them as the dictionary of stochastic coordinate coding or part of the dictionary. If the task design is set fully as a fixed dictionary *D*, the problem becomes a easy LASSO problem. But if we only fix the task designs as part of the dictionary, the dictionary will be composed of a constant part $\mathbf{D}_c$ and a learned part D_l.

$$D = [\mathbf{D}_c, D_l] \epsilon \mathbb{R}^{t\times m},\ \ \mathbf{D}_c \epsilon \mathbb{R}^{t\times m_c},\ \ D_l \epsilon \mathbb{R}^{t\times m_l}$$

Then the optimization function turns into Eq.(13).

$$\min f_i([\mathbf{D}_c, D_l], a_i) = \min \frac{1}{2} ||s_i - [\mathbf{D}_c, D_l]a_i||^2 + \lambda ||a_i||_1 \tag{13}$$

So that Eq.(10) in Algorithm will turn to Eq.(14):

$$[\mathbf{D}_c, D_l]_{i+1}^k = P_{B_m}([\mathbf{D}_c, D_l]_i^k - \eta_i^k \nabla_{D_i^k} f_i([\mathbf{D}_c, D_l]_i^k, a_i^k)) \tag{14}$$

In **Algorithm 2,** the updating process will jump over the constant dictionary part but only update the learned part. However, during each iteration the spare code of the whole dictionary will update accordingly. In this way, we will find the contribution of the task designs on each voxel, and in a global view we will find the distribution of the task designs on the brain volume.

2.3 Constrain Spatial Maps in Stochastic Coordinate Coding

In neuroscience, interested networks are usually defined in the spatial domain [15]. So it will be interesting to see what the major signal pattern is in a certain interested spatial region. The premise is as follow. The whole brain signal set $S = [s_1, \dots s_n] \in \mathbb{R}^{t \times n}$ is extracted with a certain principle, and the stochastic coordinate coding will preserve the principle, i.e., the order of voxels, in the learned sparse code matrix $A = [a_1, \dots a_n] \in \mathbb{R}^{m \times n}$. In this way, if we map each row of the sparse code back following the principle of extraction, there will be *m* spatial maps which correspond to the distributions of *m* dictionary atom signals [3]. We call these spatial maps as interested networks [3].

In this section, we will adjust the stochastic coordinate coding by restricting certain rows of the *A* matrix with the spatial distribution information. Suppose we have an interesting spatial pattern within the brain mask, the pattern itself is labeled by 1, and the rest of brain mask is labeled by 0. Then the pattern can be represented as a binary vector $V \in \{0,1\}^{1 \times n}$ with the same voxel organization of *S*. We set the pattern as constraint of the *p*-th row of *A*, in the way that *support*$(a_i)(p) = V(i)$, for $i = 1, \dots, n$. After the *support* of each voxel at the *p*-th row is set at the initialization, they will keep fixed during the whole training.

Since the a_i^0 is initialized as 0 in step 1 of **Algorithm 1,** an regularization will be made before update of a_i^{k-1}, thus if *j*=*p* the Eq.(6) turns to Eq.(15).

$$a_{i,p}^{k-1} \leftarrow \begin{cases} 0, & support(a_i^{k-1})(p) = 0 \\ h_\lambda(b_j), & support(a_i^{k-1})(p) = 1 \end{cases} \tag{15}$$

In Eq.(15), if the shrinking function $h_\lambda(b_j)$ return 0 in a certain iteration, we will update $a_{i,p}^{k-1}$ as an infinite small value, such as 1×10^{-4}. In following steps of **Algorithm 1** and **Algorithm 2**, we keep the support of a_i at the *p*-th row the same as what is initialized. With the help of restriction on the *support,* we can learn the major signal contribution and their strength distribution in the interested brain region.

2.4 Group-Wise Statistical Aanlysis of Network Spatial Maps

Individual variblility widely exsits in the learned network spatial maps. Similar to the statistical parameter mapping (SPM) [2], we can also perform group-wise statistical analysis on the spatially normalized networks across subjects with the correspondences established by D_C and A_R. In this paper, all data are registered into the MNI space before applying our method, and null hypothesis t-test was applied to generate group-wise statistical z-score maps for each corresponding networks in A_C and A_R. This is one major advantage relative to the data-driven method in [3].

However, there are still many networks in A_l which are learned automatically without any prior correspondence settled. Thus, we employ K-means clustering method to find networks which possess spatial pattern similarity among subjects, i.e., these networks consistently exist across subjects with similar spatial patterns.

3 Experimental Results

In this section, our method is evaluated on two independent task-fMRI datasets:

Working Memory (WM) Task Dataset: In an operational span (OSPAN) working memory task-based fMRI experiment under IRB approval [12], fMRI images of 28 subjects are scanned on a 3T GE Signa scanner. Briefly, acquisition parameters are as follows: fMRI: 64×64 matrix, 4mm slice thickness, 220mm FOV, 30 slices, TR=1.5s, TE=25ms, ASSET=2. Each participant performed a modified version of the OSPAN task (2 block types: OSPAN and Arithmetic,) while fMRI data was acquired.

Motor Task Dataset: In the human connectome project (HCP) [13], a motor task-based fMRI dataset was scanned for 68 subjects. The acquisition parameters of fMRI data are: 90×104 matrix, 220mm FOV, 72 slices, TR=0.72s, TE=33.1ms, flip angle = 52°, BW =2290 Hz/Px, in-plane FOV = 208 × 180 mm, 2.0 mm isotropic voxels. Six different stimulus designs, including visual cues and movements of left toe, left finger, right toe, right finger and tongue are alternated in different blocks.

The preprocessing pipeline includes motion correction, slice time correction, spatial smoothing and high-pass filtering. After pre-processing the fMRI data of all subjects are registered to the MNI space with the non-linear registration tool FNIRT [14]. In this paper, both the dictionary size in dictionary learning and the cluster number of K-means clustering are empirically determined as 200.

3.1 Detecting Task-Evoked Networks Using Supervised SCC

The stilmulus designs from both tasks in Section 3.1 are are first convolved with hemodynamic response function (HRF), as shown in the first column of Fig.2, and then set as fixed temporal features in our supervised SCC method. For comparison, the same designs are also set as design matrix of GLM based method. The second column of Fig.2 show results of our method after applying the group-wise statistical analysis (Z>2.5) in Section 2.4. In comparison, the group-wise activations (Z>2.5) from GLM method are present in the third colum of Fig.2. On average, the spatial overlap of the maps from two methods in Fig.2 is around 75%, which means they are very similar. Although variation exitsts, we could still conclude that our supervised SCC method is comparable with GLM in the performance of detecting task-related activations or networks.

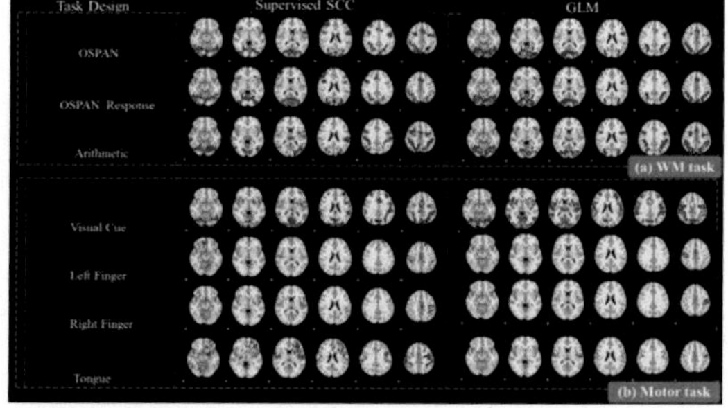

Fig.2. Task-related networks detected by our supervised SCC method. Panel (a) is the result of working memory task. Panel (b) is the result from motor task. First column of (a) and (b): Fixed task designs. Second column: Group-wise statistical z-score maps of our method (Z>2.5). Third column: Comparing activation by GLM method (Z>2.5).

3.2 Networks Detected By Restriction of Spatial Maps

Along with the setting in Section 3.1, we also set several well-established brain network templates (default mode, frontal and auditory networks) [15], which are believed to

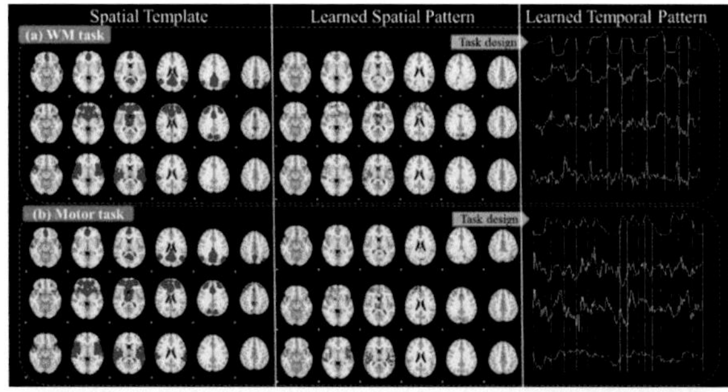

Fig. 3. The networks detected by restricting network templates in supervised SCC of one subject. Panel (a) is from working memory (WM) task dataset. Panel (b) is from motor task dataset. First column: Restricted spatial patterns. Second column: Learned spatial distribution from our method. (c) Optimized temporal patterns for the learned networks.

function in different brains and across different tasks [15], as spatial restrictions (the red regions shown in the first column of Fig.3). From the learning results shown in the second column of Fig.3, there are reasonable Gaussian-like distributions in the restricted regions. And the temporal patterns corresponding to these networks in the third columns of Fig.3 are also promising. For example, if we simply average all stimulus in one task as the global task curve (white curves in Fig.3), the temporal pattern of the default mode network tends to be anti-task [15] and that of the frontal lobe tends to peak at task change points, which are believed to correspond to action-inhibation [15].

Note that we didn't select some networks with conceptual conflict, like motor and visual networks, because motor networks should be learned with fixed task design in motor task data; Visual networks are task-related networks in both data sets.

3.3 Automatically Learned Concurrent Networks

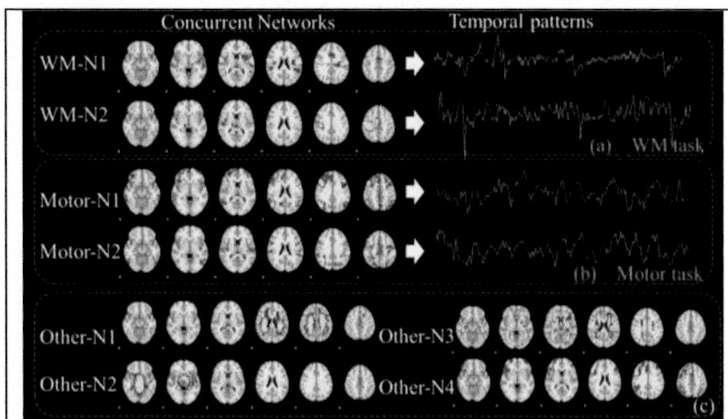

Fig. 4. Automatically learned concurrent networks. Panel (a), (b) are from the working memory task, and motor task respectively. Panel (c) shows consistent networks from both datasets.

Besides the supervised networks in the previous two sections, quantities of concurrent networks can also be learned from our method at the same time. Group consistent networks that are detectd by clustering method are shown in Fig. 4. Although the temporal response of these networks might not be directly interpreted in the second column of Fig.4a-b, it is quite interesting that some motor networks can be detected in the working memory task data, as shown in the spatial patterns of WM-N1 and WM-N2 in Fig.4a. This is reasonable because participants needed to push buttons to respond in the OSPAN task. Meanwhile, some working memory networks can also be detected in the motor task data, as shown in the spatial patterns of Motor-N1 and Motor-N2 in Fig.4b. This might be due to that participants needed to think and memorize in order to move the correct body parts. Additionally, through clustering all automatically learned networks from all subjects with spatial similarity as a metric, we could find that some networks consistently exist across subjects and datasets as shown in Fig.4c, e.g., Other-N1 mainly concentrated in the white matter, while Other-N2 and Other-N3 located on the thalamus and ventricle areas respectively, and Other-N4 majorly distributed on the left part of brain. Meaningful interpretation of these networks entails more investigations in the future.

4 Conclusion

In this paper, we proposed a novel supervised dictionary learning and sparse coding method named supervised stochastic coordinate coding (SCC) for task-base fMRI data modeling. The major advantage of this method is that temporal models and spatial templates can be supervised as constraints for network inference, and at the same time quantities of concurrent networks can also be learned automatically from data in a data-driven fashion. The applications of our method on two independent fMRI data sets have shown that our method is promising in detecting multiple concurrent and meaningful brain networks.

References

1. Logothetis, N.K.: What we can do and what we cannot do with fMRI. Nature 453(7197), 869–878 (2008)
2. Friston, K.J., et al.: Statistical parametric maps in functional imaging: a general linear approach. Human Brain Mapping 2(4), 189–210 (1994)
3. Lv, J., et al.: Holistic Atlases of Functional Networks and Interactions Reveal Reciprocal Organizational Architecture of Cortical Function. IEEE Transaction on Biomedical Engineering (2014)
4. Duncan, J.: The multiple-demand (MD) system of the primate brain: mental programs for intelligent behaviour. Trends in Cognitive Sciences 14(4), 172–179 (2010)
5. Gazzaugia, M.S. (ed.): The cognitive neurosciences III. The MIT Press (2004)
6. Pessoa, L.: Beyond brain regions: Network perspective of cognition–emotion interactions. Behavioral and Brain Sciences 35(03), 158–159 (2012)
7. Wright, J., Yang, A.Y., Ganesh, A., Sastry, S.S., Ma, Y.: Robust Face Recognition via Sparse Representation. IEEE TPAMI 31(2), 210–227 (2009)
8. Lee, K., et al.: A data-driven sparse GLM for fMRI analysis using sparse dictionary learning with MDL criterion. IEEE Transactions on Medical Imaging 30(5), 1076–1089 (2011)
9. Mairal, J., Bach, F., Ponce, J., Sapiro, G.: Online learning for matrix factorization and sparse coding. The Journal of Machine Learning Research 11, 19–60 (2010)
10. Wu, T.T., Lange, K.: Coordinate Descent Algorithms for Lasso Penalized Regression. The Annals of Applied Statistics 2(1), 224–244 (2008)
11. Jarrett, K., Kavukcuoglu, K., Ranzato, M., LeCun, Y.: What is the best multi-stage architecture for object recognition? In: ICCV, pp. 2146–2153 (2009)
12. Faraco, C.C., et al.: Complex span tasks and hippocampal recruitment during working memory. NeuroImage 55(2), 773–787 (2011)
13. Barch, D.M., et al.: Function in the human connectome: Task-fMRI and individual differences in behavior. NeuroImage 80, 169–189 (2013)
14. Andersson, J.L.R., Jenkinson, M., Smith, S.: Non-linear registration, aka spatial normalization (2010)
15. Smith, S.M., et al.: Correspondence of the brain's functional architecture during activation and rest. PNAS 106(31), 13040–13045 (2009)

Computer Assisted and Image-Guided Interventions

Autonomous Ultrasound-Guided Tissue Dissection

Philip Pratt[1], Archie Hughes-Hallett[2], Lin Zhang[1], Nisha Patel[1,2]
Erik Mayer[2], Ara Darzi[1,2], and Guang-Zhong Yang[1]

[1] Hamlyn Centre for Robotic Surgery,
Imperial College of Science, Technology and Medicine,
London SW7 2AZ, UK
[2] Department of Surgery and Cancer,
Imperial College of Science, Technology and Medicine,
London SW7 2AZ, UK
{p.pratt,a.hughes-hallett,lin.zhang11,nisha.patel2,
e.mayer,a.darzi,g.z.yang}@imperial.ac.uk

Abstract. Intraoperative ultrasound imaging can act as a valuable guide during minimally invasive tumour resection. However, contemporaneous bimanual manipulation of the transducer and cutting instrument presents significant challenges for the surgeon. Both cannot occupy the same physical location, and so a carefully coordinated relative motion is required. Using robotic partial nephrectomy as an index procedure, and employing PVA cryogel tissue phantoms in a reduced dimensionality setting, this study sets out to achieve autonomous tissue dissection with a high velocity waterjet under ultrasound guidance. The open-source da Vinci Research Kit (DVRK) provides the foundation for a novel multimodal visual servoing approach, based on the simultaneous processing and analysis of endoscopic and ultrasound images. Following an accurate and robust Jacobian estimation procedure, dissections are performed with specified theoretical tumour margin distances. The resulting margins, with a mean difference of 0.77mm, indicate that the overall system performs accurately, and that future generalisation to 3D tumour and organ surface morphologies is warranted.

1 Introduction

Many contemporary minimally invasive surgical procedures stand to benefit from intraoperative ultrasound guidance as a means of overcoming the haptic deficit imposed by having restricted access. In the context of cancerous tumour resection, the modality can provide excellent views of the interface between healthy and diseased tissues. One such case is robotic partial nephrectomy, adopted by this study as a clinical exemplar, through which the nephron-sparing approach offers the best long-term patient prognoses. However, experience tells us that the ideal paradigm of simultaneous guidance and dissection is very difficult to achieve in practice, even when registration [1] is used to co-locate endoscopic and ultrasound images. Nonetheless, rapid progress in the field of autonomous robotic surgical systems [2] points toward novel solutions to this problem. It can only be a matter of time before tumour resection requires the surgeon only in a supervisory role.

N. Navab et al. (Eds.): MICCAI 2015, Part I, LNCS 9349, pp. 249–257, 2015.
DOI: 10.1007/978-3-319-24553-9_31

Notable examples of such systems include the Probot [3], an early computer-controlled robot capable of performing transurethral resection of the prostate (TURP), successfully translated through to human clinical trials. Preoperative transrectal ultrasound, combined with a curve-fitting procedure, was used to build 3D models of the target resection volume. Recently, the open-source da Vinci Research Kit (DVRK) [4] has facilitated a 'robotic ultrasound surgical assistant' [5], whereby the imaging plane of a 'pick-up' transducer automatically follows the tips of other instruments engaged in resection tasks. These distal coordinate frames are related to each other through an initial registration of the robot arm base frames. The current proliferation of research kits promises to accelerate progress in these areas.

The use of waterjet dissection in nephron-sparing renal surgery [6] can reduce morbidity associated with intraoperative haemorrhage. The selective action of the waterjet, leading to preservation of arterial tissue, makes off-clamp dissection with precise haemostasis possible. While the use of robotic waterjet systems has seen applications in engineering [7], to date no precedents have been set in the surgical domain. Building on these separate approaches, this study aims to establish the trifecta of autonomous robotic control, guidance through ultrasound imaging and waterjet tumour resection. In comparison to the complex scissor-like action of traditional cutting tools, the linearity of the jet greatly simplifies instrument manipulation. To achieve sufficient accuracy, visual servoing is employed but with, for the first time, input from multiple imaging sources. Working in a reduced dimensionality (2D) setting ensures that the problem is tractable at the outset.

2 Materials and Methods

2.1 Experimental Setup

Having a tensile strength and elasticity similar to human renal parenchyma, bespoke polyvinyl alcohol (PVA) phantoms [8] were used to simulate 2D tumour boundaries. A shallow rectangular tray was filled to a depth of 5mm with 10% PVA solution (by weight), to which cellulose powder (2% by weight) had been added to improve echogenic contrast, and subjected to an initial freeze/thaw cycle. Curved paths were cut in this layer (figure 1, left), and the sections separated in order to make two separate phantoms. Each tray was then filled to a total depth of 10mm with cellulose-free cryogel and subjected to a final freeze/thaw cycle. The resulting phantoms represent completely endophytic lesions with boundaries invisible from the surface.

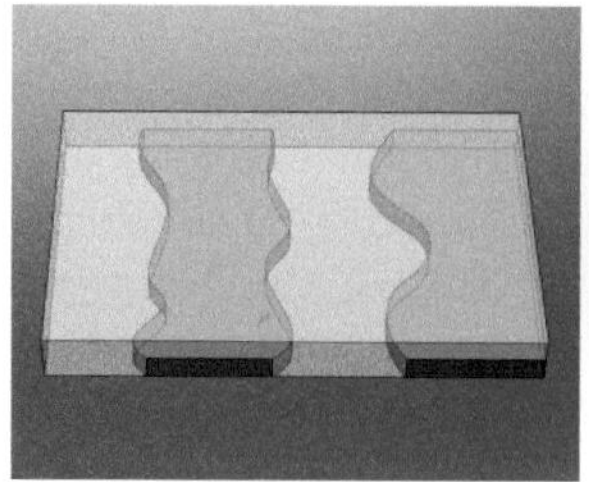
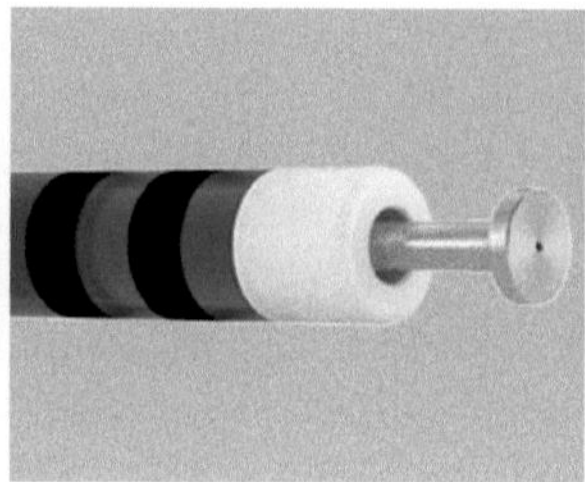
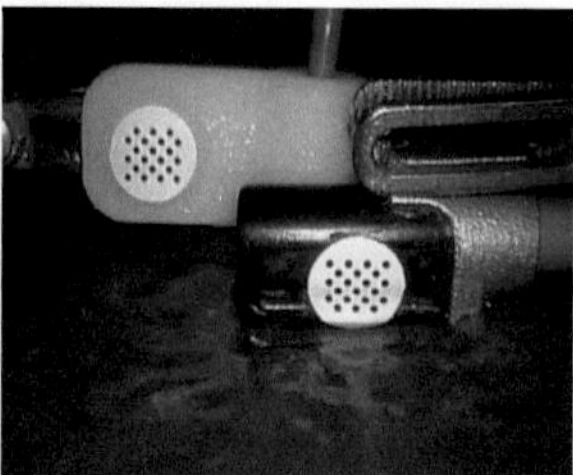

Fig. 1. Cryogel phantom (left); waterjet 'T-type' nozzle (middle); pattern mountings (right)

A 'T-type' HybridKnife (ERBE Elektromedizin, GmbH, Tuebingen, Germany), was connected to an ERBEJET2 double-piston pump cartridge and giving set with fluid bag containing 0.9% saline. The waterjet nozzle (figure 1, middle) has a diameter of 120μm, and the pump was configured with the maximum pressure setting of 80 bar. A custom mounting was 3D-printed in hard plastic material (figure 1, right), providing a platform for a KeyDot® tracking marker (KeySurgical Inc., Eden Prairie, MN, USA), and a foot allowing the nozzle to be grasped by robotic Cadiere forceps. Details regarding the ultrasound transducer, metal mounting bracket, calibration procedure, and KeyDot tracking algorithms are described in previous work [9]. To facilitate instrument identification, the two patterns were arranged in opposition.

2.2 System Architecture

The overall system architecture is illustrated in figure 2. An intact 'standard' da Vinci Surgical System (Intuitive Surgical, Sunnyvale, CA, USA) was connected to the DVRK [4], capable of controlling two patient side manipulators (PSMs). This in turn was connected to a Linux server, running various *cisst*/SAW/ROS components [4], over an IEEE-1394 Firewire link. Video feeds from the (stereo) endoscope and ultrasound cart were captured on a separate Windows machine using the Quadro digital video pipeline (Nvidia Corporation, Santa Clara, CA, USA). The tracking, visual servoing control and dissection software runs on the latter machine. Kinematic states were updated and queried continuously over a lightweight UDP network interface. The ERBEJET2 foot pedal cannot be replaced by a computer-controlled relay, and was therefore operated manually in response to visual cues from the control machine. In this study, the endoscopic camera manipulator (ECM) remains in a fixed position during dissection. The intrinsic properties and distortion coefficients of the camera were calibrated using the benchmark OpenCV implementation [10].

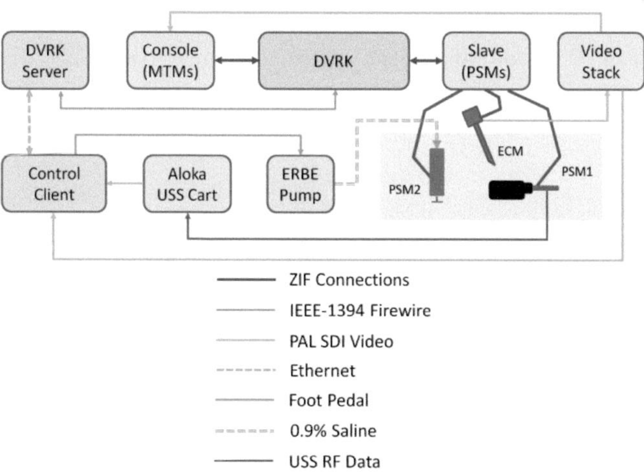

Fig. 2. Schematic diagram illustrating system architecture

2.3 Robust Jacobian Estimation

In the reduced dimensionality setting, where only end effector translations are considered, the 3-DOF Jacobian estimation is equivalent to finding the rotation matrix relating the camera and robot arm base coordinate systems. Generalisation must wait until the salient features of the overall approach are proven. Unfortunately, a simple two-sided finite difference approximation to the Jacobian matrix entries, generated by issuing orthogonal movements along the Cartesian axes in the PSM base frames B_i, was found to be very unreliable and subject to the hysteretic behaviour of the robot and its low-level control system.

Instead, 10 incremental movements were issued along each of the positive and negative X, Y and Z axes of the PSM base frame, respectively (5 outward and 5 inward), resulting in a total of 60 pose increments in the camera frame from which the Jacobian entries were estimated. For each entry, the median value was chosen in order to remove outlier motions, and then the whole matrix was subjected to the Gram-Schmidt orthogonalisation process. At the start of each dissection experiment, the end effectors were carefully teleoperated into parallel orientations orthogonal to the phantom surface. The PSM1 and PSM2 Jacobians $J_{1,2}$ were then estimated sequentially. The visual servoing loops were implemented as simple proportional controllers embedded in a finite state machine (FSM), where error signals $d\tilde{p}_i$ in the camera frames generated incremental movements $d\tilde{e}_i$ in the Cartesian robot frames, until the targets were reached within a tolerance of 0.4mm. Together with an empirically chosen gain coefficient of 0.04, an appropriate rate was set for the cutting action of the waterjet.

2.4 Coordinate Frame Relationships

Figure 3 illustrates the physical components required to perform the dissection task, their respective coordinate systems, and the relationships between incremental movements in the PSM and camera frames. The notation $T^{S \to D}$ is used to represent the transformation (constant, or otherwise) from a source coordinate frame S to the destination frame D. In addition, several constant geometric quantities were specified, either as free parameters, through measurement, or via calibration, as follows: a) the ultrasound image to probe pattern transformation $T^{U \to P_1}$ and pixel-to-millimetre scale

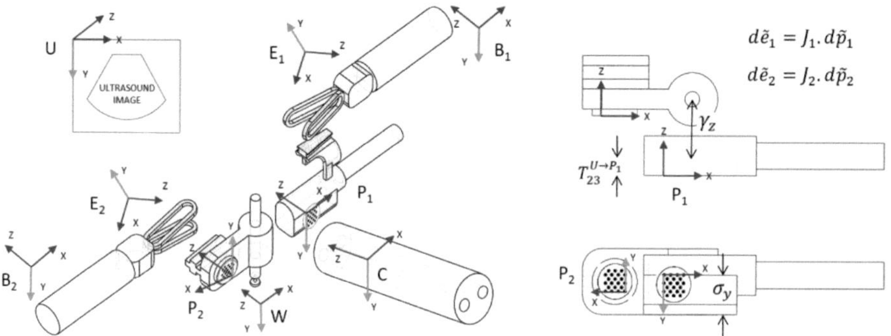

Fig. 3. Exploded view of system components and associated coordinate frames

factor s (calibrated); b) the waterjet tip to PSM2 pattern transformation $T^{W \to P_2}$ (known from the mount CAD model); c) the theoretical (i.e. intended) dissection margin μ_x; d) the Y displacement σ_y from the PSM1 pattern origin to the bottom surface of the ultrasound transducer casing; and e) the Z displacement γ_z in the probe pattern frame from the transducer to the waterjet tip.

2.5 Visual Servoing with Multimodal Inputs

Each dissection run comprises four stages: initialisation, instrument alignment, dissection path generation and waterjet engagement. During initialisation, the transducer is teleoperated (translation only) into a position crossing the tumour boundary, making contact with the phantom surface. The current state of the PSM end effectors $T^{E_1 \to B_1}$ and $T^{E_2 \to B_2}$ is queried from the DVRK. Furthermore, the target ultrasound abscissa α^{target} is stored. In subsequent movements of the probe, the visual servoing loop seeks to keep the abscissa constant. Figure 4 (left) illustrates how the region of interest is chosen (bounded by green lines), and the subsequent median filtered [10] and thresholded images. The location of the abscissa is estimated in the latter by taking the mean of the pixel X coordinates where, for each scan line left to right, the image first crosses into a non-zero intensity (yellow line).

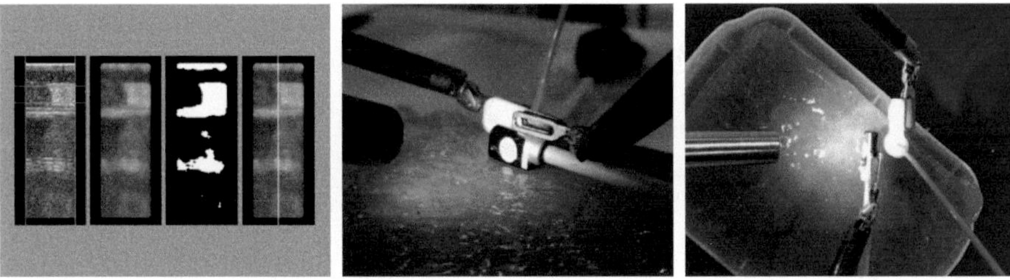

Fig. 4. Ultrasound image processing (left); side/aerial views of dissection (middle/right)

The next stage begins with teleoperation of PSM2 into an approximately correct initial position behind the transducer. Equation 1 gives the adjustment to PSM2 in the camera frame C required to bring the waterjet into alignment with the tumour boundary, taking into account the specified margin. It amounts to the difference between the desired and current positions of the waterjet tip. This vector is passed to the servoing FSM in order to move PSM2 into the required initial position.

$$T^{P_1 \to C}.\left[s.\alpha^{target} + T_{03}^{U \to P_1} - \mu_x,\ \sigma_y,\ T_{23}^{U \to P_1} + \gamma_z\right]^{\mathsf{T}} - T^{P_2 \to C}.T^{W \to P_2}.[0,0,0]^{\mathsf{T}} \quad (1)$$

2.6 Dissection Path Generation

Equation 2 describes the PSM1 adjustments in the camera frame C required to advance the probe continuously by a distance Δz in the pattern frame P_1 while accounting for movement in the ultrasound abscissa relative to the target value ($\Delta z = -1\text{mm}$ in all experiments). With reference to figure 5, PSM1 reactively follows the boundary path

$[x_i, y_i, z_i]^\top$ in the static camera coordinate frame C, but the intention is that PSM2 proactively follows the measured position of the boundary $[u_i, v_i, w_i]^\top$, while also accounting for the theoretical margin. To achieve this, the latter waterjet tip pathway is stored in the static camera frame C, leading to the sequence of PSM2 adjustments embodied in equation 3. When the tip Z position lies outside of the stored pathway, the first entry is adopted. The signal to engage the waterjet is given only when the tip reaches the start of the pathway. The spatial displacement γ_z between transducer and jet leads to a small, but inevitable delay before engagement.

$$T_i^{P_1 \to C}.[s.(\alpha_i - \alpha^{target}),\ 0,\ \Delta z]^\top - T_i^{P_1 \to C}.[0,0,0]^\top \tag{2}$$

$$[u_i, v_i, w_i]^\top - T_i^{P_2 \to C}.T^{W \to P_2}.[0,0,0]^\top \tag{3}$$

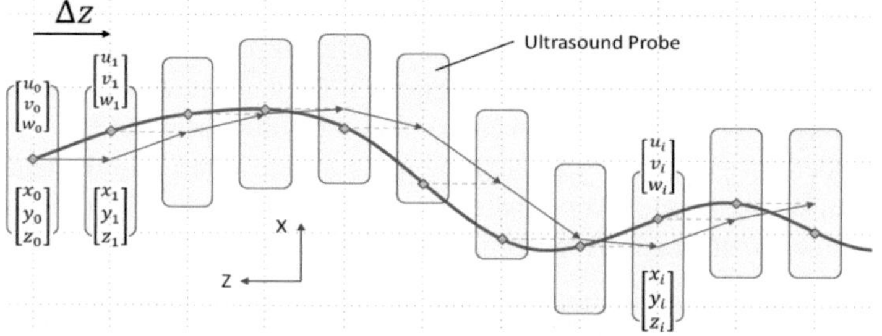

Fig. 5. Plan view: tumour boundary (blue) and its relationship to the PSM1 trajectory (red)

3 Results

3.1 Jacobian Estimation

In order to test the repeatability of the proposed multi-step 3-DOF Jacobian estimation procedure, eight runs for PSM1 were performed. For one such run, figure 6 illustrates the characteristics of the Y component of the pose changes made in response to the X/Y/Z sequence of orthogonal 1.0mm end effector increments. Median values appear as dashed lines. It is clear from this and from the observation of other runs that certain incremental motions result in significant outliers which, if ignored, render any Jacobian estimate unreliable, to the detriment of the visual servoing loop. This phenomenon explains the very poor behaviour of naïve two-sided approximations. The current DVRK control implementation does not compensate for the effects of gravity, and this is most evident in the Y pose change component (the endoscope having an upright orientation). In contrast, following analysis of the repeated multi-step runs, the largest standard deviation of each of the resulting Jacobian matrix entries is 0.01mm. The maximum range of any entry is 0.04mm, and pairwise comparison with the first run leads to a maximum Frobenius norm of 0.058. The procedure is therefore seen to be highly repeatable and capable of overcoming hardware inaccuracies.

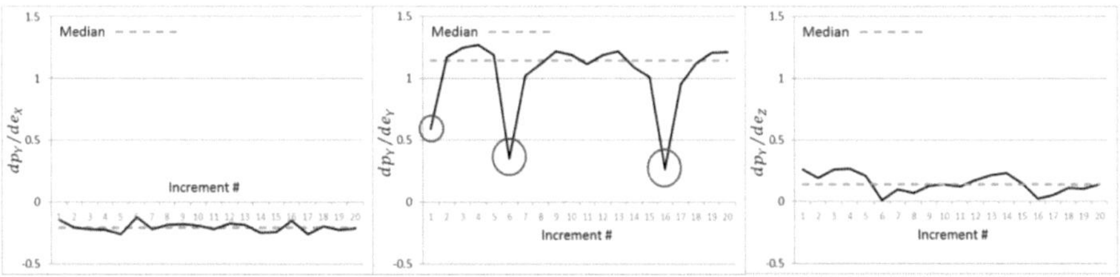

Fig. 6. The Y component of pose changes showing median values (outliers highlighted in red)

3.2 Tissue Dissection

Eight dissection experiments were performed using two theoretical margin settings and a pair of cryogel tissue phantoms. Figure 7 (left) illustrates the delayed relative motion of the ultrasound probe and waterjet during a typical run. A sequence of four video snapshots is shown, stacked top-to-bottom, and with reference to figure 5, it can be seen that the X components of the trajectories in the camera frame follow related, but temporally displaced paths. Example dissections are circled in figure 7 (middle). The fissure lengths range from 6.3mm to 14.7mm, with a mean length of 8.3mm. At present, limitations of the DVRK ECM power supply do not permit automatic control of the camera position, and thus the maximum dissection length is bounded above. Figure 7 (right) illustrates post-dissection margin measurement. A series of circle centres is identified on the fissure edge proximal to the resection target. Subsequently, the circle radii are adjusted so that they just touch the material interface. The reference measure with 1mm gradations appears on the right.

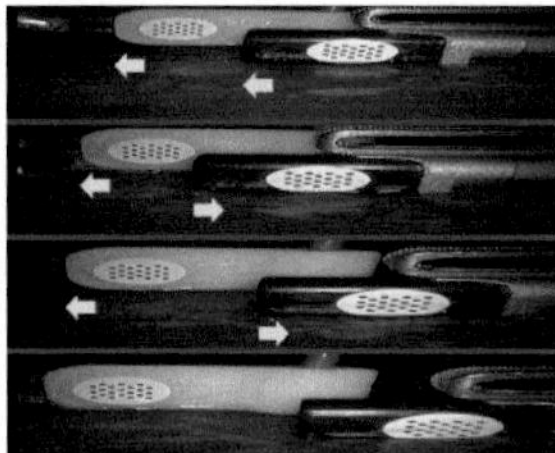
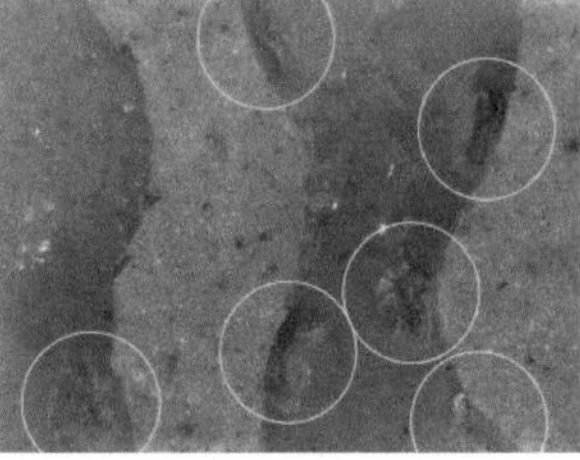
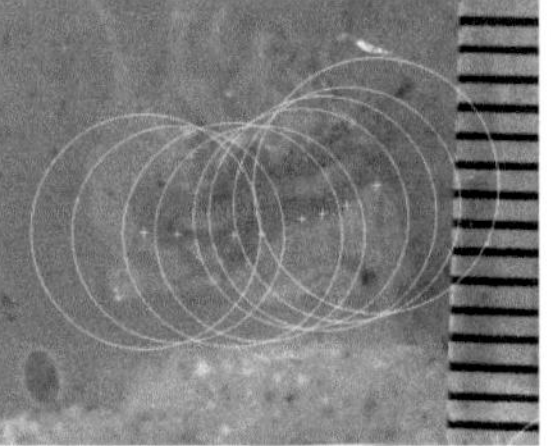

Fig. 7. Delayed relative motion of ultrasound probe and waterjet (left); phantom reverse showing dissection paths (middle); margin measurement (right)

Figure 8 show the specified theoretical margins (initial two runs at 3mm, the remainder at 3.75mm), and the measured margins with standard deviations. It also shows the margin ranges for each run, defined as the difference between maximum and minimum margin measurements. All such ranges are sub-millimetre, meaning that the deviation in the amount of ‘healthy tissue’ left behind is very small. Over all experiments, the mean difference between theoretical and measured margins is 0.77mm. Putting this into context, the widths of the fissures left by the waterjet were found to range up to 1.35mm (i.e. the maximum hole radius was approximately 0.67mm). This is due to the finite extent of the jet itself, and vibration induced by the high-velocity flow. It can be seen from the measured margin and ranges, and indeed visual inspection, that no ‘positive’ margins were present following any of the experiments.

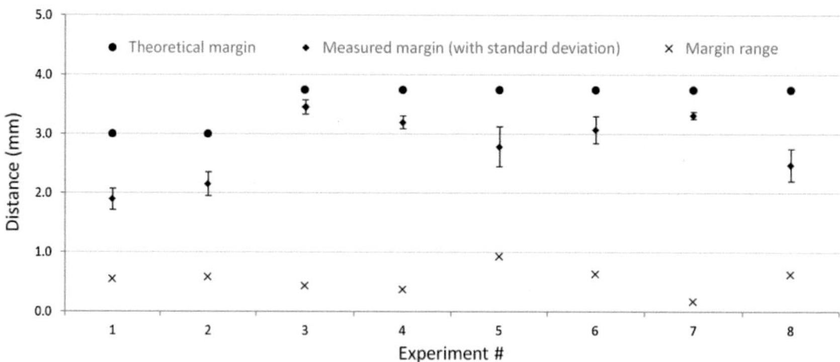

Fig. 8. Comparison of theoretical and measured margins (including ranges)

These results indicate that the cutting is sufficiently consistent and accurate, but also highlight the fact that the extent of the waterjet fissure must be calibrated for each tissue/material type, in accordance with the waterjet pressure setting, if the specified margin distance is to be met in practice.

4 Conclusion

This preliminary study sets an important precedent for the future of autonomous robotic surgical systems. Only through vision-based control can such systems ever hope to match the performance of human operators in the dynamic and variegated context of demanding surgical tasks. The machine approach has one crucial advantage over human counterparts, in that control systems can be designed to process multiple visual sources, with complementary modalities, in a contemporaneous and proportionate manner. The foundation herein evidently leads to a cumulative programme of generalisation, starting in the 2D realm but adopting dissection targets with circular topologies. Ultimately, this will lead to spherical topologies in 3D with patient-specific organ surface shapes, where real time dense stereo surface reconstruction and freehand 3D volume reconstruction will come into play. Robust methods for active 6-DOF Jacobian estimation and will be required, in addition to effector tracking algorithms reliable in the presence of occlusions. Finally, the waterjet delivery mechanism must adopt curvilinear profiles, capable of enucleation while avoiding iatrogenic injury, thereby simultaneously optimising the outcomes of cancer surgery.

References

1. Hughes-Hallett, A., Pratt, P., Mayer, E., Di Marco, A., Yang, G.-Z., Vale, J., Darzi, A.: Intraoperative ultrasound overlay in robot-assisted partial nephrectomy: first clinical experience. European Urology 65(3), 671–672 (2014)
2. Moustris, G., Hiridis, S., Deliparaschos, K., Konstantinidis, K.: Evolution of autonomous and semi-autonomous robotic surgical systems: a review of the literature. International Journal of Medical Robotics and Computer Assisted Surgery 7(4), 375–392 (2011)

3. Harris, S., Arambula-Cosio, F., Mei, Q., Hibberd, R.D., Davies, B., Wickham, J., Nathan, M., Kundu, B.: The Probot – an active robot for prostate resection. Proceedings of the Institution of Mechanical Engineers 211(H), 317–325 (1997)
4. Kazanzides, P., Chen, Z., Deguet, A., Fischer, G., Taylor, R., DiMaio, S.: An open-source research kit for the da Vinci surgical system. In: Proceedings of the IEEE International Conference on Robotics and Automation, pp. 6434–6439 (2014)
5. Mohareri, O., Salcudean, S.: da Vinci® auxiliary arm as a robotic surgical assistant for semi-autonomous ultrasound guidance during robot-assisted laparoscopic surgery. In: Proceedings of the 7th Hamlyn Symposium on Medical Robotics, pp. 45–46 (2014)
6. Basting, R., Djakovic, N., Widmann, P.: Use of water jet resection in organ-sparing kidney surgery. Journal of Endourology 14(6), 501–505 (2000)
7. Davis, D.: Robotic abrasive water jet cutting of aerostructure components. Automated Waterjet Cutting Processes, Society of Manufacturing Engineers, Detroit Michigan (1988)
8. Surry, K., Austin, J., Fenster, A., Peters, T.: Poly(vinyl alchohol) cryogel phantoms for use in ultrasound and MR imaging. Physics in Medicine and Biology 49(24), 5529–5546 (2004)
9. Pratt, P., Jaeger, A., Hughes-Hallett, A., Mayer, E., Vale, J., Darzi, A., Peters, T., Yang, G.-Z.: Robust ultrasound probe tracking: initial clinical experiences during robot-assisted partial nephrectomy. Information Processing and Computer-Assisted Interventions (2015)
10. Bradski, G., Kaehler, A.: Learning OpenCV: Computer vision with the OpenCV library. O'Reilly Media, Inc. (2008)

A Compact Retinal-Surgery Telemanipulator that Uses Disposable Instruments

Manikantan Nambi[1], Paul S. Bernstein[2], and Jake J. Abbott[1]

[1] Department of Mechanical Engineering
[2] Department of Ophthalmology and Visual Science, Moran Eye Center
University of Utah
Salt Lake City, UT, 84112, USA
{m.nambi,jake.abbott}@utah.edu, paul.bernstein@hsc.utah.edu

Abstract. We present a retinal-surgery telemanipulation system with submicron precision that is compact enough to be head-mounted and that uses a full range of existing disposable instruments. Two actuation mechanisms are described that enable the use of actuated instruments, and an instrument adapter enables quick-change of instruments. Experiments on a phantom eye show that telemanipulated surgery results in reduction of maximum downward force on the retina as compared to manual surgery for experienced users.

1 Introduction

Retinal microsurgery procedures are at the limits of human ability [1]. An error of only a few micrometers can cause the instrument to exert damaging force on the retina, causing loss of vision at the spot. The forces experienced during retinal surgeries are below what surgeons can feel, so surgeons must rely on visual feedback only [2]. The surgeon must pivot the instruments about the scleral trocars, limiting dexterity, and must use the instruments to manipulate the eye to provide better imaging through the surgical microscope. Patient movement due to breathing must be accounted for by the surgeon, and in addition, among patients who snore under monitored anesthesia (≈16% of cases [3]), half have sudden head movements during surgery, leading to a high risk of complications.

One of the most difficult retinal-surgery procedures involves the peeling of membranes on the retina. Epiretinal membranes (ERM), sheets of fibrous tissue up to 61-μm-thick [4] that distort macular anatomy and disturb vision after posterior vitreous detachment or retinal tears, and the inner limiting membrane, a naturally occurring 0.15–4-μm-thick membrane [5] that can contract with age and generate macular holes, are peeled to improve vision in affected eyes. Membrane peeling is a delicate procedure, and complications occur in the form of intraoperative hemorrhage, retinal detachment during or after surgery, regrowth of ERM, and increased rate of cataract development [6]. In some cases, a second surgery is required to remove fragments of the ERM left behind. There are opportunities for significant improvement in this and other retinal-surgery procedures in terms of safety and consistency of outcomes. Robot-assisted retinal

N. Navab et al. (Eds.): MICCAI 2015, Part I, LNCS 9349, pp. 258–265, 2015.
DOI: 10.1007/978-3-319-24553-9_32

surgery will enable surgeons to overcome their human limitations, and to extend their working life even after their manual abilities have diminished.

Prior research in robot-assisted retinal surgery has resulted in development of telemanipulated systems [7–11], co-operative manipulators [12], and active hand-held instruments [13]. The robotic systems have typically been relatively large and stiff, and thus table-mounted. The hand-held device is a clear exception, but it is primarily aimed at tremor reduction, with no ability to affect the "DC" system response. Most prior systems leave the retina at risk in the event of sudden head movement, and rhythmic head movements would need to be actively compensated. Notable exceptions are the TU Munich [10] and Columbia/Vanderbilt systems [8], which are designed to be head-mountable.

The specifications of retinal surgery are difficult to achieve using traditional mechatronic components (e.g., motors, gears), while maintaining a small form factor. In this paper, we present a manipulator for retinal surgery that utilizes piezoelectric stick-slip actuators, which were designed specifically for micromanipulation (this same style of actuator was used in [10]). The result is a manipulator with submicron resolution that is small and light enough to be head-mounted. A principal contribution of this work is an instrument adapter that enables the use of the full range of existing disposable actuated (microforceps, scissors) and non-actuated (diamond-dusted scraper (DDS), vitrector, fibre-optic light) instruments, and enables quick change of instruments, which is an important requirement in retinal surgery that has never been demonstrated in any of the prior telemanipulated systems. We also describe a custom master input device that mimics a disposable microforceps. Finally, we include some preliminary experimental demonstrations of membrane peeling in a force-sensitive phantom eye. Our complete system is shown in Fig. 1.

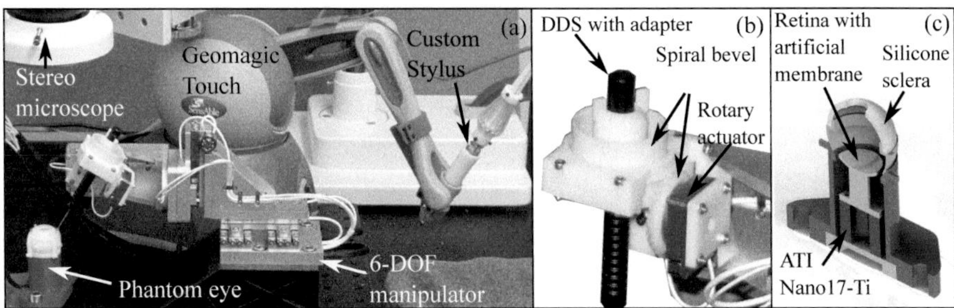

Fig. 1. Experimental setup of the retinal-surgery system. The surgeon looks in the phantom eye using a stereo microscope, and telemanipulates the end-effector of the instrument with 4-DOF (3-DOF translation, and rotation of the instrument about its axis) using a Geomagic Touch (located to enable direct access to instruments) with a custom stylus that is constrained to have the same 4-DOF by locking the wrist. (b) Yaw joint of the manipulator, which is responsible for rotation of the instrument about its axis, with an adapter that enables instruments to be attached to the manipulator. (c) Phantom eye used in experiments.

2 System Design

A six-degree-of-freedom (6-DOF) manipulator was designed using off-the-shelf piezoelectric stick-slip actuators from SmarAct GmbH (Fig. 1). It comprises a 3-DOF translation stage and a 3-DOF spherical wrist, which enables the manipulator to position the instrument inside a 20-mm-diameter circle on the retina (positioning precision measured using joint sensors: $<1\,\mu$m, max. velocity: 6 mm/s) with a virtual remote center on the surface of the eye (a sphere of 25.4-mm diameter). The linear stages have a range of 40 mm with a closed-loop resolution of 100 nm. The spherical wrist comprises three rotary actuators, with a closed-loop resolution of $25\,\mu^\circ$ for the roll and pitch actuators, and with a yaw actuator that enables open-loop rotation about the axis of the instrument with a resolution of $3\,\mathrm{m}^\circ$. The manipulator measures $200\times100\times70\,\mathrm{mm}^3$ and weighs 0.8 kg.

The manipulator was manufactured by SmarAct to our specifications, and we further modified the yaw joint of the manipulator such that it can use actuated and non-actuated instruments. The modified yaw joint was manufactured using a 3D printer (Objet Eden260). The yaw joint is designed with the yaw actuator's axis orthogonal to the instrument's axis, and the rotary motion to the instrument is transmitted using spiral bevel gears. The spiral bevel gear includes a 23-mm aperture and internal threads that enable instruments to be attached to the manipulator. The aperture size was selected such that disposable instruments of a wide range of form factors can be used with the manipulator.

From our observations in the operating room, we found that during retinal surgery, on average the surgeon changes the instrument every two minutes. It is important that a robotic system for such procedures facilitates the quick change of instruments without disturbing the flow of the procedure, so we designed an adapter that enables the surgeon to change instruments frequently, and enables the use of disposable instruments that require "pinch-grip" actuation such as microforceps and scissors, with this seventh DOF of actuation connected to the instrument rather than to the manipulator. Our mechanism utilizes adapters that are attached to disposable instruments before surgery; the adapter uses threads inspired by Luer fittings, such that the instrument can be inserted in the perfect position every time. Once the adapters are correctly affixed to the instruments (see Fig. 2a–e), the end-effector of any instrument will be at the same known location when inserted into the manipulator.

To characterize the instrument change time for our manipulator, we performed a simple experiment in which we changed the instrument from a DDS to a microforceps and then back to a DDS (5 trials), at a comfortable speed. The average time required to change an instrument was found to be 12 s.

Two different actuation mechanisms were designed to enable the use of two different families of actuated instruments that are commonly used in retinal surgery. For actuating a disposable instrument tip (e.g., Synergetics micro-forceps tip (Fig. 2a)), which requires pressing a plunger on the device, we used a linear stepper motor (LC15, HaydonKerk) with force capability of 5 N (2N is required to actuate a Synergetics microforceps). The stepper motor is attached to the microforceps tip using an adapter that enables the microforceps to be mounted

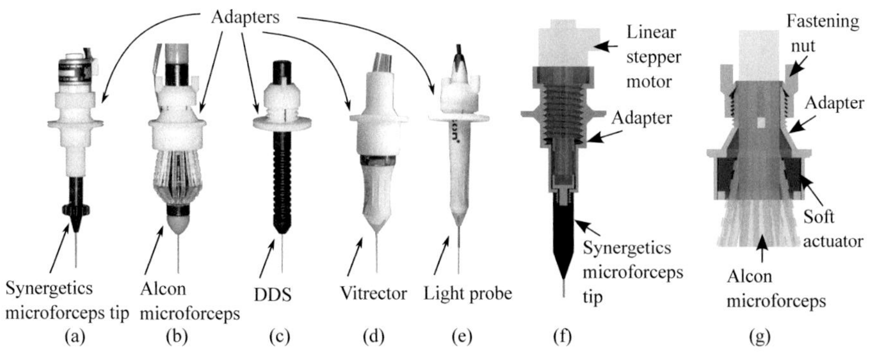

Fig. 2. (a)–(e) Disposable retinal-surgery instruments with adapters than enable quick-change mounting to the 6-DOF manipulator. (f) Section view of the Synergetics microforceps in (a) actuated by a linear stepper motor. (g) Section view of the Alcon microforceps in (b) actuated by a soft actuator.

on the manipulator (Fig. 2f). The LC15 has a linear resolution of 2.5 μm, and requires 500 steps (travel of 1.25 mm) for the complete actuation of the microforceps. The measured bandwidth for a full open-close cycle of the microforceps with the stepper motor is 2.5 Hz.

The second actuation mechanism, for use with completely disposable instruments (e.g., Alcon microforceps (Fig. 2b, 2g)), comprises a soft actuator that is inspired by a blood-pressure cuff, which squeezes the ribs on a pinch-grip device when supplied with pressurized air (already available in the operating room). The soft actuator is molded from a silicone resin (Dragon Skin 20, Smooth-on Inc.) using soft-lithography techniques. A closed-loop control system comprising two ON/OFF valves (MHJ series, Festo) and a pressure sensor is implemented, and optimized for a bandwidth of 2 Hz and a resolution of 10 discrete steps between fully closed and fully open microforceps.

A Geomagic Touch haptic interface is modified with a custom stylus to telemanipulate the retinal manipulator (Fig. 1a). The stylus is built to mimic an Alcon disposable microforceps, using components salvaged from its pinch-grip device. A linear potentiometer (ThinPot, Spectra Symbol) is used to measure the squeezing of the pinch-grip mechanism (resolution: 0.04 mm, travel: 1.25 mm), and a spring (6 N/mm) recreates the stiffness of an actual microforceps.

A master-slave position controller (software-adjustable scaling, with a deadband of 200 μm on the master) with a virtual spring-damper coupling between the master and slave positions is implemented. The gains were chosen to generate smooth and stable behavior. The remote-center-of-motion movement about the trocar is handled in software, such that the user only controls 4-DOF of instrument movement. Orbital manipulation is not implemented here, but nothing precludes it. In a telemanipulation experiment in which we attempted to generate the smallest possible instrument movement (5 trials in each of six cardinal directions), we measured, using joint sensors, a worst-case resolution of 38 μm with 8:1 scaling, and 6 μm with 100:1 scaling.

3 Membrane-Peeling Experiments and Results

To compare manual vs. telemanipulated retinal surgery (using 8:1 scaling exclusively), we performed experiments with a phantom eye shown in Fig. 1c. Trocars were inserted into the model eye as would be done in surgery. The anterior (upper portion) of the eye is made of a synthetic rubber (Phake-I, 8 mm-diameter pupil), and approximates the size, shape, and feel of the human eye. The anterior of the eye was attached to a fixture as shown in Fig. 1c, and inside the fixture, an ATI Nano17-Ti force/torque sensor (noise $< 2\,\mathrm{mN}$) was mounted with a section of a spherical surface that acts as the posterior (retinal) surface of the eye on which surgery will be performed. This mechanical isolation between the anterior and posterior of the eye ensures that only the relatively small instrument-retina interaction forces are measured by the force sensor. The retinal surface was prepared with an artificial membrane made of paper (cut to 6-mm-diameter circle, $120\,\mu$m thickness), and $10\,\mu$l of an eye lubricant gel (GenTeal) was used to achieve adhesion between the membrane and the model retina.

Three vitreoretinal surgeons with varying degrees of surgical experience—20 years (expert), 2 years (intermediate), 6 months (novice)—and a graduate student with no experience in actual surgery, performed manual and telemanipulated surgery on the phantom eye setup with an Alcon microforceps. The graduate student and expert surgeon are both authors of this paper. All the surgeons had two hours of practice on the telemanipulated system before data was recorded. The graduate student had been using the telemanipulation system for a year. Two experiments were performed by each subject. In experiment 1, subjects performed manual surgery, and in experiment 2 the surgery was performed with the telemanipulated system. The subjects had to completely peel a membrane off the retina with the microforceps. Six trials were performed in each experiment, spread across two days. Two subjects (expert and novice) performed experiment 1 followed by experiment 2 on the first day, with the order reversed on the second day, and the other subjects (intermediate and graduate student) performed the experiments in a reverse order. A fresh membrane was prepared for each trial. Although we do not purport that this pilot study is a rigorous experiment on which we can make strong claims, we do believe that the results are informative about the potential of the telemanipulated system.

To evaluate performance in our experiments, we use the maximum downward force (F_{-z}) and the completion time (T_c) in a trial as metrics; Fig. 3 shows data for all subjects and trials. The stiffness of the retina used in our experiments is higher than that of an actual retina, and hence, the forces measured can only be used for comparisons within this study. The first result we observe in the data is that the expert surgeon improves significantly from Day 1 to Day 2 with the telemanipulated system ($F(1,4) = 7.5, p = 0.05$), bringing his force level down to approximately that of his manual surgery.

Next, we observe that all four subjects perform approximately equivalently during manual surgery in terms of force, and that the expert and intermediate surgeons (which we will refer to as the *skilled* surgeons) perform substantially better than the other two subjects during manual surgery in terms of time. We also observe there are no noticeable trends (e.g., learning) from Day 1 to 2 for manual surgery, as we would expect. As a result, for all subsequent analysis we lump the two days of manual data together for a given subject to increase the power of the statistics. In addition, we lump the two days of manual data for the expert and intermediate surgeons into a single *skilled* manual data set.

Next, we observe that for the graduate student, who is an expert user with the telemanipulation system, forces are lower in telemanipulated surgery (with Days 1 and 2 lumped together) than in manual surgery ($F(1,10) = 10.9$, $p = 0.008$); however, his completion time may be slightly slower. We also find that his telemanipulated forces are lower than those of the skilled surgeons' manual forces ($F(1,16) = 11.9$, $p = 0.003$); however, his completion time is longer ($F(1,16) = 40.2$; $p < 0.001$).

Similarly, but maybe more promising, for the novice surgeon with limited surgical experience, forces are lower in telemanipulated surgery on Day 2 than in manual surgery ($F(1,7) = 3.9$, $p = 0.094$); in addition, his completion time on Day 2 may be slightly shorter than in manual surgery. We also find that the novice surgeon's telemanipulated forces on Day 2 are lower than those of the skilled surgeons' manual forces ($F(1,13) = 11.6$, $p = 0.005$); however, his completion time is longer ($F(1,13) = 38.5$, $p < 0.001$).

Finally, we observed that the high positioning resolution in telemanipulated surgery sometimes resulted in the membrane being peeled off in layers, and multiple grasping actions were required to peel the membrane, which contributed to a higher T_c. It may be necessary to train users of the telemanipulator to penetrate *deep enough* into the retina to grasp the entire membrane.

4 Discussion

In terms the achievable precision and velocity at the instrument's end-effector, our manipulator compares well with other retinal-surgery manipulators (Table 1).

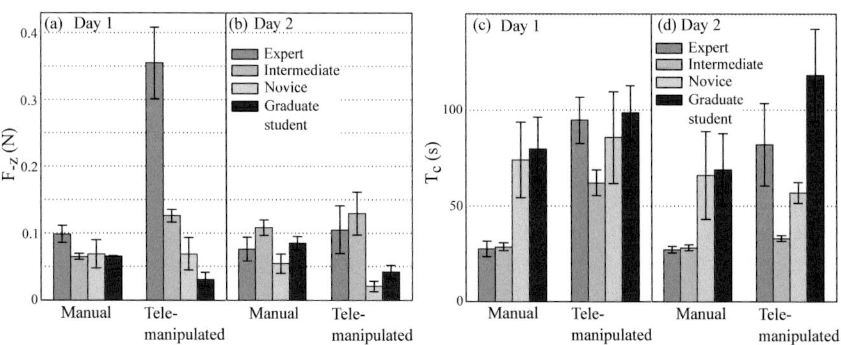

Fig. 3. Experimental results comparing manual and telemanipulated membrane peeling with a microforceps. (a)–(b) shows maximum downward force (F_{-z}), and (c)–(d) shows completion time (T_c). Data is divided according to subject, day, and mode of experiment. Error bars indicate standard deviation.

Table 1. Comparison of robot-assisted retinal-surgery systems.

System	Precision	Velocity	Head-mountable	Quick-change/existing actuated instruments
Northwestern [7]	0.2 μm	NA	No	No/No
Johns Hopkins [12]	< 1 μm	5 mm/s	No	Yes/No
Univ. of Tokyo [9]	5 μm	NA	No	No/Yes
TU Eindhovan [11]	10 μm	NA	No	Yes/No
Columbia/Vanderbilt [8]	< 5 μm	NA	Yes	No/Yes
TU Munich [10]	5 μm	40 mm/s	Yes	NA/NA
Our System	**< 1 μm**	**6 mm/s**	**Yes**	**Yes/Yes**

During actual membrane peeling, instrument velocities have been measured in the range of 0.1–0.5 mm/s [14], which our manipulator is easily capable of achieving. However, during repositioning tasks, velocities higher than our maximum of 6 mm/s would be desirable, if the goal is to recreate instrument movements similar to manual surgery. Different kinematics could be used to modify the resolution-velocity trade-off. Regardless, the quick-change adapter, disposable-instrument actuators, and custom stylus presented here could be utilized with any manipulator kinematics, including existing manipulators (Table 1). Our system could also incorporate force-sensing instruments [14] for improved safety.

Due to the underactuation of our inexpensive haptic interface (6-DOF with only 3-DOF actuation), we constrained our haptic interface to have the same 4-DOF as the instrument by locking the wrist angle of the haptic stylus. Also, because of the fixed trocar point in telemanipulated surgery, orbital movement of the eye was not possible. As a result, the hand motions required in telemanipulated surgery with our haptic interface was fundamentally different than in manual surgery. The two subjects who perform better than manual surgery with the telemanipulated system also have the least experience in real surgery. Moving to a haptic master that more closely matches hand motions observed in real surgery may be important for improving performance with the system, and for enabling intuitive orbital manipulation.

In our experiments, subjects manually manipulated a light-probe in the phantom eye with their left hand while telemanipulating the instrument with their right hand. This leads to bending of delicate instruments when both instruments do not work in concert, resulting in unintended motion at the end-effector. To truly demonstrate the precision capabilities of the telemanipulated system, all manual interaction should be removed by telemanipulating both instruments. Additionally, we expect that a phantom that mimics human head/eye movement during surgery would highlight the benefits of a head-mounted manipulator.

Acknowledgements. This project was funded by two Intuitive Surgical Technology Research Grants.

References

1. Riviere, C.N., Rader, R.S., Khosla, P.K.: Characteristics of hand motion of eye surgeons. In: Int. Conf. IEEE. Engineering in Medicine and Biology Society, pp. 1690–1693 (1997)
2. Gupta, P.K., Jensen, P.S., de Juan Jr., E.: Surgical forces and tactile perception during retinal microsurgery. In: Taylor, C., Colchester, A. (eds.) MICCAI 1999. LNCS, vol. 1679, pp. 1218–1225. Springer, Heidelberg (1999)
3. McCannel, C.A., Olson, E.J., Donaldson, M.J., Bakri, S.J., Pulido, J.S., Mueller, D.: Snoring is associated with unexpected patient head movement during monitored anesthesia care vitreoretinal surgery. Retina 32(7), 1324–1327 (2012)
4. Wilkins, J.R., Puliafito, C.A., Hee, M.R., Duker, J.S., Reichel, E., Coker, J.G., Schuman, J.S., Swanson, E.A., Fujimoto, J.G.: Characterization of epiretinal membranes using optical coherence tomography. Ophthalmology 103(12), 2142–2151 (1996)
5. Henrich, P.B., Monnier, C.A., Loparic, M., Cattin, P.C.: Material properties of the internal limiting membrane and their significance in chromovitrectomy. Ophthalmologica 230(2), 11–20 (2013)
6. Donati, G., Kapetanios, A.D., Pournaras, C.J.: Complications of surgery for epiretinal membranes. Graefe's Archive for Clinical and Experimental Ophthalmology 236(10), 739–746 (1998)
7. Jensen, P.S., Grace, K.W., Attariwala, R., Colgate, J.E., Glucksberg, M.R.: Toward robot-assisted vascular microsurgery in the retina. Graefe's Archive for Clinical and Experimental Ophthalmology 235(11), 696–701 (1997)
8. Wei, W., Popplewell, C., Chang, S., Fine, H.F., Simaan, N.: Enabling technology for microvascular stenting in ophthalmic surgery. J. Medical Devices 4(1), 14503 (2010)
9. Ida, Y., Sugita, N., Ueta, T., Tamaki, Y., Tanimoto, K., Mitsuishi, M.: Microsurgical robotic system for vitreoretinal surgery. Int. J. Computer Assisted Radiology and Surgery 7(1), 27–34 (2012)
10. Nasseri, M., Eder, M., Nair, S., Dean, E., Maier, M., Zapp, D., Lohmann, C., Knoll, A.: The introduction of a new robot for assistance in ophthalmic surgery. In: Int. Conf. IEEE Engineering in Medicine and Biology Society, pp. 5682–5685 (2013)
11. Meenink, H., Hendrix, R., Naus, G., Beelen, M., Nijmeijer, H., Steinbuch, M., Oosterhout, E., Smet, M.: Robot-assisted vitreoretinal surgery. In: Medical Robotics: Minimally Invasive Surgery, pp. 185–209 (2012)
12. Uneri, A., Balicki, M.A., Handa, J., Gehlbach, P., Taylor, R.H., Iordachita, I.: New steady-hand eye robot with micro-force sensing for vitreoretinal surgery. In: IEEE Int. Conf. Biomedical Robotics and Biomechatronics, pp. 814–819 (2010)
13. MacLachlan, R.A., Becker, B.C., Cuevas Tabarés, J., Podnar, G.W., Lobes, L.A., Riviere, C.N.: Micron: an actively stabilized handheld tool for microsurgery. IEEE Trans. Robotics 28(1), 195–212 (2012)
14. Balicki, M., Uneri, A., Iordachita, I., Handa, J., Gehlbach, P., Taylor, R.: Micro-force sensing in robot assisted membrane peeling for vitreoretinal surgery. In: Jiang, T., Navab, N., Pluim, J.P.W., Viergever, M.A. (eds.) MICCAI 2010, Part III. LNCS, vol. 6363, pp. 303–310. Springer, Heidelberg (2010)

Surgical Tool Tracking and Pose Estimation in Retinal Microsurgery

Nicola Rieke[1], David Joseph Tan[1], Mohamed Alsheakhali[1], Federico Tombari[1,3], Chiara Amat di San Filippo[2], Vasileios Belagiannis[1], Abouzar Eslami[2], and Nassir Navab[1]

[1] Computer Aided Medical Procedures, Technische Universität München, Germany
[2] Carl Zeiss Meditec AG, München, Germany
[3] DISI, University of Bologna, Italy
Nicola.Rieke@tum.de

Abstract. Retinal Microsurgery (RM) is performed with small surgical tools which are observed through a microscope. Real-time estimation of the tool's pose enables the application of various computer-assisted techniques such as augmented reality, with the potential of improving the clinical outcome. However, most existing methods are prone to fail in *in-vivo* sequences due to partial occlusions, illumination and appearance changes of the tool. To overcome these problems, we propose an algorithm for simultaneous tool tracking and pose estimation that is inspired by state-of-the-art computer vision techniques. Specifically, we introduce a method based on regression forests to track the tool tip and to recover the tool's articulated pose. To demonstrate the performance of our algorithm, we evaluate on a dataset which comprises four real surgery sequences, and compare with the state-of-the-art methods on a publicly available dataset.

1 Introduction

Retinal Microsurgery (RM) is a delicate medical operation which requires extremely high handling precision of the utilized surgical instruments. Usually, the visual control for the surgeon is restricted to a limited 2D field of view through a microscope. Problems such as lens distortions and the lack of depth information or haptic feedback complicate the procedures further. Recent research aimed at assisting the surgeon by introducing smart imaging such as the Optical Coherence Tomography (OCT) [1], which visualizes subretinal structure information. In the current workflow, these devices have to be manually positioned on the region of interest, which is usually close to the tool tip. The ability of extracting the position of the surgical tool tip in real-time allows to carry out this positioning automatically. Other applications that require tool tracking include surgical motion analysis and visual servoing. The estimation of the articulated pose of the tool rather than its position alone allows us to measure the size of the anatomical structures in the video sequence. Additionally, it paves the way for advanced augmented reality applications which provide, for example, proximity

N. Navab et al. (Eds.): MICCAI 2015, Part I, LNCS 9349, pp. 266–273, 2015.
DOI: 10.1007/978-3-319-24553-9_33

information of the tool tips to the retina. Despite recent advances, the vision based tracking of the tool tip's location in *in-vivo* is still challenging, mainly due to lighting variation and variable instrument appearances. Moreover, tracking has to be real-time capable in order to be employed during a surgical procedure. These challenges have been addressed with different approaches, including color-based [2] and geometry-based methods [3–5]. Other relevant works [6–8] focus on a specific tool model (e.g. vitrectomy or closed forceps). The learning-based approach from Sznitman et al. [9] introduces the combination of a tool detector, which relies on deformable feature learning, and a simple gradient tracker. Li et al. [10] present an instrument tracking method based on online learning. Both methods [9, 10] achieve accurate results for *in-vivo* RM sequences and their implementation runs at video frame-rate. However, the tracking is restricted to the center joint of the surgical forceps and does not localize the two tips of the instrument, which are extremely important for the surgeon. In contrast, the learning-based method published by Pezzementi et al. [11] yields the pose of the surgical tool, but relies on a high amount of labeled data in order to capture the appearance changes of the instrument.

This paper introduces an alternative visual tracking approach that goes beyond phantom data. It can handle incomplete and noisy data by building on regression forests to yield the positions of the tool tips as well as the center point of the forceps in *in-vivo* RM sequences in real-time. First, the tracking algorithm finds a bounding box around the tool tip by estimating the relation between the instrument motion and changes induced in the image intensities. Successively, the pose estimation localizes the points of interest within this region by evaluating a learned mapping between image patches and the articulated pose. To the best of our knowledge, modeling the localization of articulated surgical forceps as simultaneous tracking and pose estimation, is a novel approach in real *in-vivo* microscopic surgery. Throughout experimental results, we demonstrate how the proposed method is able to withstand challenging environments characterized by variable illumination and noise, as well as to yield the pose of various forceps types in real-time. A comparison with the state of the art on a public benchmark demonstrates further the performance of our method.

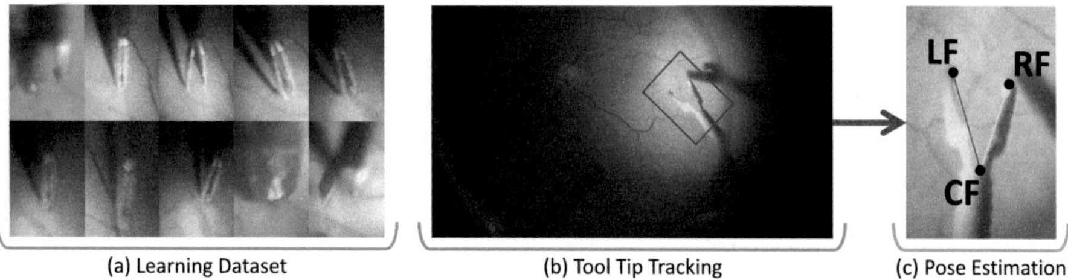

Fig. 1. Left: Learning set with various templates including open and closed forceps. Right: Tracking in the frame and pose estimation within the reduced region.

2 Proposed Method

The overall goal is to localize the three joint points of the forceps for every frame in real-time. As the image quality is poor in general, tracking the three points independently is prone to fail. We propose a method that breaks down the difficulty into two separate tasks. Our pipeline begins with a template tracking algorithm (Sec. 2.2) that estimates a bounding box around the tool tip in the current frame. In the second step, a pose estimation algorithm (Sec. 2.3) localizes the three points of interest within this region. Both algorithms are based on regression forests (Sec. 2.1). In case of tracking, the objective is to regress the location of the bounding box, while during pose estimation the task is to regress the points of interest. The typical input and output data of the entire algorithm is shown in Fig. 1.

2.1 Regression Forest

From a generic input $\mathbf{X}$ and output $\mathbf{Y}$, the regression forest is used to learn the relation of $\mathbf{X}$ and $\mathbf{Y}$ such that, given the input $\mathbf{X}$, the forest can predict the output $\mathbf{Y}$. Every tree of the forest is defined by a set of branches and leaves. At each branch, a binary splitting function θ determines if a training sample of $\mathbf{X}$ goes to the left P_l or right P_r subset of samples. During *training* the splitting functions are selected in a way that maximizes the information gain $g(\theta)$ by optimally splitting the training samples of the node. The information gain is given as:

$$g(\theta) = H(P) - \sum_{i \in \{l,r\}} \frac{|P_i(\theta)|}{|P|} H(P_i(\theta)), \tag{1}$$

where $H(\cdot)$ is the entropy. Splitting aims to divide the learning dataset into smaller subsets through $\mathbf{X}$ while optimizing for $\mathbf{Y}$ by making the parameters of the individual subsets more coherent. Based on the above rule, the tree grows by iteratively applying the same splitting process and stops when the number of samples $|\mathcal{P}|$ is less than a threshold, the best information gain is less than a threshold or the maximum depth is reached. All final nodes are considered as leaves and store the prediction, i.e. a statistical representation of all $\mathbf{Y}$ that reached this node. The same scheme is followed for a number of trees in order to build a forest. During *prediction*, the branches look at the splitting function to navigate a sample of $\mathbf{X}$ towards the left or right child until it reaches a leaf that gives the corresponding prediction. After taking the predictions from different trees, an average prediction is computed as the final output.

2.2 Tracking

Given a sequence of images $\{I_t\}_{t=0}^{n_t} = \{I_0, I_1, \ldots, I_{n_t}\}$, the proposed tracking approach learns from the initial image I_0 — where we assume to be given a rectangular template around the tool tip — and then propagates the learned model of the template in the following frames. In more detail, within such template,

n_s sample points $\{\mathbf{x}_0^s\}_{s=1}^{n_s}$ are randomly selected such that the template can be described using the intensity vector $\mathbf{i}_0 = [I_0(\mathbf{x}_0^s)]_{s=1}^{n_s}$. The objective of frame-to-frame tracking is to find the 2D translation vector $\delta\boldsymbol{\mu}$ that updates the location of the tool based on the intensities in the current frame $\mathbf{i}_t = [I_t(\mathbf{x}_{t-1}^s)]_{s=1}^{n_s}$ using the location of sample points from the previous frame $\{\mathbf{x}_{t-1}^s\}_{s=1}^{n_s}$. The tracker [12] learns the relation of the changes in the intensities $\delta\mathbf{i} = \mathbf{i}_t - \mathbf{i}_0$ and the transformation parameters $\delta\boldsymbol{\mu}$. To model the structure of the forest based on Sec. 2.1, we set the input $\mathbf{X} = \delta\mathbf{i}$, the parameters $\mathbf{Y} = \delta\boldsymbol{\mu}$ and the function $H(\cdot)$ as the standard deviation, while the leaves store the mean and standard deviation of the parameters that arrive on that node. It is noteworthy to mention that since $\mathbf{i}_0$ is constant and the branch only compares an index of the vector $\delta\mathbf{i}$, we can simplify the forests by learning the relation of $\mathbf{i}$ and $\delta\boldsymbol{\mu}$ instead of $\delta\mathbf{i}$ and $\delta\boldsymbol{\mu}$. This enables the tracker to directly look at the intensities $\mathbf{i}$, without explicitly taking into account the intensities of the template $\mathbf{i}_0$. This brings in an important benefit, since it allows the tracker to alleviate from the restriction of tracking a single template, and to use multiple templates within the same forests. Therefore, differently from [12], we propose here to correlate multiple templates to compensate for the motion of the tool tip as it opens and closes, as well as for the strong illumination changes and photometric distortions that are typically present in such working conditions. Nevertheless, the proposed approach is still able to yield an efficiency of less than 2 ms per frame, using only one CPU core. To compensate for a possible loss in tracking, we impose a confidence measure using the average standard deviation of the predicted leaves from different trees of the forest. During learning, a tree recursively splits the dataset into two subsets such that the parameters in each subset have a lower standard deviation. Henceforth, a confident prediction must have an average standard deviation less than a threshold τ_σ. If the prediction is confident, the location of the template is updated using $\delta\boldsymbol{\mu}$; otherwise, its previous location is propagated to the next frame.

2.3 Pose Estimation

Given the bounding box $I_B \subset I_t$ around the tool tip from the tracking, the pose estimation algorithm localizes three joints within this region. By considering the surgical tool as an articulated object, we can transform the problem of localizing the tool parts into a task that was successfully addressed in the area of human pose estimation [13], which can predict the pose in very challenging scenarios with occlusion and noisy data. In order to integrate this method in the tool pose estimation, we define the set of joints as the tip of the left part of the fork (LF), the tip of the right part of the fork (RF) and the connecting center part of the fork (CF) (compare Fig. 1): $\mathbf{Y} = \{LF, RF, CF\} \subset \mathbb{R}^2 \times 3$. As the input space for the tree, we set $\mathbf{X}$ to be the HOG features of randomly selected image patches with associated joint offsets. The binary split function θ divides the samples based on a threshold in one dimension of $\mathbf{X}$. The function $H(\cdot)$ is chosen to be the sum-of-squared-differences. As a result, the offsets of all instrument joints $y \in \mathbf{Y}$ are stored in each leaf of each tree. During the prediction, image patches

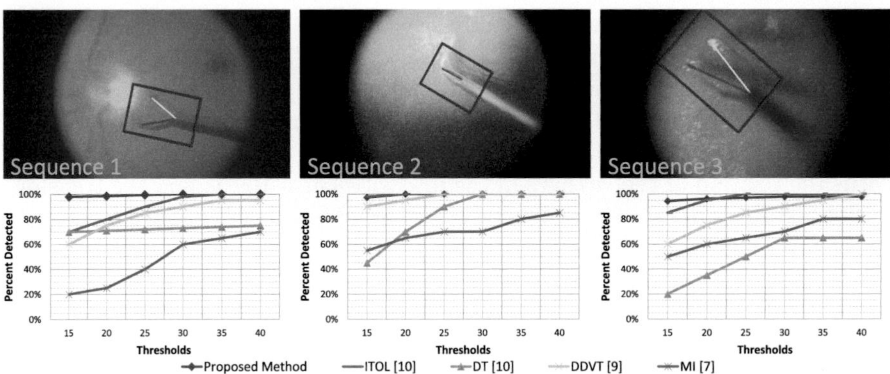

Fig. 2. Results for each sequence of the *public* dataset, when learned and tested on separate sequences, in terms of Threshold Score, as performed in [10]. Top: a qualitative example of detected bounding box and tool pose for each sequence.

are extracted from random pixel positions within the bounding box I_B. In order to combine the votes of the different trees and to find the most probable location of the joint, a greedy dense-window algorithm is applied, as in [13]. The final output of the pose estimation step are the 2D coordinates of each joint in $\mathbf{Y}$.

3 Experiments and Results

The experimental validation of the proposed algorithm is carried out on two different Retina Microsurgery (RM) datasets: the first one, referred to as the *public* dataset [9], is a fully annotated dataset of three different sequences of *in-vivo* vitreoretinal surgery. It comprises 1171 images with a resolution of 640x480 pixels each. The main difficulty of this dataset consists in the presence of noise and shadow as well as variable illumination conditions. The forceps type is the same in all sequences. The second one, referred to as the *appearance* dataset, is a new dataset comprising four real *in-vivo* RM surgeries with 200 manually annotated consecutive images at 1920x1080 pixels of resolution each. This dataset is challenging since it includes different types of forceps, as well as different illumination conditions and microscope zoom factors.

The performance of the algorithm on these datasets was evaluated by means of two different metrics: the strict Percentage of Correct Parts (strict PCP) [14] and the Threshold Score used by Sznitman et al. [9]. The Threshold Score recovers the pixel-wise aspect of the quality for the predicted localizations, i.e. a prediction for the position of a joint is evaluated as correct if the pixel distance to the ground truth is smaller than a threshold. The strict PCP score is a standard metric in human pose estimation and addresses the length of the connected joints of the model. Considering two connected joints, a prediction is evaluated as correct if the distances between the predicted localization and the ground truth for the joints are both smaller than $\alpha \in \mathbb{R}$ times the corresponding ground

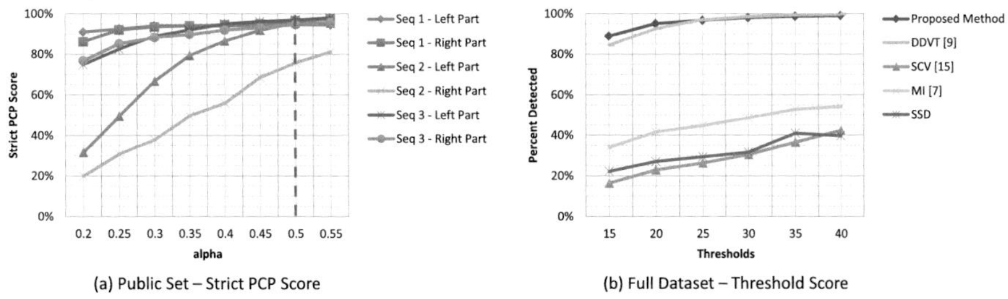

Fig. 3. Left: Strict PCP scores for testing on separate sequences of the *public* dataset. The vertical line indicates the standard α value in human pose estimation [14]. Right: Threshold Score comparison to other methods when tested on full dataset. Results for referenced methods are given by [9].

truth length of the connection (in the field of human pose estimation, usually $\alpha = 0.5$ [14]). Our method is implemented in C++ and runs at 30 fps on an off-the-shelf computer. For the tracker we used 500 sample points and 90 trees for the *public* dataset and 100 trees for the *appearance* dataset. Based on the results in [13], we have set the number of trees for the pose estimation to 15, the HOG features bin size to 9 and the patch size resolution to 50x50 pixels.

3.1 Public Dataset Evaluation

We compare our method with the state-of-the-art methods DDVT [9], MI [7], SCV [15] and ITOL [10]. Analogously to results presented on such works for this dataset [9, 10], we evaluated the pixel-wise measure for the center joint for thresholds between 15 and 40 pixels. First, we evaluated the algorithm for every sequence separately by training the regression trees on the first half of the sequence and testing on the second half. Our method outperforms the baseline methods, reaching over 94% prediction rate in every sequence (Fig. 2). Even the inclusion of all the first halves of the sequences in one training dataset results in higher detection rates of our method than the state-of-the-art methods when tested on the unseen halves (Fig. 3a). In terms of strict PCP score, it can be observed that the length of the forceps parts, thus also the tool tip joints, are predicted correctly even for α values below the standard measure. In contrast to the other methods, our algorithm is able to reliably track the instrument over the entire sequence without the need of reinitialisation.

Table 1. Strict PCP for Appearance Dataset for $\alpha = 0.5$.

	Set 1	Set 2	Set 3	Set 4
Left Part	69.70	93.94	94.47	46.46
Right Part	58.58	93.43	94.47	57.71

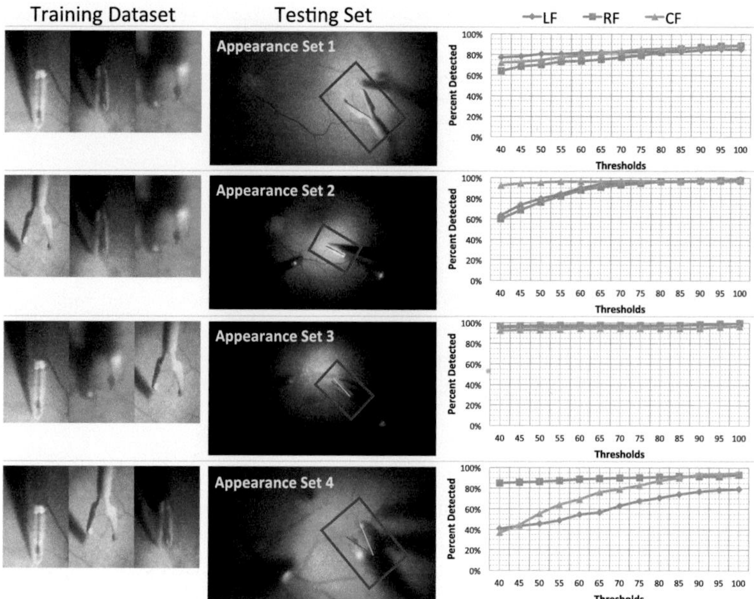

Fig. 4. Results for the cross-validation experiment on the *appearance* dataset. The first column shows examples of the respective training dataset and the second shows one image from the testing set. The threshold score on the right indicates the percentage of correctly predicted locations for the different joints.

3.2 Appearance Dataset Evaluation

Learning-based methods tend to fail on data which comprises image content that is not seen in the training dataset. In this section we show that the proposed method can generalize from different illumination conditions, zoom factors and noise levels. In contrast to the *public* dataset, this dataset includes various forceps types. The experiment was performed in a 4-fold leave-one-out fashion, i.e. training the forests each time on three sequences and testing on the remaining one. Since the average tool shaft diameter is 50 pixel for this dataset, we evaluated the threshold measure for values between 40 and 100 pixels. The results are summarized in Fig. 4. For every sequence, the tracker only had to be reinitialized once. The strict PCP results for $\alpha = 0.5$ are depicted in Table 1 with a mean strict PCP score of 76% for both the left and right part of the forceps.

4 Conclusions

We presented a novel approach that simultaneously predicts location and pose of surgical forceps in *in-vivo* RM sequences at 30 fps. This paper demonstrates the algorithm's capability to estimate the correct locations even in challenging situations as well as to generalize to unseen tools. Moreover, our experimental results indicate that our approach outperforms state-of-the-art methods.

References

[1] Balicki, M., Han, J.-H., Iordachita, I., Gehlbach, P., Handa, J., Taylor, R., Kang, J.: Single fiber optical coherence tomography microsurgical instruments for computer and robot-assisted retinal surgery. In: Yang, G.-Z., Hawkes, D., Rueckert, D., Noble, A., Taylor, C. (eds.) MICCAI 2009, Part I. LNCS, vol. 5761, pp. 108–115. Springer, Heidelberg (2009)

[2] Allan, M., Ourselin, S., Thompson, S., Hawkes, D.J., Kelly, J., Stoyanov, D.: Toward detection and localization of instruments in minimally invasive surgery. IEEE Transactions on Biomedical Engineering 60, 1050–1058 (2013)

[3] Baek, Y.M., Tanaka, S., Kanako, H., Sugita, N., Morita, A., Sora, S., Mochizuki, R., Mitsuishi, M.: Full state visual forceps tracking under a microscope using projective contour models. In: Proc. of IEEE ICRA, pp. 2919–2925 (2012)

[4] Reiter, A., Allen, P.K., Zhao, T.: Feature classification for tracking articulated surgical tools. In: Ayache, N., Delingette, H., Golland, P., Mori, K. (eds.) MICCAI 2012, Part II. LNCS, vol. 7511, pp. 592–600. Springer, Heidelberg (2012)

[5] Wolf, R., Duchateau, J., Cinquin, P., Voros, S.: 3d tracking of laparoscopic instruments using statistical and geometric modeling. In: Fichtinger, G., Martel, A., Peters, T. (eds.) MICCAI 2011, Part I. LNCS, vol. 6891, pp. 203–210. Springer, Heidelberg (2011)

[6] Sznitman, R., Basu, A., Richa, R., Handa, J., Gehlbach, P., Taylor, R.H., Jedynak, B., Hager, G.D.: Unified detection and tracking in retinal microsurgery. In: Fichtinger, G., Martel, A., Peters, T. (eds.) MICCAI 2011, Part I. LNCS, vol. 6891, pp. 1–8. Springer, Heidelberg (2011)

[7] Richa, R., Balicki, M., Meisner, E., Sznitman, R., Taylor, R., Hager, G.: Visual tracking of surgical tools for proximity detection in retinal surgery. In: Taylor, R.H., Yang, G.-Z. (eds.) IPCAI 2011. LNCS, vol. 6689, pp. 55–66. Springer, Heidelberg (2011)

[8] Sznitman, R., Becker, C., Fua, P.: Fast part-based classification for instrument detection in minimally invasive surgery. In: Golland, P., Hata, N., Barillot, C., Hornegger, J., Howe, R. (eds.) MICCAI 2014, Part II. LNCS, vol. 8674, pp. 692–699. Springer, Heidelberg (2014)

[9] Sznitman, R., Ali, K., Richa, R., Taylor, R.H., Hager, G.D., Fua, P.: Data-driven visual tracking in retinal microsurgery. In: Ayache, N., Delingette, H., Golland, P., Mori, K. (eds.) MICCAI 2012, Part II. LNCS, vol. 7511, pp. 568–575. Springer, Heidelberg (2012)

[10] Li, Y., Chen, C., Huang, X., Huang, J.: Instrument tracking via online learning in retinal microsurgery. In: Golland, P., Hata, N., Barillot, C., Hornegger, J., Howe, R. (eds.) MICCAI 2014, Part I. LNCS, vol. 8673, pp. 464–471. Springer, Heidelberg (2014)

[11] Pezzementi, Z., Voros, S., Hager, G.D.: Articulated object tracking by rendering consistent appearance parts. In: ICRA 2009, pp. 3940–3947 (2009)

[12] Tan, D.J., Ilic, S.: Multi-forest tracker: a chameleon in tracking. In: CVPR 2014, pp. 1202–1209 (2014)

[13] Belagiannis, V., Amann, C., Navab, N., Ilic, S.: Holistic human pose estimation with regression forests. In: Perales, F.J., Santos-Victor, J. (eds.) AMDO 2014. LNCS, vol. 8563, pp. 20–30. Springer, Heidelberg (2014)

[14] Ferrari, V., Marin-Jimenez, M., Zisserman, A.: Progressive search space reduction for human pose estimation. In: CVPR, pp. 1–8 (2008)

[15] Pickering, M.R., Muhit, A.A., Scarvell, J.M., Smith, P.N.: A new multi-modal similarity measure for fast gradient-based 2D-3D image registration. In: EMBC 2009, pp. 5821–5824 (2009)

Direct Calibration of a Laser Ablation System in the Projective Voltage Space

Adrian Schneider[1,2], Simon Pezold[1], Kyung-won Baek[1], Dilyan Marinov[2], and Philippe C. Cattin[1,2]

[1] Department of Biomedical Engineering, University of Basel, Switzerland
[2] Advanced Osteotomy Tools AG, Basel, Switzerland

Abstract. Laser ablation is a widely adopted technique in many contemporary medical applications. However, it is new to use a laser to cut bone and perform general osteotomy surgical tasks with it. In this paper, we propose to apply the *direct linear transformation* algorithm to calibrate and integrate a laser deflecting tilting mirror into the affine transformation chain of a sophisticated surgical navigation system, involving next generation robots and optical tracking. Experiments were performed on synthetic input and real data. The evaluation showed a *target registration error* of 0.3 mm ± 0.2 mm in a working distance of 150 mm.

Keywords: Robotics, Navigation, Laser, Mirror, DLT.

1 Introduction

Laser ablation is a tissue cutting technique that is widely adopted in ophthalmology and dentistry. Although such a *contact-free* cutting method would also be beneficial when cutting bones, i.e. in osteotomy, only little research has been invested in this area so far. One major reason for this was the lack of a compact laser source able to efficiently cut bone without carbonizing it.

With the proposed laser osteotome, see Fig. 1, we try to bridge this gap. To guarantee a high cutting precision, the laser source is directly mounted on a robot's end effector and is optically tracked using a stereo optical tracking device. A reflective mirror mounted on a 2-axes tilting mirror stage was introduced to deflect the laser beam. This tilting mirror permits quickly changing the direction of the laser beam. Large displacements are covered by the robot arm, whereas the small changes in the target location are handled by the tilting mirror. The question remains on how to align a voltage controlled mirror with the coordinate systems (CS) of the optical tracker, patient, and robot.

In this paper, we present a robust method to calibrate the tilting mirror and integrate it into the affine transformation chain. The essence of our approach is to apply a projective camera model to the given situation. In reference to Fig. 2, the camera center C corresponds to the mirror's laser deflecting spot D, from where light rays are received or emitted in a conical manner. In the case of an

N. Navab et al. (Eds.): MICCAI 2015, Part I, LNCS 9349, pp. 274–281, 2015.
DOI: 10.1007/978-3-319-24553-9_34

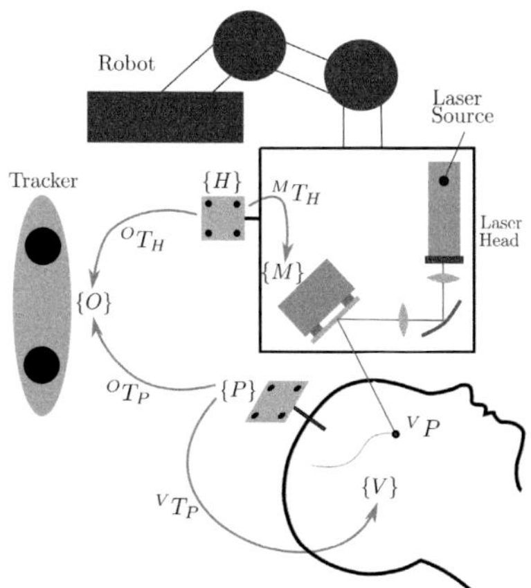

Fig. 1. Navigated laser system. Arrows denote affine transformations.

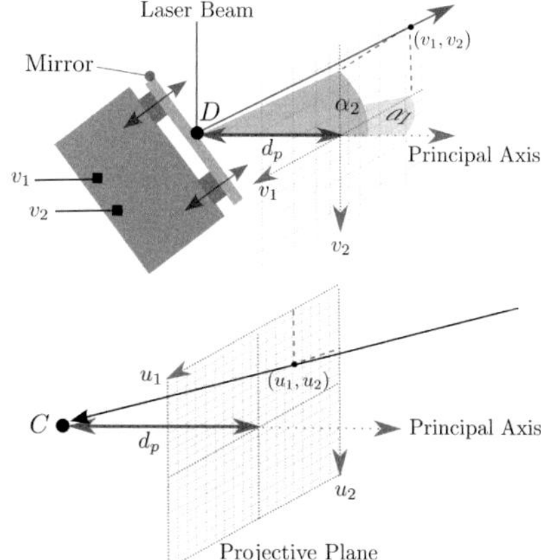

Fig. 2. Analogy of a laser tilting mirror (top) and a camera (below).

actual digital camera, the projective plane is an equidistant grid of photosensors u_1, u_2, whereas the mirror operates in a *virtual* voltage space v_1, v_2.

In the field of computer vision, well established camera calibration methods exist. In 1971, Abdel-Aziz and Karara introduced the *Direct Linear Transformation* (DLT) [1], which was a commonly used but rudimentary calibration technique. The main difference to contemporary calibration algorithms is that DLT does not consider nonlinear lens distortion effects, such as radial or tangential distortion. However, this is not required in the case of reflective optics as only mirrors and no lenses are involved. An interesting property of the DLT is that the extrinsic and intrinsic mirror parameters can be determined simultaneously.

In robotics, comparable work has been done on laser rangefinders, which perform depth measurements by triangulation of a moving laser beam and a camera [5]. Unfortunately, they focus only on extrinsic parameters and take the laser's steering properties (intrinsic) as given. The same pattern can be observed in many other applications. Often, the optical path and the mechanics, such as the steering mirror, are known very accurately. It makes sense to use this information and lock as many degrees of freedom as possible. In our system, the intrinsic parameters of the tilting mirror are known as well. But for two reasons we cannot use them: First, the optical setup of our prototype laser head is changing frequently. Second and more importantly, the regulatory authorities require the system to be calibrated on a regular basis when used in clinical practice, which certainly involves the determination of the mirror's overall properties.

Interesting related publications can be found in the field of catadioptric systems. From there we learned that it is common to apply a pinhole model to describe a moving mirror with a fixed center of reflection. A comparable situation is described in [4]. However, the setup there involves a hyperbolic mirror and a camera, which has to be calibrated with a non-linear approach. Our situation is comparably simple and we show that applying the DLT is appropriate.

2 Methods

2.1 Tilting Mirror Calibration with the DLT

As an input, the DLT algorithm requires several 2D–3D point correspondences. Using the pinhole camera model (Fig. 2), the projection of the i-th point from 3D spatial coordinates ${}^{H}X_i = [x, y, z, 1]_i^T$ to 2D pixel coordinates $u_i = [u_1, u_2, 1]_i^T$ on the projection plane is generally given by

$$\kappa u_i = \tilde{K} \cdot {}^{M}T_H \cdot {}^{H}X_i \Leftrightarrow \kappa \begin{bmatrix} u_1 \\ u_2 \\ 1 \end{bmatrix}_i = \begin{bmatrix} \tilde{f}_1 & 0 & \tilde{c}_1 \\ 0 & \tilde{f}_2 & \tilde{c}_2 \\ 0 & 0 & 1 \end{bmatrix} \cdot \begin{bmatrix} r_{11} & r_{12} & r_{13} & t_1 \\ r_{21} & r_{22} & r_{23} & t_2 \\ r_{31} & r_{32} & r_{33} & t_3 \end{bmatrix} \cdot \begin{bmatrix} x \\ y \\ z \\ 1 \end{bmatrix}_i, \quad (1)$$

with the intrinsic parameter matrix $\tilde{K}$ and the affine transformation ${}^{M}T_H$, where $\tilde{K}$ holds the focal distances $\tilde{f}_j$ and the principal point coordinates $\tilde{c}_j$ $(j = 1, 2)$, ${}^{M}T_H$ consists of a rotation part $r_{11}, \ldots, r_{33}$ and a translation part t_1, t_2, t_3, and κ is a normalization constant. In our model, ${}^{M}T_H$ represents the rigid transformation of the mirror's CS $\{M\}$ with respect to the optical marker's CS $\{H\}$ (Fig. 1). The corresponding spatial coordinate ${}^{H}X_i$ is expressed in the $\{H\}$ CS and denotes the 3D point where the laser beam impacts.

Choosing the distance from the projective center to the projective plane $d_p = 1$, u_j $(j = 1, 2)$ can be rewritten as $u_j = \tan(\alpha_j)$, where α_j denotes the angles of the two axes in which the deflection mirror is tilted. The angles are unknown, but they are linear to the known applied voltages v_j, enabling us to rewrite them as $\alpha_j = a_j v_j + b_j$ with the linearity parameters a_j, b_j. Putting these reformulations together, we can rewrite the projection as

$$\kappa \begin{bmatrix} \tan(a_1 v_1 + b_1) \\ \tan(a_2 v_2 + b_2) \\ 1 \end{bmatrix}_i = \tilde{K} \cdot {}^{M}T_H \cdot {}^{H}X_i. \quad (2)$$

The small-angle approximation enables us to simplify $\tan(\alpha_j) \approx \alpha_j$ $(\alpha_j < 10°)$, thus $\tan(a_j v_j + b_j) \approx a_j v_j + b_j$, which we use to simplify the projection as

$$\kappa \hat{C} \begin{bmatrix} v_1 \\ v_2 \\ 1 \end{bmatrix}_i \approx \tilde{K} \cdot {}^{M}T_H \cdot {}^{H}X_i \quad \text{with} \quad \hat{C} = \begin{bmatrix} a_1 & 0 & b_1 \\ 0 & a_2 & b_2 \\ 0 & 0 & 1 \end{bmatrix}. \quad (3)$$

Combining $\hat{C}$ and $\tilde{K}$ leads to the final approximative projection from spatial coordinates to voltage space:

$$\kappa v_i = \kappa \begin{bmatrix} v_1 \\ v_2 \\ 1 \end{bmatrix}_i \approx K \cdot {}^{M}T_H \cdot {}^{H}X_i \quad \text{with} \quad K = \hat{C}^{-1}\tilde{K} = \begin{bmatrix} f_1 & 0 & c_1 \\ 0 & f_2 & c_2 \\ 0 & 0 & 1 \end{bmatrix}, \quad (4)$$

where K holds the new intrinsic parameters f_j $(= \frac{\tilde{f}_j}{a_j})$ and c_j $(= \frac{\tilde{c}_j}{a_j} - \frac{b_j}{a_j})$.

We would like to point out two important aspects of the final model. First, it is feasible for small tilting angles only. This holds in our case, as our mirror is operated in a range of $\pm 6°$, resulting in a relative approximation error of 0.4%. Second, the actual angle–voltage relation need not be known, in fact: K and ${}^{M}T_{H}$ are calculated solely from correspondences between voltage pairs v_i and 3D points ${}^{H}X_i$, both of which are known. Showing the relationship between v_i, K and $u_i, \tilde{K}$ was only necessary to establish the model.

The vector v_i is proportional to the vector $[K \cdot {}^{M}T_{H} \cdot {}^{H}X_i]$, see Eq. (4). As a consequence, their crossproduct ($\times$) is 0. Applying the DLT, we find K and ${}^{M}T_{H}$ by solving for their product $P = K \cdot {}^{M}T_{H}$, which leads to

$$v_i \times \left(P \cdot {}^{H}X_i\right) = 0 \quad \Leftrightarrow \quad \begin{bmatrix} v_1 \\ v_2 \\ 1 \end{bmatrix}_i \times \left(\begin{bmatrix} p_{11} & p_{12} & p_{13} & p_{14} \\ p_{21} & p_{22} & p_{23} & p_{24} \\ p_{31} & p_{32} & p_{33} & p_{34} \end{bmatrix} \cdot \begin{bmatrix} x \\ y \\ z \\ 1 \end{bmatrix}_i \right) = 0, \tag{5}$$

with $p_{11} \dots p_{34}$ as unknowns and $[v_1, v_2]_i^T$, $[x, y, z]_i^T$ given by the point correspondences. This can be converted into a linear system of equations

$$A \cdot \begin{bmatrix} p_{11} \\ \vdots \\ p_{34} \end{bmatrix} = 0 \quad \text{with} \quad A = \begin{bmatrix} 0 & 0 & 0 & 0 & -x_0 & -y_0 & -z_0 & 1 & v_{2_0}x_0 & v_{2_0}y_0 & v_{2_0}z_0 & v_{2_0} \\ x_0 & y_0 & z_0 & 1 & 0 & 0 & 0 & 0 & -v_{1_0}x_0 & -v_{1_0}y_0 & -v_{1_0}z_0 & -v_{1_0} \\ \dots \\ 0 & 0 & 0 & 0 & -x_i & -y_i & -z_i & 1 & v_{2_i}x_i & v_{2_i}y_i & v_{2_i}z_i & v_{2_i} \\ x_i & y_i & z_i & 1 & 0 & 0 & 0 & 0 & -v_{1_i}x_i & -v_{1_i}y_i & -v_{1_i}z_i & -v_{1_i} \\ \dots \\ 0 & 0 & 0 & 0 & -x_N & -y_N & -z_N & 1 & v_{2_N}x_N & v_{2_N}y_N & v_{2_N}z_N & v_{2_N} \\ x_N & y_N & z_N & 1 & 0 & 0 & 0 & 0 & -v_{1_N}x_N & -v_{1_N}y_N & -v_{1_N}z_N & -v_{1_N} \end{bmatrix}. \tag{6}$$

Each correspondence results in three equations, one of which is redundant due to linear dependence. Thus, a number of $N \geq 6$ correspondences is required to solve for the 12 unknowns. The resulting product P can then be decomposed into K and ${}^{M}T_{H}$ as described in [3].

Input Data Normalization: The algorithm described above is the basic DLT. To enhance the numerical stability, we first transform the 2D–3D point correspondences in order to reach certain spatial properties. In [3], this can be found as *Normalized DLT*. In the presence of measurement noise, it is highly recommended to normalize the input data.

2.2 Calibration Errors

Due to the small-angle approximation and measurement noise, the computed solution K, ${}^{M}T_{H}$ will not map the given N input 2D–3D correspondences perfectly. Several error measures can be applied to quantify the quality of the calibration procedure. The *algebraic error* is the residual of the underlying least squares problem in Eq. (6). The *backprojection error* E is a geometric error quantity in the voltage plane. With the computed calibration result, the acquired 3D points ${}^{H}X_i$ are virtually projected as v_i' and compared with corresponding voltage pairs v_i by computing their Euclidean distances, as

$$E_i = \left\| v_i - v_i' \right\| \quad \text{with} \quad v_i' \propto K \cdot {}^{M}T_{H} \cdot {}^{H}X_i \quad \text{for} \quad i = 1, \dots, N. \tag{7}$$

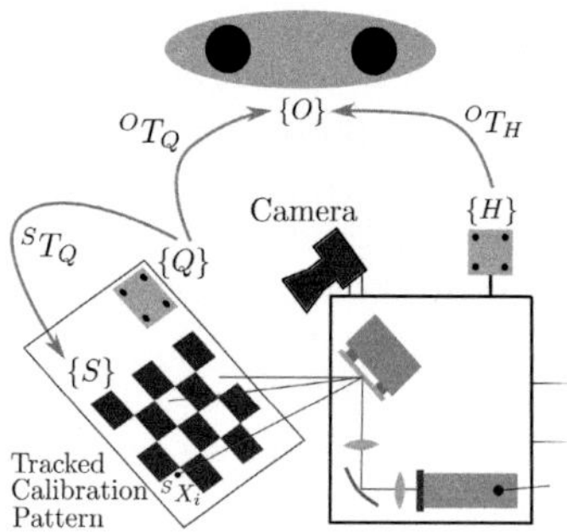

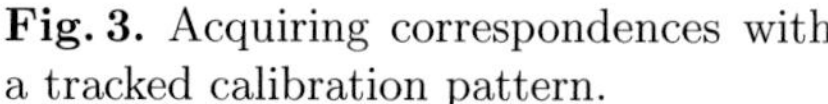
Fig. 3. Acquiring correspondences with a tracked calibration pattern.

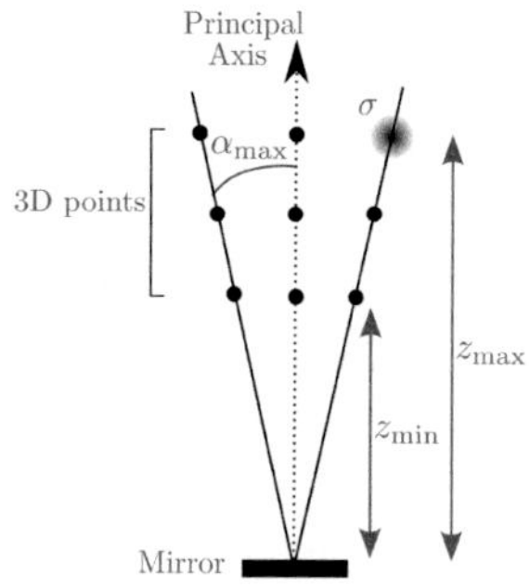

Fig. 4. Synthetic input data generation for the calibration.

The most important error measure for surgeons is the deviation from the planned location on the target site, i.e. on the patient herself and in millimetre, the so called *target registration error* (TRE). An error in the voltage plane E_i can be extrapolated with the distance between tilting mirror and target d_i, which is easy to determine after transforming the 3D points into the mirror CS. The TRE T_i is then computed for all N point correspondences as

$$T_i = d_i \left\| K^{-1} \cdot [E_i, 0, 0]^T \right\| \quad \text{with} \quad d_i = \left\| {}^{M}T_H \cdot {}^{H}X_i \right\| \quad \text{for} \quad i = 1, \ldots, N. \quad (8)$$

2.3 Acquiring 2D–3D Correspondences

The accuracy of the mirror calibration depends strongly on the quality of its input data. Figure 3 illustrates our acquisition setup. The robot is driven into an appropriate position. Then $N_v \geq 1$ predefined voltage pairs v_i $(i = 1, \ldots, N_v)$ are applied to the tilting mirror. Their laser impact on a chessboard is recorded with a camera, and the standard blob-detector of *OpenCV* is used to recover their pixel positions, which can be easily transformed into the given chessboard CS ${}^{S}X_i$. It is important to notice that recovering ${}^{S}X_i$ with the camera is an independent process. Neither the relative position of the camera to the tilting mirror nor the rest of the system matters. However, a focused image preferably orthogonal to the chessboard enhances the accuracy of acquired positions.

In order to transform the laser position from the chessboard CS $\{S\}$ into the laser head CS $\{H\}$, first one has to resolve the transformation from the chessboard to its tracked marker ${}^{S}T_Q$. A common method based on fitting two 3D point sets [2] was applied for that purpose. The final transformation is

$${}^{H}X_i = \left({}^{O}T_H\right)^{-1} \cdot {}^{O}T_Q \cdot \left({}^{S}T_Q\right)^{-1} \cdot {}^{S}X_i, \quad (9)$$

where ${}^{O}T_Q$ and ${}^{O}T_H$ are given by the optical tracking system.

These steps are repeated from N_p different robot positions. Therefore, the total amount of collected 2D–3D correspondences is $N = N_v N_p$. A simple robot trajectory is orthogonal to the chessboard surface.

2.4 Integration of the Tilting Mirror

Using the notation introduced in Fig. 1, the transformations ${}^{O}T_H$ and ${}^{O}T_P$ are given by the tracking system. The 3D–3D registration ${}^{V}T_P$ from the patient marker to the operation planning data (CT, MR) can be performed with the method described in [2]. Given a cutting position ${}^{V}P$ on the patient, the two voltages (v_1, v_2) for the mirror can be computed by

$$\left[v_1, v_2, 1\right]^T \propto K \cdot {}^{M}T_H \cdot \left({}^{O}T_H\right)^{-1} \cdot {}^{O}T_P \cdot \left({}^{V}T_P\right)^{-1} \cdot {}^{V}P, \tag{10}$$

which finally forms the complete transformation chain.

3 Experiments and Results

In this section, the performance of the described calibration approach is examined in detail based on synthetic and real input data. These experiments were performed by applying the normalized DLT approach.

Error Analyses with Synthetic Input Data: In these experiments, synthetic data was produced to analyze the presented method in terms of error behavior. As illustrated in Fig. 4, the calibration data generation can be configured by the four parameters $\alpha_{\max}$ (maximum angle for both mirror axes), $z_{\min}$ and $z_{\max}$ (distance in principal direction between the mirror and the 3D points), N_v (number of different voltage pairs applied in each robot position), N_p (number of different robot positions), and σ (standard deviation of zero-mean Gaussian noise applied to the 3D points). The point correspondences are generated in a deterministic way. For our simulated tilting mirror, v_1, v_2 are chosen to be equal to α_1, α_2 (1°/voltage). Based on a given $\alpha_{\max}$, an equidistant voltage array of size N_v is generated, where values of both axes α_1, α_2 are in the range of $-\alpha_{\max} \leq \alpha_{1,2} \leq \alpha_{\max}$. These are the 2D points. Their corresponding 3D coordinates are generated by applying this voltage array to the mirror and projecting to N_p different orthogonal planes with distance z_p, so that $z_0 = z_{\min}, \ldots, z_{N_p} = z_{\max}$. As already mentioned, this leads to a total number of $N = N_v N_p$ point correspondences. To simulate the presence of noise, zero-mean Gaussian noise σ is added in all three dimensions to each 3D coordinate.

Maximum Deflection Angle Influence: Since the proposed method is based on the small-angle approximation, calibrations with increasing maximum deflection angle were performed. In particular, synthetic data sets with varying $\alpha_{\max} = 2^\circ, \ldots, 8^\circ$ were generated, whereas the other parameters were kept constant at $z_{\min}$ =140 mm and $z_{\max}$ =160 mm, $\sigma = 0$, $N_v = 25$, and $N_p = 5$. Of each of these data sets, the mirror calibration was computed and the TRE T_i was determined and presented as a box plot, where the central mark is the median, the edges of the box are the 25th and 75th percentiles and the whiskers extend to the minimum and maximum errors. Figure 5 shows the results.

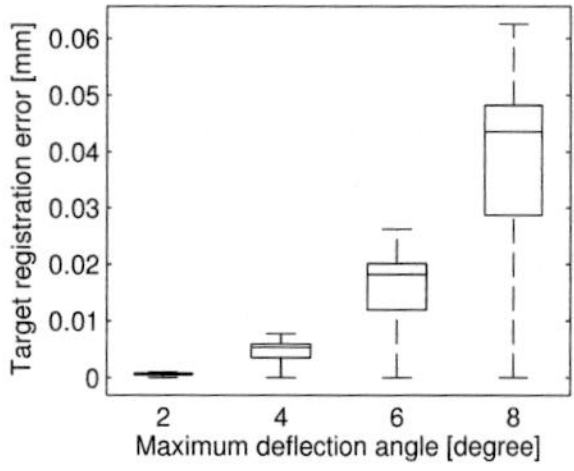

Fig. 5. TRE with increasing maximum mirror angle $\alpha_{\max}$.

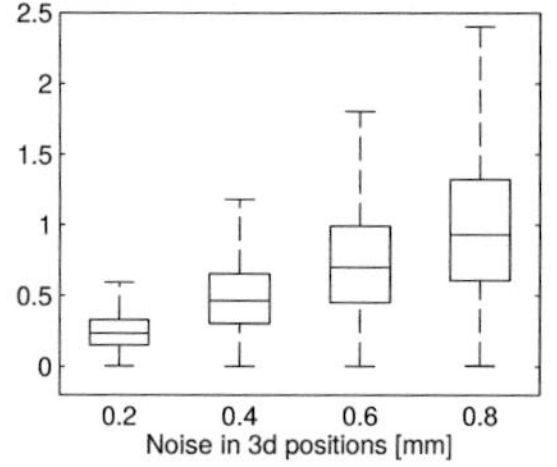

Fig. 6. TRE with increasing Gaussian noise σ.

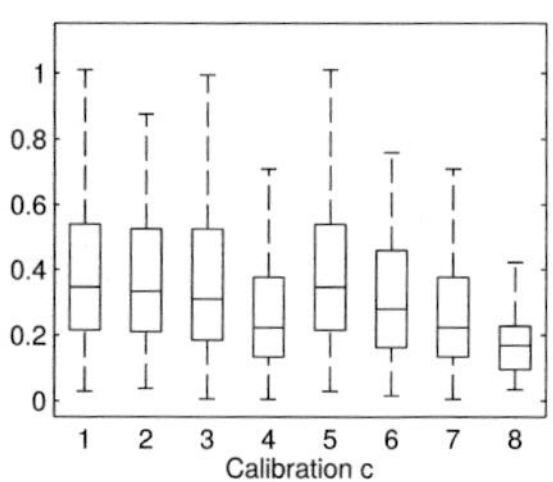

Fig. 7. TRE for real acquired correspondences.

Impact of Noise: In this experiment, calibrations with increasing Gaussian noise $\sigma = 0.2\,\text{mm}, \ldots, 0.8\,\text{mm}$ were made. Other parameters remained constant at $\alpha_{\max} = 6°$, $z_{\min}$ =140 mm, $z_{\max}$ =160 mm, $N_v = 25$, and $N_p = 5$. For each noise level, $N_c = 100$ calibrations were made. Figure 6 shows the resulting TRE.

Results: One can clearly see that the tangent approximation for small angles is unproblematic. In our system, the maximum deflection angle $\alpha_{\max}$ is 6°, which corresponds to a maximum TRE of about 30 µm. Measurement noise, however, is an issue. The reported accuracy of our used tracking system is 0.25 mm. Based on the simulation, this corresponds to a TRE of about 0.5 mm.

Calibration with Real Data: In this experiment, the proposed calibration method was tested within the actual laser ablation system. As a tilting mirror, the OIM5001 (Optics In Motion) was used. The used optical tracking system was the CamBar B2 (AXIOS 3D Services) and the robot was the iiwa (KUKA Laboratories). The distance z between the chessboard and the tilting mirror was around 150 mm. The maximum deflection angle $\alpha_{\max}$ was about 6°. However, since the extrinsic and intrinsic mirror properties ${}^{M}T_{H}$, K are unknown at this time, the exact values of z and α can be determined only afterwards.

In the following, $N_c = 8$ independent tilting mirror calibrations were done. For each calibration c, $N_p = 5$ different robot positions along the chessboard normal were used. In each position, $N_v = 25$ voltage pairs were applied. Therefore, the maximum number of 2D–3D correspondences for each calibration c was $N = 125$. But due the regularly failure of the visual blob-detection within black chessboard fields, N showed to easily drop to 80.

Results: The results of the 8 calibrations can be seen in Fig. 7. The average TRE is 0.3 mm, with a standard deviation of 0.2 mm. The maximum error is 1.0 mm. The average distance z between the mirror and all involved correspondences was 141 mm and the average $\alpha_{\max}$ was 6.8°. When comparing the measured error with the results of noisy synthetic input data, this meets the expected error when using an optical tracking device with a spatial accuracy of 0.25 mm.

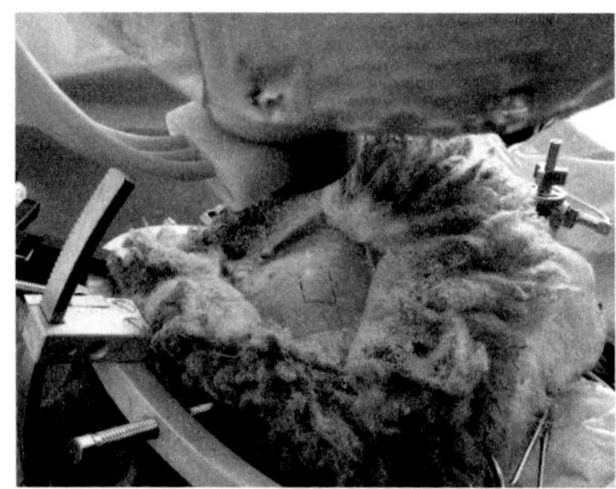

Fig. 8. The laser system performing a navigated cut on a sheep head.

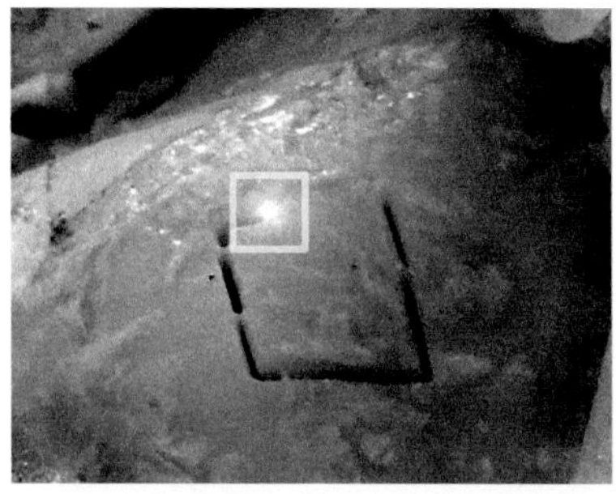

Fig. 9. Enlarged view of the cutting region. The bright spot is the laser.

4 Conclusion

We showed that a voltage controlled tilting mirror can be accurately calibrated by using the pinhole camera model and the *direct linear transformation* approach to solve it. With a *target registration error* of $0.3\,\mathrm{mm} \pm 0.2\,\mathrm{mm}$ at a working distance of 150 mm, our laser ablation system not only exceeds general osteotomy requirements, but also opens up new surgical possibilities in terms of cutting shapes. Although a maximum cutting error of 1.0 mm is tolerable, it does not meet our own demands. Currently we are designing non-planar optical markers to increase the tracking accuracy. Preliminary results are promising.

To conclude, we would like to give the reader an impression of the presented laser system in action. Figures 8 and 9 show a navigated cut on a sheep skull.

References

1. Abdel-Aziz, Y., Karara, H.: Direct Linear Transformation from Comparator Coordinates Into Object Space Coordinates in Close-range Photogrammetry (1971)
2. Arun, K.S., Huang, T.S., Blostein, S.D.: Least-squares fitting of two 3-D point sets. IEEE Trans. on Pattern Analysis and Machine Intelligence (5), 698–700 (1987)
3. Hartley, R., Zisserman, A.: Multiple view geometry in computer vision. Cambridge Univ Press (2010)
4. Orghidan, R., Salvi, J., Mouaddib, E.M.: Calibration of a structured light-based stereo catadioptric sensor. In: Conference on Computer Vision and Pattern Recognition Workshop, CVPRW 2003, vol. 7, p. 70. IEEE (2003)
5. Zhang, Q., Pless, R.: Extrinsic calibration of a camera and laser range finder. In: Proceedings of the 2004 IEEE/RSJ International Conference on Intelligent Robots and Systems (IROS 2004), vol. 3, pp. 2301–2306. IEEE (2004)

Surrogate-Driven Estimation of Respiratory Motion and Layers in X-Ray Fluoroscopy

Peter Fischer[1], Thomas Pohl[2], Andreas Maier[1], and Joachim Hornegger[1]

[1] Pattern Recognition Lab and Erlangen Graduate School in Advanced Optical Technologies (SAOT), FAU Erlangen-Nürnberg, Erlangen, Germany,
peter.fischer@fau.de

[2] Siemens Healthcare, Forchheim, Germany

Abstract. Dense motion estimation in X-ray fluoroscopy is challenging due to low soft-tissue contrast and the transparent projection of 3-D information to 2-D. Motion layers have been introduced as an intermediate representation, but so far failed to generate plausible motions because their estimation is ill-posed. To attain plausible motions, we include prior information for each motion layer in the form of a surrogate signal. In particular, we extract a respiratory signal from the images using manifold learning and use it to define a surrogate-driven motion model. The model is incorporated into an energy minimization framework with smoothness priors to enable motion estimation.

Experimentally, our method estimates 48% of the 2-D motion field on XCAT phantom data. On real X-ray sequences, the target registration error of manually annotated landmarks is reduced by 52%. In addition, we qualitatively show that a meaningful separation into motion layers is achieved.

1 Introduction

X-ray fluoroscopy is an important modality for guidance of minimally-invasive interventions. It has good spatial and temporal resolution and clearly visualizes interventional devices and bones. However, the contrast of soft tissue is low and 3-D information is lost due to the transparent projection to 2-D. In this paper, we deal with dense motion estimation in X-ray images. There are many clinical applications of fluoroscopy for which this is beneficial. Temporal denoising algorithms depend on accurate motion estimates [1]. Coronary DSA requires the compensation of cardiac and respiratory motion occurring between the mask and the contrasted image [14]. In thoracic and abdominal interventions, fusion of X-ray images with previously acquired roadmap overlays, created from contrasted images, CT, MR, or C-arm CT, requires motion compensation to correctly display the overlays on the live fluoroscopic images [4,15].

There are two major challenges for motion estimation in fluoroscopy. First, the low soft-tissue contrast complicates intensity-based image registration, because common similarity measures are dominated by high-contrast structures. Second, the estimation of 2-D motion in X-ray fluoroscopy is ill-posed due to the

N. Navab et al. (Eds.): MICCAI 2015, Part I, LNCS 9349, pp. 282–289, 2015.
DOI: 10.1007/978-3-319-24553-9_35

transparent projection of differently moving 3-D structures to 2-D. To alleviate the transparency problem, motion layers have been introduced [11]. The goal of motion estimation is then to compute a separate 2-D motion field for each layer.

Two approaches have been proposed for this problem. The first approach avoids to compute motion layers and directly estimates multiple 2-D motions for each pixel. Assuming locally constant motion in space and time in each layer, the common brightness constancy assumption can be extended to the transparent setting [1,11]. Alternatively, certain special motion types can be estimated in transparency, e.g., parametric motions [3] or a single non-static layer [15]. However, these assumptions are restrictive and cumbersome for more than two layers. The second approach is estimation of layers and motions. This leads to a chicken-and-egg problem, i.e., it is easy to compute the layers when the motion is known and vice versa. Szeliski et al. assume parametric motion to simplify the problem [12]. Preston et al. introduce a layer gradient penalty for the layers and a smoothness prior for the motions [9]. However, the motions and layers are not physiologically meaningful, restricting their usefulness to applications where the layers and motions are recombined, e.g., frame interpolation or denoising. Surrogate signals are commonly used in respiratory motion models [8]. For example, Martin et al. estimate a surrogate-driven 3-D motion field in motion-compensated C-arm CT reconstruction [7] .

In this work, we propose to enhance layered motion estimation using a separate surrogate signal for each layer. In particular, we use a static layer without motion and a respiratory layer with motion proportional to a respiratory surrogate signal. The respiratory surrogate signal is extracted from the X-ray sequence using manifold learning. Together with smoothness priors for layers and motions, this enables us to retrospectively estimate physiologically plausible layers and motions in an energy formulation. The proposed method is especially suited for building 2-D respiratory motion models, as the dependence of the motion on the surrogate signals is required anyways. We quantify the estimation error of the proposed method on simulated X-ray images by comparing the estimated to the ground truth motion. On clinical sequences, we evaluate quantitatively using manual annotations and qualitatively show that the respiratory motion is accurately captured and that the motion layers are separated.

2 Methods

2.1 Image Formation Model

We are interested in separating X-ray images $I\left(\boldsymbol{x},t\right)$, $t \in \{1,\ldots,T\}$ into different motion layers $L_l\left(\boldsymbol{x}\right)$, where each layer may undergo independent non-parametric 2-D motion $\boldsymbol{v}_l\left(\boldsymbol{x},t\right) \in \mathbb{R}^2$. $\boldsymbol{x} \in \mathbb{R}^2$ is the image pixel position. A motion layer can roughly be assigned to each source of motion, e.g., breathing, heartbeat, and background. The images are created additively from the transformed layers as

$$I\left(\boldsymbol{x},t\right) = \sum_{l=1}^{N} L_l\left(\boldsymbol{x} - \boldsymbol{v}_l\left(\boldsymbol{x},t\right)\right) + \eta \ , \tag{1}$$

where $\eta \in \mathbb{R}$ is introduced to account for model errors and observation noise in the log-transformed X-ray model [9]. In this paper, we restrict the number of layers in the image sequence to $N = 2$, a static and a respiratory layer.

2.2 Surrogate-Driven Motion Model

The surrogate-driven model for layered motion is defined as

$$\boldsymbol{v}_l(\boldsymbol{x}, t) = s_l(t) \cdot \boldsymbol{\nu}_l(\boldsymbol{x}) \ , \tag{2}$$

where $s_l(t) \in \mathbb{R}$ is a surrogate signal that is used to scale the base motion $\boldsymbol{\nu}_l(\boldsymbol{x}) \in \mathbb{R}^2$. The surrogate-driven motion model is crucial to achieve physiologically plausible motions. It reduces the number of motion parameters by a factor of $T-1$ compared to unconstrained motion fields, because $\boldsymbol{\nu}_l(\boldsymbol{x})$ is defined only for one point in time and extended to other times using Eq. (2), whereas unconstrained motion fields are defined for all points in time except $t = 0$. Thus, the parameter space is constrained to the subspace where the motion fields agree with the surrogate signals and thus with the underlying physiological processes.

In our application, the static layer with a constant surrogate signal $s_1(t) = 0$ is required to describe the static components of the X-ray sequence. The respiratory surrogate signal $s_2(t)$ can in principle be acquired by any means, e.g., spirometry or respiratory belt. In this work, we derive the respiratory signal directly from the intensities of the X-ray images using manifold learning. It has proven to be effective for X-ray fluoroscopy [5]. The advantage for our application is that the signal is based on the same images that are used for motion estimation, thus facilitating the proportionality assumption in Eq. (2).

2.3 Motion and Layer Estimation

To define a tractable optimization problem for joint motion and layer estimation, we include Eq. (1) and Eq. (2) into an energy formulation

$$E(\mathcal{L}, \mathcal{V}) = D(\mathcal{L}, \mathcal{V}) + \lambda_L R(\mathcal{L}) + \lambda_\nu R(\mathcal{V}) \ , \tag{3}$$

where $D(\mathcal{L}, \mathcal{V})$ is the data term, $R(\mathcal{L})$ and $R(\mathcal{V})$ are regularization terms for the layers and motions and $\lambda_L, \lambda_\nu \in \mathbb{R}$ are their weights. $\mathcal{L}$ is the set of all layers L_l and $\mathcal{V}$ is the set of all base motions $\boldsymbol{\nu}_l$.

The data term penalizes deviations from Eq. (1). Since the image formation model is only an inaccurate representation of the true X-ray generation process, robustness to outliers in the data term

$$D(\mathcal{L}, \mathcal{V}) = \sum_{t=1}^{T} \int_{\Omega} \psi\left(I(\boldsymbol{x}, t) - \sum_{l=1}^{N} L_l(\boldsymbol{x} - \boldsymbol{v}_l(\boldsymbol{x}, t)) \right) \mathrm{d}\boldsymbol{x} \tag{4}$$

is mandatory, where Ω is the image domain and ψ is a robust penalty function. We use the Charbonnier penalty $\psi(z) = \sqrt{(\epsilon^2 + z^2)} - \epsilon$ with $\epsilon = 0.01$ as a differentiable approximation of the L_1-norm.

The regularization term for the layers is designed to favor spatially smooth layers, while still allowing for edges. Similar to denoising and reconstruction, we use a differentiable approximation of the isotropic total variation (TV) regularization

$$R(\mathcal{L}) = \sum_{l=1}^{N} \int_{\Omega} \psi\left(\|\nabla L_l(\boldsymbol{x})\|_2\right) \mathrm{d}\boldsymbol{x} \ , \tag{5}$$

where $\nabla = (\partial_x, \partial_y)^T$ is the spatial gradient. Preston et al. adapt the TV regularization to the image gradients [9]. In our experience, this does not improve the results, because Eq. (5) is already edge-preserving, and is much more expensive to compute, because all images must be warped to $t = 1$.

A similar spatial smoothness constraint is employed for the motions

$$R(\mathcal{V}) = \sum_{l=1}^{N} \int_{\Omega} \psi\left(\sqrt{\|\nabla \nu_l^x(\boldsymbol{x})\|_2^2 + \|\nabla \nu_l^y(\boldsymbol{x})\|_2^2}\right) \mathrm{d}\boldsymbol{x} \ , \tag{6}$$

where ν_l^x, ν_l^y are the horizontal and vertical motions, respectively. Here, the robust penalty allows for motion boundaries. In addition, it is computationally less expensive than regularizing a full 2-D+t motion field for each layer, because it must be computed only for one point in time. In general, motion estimation benefits from regularization along the time-domain. However, this is already covered by the surrogate-driven motion model. In this sense, Eq. (2) is a strong regularization of the motion field along the surrogate signal.

2.4 Implementation

As the manifold learning method to extract the respiratory signal from the intensities of the entire X-ray image, we use Isomap [5,13], with $k = 20$ neighbors to construct the k-nearest-neighbors graph. To reduce noise and the influence of other motions, a third-order Butterworth low-pass filter with a cut-off frequency of 1.5 Hz is applied to the surrogate signal retrospectively.

The energy function Eq. (3) is minimized in a coarse-to-fine pyramid. This speeds up the optimization and avoids local minima. We use a downsampling factor of 0.5 and choose the number of levels such that the coarsest level has a size of ~ 20 pixels in each dimension. The base motions $\mathcal{V}$ and layers $\mathcal{L}$ are initialized randomly at the coarsest level. At each level, the energy function is minimized in an alternation scheme, i.e., minimization w.r.t. $\mathcal{V}$ while keeping $\mathcal{L}$ fixed, and then vice versa. This scheme is repeated 10 times on each level. A L-BFGS-B optimizer with up to 1000 iterations is used in each minimization. It is initialized with the solution of the previous alternation. The layers are constrained to be non-negative and bounded above by the image intensity maximum [12]. For non-integer positions $\boldsymbol{x}$, bilinear interpolation is used to compute intensities.

Note that $\boldsymbol{v}_l(\boldsymbol{x}, t)$ is defined in the time-dependent coordinate system of $I(\boldsymbol{x}, t)$ in Eq. (2). Intuitively, it would be preferable to model the motion of a certain structure over time as scaled versions of a base motion by defining it in the fixed coordinate system of $L_l(\boldsymbol{x})$. However, this would require the inversion of $\boldsymbol{v}_l(\boldsymbol{x}, t)$ in each optimizer iteration to evaluate Eq. (4), which is very inefficient.

3 Experiments and Results

In the experiments, we evaluate the proposed method (REG-SL) on simulated and clinical X-ray sequences. The baseline method is a static layer (STAT), i.e., no motion. As alternatives, conventional 2-D/2-D registration (REG-2D) and layered motion estimation without surrogate signals (REG-L) are employed. All methods optimize the same energy Eq. (3). However, for REG-L and REG-2D, Eq. (6) is computed for each point in time and the curvature of the motion fields is regularized over time, with the weight parameter $\lambda_{\mathcal{T}} \in \mathbb{R}$. This reduces potential bias in the evaluation, because it substitutes the inherent smoothness of the proposed surrogate-driven motion model. The parameters are empirically set to $\lambda_L = 0.05$, $\lambda_{\nu} = 0.025$, and $\lambda_{\mathcal{T}} = 0.001$ such that the computed motions are visually reasonable for all methods in a pilot experiment.

3.1 Simulated Data

In order to densely evaluate the computed motion, simulated X-ray sequences are created by transforming two layers using known 2-D motion fields. The layers are rendered using the XCAT phantom [10] with a material-resolved renderer from CONRAD [6], where each material is assigned to a single layer. The 4-D XCAT phantom is not used directly, because then no ground truth 2-D motions would be known. The 2-D motion field of the respiratory layer is created using Eq. (2), where the base motion $\boldsymbol{\nu}_2$ is a thin-plate spline interpolation of manually annotated point motions. In the end, Gaussian and Laplacian noise with standard deviation of 1% of the image intensity range is added. The eight simulated sequences each consist of $T = 10$ images of 128×128 pixels with different layers and motions. An exemplary sequence with its constituents is shown in Figs. 1b to 1d. The ground truth motion of the respiratory layer is compared to the computed motion using the endpoint error (EE) [2]. Pixels with zero intensity in the ground-truth layer are excluded due to their unidentifiable motion, see Fig. 1c.

Table 1 shows the results of this experiment. The proposed REG-SL has the lowest EE of 2.0 mm averaged over all sequences and compensates 48% of the total motion in the images, which is represented by STAT. REG-2D and REG-L are only able to slightly decrease the EE compared to STAT. We additionally estimate the motion using the ground truth respiratory signal in the surrogate-driven motion model (REG-SL-GT), see Fig. 1a. As the EE is not substantially reduced further, the chosen method for surrogate signal extraction is validated for this application. The runtime of the methods, implemented in Python and C++, was measured on a notebook with a Core i7-3720QM processor. STAT is of course fastest, because it requires no processing. Among the registration methods, REG-2D is faster than the others with an average runtime of 33 s, because it does not need to iterate between layer and motion estimation.

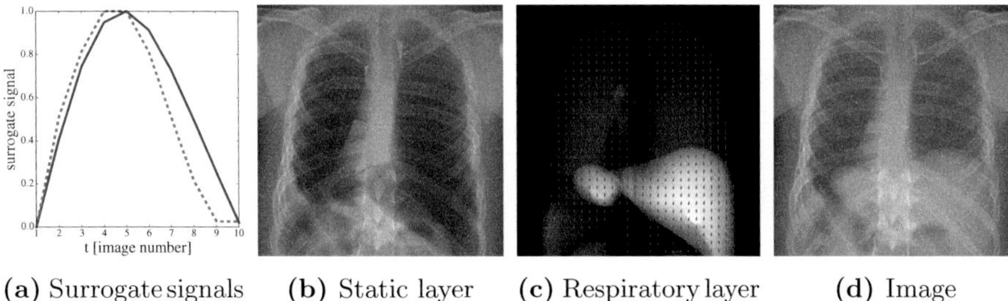

(a) Surrogate signals (b) Static layer (c) Respiratory layer (d) Image

Fig. 1. Surrogate signals (true - -, estimated –), layers with overlaid motion (↑), and simulated image of XCAT experiments (best viewed in color).

Table 1. Evaluation of motion estimation methods on simulated data using runtime and endpoint error (EE) and on clinical data using TRE (mean ± std).

	STAT	REG-2D	REG-L	REG-SL	REG-SL-GT
Runtime [s]	**0.0**	33 ± 3.5	136 ± 46	48 ± 6.8	54 ± 18
EE [mm]	3.8 ± 5.0	3.1 ± 3.9	3.5 ± 4.1	2.0 ± 2.5	$\mathbf{1.9} \pm \mathbf{3.0}$
TRE [mm]	4.6 ± 4.9	3.9 ± 5.2	3.8 ± 4.3	$\mathbf{2.2} \pm \mathbf{3.0}$	-

3.2 Clinical Data

On clinical X-ray data, quantitative evaluation of dense 2-D motion fields or layers is challenging due to the absence of ground truth. Therefore, we resort to measuring the target registration error (TRE) at certain structures of interest. This has the drawback that the validity of the 2-D motion fields is measured only sparsely. As the target anatomy, we manually annotate structures that are known to correspond to respiratory motion, e.g., diaphragm or guidewires. The TRE is measured as the tracking error $\min_k \|C(s) - C_{\text{GT}}(k)\|_2$ between each point s on the computed curve C and the annotated curve C_{GT} in mm on the detector. This experiment is performed on 6 sequences of in total 818 images with sizes of $193 - 1024$ pixels and pixel size of $0.18 - 0.43$ mm in each dimension. The images are downsampled by a multiple of two to ~ 128 pixels for lower runtime and memory requirements, but the error is measured in the full resolution.

The results are shown in the last row of Table 1. The total motion of the annotated structures is 4.6 ± 4.9 mm as represented by STAT. 2-D registration and layered motion estimation reduce the motion to 3.9 and 3.8 mm, respectively. For these methods, the extent of the reduction heavily depends on the image content. If there are few X-ray transparency effects in the region of the annotated structure, the motion is correctly estimated with REG-2D. The success of REG-L depends on the computed local minimum of the non-convex energy. REG-SL has a residual motion of 2.2 ± 3.0 mm, so 52% of the motion is compensated.

In the sequence of Fig. 2, our REG-SL is superior to the other methods. Transparency effects of the skin markers and the ribs deteriorate the results of REG-2D. For REG-L, neither discovered layer is anatomically plausible and thus the motions are implausible as well. In REG-SL, static structures are suppressed

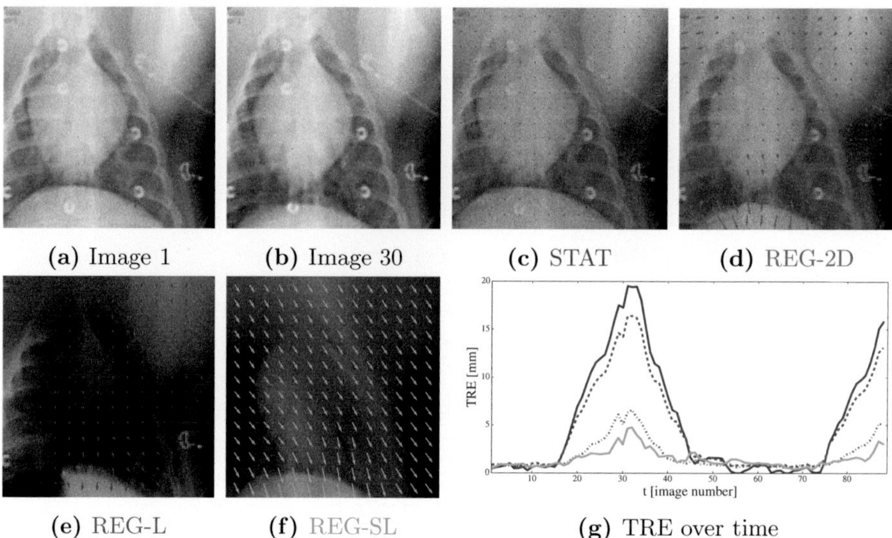

(a) Image 1 (b) Image 30 (c) STAT (d) REG-2D

(e) REG-L (f) REG-SL (g) TRE over time

Fig. 2. Respiratory layer and motion (Figs. 2c to 2f) between two images (Figs. 2a and 2b) and TRE (Fig. 2g) on a real X-ray sequence (best viewed in color).

in the respiratory layer, but the diaphragm and some soft tissue is preserved. The TRE over time in Fig. 2g is most reduced by REG-SL in case of large motion.

4 Conclusion and Outlook

We propose a surrogate-driven motion model for layered motion estimation in X-ray fluoroscopy. The surrogate signal constrains the ill-posed optimization problem such that physiologically plausible dense 2-D motion can be estimated from X-ray images. In general, the method has little requirements. The surrogate signals can be extracted directly from the images using manifold learning, so no additional devices or synchronization are necessary. Motion estimation is independent of C-arm and table position. It can be used for thoracic or abdominal sequences, but should cover at least one breathing cycle, such that the manifold learning gives a useful respiratory signal. A restriction is the linear relationship between surrogate signal and motion. Nevertheless, its results are superior to previous approaches in our experiments. The error of 2.2 mm is in a clinically acceptable scale, e.g., for overlay navigation [4].

In future work, a more complex motion model could relax the linearity assumption, e.g., more surrogate signals per layer or a non-linear dependency between signal and motion. Another interesting point is to extend the method for estimating more than two layers. In particular, a layer with cardiac motion would be beneficial. The runtime is still too long for real-time or interactive use and should be reduced, e.g., using a GPU implementation. Furthermore, the usefulness of the computed motion must be validated for a potential clinical application, since it is only a 2-D approximation of the true 3-D motion.

Acknowledgments. The authors gratefully acknowledge funding of the Erlangen Graduate School in Advanced Optical Technologies (SAOT) by the German Research Foundation (DFG) in the framework of the German excellence initiative and by Siemens Healthcare. The concepts and information presented in this paper are based on research and are not commercially available.

References

1. Auvray, V., Liénard, J., Bouthemy, P.: Multiresolution parametric estimation of transparent motions and denoising of fluoroscopic images. In: Duncan, J.S., Gerig, G. (eds.) MICCAI 2005. LNCS, vol. 3750, pp. 352–360. Springer, Heidelberg (2005)
2. Baker, S., Scharstein, D., Lewis, J., Roth, S., Black, M.J., Szeliski, R.: A database and evaluation methodology for optical flow. Int. J. Comput. Vis. 92(1), 1–31 (2011)
3. Black, M.J., Anandan, P.: The robust estimation of multiple motions: Parametric and piecewise-smooth flow fields. Comput. Vis. Image Underst. 63(1), 75–104 (1996)
4. Brost, A., Liao, R., Strobel, N., Hornegger, J.: Respiratory motion compensation by model-based catheter tracking during EP procedures. Med. Image Anal. 14(5), 695–706 (2010)
5. Fischer, P., Pohl, T., Hornegger, J.: Real-time respiratory signal extraction from x-ray sequences using incremental manifold learning. In: ISBI, pp. 915–918. IEEE (2014)
6. Maier, A., Hofmann, H., Berger, M., Fischer, P., Schwemmer, C., Wu, H., Müller, K., Hornegger, J., Choi, J.H., Riess, C., Keil, A., Fahrig, R.: CONRAD - a software framework for cone-beam imaging in radiology. Med. Phys. 40(11), 111914 (2013)
7. Martin, J., McClelland, J., Champion, B., Hawkes, D.J.: Building surrogate-driven motion models from cone-beam CT via surrogate-correlated optical flow. In: Stoyanov, D., Collins, D.L., Sakuma, I., Abolmaesumi, P., Jannin, P. (eds.) IPCAI 2014. LNCS, vol. 8498, pp. 61–67. Springer, Heidelberg (2014)
8. McClelland, J.R., Hawkes, D.J., Schaeffter, T., King, A.P.: Respiratory motion models: a review. Med. Image Anal. 17(1), 19–42 (2013)
9. Preston, J., Rottman, C., Cheryauka, A., Anderton, L., Whitaker, R., Joshi, S.: Multi-layer deformation estimation for fluoroscopic imaging. In: Gee, J.C., Joshi, S., Pohl, K.M., Wells, W.M., Zöllei, L. (eds.) IPMI 2013. LNCS, vol. 7917, pp. 123–134. Springer, Heidelberg (2013)
10. Segars, W., Mahesh, M., Beck, T., Frey, E., Tsui, B.: Realistic CT simulation using the 4D XCAT phantom. Med. Phys. 35(8), 3800–3808 (2008)
11. Shizawa, M., Mase, K.: Simultaneous multiple optical flow estimation. In: ICPR, vol. 1, pp. 274–278. IEEE (1990)
12. Szeliski, R., Avidan, S., Anandan, P.: Layer extraction from multiple images containing reflections and transparency. In: CVPR, vol. 1, pp. 246–253. IEEE (2000)
13. Tenenbaum, J.B., de Silva, V., Langford, J.C.: A global geometric framework for nonlinear dimensionality reduction. Science 290(5500), 2319–2323 (2000)
14. Zhu, Y., Prummer, S., Wang, P., Chen, T., Comaniciu, D., Ostermeier, M.: Dynamic layer separation for coronary DSA and enhancement in fluoroscopic sequences. In: Yang, G.-Z., Hawkes, D., Rueckert, D., Noble, A., Taylor, C. (eds.) MICCAI 2009, Part II. LNCS, vol. 5762, pp. 877–884. Springer, Heidelberg (2009)
15. Zhu, Y., Tsin, Y., Sundar, H., Sauer, F.: Image-based respiratory motion compensation for fluoroscopic coronary roadmapping. In: Jiang, T., Navab, N., Pluim, J.P.W., Viergever, M.A. (eds.) MICCAI 2010, Part III. LNCS, vol. 6363, pp. 287–294. Springer, Heidelberg (2010)

Robust 5DOF Transesophageal Echo Probe Tracking at Fluoroscopic Frame Rates

Charles R. Hatt[1,2], Michael A. Speidel[1,2], and Amish N. Raval[2]

[1] Department of Medical Physics, University of Wisconsin - Madison, USA
[2] Division of Cardiovascular Medicine, University of Wisconsin - Madison, USA

Abstract. Registration between transesophageal echocardiography (TEE) and x-ray fluoroscopy (XRF) has recently been introduced as a potentially useful tool for advanced image guidance of structural heart interventions. Algorithms for registration at fluoroscopic imaging frame rates (15-30 fps) have yet to be reported, despite the fact that probe movement resulting from cardiorespiratory motion and physician manipulation can introduce non-trivial registration errors during untracked image frames. In this work, we present a novel algorithm for GPU-accelerated 2D/3D registration and apply it to the problem of TEE probe tracking in XRF sequences. Implementation in `CUDA C` resulted in an extremely fast similarity computation of $< 80\ \mu s$, which in turn enabled registration frame rates ranging from 23.6-92.3 fps. The method was validated on simulated and clinical datasets and achieved target registration errors comparable to previously reported methods but at much faster registration speeds. Our results show, for the first time, the ability to accurately register TEE and XRF coordinate systems at fluoroscopic frame rates without the need for external hardware. The algorithm is generic and can potentially be applied to other 2D/3D registration problems where real-time performance is required.

1 Introduction

Image registration between transesophageal echocardiography (TEE) and x-ray fluoroscopy (XRF) has generated interest in recent years [1] as a tool for enhancing image guidance during structural heart interventions. XRF is considered the primary imaging modality for real-time visualization of devices, while TEE can image soft-tissue structures in real-time. Combining these two modalities in a single visualization framework has the potential to provide the best of both worlds: simultaneous imaging of devices and cardiac anatomy.

Registration can be accomplished by estimating the 3D pose of the TEE probe in the XRF imaging space using a variety of methods. 2D/3D registration methods are capable of accurately estimating all pose parameters by iteratively matching a 3D model of the probe to the XRF image. In [2,3], this was accomplished by generating a digitally reconstructed radiograph (DRR) and computing a similarity metric between the DRR and the XRF image. DRR generation was significantly accelerated using a GPU-based raycasting algorithm, but the overall registration frame rate was still on the order of $0.3 - 2.0$ frames-per-second

N. Navab et al. (Eds.): MICCAI 2015, Part I, LNCS 9349, pp. 290–297, 2015.
DOI: 10.1007/978-3-319-24553-9_36

(fps) for a single plane XRF system. During a cardiac procedure, the probe can move around quickly due to cardiorespiratory motion or physician manipulation. There is therefore a need for a registration method that performs at a typical XRF imaging frame rate (e.g. 15 fps).

In [4], accurate, 20 fps registration was accomplished by attaching radio-opaque fiducials to the TEE probe. Aside from the need for custom modification, this solution was undesirable due to its potential to increase the risk of esophageal injury. In [5], DRR generation was accelerated by modeling the TEE probe as a mesh and using `OpenGL` based rendering. DRR computation was significantly accelerated, but the overall similarity metric computation time (1 ms per iteration) is still not fast enough to perform registration at imaging frame rates based on results reported in this paper.

In this work, we report on a novel 2D/3D registration algorithm that can operate at between 23.6 and 92.3 fps. Similar to the work presented in [6], our algorithm efficiently computes an image similarity metric without explicitly generating any DRRs. In simulated and clinical datasets, our method performed similarly in terms of target registration error to standard methods combining ray-casting with normalized cross-correlation (NCC) and gradient correlation (GCC) similarity metrics, but operated at much higher frame rates.

2 Methods

2.1 Algorithm

Image-based 2D/3D registration is accomplished by estimating the 3D location and orientation (pose) of an object, generating a DRR based on this estimate, and comparing the DRR to the XRF image using a computed image similarity metric. Using non-linear optimization, this process is repeated until the similarity converges to an optimal value. Since this is an iterative process, a key determinant of overall registration time is the time needed to generate the DRR at each step of the optimization. For our application, optimization typically requires 150-300 similarity computations, depending on how close the initial pose is to the final solution. This means that both DRR generation and similarity computation need to be completed in roughly 300 μs on average for 15 fps registration. DRRs are typically generated using raycasting techniques. These methods compute line integrals, at each DRR pixel, along simulated x-rays passing through a volume of interest. An alternative method is splatting, where a DRR is generated by spatially transforming a 3D point-cloud model, projecting the transformed points onto the detector plane, and summing up values at discrete detector pixel positions. The point model is often generated from a CT scan. Mathematically, the DRR can be expressed as:

$$D(u_i) = \sum_{j \in S_i} -V(x_j),\ S_i = \{\ j \mid \lfloor P \cdot T \cdot x_j \rceil = u_i\ \} \tag{1}$$

Here, S_i refers to the set of points that project onto pixel i after the model has been spatially transformed, x_j is the 3D coordinate of the jth model point, $V(x_j)$ is the intensity value associated with the jth model point, T is the spatial transformation matrix describing 6DOF translation and rotation, and P is the projection matrix modeling the imaging process. Fig. 1 demonstrates a comparison of TEE probe DRRs generated using raycasting and splatting.

When using only a CPU for computation, splatting can be more computationally efficient than raycasting, especially when the size of the point cloud is small compared to the size of the data volume it was derived from. However, splatting does not necessarily translate well to the GPU, because every projected point must perform an *indirect write* operation at a random pixel (see Fig. 2, left, line 3). However, it can be shown that the correlation similarity metric can be reformulated so that all of the write operations are replaced with extremely fast texture reads on the GPU.

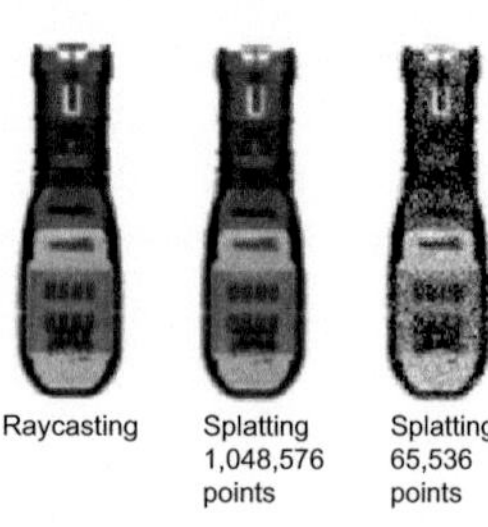

Fig. 1. Methods for generating probe DRRs.

Consider the correlation (CC) between an XRF image $I(u)$ and a DRR $D(u)$:

$$CC = \sum_i I(u_i)D(u_i) \tag{2}$$

For a splat-generated DRR, we can substitute the $D(u)$ term to obtain:

$$CC = \sum_i I(u_i)(\sum_{j \in S_i} -V(x_j)) = -\sum_i \sum_{j \in S_i} I(P \cdot T \cdot\ x_j)V(x_j) \tag{3}$$

Finally, this simplifies to a sum over all 3D points:

$$CC = -\sum_j I(P \cdot T \cdot\ x_j)V(x_j) \tag{4}$$

This expression simply states that the correlation is equal to the sum, over all 3D points, of the point intensity times the value of the pixel that it projects onto. Equation 4 shows that the DRR does not need to be explicitly generated to compute the similarity, enabling more efficient computation (Fig. 2).

```
//Splat correlation w/ DRRs
1  for each point x
2     u = P*T*x
3     DRR[u]=DRR[u] + -V[x]
4  for each pixel u
5     cc+=DRR[u]*I[u]
```

```
//Direct method w/o DRRs
1  for each point x
2     u = P*T*x
3     cc+=I[u] * -V[x]
4
5
```

Fig. 2. Pseudo-code for computation of correlation for explicit DRR generation (left) and the proposed method (right).

Because this similarity is inspired by splatting and is directly computed from the image, without the explicit generation of a DRR, we refer to it as "direct splat correlation" (DSC).

2.2 Experiments

3D TEE Model A Philips X7-2t TEE probe was used in this study. The 3D model of the TEE probe was generated from a cone beam CT image (Philips FD20). A point cloud representation of the probe was created using the following procedure:

1. Features in the probe CT that were visually classified as having high-intensities were manually segmented.
2. 2^{16} points were randomly generated within the segmented region. This was the smallest number of points that fit the criteria for both computational efficiency and accuracy.
3. Linear interpolation was used to assign an intensity value to each point.

Computer Hardware and Software. All experiments were run on a Dell Precision T7500 work station running Ubuntu Linux with a 3.47 GHz Intel Xeon processor and a NVIDIA Tesla K20 GPU. VNL libraries were used for optimization, and all similarity functions were implemented in `CUDA C`. Retrospective clinical dataset processing was approved by the local institutional review board.

Simulations. The first set of experiments tested the accuracy and speed of the algorithm *in silico* compared to standard methods for XRF/TEE registration reported in [2,3]. Simulation images (I_{sim}) were a hybrid of real background anatomy (I_{xrf}) and synthetic DRRs (I_{drr}).

Synthetic DRRs were rendered using the splatting method with a point cloud large enough to generate high quality DRRs (2^{21} points). The background anatomy was obtained using images from transcatheter aortic valve implantation (TAVI) procedures and the hybrid image was formulated as:

$$I_{sim} = I_{xrf} \cdot e^{-\alpha I_{drr}} \tag{5}$$

The parameter α controlled the probe to background contrast and was randomly varied to generate a contrast ratio ranging from 0.45 to 0.85 for each experiment. Fig. 3 shows a few examples of the simulated images.

For each experiment, the TEE probe was placed at a random location and orientation within the XRF C-arm image space. Based on our observations from an image database of TAVI cases, the TEE probe rarely has Euler angle rotations outside the range of -75° to 75° about its primary axis (y-axis), -30° to 30° about the x-axis of the image detector, and -45° to 45° about the source-detector axis (z-axis). Once an initial pose was created, a random mis-registration was applied, which the experiments attempted to recover. The random mis-registration was

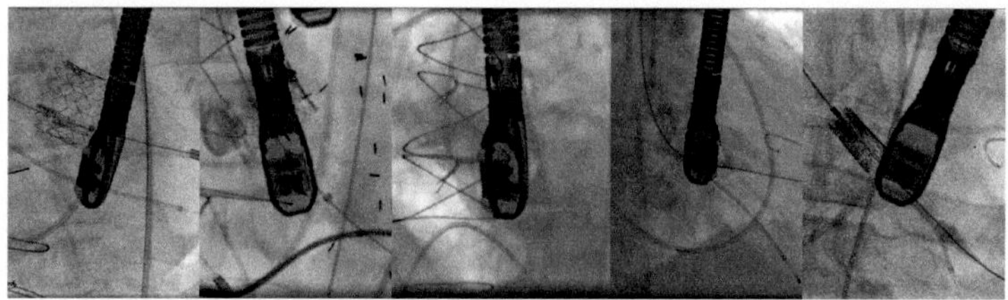

Fig. 3. Examples of simulated images

chosen from a zero mean uniform distribution over ranges of 3.0 mm, 3.0 mm, 5.0 mm, 30°, 30°, 6° for the parameters $t_x, t_y, t_z, \theta_x, \theta_y, \theta_z$, respectively.

Once the simulated image and mis-registration was generated, 3 different algorithms and 2 optimizers were tested. The first algorithm was the proposed algorithm (DSC), and the second and third were normalized cross-correlation and gradient correlation using raycasted DRRs (rcNCC, rcGCC, see [7] for details). The two optimizers tested were the Nelder-Mead (nm) and Powell (pwl) methods, both of which work well for low-dimensional optimization problems that do not have analytical cost function gradients.

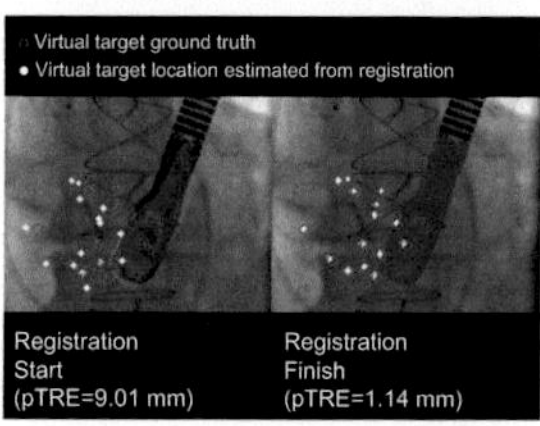

Fig. 4. Virtual targets used to compute pTRE before and after registration

The simulation experiments assumed a single x-ray projection, which typically results in inaccurate estimates of t_z. Therefore, we focused on optimization of the other five parameters, which resulted in a faster, more accurate optimization problem. Furthermore, when projecting echo data onto the XRF image, the errors in the estimation of t_z have little effect on target projection errors (for the same reason that t_z is difficult to estimate in the first place). Therefore, our accuracy metric was projection target registration error (pTRE), which was the root-mean-square error between known target points in XRF and estimated target points from echo following registration and projection to the XRF image:

$$\text{pTRE} = \sqrt{\frac{1}{N}\sum_n \left(\left\| \frac{1}{m_n}(p_n^{(xrf)} - P \cdot T \cdot p_n^{(echo)}) \right\|_2 \right)^2} \quad (6)$$

where m_n is the projective magnification of point $T \cdot p_n^{(echo)}$.

pTRE, % of successful registrations, and frame rate were reported for each experiment. We chose to define a successful registration as a pTRE < 5.0 mm based on results from [3] where pTRE of 2.9 mm was the average error, but in reality this measure is application dependent. pTRE is only computed for successful registrations, to avoid large registration errors skewing the statistics. 5000 experiments were performed.

For all experiments, virtual target points were used to compute pTRE. The virtual target points were randomly generated from within the center of a virtual ultrasound volume emanating from the TEE probe, at a mean distance of 50 mm from the probe face (Fig. 4). Errors from the probe model to echo volume calibration (${}^{echo}T_{probe}$) were not considered in the analysis.

Clinical Datasets. Validation was also performed on real images from TAVI procedures. 39 image sequences from 19 cases (3635 frames) were identified as containing significant probe movement due to physician manipulation or cardiorespiratory motion. Due to a lack of ground truth, a surrogate ground truth was created for each sequence using the following procedure:

1. Manual registration was performed for the first frame of each sequence.
2. The initial manual registration was refined using the rcGCC-pwl method.
3. rcGCC-pwl was used to define the ground truth registration at each consecutive frame. Each sequence was then visually checked, frame-by-frame, for errors. The probe could not be tracked in four sequences and they were removed from the analysis.

For the clinical datasets, we examined the tracking accuracy and robustness under real clinical conditions where both image streaming and registration delays must be considered. Assuming 15 fps image streaming, the registration lag was calculated as $n_{lag} = ceil(15 \times t_{registration})$ frames. Each skipped frame was only allowed to use the most recently finished registration result for its pTRE calculation, and every registration (T_n) was initialized with the most recently processed registration result ($T_{n-n_{lag}}$). Note that slower registration times resulted in increased pTRE due to not only more skipped frames but also less accurate frame-to-frame initialization.

3 Results

Simulations Results for the simulation studies are shown in Fig. 5. In terms of pTRE, the rcNCC and rcGCC both slightly outperformed the DSC method, with the rcGCC-pwl combination having roughly half the error of the DSC-nm method. However, the mean and standard deviation of all methods fell within the range of clinical acceptability (< 2.0 mm). Furthermore, the DSC-nm combination outperformed the other methods in terms of success rate, indicating that, although the other methods are slightly more accurate, the DSC-nm method is more robust. The average frame rate for DSC was 33.0 ± 9.4 fps (mean $\pm$ std). This is over an order of magnitude faster than the other methods, which were 3.0 ± 1.2 and 2.2 ± 0.9 fps for rcNCC-nm and rcGCC-nm, respectively.

Clinical Datasets Fig. 6 shows results for all clinical sequences. It can be seen that the lowest average pTRE was found using the rcGCC method, but the meaning of this result is unclear due to the fact that rcGCC was used as a proxy measure for the ground truth. Frame-rate increased compared to simulations, averaging 73.1 ± 19.2 fps for DSC-nm, 8.9 ± 2.2 fps for rcNCC-nm, and 5.9

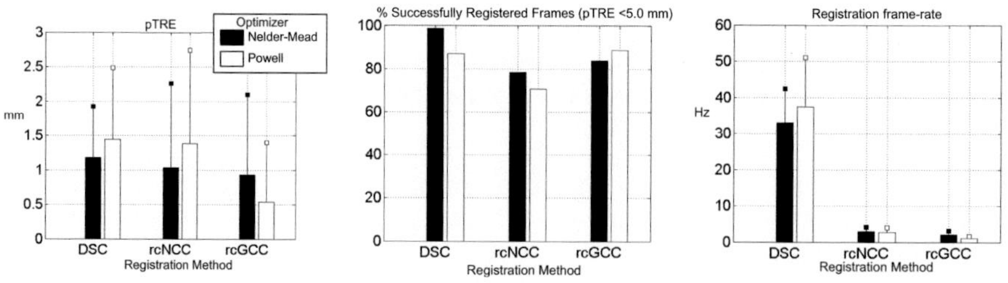

Fig. 5. Simulations. Left: Average pTRE for successful registrations. Comparisons between methods were all statistically significant ($p < 0.001$). Middle: Percentage of successfully registered frames (pTRE<5.0 mm). Right: Average frame rate.

$\pm$ 1.5 fps for rcGCC-nm. This was due to the fact that the difference in pose parameters between frames was generally smaller for the clinical datasets and therefore roughly half of the similarity function computations were needed for convergence.

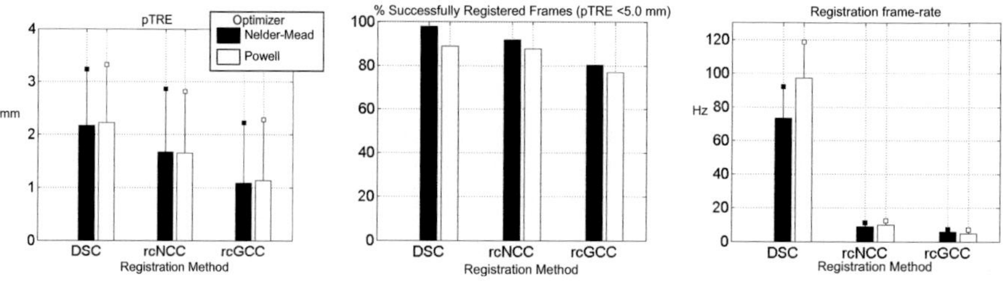

Fig. 6. Clinical datasets. Left: Average pTRE for successful registrations. Comparisons between methods were all statistically significant ($p < 0.001$). Middle: Percentage of successfully registered frames (pTRE<5.0 mm). Right: Average frame rate.

4 Discussion

The presented DSC method is an order of magnitude faster than the rcNCC and rcGCC methods, and is the only method that is able to reliably track the TEE probe without skipping frames. The frame rate increase comes at the cost of an increase in pTRE, which may be due to the lack of normalization by the DRR standard deviation used for the NCC and GCC metric computations. However, results indicate that the increase in error is still clinically acceptable. Results from the simulations and clinical datasets both show that the DSC method results in fewer failed registrations, indicating that the DSC metric may have a wider basin of convergence than the other similarity functions and therefore is more robust to poor initialization. In the future we will explore a hybrid registration approach combining the DSC and rcGCC methods, using DSC to obtain a fast, robust initial result and then refining the registration with rcGCC for better accuracy. Validation in bi-plane XRF is another topic for future work. We believe that the DSC method has the potential to work well as a real-time 5DOF/6DOF device tracking algorithm. In particular, the algorithm may be well suited for tracking relatively small, high contrast objects such as a recently proposed fiducial embedded intracardiac echo catheter [8]. Future work will focus on integration with echo image processing for real-time multimodal visualization during cardiac interventions.

5 Conclusion

A method for fast 2D/3D registration of devices in XRF images is presented. Average registration frame rates were 33.0 ± 9.4 fps and 73.1 ± 19.2 fps for simulated and clinical datasets, respectively. Results also indicate that the proposed method converges to a clinically acceptable target registration error more often than prior methods. Future work will focus on clinical implementation and application of the algorithm to other devices.

References

1. Fagan, T.E., Truong, U.T., Jone, P.N., Bracken, J., Quaife, R., Hazeem, A.A.A., Salcedo, E.E., Fonseca, B.M.: Multimodality 3-dimensional image integration for congenital cardiac catheterization. Methodist DeBakey Cardiovascular Journal 10(2), 68 (2014)
2. Gao, G., Penney, G., Ma, Y., Gogin, N., Cathier, P., Arujuna, A., Morton, G., Caulfield, D., Gill, J., Aldo Rinaldi, C., et al.: Registration of 3D trans-esophageal echocardiography to X-ray fluoroscopy using image-based probe tracking. Medical Image Analysis 16(1), 38–49 (2012)
3. Housden, R.J., et al.: Evaluation of a Real-Time Hybrid Three-Dimensional Echo and X-Ray Imaging System for Guidance of Cardiac Catheterisation Procedures. In: Ayache, N., Delingette, H., Golland, P., Mori, K. (eds.) MICCAI 2012, Part II. LNCS, vol. 7511, pp. 25–32. Springer, Heidelberg (2012)
4. Lang, P., Seslija, P., Chu, M.W., Bainbridge, D., Guiraudon, G.M., Jones, D.L., Peters, T.M.: US–fluoroscopy Registration for Transcatheter Aortic Valve Implantation. IEEE Transactions on Biomedical Engineering 59(5), 1444–1453 (2012)
5. Kaiser, M., John, M., Borsdorf, A., Mountney, P., Ionasec, R., Nöttling, A., Kiefer, P., Seeburger, J., Neumuth, T.: Significant acceleration of 2D-3D registration-based fusion of ultrasound and x-ray images by mesh-based DRR rendering. In: Medical Imaging, International Society for Optics and Photonics, p. 867111 (2013)
6. Wein, W., Röper, B., Navab, N.: 2D/3D registration based on volume gradients. In: Medical Imaging, International Society for Optics and Photonics, pp. 144–150 (2005)
7. Penney, G.P., Weese, J., Little, J.A., Desmedt, P., Hill, D.L., Hawkes, D.J.: A comparison of similarity measures for use in 2D-3D medical image registration. IEEE Transactions on Medical Imaging 17(4), 586–595 (1998)
8. Ralovich, K., John, M., Camus, E., Navab, N., Heimann, T.: 6DoF catheter detection, application to intracardiac echocardiography. In: Golland, P., Hata, N., Barillot, C., Hornegger, J., Howe, R. (eds.) MICCAI 2014, Part II. LNCS, vol. 8674, pp. 635–642. Springer, Heidelberg (2014)

Rigid Motion Compensation in Interventional C-arm CT Using Consistency Measure on Projection Data

Robert Frysch and Georg Rose

Institute for Medical Engineering, University of Magdeburg, Germany
robert.frysch@ovgu.de

Abstract. Interventional C-arm CT has the potential to visualize brain hemorrhages in the operating suite and save valuable time for stroke patients. Due to the critical constitution of the patients, C-arm CT images are frequently affected by patient motion artifacts, which often makes the reliable diagnosis of hemorrhages impossible. In this work, we propose a geometric optimization algorithm to compensate for these artifacts and present first results. The algorithm is based on a projection data consistency measure, which avoids computationally expensive forward- and backprojection steps in the optimization process. The ability to estimate movements with this measure is investigated for different rigid degrees of freedom. It was shown that out-of-plane parameters, i. e. geometrical deviations perpendicular to the plane of rotation, can be estimated with high precision. Movement artifacts in reconstructions are consistently reduced throughout all analyzed clinical datasets. With its low computational cost and high robustness, the proposed algorithm is well-suited for integration into clinical software prototypes for further evaluation.

1 Introduction

The soft tissue contrast resolution of C-arm based computed tomography (CT) has been continuously improved over the past decade. Recent publications already demonstrate good visibility of brain hemorrhages [11]. However, the application of the interventional C-arm for the acute stroke assessment, providing the ability for stroke diagnosis in the operating room, requires a reliable detection of even very small bleedings also in the vicinity of bones. In order to meet these requirements, one has to overcome image quality disturbances caused by beam hardening, poor scatter compensation and particularly motion of the patients during the long acquisition times.

We are targeting a motion compensation method for C-arm CT which neither depends on additional measurements nor requires assumptions or information about the object's shape. Various methods can be found in the literature discussing geometric calibration and motion compensation, which are closely related. Certain approaches are based on volumetric reconstructions in the optimization processes. Either the objective function determines the similarity of

N. Navab et al. (Eds.): MICCAI 2015, Part I, LNCS 9349, pp. 298–306, 2015.
DOI: 10.1007/978-3-319-24553-9_37

simulated and measured projections (2D-3D registration) [8] or operates in the volume domain quantifying geometric misadjustment with an artifact measure ("symptomatical approach") [5]. Other approaches, like the proposed, operate only on the redundancies in the projection images. Therefore, computationally intensive reconstruction within the optimization procedure becomes obsolete, allowing for very short overall processing time. Epipolar geometry is typically used to identify redundancies [12,7]. Debbeler et al. [3] introduced a novel online geometric calibration approach for industrial CT using a global optimization of several geometric parameters of the CT alignment (e. g. detector shift). This approach was extended in Maass et al. [6] to a local adaption of the geometry of each projection image. It benefits from a robust consistency measure, which exploits redundancies in the complete acquired projection data based on Grangeat's fundamental relation for cone-beam CT [4]. A reformulation of this consistency measure for the context of epipolar geometry is provided by Aichert et al. [2,1]. Therein, a simulation study was performed for the compensation of artificial geometry shifts in small sets of cone-beam projections. In this work, we adapt this strategy to real C-arm short scans, i. e. a cone-beam geometry with semicircle trajectory. We present first reconstruction results of rigid motion compensation for real patient data based on the consistency measure.

At first, we investigated the ability of this approach to estimate the motion parameters for several degrees of freedom. Based on these insights, we applied a customized geometry optimization procedure to projections from five clinical datasets. This geometric adaptation was followed by a standard reconstruction (FDK). Reconstructed images without motion compensation were used for comparison.

2 Methods

2.1 Objective Function

One can define a consistency measure based on redundancies occurring in CT projection datasets. For this, we consider a plane $\{\mathbf{n}, l\}$: $\{\mathbf{x} \in \mathbb{R}^3 \,|\, \mathbf{n} \cdot \mathbf{x} = l\}$ in the patient's world coordinate system with the normal unit vector $\mathbf{n}$ and the distance l to the origin. The projection's redundancies manifest in Grangeat's fundamental relation which connects the 3D Radon transform[1] $r(\mathbf{n}, l)$ with an intermediate function $S_i(\mathbf{n})$ (cf. Defrise et al. [4]):

$$S_i(\mathbf{n}) := -\int_{S^2} \mathbf{dm}\, \delta'(\mathbf{m} \cdot \mathbf{n}) g_i(\mathbf{m}) = \frac{\partial}{\partial l}\, r(\mathbf{n}, l)|_{l=\mathbf{C}_i \cdot \mathbf{n}} \,. \tag{1}$$

$\mathbf{C}_i$ denotes the vector to the point of the i'th x-ray source position lying on the plane. The intermediate function $S_i(\mathbf{n})$ is a transformation of the cone-beam projections $g_i(\mathbf{m})$ (also called X-ray transform; alternative representation of the 2D projection images $g_i(x, y)$), where $\mathbf{m}$ is the direction of a ray starting from $\mathbf{C}_i$. The integration is over the unit 2-sphere and $\delta'(x)$ is the derivative of the

[1] 3D radon transform: integrals over 2D planes of a three-dimensional scalar field.

Dirac delta distribution. Thus, there are only contributions from $g_i(\mathbf{m})$, when $\mathbf{m}$ is perpendicular to $\mathbf{n}$. In other words the integration is reduced to an 1D manifold considering only x-rays which lie within the plane $\{\mathbf{n}, l = \mathbf{C}_i \cdot \mathbf{n}\}$, i. e. add up projection values located at the line of intersection between this plane and the detector plane. As a consequence, it is appropriate to identify the plane $\{\mathbf{n}, l\}$ with the intersection line in the i'th detector coordinate system using conventional 2D Radon parametrization $\{\vartheta, s\}$ (ϑ denotes the angle of the line's normal and s the distance to origin). The coordinate transformation to Radon parameters of the i'th local system $\{\mathbf{n}, l\} \to \{\vartheta, s\}_i$ in the integral (1) can also be found in Defrise et al. [4]. Its rewritten result is:

$$S_i(\vartheta, s) = \frac{s^2 + D^2}{D^2} \cdot \frac{\partial}{\partial s} \Re\left[\tilde{g}_i\right](\vartheta, s), \text{ with } \tilde{g}_i(x, y) = \frac{D}{\sqrt{x^2 + y^2 + D^2}} \cdot g_i(x, y)\,. \tag{2}$$

D is the source-detector distance and $\Re\,[\,.\,](\vartheta, s)$ the 2D Radon transform (parallel beam) which has to be applied to cosine weighted projections $\tilde{g}_i(x, y)$.

Assuming a static object, the expression at the right-hand side of Grangeat's equation (1) depends only on the plane $\{\mathbf{n}, l\}$. By selecting another projection g_j with source position $\mathbf{C}_j$ which also fulfills $l = \mathbf{C}_j \cdot \mathbf{n}$, i. e. it is located in the same plane, one can conclude that the intermediate function values $S_i(\mathbf{n}) = S_i(\vartheta_i, s_i)$ and $S_j(\mathbf{n}) = S_j(\vartheta_j, s_j)$ are equal. Now, we can fix the source positions and consider N different planes with normal vectors $\mathbf{n}^n$ for which $\mathbf{C}_i \cdot \mathbf{n}^n = \mathbf{C}_j \cdot \mathbf{n}^n$ holds true. For each of these planes redundant pairs $S_i(\vartheta_i^n, s_i^n) \overset{!}{=} S_j(\vartheta_j^n, s_j^n)$ from two projections can be found.

We define the following error matrix (norm type) describing the consistency of each combination of two projection images:

$$\varepsilon_{ij} := \frac{1}{N} \sum_{n=1}^{N} \left| S_i(\vartheta_i^n, s_i^n) - S_j(\vartheta_j^n, s_j^n) \right|^p, \quad N \overset{\text{gen.}}{=} N_{ij}\,.$$

The parameter p controls properties of this metric like smoothness, detectability of inconsistencies or consideration of outliers and has to be chosen empirically. We figured out a reliable value of $p = 0.3$ in simulations and used it throughout all experiments. In general, the number of available mutual planes N containing $\mathbf{C}_i$ and $\mathbf{C}_j$ depends on i and j. This is due to divergent geometric situations of combinations of two C-arm positions and the finiteness of the detector (more detailed in section 2.3). A summation of the error function ε_{ij} enables us to quantify the consistency of a set of projections with indices $\mathbf{I} = \{i_1, \ldots, i_I\}$ with respect to all the other J existing projections:

$$E_{\mathbf{I}} := \sum_{i \in \mathbf{I}} \sum_{j \notin \mathbf{I}} \varepsilon_{ij}\,.$$

Thus, we obtain an objective function for a given set of I projection images containing $\overline{N} \times I \times J$ redundant pairs of values (with $\overline{N}$ as a corresponding average of N_{ij}). In the special case of considering only one projection angle i, we obtain $E_i = \sum_{j \neq i} \varepsilon_{ij}$. The high quantity of redundant pairs provides a good basis for an optimization which is robust in terms of noise.

2.2 Optimization Procedure

We define a world coordinate system which is orientated in such a way that the z-axis is parallel to the C-arm's rotational axis. Our optimization approach for a rigid geometric modification is based on the following parameter set

$$\triangle\mathbf{p} := \begin{bmatrix} \boldsymbol{\alpha} \\ \boldsymbol{\tau} \end{bmatrix}, \text{with } \boldsymbol{\tau} = \begin{bmatrix} \tau_x \\ \tau_y \\ \tau_z \end{bmatrix}, \ \boldsymbol{\alpha} = \begin{bmatrix} \alpha_x \\ \alpha_y \\ \alpha_z \end{bmatrix},$$

thus including a shift of the world coordinate system by a vector $\boldsymbol{\tau}$ as well as a rotation w.r.t. the axis $\boldsymbol{\alpha}$ by an angle $\|\boldsymbol{\alpha}\|$. It defines a useful dependency of the objective function $E_{\mathbf{I}} = E_{\mathbf{I}}(\triangle\mathbf{p})$ without ambiguous points in the 6D optimization space. Moreover, we can separate these geometric changes into two distinctive groups:

$$\text{out-of-plane parameters: } \triangle\mathbf{p}_{\mathsf{OP}} = \begin{bmatrix} \alpha_x \\ \alpha_y \\ t_z \end{bmatrix}, \text{ in-plane parameters: } \triangle\mathbf{p}_{\mathsf{IP}} = \begin{bmatrix} \alpha_z \\ t_x \\ t_y \end{bmatrix}.$$

Due to the semicircle geometry of the short scan, most projections do not have opposing views. Therefore, planes including X-ray sources of such projections and hitting the (limited) detector can only be slightly tilted from the plane of rotation. It was expected that the intermediate function values of those would not be susceptible to modifications of in-plane (IP) parameters, because the according 3D Radon transform value is not affected by translations/rotations within those planes (or planes parallel to them). On the contrary, geometric variations stepping out of the plane of rotation should significantly change the consistency error ε_{ij}.

This expectation was confirmed by simulations with a 3D Shepp-Logan phantom. In figure 1, only one of the six parameters $\triangle\mathbf{p}$ is changed from a perfect semicircle trajectory for each angle (row) and its consistency error ε_{ij} is determined by the unaltered other angles (columns). One can observe significant increases in the error function throughout all projections when changing one of the out-of-plane (OP) parameters $\triangle\mathbf{p}_{\mathsf{OP}}$. In contrast, when modifying IP parameters $\triangle\mathbf{p}_{\mathsf{IP}}$, the consistency measure is only sensible for the first and last projections, which represent opposite views and offer the most redundancy. To be more precise, this includes all projections containing identical rays (angular range equals to two times of the opening angle of the fan). In the following these projections will be referred to as the "fan angle sector".

Considering these findings, a separate optimization of the three OP parameters was performed for each single projection. If required, optimization can be extended to the full 6D $\triangle\mathbf{p}$ inside the fan angle sector as well as the inter-fan angle sector, if we increase the angle block length I, e. g. $I = 2$ (for fan angle

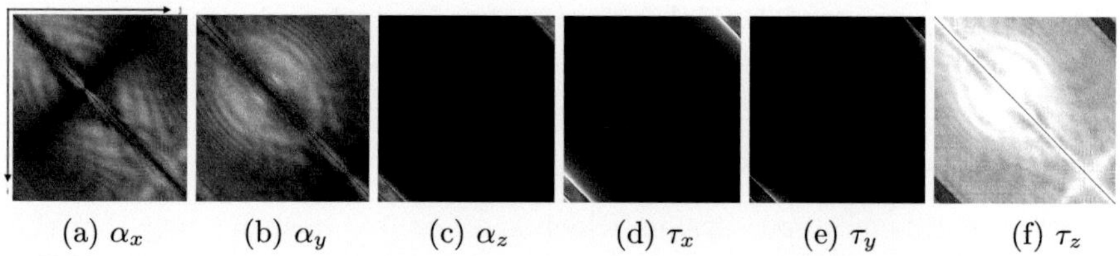

(a) α_x (b) α_y (c) α_z (d) τ_x (e) τ_y (f) τ_z

Fig. 1. Consistency measure ε_{ij} of each single rigid degree of freedom. For each defined geometry parameter, the increase of the error matrix ε_{ij} is depicted for misadjustments between two projections at row i and column j of 0.5 ° or 0.5 mm, respectively. The same grey scale window is used for each matrix. The largest increase of the error can be observed for the OP parameter in (a), (b) and (f).

sector) and $I = 15$ (for inter-fan angle sector). Optimizing a larger block of $\mathbf{I}$ results in a higher number of redundant pairs in the objective function leading to more support. However, a further consequence of the increased block size, the estimation of the geometry of projections with rapid patient motion is hampered.

2.3 Implementation

The intermediate function was computed on the CPU before the actual optimization routine. This function was then sampled and stored for the optimization process in the GPU's video RAM:

1. cosine weighting of $g_i(x, y)$
2. Radon transformation based on the model of Siddon [10] with a sampling rate of $\Delta s = 1$ Pixel and $\Delta\vartheta = 0.5\,°$
3. numerical differentiation with respect to s (centered derivative filter $[-1, 0, 1]$) and weighting according to (2)

The weightings in steps 1. and 2. could be computed as pre-processing steps since the intrinsic parameter of the C-arm system were fixed within the optimization routine. The sampling rates Δs und $\Delta\vartheta$ of the Radon transformation were determined empirically by selecting the configuration with the lowest numerical error in the simulations.

The essential part of the optimization represents the search for the redundant Radon pairs $(\vartheta_i, s_i) \leftrightarrow (\vartheta_j, s_j)$ of two projections required to determine the ε_{ij}. For that, we used the constraint that two source positions $\mathbf{C}_i$ and $\mathbf{C}_j$ are on the same plane. An intuitive way of gathering the related set of planes is to rotate an initial plane around a line connecting the two sources by an angle ϕ. Using this strategy, we were able to estimate several redundant pairs of intermediate function values by a fast linear interpolation on video the GPU's RAM. Thereby, only those planes with intersection lines $\{\vartheta, s\}_{i/j}$ located inside both detector areas were considered. The smallest reasonable change $\Delta\phi$ of the plane rotation is given by the sampling of the Radon transformation. It was estimated through geometric consideration (not shown here). Using the above parameters and the geometry of a Siemens Artis Q C-arm with source-detector distance $D = 1.2\,\text{m}$, detector resolution of 0.308×0.308 mm and 1240×960 pixels, we estimated a lower bound of $\Delta\phi \approx 0.015\,°$, resulting in a maximum number of redundant pairs $N_{\text{max}} = \frac{180\,°}{\Delta\phi} \approx 12,000$. As already mentioned in section 2.1, this amount is not attainable for all projection combinations when using equidistant rotational steps. Especially, the overall amount for each angle is not equally distributed, due to limited angle of rotation (approx. 200 °) in short scans (in connection with limited detector size). The number of usable planes (associated with available redundant values) is shown in figure 2.

The computation of the objective function $E_{\mathbf{I}}$ was performed for each ε_{ij} in parallel on GPU using OpenCL programming language. For minimization of the objective function, we used a nonlinear optimization algorithm from the open-source library NLopt[2] which is based on T. Rowan's "Subplex" [9] implementation.

In summary, the main methodical differences to the work of Maass et al. [6] are: nonlinear optimizer instead of grid search, multidimensional optimizing of the world coordinate system instead of single intrinsic CT geometry parameters (motion instead of calibration), $p = 0.3$ instead of $p = 2$ (smoothing the objective function), $N_{\text{max}} = 12,000$ instead of $N_{\text{max}} = 768$.
With these adaptions, we tried to overcome the inferior preconditions of the C-arm in terms of data quality (e. g. partial overexposure) and short-scan geometry.

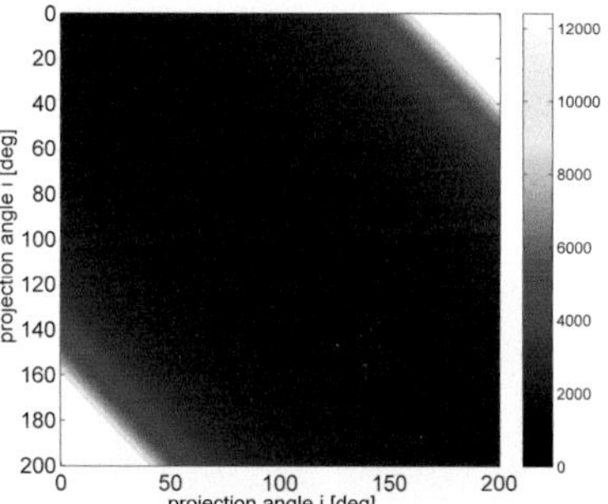

Fig. 2. Number of usable redundant Radon planes for each X-ray image pair of a short scan (0 ° . . . 200 °). Most of the planes are concentrated at the fan angle sector containing opposite views.

3 Results

A Siemens Artis Q system has been used to acquire the clinical data using a 20 sec protocol with 496 projection images. Figure 3 depicts the effect of the optimization on the error matrix ε_{ij}. In this example, the acquisition of a patient head with distinct movements was used. One can notice an increase of the consistency error ε_{ij} as well the totalized $E_i = \sum_j \varepsilon_{ij}$ for the misadjusted projections. The peaks in figure 3b are correlated with the amount of geometric changes after the optimization. The optimization was performed sequentially through all images, but was applied for all three OP parameter at once. Figure 4 depicts the improvement of the reconstruction (via FDK) in four datasets after the 3D OP optimization which was already sufficient in most cases. However, Figure 5

[2] Steven G. Johnson, The NLopt nonlinear-optimization package.

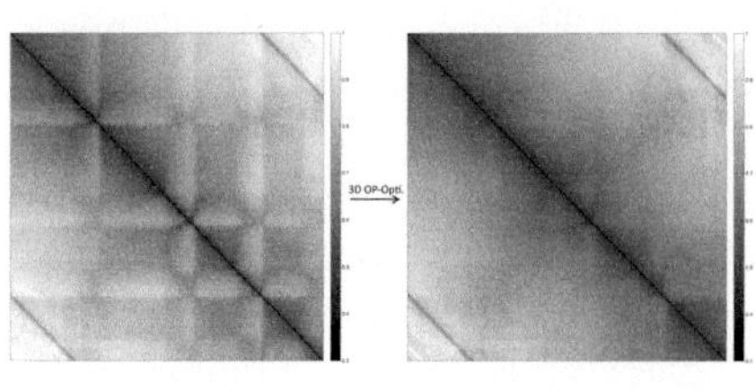

(a) Error matrix ε_{ij} before (left) and after (right) the optimization. Reconstructions are shown in the upper right in figure 4.

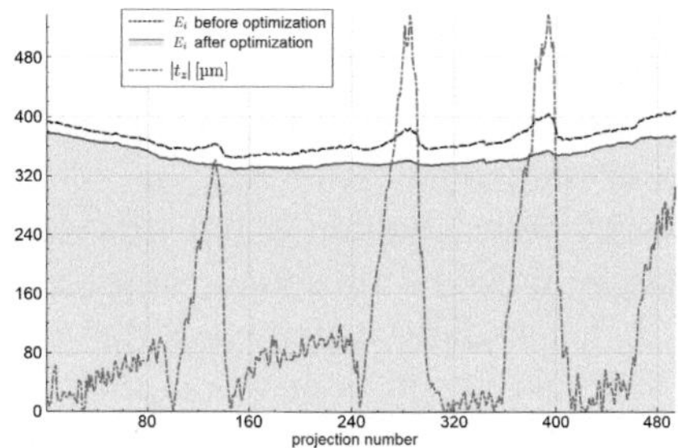

(b) Totalized Error E_i before and after the 3D OP optimization and the absolute value of the resulting OP parameter t_z.

Fig. 3. Impact of a sequential 3D OP parameter optimization on the consistency metric ε_{ij}, its summation E_i over columns and the translations $\{t_z\}_i$ in $\triangle \mathbf{p}_{\mathrm{OP}}$

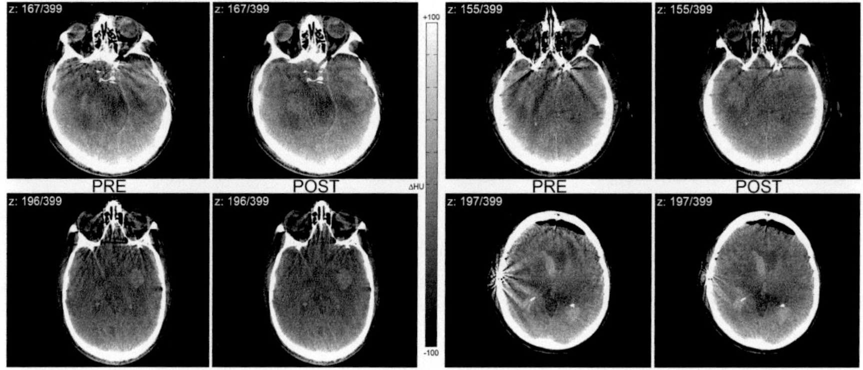

Fig. 4. Reconstructions of four clinical datasets before and after a sequential 3D OP motion compensation (very robust). Computation time per patient is about 30 sec using a standard gaming videocard AMD Radeon R9 280.

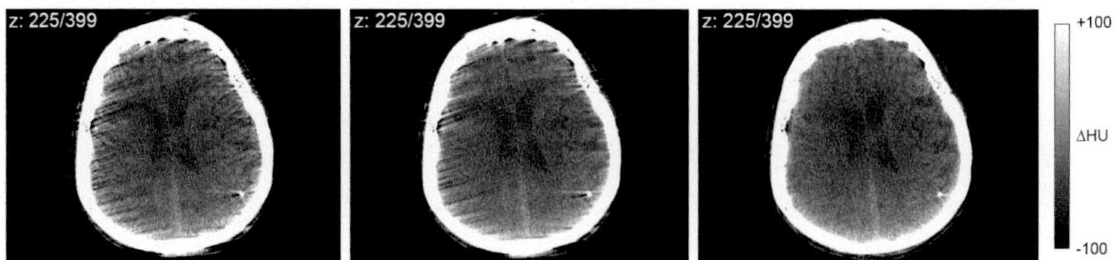

Fig. 5. Reconstruction with uncorrected geometry (left), after a sequential 3D OP motion compensation (center) and subsequent full 6D optimization (OP+IP).

presents a case where a 6D optimization of the whole parameter vector $\triangle \mathbf{p}$ provides further improvoment of image quality. Note that the 6D optimization is unstable in general and does not improve image quality in every case. This will be subject of future work.

4 Conclusions

In this work we show the possibility to compensate rigid patient motion in the out-of-plane parameters, which can be performed in a robust manner. These parameters can be separated from the other geometric directions and optimized in a 3D nonlinear minimization procedure. This leads to a robust motion compensation of the reconstructed images at a relatively low computational cost. In most cases, it was sufficient to neglect the in-plane parameters which are, in general, difficult to optimize. However, assumably, they have minor influence on the image quality. In one case, it was beneficial to consider all six degrees of freedom which was realized by optimizing a larger block of projections at once. Limitations may occur, if there are further artefacts within the projections due to truncation, detector overexposure or beam hardening. A refinement of the optimization strategy, e. g. the detection of motion based on pattern recognition in the error matrix ε_{ij}, can reduce the computational cost.

Acknowledgment. The work of this paper is partly funded by the German BMBF within the Forschungscampus *STIMULATE* (13GW0095A).

References

1. Aichert, A., Berger, M., Wang, J., Maass, N., Doerfler, A., Hornegger, J., Maier, A.: Epipolar consistency in transmission imaging. IEEE TMI (2015). Epub ahead of print, doi:10.1109/TMI.2015.2426417
2. Aichert, A., Maass, N., Deuerling-Zheng, Y., Berger, M., Manhart, M., Hornegger, J., Maier, A., Doerfler, A.: Redundancies in x-ray images due to the epipolar geometry for transmission imaging. In: Third CT Meeting, pp. 333–337 (2014)
3. Debbeler, C., Maass, N., Elter, M., Dennerlein, F., Buzug, T.M.: A new CT rawdata redundancy measure applied to automated misalignment correction. In: 12th Fully 3D, pp. 264–267 (2013)
4. Defrise, M., Clack, R.: A cone-beam reconstruction algorithm using shift-variant filtering and cone-beam backprojection. IEEE TMI 13(1), 186–195 (1994)
5. Kyriakou, Y., Lapp, R.M., Hillebrand, L., Ertel, D., Kalender, W.A.: Image-based online correction of misalignment artifacts in cone-beam CT. In: SPIE, vol. 7258, pp. 72581V–72581V–10 (2009)
6. Maass, N., Dennerlein, F., Aichert, A., Maier, A.: Geometrical jitter correction in computed tomography. In: Third CT Meeting, pp. 338–342 (2014)
7. Meng, Y., Gong, H., Yang, X.: Online geometric calibration of cone-beam computed tomography for arbitrary imaging objects. IEEE TMI 32(2), 278–288 (2013)
8. Muders, J., Hesser, J.: Stable and robust geometric self-calibration for cone-beam CT using mutual information. IEEE TNS 61(1), 202–217 (2014)
9. Rowan, T.: Functional Stability Analysis of Numerical Algorithms. Ph.d. thesis, University of Texas at Austin, Department of Computer Sciences (1990)

10. Siddon, R.L.: Fast calculation of the exact radiological path for a three-dimensional CT array. Medical Physics 12, 252–255 (1985)
11. Söderman, M., Babic, D., Holmin, S., Andersson, T.: Brain imaging with a flat detector C-arm. Neuroradiology 50, 863–868 (2008)
12. Wein, W., Ladikos, A.: Detecting patient motion in projection space for cone-beam computed tomography. In: Fichtinger, G., Martel, A., Peters, T. (eds.) MICCAI 2011, Part I. LNCS, vol. 6891, pp. 516–523. Springer, Heidelberg (2011)

Hough Forests for Real-Time, Automatic Device Localization in Fluoroscopic Images: Application to TAVR

Charles R. Hatt[1,2], Michael A. Speidel[1,2], and Amish N. Raval[2]

[1] Department of Medical Physics, University of Wisconsin, Madison, USA
[2] Division of Cardiovascular Medicine, University of Wisconsin, Madison, USA

Abstract. A method for real-time localization of devices in fluoroscopic images is presented. Device pose is estimated using a Hough forest based detection framework. The method was applied to two types of devices used for transcatheter aortic valve replacement: a transesophageal echo (TEE) probe and prosthetic valve (PV). Validation was performed on clinical datasets, where both the TEE probe and PV were successfully detected in 95.8% and 90.1% of images, respectively. TEE probe position and orientation errors were 1.42 ± 0.79 mm and $2.59^\circ \pm 1.87^\circ$, while PV position and orientation errors were 1.04 ± 0.77 mm and $2.90^\circ \pm 2.37^\circ$. The Hough forest was implemented in CUDA C, and was able to generate device location hypotheses in less than 50 ms for all experiments.

1 Introduction

Detection and pose estimation of devices in x-ray fluoroscopic (XRF) images is a challenging but important task for enabling multimodal image fusion in cardiac interventional procedures. For example, catheter detection and tracking can be used to provide motion compensation of anatomical roadmaps used to help guide electrophysiology procedures [1]. Another application which has recently gained interest is transesophageal echo (TEE) to XRF registration [2]. TEE/XRF registration allows anatomical information from echo to be combined with device imaging from XRF.

A procedure that may benefit from a smart integration of XRF and TEE imaging is transcatheter aortic valve replacement (TAVR). For example, obtaining the optimal 3D echo cut-planes for anatomical and device visualization is non-trivial, even for experienced echocardiographers. Furthermore, once the optimal echo view is obtained, the device is not necessarily easy to visualize. By registering the two modalities, a prosthetic valve (PV) can be detected in XRF, and its position and orientation may be used to compute the optimal echo cut-planes for visualization. The PV can then potentially be rendered within the 3D echo volume (Fig. 1) as an alternate imaging tool for guiding PV deployment.

A key component of the clinical workflow is automatic localization of the devices at the beginning of an image sequence. In this paper, we describe a common framework for TEE and PV localization in XRF images. A Hough

N. Navab et al. (Eds.): MICCAI 2015, Part I, LNCS 9349, pp. 307–314, 2015.
DOI: 10.1007/978-3-319-24553-9_38

forest (HF) detector was trained that can detect multiple parts of each device, allowing for estimation of in-plane pose parameters. The data was validated on 1077 clinical images of the TEE probe and 388 of the PV.

Previous Work. In [3], the TEE probe was detected using the probabilistic boosting-tree approach with Haar wavelets and steerable features. Out-of-plane rotations were estimated using an oriented gradient binary template library. Average detection time was 0.53 seconds. In [4], the work from [3] was extended by focusing on a framework for adapting a classifier generated with *in silico* training data to perform better on *in-vivo* test data. Impressive results for detection of in-plane TEE pose parameters were obtained in terms of localization accuracy, low false positive rate, and detection speed.

In [5], the PV was manually segmented and then automatically tracked using template matching. To eliminate the need for manual interaction during computed-aided interventions, the method presented in this paper focuses on automatic device localization using a HF framework. Previously, this framework was used for anatomy localization in CT volumes [6]. To the best of our knowledge, our work is the first to employ a real-time HF for device localization during image guided interventions.

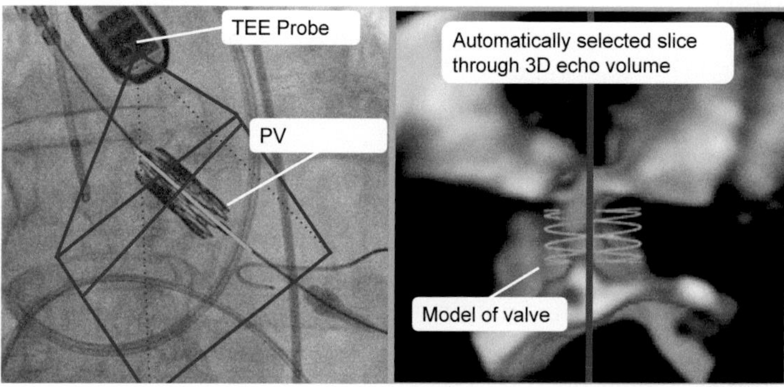

Fig. 1. Potential workflow enabled by TEE/XRF registration and PV detection. In the XRF image, the red line perpendicular to the PV corresponds to a plane through the echo image. The green line matches the viewing plane of the echo image.

2 Methods

2.1 Algorithm

We employ the HF framework for object localization [7]. A key component of our implementation is the simultaneous detection of multiple object parts, which allows for estimation of device pose under varying orientations. In the following section, a review of the HF object detection framework is presented in context of our application.

Hough Forest Detector. A HF is a specific type of random forest that is designed for object detection. A random forest is a collection of decision trees that perform classification and/or regression. A HF takes image patches as input, and simultaneously performs both classification (is it part of an object?) and regression (where is the object?). The term "Hough" comes from the idea that each input image patch classified as part of the object votes for the object center. Votes are added in an accumulator image ("Hough" image, Fig. 3), and peaks are considered as object detection hypotheses. In our implementation, we designed a HF that locates two ends of a device, referred to as the "tip" and "tail" (Fig. 3).

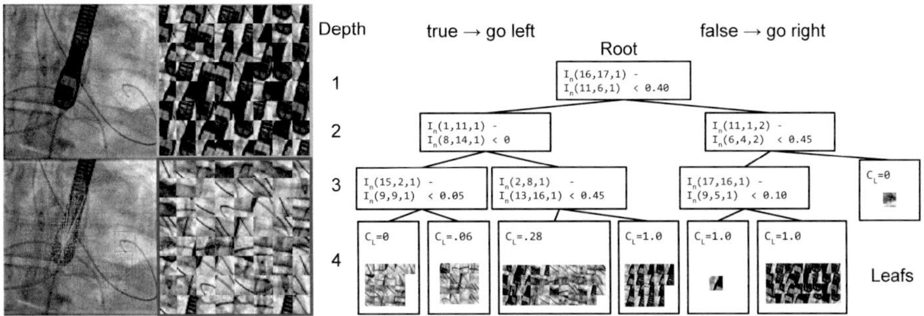

Fig. 2. A simple example of a decision tree trained on a single image of the TEE probe. Left: Example simulated TEE probe image, with locations of background (red) and device (green) training patches. Right: Example of a simple decision tree. Input data traverses the nodes based on binary test results and arrives at leaf nodes. In this example, all of the patches from the training image are shown in their destination leaf nodes.

A decision tree is an acyclic directed graph where each node contains a single input edge (except the root node) and two output edges (except the terminal nodes). During testing, data is input into the root node, and rules based on binary tests (aka features) determine which edge to travel down. For image patches, these binary tests typically encode patch appearance. Eventually the data will arrive at a terminal "leaf" node. The leaf node contains data, learned during training, about how to classify (or regress) the input data.

Each tree is trained by computing a set of binary tests on labeled training data, which are used to establish splitting rules. The splitting rules are chosen to maximize class discrimination at each node. In this work, binary pixel comparison tests are used due to their computational efficiency. Multi-channel image patches are used as input data, where a channel can be the raw pixel intensities or some operation computed on the intensities, e.g. gradient magnitude, blobness filter, etc... For each multi-channel input training patch I_n, a set of K binary tests are computed as follows:

$$F_{k,n}(p_k, q_k, r_k, s_k, \tau_k, z_k) = I_n(p_k, q_k, z_k) - I_n(r_k, s_k, z_k) < \tau_k \tag{1}$$

Where (p, q) and (r, s) are patch pixel coordinates, τ is a threshold used for detecting varying contrast, and z is the channel index. Image channels used in this work were image intensity, the x-gradient and the y-gradient. Each channel of each patch is normalized to have a range of 1 ($I_z(u, v) = \frac{I_z(u,v)}{max(I_z)-min(I_z)}$) , I_z is the patch for channel z).

Training begins by inputing a $K \times N$ training matrix with N training patches and K tests into the root node (Fig. 2). For classification, a metric is computed for each test k over all samples. In this work, the metric used for classification is the information gain:

$$G_k^c = H(S) - \frac{|S_1|}{|S|}H(S_1) - \frac{|S_0|}{|S|}H(S_0) \tag{2}$$

$$H(S) = -\sum_{c \in C} p(c)log(p(c)) \tag{3}$$

Where S is the entire set of training data, S_0 is the set of training data where F_k is false and S_1 is the set of training data where F_k is true, and $H(S)$ is the Shannon entropy over all classes (device or background) in the set S.

Alternatively, for regression of continuous variables, the metric is:

$$G_k^r = |S|var(S) - |S_1|var(S_1) - |S_0|var(S_0) \tag{4}$$

Where $var(S)$ is the variance of continuous data describing the device orientation or offset vectors within each set (non-device patches are ignored for this calculation).

A random decision is made at each node on which attribute to base the splitting rule on: class, offsets, or device orientation. If the offsets are chosen, a random choice about which offsets to regress ("tip" or "tail") is made. The test that gives the maximum value of G_k^c or G_k^r is stored as the splitting rule for that node, and the training data is passed onto the left or right child node according to the splitting rule. The same process is completed until a maximum tree depth D is reached or all of the samples in a node belong to the background class. The terminal node is termed a "leaf" node, and it stores the classes labels and offsets associated with all of the training data that arrived at that node. In order to speed up run-time, offsets in each leaf node are partitioned into 16 clusters using k-means and the cluster means replace the original offsets.

A key feature of HFs is the use of randomness during training, which helps prevent over-fitting the classifier to the training data. This is accomplished by only generating a small random subset of binary pixel tests for each tree, as well as randomizing whether each node will build a splitting rule based on class, offset vector, or device orientation. For example, in our implementation for the TEE probe, 8192 out of over 1 million binary tests are available to each tree.

During testing, a new image patch centered on (u_p, v_p) is fed into the root node of each tree and traverses the tree according to the splitting rules established during training. When it arrives at a leaf node, each offset (u_o, v_o) in the leaf node votes for the device parts in the Hough image accordingly:

$$I_H(u_H, v_H) \rightarrow I_H(u_H, v_H) + \frac{C_L}{|D_L|} \tag{5}$$

Where $(u_H, v_H) = (u_p, v_p) + (u_o, v_o)$, C_L is the proportion of device samples in the leaf node, and $|D_L|$ is the number of offsets in the leaf node.

This process is then repeated at every patch and for every tree in the HF. The final I_H is blurred with a gaussian kernel and peaks are classified as tip and tail detection hypotheses (Fig. 3).

HF input patches can be sampled densely at random locations or sparsely at salient key-points. For our application, we found that device detection was faster and more reliable using densely sampled patches at random locations.

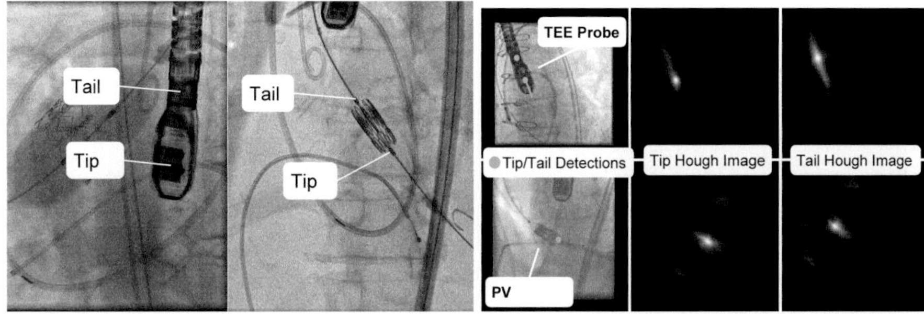

Fig. 3. Left: TEE probe and PV, with tip and tail labeled. Right: TEE probe and valve detection hypotheses with corresponding Hough images showing clearly defined peaks at the tip and tail of the devices.

Hypothesis Scoring. A Hough image peak was considered a valid hypothesis if it was $> 0.8 * max(I_H)$ following non-maximum suppression. At most, the top 10 peaks were retained as part hypotheses, but in practice usually only a few peaks survived the first criteria. All L tail and M tip hypotheses are combined to form $L \times M$ tip-tail pair hypotheses.

Next, unfeasible tail-tip pair hypotheses were removed. This was done by creating tail-tip pair distance and orientation matrices, and removing pair hypotheses that fell outside of the ranges of distance and orientation seen in the training datasets. Remaining tip-tail hypotheses are then given a score $S_{lm} = I_{H_{tip}}(u_l, v_l) \cdot I_{H_{tail}}(u_m, v_m)$. The tip-tail pair with the highest score is selected as the detected device.

2.2 Experiments

Computer Hardware and Software. All experiments were run on a Dell Precision T7500 work station running Ubuntu Linux with a 3.47 GHz Intel Xeon processor and a NVIDIA Tesla K20 GPU. HF code was written in CUDA C. Retrospective clinical dataset processing was approved by the local institutional review board. The Philips X2-7t probe and the Edwards Sapien valve were used in this study.

Training Datasets. For the TEE probe, the classifier was trained on simulated XRF images. Similar to the method from [4], hybrid images were created by blending anatomical background images from TAVR cases with digitally reconstructed radiographs (DRRs) of the TEE probe. For the PV, 389 clinical images from TAVR cases were manually annotated and used for training. In order to increase the size of the training dataset for the PV detector, each training image was randomly rotated and re-used as if it were a new image. The PV was only trained and detected in the pre-deployment state.

Table 1. HF parameters for the TEE and PV. N = number of training samples. K = number of tests per tree. T = number of trees. D = tree depth.

	Patch size	N	K	T	D	Image resolution	Patches at run-time
TEE	17×17	65536	8192	32	10	1.0 mm	16384
PV	25×25	16384	8192	64	8	0.5 mm	16384

Validation. The TEE and PV detector were tested on 1077 and 388 clinical XRF images, respectively. Ground truth data for the TEE images was obtained by manually registering a model of the TEE probe to the image, followed by 2D/3D registration based refinement using the method from [2], which reported sub-millimeter in-plane position accuracy. The PV ground truth was obtained by manual annotation of the tip and tail in the test images.

For validation, we measured the rate of successful detections, the mean localization error for successful detections, and the orientation error for successful detections. HF run-time was also reported, which was the amount of time it took for the HF to process all patches for each tree and create the Hough images. A detection was considered successful if the distance error was less than 5 mm and the orientation error was $< 10°$. Localization error was the Euclidean distance between the true device center and the measured device center computed at the detector (i.e. projection magnification was not considered.)

3 Results

Results are summarized in Table 2. The rate of successful detections was 95.8% for the TEE probe and 90.1% for the PV. This was competitive with previously reported results for the TEE probe [3,4], especially when considering that the HF was trained on simulated images. For successful detections, both devices resulted in localization errors less than 1.5 mm on average, and orientation errors less than 3.0°.

Table 2. Detection results for the HF device detector.

	# Test images	Successful Detection Rate (%)	Localization Error (mm)	Orientation Error ($^{\circ}$)	Run-time for HF (ms)
TEE	1077	95.8	1.42 ± 0.79	2.59 ± 1.87	38.8 ± 5.00
PV	388	90.1	1.04 ± 0.77	2.90 ± 2.37	37.0 ± 2.29

4 Discussion

The presented method was able to accurately detect both the TEE probe and the PV in over 90% of images. Most of the failed detections were due to occlusion from x-ray contrast during aortagraphy. The success rate for the PV was higher than expected, because a large percentage of the PV test images were recorded during contrast infusion. Furthermore, the PVs in the training and testing images varied greatly in size and appearance due to different patient sizes and valve models. This indicates that the HF classifier is robust to appearance variation and that greater detection performance may be possible using a classifier trained on single specific valve size and model.

The real-time performance of the method is contingent on the full image processing workflow. However, we expect that the bulk of processing is required by the HF, which we have shown has a maximum run-time less than 50 ms. The other steps, which comprise random patch location generation and extraction, can be implemented very efficiently on the GPU using texture reads. We expect that the full image processing workflow can be completed in less than 60 ms, which is sufficient for typical fluoroscopic imaging frame rates (15 fps)

The main application of these methods is to enable XRF/Echo image fusion, where the device will either be rendered in the echo image, or soft-tissue information from echo will be projected onto the XRF image. It is expected that these tools will minimize the need for use of x-ray contrast, which is not only healthier for the patient, but also decreases the risk of device detection failure. For the TEE probe, future work will focus on detection of the out-of-plane pose parameters, which is often a necessary step for fully automatic initialization of 2D/3D registration. For the PV, future work will focus on not only detecting the PV prior to deployment, but also during and after. This will allow a dynamic model of the PV to be rendered in echo images, potentially resulting in new image guidance tools for TAVR deployment.

5 Conclusion

A method for real-time, automatic detection of devices in fluoroscopic images is presented. Based on the Hough forest object detection framework, the method is fully automatic, and has the potential to operate at fluoroscopic frame rates. The percentage of successful device detections was 95.8% for the TEE probe and 90.1% for the prosthetic valve, despite the presence of x-ray contrast in many of the image frames. Future work will focus on detecting PV deformation during and after valve deployment for enhanced multi-modal guidance of TAVR.

References

1. Brost, A., Wimmer, A., Liao, R., Bourier, F., Koch, M., Strobel, N., Kurzidim, K., Hornegger, J.: Constrained registration for motion compensation in atrial fibrillation ablation procedures. IEEE Transactions on Medical Imaging 31(4), 870–881 (2012)
2. Gao, G., Penney, G., Ma, Y., Gogin, N., Cathier, P., Arujuna, A., Morton, G., Caulfield, D., Gill, J., Rinaldi, C.A., Hancock, J., Redwood, S., Thomas, M., Razavi, R., Gijsbers, G., Rhode, K.: Registration of 3D trans-esophageal echocardiography to x-ray fluoroscopy using image-based probe tracking. Medical Image Analysis 16(1), 38–49 (2012)
3. Mountney, P., et al.: Ultrasound and Fluoroscopic Images Fusion by Autonomous Ultrasound Probe Detection. In: Ayache, N., Delingette, H., Golland, P., Mori, K. (eds.) MICCAI 2012, Part II. LNCS, vol. 7511, pp. 544–551. Springer, Heidelberg (2012)
4. Heimann, T., Mountney, P., John, M., Ionasec, R.: Real-time ultrasound transducer localization in fluoroscopy images by transfer learning from synthetic training data. Medical Image Analysis 18(8), 1320–1328 (2014). Special Issue on the 2013 Conference on Medical Image Computing and Computer Assisted Intervention
5. Karar, M., Merk, D., Chalopin, C., Walther, T., Falk, V., Burgert, O.: Aortic valve prosthesis tracking for transapical aortic valve implantation. International Journal of Computer Assisted Radiology and Surgery 6(5), 583–590 (2011)
6. Criminisi, A., Shotton, J., Robertson, D., Konukoglu, E.: Regression forests for efficient anatomy detection and localization in CT studies. In: Menze, B., Langs, G., Tu, Z., Criminisi, A. (eds.) MICCAI 2010. LNCS, vol. 6533, pp. 106–117. Springer, Heidelberg (2011)
7. Gall, J., Lempitsky, V.: Class-specific hough forests for object detection. In: Criminisi, A., Shotton, J. (eds.) Decision Forests for Computer Vision and Medical Image Analysis. Advances in Computer Vision and Pattern Recognition, pp. 143–157. Springer, London (2013)

Hybrid Utrasound and MRI Acquisitions for High-Speed Imaging of Respiratory Organ Motion

Frank Preiswerk, Matthew Toews, W. Scott Hoge, Jr-yuan George Chiou, Lawrence P. Panych, William M. Wells III, and Bruno Madore

Brigham and Women's Hospital, Harvard Medical School
frank@bwh.harvard.edu

Abstract. Magnetic Resonance (MR) imaging provides excellent image quality at a high cost and low frame rate. Ultrasound (US) provides poor image quality at a low cost and high frame rate. We propose an instance-based learning system to obtain the best of both worlds: high quality MR images at high frame rates from a low cost single-element US sensor. Concurrent US and MRI pairs are acquired during a relatively brief offline learning phase involving the US transducer and MR scanner. High frame rate, high quality MR imaging of respiratory organ motion is then predicted from US measurements, even after stopping MRI acquisition, using a probabilistic kernel regression framework. Experimental results show predicted MR images to be highly representative of actual MR images.

1 Introduction

Magnetic Resonance (MR) imaging has gained considerable traction in the last two decades as a modality of choice for image-guided therapies [1,2], primarily due to its excellent soft-tissue contrast and its non-invasive nature. However, major challenges include relatively slow frame rates and limited physical patient access within the MR bore. Perhaps the most notable effort made toward scanner design and providing patient access has been the (now discontinued) double-doughnut 0.5 T SIGNA SP/i design [3], whereby the interventionist could step in-between two physically-separate magnets and gain direct access to the patient. Other interventional MR systems have also been developed and commercialized but patient access, MR-compatibility of instruments and overall costs have remained considerable hurdles. In contrast to MR imaging, ultrasound (US) imaging provides fast frame rates and nearly-unhindered physical access to the patient. US imaging systems are cheaper and faster than MR, yet produce images that are often found lacking in terms of contrast and overall quality. As a consequence, several noteworthy efforts have been made to combine the two complementary imaging modalities and a body of work has emerged on developing hybrid methods [4,5,6,7,8,9,10]. In [4,5], hybrid 2D US/MR systems were proposed where orientation information extracted from US data was used to update the image slice position of an SSFP sequence in real time, for prospective

N. Navab et al. (Eds.): MICCAI 2015, Part I, LNCS 9349, pp. 315–322, 2015.
DOI: 10.1007/978-3-319-24553-9_39

motion compensation in a motion phantom. A similar hybrid system was presented in [7], where a clinical US imaging system was integrated with 1.5 T and 3 T clinical MR scanners for simultaneous 4D MRI and US imaging.

The present work involves a small 8 mm-diameter single-element MR-compatible ultrasonic transducer applied to the skin of the abdomen and held in place using a simple adhesive bandage (Figure 1). A regular flexible MR coil array can readily be wrapped over this small US probe, at no detectable penalty in MR image quality. The emitted US field is not focused, it is expected to penetrate and reflect possibly several times within the abdomen. A-mode ultrasound raw data signals (USrd) are acquired at a very high frame rate during regular MR image acquisition, and these signals act as a unique signature for the internal organ configuration, including respiratory state. This is in sharp contrast with more traditional US imaging whereby the imaging probe would consist of an array of transducer elements, hand-held over the anatomy of interest to capture images. While the simple and convenient USrd sensor used here is insufficient to produce spatially resolved US images, it provides a 1D trace rich in information that can be correlated with simultaneously-acquired and spatially-resolved MR images. It was previously shown that such a 1D USrd signal might be suitable as a biometric navigator [8]. Here, we use a hybrid US-MR system to achieve two goals within the realm of abdominal imaging under respiratory organ motion: First, the temporal resolution of the MR image sequence is artificially boosted by orders of magnitude using an algorithm that learns from a stream of simultaneous MR and US data, providing the interventionist with a real-time view of abdominal organ motion. Second, after a learning phase the algorithm can be applied to the US data alone, allowing high-rate image reconstructions even when the patient is outside the scanner, thus offering a new take on the problem of intra-procedural imaging. A distinguishing feature of the proposed approach comes from the low cost of the US system and the simplicity of the generated US signal.

2 Materials and Methods

2.1 Hardware Setup and Data Acquisition

An MR-compatible, single-element USrd sensor (Imasonics, 8-mm diameter, 5.8 MHz) was inserted into a specially-carved rubber disc (3.5 cm diameter, 1.4 cm thickness), positioned onto the abdomen of the subject and held in place using an adhesive bandage (Walgreens, bordered gauze 10.2×10.2 cm). MR images were acquired using a 3 T General Electric system (Signa HDxt Twin Speed, 40 mT/m, 150 T/m/s) and a regular 8-element flexible cardiac array coil. Every TR interval, the MR scanner generated a trigger pulse for a pulser/receiver (Olympus 5072) to fire the USrd transducer. The resulting USrd data were recorded on a server via a sampling card (NI PCI-5122, National Instruments). The server also fetched the acquired MR raw data via a product raw-data server connection. Both incoming data streams, MR and US, were time-stamped and saved for processing. Figure 1 shows an overview of the experimental setup.

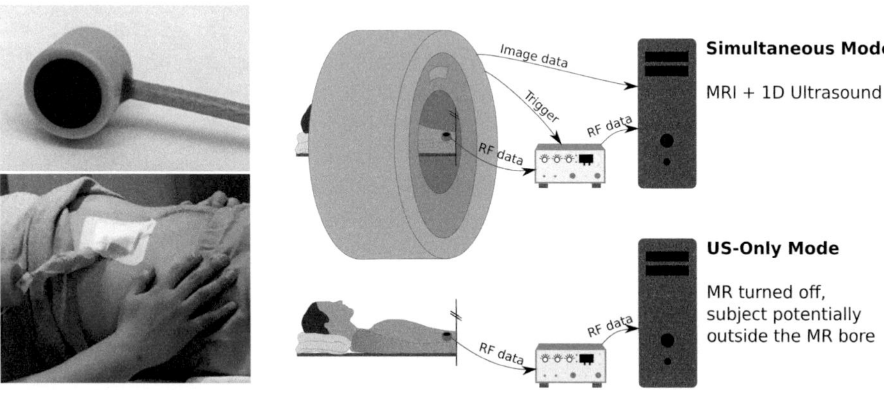

Fig. 1. Overview of the hardware setup. Left: MR-compatible USrd sensor (top), placed on the volunteer using adhesive bandage (bottom). Right: The system operates in two modes. First, the subject is placed inside the MR scanner for combined MRI and USrd acquisition (top). In this mode the system estimates MR images at high-speed while still learning from incoming MR data. In scanner-less mode, only USrd data are acquired but high-speed MR images are still synthesized based on the data from the training phase. No MR scanner is required in this case.

Table 1. Overview of acquired datasets. S means 'sagittal' and C means 'coronal'

Id	Mode	Acquisition length [s]	TR [ms]	f_I [Hz]	f_{US} [Hz]	Number of MR images	Number of US traces
1.1	S	64	7	1.5	142.9	95	9120
2.1	S	198	7	1.5	142.9	295	28 320
3.1	S	116	10	0.8	100	91	11 520
4.1-4.2	S	109-122	8-10	0.8-1.3	100-125	95-155	12160-14880
5.1-5.6	S+C	50-111	18	1.7	55.6	86-192	2624-6144

Three human subjects were recruited and imaged following informed consent, over the course of four distinct scanning sessions (i.e. one of the subjects volunteered for two sessions). For the first three sessions a simpler MR protocol involving a single sagittal (S) plane was employed, while for the last session a more involved sagittal-coronal (S+C) two-plane protocol was employed instead (75 % partial-Fourier, two-fold parallel imaging scheme). Imaging parameters are listed in Table 1 and in the following: Flip angle = 30°, matrix size = 128×96 or 128×128 (S) / 192×192 (S+C), slice thickness = 5 mm, FOV = 20 cm (S) / 38 cm (S+C).

2.2 Algorithm - Simpler Case: Single-Plane MR Acquisition

Typical US image reconstruction algorithms, based on a delay-and-sum beamforming operation, are designed to discard much of the received US signals as they may have failed the basic US spatial encoding process; in contrast, the proposed algorithm utilizes raw US data without discarding any of them. While there is nothing special about the MR or the USrd signals obtained here, interesting behaviors appear as correlations are found between them, allowing USrd signals to become a surrogate for MR data. Given enough data is acquired for these correlations to be learned from, it becomes possible to boost the temporal resolution of a sequence of MR images by orders of magnitude. The overall proposed approach is made particularly interesting by the fact that the generation of MR-like images can be continued even after the subject is taken out of the MR scanner, solely based on the USrd signal.

The majority of temporal models are based on the Markovian dependency assumption, i.e. the current state is dependent only on its immediate predecessor. Temporal modeling, either short term Markovian or cyclical motion, faces the difficulty of estimating motion in the presence of irregularities, such as irregular breathing, gasping or coughing. Instance-based learning (IBL), on the other hand, operates by storing a potentially large number of training data samples in memory, then performing inference on new data based directly on previously-seen instances. This non-parametric approach is fundamentally different to training a parametric model from data instances and has many advantages: It can be adopted in situations where parametric models are unknown or difficult to specify accurately and it scales to the granularity of the data space. Furthermore, it is known [11] that IBL is in probabilistic terms equivalent to averaging over all the (possibly infinitely many) models of a fixed model family. Thus, IBL will become increasingly relevant as data acquisition, storage and retrieval systems increase in size and speed.

Let U_t represent the observed ultrasound vector at time t and let I_t be a random variable representing the estimated MR image at time t. Let further $D = \{I, U\}$ be the collection of all previously acquired MR and US data I and U, respectively. Our method seeks to estimate I_t from U_t, i.e. to estimate an MR image for each USrd signal coming in at a frequency much beyond that of the MR image acquisition process. For this purpose we propose computing the expected value of I_t conditioned on U_t,

$$\mathop{\mathbb{E}}_{I_t}[I_t|U_t, D] = \int I_t \; p(I_t|U_t, D)dI_t = \frac{\int I_t \; p(I_t, U_t|D)dI_t}{p(U_t|D)}. \tag{1}$$

The second equality results from applying the Bayes rule, where $p(I_t, U_t|D)$ is the joint density of observed US trace U_t and MR image I_t, conditioned on previously seen data D. We propose an instance-based method for computing Equation (1), as follows. The joint density in the numerator is estimated using Kernel Density Estimation (KDE)[12] of the form

$$p(a, b) \approx \frac{1}{N} \sum_i k_a(a - a_i) k_b(b - b_i). \tag{2}$$

Let $\{(I_i, U_i)\}$ be a set of training instances, consisting of N concurrently acquired MRI and US pairs (I_i, U_i). As a modeling choice, we define k_a to be the

Dirac delta function centered at I_i and k_b to be a Gaussian centered around U_i with isotropic covariance matrix $\Sigma = c \cdot \mathbb{I}$, where $\mathbb{I}$ is the identity matrix. The numerator in Equation (1) then becomes

$$\int I_t \; p(I_t, U_t|D) dI_t \approx \frac{1}{N} \int I_t \sum_i \delta(I_t - I_i) \mathcal{N}(U_t; U_i, \Sigma) dI_t \tag{3}$$

$$= \frac{1}{N} \sum_i I_i \; \mathcal{N}(U_t; U_i, \Sigma). \tag{4}$$

The normalizing factor $p(U_t|D)$ in the denominator of Equation (1) is unimportant in maximum a-posteriori estimation, however it is required for computing the expectation. It can be estimated in a similar manner to the numerator as follows:

$$p(U_t|D) \approx \frac{1}{N} \sum_i \mathcal{N}(U_t; U_i, \Sigma). \tag{5}$$

Combining Equations (4) and (5), the final computational form of the estimator in Equation (1) becomes

$$\mathbb{E}[I_t|U_t, D] \approx \frac{\sum_i I_i \; \mathcal{N}(U_t; U_i, \Sigma)}{\sum_i \mathcal{N}(U_t; U_i, \Sigma)}. \tag{6}$$

Note that the forms of the numerator and denominator in Equation (6) are equivalent to Nadaraya-Watson Kernel Regression [13].

Evaluating $\mathbb{E}[I_t|U_t, D]$ requires a computationally expensive sum over a potentially large number of training samples. However with a suitably small c, the sum is dominated by small number of 'nearest neighbors' for U_t. A search can performed to identify a set of k-nearest neighbors $\{U_i\}$ of the current US observation U_t within the training data set. This search can be performed efficiently with fast approximate search methods, e.g. k-d-trees. Equation (6) can then be computed from elements within this subset. Note that with $k = 1$, the expectation is equivalent maximum a-posteriori estimation, which in our experiments leads to noisy estimates in the case of discrete data. Computing the expectation with $k > 1$ leads to smoother estimates of I_t via considering a weighted average of similar observations. Note also that a low posterior probability generally indicates an outlier U_t that has not previously been observed, which can be used to detect unexpected organ configurations.

2.3 Algorithm - Extension to Multiple-Plane MR Acquisition

An interesting extension to the algorithm is to work on MR sequences that acquire multiple intersecting slices and to estimate a coherent volumetric image. This means the probabilistic formulation must be adapted to take into account how well the matches of different planes agree. For the simplest case of two alternating slice positions, the expectation now becomes

$$\mathop{\mathbb{E}}_{I_t,J_t}[[I_t,J_t]|U_t,D] = \int\int [I_t,J_t]\; p(I_t,J_t|U_t,D) dI_t\, dJ_t, \tag{7}$$

where $[I_t, J_t]$ is a concatenation of the two images.

Let $[I_t]_L$ and $[J_t]_L$ be all pixels from I_t and J_t, respectively, that are located at the intersection between the two planes. $[I_t]_{\bar{L}}$ and $[J_t]_{\bar{L}}$ represent all other locations. The joint distribution $p(I_t, J_t, U_t|D)$ can be factorized into conditionally independent regions of I and J given U_t, and a dependent region where they intersect,

$$p(I_t,J_t|U_t,D) = p([I_t]_{\bar{L}}|U_t,D)p([J_t]_{\bar{L}}|U_t,D)p([I_t]_L,[J_t]_L|U_t,D). \tag{8}$$

We model $p([I_t]_L, [J_t]_L|U_t, D)$ with a Gaussian $\mathcal{N}([I_t]_L; [J_t]_L, \Sigma_L)$ with empirically-determined covariance matrix Σ_L and arbitrarily choosing $[I_t]_L$ (or $[J_t]_L$) as the mean. Putting everything together and again applying KDE as done in Equation (6) leads to

$$\mathop{\mathbb{E}}_{I_t,J_t}[[I_t,J_t]|U_t,D] \approx \frac{\sum_i \sum_j [I_i,J_j]\; \mathcal{N}(U_t;U_i,\Sigma)\mathcal{N}(U_t;U_j,\Sigma)\mathcal{N}([I_t]_L;[J_t]_L,\Sigma_L)}{\sum_i \sum_j \mathcal{N}(U_t;U_i,\Sigma)\mathcal{N}(U_t;U_j,\Sigma)\mathcal{N}([I_t]_L;[J_t]_L,\Sigma_L)}, \tag{9}$$

where U_i and U_j are the USrd signals corresponding to images I_i and J_i, respectively. The generalization to an arbitrary number of image planes parallel to I_t and J_t is straight forward by repeated application of the product rule in Equation (8). Allowing for arbitrary plane orientations involves higher-order terms but follows the same principle.

3 Results and Discussion

Figure 2 shows examples of estimated images for times when an MR image was also acquired. This allows to compare the estimates to their ground-truth images. As the figure shows, estimates at both exhale and inhale are very similar to the actual MR images acquired. In order to better visualize time, Figure 3 shows plots of a single line of pixels in superior-inferior direction over time (m-mode) for dataset 6.1. At the beginning, neither the acquired images nor their predictions reflect the temporally highly-resolved USrd signal. However, after a short training period the estimated MR sequence runs at the same speed as the ultrasound. Notably, after the MR acquisition is stopped, the algorithm continues to give estimated MR frames that are very well in agreement with the USrd signal. For datasets 1.1-4.2, the location of a clearly visible vessel was manually selected in 10 MR images after one minute of learning. An average error of 1.19 px (standard deviation 0.8 px) was determined, which shows that the algorithm in fact estimates MR images that accurately represent respiratory motion.

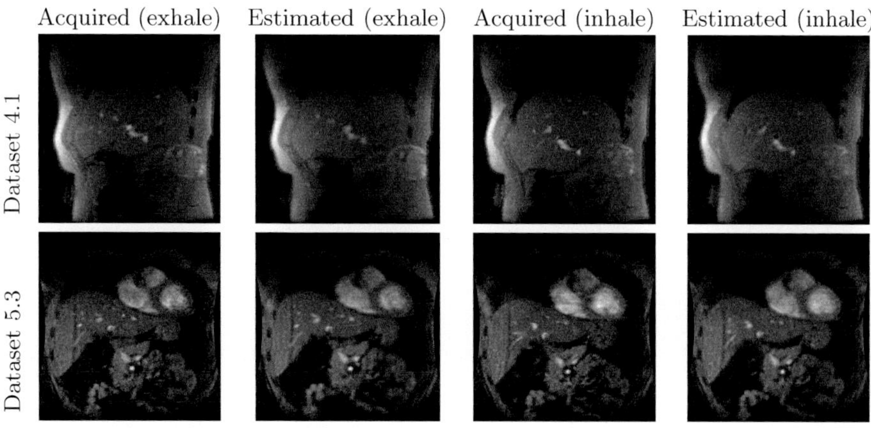

Fig. 2. Comparison of acquired MR images and their estimates.

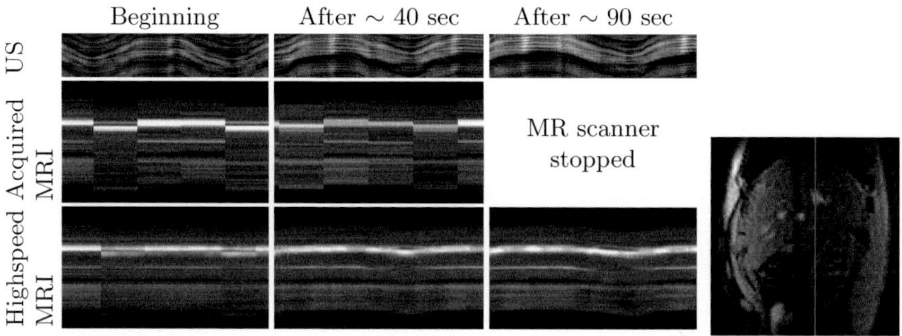

Fig. 3. M-mode visualizations of dataset 6.1. The image on the right shows the position of the m-mode line.

The proposed system could potentially be used to track lesions during image-guided therapy. Compared to MR, it is extremely simple and cheap; even so, it allowed temporal resolution to be improved by orders of magnitude compared to MR alone. Limitations of the present study included the small number of human subjects recruited so far, the fact they were healthy volunteers rather than patients, and the off-line nature of the currently-implemented reconstruction chain. While all aspects of the processing did execute fast enough on an off-the-shelf PC to be compatible with a real-time application, individual components have not yet all been implemented and linked for truly real-time reconstruction and display to occur. Future work further includes the development of problem detectors to identify and gracefully handle all time periods when motion might momentarily become too rapid and unpredictable, such as during violent coughing or gasping.

Acknowledgment. This work was supported by grants from NIH (R01CA149342, P41EB015898 and R01EB010195) and SNSF (P2BSP2_155234).

References

1. Silverman, S.G., Collick, B.D., Figueira, M.R., Khorasani, R., Adams, D.F., Newman, R.W., Topulos, G.P., Jolesz, F.A.: Interactive MR-guided biopsy in an open-configuration MR imaging system. Radiology 197(1), 175–181 (1995)
2. Morrison, P.R., Silverman, S.G., Tuncali, K., Tatli, S.: MRI-guided cryotherapy. Journal of Magnetic Resonance Imaging 27(2), 410–420 (2008)
3. Schenck, J.F., Jolesz, F.A., Roemer, P.B., Cline, H.E., Lorensen, W.E., Kikinis, R., Silverman, S.G., Hardy, C.J., Barber, W.D., Laskaris, E.T.: Superconducting open-configuration MR imaging system for image-guided therapy. Radiology 195(3), 805–814 (1995)
4. Günther, M., Feinberg, D.A.: Ultrasound-guided MRI: Preliminary results using a motion phantom. Magnetic Resonance in Medicine 52(1), 27–32 (2004)
5. Feinberg, D.A., Giese, D., Bongers, D.A., Ramanna, S., Zaitsev, M., Markl, M., Günther, M.: Hybrid ultrasound MRI for improved cardiac imaging and real-time respiration control. Magnetic Resonance in Medicine 63(2), 290–296 (2010)
6. Arvanitis, C.D., Livingstone, M.S., McDannold, N.: Combined ultrasound and MR imaging to guide focused ultrasound therapies in the brain. Physics in Medicine and Biology 58(14), 4749–4761 (2013)
7. Petrusca, L., Cattin, P., De Luca, V., Preiswerk, F., Celicanin, Z., Auboiroux, V., Viallon, M., Arnold, P., Santini, F., Terraz, S., et al.: Hybrid ultrasound/magnetic resonance simultaneous acquisition and image fusion for motion monitoring in the upper abdomen. Investigative Radiology 48(5), 333–340 (2013)
8. Schwartz, B.M., McDannold, N.J.: Ultrasound echoes as biometric navigators. Magnetic Resonance in Medicine 69(4), 1023–1033 (2013)
9. Matthew Toews, C.S., Mei, R., Chu, W.S., Hoge, L.P.: Panych: Detecting rapid organ motion using a hybrid MR-ultrasound setup and Bayesian data processing. Proc. Intl. Soc. Mag. Reson. Med. (ISMRM), 7309 (2014)
10. Preiswerk, F., Hoge, W.S., Toews, M., Yuan George Chiou, J., Chauvin, L., Panych, L.P., Madore, B.: Speeding-up MR acquisitions using ultrasound signals, and scanner-less real-time MR imaging. Proc. Intl. Soc. Mag. Reson. Med. (ISMRM), 863 (2015)
11. Kontkanen, P., Myllymdki, P., Silander, T., Tirri, H.: Bayes optimal instance-based learning. In: Nédellec, C., Rouveirol, C. (eds.) ECML 1998. LNCS, vol. 1398, pp. 77–88. Springer, Heidelberg (1998)
12. Parzen, E.: On estimation of a probability density function and mode. The Annals of Mathematical Statistics, 1065–1076 (1962)
13. Nadaraya, E.A.: On estimating regression. Theory of Probability & Its Applications 9(1), 141–142 (1964)

A Portable Intra-Operative Framework Applied to Distal Radius Fracture Surgery*

Jessica Magaraggia[1,2,3], Wei Wei[2], Markus Weiten[2], Gerhard Kleinszig[2], Sven Vetter[4], Jochen Franke[4], Karl Barth[2], Elli Angelopoulou[1,3], and Joachim Hornegger[1,3]

[1] Pattern Recognition Lab, FAU Erlangen-Nürnberg, Erlangen, Germany
[2] Siemens Healthcare GmbH, Erlangen, Germany
[3] Research Training Group 1773 "Heterogeneous Image Systems", Erlangen, Germany
[4] BG Trauma Center, Ludwigshafen am Rhein, Germany

Abstract. Fractures of the distal radius account for about 15% of all extremity fractures. To date, open reduction and internal plate fixation is the standard operative treatment. During the procedure, only fluoroscopic images are available for the planning of the screw placement and the monitoring of the instrument trajectory. Complications arising from malpositioned screws can lead to revision surgery. With the aim of improving screw placement accuracy, we present a prototype framework for fully intra-operative guidance that simplifies the planning transfer. Planning is performed directly intra-operatively and expressed in terms of screw configuration w.r.t the used implant plate. Subsequently, guidance is provided solely by a combination of locally positioned markers and a small camera placed on the surgical instrument that allows real-time position feedback. We evaluated our framework on 34 plastic bones and 3 healthy forearm cadaver specimens. In total, 146 screws were placed. On bone phantoms, we achieved an accuracy of 1.02 ± 0.57mm, $3.68 \pm 4.38°$ and $1.77 \pm 1.38°$ in the screw tip position and orientation (azimuth and elevation) respectively. On forearm specimens, we achieved a corresponding accuracy of 1.63 ± 0.91mm, $5.85 \pm 4.93°$ and $3.48 \pm 3.07°$. Our analysis shows that our framework has the potential for improving the accuracy of the screw placement compared to the state of the art.

1 Introduction

Fractures of the distal radius account for up to 15% of all extremity fractures. Open reduction and internal plate fixation is the most common operative treatment. During the procedure, intra-operative correct estimation of screw length and position under fluoroscopic control still represents a challenge. Among the reported complications (ranging from 6% to 80% [9]), several studies describe how the irregular anatomy of the distal radius leads to unrecognized cortical

* The presented method is investigational use and is limited by law to investigational use. It is not commercially available and its future availability cannot be ensured.

N. Navab et al. (Eds.): MICCAI 2015, Part I, LNCS 9349, pp. 323–330, 2015.
DOI: 10.1007/978-3-319-24553-9_40

perforation by screw tips, regardless of the art of locking plating: dorsal, palmar or volar [2, 11]. Sugun et al. [11] reported a screw prominence rate of 25.65%, ranging from 0.5 to 6.1mm. In fact, depending on the type of view used (lateral, anterior-posterior, supinated, pronated, etc.) protrusions ranging from 3 to 6.5mm on average are required before protruding screws can be detected. It was also suggested that screw prominence greater than 1.5mm is likely to lead to complications [11]. Aurora et al. [2] reported that 9% of all complications are related to protruding screws, like plunging the drill bit into undesired soft-tissue structures and tendon rupture.Typically, revision surgery and implant removal are advised at the first sign of tendon irritation. Post-operatively, the severity of the complications associated with prominent screws is well recognized. An additional critical aspect is the intra-operative damage caused by perforation of the articulation compartments by the drill bit while preparing the insertion hole. In an extensive study conducted on cadaver forearms, Pichler et al. [10] reported a 43% incidence of drill bit violations of the third extensor compartment.

This leads to both a trial-and-error process during surgery for correct drilling and screw positioning, and to empty drill traces injuring soft tissue compartments [1]. Hence, practice advocates for solutions providing better intra-operative position control. Researchers continue investigating guidance techniques for orthopedic and trauma procedures. Although the usage of navigation solutions may increase the procedure time or involve some additional learning time, they successfully improve accuracy and reduce inter-user variability [6]. Commercial solutions like VectorVision (BrainLab) use an infrared stereo-camera and related markers. More recently, promising solutions for accurate screw placement have been proposed [3, 7], which, however require either a robotic arm or an augmented C-arm. Lately, Vetter et al. [12] presented the first clinical study on the use of an intra-operative planning application. However, in [12] plan transfer still strongly relied solely on the skills of the surgeon.

To support the surgeon in more accurate screw positioning, we developed a framework for combined intra-operative planning and guidance. For the planning, X-ray intra-operative images are acquired after fixing the plate onto the bone shaft. The plate model is then registered and an augmented view of the implant plate onto the acquired images supports the physician in deciding screw length and orientation. The core of our approach is the translation of the planning in a series of local plans for each screw. This allows the planning to be transferred under guidance support, which is provided solely by a combination of local markers fixed onto a conventional drill guide used for drilling (see Fig 1). Our augmented drill guide provides a local reference system onto the fixation plate. During the procedure, camera images are processed and correspondences are built between the detected marker-features and the real marker geometry. This allows the reconstruction of the position of the camera, and consequently of the attached instrument, in real-time w.r.t the plate, which was previously registered to the acquired X-ray images. Our method bypasses the need for bulky markers to be fixed onto the patient to provide a global patient reference as in conventional navigation systems [5]. Only small additional components such as

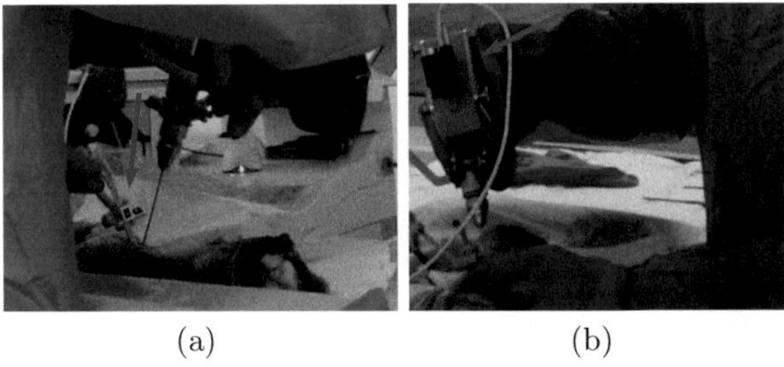

(a) (b)

Fig. 1. The hardware components of our design: (a) the drill guide with the attached markers and (b) the drill with the mounted camera.

markers and a video camera are required to be attached onto instrumentation already belonging to the standard clinical workflow. Our framework is general enough to adapt to several surgical fracture treatments, where precise screw positioning is required but bulky standard navigation systems are not applicable. In this study, the feasibility of our portable framework is shown. A prototype for reduction of distal radius fracture was built using standard surgical instrumentation. Extensive evaluation was performed on distal radius phantoms. First tests on forearm cadaver specimens were also carried out.

2 Methods

Our framework first allows the planning of the screw configuration required for fracture repositioning. Afterwards, the physician is supported during planning transfer via a flexible guidance solution that provides real-time position feedback of the drill. The current instrument position and its offset from the planned trajectory is visualized w.r.t the employed fixation plate and the patient anatomy.

2.1 Intra-Operative Planning

Similarly to Vetter et al. [12] we also perform the planning intraoperatively. After fixing the plate onto the bone shaft, two X-ray images, a lateral, $\mathrm{I_{LAT}}$, and an anterior-posterior, $\mathrm{I_{AP}}$, are acquired using a mobile C-arm. An automatic 2D/3D registration is then performed to register the plate model, $\mathrm{P_L}$, to $\mathrm{I_{LAT}}$ and $\mathrm{I_{AP}}$. The registration result is described by the transformation matrices $\mathbf{T}_{\mathrm{LAT}}^{\mathrm{P_L}}$ and $\mathbf{T}_{\mathrm{AP}}^{\mathrm{P_L}}$. After registration, the plate model is overlaid to $\mathrm{I_{LAT}}$ and $\mathrm{I_{AP}}$. Using a comprehensive augmented overview of the complete plate-screw configuration, the physician determines the number of fixing screws, their orientation and length. The planning is then expressed as a set $\mathrm{X} = \{(\mathbf{P}_{\mathrm{T_i}}, \mathbf{v}_{\mathrm{A_i}})_{\mathrm{H_i}}\}$, where $(\mathbf{P}_{\mathrm{T_i}}, \mathbf{v}_{\mathrm{A_i}})_{\mathrm{H_i}}$ represent the screw tip position and the screw direction versor, respectively, in the local coordinate system of the i-th hole, $\mathrm{S_{H_i}}$, of the employed plate (see Fig. 2(a)). The transformation $\mathbf{T}_{\mathrm{P_L}}^{\mathrm{H_i}}$ is known by construction.

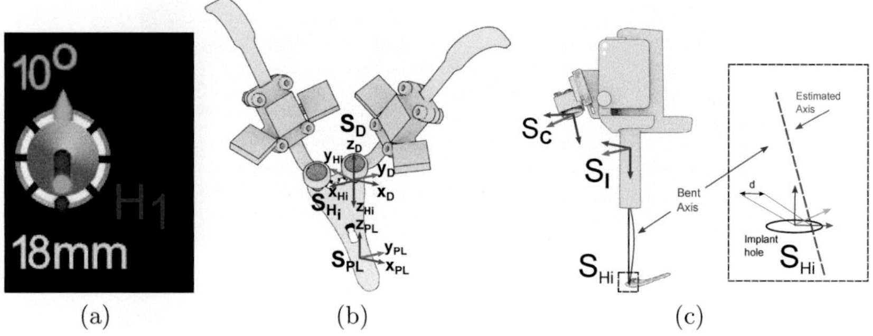

Fig. 2. (a) Local visualization of a screw plan. (b) A schematic representation of our augmented drill guide positioned on an implant plate. (c) Graphic depiction of the problem of the axis offset due to axis bending.

2.2 Intra-Operative Guidance

The plate registration and parametrization of the planning in terms of the local set of coordinates X allow the guidance pipeline to be decoupled from a global patient reference. As we proposed in [8], we augment the drill guide, which is used for drilling support, with optical markers that can be seen from a small video camera mounted on a surgical drill. Holders for markers and camera were designed and then realized using rapid prototyping. They are mounted on standard surgical instrumentation (see Fig 1). The calibration of the camera-drill system, expressed by the transformation $\mathbf{T}_{\mathrm{C}}^{\mathrm{I}}$, allows us to express the position and orientation of the drill bit w.r.t the camera coordinate system $\mathrm{S_C}$. Before drilling, the physician is asked to position the calibrated collection of drill guide-markers, $\mathrm{S_D}$, onto the plate, as depicted in Fig. 2(b). Thus, $\mathrm{S_D}$ does coincide with the local coordinate system of the current hole $\mathrm{S_{H_i}}$.

While drilling, the markers placed onto the drill guide are inside the Field of View (FoV) of the camera. Marker detection and subsequent camera pose estimation, expressed by $\mathbf{T}_{\mathrm{D}}^{\mathrm{C}}$, are performed in real-time. Unlike our prior work [8], we employ binary encoded markers based on code redundancy similar to [13] and [4] in order to increase the robustness of marker identification especially w.r.t inhomogeneous illumination.

The geometric relations between plate hole, drill guide-markers, camera, and drill allow us to calculate the transformation $\mathbf{T}_{\mathrm{H_i}}^{\mathrm{I}}$, from $\mathrm{S_I}$ to $\mathrm{S_{H_i}}$, and hence the instrument position in real-time w.r.t $\mathrm{S_{H_i}}$ as $(\mathbf{P}_{\mathrm{I}}, \mathbf{v}_{\mathrm{I}})_{\mathrm{H_i}}$. Depending on the selected drill guide position, a known transformation $\mathbf{T}_{\mathrm{D}}^{\mathrm{H_i}}$ exists between the two coordinate systems $\mathrm{S_{H_i}}$ and $\mathrm{S_D}$ (see Eq. 1). In our previous work [8], we showed that the accuracy of the estimated position is affected by the vibration of the instrument, that negatively impacts the image quality. A reported cause was the instrument contact with the surrounding components in particular during the perforation of the bone surface. By quantifying the image blur at the edges of the markers we can exclude highly blurred images from our computations. Moreover, the user is advised to follow the natural sequence of 2 steps: 1) Targeting and 2) Drilling. Thus, motion blur is minimized during targeting.

$$\mathbf{T}^{\mathrm{I}}_{\mathrm{H_i}} = \mathbf{T}^{\mathrm{D}}_{\mathrm{H_i}} \mathbf{T}^{\mathrm{C}}_{\mathrm{D}} \mathbf{T}^{\mathrm{I}}_{\mathrm{C}} \tag{1}$$

$$\mathbf{T}^{\mathrm{I}}_{\mathrm{AP}} = \mathbf{T}^{\mathrm{P_L}}_{\mathrm{AP}} \mathbf{T}^{\mathrm{H_i}}_{\mathrm{P_L}} \mathbf{T}^{\mathrm{I}}_{\mathrm{H_i}} \tag{2}$$

The previously performed 2D/3D registration between the plate model and the intra-operative X-rays allows us to report the instrument position directly onto $\mathrm{I_{AP}}$ (see the final transformation, $\mathbf{T}^{\mathrm{I}}_{\mathrm{AP}}$, in Eq. 2). The same can be done for $\mathrm{I_{LAT}}$. Hence, our guidance design reports the instrument position w.r.t the patient anatomy without the need for additional marker reference to be fixed onto the patient, as traditional navigation systems would require.

2.3 Instrument Visualization

Visualization of the instrument position is performed 1) on a simplified but comprehensive scene focusing on the local visualization w.r.t the drill guide $\mathrm{S_D}$ and 2) as a 3D overlay onto $\mathrm{I_{LAT}}$ and $\mathrm{I_{AP}}$. As with all hand-held instruments, depending on the diameter and length of the drill bit, bending of the drill axis can occur during the operation. However, our instrument calibration is expressed by the rigid transformation $\mathbf{T}^{\mathrm{I}}_{\mathrm{C}}$. A bending of the axis undermines our rigidity assumption (see Fig. 2(c)). Although no modeling for the axis bending can be applied, safety concerns require the recognition of these critical cases. Recall that the drill bit trajectory is constrained to pass through the origin $\mathrm{O_{H_i}}$ of $\mathrm{S_{H_i}}$. The intersection $\mathrm{P_{A_i}}$ between the estimated axis trajectory and the plane orthogonal to hole axis is calculated. Values of the distance $d = \overline{\mathrm{O_{H_i}}, \mathrm{P_{A_i}}} \neq 0$ are considered as an indication of the axis bending. A warning is given to the user, suggesting that attention should be paid while holding the instrument.

3 Experiments

Extensive experiments were conducted both on distal radius bone phantoms and on healthy forearm cadaver specimens. A total of 34 (15 rights and 19 left)

Table 1. Mean and median values for tip distance ($\mathrm{d_T}$), and for errors in azimuth (α), elevation (β) and total (ψ) angles for plastic bones: 1) All users (AU), 15 right bones (60 screws) and 19 left bones (75 screws); 2) Engineering experts (EE), 13 right bones (52 screws) and 17 left bones (67 screws); 3) Medical experts, (ME) 2 right bones (8 screws) and 2 left bones (8 screws). The last row refers to the forearm specimens (FS).

	$\mathrm{d_T}$ (mm)		α (°)		β (°)		ψ (°)	
AU	1.02 ± 0.57	0.89	3.68 ± 4.38	2.60	1.77 ± 1.38	1.49	2.52 ± 1.62	2.18
EE	0.97 ± 0.47	0.89	3.29 ± 4.02	2.45	1.76 ± 1.34	1.52	2.43 ± 1.37	2.18
ME	1.34 ± 1.02	1.06	5.86 ± 6.18	3.18	1.85 ± 1.73	1.21	3.21 ± 2.87	2.39
FS	1.63 ± 0.91	1.40	5.85 ± 4.93	4.07	3.48 ± 3.07	2.17	4.54 ± 2.77	4.37

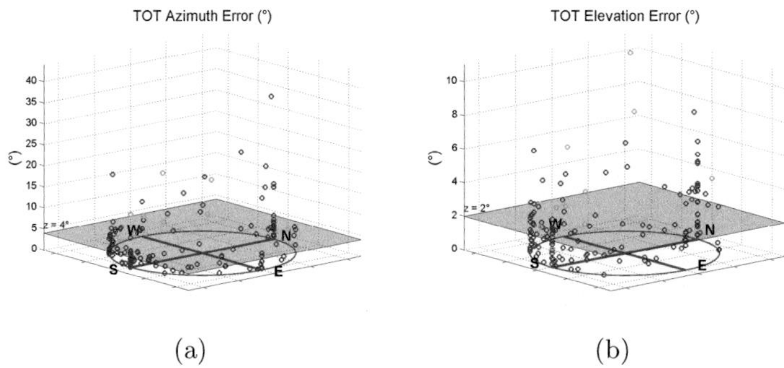

Fig. 3. Error distribution for the 4 angular sectors for phantoms (blue) and specimens (green): (a) azimuth and (b) elevation. North relates to the distal side of the plate.

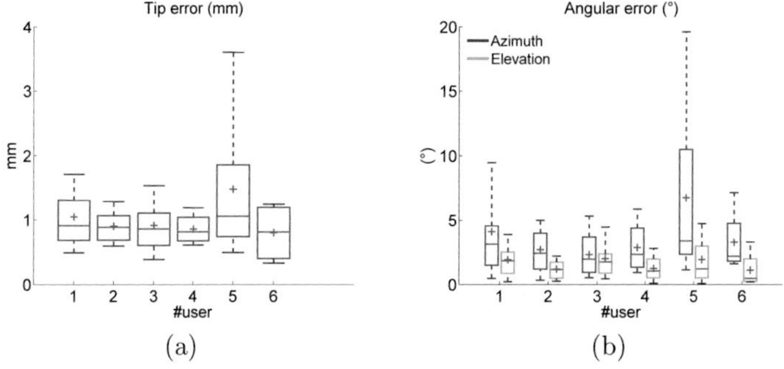

Fig. 4. Inter-user variability for the bone phantoms in terms of (a) the tip error, and (b) the angular error in azimuth and elevation. Users 1 to 4 are engineering experts, while 5 and 6 are medical experts. Users 4 and 6 operated each on a single phantom.

phantoms (involving 135 screws) and 3 specimens (2 rights and 1 left involving 11 screws for which the drill guide was correctly oriented) were used in our evaluation. The length of the screws ranged from 14 to 24mm. Two user groups (4 users with engineering expertise and 2 medical experts) operated on the phantoms. The specimens were operated by just one medical expert. According to the proposed workflow, for each test, the operator was asked to: 1) fix the implant to the test-body, 2) acquire 2 radio-graphic images for implant registration, 3) plan the desired screw configuration, 4) select the current screw hole and accordingly position our marker-drill guide, 5) transfer the plan guided by the real-time feedback of our software, and 6) place the screws and acquire a 3D volume (Arcadis® Orbic 3D, Siemens; Volume: 256^3 voxels; Spacing: 0.485mm). After manual registration of the plate to the 3D volume, we evaluated the accuracy of the transferred plan in terms of the Euclidean distance of the screw tip, d_T, and of the absolute errors in the screw axis orientation, expressed in azimuth, α, elevation, β, as well as total, ψ, angles (see Table 1). Our error estimates contain all 6 process steps. Our ANOVA analysis showed significant ($p < 0.05$) difference in d_T and no significant difference ($p > 0.05$) in ψ between EE and ME.

4 Discussion and Conclusions

Our portable framework for intra-operative planning and guidance for distal radius fracture surgery does not require the fixation of any navigation markers onto the patient. The patient reference is provided directly by the plate registration onto the images acquired intra-operatively. For guidance, minimal additional instrumentation is required. The feasibility of our framework and its impact on screw positioning accuracy were investigated. For performance comparison, we recall the closest related work [12], a clinical study conducted using solely intra-operative planning. Though their results refer to real cases, we can still use them as a point of reference for the expected accuracy without a guidance system: their reported errors in d_T, α and β are 2.24±0.97mm, 18.69±29.84° and 1.66±4.46° respectively. The series of our evaluations conducted in a lab environment on phantoms (see Table 1), showed overall a significant increase in screw placement accuracy and robustness. The mean error in d_T and α was reduced by 54% and 80% respectively, while the standard deviation dropped by 41% and 85% accordingly. The mean error in β increased from 1.66° to 1.77°, while the standard deviation was more than halved. As expected, the error distribution (see Fig. 3) shows that higher error occurs when drilling in the north sector, i.e. close to the marker holder, since this reduces marker visibility. In these specific cases, appropriate drill guide rotation is expected to increase accuracy.

A similar performance was observed in the experiments conducted on forearm specimens. The mean error in d_T and α was reduced by 27% and 69% respectively, while the standard deviation was decreased by 6% and 83% accordingly. The mean error in β increased from 1.66° to 3.48°, while the standard deviation was decreased by 31%. In one of the right forearms, the drill guide for one of the screws was rotated 90° w.r.t the planned position. Although our software allows selecting the drill guide orientation for planning transfer, in this case the change in orientation was not conveyed by the user. Even under such circumstances, our guidance framework helped keep mean error values for both α and β below 10° and 4° respectively. Introducing the above mentioned case of incorrectly positioned drill guide into our quantitative evaluation, results in errors in d_T, α and β of 1.94±1.37mm, 9.00±11.89° and 3.32±2.98° respectively. Moreover, our sequential analysis showed that the performance of user 5 improved over time for both phantoms and forearm specimens. A fourth specimen was excluded from the quantitative evaluation, since plate rotation occurred during the procedure. Our results show that our framework is expected to increase the accuracy in screw positioning and to improve robustness. Further testing is to be performed on specimens presenting common fracture types.

Acknowledgements. This work was supported by the Research Training Group 1773 "Heterogeneous Image Systems", funded by the German Research Foundation (DFG).

References

1. Al-Rashid, M., Theivendran, K., Craigen, M.: Delayed ruptures of the extensor tendon secondary to the use of volar locking compression plates for distal radial fractures. Journal of Bone & Joint Surgery, British 88(12), 1610–1612 (2006)
2. Arora, R., Lutz, M., Hennerbichler, A., Krappinger, D., Espen, D., Gabl, M.: Complications following internal fixation of unstable distal radius fracture with a palmar locking-plate. Journal of Orthopaedic Trauma 21(5), 316–322 (2007)
3. Diotte, B., Fallavollita, P., Wang, L., Weidert, S., Thaller, P.H., Euler, E., Navab, N.: Radiation-free drill guidance in interlocking of intramedullary nails. In: Ayache, N., Delingette, H., Golland, P., Mori, K. (eds.) MICCAI 2012, Part I. LNCS, vol. 7510, pp. 18–25. Springer, Heidelberg (2012)
4. Fiala, M.: Artag fiducial marker system applied to vision based spacecraft docking. In: IROS, Workshop on Robot Vision for Space Applications, pp. 35–40 (2005)
5. Frank, J., Gritzbach, B., Winter, C., Maier, B., Marzi, I.: Computer-assisted femur fracture reduction. European Journal of Trauma and Emergency Surgery 36(2), 151–156 (2010)
6. Jenny, J.Y., Miehlke, R.K., Giurea, A.: Learning curve in navigated total knee replacement. a multi-centre study comparing experienced and beginner centres. The Knee 15(2), 80–84 (2008)
7. Koutenaei, B.A., Guler, O., Wilson, E., Thoranaghatte, R.U., Oetgen, M., Navab, N., Cleary, K.: Improved screw placement for slipped capital femoral epiphysis (SCFE) using robotically-assisted drill guidance. In: Golland, P., Hata, N., Barillot, C., Hornegger, J., Howe, R. (eds.) MICCAI 2014, Part I. LNCS, vol. 8673, pp. 488–495. Springer, Heidelberg (2014)
8. Magaraggia, J., Kleinszig, G., Wei, W., Weiten, M., Graumann, R., Angelopoulou, E., Hornegger, J.: On the accuracy of a video-based drill-guidance solution for orthopedic and trauma surgery: preliminary results. In: SPIE Medical Imaging, pp. 903610–903610. International Society for Optics and Photonics (2014)
9. McKay, S.D., MacDermid, J.C., Roth, J.H., Richards, R.S.: Assessment of complications of distal radius fractures and development of a complication checklist. Journal of Hand Surgery 26(5), 916–922 (2001)
10. Pichler, W., Grechenig, W., Clement, H., Windisch, G., Tesch, N.: Perforation of the third extensor compartment by the drill bit during palmar plating of the distal radius. Journal of Hand Surgery (European Volume) 34(3), 333–335 (2009)
11. Sügün, T., Karabay, N., Gürbüz, Y., Özaksar, K., Toros, T., Kayalar, M.: Screw prominences related to palmar locking plating of distal radius. Journal of Hand Surgery (European Volume) 36(4), 320–324 (2011)
12. Vetter, S., Mühlhäuser, I., von Recum, J., Grützner, P.A., Franke, J.: Validation of a virtual implant planning system (VIPS) in distal radius fractures. Bone & Joint Journal Orthopaedic Proceedings Supplement 96(Supp 16), 50–50 (2014)
13. Wagner, D., Schmalstieg, D.: Artoolkitplus for pose tracking on mobile devices. In: CVWW 2007, 12th Computer Vision Winter Workshop, Sankt Lambrecht, Austria (2007)

Image Based Surgical Instrument Pose Estimation with Multi-class Labelling and Optical Flow

Max Allan[1], Ping-Lin Chang[1], Sébastien Ourselin[1], David J. Hawkes[1], Ashwin Sridhar[2], John Kelly[2], and Danail Stoyanov[1]

[1] Centre for Medical Image Computing, University College London, UK
[2] Division of Surgery and Interventional Science, UCL Medical School, UK

Abstract. Image based detection, tracking and pose estimation of surgical instruments in minimally invasive surgery has a number of potential applications for computer assisted interventions. Recent developments in the field have resulted in advanced techniques for 2D instrument detection in laparoscopic images, however, full 3D pose estimation remains a challenging and unsolved problem. In this paper, we present a novel method for estimating the 3D pose of robotic instruments, including axial rotation, by fusing information from large homogeneous regions and local optical flow features. We demonstrate the accuracy and robustness of this approach on ex vivo data with calibrated ground truth given by surgical robot kinematics which we will also make available to the community. Qualitative validation on in vivo data from robotic assisted prostatectomy further demonstrates that the technique can function in clinical scenarios.

1 Introduction

Robotic minimally invasive surgery can facilitate procedures in confined and difficult to access anatomical regions. However, accessing the anatomy with robotic instruments reduces the surgeon's ability to sense force feedback from instrument-tissue interactions and the limited field of view of the surgical camera makes localization with respect to preoperative patient data challenging. Computer assisted interventions (CAI) can integrate additional information during the operation to help the surgeon and knowing the 3D position and orientation of the surgical instruments during surgery is a critical CAI element. The instrument pose can additionally be used in robotic surgery to provide control enhancements with dynamic motion constraints or to detect tool-tissue interactions and provide force feedback [13].

Image-based methods can potentially estimate instrument pose in the reference frame of the laparoscope without requiring electromagnetic or optical sensors [6,12]. This usually involves extracting image features such as edges, points or regions and then solving alignment cost functions which measure the agreement with parametrized models of the tool [10]. Gradient based methods

N. Navab et al. (Eds.): MICCAI 2015, Part I, LNCS 9349, pp. 331–338, 2015.
DOI: 10.1007/978-3-319-24553-9_41

are often preferred but it is challenging to develop cost functions that do not easily become trapped in local minima and fail to find the correct pose [15,1]. [9] used gradient free optimization from color and texture features for articulated instruments but the chosen cost can be complex to optimize resulting in slow and often inaccurate solutions. Another alternative is to use Random Forests (RF) to detect instrument parts [14] which gives promising results and low computational cost but is only shown as a 2D tracking method. Using robot kinematic information from the joint encoders has been investigated but accumulation of errors can result in significant error and bounded brute-force template-matching has been employed to reduce the offset [3]. Region based methods for surgical instruments were proposed in [1] where bag-of-pixel based object appearance models were used to demonstrated pose estimation that is robust to viewpoint and illumination changes [4]. However disregarding all spatial information within the object boundary makes it challenging to recover the instrument roll axis and the yaw axis which is usually strongly affected by the foreshortening visual cue. Additional cues have been fused with region features to obtain more stable tracking but did not address the correspondence problem when dealing with multiple point detections on the instrument tip [2].

In this paper, we present a novel image-driven pose estimation technique for robotic instruments in minimally invasive surgery (MIS). This is achieved by fusing large scale region based constraints with low level optical flow information. The interior homogeneous-intensity regions of the instruments are described with separate appearance models and this is used to formulate region based alignment as a multi region problem rather than using a binary silhouette. The interior instrument appearance is a strong regional cue on robotic instruments and helps to solve the foreshortening problem by introducing a full visible boundary in the image plane. We focus on estimating rigid 3D pose without the full articulation of the robotic instruments. Quantitative validation is shown on calibrated ex vivo data collected using the da Vinci® research kit (DVRK) and API [8] and qualitative validation is demonstrated on challenging in vivo data.

2 Method

Our method works by fusing large-scale region features, which are based on the output of multi-label probabilistic classification, with small-scale flow features. The region features drive coarse pose estimation through the alignment of predicted regions generated from the projection of the instrument, given a particular pose estimate, with the detected regions on the classification map. To improve fine scale estimation, salient features on the instrument surface are tracked from frame-to-frame using optical flow.

2.1 Multi-label Probabilistic Classification

We use RFs to provide probabilistic region classification an image, assigning pixel to one of K object classes, where in a typical image there will be $K-1$

regions for an instrument and 1 region for the background (see Fig. 1a. When applied to classification, each RF is an ensemble of decision trees which each vote on a labelling for the input pixel. The vote of a single tree is decided by directing an input sample $\mathbf{x}$ from a root node $\S_{parent}$ to one of its two child nodes $\S_{child}$ according to a linear model $y = \mathbf{wx}$ where the left child is chosen if $y < T_i$ and to the right node if $y \geq T_i$ where T_i is a node specific threshold value. This root to child splitting is applied recursively on the sample until it reaches a terminating node, known as a *leaf node* where it is given a label according to a probability distribution $p(C|\mathbf{x})$ stored in that node. Each tree in the forest applies a classification vote and then these votes are averaged across all the trees to obtain the output of the forest.

Training our forest involved the manual segmentation of a single frame containing instruments positioned in front of a tissue background into the specified K classes however, in principal a large background library of possible tissue types and foreground models would be learned offline to allow the system to operate in different surgical setups without re-training. We use a simple color based feature set of Hue, Saturation, Opponent 1 and Opponent 2 which were shown to have good classification on MIS images [1].

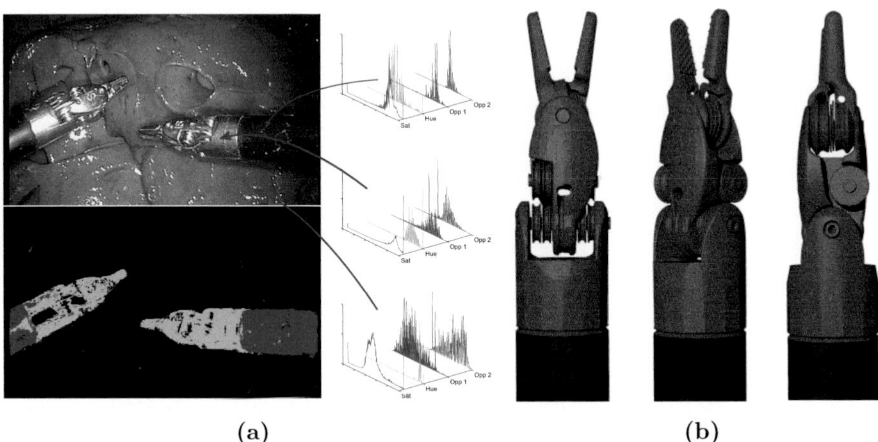

(a) (b)

Fig. 1. (a) shows the feature distribution for each of the $K = 3$ classes with output classification and (b) shows example renderings of a robotic instrument CAD model from Intuitive Surgical Inc.

2.2 Multi-region Segmentation with Level Sets

Statistical region-based 3D pose estimation is formulated as a segmentation problem, where the pose parameters which enable the silhouette of the projection of a geometric model to optimally divide an image into two regions are estimated. For robotic instruments, modelling internal homogeneous regions separately can be used to create strong delineating contours, which can improve the estimated pose over modelling the interior with a single distribution and using only the silhouette. We therefore model an instrument's appearance with $K-1$ statistical models so, given a single background model, we describe the image with K statistical models. Pose estimation then becomes a problem of finding the $K-1$ contours which divide the image plane up into K regions such that the pixels within the ith region agree maximally with the ith statistical model.

We describe the segmenting contours using level sets of signed distance functions [7,4] as they avoid the problem of an explicitly parametrized curve while elegantly applying implicit correspondences between the region-based data contours and the model projection contours. Finding the contours which optimally assign each of the K models to the image becomes a variational problem which is described using the the following cost:

$$E_{region}(\Theta) = -\sum_{i}^{K}\sum_{\mathbf{x}\in\Omega} \log\left(H(\phi^i(\mathbf{x},\Theta))P_f^{\Omega_i} + (1 - H(\phi^i(\mathbf{x},\Theta)))P_b^{\Omega_i}\right) \quad (1)$$

where $\phi^i(\mathbf{x},\Theta)$ is the Euclidean distance between at the pixel $\mathbf{x}$ and the closest point on the contour generated from the ith model projection at pose Θ. $\phi(.)$ is set to the negative distance outside the contour and positive inside. We represent pose as translation and rotation for which we use the quaternion representation. $H(.)$ is a smoothed Heaviside function which truncates the values of ϕ into a spatial prior on the model assignment. Ω_i are the pixels within the ith region of the image Ω and $P_{f,b}^{\Omega_i}$ are the learned distributions for the pixels inside (foreground) and outside (background) the ith contour. Rather than performing one-against-all for the background distribution, we instead use the expected neighbour class of the pixel $\mathbf{x}$ as the chosen background distribution.

2.3 Optimization and Tracking

The level set segmentation provides accurate pose estimation but in the presence of fast motion and noise errors can appear especially around the roll axis of the instrument where the contour cues may not provide sufficient constraints. However, low level interior features and optical flow in the image can provide strong cues about the motion of the instrument from frame-to-frame. We use simple gradient-based salient features [11] and assuming the first frame contains the correct pose, backproject the tracked points onto the object model and do frame-to-frame tracking using the Lucas-Kanade method [5]. The optimization of this functional involves the joint minimization of the region based cost which we perform over both frames, if available, and the flow based cost solving for a single set of pose parameters to obtain stereo constraints.

$$E(\Theta) = \min_{\Theta} \sum_{j} E^{j}_{region}(\Theta) + \lambda \sum_{i}^{N} ||\mathbf{y}'_i - P(\mathbf{y}_i, \Theta)||^2 \tag{2}$$

where $\mathbf{y}'_i$ is the position of the ith optical flow tracked point in the image frame and $P(\mathbf{y}_i, \Theta)$ represents our estimate of where the point $\mathbf{y}_i$ projects to from the surface of our model. In essence this is 2D-3D registration. The sum over j is over the left and right frames of the stereo pair where E^{j}_{region} refers to the energy function from the left or right frame. λ is the usual weighting factor between our two cost functions and is set experimentally. We use gradient descent to find the minimum for each frame and combine with a Kalman filter for temporal consistency. Initialization is assumed to be correct for the first frame and can be achieved within a few seconds using a manual positioning of the instrument.

3 Results

Our algorithm is written in C++ and OpenGL using OpenCV[1]. Processing time measured on a single core of a 1.9GHz processor for classification of a single stereo frame using a RF is ≈ 0.83 seconds, for a gradient descent step on one stereo frame is ≈ 0.3 seconds (typically 10-20 steps required) and processing time for the flow tracking is ≈ 0.006 seconds per frame. The most computationally expensive component is the region based cost for which each pixel is computed independently allowing for real time speeds when using a GPU implementation [10]. Furthermore, RFs are suitable for GPU parallelisation and by only performing classification in regions where the derivatives are non-zero, we can greatly reduce the number of pixels which require classification to around 0.5% of the image. The source code and data from our method are available online[2].

3.1 Quantitative Validation

Using the da Vinci® API it is possible to estimate the position and orientation of each robotic instrument by reading the motor joint encoder values and then using the Denavit Hartenberg (DH) chain to compute the relative orientations of the instruments and the camera. The encoder values accumulate errors over time resulting in joints being offset from the camera frame, which is why image-based estimation is important even when encoder information is available. The majority of this error can be calibrated out with a fixed offset to obtain a ground truth pose in the camera frame with high accuracy. We constructed an ex vivo sequence of 1000 frames with a lamb liver tissue and computed the pose of the instruments in each frame using our method and also computed a ground truth pose using the robot forward kinematics. To assess our method, we compare

[1] `http://opencv.org`

[2] `http://www.surgicalvision.cs.ucl.ac.uk/code`

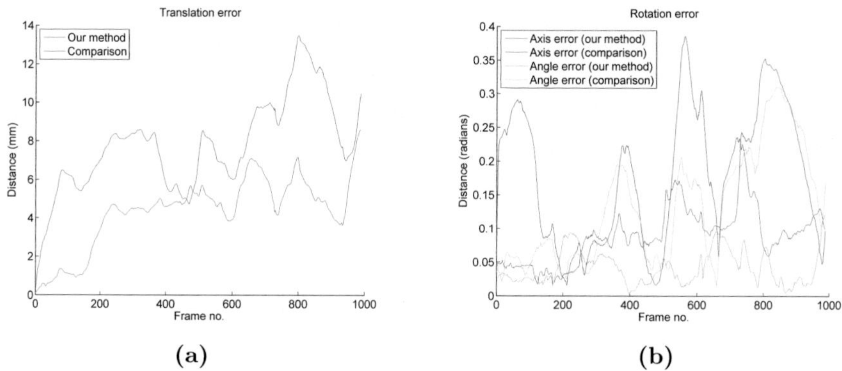

Fig. 2. (a) RMS error in measuring translation from the camera center to the origin of the model coordinates (near the head) from our algorithm and from the comparison method when compared to the ground truth estimates using ex vivo data. (b) Similar to (a) but showing angular distance between axis and angular error when using the angle-axis representation of the instrument pose.

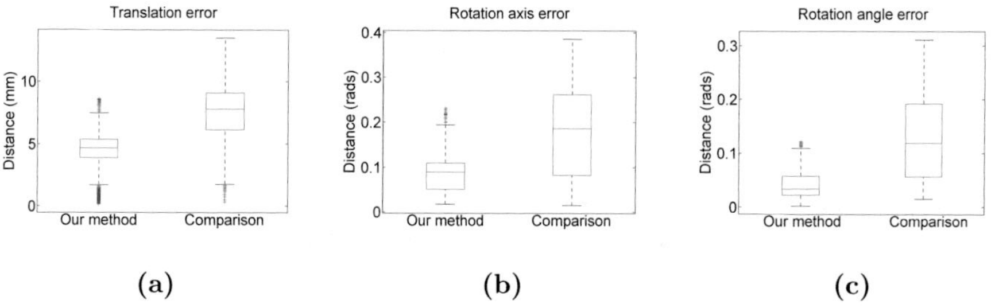

Fig. 3. Error distribution for data in Fig. 2. Red line shows median error while the top and bottom of the box show the 25th and 75th percentiles, the whiskers extend to the most extreme data points not considered outliers, and outliers are plotted individually.

it with a our previous silhouette based tracking technique [2] which does not use interior contours or the low level flow features.

We report errors for rotation using the angle-axis representation, computing angular distance between the axes and also the difference between the angular rotation around those axes, and translation between the camera and instrument coordinate system, where we average the error at each frame across both instruments. Trajectory errors are shown in Fig. 2 and error distributions are show in a box plot in Fig. 3. Translational error is broken down into each axis in numerical form in Table 1.

Table 1. The mean error ± std deviation of each translational degree of freedom and the rotational angle/axis of the robotic instruments for the ex vivo data. Top row is our method and bottom is the comparison method.

	x (mm)	y (mm)	z (mm)	axis (rads)	angle (rads)
This work	0.70 ± 0.31	0.50 ± 0.27	4.09 ± 1.82	0.08 ± 0.04	0.04 ± 0.03
[2]	1.09 ± 0.65	0.59 ± 0.29	7.48 ± 2.32	0.18 ± 0.10	0.13 ± 0.08

3.2 Qualitative Validation

We show qualitative validation for both ex vivo and in vivo sequences in Fig. 4 where the overlap between the projected model and the underlying image demonstrates the accuracy of our method.

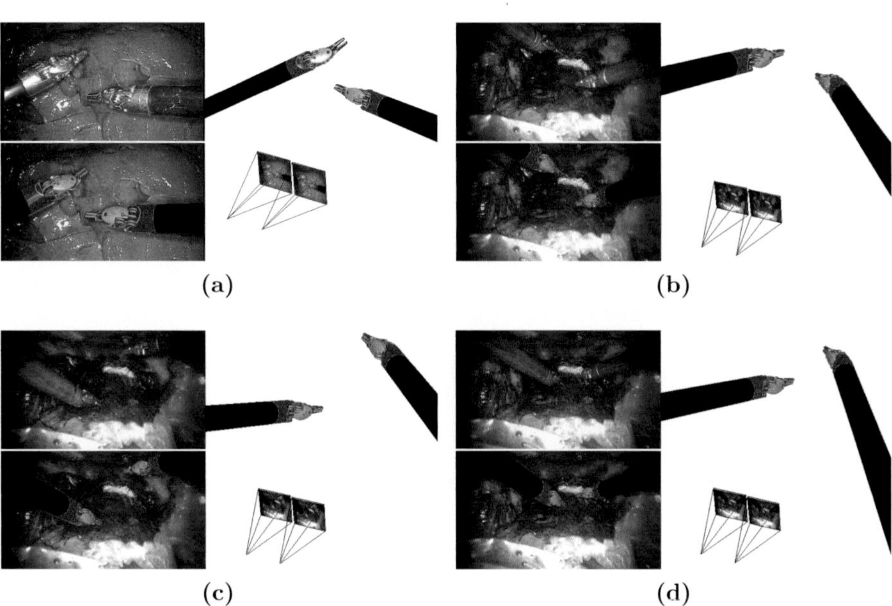

Fig. 4. Qualitative validation on a challenging ex vivo (a) and in vivo (b-d) sequence showing an example left camera image, the same frame with instruments overlaid at the current pose estimate and a 3D plot of the instruments in front of the stereo camera pair.

4 Conclusion and Discussion

The results from Fig. 2 and Table 1 demonstrate the significant quantitative improvements in our algorithm in comparison to the state-of-the-art method [2], in particularly with respect to the rotational parameters, which is the result of using frame-to-frame low level flow features to estimate the instrument roll. Results in the x and y direction are very stable with errors below ≤ 0.7 mm with increased error in the z direction. This is typically the largest source of error as, even when using stereo constraints larger differences in 3D position only reveal themselves as small inaccuracies in the 2D data/model alignment. Additionally we observe that the errors increase over the duration of the experiment which is common in model based tracking as errors from previous frames gradually cause the correct estimate to drift away from the true solution. Future improvements to our method will involve solving our cost function for all degrees of freedom of the articulated robotic instrument rather than using $SE(3)$.

Acknowledgements. The authors would like to acknowledge Simon Di-Maio and Dale Bergman at Intuitive Surgical Inc. for supplying the CAD models.

References

1. Allan, M., Ourselin, S., Thompson, S., Hawkes, D.J., Kelly, J., Stoyanov, D.: Toward detection and localization of instruments in minimally invasive surgery. IEEE Transactions on Biomedical Engineering 60(4), 1050–1058 (2013)
2. Allan, M., Thompson, S., Clarkson, M.J., Ourselin, S., Hawkes, D.J., Kelly, J., Stoyanov, D.: 2d-3d pose tracking of rigid instruments in minimally invasive surgery. In: Stoyanov, D., Collins, D.L., Sakuma, I., Abolmaesumi, P., Jannin, P. (eds.) IPCAI 2014. LNCS, vol. 8498, pp. 1–10. Springer, Heidelberg (2014)
3. Austin, R.: K, A.P., Tao, Z.: Articulated surgical tool detection using virtually-rendered templates. In: Computer Assisted Radiology and Surgery (2012)
4. Bibby, C., Reid, I.: Robust Real-Time visual tracking using Pixel-Wise posteriors. In: ECCV, pp. 831–844 (2008)
5. Bouguet, J.Y.: Pyramidal implementation of the lucas kanade feature tracker. Intel Corporation, Microprocessor Research Labs (2000)
6. Chmarra, M.K., Grimbergen, C.A., Dankelman, J.: Systems for tracking minimally invasive surgical instruments. Minimally Invasive Therapy & Allied Technologies 16(6), 328–340 (2007)
7. Cremers, D., Rousson, M., Deriche, R.: A review of statistical approaches to level set segmentation. IJCV 72(2), 195–215 (2007)
8. DiMaio, S., Hasser, C.: The da vinci research interface (July 2008)
9. Pezzementi, Z., Voros, S., Hager, G.D.: Articulated object tracking by rendering consistent appearance parts. In: ICRA 2009, pp. 3940–3947 (May 2009)
10. Prisacariu, V.A., Reid, I.D.: PWP3D: Real-Time segmentation and tracking of 3D objects. Int. J. Computer Vision 98(3), 335–354 (2012)
11. Shi, J., Tomasi, C.: Good features to track. In: CVPR 1994, pp. 593–600 (June 1994)
12. Speidel, S., Sudra, G., Senemaud, J., Drentschew, M., Müller-Stich, B.P., Gutt, C., Dillmann, R.: Recognition of risk situations based on endoscopic instrument tracking and knowledge based situation modeling. In: Medical Imaging 2008: Visualization, Image-Guided Procedures, and Modeling, vol. 6918 (2008)
13. Stoyanov, D.: Surgical vision. Annals of Biomedical Engineering 40(2) (2012)
14. Sznitman, R., Becker, C., Fua, P.: Fast part-based classification for instrument detection in minimally invasive surgery. In: Golland, P., Hata, N., Barillot, C., Hornegger, J., Howe, R. (eds.) MICCAI 2014, Part II. LNCS, vol. 8674, pp. 692–699. Springer, Heidelberg (2014)
15. Sznitman, R., Ali, K., Richa, R., Taylor, R.H., Hager, G.D., Fua, P.: Data-driven visual tracking in retinal microsurgery. In: Ayache, N., Delingette, H., Golland, P., Mori, K. (eds.) MICCAI 2012, Part II. LNCS, vol. 7511, pp. 568–575. Springer, Heidelberg (2012)

Adaption of 3D Models to 2D X-Ray Images during Endovascular Abdominal Aneurysm Repair

Daniel Toth[1,2], Marcus Pfister[1], Andreas Maier[2], Markus Kowarschik[1], and Joachim Hornegger[2]

[1] Siemens Healthcare GmbH, Forchheim, Germany
[2] Pattern Recognition Lab., Friedrich-Alexander-University Erlangen-Nuremberg, Erlangen, Germany

Abstract. Endovascular aneurysm repair (EVAR) has been gaining popularity over open repair of abdominal aortic aneurysms (AAAs) in the recent years. This paper describes a distortion correction approach to be applied during the EVAR cases. In a novel workflow, models (meshes) of the aorta and its branching arteries generated from preoperatively acquired computed tomography (CT) scans are overlayed with interventionally acquired fluoroscopic images. The overlay provides an arterial roadmap for the operator, with landmarks (LMs) marking the ostia, which are critical for stent placement. As several endovascular devices, such as angiographic catheters, are inserted, the anatomy may be distorted. The distortion reduces the accuracy of the overlay. To overcome the mismatch, the aortic and the iliac meshes are adapted to a device seen in uncontrasted intraoperative fluoroscopic images using the skeleton-based as-rigid-as-possible (ARAP) method. The deformation was evaluated by comparing the distance between an ostium and the corresponding LM prior to and after the deformation. The central positions of the ostia were marked in digital subtraction angiography (DSA) images as ground truth. The mean Euclidean distance in the image plane was reduced from 19.81 ± 17.14 mm to 4.56 ± 2.81 mm.

Keywords: computational geometry, as-rigid-as-possible, mesh deformation, abdominal aortic aneurysm, EVAR.

1 Introduction

The abdominal aortic aneurysm (AAA) is one of the most frequent aortic diseases. It is a dilatation of the abdominal aorta. AAAs, such as cardiac diseases, are becoming increasingly more common due to the continuous aging of the population. In the case of aneurysm rupture, 60% of the patients reach the hospital alive and 65% of these patients die during elective repair [1]. Detection of AAAs prior to rupture is challenging. They are mostly asymptomatic, thus often found accidentally. If the aneurysm diameter exceeds 5.5 cm or its expansion is rapid, it is decided for elective repair [9]. Endovascular aneurysm repair (EVAR) represents a more novel approach than open surgery. During an EVAR intervention,

N. Navab et al. (Eds.): MICCAI 2015, Part I, LNCS 9349, pp. 339–346, 2015.
DOI: 10.1007/978-3-319-24553-9_42

the operating physician inserts endovascular instruments through minor incisions at the groins and places a stent graft into the body of the aneurysm to exclude the weakened wall of the aorta from the blood flow. EVAR causes less trauma to the patient and the recovery times are significantly shorter compared to open repair. There is no difference in long-term mortality rates, but the short-term death rate of EVAR is significantly lower [10].

EVAR procedures are navigated by X-ray fluoroscopic images. To visualize vascular structures during the intervention, iodinated contrast agent is injected. However, as the patients are in advanced age, their renal functions may not be sufficient to process the injected contrast medium. In a more novel workflow, a preoperatively acquired computed tomography (CT) volume is segmented [8]. The resulting surface meshes of the aorta and the branching arteries are used for preinterventional planning. Landmarks (LMs) of the main branching artery ostia are calculated automatically and the physician may set further LMs manually. After the LM calculation, optimal angulations of the interventional C-arm system are calculated to be recalled during the intervention.

During the intervention, the preoperative CT dataset is registered to the C-arm system [2] and the mesh models of the aorta and its branching arteries are projected onto the fluoroscopic images which provides an arterial roadmap for the operator and potentially leads to a reduction in contrast agent load. However, the inserted endovascular devices may distort the anatomy and reduce the accuracy of the overlay. To compensate for the mismatch, several approaches have been developed previously. Non-rigid registration approaches were implemented by Liao et al. [7] and Guyot et al. [3], which require intense contrast agent usage. Another approach is based on the implementation of a finite element method (FEM) [6]. The FEM has a high computational complexity and current implementations only simulate the deformation prior to the intervention.

In this paper, the application of the skeleton-based variant of the as-rigid-as-possible (ARAP) mesh deformation for endovascular distortion correction is presented. The ARAP method was developed by Igarashi et al. for 2D surface deformations [5] and reformulated by Sorkine and Alexa to handle 3D surface meshes [11]. The 3D ARAP method can be considered as the successor of the Laplacian surface editing method developed by Sorkine et al. [12]. The 3D surface mesh ARAP framework was extended by Zhang et al. with a skeletal constraint to result in better volume preservation [13]. We implemented this skeleton-based variant of the ARAP surface mesh deformation with a control point selection and transformation algorithm. The evaluation revealed that the implemented method was able to increase the accuracy of the arterial roadmap significantly in the case of anatomical distortion.

2 Methods

The idea is to adapt the mesh model to the reconstructed 3D device such that it smoothly deforms to the new position. Due to the knowledge of the position of the 3D device, the new position of some of the vertices can be determined. Due

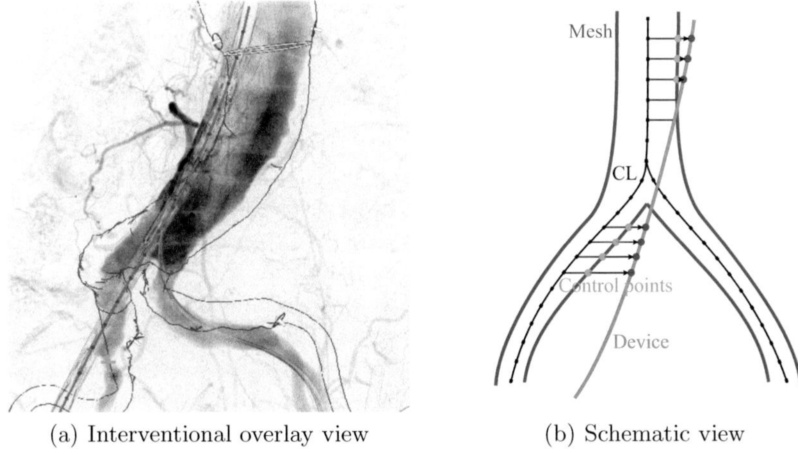

(a) Interventional overlay view (b) Schematic view

Fig. 1. (a) The interventional view shows an overlay of a preoperative CT and a DSA image with the reconstructed device. (b) Rays are cast between the mesh centerline (CL) and the device. If a ray hits the mesh, the hit point is designated as a control point, which will be moved to the device points.

to anatomical constraints, the position of some other vertices can be fixed. The known vertices represent the control points of the applied method, see Figure 1.

The ARAP method ensures that the deformed shape matches the control points on one hand and, on the other hand, the remaining vertices are displaced with as minimal transformations as possible.

2.1 Skeleton-Based As-Rigid-As-Possible Mesh Deformation

A triangular surface mesh, in the following shape $\mathcal{S}$, is characterized by its vertices $\mathbf{v}_i \in \mathbb{R}^3$ and edges $\mathbf{e}_{ij} = \mathbf{v}_i - \mathbf{v}_j$ connecting the vertices. A deformed surface mesh is denoted by $\mathcal{S}'$ in the following, with deformed vertex positions $\mathbf{v}'_i$ and deformed edges $\mathbf{e}'_{ij}$. Shapes $\mathcal{S}$ and $\mathcal{S}'$ may have different geometries, but must have the same topology after deformation.

For the non-rigid deformation between the shapes $\mathcal{S}$ and $\mathcal{S}'$, an energy function was formulated by Sorkine and Alexa [11]:

$$E(\mathcal{S}, \mathcal{S}') = \sum_{i=1}^{n} \sum_{j \in \mathcal{N}(i)} w_{ij} ||\mathbf{e}'_{ij} - \mathbf{R}_i \mathbf{e}_{ij}||_2^2, \tag{1}$$

where n denotes the number of vertices, the w_{ij} represent edge weights and $\mathbf{R}_i$ denotes the rotation matrix of a cell, i.e., the vertex $\mathbf{v}_i$ and its one-ring neighborhood $\mathcal{N}(i)$. To compensate for possible mesh non-uniformities, the w_{ij} were chosen to be cotangent weights [11]. This formulation guarantees maximal rigidity, if optimized for minimal rotations. The minimization and reordering results for all vertices i in

$$\sum_{j\in\mathcal{N}(i)} w_{ij}(\mathbf{v}'_i - \mathbf{v}'_j) = \sum_{j\in\mathcal{N}(i)} \frac{w_{ij}}{2}(\mathbf{R}_i + \mathbf{R}_j)(\mathbf{v}_i - \mathbf{v}_j) \Longrightarrow \mathbf{L}\mathbf{v}' = \mathbf{b}(\mathbf{R}), \quad (2)$$

where $\mathbf{L}$ is a weighted Laplacian matrix and $\mathbf{b}(\mathbf{R})$ denotes the right hand side of the resulting linear system of equations depending on the local rotations.

The ARAP transformation is controlled by a subset of vertices with known new positions. These positions may either be kept identical to their previous ones (anchor points) or transformed into explicitly defined new ones (handle points). The union of these designated vertices is called control points. In [12] these m control points $\mathbf{v}_{c_i}$ are taken into account in the previously derived Laplacian surface editing energy formulation

$$E_L(\mathcal{S}, \mathcal{S}') = ||\mathbf{L}\mathbf{v}' - \delta||_2^2 + \sum_{i=1}^{m} ||\mathbf{v}'_{c_i} - \mathbf{v}_{c_i}||_2^2 \Longrightarrow \mathbf{L}\mathbf{v}' = \mathbf{b}, \quad (3)$$

where $\delta = \mathbf{L}\mathbf{v}$.

The similarity between Equation 2 and Equation 3 is apparent. The control point constraint can easily be added to the ARAP energy formulation and system matrix as well. The left hand side, the system matrix, is identical, but the right hand side is dependent on the local rotations $\mathbf{R}_i$ in the ARAP method.

The linear system of equations of the ARAP approach can be solved with a two-step iteration. Prior to the iteration, the edge weights w_{ij} are computed and the system matrix $\mathbf{L}$ is assembled and prefactorized. As the matrix $\mathbf{L}$ is sparse, symmetric and positive definite, a sparse Cholesky decomposition, as proposed in [11], is used. Next, an initial guess, the Laplacian surface editing solution, $\mathbf{v}'_{(0)}$ is calculated by solving Equation 2 with all rotations $\mathbf{R}_i$ set to identity.

In the first step, the iteration calculates the optimal local rotations $\mathbf{R}_i$ by minimizing Equation 1 with the calculated previous solution $\mathbf{v}'_{(0)}$. In the second step, the rotations $\mathbf{R}_i$ are substituted into the right hand side of Equation 2 and the next solution $\mathbf{v}'_{(1)}$ is calculated by solving the equation system. These two iteration steps are repeated until convergence.

We implemented the extended ARAP framework developed by Zhang et al. to account for possible volume deflations [13]. For volume preservation, a skeletal constraint was incorporated. The constraint can be formulated as an additional term in the Laplacian energy function:

$$E_{skel}(\mathcal{S}, \mathcal{S}') = ||\mathbf{L}\mathbf{v}' - \delta||_2^2 + ||\mathbf{L}_s\mathbf{v}'_{all} - \delta_s||_2^2 + \sum_{i=1}^{m} ||\mathbf{v}'_{c_i} - \mathbf{v}_{c_i}||_2^2, \quad (4)$$

where $\mathbf{L}_s$ denotes the Laplacian matrix of the skeleton points, $\mathbf{v}'_{all} = [\mathbf{v}', \mathbf{v}'_s]^T$ with $\mathbf{v}'_s$ as the added skeleton points and $\delta_s = \mathbf{L}_s\mathbf{v}_{all}$. In matrix form, this reads

$$\begin{bmatrix} \mathbf{L} & | & \mathbf{0} \\ \mathbf{I}_c & | & \mathbf{0} \\ & \mathbf{L}_s & \end{bmatrix} \begin{bmatrix} \mathbf{v}' \\ \mathbf{v}'_s \end{bmatrix} = \begin{bmatrix} \delta \\ \mathbf{v}_c \\ \delta_s \end{bmatrix}, \quad (5)$$

where $\mathbf{I}_c$ denotes the mapping between $\mathbf{v}$ and $\mathbf{v}_c$.

The additional rows in the system matrix do not increase the computational complexity significantly, as $m \ll n$. The resulting linear system of equations can be solved by applying the previously described two-step iterative scheme.

2.2 Control Point Selection

To determine whether and where to deform the aortic or an iliac surface mesh, rays are cast from the centerline of the vessel mesh to the reconstructed endovascular device in 3D. If a cast ray hits the mesh, this indicates that the device line is outside of the mesh, thus the mesh has to be deformed around the hit point $\mathbf{h}$. The hit point is selected as a handle point and its shift $\mathbf{s}$ is calculated by

$$\mathbf{s} = \mathbf{d} - \mathbf{h} + \Delta d \frac{(\mathbf{d} - \mathbf{h})}{||\mathbf{d} - \mathbf{h}||}, \tag{6}$$

where $\mathbf{d}$ denotes the respective device point and Δd represents the device thickness. In case of tortuous vessels, a resampling of the control points is performed to ensure a more equally distributed sampling. To account for the large flexibility of the abdominal aorta, no anchor points were defined explicitly.

2.3 Mesh Deformation

The aortic and iliac meshes are deformed independently of each other. First, the inserted device is reconstructed in 3D from two views [4]. Next, the control points for the aortic and the iliac mesh to be deformed are defined.

As the skeleton-based ARAP deformation is used, a skeleton has to be generated, which is simple as the vessel meshes are rather tubular. Each mesh is sliced by planes every 5 mm along the centerline perpendicular to it. Along each slicing plane, six equiangular rays are cast. The ray-mesh hit points are defined as skeleton points. First, the aortic mesh is deformed by translating the control points and executing the two-step iteration. Second, the selected iliac mesh is deformed by translating its control points by the calculated shifts, and the top control points are moved to the previously found nearest aortic vertices. After the deformation, the vertices of the aortic mesh below the bound iliac points are erased for the sake of consistency. The complete deformation (prefactorization and iteration) is performed within one second for a typical mesh size of 7500 vertices on an Intel i7 - 3720QM with 8 GB RAM.

3 Results and Evaluation

3.1 Data Description

The evaluation of the implemented method was performed on real clinical data. The data was provided by two clinical collaboration sites, Universitätsklinikum Heidelberg (HD) and Centre Hospitalier de l'Université de Montréal (CHUM).

Each of the datasets covered a CT volume with sufficient quality for segmentation, data for registration and DSA images of the iliac bifurcation. Optimally, each patient has two 2D images of each iliac bifurcation to be able to reconstruct the endovascular device in 3D. 17 datasets with 31 distinct DSA images (excluding images for device reconstruction) were found eligable for evaluation.

3.2 Qualitative Results

First, the deformation was evaluated qualitatively by clinical experts. The segmented models were registered to the renal arteries and the overlay images before and after the deformation were compared visually. As the aorta is rather stiff, the deformation is mostly minor. The deformation corrects for the distortion of the anatomy by the device, while preserving the LM positions, such as those of the renals. The correspondence between the deformed mesh and the contrast agent flow in the DSA images is higher.

In the case of the highly tortuous iliac arteries, even larger improvements can be observed. The part of the reconstructed devices located outside of the mesh is mostly larger than in the aortic case. The distances between the internal iliac artery LMs and the observed ostium positions may also be larger. The overlayed deformed meshes show high correspondence to the contrast agent flow in the DSA images. The new LM positions also show an improvement, see Figure 2.

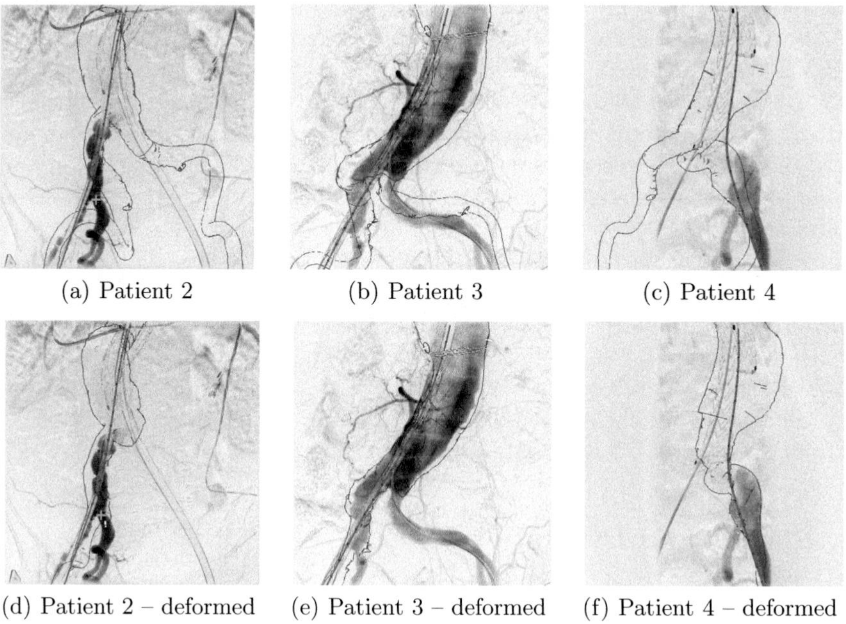

(a) Patient 2 (b) Patient 3 (c) Patient 4

(d) Patient 2 – deformed (e) Patient 3 – deformed (f) Patient 4 – deformed

Fig. 2. Iliac overlay images of three patients before (a)(b)(c) and after distortion correction (d)(e)(f) by the skeleton-based ARAP deformation method. Medical data courtesy of HD and CHUM.

3.3 Quantitative Results

The visual impressions of the qualitative evaluation were also proven by quantitative measures. Since there is no possibility to evaluate in 3D, the central positions of the internal iliac artery ostia were marked in the 2D DSA images as ground truth. The corresponding projections of the LM positions were compared to the ground truth prior to and after the deformation, see Table 1.

First, the Euclidean distances between the ostia and the corresponding LMs were measured. The mean initial (undeformed) distance between the ostia and the corresponding LMs was 19.81 mm with a standard deviation of 17.14 mm. After deformation, the mean distance was reduced to 4.56 mm and the standard deviation to 2.81 mm. The median was initially slightly lower than the mean and was also reduced significantly from 15.79 mm to 3.65 mm.

As the characteristic direction of the iliac arteries is vertical, during stent placement the height of the stent endings is critical. Thus, a second distance measure, the vertical distance (difference of z-coordinates), was also considered. The mean initial distance was 11.33 mm with a standard deviation of 8.21 mm. It was reduced to 2.73 mm with a standard deviation of 2.20 mm.

Table 1. Distances between ostia and the corresponding LMs.

	Euclidean dist.		**Vertical dist.**	
	Initial	Deformed	**Initial**	Deformed
Mean (mm)	19.81	4.56	11.33	2.73
Std. dev. (mm)	17.14	2.81	8.21	2.20
Median (mm)	15.79	3.65	9.33	2.25

4 Conclusion and Outlook

This paper proposes an approach towards distortion correction during endovascular AAA repair procedures. The method accounts for distortions caused by inserted endovascular devices by adapting the segmented models of the aorta and the iliac arteries using the skeleton-based ARAP mesh deformation. Evaluation shows that the distortion correction increases the accuracy of the overlay of the projected surface meshes with interventionally acquired fluoroscopic images.

The method could be extended to account for multiple inserted devices, thus increasing the accuracy of the deformation. Additionally, both iliacs may be deformed simultaneously. Furthermore, the range of applications can be extended by applying the method for thoracic aortic aneurysm (TAA) repairs.

Acknowledgements and Disclaimer. The authors gratefully acknowledge the help of the group of Prof. Dr. med. D. Böckler from HD, the group of Dr. G. Soulez MD, Msc from CHUM and the group of Dr. med M. Austermann from the Universitätsklinikum Münster for providing the clinical data and evaluating qualitatively. The concepts and information presented in this paper are based on research and are not commercially available.

References

1. Basnyat, P.S., Biffin, A.H.B., Moseley, L.G., Hedges, A.R., Lewis, M.H.: Mortality from ruptured abdominal aortic aneurysm in wales. British Journal of Surgery 86(6), 765–770 (1999)
2. Douane, F., Kauffmann, C., Thérasse, E., Lessard, S., Beaudouin, N., Blair, J.F., Oliva, V., Pfister, M., Soulez, G.: Accuracy of rigid registration between CT angiography and fluoroscopy during endovascular repair of abdominal aortic aneurysm (AAA). In: Haage, P., Morgan, R.A. (eds.) CIRSE, Barcelona, Spain, September 14–18 (2013)
3. Guyot, A., Varnavas, A., Carrell, T., Penney, G.: Non-rigid 2D-3D registration using anisotropic error ellipsoids to account for projection uncertainties during aortic surgery. In: Mori, K., Sakuma, I., Sato, Y., Barillot, C., Navab, N. (eds.) MICCAI 2013, Part III. LNCS, vol. 8151, pp. 179–186. Springer, Heidelberg (2013)
4. Hoffmann, M., Brost, A., Jakob, C., Bourier, F., Koch, M., Kurzidim, K., Hornegger, J., Strobel, N.: Semi-automatic catheter reconstruction from two views. In: Ayache, N., Delingette, H., Golland, P., Mori, K. (eds.) MICCAI 2012, Part II. LNCS, vol. 7511, pp. 584–591. Springer, Heidelberg (2012)
5. Igarashi, T., Moscovich, T., Hughes, J.F.: As-rigid-as-possible shape manipulation. ACM Transactions on Graphics (TOG) 24(3), 1134–1141 (2005)
6. Kaladji, A., Dumenil, A., Castro, M., Cardon, A., Becquemin, J.-P., Bou-Saïd, B., Lucas, A., Haigron, P.: Prediction of deformations during endovascular aortic aneurysm repair using finite element simulation. Computerized Medical Imaging and Graphics 37(2), 142–149 (2013)
7. Liao, R., Tan, Y., Sundar, H., Pfister, M., Kamen, A.: An efficient graph-based deformable 2D/3D registration algorithm with applications for abdominal aortic aneurysm interventions. In: Liao, H., Edwards, P.J.E., Pan, X., Fan, Y., Yang, G.-Z. (eds.) MIAR 2010. LNCS, vol. 6326, pp. 561–570. Springer, Heidelberg (2010)
8. Pfister, M., Toth, D.: Clinical prototype of an integrated workflow for EVAR using surface meshes of pre-operative CT data. In: Proceedings of the 1st Conference on Image-Guided Interventions (2014)
9. Sakalihasan, N., Limet, R., Defawe, O.D.: Abdominal aortic aneurysm. The Lancet 365(9470), 1577–1589 (2005)
10. Schanzer, A., Messina, L.: Two decades of endovascular abdominal aortic aneurysm repair: Enormous progress with serious lessons learned. Journal of the American Heart Association 1(3), e000075 (2012)
11. Sorkine, O., Alexa, M.: As-rigid-as-possible surface modeling. In: Proceedings of the Fifth Eurographics Symposium on Geometry Processing, Barcelona, Spain, July 4-6, pp. 109–116 (2007)
12. Sorkine, O., Cohen-Or, D., Lipman, Y., Alexa, M., Rössl, C., Seidel, H.: Laplacian surface editing. In: Second Eurographics Symposium on Geometry Processing, Nice, France, July 8-10, pp. 175–184 (2004)
13. Zhang, S., Nealen, A., Metaxas, D.: Skeleton based as-rigid-as-possible volume modeling. Eurographics 2010–Short Papers, pp. 21–24 (2010)

Projection-Based Phase Features for Localization of a Needle Tip in 2D Curvilinear Ultrasound

Ilker Hacihaliloglu[1], Parmida Beigi[1], Gary Ng[3], Robert N. Rohling[1,2], Septimiu Salcudean[1], and Purang Abolmaesumi[1]

[1] Electrical and Computer Engineering, University of British Columbia, Canada
[2] Mechanical Engineering, Universtiy of British Columbia, Canada
[3] Philips Research, Bothell, Washington, United States

Abstract. Localization of a needle's tip in ultrasound images is often a challenge during percutaneous procedures due to the inherent limitations of ultrasound imaging. A new method is proposed for tip localization with curvilinear arrays using local image statistics over a region extended from the partially visible needle shaft. First, local phase-based image projections are extracted using orientation-tuned Log-Gabor filters to coarsely estimate the needle trajectory. The trajectory estimation is then improved using a best fit iterative method. To account for the typically discontinuous needle shaft appearance, a geometric optimization is then performed that connects the extracted inliers of the point cloud. In the final stage, the enhanced needle trajectory points are passed to a feature extraction method that uses a combination of spatially distributed image statistics to enhance the needle tip. The needle tip is localized using the enhanced images and calculated trajectory. Validation results obtained from 150 *ex vivo* ultrasound scans show an accuracy of 0.43 ± 0.31 mm for needle tip localization.

Keywords: Ultrasound, local phase, epidurals, needle enhancement.

1 Introduction

Ultrasound (US) guidance is useful for many needle insertions, including biopsy, therapy and anesthesia. The key is to observe the advancement of a needle tip towards the target. Unfortunately, needle visualization in US images is strongly dependent on the orientation of the specularly reflecting needle to the US beam and is poorest when performing blocks with a steep needle insertion angle, such as, typically femoral blocks in obese patients [1]. Medium frequency curvilinear transducers are used to achieve the necessary depth of penetration and field of view, but only a small portion or none of the needle gives a strong reflection. Needle visibility can be successfully enhanced by beam steering on linear transducers, seen on commercial machines, but only a portion of the needle is enhanced with curvilinear arrays so the tip is still indistinguishable. A solution

N. Navab et al. (Eds.): MICCAI 2015, Part I, LNCS 9349, pp. 347–354, 2015.
DOI: 10.1007/978-3-319-24553-9_43

is needed for enhancing and localizing a needle in US images obtained using curvilinear transducers.

The following papers provide a brief overview of the general history of needle enhancement in US. Methods based on Radon transform and variants of Hough transform were proposed by different groups [2, 3]. The needle tip localization error results varied between 0.45 mm and 1.92 mm for *ex vivo* or phantom scans. In [2], validation on clinical scans achieved a mean needle targeting error value of 0.19 mm. However, tip localization accuracy was not reported. Parallel integral projection based algorithms, based on the fact that needles appear as the highest intensity line-like features in US images, were used in [4–6]. The reported needle tip localization results on turkey breast [4], gel phantom [5] and *in vivo* animal study [6] were 0.69 mm, 0.26 mm and 1.4 mm respectively. Uhercik *et al.* [7] used intensity thresholding, a robust randomized search procedure using random sample consensus (RANSAC), and tool axes optimization for needle shaft localization. The tissue-mimicking phantom experiment resulted with a mean tip localization accuracy of 0.64 mm. In recent work, Wu *et al.* [8] used gradient orientation and magnitude information for localizing needles. Chicken breast phantom experiments achieved a minimum tip localization error of $<$ 0.85 mm. On *In vivo* patient scans the method achieved a needle tip localization accuracy of 1.15 mm [8].

This paper focuses on the challenge of guiding a needle for epidurals, particularly for lumbar blocks, where the needle shaft is poorly visible due to the steep trajectory and variable strength reflections due to range of beam angles from the curvilinear transducer. Our proposed method for needle trajectory estimation is based on the extraction of local phase needle image projections obtained using orientable Log-Gabor filters. The key innovation for extracting the needle tip, is a new feature extraction method based on the combination of spatially distributed image statistics into a compact feature descriptor using the information extracted from the needle trajectory. We show qualitative and quantitative validation results on *ex vivo* US scans obtained from bovine and porcine tissue samples using a relative needle and transducer geometry suitable for lumbar in-plane US guided needle insertion.

2 Methods

The proposed enhancement method is based on our previous experience with in-plane guidance of lumbar injections *in vivo* where (i) the needle is inserted in-plane and the insertion side (left or right) is known, (ii) the needle tip appears as a characteristic but variable intensity echo, and (iii) only the portion of the needle shaft close to the transducer surface is visible. Specifically, we focus on the enhancement of in-plane needles with mid to steep insertion angles from 2D US images obtained using a curvilinear transducer (Fig. 1 (a)). In this work, we investigate needle insertion angles (α) ranging from 40° to 70°, to the skin surface. Due to the convex shape of the transducer and the mid to steep insertion angle, the only visible part of the needle shaft is the part that is close to the

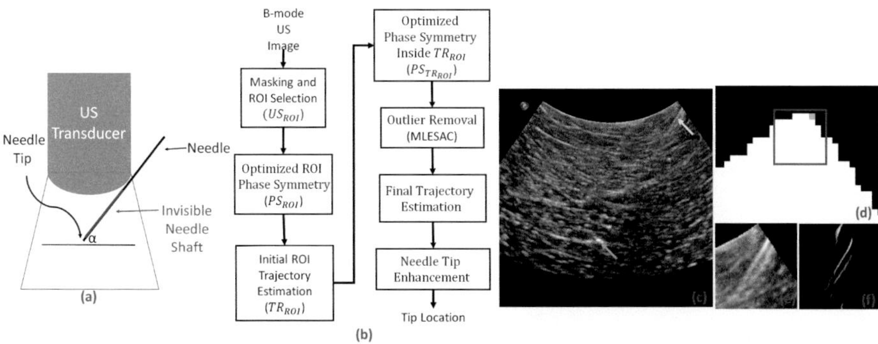

Fig. 1. (a) Schematic drawing of the experimental imaging setup. The insertion angle (α) is measured in relation to the phantom/skin surface ($\alpha = 0°$ is parallel to the skin surface). (b) Flowchart of the proposed method. (c) B-mode US image. The yellow arrow points to the partially visible needle shaft and the blue arrow points the needle tip. (d) Zoom in of the upper right side of the mask image where ROI selected mask image is shown in the red square. (e) B-mode US image corresponding to the selected ROI (US_{ROI}). (f) Optimized local phase image of (e) (PS_{ROI}).

transducer surface where the needle is nearly perpendicular to the US beam (Fig. 1 (c)). In the next section we provide an explanation how these imaging features are used in our proposed method. The flowchart of the proposed method is provided in Fig. 1 (b).

2.1 Needle Tip Localization Using Projection-Based Image Phase Features

Optimized Phase Projections: The first step of the proposed method is to automatically extract a region of interest (ROI) that covers that visible needle section. This is achieved by producing a mask from the B-mode US image using simple thresholding and selecting the pixel that is located on the far right top corner of this mask image (Fig. 1 (d) green pixel). We define our ROI by creating a rectangular region around this pixel where the pixel location is the centre of the top side of the rectangle. The ROI US image will be denoted as US_{ROI} (Fig. 1 (e)). In all the collected scans, the needle was inserted from the right side of the B-mode image. *A priori* knowledge of the needle insertion side is used during this step. Accurate selection of this ROI is not critical for the algorithm; it only needs to contain a portion of the needle shaft.

Recently, intensity-invariant, local phase-based image processing methods, based on filtering the US data with band-pass Log-Gabor filters, have shown promising results for extraction of soft tissue and bone interfaces [9]. Phase-based features are designed to be intensity-invariant and therefore insensitive to US imaging parameters such as imaging depth, as evidenced in previous work on bone detection [9]. In order to extract the needle shaft, we filter the

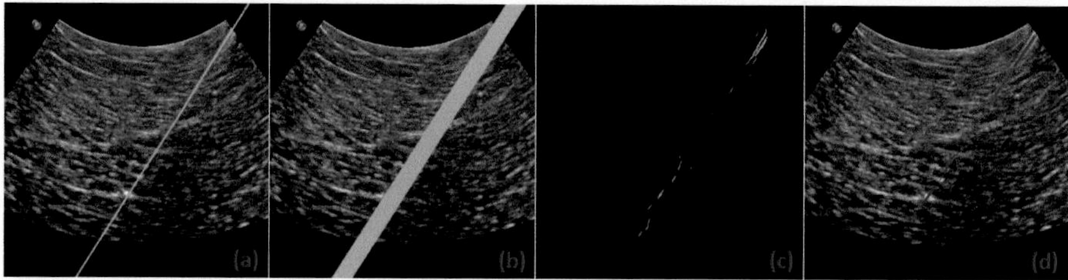

Fig. 2. (a) Estimated initial trajectory (green line) overlaid on the B-mode US image. (b) The extended ROI trajectory(TR_{ROI}) overlaid on the B-mode US image. (c) The $PS_{TR_{ROI}}$ image calculated from the B-mode US image by limiting the local phase feature extraction to the region defined by TR_{ROI}. (d) Inliers detected using the MLESAC algorithm (blue pixels) overlaid on top of the B-mode US image.

US_{ROI} image with a Log-Gabor filter whose transfer function is defined as $LG(\omega, \theta) = exp(\frac{-log(\omega/\kappa)^2}{2log(\sigma_\omega)^2})exp(\frac{-(\theta-\theta_m)^2}{2(\sigma_\theta)^2})$. Here ω and θ are related to the scale and orientation of the filter. κ is the centre frequency of the filter, σ_ω is related to the spread of the frequency spectrum in a logarithmic function, and σ_θ defines the angular bandwidth of the filter. θ_m is the specific orientation of the filter. These filter parameters were selected automatically using the framework proposed by Hacihaliloglu *et al.* [9]. The output of this filtering operation is used to construct a phase-based descriptor called phase symmetry (PS) [9]. The PS_{ROI} image extracted by processing the US_{ROI} image shows a distinct local phase feature for the needle shaft (Fig. 1 (f)).

Initial Trajectory Estimation: In order to estimate the initial trajectory we calculate the Radon Transform (RT) of the PS_{ROI} image. The initial needle trajectory is estimated by performing an inverse RT operation using only the peak RT value (Fig. 2 (a)). In order to account for a possible bending of the needle during the insertion and provide a more accurate initial trajectory estimate, we extend this estimated trajectory to an initial trajectory ROI which we call TR_{ROI}. TR_{ROI} is calculated by keeping the maximum RT and its angle value constant but expanding the corresponding distance (ρ) by $\Delta\rho$ pixels in each direction in the RT space and calculating the inverse RT (Fig. 2 (b)). The diameter of the needle used in this study is 1.47 mm; to select a safe zone we expand this diameter value to 5.47 mm (2 mm from each side) which accounts for a $\Delta\rho$ value of 20 pixels, accommodating common anesthesia needles.

Final Trajectory Estimation: The TR_{ROI}, calculated in the previous step, provides a region in the B-mode US image which includes the needle shaft and tip. To enhance these two features, the local phase-based PS calculation is performed on the full sized US image but by limiting the extraction process to the region defined by TR_{ROI}. We define this new PS image as $PS_{TR_{ROI}}$. Limiting the PS calculation to the TR_{ROI} eliminates the extraction of unwanted soft tissue interfaces and focuses on the ROI where the needle shaft and the tip is expected

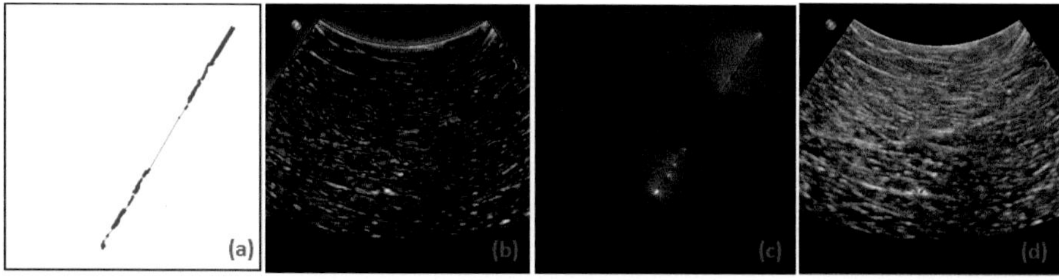

Fig. 3. (a) Final needle trajectory, (shown in red) obtained after geometric optimization approach, overlaid on the disconnected MLESAC point cloud (shown in blue). The line segments 'a','b' and the black circle (knot) are used during the needle tip detection. (b) Band-pass filtered B-mode US image used as input for tip estimation. (c) Output obtained from the needle tip enhancement approach.(d) Enhanced needle tip (shown in red) overlaid on the B-mode US image.

to be (Fig. 2 (c)). Investigating Fig. 2 (c) we can see that there are still some false positive local phase features in the $PS_{TR_{ROI}}$ image. In order to eliminate the final remaining false positive local phase features we perform a randomized search procedure by modifying the traditional RANSAC (Random Sample Consensus) algorithm. The traditional RANSAC approach fits a model the point cloud based on a threshold value. Therefore, the accuracy of the RANSAC algorithm, for needle axis localization, is limited to this selected threshold value [7]. In order to overcome this problem we propose to use a new method called Maximum Likelihood Estimation SAmple Consensus (MLESAC)[10]. MLESAC evaluates the likelihood of the hypothesis, representing the error distribution as a mixture model. The error is modeled as a mixture model of Gaussian and uniform distribution $p(e) = (\gamma(\frac{1}{\sqrt{2\pi}\sigma})exp(-\frac{e^2}{2\sigma^2}) + \frac{(1-\gamma)}{\nu})$. Here ν is the diameter of the search window, γ is the mixing parameter and σ is the standard deviation of the error on each coordinate. The final step is to find the best estimate which minimizes the negative log likelihood of the error function [10] using expectation maximization (EM) algorithm. Parameter γ is estimated during the EM part and ν is dependent on the data size. The MLESAC algorithm results are shown in Figure 2 (d) where we can see a clear overlap of the detected inliers with the needle shaft as well as the needle tip. The final trajectory estimate is obtained by connecting these extracted inliers using a geometric optimization approach [11]. Given a collection of F curves and n inlier points (x_i, y_i), $i = 1, ..., n$, the optimization approach tries to find the size of the largest subset of points $(N_n(F))$ lying on a curve in F. Based on the *a priori* knowledge that the needle shaft is a rigid object and should follow a straight path with minimal bending, we define the curve as a monotonic Lipschitz function. If we define $M(i)$ as the maximum number of points from $(x_1, y_1), ..., (x_i, y_i)$ on a curve ending at (x_i, y_i), during the optimization, we compute $M(i) = 1 + max_{j<i, y_j<y_i} M(j)$ and then $N_n(F) = max[M(i)]$. The estimated final trajectory obtained is shown in Fig. 3 (a) as a red line.

Needle Tip Enhancement and Localization Using Spatially Distributed Image Statistics: The needle tip estimation is based on the RT, but instead of integrating the US image intensity values along a line L, they are distributed among various line segments along L (e.g. Fig. 3 (a) segments 'a' and 'b') [12]. The line segments are defined by a set of salient points, called knots (Fig. 3 (a) black circle), along L which are the intersection points of L and the trajectory estimated in the previous step. By using the trajectory we eliminate the extraction/enhancement of the soft tissue interfaces that have similar intensity values as the needle tip, but are not aligned with the trajectory. Similar to the original RT method, each line also has an associated direction, which is given by an angle θ. However, the output for each angle is an image, which is the main difference from the traditional RT where the output in such a case is a 1D function. If the set of knots along L is given as $(t_1, ..., t_n)$, the value of the new extracted feature is given by:

$$US_{needle}(US_B, L(t)) = \frac{\int_{t_i}^{t_{i+1}} US_B(L(t))dt}{\|L(t_{i+1}) - L(t_i)\|_2}; t \in [t_i, t_{i+1}]. \quad (1)$$

Here, US_B represents the band-pass filtered US image (Fig. 3 (b)). We obtain US_B using the Log-Gabor filter without the orientation selectivity $LG(\omega) = exp(-log(\omega/\kappa)^2/2log(\sigma_\omega)^2)$. L is the line along which features are obtained. The function US_{needle} assigns all the pixels between the knots t_1 and t_{i+1} along L, the mean value of function US_{needle} along L, between the same two knots. Investigating the calculated US_{needle} image we can see that the pixel corresponding to the estimated needle tip is enhanced after this feature extraction operation (Fig. 3 (c)). Fig. 3 (d) shows the overlay of the maximum intensity pixels of US_{needle} (colour coded in red) on the B-mode US image. The needle tip localization was achieved by selecting the first maximum intensity needle tip pixel, lying along the calculated final needle trajectory and outside of US_{ROI}, from the enhanced needle images.

2.2 Data Acquisition and Experiments

The US images used in the evaluation of the proposed method were obtained using an iU22 ultrasound system (Philips Ultrasound, Bothell, WA) with a 2D curvilinear transducer (C5-1). Freshly excised *ex vivo* porcine and bovine tissue samples, obtained from a local butcher, were used as the imaging medium. Standard 17 gauge Tuohy anesthesia needles (Arrow International, Reading, PA, USA) were inserted to this setup. A total of individual 150 2D US images (75 porcine and 75 bovine) were collected where the imaging depth setting varied from 5 cm up to 9 cm. The needle was inserted at different angles ($40° - 70°$), and various insertion depths (2 cm - 9 cm). In all the collected images the insertion angle was steep enough so that the only visible portion of the needle in the collected US image was the end part of the shaft and the needle tip. Quantitative validation was obtained by comparing the segmented needle tip, performed using the proposed method, against the gold standard manual segmentation. The manual segmentation was also confirmed by the known depth at which the needle was inserted. "The error was calculated by measuring the Euclidean distance (ED) between these points and calculating root-mean-square (RMS) and 95% confidence intervals. The proposed method was implemented in MATLAB. The Log-Gabor filter parameters were automatically optimized using the framework proposed in [9]. For the MLESAC algorithm $\sigma = 1$ provided successful inlier estimation results while avoiding the estimation of unwanted outliers. The angle θ for the needle tip enhancement ranged from $0° - 300°$ with $6°$ increments. Throughout the experimental validation these parameters were not changed.

3 Results

Figure 4 shows sample results. Investigating the B-mode US images, we can see that the proposed method successfully enhances the needle tip in the presence of disconnected and partially visible needle shaft. Due to the directionally optimized local phase features, the proposed method is not affected by the soft tissue interfaces with higher intensity values (Fig. 4 (a) second row). Furthermore, the method appears unaffected by the intensity variations present in different US scans. If the needle shaft has a similar intensity value as the tip the proposed method results in the enhancement of both features (Fig. 4 (a) second row). The processing time in MATLAB was 0.8 seconds for a 450×450 2D image. Needle scans inside the bovine and porcine tissue resulted with an overall mean ED error value of 0.43 mm (RMS 0.53 mm SD 0.31 mm and 95% CI 0.51 mm) and 0.4 mm (RMS 0.49 mm SD 0.29 mm 95% CI 0.47 mm), respectively (Fig. 4 (b)). The maximum localization errors were 1.19 mm and 1.24 mm for bovine and porcine scans, respectively.

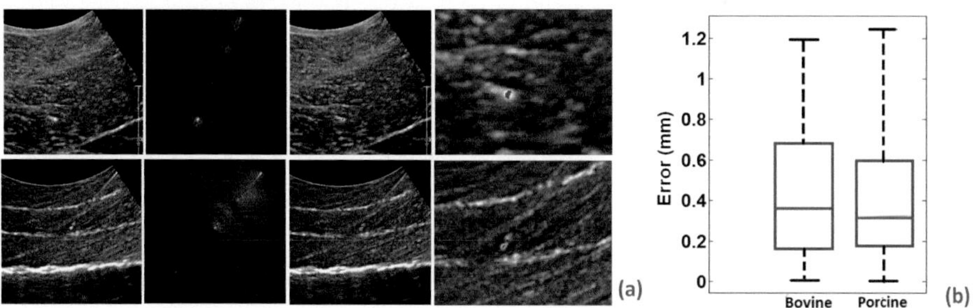

Fig. 4. (a) Sample results of porcine tissue *ex vivo*. First column: B-mode US images. Second column: Result of needle tip enhancement. Third column: Overlay of enhanced needle tip on top of the B-mode US image. Fourth column: Expanded view of the third column.(b) Quantitative results for needle tip localization.

4 Discussions and Conclusions

We propose a method to localize the tip using both echo information from the tip and the partially visible needle shaft. The quantitative experiments indicate a mean RMS error of 0.53 mm and 0.49 mm for for bovine and porcine tissue respectively. The accuracy of the method is improved using the available prior information before the insertion of the needle. The method is tested on epidural needles with no or minimal bending. For situations where needle bending occurs, tool models incorporating this bending information can be incorporated to the framework. If the US transducer is placed further from the needle, the ROI selection step can be eliminated since for these situations the visible section of the needle shaft would be longer. Future work will focus on validation of the method on *in vivo* scans and different application of image guided interventions where visualization of needles from US data is of importance.

References

[1] Schafhalter-Zoppoth, I., McCulloch, C.E., Gray, A.T.: Ultrasound visibility of needles used for regional nerve block: An in vitro study. Reg. Anes. and Pain Medicine 29(5), 480–488 (2004)

[2] Hatt, C.R., Ng, G., Parthasarathy, V.: Enhanced needle localization in ultrasound using beam steering and learning-based segmentation. Comp. Med. Imag. and Grap. 14, 45–54 (2015)

[3] Zhou, H., Qiu, W., Ding, M., Zhang, S.: Automatic needle segmentation in 3D ultrasound images using 3D improved Hough transform. In: Proc. SPIE Med. Imag., pp. 691821-1-691821-9 (2008)

[4] Ding, M., Fenster, A.: Projection-based needle segmentation in 3D ultrasound images. In: Ellis, R.E., Peters, T.M. (eds.) MICCAI 2003. LNCS, vol. 2879, pp. 319–327. Springer, Heidelberg (2003)

[5] Barva, M., Uhercik, M., Mari, J.M., Kybic, J., Duhamel, J.R., Liebgott, H., Hlavac, V., Cachard, C.: Parallel integral projection transform for straight electrode localization in 3-D ultrasound images. IEEE Trans. UFFC 55(7), 1559–1569 (2008)

[6] Novotny, P.M., Stoll, J.A., Vasilyev, N.V., del Nido, P.J., Dupont, P.E., Howe, R.D.: GPU based real-time instrument tracking with three dimensional ultrasound. Med. Imag. Anal. 11(5), 458–464 (2007)

[7] Uhercik, M., Kybic, J., Liebgott, H., Cachard, C.: Model fitting using ransac for surgical tool localization in 3D ultrasound images. IEEE Trans. on Biomed. Eng. 57(8), 1907–1916 (2010)

[8] Wu, Q., Yuchi, M., Ding, M.: Phase Grouping-Based Needle Segmentation in 3-D Trans-rectal Ultrasound-Guided Prostate Trans-perineal Therapy. Ultrasound in Med. and Biol. 40(4), 804–816 (2014)

[9] Hacihaliloglu, I., Abugharbieh, R., Hodgson, A., Rohling, R.N.: Automatic adaptive parameterization in local phase feature-based bone segmentation in ultrasound. Ultrasound in Med. and Biol. 37(10), 1689–1703 (2011)

[10] Torr, P.H.S., Zisserman, A.: MLESAC: A New Robust Estimator with Application to Estimating Image Geometry. Journal of Computer Vision and Image Under 78(1), 138–156 (2000)

[11] Arias-Castro, E., Donoho, D.L., Huo, X., Tovey, C.: Connect-the-dots: how many random points can a regular curve pass through. Adv. Adv. in Appl. Prob., 37(3), 571–603 (2005)

[12] Kumar, R., Vazquez-Reina, A., Pfister, H.: Radon-Like features and their application to connectomics. In: IEEE CVPR Workshop, pp. 186–193 (2010)

Inertial Measurement Unit for Radiation-Free Navigated Screw Placement in Slipped Capital Femoral Epiphysis Surgery

Bamshad Azizi Koutenaei[1,2], Ozgur Guler[1], Emmanuel Wilson[1], Matthew Oetgen[1], Patrick Grimm[1], Nassir Navab[2,3], and Kevin Cleary[1]

[1] Children's National Medical Center, Washington D.C, United States
{bazizi,oguler,ewilson,moetgen,pgrimm,kcleary}@cnmc.org
[2] Chair for Computer Aided Medical Procedures (CAMP), TUM, Munich, Germany
[3] Computer Aided Medical Procedures (CAMP), Johns Hopkins University, USA
nassir@cs.tum.edu

Abstract. Slipped Capital Femoral Epiphysis (SCFE) is a common pathologic hip condition in adolescents. In the standard treatment, a surgeon relies on multiple intra-operative fluoroscopic X-ray images to plan the screw placement and to guide a drill along the intended trajectory. More complex cases could require more images, and thereby, higher radiation dose to both patient and surgeon. We introduce a novel technique using an Inertial Measurement Unit (IMU) for recovering and visualizing the orthopedic tool trajectory in two orthogonal X-ray images in real-time. The proposed technique improves screw placement accuracy and reduces the number of required fluoroscopic X-ray images without changing the current workflow. We present results from a phantom study using 20 bones to perform drilling and screw placement tasks. While dramatically reducing the number of required fluoroscopic images from 20 to 4, the results also show improvement in accuracy compared to the manual SCFE approach.

Keywords: Slipped Capital Femoral Epiphysis (SCFE), Computer-assisted Orthopedic Surgery, Computer-aided Intervention, Inertial Measurement Unit.

1 Introduction

Computer-assisted surgery (CAS) has been used in various clinical procedures. Surgical planning methods for image guidance fall within two broad categories: volumetric image-based navigation (primarily, CT and MRI) and intraoperative fluoroscopic navigation [1]. Both methods could be used in passive and active CAS systems [2]. CAS systems have found increased use particularly in orthopedic surgery, where surgeon interaction is largely with rigid anatomy that is immobilized with relative efficacy. In many orthopedic procedures, the surgeon relies heavily on intra-operative fluoroscopic images; from planning implant trajectory, to guiding intra-operative positioning, and finally, to confirming implant position at completion. Antirotator proximal femoral nailing and intramedullary nailing of femur fracture are examples of

N. Navab et al. (Eds.): MICCAI 2015, Part I, LNCS 9349, pp. 355–362, 2015.
DOI: 10.1007/978-3-319-24553-9_44

orthopedic procedures that broadly follow this approach with regards to image acquisition. The pre-operative fluoroscopic images are crucial in planning the procedure, and post-operative images are needed to validate procedural accuracy. The number of additional images acquired during the procedure to orient and reposition a tool depend on surgeon skill and experience, and leads to increased radiation dose and procedure times. For instance, the average number of fluoroscopy images used for distal locking was 48.27 that causes significant radiation exposure [3]. Therefore many augmented reality systems proposed to reduce radiation exposure during the surgery for instance: half-mirror display devices [4], single laser-beam pointers [5], video see-through binocular systems [6] visualization based on IMU [7], systems that directly project images onto the patient's body [8], and other radiation-free drill guidance for orthopedic surgery [9][10][11][12].

Therefore we introduce a system in this paper that could reduce radiation dose, while improving implant accuracy with applicability in many orthopedic procedures. As a case study we chose slipped capital femoral epiphysis (SCFE) surgery.

SCFE is a common hip disorder that causes displacement of the proximal femoral epiphysis. Traditional surgical treatment requires placing screws from the proximal femoral metaphysis into the femoral head for stabilization of the proximal femoral epiphysis (Fig. 1). In the conventional approach to SCFE, the surgeon uses intra-operative fluoroscopic imaging as visualization aid to guide the screw placement and confirm the drill trajectory.

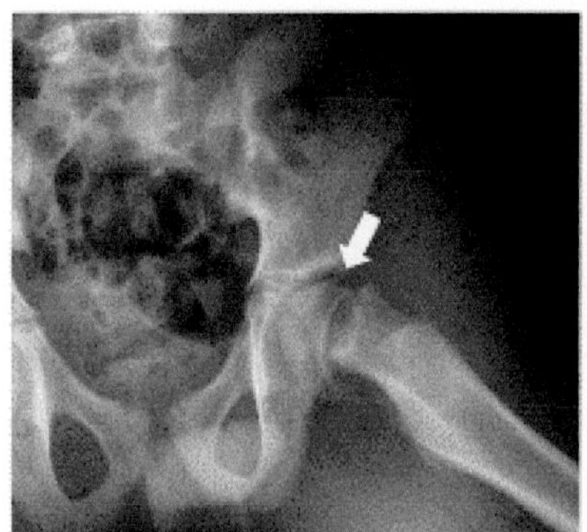
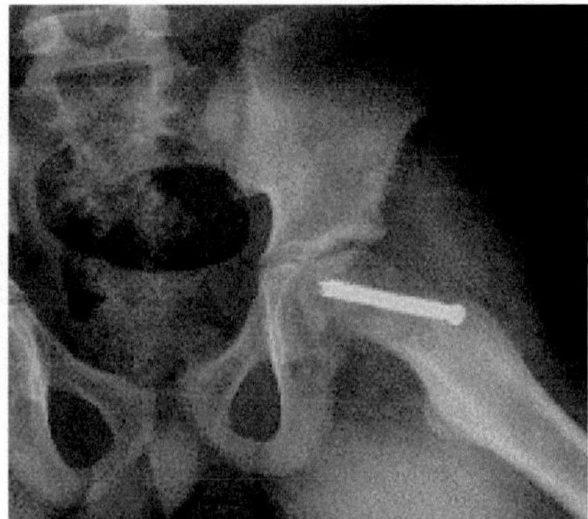

Fig. 1. (Left) radiograph of a SCFE case (arrow). (Right) fixation of the SCFE

In regards to the placement of implants to treat SCFE, a navigation system based on inertial measurement unit (IMU) could help reduce both radiation dose and procedure time. Therefore we implemented a system that superimposes IMU information onto two orthogonal fluoroscopic images.

2 Methodology

A conventional SCFE procedure uses intra-operative fluoroscopic images for visualization to accurately place the screw. This causes significant radiation exposure for both surgeon and patient. A typical work-flow involves the surgeon extrapolating a tool entry point based on target site and optimal tool orientation using fluoroscopic images. Once an optimal tool trajectory is evaluated, additional X-ray images are acquired to confirm that the tool is being inserted along this planned path. On average, about 20 x-ray images are acquired to deduce the best orientation and guide the tool during the procedure. The question we asked is: "What new information of clinical utility are these additional x-ray images providing?" Once a surgeon has mapped out the procedural workflow using pre-operative planning images, these additional images serve no clinical utility beyond confirming tool orientation. Our approach was to use a relatively inexpensive hardware device to augment this information in lieu of x-ray image. We were able to register and super-impose the real-time tool trajectory on two pre-operative orthogonal x-ray images. This results in improving screw placement and greatly decreased radiation exposure.

We chose an Inertial Measurement Unit (IMU) because of its compact size, low cost, and accurate orientation representation. The IMU used for this system is an X-IMU (x-io Technologies, Bristol, UK). The device consists of a 3-axis gyroscope, 3-axis accelerometer, and a 3-axis magnetometer. It sends combined data from the various sensors encapsulated in each data packet. Data transfer is done over Bluetooth LowEnergy (BLE) wireless protocol to our application running on a laptop at a rate of 512 packets per second. The laptop application uses a sensor fusion algorithm [13] to calculate the current orientation. We designed a 3D-printed fixture which mounts to the drill base and houses the IMU device. This provides a fixed, known relation between the drill bit and IMU. We used an Epiphan DVI2USB3.0 frame-grabber (Epiphany Systems Inc., Palo Alto, CA) to frame-grab the x-ray images from the Siemens Zeego system. To facilitate a more ergonomic surgeon experience, we streamed the laptop visualization to a Samsung tablet placed next to the surgeon.

In this paper, we introduce two different methods to assist the surgeon. In method (A) we use one image, one pivot point placed on the bone to identify an entry point, and a calibrated IMU placed within the image plane. In method (B) we use two orthogonal x-ray images and four points (1 pivot point and three fiducials for coordinate registration). No additional calibration of the IMU is required in the latter approach.

Pre-operative Set-up: In method (A), we used a 3D-printed calibration fixture to align the IMU to the patient table coordinate, shown in Fig 2a. During the procedure, we used a second 3D-printed fixture to affix the IMU to the drill, shown in Figure 2b. The IMU calibration fixture orients the IMU XY-plane with the A-P fluoroscopic image plane, and IMU YZ-plane with the lateral fluoroscopic plane. The patient table position and Zeego robot coordinates are inherently calibrated. Therefore, by orienting the IMU coordinate frame with respect to the patient table, we have a calibration between fluoroscopic image plane and the IMU coordinates. For method (B), the registration between IMU and fluoroscopic image coordinates is done based on selection of four corresponding points in each pair of orthogonal x-ray images. The four points are comprised of the drill tip and three 8mm diameter metal sphere fiducials, shown in Fig 2c.

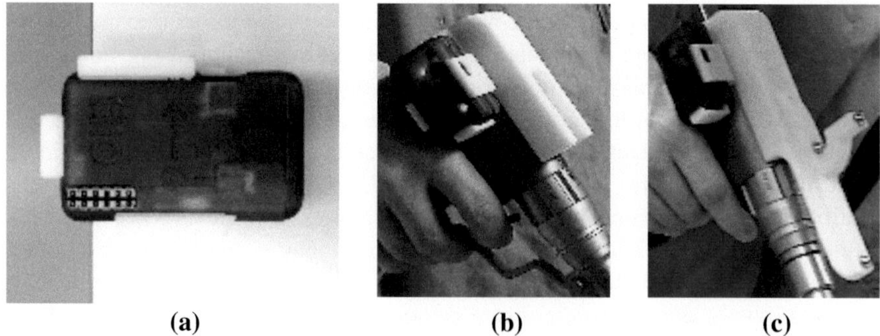

Fig. 2. (a) Calibration fixture (b) Drill fixture (c) Fiducial spheres for coordinate registration

Intra-Operative Planning: Here we explain the two methods employed to register the drill coordinates to image space in real-time.

Method (A): The surgeon identifies an entry point by drilling a small divot at the bone surface. Two orthogonal x-rays images are acquired (in A-P and Lateral orientations). As mentioned before, in this method navigation can be based off one image alone. However, image augmentation and navigation was done using both the A-P and Lateral images, as this approach is clinically most relevant. After loading those images in our application, we define the drill tip as a pivot point. We use seed based region growing segmentation to choose the best possible pivot point in a semi-automatic manner. Subsequently, the IMU is placed within the calibration fixture and placed at the edge of the patient table. The calibration fixture was designed such that it orients the IMU coordinates in a known configuration with respect to image coordinates. Based on our setting, the IMU X-Y plane maps to the A-P image plane and the IMU Y-Z frame maps to the lateral image (Error < 0.6 mm). Afterward, our method projects the updated orientation to two orthogonal images. These two projections are calculated by the following chain of transformations, and shown in Figure 3.

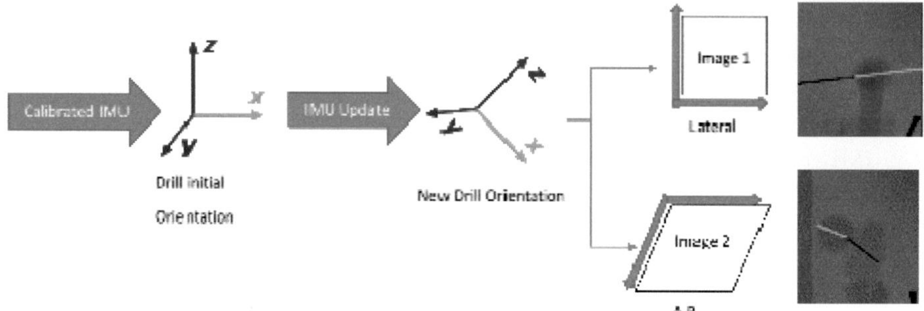

Fig. 3. Flow chart of method (A) transformation chain

T is a 4x4 transformation matrix, P is a projection matrix, and Tr is a translation matrix. (IMU = device, WRD = World defined by IMU, IMG = C-arm)

$$^{Pivot}Tr_{XY} * {}^{XY}P_{IMG} * {}^{IMG}T_{WRD} * {}^{WRD}T_{IMU} \quad (1)$$

$$^{Pivot}Tr_{YZ} * {}^{YZ}P_{IMG} * {}^{IMG}T_{WRD} * {}^{WRD}T_{IMU} \quad (2)$$

Method (B): The surgeon defines the entry point and drills into the bone surface to create an identifying divot point. The drill is fixed besides the table using a passive arm such that the drill tip is within the divot. Two orthogonal x-ray images (AP and Lateral) that visualize the drill tip and the three fiducials are acquired. After loading the images in our application, the three fiducials and drill tip are identified in commensurate order in both AP and Lateral images. We used a seed based region growing segmentation to choose the best possible pivot point and also center of the spheres in a semi-automatic manner. The application calculates the 3D position of those fiducial points by combining selected point positions in the two images (we obtain x and y coordinates from AP, and z coordinate from the Lateral image). With this we calculate the transformation between world coordinates to image coordinates. Since the drill bit is aligned precisely to the X-axis of the IMU, our application projects the x-axis of the IMU in the AP and Lateral images (Error < 0.8 mm). These two projections are calculated by the following chain of transformation, shown in Figure 4.

T is a 4x4 transformation matrix, P is a projection matrix, and Tr is a translation matrix. (IMU = device, WRD = World defined by IMU, IMG = C-arm)

$$^{Pivot}Tr_{XY} * {}^{XY}P_{IMG} * {}^{IMG}T_{Drill} * {}^{Drill}T_{IMUi} * {}^{IMUi}T_{WRD} * {}^{WRD}T_{IMUup} \quad (3)$$

$$^{Pivot}Tr_{YZ} * {}^{YZ}P_{IMG} * {}^{IMG}T_{Drill} * {}^{Drill}T_{IMUi} * {}^{IMUi}T_{WRD} * {}^{WRD}T_{IMUup} \quad (4)$$

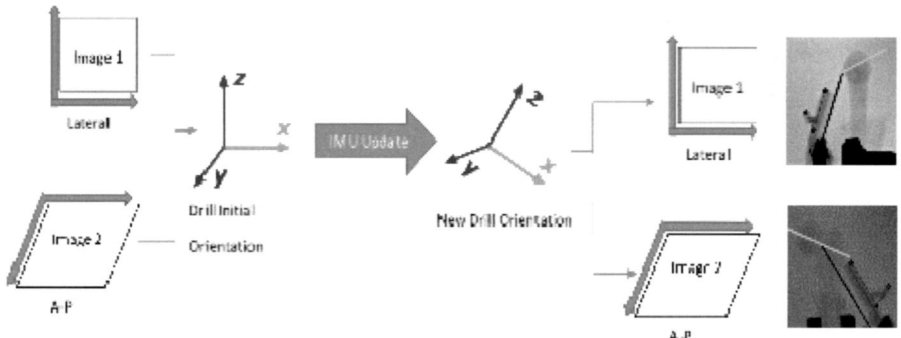

Fig. 4. Flow chart of method (B) transformation chain

Post-Operative Verification: Once the surgeon plans a path, the application collects and logs IMU orientation data until the surgeon has drilled to the target location. Once at the target location, a pair of confirmatory AP and Lateral images are acquired to correctly identify actual drill position. Post-operative validation is achieved by comparing the planned drill trajectory to actual, as shown in Fig 5.

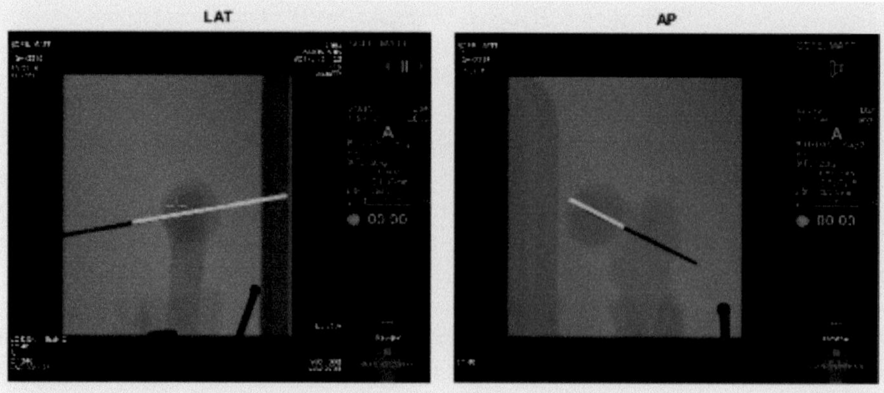

Fig. 5. Post x-ray evaluation in Lateral and A-P (yellow line is the trajectory before drilling)

3 Results

We started the study by assessing the accuracy of the x-IMU device using a Polaris optical tracker (Northern Digital Inc., Waterloo, Canada). In addition, the internal report of X-IMU shows the IMU device and algorithm we used is highly accurate[1]. The first proof-of-concept test in the lab used two orthogonal images with a standard smartphone camera to assess the efficacy of this approach. These tests confirmed the validity of our concept. Following lab tests, we completed a study in the operating room, including image acquisition from the Siemens Zeego C-arm system.

Left femur bone models with slipped capital epiphysis deformity (Model # 1161, Sawbones Worldwide, Vashon Island, WA) were used to perform the drilling and screw placement tasks, shown in Figure 6. 10 manual procedures were performed by the experienced surgeon, which served as baseline assessment of the procedural accuracy and completion time. Subsequently, 30 assisted trials were performed by the experienced orthopedic surgeon, and another 10 assisted trials performed by an orthopedic resident with no experience in SCFE surgery. For each trial, the total procedure time and number of fluoroscopic images acquired were logged, and the final placement accuracy computed from confirmatory orthogonal images acquired at the end of each trial. Average procedure time for the manual trials was 2:46 (mm:ss). Average procedure time was 1:51 (mm:ss) for the assisted trials for the experienced surgeon and 4:31 (mm:ss) for the non-experienced surgeon. The longer procedure time for the assisted trials for the non-experienced surgeon can be in part attributed to considerations given to learning curve and set-up time. The accuracy results show clear improvement with the assisted trials. Pending a study on a larger number of data samples, this shows sufficient accuracy in comparison to the conventional [14] and robotic-assisted approach [15]. The results are shown in Table 1.

---

[1] http://www.x-io.co.uk/res/doc/madgwick_internal_report.pdf

Table 1. 10 manual and 40 navigated trials conducted by experienced and non-experienced surgeon. Total error is measured for target points based on distance of desired and drilled points (Statistical Significance: $p < 0.05$, Registration Error: Err < 0.8 mm).

	Skill in SCFE	Total time	# of images	Total error
10 Manual	Experienced	2:46	20.4	7.6 mm
30 Assisted	Experienced	1:51	4	3.59 mm
10 Assisted	Non-Experienced	4:31	4	6.35 mm

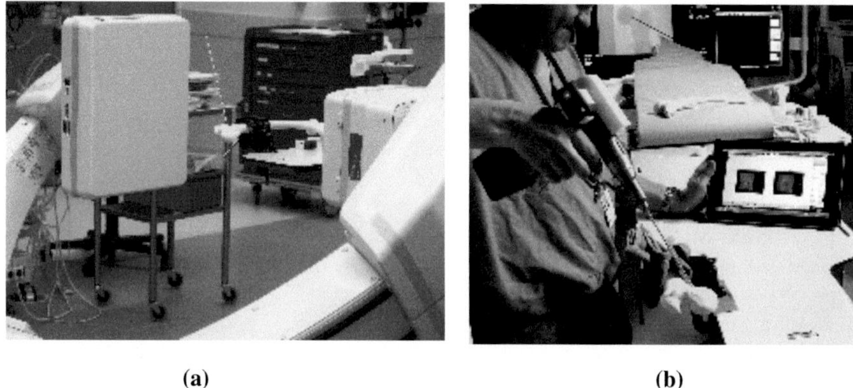

(a) (b)

Fig. 6. Phantom study in interventional suite. (a) Setup for lateral exposure (b) Surgeon using the visualization for planning optimal tool path

4 Conclusion and Future Work

Slipped capital femoral epiphysis is a relatively common orthopedic procedure in children where the accurate placement of the fixation screw often requires 20 x-ray images or a CT dataset in a conventional approach. This paper introduces a simple, cost-effective system to assist surgeons in intra-operative path planning in a real-time manner based on an IMU device. With this device setup, and reliance on only two orthogonal x-ray images, we were able to streamline the SCFE procedure. In addition, these techniques could be extended to many other orthopedic procedures that follow a similar clinical workflow. This preliminary study shows promising results, both in overall radiation exposure reduction and improved accuracy to the conventional approach in a phantom study. In future, the system could be complemented by using a head mounted display and more sophisticated navigation and visualization tools. Our long term goal is to pursue a clinical trial to determine if this approach could lead to a more accessible SCFE workflow and improved clinical outcome for patients.

References

1. Sugano, N.: Computer-assisted orthopedic surgery. Journal of Orthopaedic Science 8(3), 442–448 (2003)
2. Musahl, V., Plakseychuk, A., Fu, F.H.: Current opinion on computer-aided surgical navigation and robotics: role in the treatment of sports-related injuries. Sports Med. 32(13), 809–818 (2002)
3. Rohilla, R., Singh, R., Magu, N., Devgan, A., Siwach, R., Sangwan, S.: Simultaneous use of cannulated reamer and schanz screw for closed intramedullary femoral nailing. ISRN Surg. (2011) (published online)
4. Liao, H., Ishihara, H., Tran, H.H., Masamune, K., Sakuma, I., Dohi, T.: Fusion of Laser Guidance and 3-D Autostereoscopic Image Overlay for Precision-Guided Surgery. In: Dohi, T., Sakuma, I., Liao, H. (eds.) MIAR 2008. LNCS, vol. 5128, pp. 367–376. Springer, Heidelberg (2008)
5. Marmurek, J., Wedlake, C., Pardasani, U., Eagleson, R., Peters, T.: Image-Guided Laser Projection for Port Placement in Minimally Invasive Surgery. Stud. Health Technol. Inform. 119, 367–372 (2006)
6. Fuchs, H., State, A., Pisano, E.D., Garrett, W.F., Hirota, G., Livingston, M., Whitton, M.C., Pizer, S.: Towards Performing Ultrasound-Guided Needle Biopsies from within a Head-Mounted Display. In: Höhne, K.H., Kikinis, R. (eds.) VBC 1996. LNCS, vol. 1131, pp. 591–600. Springer, Heidelberg (1996)
7. Walti, J., Jost, G.F., Cattin, P.C.: A New Cost-Effective Approach to Pedicular Screw Placement. In: Linte, C.A. (ed.) AE-CAI 2014. LNCS, vol. 8678, pp. 90–97. Springer, Heidelberg (2014)
8. Volonte, F., Pugin, F., Bucher, P., Sugimoto, M., Ratib, O., Morel, P.: Augmented Reality and Image Overlary Navigation with OsiriX in Laparoscopic and Robotic Surgery: Not Only a Matter of Fashion. J. Hepatobiliary Pancreat Sci. 18, 506–509 (2011)
9. Diotte, B., Fallavollita, P., Wang, L., Weidert, S., Thaller, P.-H., Euler, E., Navab, N.: Radiation-free drill guidance in interlocking of intramedullary nails. In: Ayache, N., Delingette, H., Golland, P., Mori, K. (eds.) MICCAI 2012, Part I. LNCS, vol. 7510, pp. 18–25. Springer, Heidelberg (2012)
10. Hoffmann, M., et al.: Next generation distal locking for intramedullary nails using an electromagnetic X-ray-radiation-free real-time navigation system. Journal of Trauma and Acute Care Surgery 73, Jg., Nr. 1, 243–248 (2012)
11. Stathopoulos, I., et al.: Radiation-free distal locking of intramedullary nails: Evaluation of a new electromagnetic computer-assisted guidance system. Injury, 44. Jg., Nr. 6, 872–875 (2013)
12. Arlettaz, Y., et al.: Distal locking of femoral nails: evaluation of a new radiation independent targeting system. Journal of Orthopaedic Trauma 26. Jg., Nr. 11, S. 633–637 (2012)
13. Madgwick, S.O.H., Harrison, A.J.L., Vaidyanathan, R.: Estimation of IMU and MARG orientation using a gradient descent algorithm. In: 2011 IEEE International Conference Rehabilitation Robotics (ICORR), pp. 1–7 (2011), doi:10.1109/ICORR.2011.5975346
14. Pring, E.M., Adamczyk, M., Hosalkar, H.S., Bastrom, T.P., Wallace, C.D., Newton, P.O.: In situ screw fixation of slipped capital femoral epiphysis with a novel approach: a double-cohort controlled study. Journal of Children's Orthopaedics 4(3), 239–244 (2010)
15. Azizi Koutenaei, B., Guler, O., Wilson, E., et al.: Improved Screw Placement for Slipped Capital Femoral Epiphysis (SCFE) using Robotically-Assisted Drill Guidance. In: International Conference on Medical Image Computing and Computer-Assisted Intervention, vol. 17(01), pp. 488–495 (2014)

Pictorial Structures on RGB-D Images for Human Pose Estimation in the Operating Room

Abdolrahim Kadkhodamohammadi[1], Afshin Gangi[1,2], Michel de Mathelin[1], and Nicolas Padoy[1]

[1] ICube, University of Strasbourg, CNRS, IHU Strasbourg, France
{kadkhodamohammad,gangi,demathelin,npadoy}@unistra.fr
[2] Radiology Department, University Hospital of Strasbourg, France

Abstract. Human pose estimation in the operating room (OR) can benefit many applications, such as surgical activity recognition, radiation exposure monitoring and performance assessment. However, the OR is a very challenging environment for computer vision systems due to limited camera positioning possibilities, severe illumination changes and similar colors of clothes and equipments. This paper tackles the problem of human pose estimation in the OR using RGB-D images, hypothesizing that the combination of depth and color information will improve the pose estimation results in such a difficult environment. We propose an approach based on pictorial structures that makes use of both channels of the RGB-D camera and also introduce a new feature descriptor for depth images, called histogram of depth differences (HDD), that captures local depth level changes. To quantitatively evaluate the proposed approach, we generate a novel dataset by manually annotating images recorded from different camera views during several days of live surgeries. Our experiments show that the pictorial structures (PS) approach applied on depth images using HDD outperforms the state-of-the art PS approach applied on the corresponding color images by over 11%. Furthermore, the proposed HDD descriptor has superior performance when compared to two other classical descriptors applied on depth images. Finally, the appearance models generated from the depth images perform better than those generated from the color images, and the combination of both improves the overall results. We therefore conclude that it is highly beneficial to use depth information in the pictorial structure model and also for human pose estimation in operating rooms.

Keywords: Body pose estimation, Pictorial structures, RGB-D images, Surgical workflow analysis.

1 Introduction

Recognizing and estimating the poses of clinical staff can provide invaluable input for many applications in the operating room (OR), for example surgical

N. Navab et al. (Eds.): MICCAI 2015, Part I, LNCS 9349, pp. 363–370, 2015.
DOI: 10.1007/978-3-319-24553-9_45

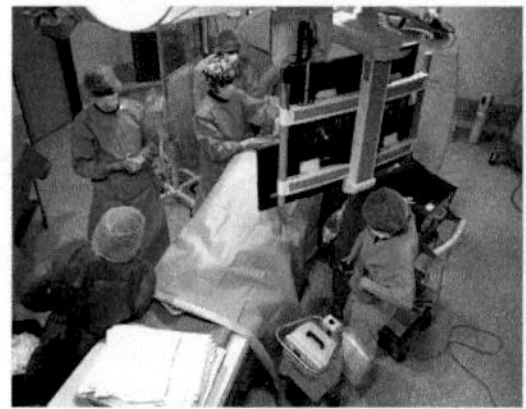
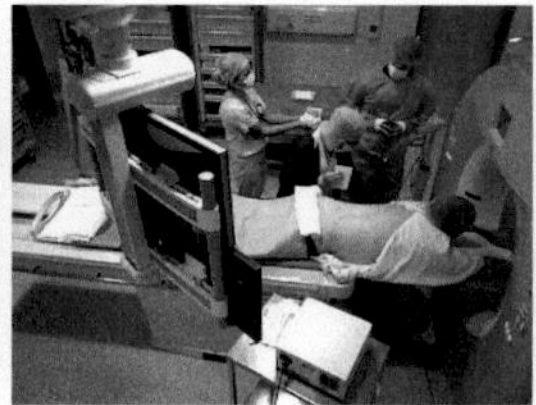
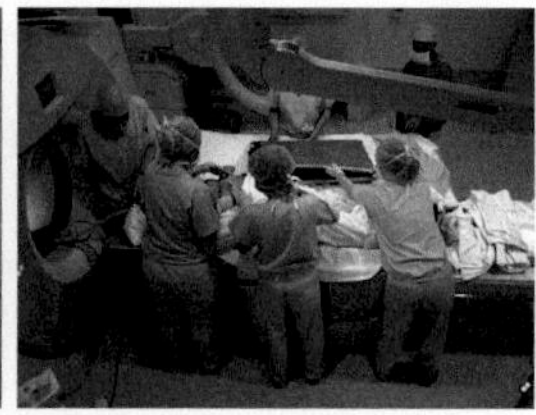

Fig. 1. Sample images of the clinician pose dataset acquired during live surgeries. Each image shows the OR from one of three different views used to capture the environment.

activity recognition [8,4], performance assessment [6], context-aware user interfaces [9,7] and radiation safety monitoring [5].

Human pose estimation (HPE) is also one of the fundamental problems of computer vision and has produced a vast literature over the last few decades. HPE is mainly addressed by part based approaches thanks to [2] that has made exact inference tractable on pictorial structures (PS) with tree-structured graphs by using the generalized distance transform algorithm. Recently, Yang and Ramanan [13] proposed an approach based on structured support vector machines (SVM) and PS that jointly learns mixtures of parts and a loosely coupled pairwise dependency model to capture different part appearances and their co-occurrences. Other works have tried to improve PS by enhancing its underlying graphical model to capture higher order relationships between parts, such as temporal consistency [3] and repulsive factors between left and right parts [1], with the penalty of approximate inference. Toshev at al. [12] also proposed a holistic method based on deep neural networks to regress for body joints, which requires a very large training set. In contrast to previous works that are only relying on color images to model body part appearances, [10] proposed to use random forests on depth images alone and reported promising result for human pose estimation in scenarios where a foreground mask can be obtained. However, obtaining foreground masks in the cluttered scenes of the OR, as shown in figure 1, is not a trivial task.

Even though many HPE methods are proposed in the vision literature, they cannot be directly applied to the OR due to the numerous difficulties implied by such an environment. First of all, the safety requirements of the OR and the multiple articulated arms mounted on the ceiling constrain camera positioning. Second, the illumination can change severely. Finally, most equipments and clinical clothes have the same color. [3] proposes an approach for 3D human pose estimation in the OR using discrete optimization over RGB-D sequences. A generic body part detector was used, similar to [10], that had not been trained for the OR environment. To cope with the misdetections of the detector and to enforce temporal consistency, [3] proposes an optimization over a connected graph modeling the whole sequence. Ground-truth initializations for the first and last frame are needed. These requirements make the approach unsuitable for real-time applications. Moreover, the dataset used for evaluation has been recorded in real interventional rooms but not during real surgeries. Thus, it does not include all the visual challenges occurring during live operations.

In this work, we address the challenging problem of human pose estimation in the OR. We base our approach upon [13] due to four main reasons: first, it is the state-of-the-art method for human pose estimation; second, by using mixtures of parts, the approach tolerates appearance changes and part foreshortening, which are common in the OR; third, the method performs exact inference in a tractable manner on tree-structured pairwise dependency models; and finally, all parameters are learned using a structured SVM solver, thus eliminating the need for further manual adjustments.

The body part appearance models in [13] are built using intensity images only. The histogram of oriented gradient (HOG) descriptor, referred to as I-HOG in this paper when applied on intensity images, is used to build the part models. However, in a complex environment such as the OR, color images might not always carry enough descriptive information due to severe illumination changes and high color similarities. With the advent of affordable RGB-D sensors, it is now possible to capture both color and depth images simultaneously. The depth image is computed by decoding the deformation of a known pattern that is projected onto a scene using infrared light. Thus, the depth accuracy is not affected by brightness or contrast changes. We therefore propose to construct robust and discriminative body part appearance models by combining both color and depth features.

We also introduce a new descriptor for depth images, named histogram of depth differences (HDD), that encodes surface level changes. We compare it with two other descriptors for depth images: the aforementioned HOG descriptor that we apply on depth images for comparison (D-HOG), and the histogram of oriented normal vectors (HONV) [11] that has been reported to perform well for object detection in depth images.

In summary, we propose an approach for human body pose estimation in the OR that relies jointly on color and on depth images. To the best of our knowledge, this is the first PS-based approach on RGB-D data and also the first single frame human pose estimation approach that has been proposed for the OR. We additionally introduce the HDD descriptor for depth images and compare it with two other classical descriptors. Finally, we quantitatively evaluate our approach on a novel dataset recorded during several days of live surgeries.

2 Method

In this section, we briefly describe the flexible mixtures of parts (FMP) approach [13] that serves as a basis for our human pose estimator. We also present the HONV descriptor and introduce the HDD descriptor for depth images.

2.1 Flexible Mixtures of Parts

The flexible mixtures of parts approach [13] represents the human body as a set of rigid body parts that are loosely coupled with each other using springs. The state of each body part i is specified by the pixel position l_i of its joint and by its

0	0	0
-1	0	1
0	0	0

-1	0	0
0	0	0
0	0	1

0	-1	0
0	0	0
0	1	0

0	0	-1
0	0	0
1	0	0

Fig. 2. Four different kernels that capture local level changes in depth images.

body part type t_i. This type can be defined based on low level information, such as part position, or high level information, such as the state of the part (e.g. open versus closed hand). We write $i \in \{1, ..., K\}, l_i \in \{1, ..., L\}$ and $t_i \in \{1, ..., T\}$. Let $G = (V, E)$ be a relational graph whose K nodes represent body parts and whose edges define connections between body parts to enforce body kinematics.

$$S(I, D, l, t) = \sum_{i \in V} w_i^{t_i}.\phi(I, D, l_i) + \sum_{ij \in E} w_{ij}^{t_i,t_j}.\psi(l_i - l_j) + \sum_{i \in V} b_i^{t_i} + \sum_{ij \in E} b_{ij}^{t_i,t_j} \quad (1)$$

is a score function, where I denotes the input image and D is the aligned depth image. The first term in eq. 1 is the part appearance model that computes the score of placing a part i at location l_i based on the part appearance template $w_i^{t_i}$ and the feature vector $\phi(I, D, l_i)$. The second term computes the deformation score based on relative displacements between parts that are encoded by $\psi(l_i - l_j) = [dx\ dx^2\ dy\ dy^2]^T$, where (dx, dy) is the relative location of part i w.r.t. part j. The last two terms are computing the part type compatibility score, where b_i is the score of choosing a particular mixture for part i and $b_{ij}^{t_i,t_j}$ encodes the co-occurrence compatibility of part types.

Inference and Learning: Estimating the body pose in this model corresponds to finding $(l^*, t^*) = \text{argmax}_{l,t}\ S(I, l, t)$. For a tree-structured relational graph G, this optimization can be solved efficiently and exactly with dynamic programming. In a supervised learning setup, we assume that a set of labeled positive and negative examples is available. The model parameters can then be learned using structural SVM. For more details, we refer to the original paper [13].

2.2 Appearance Model

We now focus on the different feature descriptors that can be used to build the body part appearance model. To construct ϕ, we uniformly divide images into non overlapping windows, called cells, in which the descriptors are computed. Following the same avenue as [13], I-HOG is used on color images and serves as our baseline. The D-HOG descriptor applies HOG on depth images. The two other depth-based descriptors used in this paper are described below.

Histogram of Oriented Normal Vectors (HONV): This descriptor represents object surfaces using a histogram of normal vectors. The gradient of the depth image is first used to compute the normal vectors in spherical coordinates. Each normal vector is then represented by a pair of azimuth and zenith angles and quantized to vote into a 2D histogram; more details can be found in [11].

Histogram of Depth Differences (HDD): A depth image encodes in each pixel the distance between the depth sensor and the surfaces of the scene. In [10], a simple depth operator is proposed that performs well for body part detection. This operator is able to distinguish between different body parts by capturing part depth differences and is learned during the training of a deep random forest. Inspired by this operator, we introduce a simple yet efficient new descriptor that captures local level changes in a depth image using the kernels shown in figure 2. Let K_k be one of the HDD kernels with $k \in \{1, ..., 4\}$. We define the normalized convolution response at position (x, y) as

$$C_{ks}(x, y) = (K_k \ * \ P_s(x, y))/D_s(x, y), \tag{2}$$

where $s \in \{1, ..., n\}$ is the scale of the depth image and $P_s(x, y)$ is the depth image patch at location (x, y) for scale s. The convolution is applied over a scale space to capture the changes in different spatial neighborhoods. The responses are also normalized by the depth value at the center of each patch for depth invariance. For each cell, the descriptor is then built by quantizing all the responses and by binning them into a 3D histogram of kernel, scale and quantization levels.

3 Experimental Results and Discussions

We evaluate our approach on a new RGB-D dataset recorded in an operating room using an *Asus Xtion Pro Live* camera. To capture different views of the room, the camera position is changed among three possible locations, as shown in figure 1. All activities happening in the OR are recorded for seven half days at 20fps. Due to the large number of frames and the similarity of consecutive frames, we manually annotate every 500th frame to provide ground truth positions for the upper body parts. Ultimately, we obtain a dataset that includes 1451 frames containing 1991 annotated persons and that is balanced across the half days. We have also selected 173 frames that do not contain any human to serve as negative examples. Since the distances of the annotated persons with respect to camera vary in the range of $[1.2 - 4.5]$ meters, body parts at multiple scales are present in this dataset. Different individuals including surgeons, nurses and anesthesiologists wearing various clothes, such as scrub suits, surgical gowns and radiation protection aprons have been annotated. We have divided the dataset into seven disjoint sets where all frames in a set belong to the same half day recording. A leave-one-out scheme is applied so that one set is used as test set and the rest as training set. We report the average results of seven-fold cross validation during the evaluation.

Following current practice in the literature, we use the probability of correct keypoint (PCK) as evaluation metric [13]. A tight bounding box is obtained from the annotated upper body pose of each person. Given the bounding box, the pose estimator returns a set of keypoints indicating the body joint locations. A keypoint is correct if it falls within $\alpha \, . \, max(w, h)$ pixels of the ground truth, where w and h are respectively the width and height of the bounding box, and α specifies the relative threshold used to consider a keypoint as a correct detection.

Table 1. PCK results for different appearance models on the clinician pose dataset.

Color Desc.	Depth Desc.	Head	Shoulder	Elbow	Wrist	Hip	Total
I-HOG	-	84.12	72.70	56.98	56.53	45.91	63.25
-	D-HOG	90.87	83.30	65.15	66.21	57.12	72.53
I-HOG	D-HOG	**93.92**	84.75	70.26	67.80	59.54	75.25
-	HONV	84.80	80.20	58.64	56.81	47.52	65.60
I-HOG	HONV	92.52	**85.89**	69.31	68.91	60.27	75.38
-	HDD	91.18	82.89	67.35	69.93	62.12	74.69
I-HOG	HDD	92.76	84.10	**71.12**	**71.62**	**63.62**	**76.64**

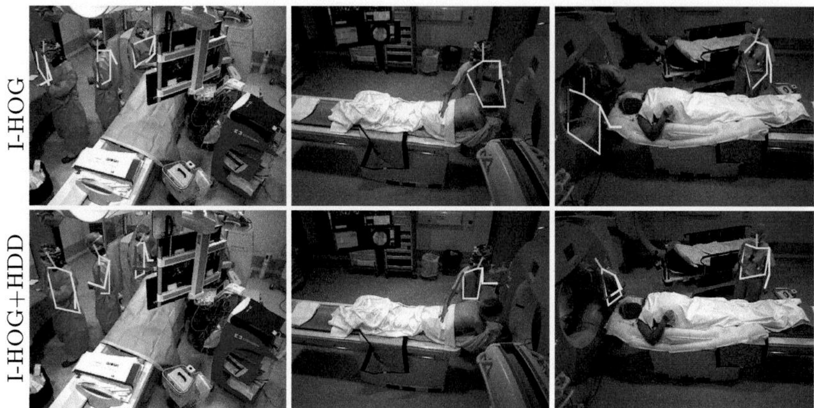

Fig. 3. Examples of pose estimation using I-HOG and I-HOG+HDD.

We set $\alpha = 0.2$ as proposed by [13]. In table 1, we present the evaluation results for the different appearance models on the clinician pose dataset. To combine different appearance models, we concatenate their descriptors. A cell size of 6×6 pixels has been set to stay consistent with the one commonly used with HOG.

HOG: We construct the body part appearance models using the HOG descriptor in three different ways. We first evaluate HOG on color images (I-HOG) to generate the baseline using the same parameters as in [13]. Second, we apply the same descriptor on the depth images and follow the same pipeline (D-HOG). Finally, both I-HOG and D-HOG are used to jointly learn body part models. D-HOG improves the results over the baseline significantly (+9.28%), which indicates the strength of depth-based appearance models as compared to the original color-based one. Since the same descriptor is used for both I-HOG and D-HOG, it highlights that the intensity gradient is not always reliable in such an environment due to the high color similarity of the clothes and equipments as well as the severe illumination changes, while depth gradients provide more robust representations. The representation based on I-HOG+D-HOG boosts the performance even more (+12%) by building a strong appearance model that combines the complementary information provided by the color and depth sensors.

HONV: To evaluate the performance of HONV, a normalization scheme is needed for the descriptor. We have compared the L2-norm and L2-Hys normalization schemes, where L2-Hys is similar to L2-norm but limits the maximum value to 0.2. Since both normalization methods show similar performance and L2-Hys is used with HOG, only the results with the L2-Hys normalization scheme are reported. HONV improves the results (+2.35%) over the baseline and its combination with I-HOG enhances the performance (+12.13%).

HDD: We compute the HDD descriptor in three scales and coarsely quantize the kernel responses into 10 levels to be robust to noise and spatial distortions. Thus, we obtain a descriptor of size $4 \times 3 \times 10$ per cell. Since L2-norm and L2-Hys normalizations show similar performance, following the same reasoning as before, we report the results with L2-Hys normalization. As shown in table 1, the HDD descriptor significantly improves the results over the baseline (+11.44%). Combining both HDD and I-HOG further boosts the performance (+13.39%).

In summary, the experiments show that the color descriptor I-HOG is not always reliable due to the lack of texture on the surgical clothes and to the color similarities of clothes and equipments, while the depth descriptors provide more robust body part representations. Table 1 also shows the results per body part. High improvements on shoulder detection are obtained using all depth descriptors. This can be explained by the very distinctive depth changes on shoulders that are often not captured by the color images due to color similarities or illumination changes. However, noisy depth maps can heavily distort edges and surface normals, especially when body parts are close to each other. The consistent performance improvement of HDD over the other depth descriptors on the most challenging parts, namely elbow and wrist, shows the benefits of its coarse representation in such cases. Finally, the combination of color and depth descriptors improves the body part models and the best performance is obtained using I-HOG+HDD. Figure 3 shows the overlaid skeletons for several frames using I-HOG and I-HOG+HDD. The first two columns illustrate cases where the color-based body part detector is confused by intensity changes while the HDD-based detector correctly localizes the body parts. The last column shows failure cases for both descriptors that indicate the need for better occlusion handling and 3D inference.

4 Conclusions

In this paper, we propose an approach based on pictorial structures for human pose estimation in the operating room. We first extend the appearance representations used in PS to RGB-D images by constructing strong and discriminative body part detectors using both color and depth images to deal with the visual challenges present in the room. We also propose a new descriptor for depth images that encodes the local level changes in a 3D histogram. Since this descriptor is computed over a scale space and coarsely discretized, it is robust to local geometric distortions. Furthermore, to quantitatively evaluate our approach, we generate a novel RGB-D dataset in which upper body poses of clinicians are manually annotated. We then conduct a series of experiments that compare the different appearance representation approaches. We show that depth descriptors are performing better than the color descriptor. Furthermore, the combination of the color and depth descriptors always improves the body part detections. Finally, the proposed HDD descriptor improves the performance by 13.39% over the baseline and significantly enhances the elbow, wrist and hip detections.

Acknowledgements. This work was supported by French state funds managed by the ANR within the Investissements d'Avenir program under references ANR-11-LABX-0004 (Labex CAMI), ANR-10-IDEX-0002-02 (IdEx Unistra) and ANR-10-IAHU-02 (IHU Strasbourg).

References

1. Andriluka, M., Roth, S., Schiele, B.: Discriminative appearance models for pictorial structures. Int. J. Comput. Vision 99(3) (2012)
2. Felzenszwalb, P.F., Huttenlocher, D.P.: Pictorial structures for object recognition. Int. J. Comput. Vision 61(1), 55–79 (2005)
3. Kadkhodamohammadi, A., Gangi, A., de Mathelin, M., Padoy, N.: Temporally consistent 3D pose estimation in the interventional room using discrete MRF optimization over RGBD sequences. In: Stoyanov, D., Collins, D.L., Sakuma, I., Abolmaesumi, P., Jannin, P. (eds.) IPCAI 2014. LNCS, vol. 8498, pp. 168–177. Springer, Heidelberg (2014)
4. Lea, C., Facker, J.C., Hager, G.D., Taylor, R.H., Saria, S.: 3D sensing algorithms towards building an intelligent intensive care unit. In: AMIA CRI (2013)
5. Loy Rodas, N., Padoy, N.: Seeing is believing: increasing intraoperative awareness to scattered radiation in interventional procedures by combining augmented reality, monte carlo simulations and wireless dosimeters. International Journal of Computer Assisted Radiology and Surgery, 1–11 (2015)
6. Mason, J., Ansell, J., Warren, N., Torkington, J.: Is motion analysis a valid tool for assessing laparoscopic skill? Surgical Endoscopy 27(5), 1468–1477 (2013)
7. Noonan, D.P., Mylonas, G.P., Darzi, A., Yang, G.Z.: Gaze contingent articulated robot control for robot assisted min. invasive surgery. In: IROS (2008)
8. Padoy, N., Mateus, D., Weinland, D., Berger, M.O., Navab, N.: Workflow Monitoring based on 3D Motion Features. In: VOEC-ICCV, pp. 585–592 (2009)
9. Schwarz, L., Bigdelou, A., Navab, N.: Learning gestures for customizable human-computer interaction in the operating room. In: Fichtinger, G., Martel, A., Peters, T. (eds.) MICCAI 2011, Part I. LNCS, vol. 6891, pp. 129–136. Springer, Heidelberg (2011)
10. Shotton, J., Fitzgibbon, A.W., Cook, M., Sharp, T., Finocchio, M., Moore, R., Kipman, A., Blake, A.: Real-time human pose recognition in parts from single depth images. In: CVPR, pp. 1297–1304 (2011)
11. Tang, S., Wang, X., Lv, X., Han, T., Keller, J., He, Z., Skubic, M., Lao, S.: Histogram of oriented normal vectors for object recognition with a depth sensor. In: Lee, K.M., Matsushita, Y., Rehg, J.M., Hu, Z. (eds.) ACCV 2012, Part II. LNCS, vol. 7725, pp. 525–538. Springer, Heidelberg (2013)
12. Toshev, A., Szegedy, C.: DeepPose: Human pose estimation via deep neural networks. In: CVPR (2014)
13. Yang, Y., Ramanan, D.: Articulated human detection with flexible mixtures of parts. PAMI 35(12), 2878–2890 (2013)

Interventional Photoacoustic Imaging of the Human Placenta with Ultrasonic Tracking for Minimally Invasive Fetal Surgeries

Wenfeng Xia[1], Efthymios Maneas[2], Daniil I. Nikitichev[1], Charles A. Mosse[1], Gustavo Sato dos Santos[2], Tom Vercauteren[2], Anna L. David[3], Jan Deprest[4], Sébastien Ourselin[2], Paul C. Beard[1], and Adrien E. Desjardins[1]

[1] Department of Medical Physics and Biomedical Engineering, University College London, Gower Street, London WC1E 6BT, United Kingdom
[2] Translational Imaging Group, Centre for Medical Image Computing, Department of Medical Physics and Biomedical Engineering, University College London, Wolfson House, London WC1E 6BT, United Kingdom
[3] Institute for Women's Health, University College London, 86-96 Chenies Mews, London WC1E 6HX, United Kingdom
[4] Department of Obstetrics and Gynecology, University Hospitals KU Leuven, Leuven, Belgium

wenfeng.xia@ucl.ac.uk

Abstract. Image guidance plays a central role in minimally invasive fetal surgery such as photocoagulation of inter-twin placental anastomosing vessels to treat twin-to-twin transfusion syndrome (TTTS). Fetoscopic guidance provides insufficient sensitivity for imaging the vasculature that lies beneath the fetal placental surface due to strong light scattering in biological tissues. Incomplete photocoagulation of anastamoses is associated with postoperative complications and higher perinatal mortality. In this study, we investigated the use of multi-spectral photoacoustic (PA) imaging for better visualization of the placental vasculature. Excitation light was delivered with an optical fiber with dimensions that are compatible with the working channel of a fetoscope. Imaging was performed on an *ex vivo* normal term human placenta collected at Caesarean section birth. The photoacoustically-generated ultrasound signals were received by an external clinical linear array ultrasound imaging probe. A vein under illumination on the fetal placenta surface was visualized with PA imaging, and good correspondence was obtained between the measured PA spectrum and the optical absorption spectrum of deoxygenated blood. The delivery fiber had an attached fiber optic ultrasound sensor positioned directly adjacent to it, so that its spatial position could be tracked by receiving transmissions from the ultrasound imaging probe. This study provides strong indications that PA imaging in combination with ultrasonic tracking could be useful for detecting the human placental vasculature during minimally invasive fetal surgery.

N. Navab et al. (Eds.): MICCAI 2015, Part I, LNCS 9349, pp. 371–378, 2015.
DOI: 10.1007/978-3-319-24553-9_46

1 Introduction

Image guidance is a central component of minimally invasive fetal surgery for treatment of twin-to-twin transfusion syndrome (TTTS). The gold standard for treatment involves laser photocoagulation of anastamosing vessels on the fetal side of the placenta [1]. In current practice, anastomosing vessels are identified with vessels along the equator using a fetoscope. Due to the limitations of this modality, there is a risk that sub-surface vessels that are small and those that are at the periphery of the placenta are missed, so that treatment is incomplete. Ultrasound (US) imaging with a probe positioned at the external surface of the mother provides inadequate visualization for small placental vessels. Visualization with US can be particularly poor when the placenta is on the posterior part of the uterus, at a large distance from the imaging probe so that low US frequencies are required. Power Doppler (PD) was also proposed by several groups to visualize the placenta vasculature [2,3]. One challenge with PD is that successful vessel identification is strongly dependent on the skill of the operator and the vessel orientation; additionally, this technique lacks sensitivity for small vessels due to low US contrast for soft tissues.

Photoacoustic (PA) imaging has strong potential to provide guidance information during TTTS that is complementary to fetoscopy and external US imaging. With PA imaging, pulsed or temporally modulated excitation light is absorbed in tissue, which causes temperature rises and subsequent generation of US waves [4]. These US waves can be received with an imaging probe at the surface of a patient and reconstructed to form 2D or 3D images with contrast for tissue chromophores. Multispectral PA images, which are acquired by varying the wavelength of excitation light, can be used to provide quantitative information about chromophore concentrations [5].

Conventional implementations of PA imaging, in which excitation light is delivered at the surface of the patient, may be suboptimal in the context of TTTS. As placental vessels typically lie more than five centimeters below the surface of the patient, the PA signals may be very low or undetectable due to the prominence of scattering and absorption of excitation light [6]. In this study, light is delivered directly to the placental surface using an optical fiber that is sufficiently small to be inserted into the instrument channel of a fetoscope. The generated PA signals were detected by a commercial linear array US imaging probe.

The PA imaging system in this study was extended to allow for real-time in-plane ultrasonic tracking of the optical fiber that delivers excitation light. Ultrasonic tracking was implemented with a fiber-optic hydrophone that was positioned alongside the delivery fiber. Multispectral PA imaging and ultrasonic tracking were performed on a human placenta *ex vivo*, and the measured photoacoustic spectrum from a vein was compared with the optical spectra of oxy- and deoxy-hemoglobin.

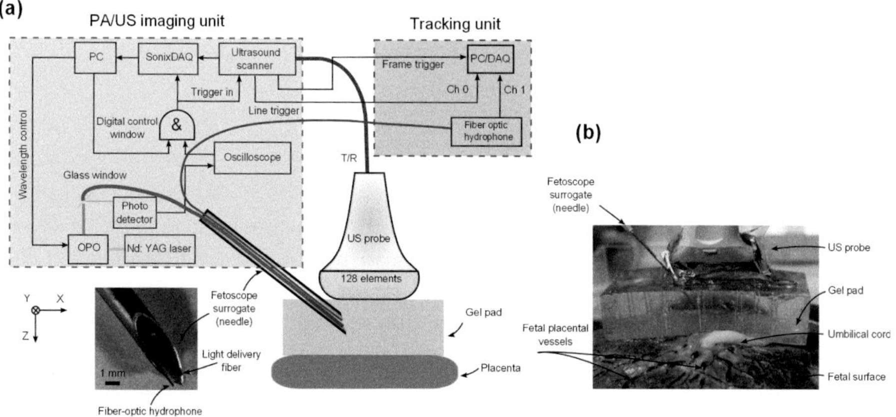

Fig. 1. (a) Schematic illustration of the photoacoustic imaging and ultrasonic tracking system. (b) Photograph of the fetal surface of a human placenta under the imaging probe.

2 Materials and Methods

2.1 PA Imaging and Ultrasonic Tracking System

The system that was used for PA imaging and tracking was based on a clinical US imaging system with a 128-element, 10 MHz linear-array US probe (SonixMDP, Analogic Ultrasound, Richmond, BC, Canada) as shown in Figure 1a. It was operated in research mode, which provides the access to low-level libraries for acquisition of B-mode images, transmission of US pulses for tracking, and collection of pre-beamformed RF data through a 128 channel DAQ system (Sonix-DAQ, Analogic Ultrasound, Richmond, BC, Canada) for PA imaging.

PA Imaging. Pulsed light with multiple wavelengths was provided by an optical parametric oscillator (OPO) system (VersaScan L-532, GWU-Lasertechnik, Erftstadt, Germany) pumped by a Nd:YAG laser (pulse width 6 ns, repetition rate 10 Hz, Quanta-Ray, INDI-40-10, Spectra-Physics, Santa Clara, CA). The signal and the idler from the OPO provided two wavelength ranges: 700-900 nm and 1100-2200 nm respectively. In this study, only the signal output was used (Figure 1a). The OPO output was coupled into an optical fiber with a 910 μm core diameter (FG910LEC, Thorlabs, Newton, NJ). A small portion of this output (4%) was deflected to a photodetector (DET10A, Thorlabs, Newton, NJ) to compensate for pulse-to-pulse energy fluctuations and to provide optical triggering. A maximum pulse energy of 6 mJ was used in this study was delivered from the distal end of the fiber (flat-cleaved at normal incidence). Control of PA image acquisition was realized using a logic AND gate with two inputs: the optical trigger and a digital control window provided by a LabView control program via a digital I/O card (NI-USB-6501, National Instruments, Berkshire, UK). PA image reconstruction was performed in real-time using a custom delay-and-sum beam-forming algorithm; offline, a more accurate Fourier-domain reconstruction algorithm [7] was used.

Ultrasonic Tracking. A fiber-optic hydrophone (125 μm cladding, Precision Acoustics, Dorchester, UK) [8] was used to receive US transmissions from the linear array probe (Figure 1a). Each element of the linear array was excited by a bipolar electrical pulse (Figure 2a). The fiber-optic hydrophone (FOH) data collection were synchronized with the US tracking transmissions using two output triggers: a frame trigger corresponding to the start of each image frame, and a line trigger corresponding to the start of each transmission. Using the frame trigger, the line trigger signal and the FOH data was digitized using a DAQ card (USB-5132, National Instrument, Austin, Texas) as illustrated in Figure 1a. The line triggers were used to parse the FOH data according to the start of each US tracking transmission. With knowledge of the sound speed in the medium, the time-of-flights of the US pulses determine the distance between the hydrophone tip and the centers of the transmitting elements (Figure 2a). The peaks of the time-gated signals form a parabolic shape (Figure 2b). A received transmission from transducer element number 30 is shown in Figure 2c. An image of the hydrophone tip was reconstructed by applying a Fourier-domain reconstruction algorithm which was developed initially for PA imaging [7] (Figure 2d). An important advantage of the ultrasonic tracking images is that they are inherently co-registered with the conventional B-mode US images and the PA images.

The fiber-optic hydrophone and the excitation light delivery fiber were inserted into the cannula of a 14 gauge spinal needle (Terumo, Surrey, UK), which served as a surrogate for the fetoscope. The distal ends of the fibers were flush with the bevel surface of the needle (Figure 1a).

2.2 Imaging and Tracking with a Human Placenta

A term human placenta was collected after a caesarean section delivery at the University College London Hospital (UCLH). The study was approved by a Joint Committees of UCL and UCLH on the Ethics of Human Research and the placenta was collected after written informed consent from the mother. Following delivery, the umbilical cord was clamped immediately to preserve the maximum amount of blood inside the placental fetal vasculature.

PA imaging of the placenta was performed with a block of gel positioned between the US probe and the fetal surface of the placenta. This gel, which was optically and acoustically transparent, served to simulate the amniotic fluid within the gestation sac (Figure 1b). During PA imaging, it was chosen in place of saline or similar aqueous solutions to limit diffusion of blood out of the placenta. With ultrasonic tracking, gel was not used as its acoustic coupling with the hydrophone was poor; the placenta was immersed in a saline and the fetoscope surrogate was inserted to the placenta surface at an angle of 62 degrees (measured relative to the US probe surface).

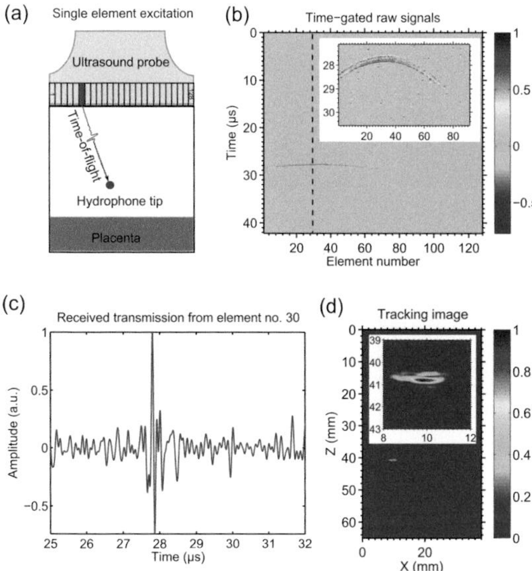

Fig. 2. (a) Schematic illustration of single-element excitation of the linear array imaging probe to acquire a tracking image. (b) Time-gated transmissions received by the hydrophone. (c) The received transmission from transducer element number 30. (d) The reconstructed tracking image.

3 Results and Discussion

With PA imaging, a portion of the placental surface that was illuminated with excitation light was visualized (Figure 3a-c). A circular region with high signal amplitudes, which corresponded to a major vein on the placental surface, featured prominently in the PA images. A decrease in the average PA signal amplitude across the wavelength range of 760 nm to 840 nm (Figure 3d) was also apparent in the images (Figure 3a-c). Across the wavelength range of 750 to 900 nm, good correspondence between the average PA signal and the optical absorption spectrum of deoxygenated blood was observed (Figure 4d). Absorbing structures at a depth in tissue of approximately 5 mm were apparent, which were attributed to small blood vessels. The appearance of the fetoscope surrogate (needle), which is consistent with previous studies [9,10], can be attributed to photoacoustic excitation from back-scattered excitation light. The PA signal from the fiber could be used to provide an indication of the fiber location relative to B-mode US images; however, severe artifacts resulting from US reflections within the fetoscope surrogate are likely to limit the accuracy of this method.

With ultrasonic tracking, the hydrophone tip was clearly visualized (Figure 4). At two depths (25 mm and 41 mm), the US (Figure 4a,d) and tracking (Figure 4b,e) images of the tip of the fetoscope surrogate had excellent spatial agreement. High SNRs were achieved for the tracking images (490 and 480, respectively). The full width at half maximum values of the axial and lateral profiles, which

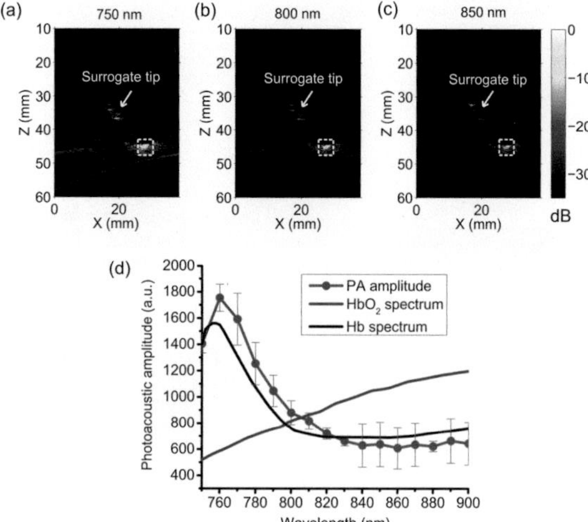

Fig. 3. Photoacoustic images of the placenta at wavelengths of (a) 750 nm, (b) 800 nm and (c) 850 nm. The averaged photoacoustic amplitude over the region of interest (white box) as a function of excitation light wavelengths are shown in (d), with the optical absorption spectra of oxygenated and deoxygenated blood scaled to the averaged photoacoustic amplitude at 750 nm.

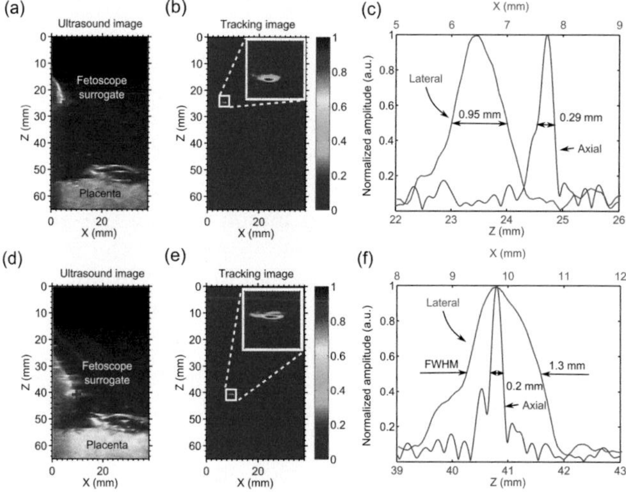

Fig. 4. The hydrophone tip tracked at two locations within the ultrasound image plane. Two ultrasound images are shown in (a) and (d) with corresponding tracking images shown in (b) (e) respectively. The axial and lateral profiles for the hydrophone tip image at two locations are shown in (c) and (f) with the full width at half maximum values indicating the accuracy of the tracking method.

can be taken as measures of the tracking accuracy, were consistently in a submillimeter level (Figure 4c,f).

In the context of minimally invasive fetal surgery, there are several potential benefits of ultrasonic tracking. First, knowledge of the position of the fiber that delivers excitation light relative to the US imaging probe could be used to model the light and US propagation, and further to facilitate the accurate recovery of optical absorption spectra of chromophores. Ultrasonic tracking of the fetoscope tip, which would be possible if the hydrophone were integrated directly to the fetoscope, could facilitate fusion of fetoscopic and US images, as well as mosaicing of fetoscopic images. Furthermore, the orientation of the fetoscope relative to the US probe could be tracked using multiple hydrophone sensors distributed along it.

In the context of medical device tracking, an optical hydrophone as an US sensor has several advantages relative to a conventional piezoelectric US transducer [8,11]. First, it is narrow and flexible, which facilitates integration into devices. Second, it provides sufficient sensitivity for tracking, as demonstrated with a high SNR (Figure 4). Finally, it possesses nearly omnidirectional sensitivity below 25 MHz, which allows the tracking with steep insertion angles.

The experimental paradigm in this study has several limitations. First, while the gel block phantom was designed to represent typical experiences encountered in clinical practice, it did not allow for very large distances between the US imaging probe and the placenta such as those that may be encountered with obese patients. Second, it would have been useful to have co-registration with other modalities such as MRI and CT, but the accuracy would be limited by placental deformations. Third, follow-on studies are required to thoroughly compare the tracking method used in this paper with others. An alternative tracking method to consider is the use of an US reflector on the fetoscope.

Interventional photoacoustic imaging has attracted great attention in recent years [10,12,13,14,15]. However, to the authors knowledge, this proof-of-concept study is the first to provide multispectral photoacoustic imaging of the human placenta, and also the first to provide ultrasonic tracking in a fetoscopic context. It sets the stage for comprehensive PA imaging across the surface of the placenta in both normal and pathological cases in concert with histology. In future studies, perfusion models that incorporate mechanisms for modifying the blood oxygenation could be used to assess the sensitivity of PA images to blood flow [16] and oxygen saturation [5]. Further multispectral PA imaging could be used to discriminate between coagulated and non-coagulated blood during the treatment of TTTS, based on their absorption spectra [17]. Photoacoustic imaging has strong potential to improve visualization of placental vasculature during minimally invasive treatment of TTTS, and thereby to improve procedural outcomes.

Acknowledgments. This work was supported by an Innovative Engineering for Health award by the Wellcome Trust [WT101957] and the Engineering and Physical Sciences Research Council (EPSRC) [NS/A000027/1], by a Starting Grant from the European Research Council [ERC-2012-StG, Proposal 310970 MOPHIM], and by an EPSRC First Grant [EP/J010952/1]. The authors acknowledge support from the Biomedical Research Centre of the United Kingdom National Institute for Health Research (NIHR).

References

1. Slaghekke, F., et al.: Fetoscopic laser coagulation of the vascular equator versus selective coagulation for twin-to-twin transfusion syndrome: an open-label randomised controlled trial. Lancet 383, 2144–2151 (2014)
2. Pretorius, D.H., et al.: Imaging of placental vasculature using three-dimensional ultrasound and color power Doppler: a preliminary study. Ultrasound Obstet. Gynecol. 21(1), 45–49 (1998)
3. Noguchi, J., et al.: Placental vascular sonobiopsy using three-dimensional power Doppler ultrasound in normal and growth restricted fetuses. Placenta 30(5), 391–397 (2009)
4. Beard, P.C.: Biomedical photocoustic imaging. Interface Focus 1(4), 602–631 (2011)
5. Cox, B., et al.: Quantitative spectroscopic photoacoustic imaging: a review. J. Biomed. Opt. 17(6), 061202 (2012)
6. Xia, W., et al.: An optimized ultrasound detector for photoacoustic breast tomography. Med. Phys. 40(3), 032901 (2013)
7. Treeby, B.E., Cox, B.T.: k-Wave: MATLAB toolbox for the simulation and reconstruction of photoacoustic wave fields. J. Biomed. Opt. 15(2), 021314 (2010)
8. Morris, P., et al.: A Fabry-Pérot fiber-optic ultrasonic hydrophone for the simultaneous measurement of temperature and acoustic pressure. J. Acoust. Soc. Am. 125(6), 3611–3622 (2009)
9. Su, J., et al.: Photoacoustic imaging of clinical metal needles in tissue. J. Biomed. Opt. 15(2), 021309 (2010)
10. Piras, D., et al.: Photoacoustic needle: minimally invasive guidance to biopsy. J. Biomed. Opt. 18(7), 070502 (2013)
11. Mung, J., Vignon, F., Jain, A.: A non-disruptive technology for robust 3D tool tracking for ultrasound-guided interventions. In: Fichtinger, G., Martel, A., Peters, T., et al. (eds.) MICCAI 2011, Part I. LNCS, vol. 6891, pp. 153–160. Springer, Heidelberg (2011)
12. Lediju Bell, M.A., et al.: in vivo visualization of prostate brachytherapy seeds with photoacoustic imaging. J. Biomed. Opt. 19(12), 126011 (2014)
13. Lediju Bell, M.A., et al.: Transurethral light delivery for prostate photoacoustic imaging. J. Biomed. Opt. 20(3), 036002 (2015)
14. Tavakoli, B., et al.: Detecting occlusion inside a ventricular catheter using photoacoustic imaging through skull. In: Proc. SPIE 8943, p. 89434O (2014)
15. Lin, L., et al.: in vivo deep brain imaging of rats using oral-cavity illuminated photoacoustic computed tomography. J. Biomed. Opt. 20(1), 016019 (2015)
16. Brunker, J., Beard, P.: Pulsed photoacoustic Doppler flowmetry using time-domain cross-correlation: Accuracy, resolution and scalability. J. Acoust. Soc. Am. 132(3), 1780–1791 (2012)
17. Talbert, R., et al.: Photoaoustic discrimination of viable and thermally coagulated blood using a two-wavelength method for burn injury monitoring. Phys. Med. Biol. 52, 1815–1829 (2007)

Automated Segmentation of Surgical Motion for Performance Analysis and Feedback

Yun Zhou[1], Ioanna Ioannou[2], Sudanthi Wijewickrema[2] James Bailey[1], Gregor Kennedy[3], and Stephen O'Leary[2]

[1] Department of Computing and Information Systems, University of Melbourne
[2] Department of Otolaryngology, University of Melbourne
[3] Centre for the Study of Higher Education, University of Melbourne

Abstract. Advances in technology have motivated the increasing use of virtual reality simulation-based training systems in surgical education, as well as the use of motion capture systems to record surgical performance. These systems have the ability to collect large volumes of trajectory data. The capability to analyse motion data in a meaningful manner is valuable in characterising and evaluating the quality of surgical technique, and in facilitating the development of intelligent self-guided training systems with automated performance feedback. To this end, we propose an automatic trajectory segmentation technique, which divides surgical tool trajectories into their component movements according to spatio-temporal features. We evaluate this technique on two different temporal bone surgery tasks requiring the use of distinct surgical techniques and show that the proposed approach achieves higher accuracy compared to an existing method.

Keywords: Motion analysis, Surgical simulation.

1 Introduction

Interest in the analysis of surgical motion has flourished in recent years with the development and use of an ever expanding range of motion capture technologies. Virtual reality (VR) simulators are becoming an increasingly important component of surgical training programs, and the use of motorised haptic devices in these simulators readily enables the capture of surgical motion. Efforts have also been made to record surgical motion in the operating theatre, as increasingly accurate and unobstructive sensors become available.

Consequently, the analysis of surgical motion has become an active field of research. In the surgical domains that involve drilling - such as temporal bone surgery, orthopedic surgery and dental surgery - good technique is encompassed in the way a surgeon utilises their drill to remove tissue. Expert surgeons often describe good technique by delineating the desired characteristics of drilling strokes. For example, in a mastoidectomy procedure the use of long strokes parallel to sensitive anatomical structures is considered good technique.

The aim of this paper is to develop an automated method of segmenting drilling trajectories into a sequence of clinically meaningful component motions,

N. Navab et al. (Eds.): MICCAI 2015, Part I, LNCS 9349, pp. 379–386, 2015.
DOI: 10.1007/978-3-319-24553-9_47

which we refer to as strokes. The characteristics of these strokes (e.g. distance, shape, applied force) can be analysed to quantify the differences between expert and trainee surgeons, evaluate the quality of their surgical technique, and even provide automated feedback during training. Trajectory segmentation using spatio-temporal features has been studied widely in other application areas, such as handwriting recognition [1,8] and geographic information systems [2].

In this work, we propose a classification approach based on spatio-temporal features to automatically segment surgical drilling trajectories. We begin with a description of the dataset used to train and evaluate the classifiers, followed by the steps of the proposed approach and the chosen set of spatio-temporal features. We proceed to define the baseline method and our classification-based method. Finally we define the evaluation metrics used to measure the quality of the segmentation, followed by the results of the evaluation.

2 Method

We begin with a formal definition of trajectory and stroke. The trajectory of a moving tool is defined as a sequence of pairs, $\tau = [(p_1, t_1), (p_2, t_2), ..., (p_n, t_n)]$, where p_i is a three-dimensional vector representing the position observed at time t_i, $i \in [1, n]$ and n is the number of data points in the trajectory. We denote a stroke from time t_i to time t_j as a sequence of points in τ: $s = \tau[t_i, t_j]$.

Experiment Data: The trajectory data used to build segmentation models in this experiment was collected on a VR temporal bone surgery simulator. The data consisted of 16 expert and 10 trainee performances conducted by 7 experts and 6 trainees. Each performance included the full preparation of the temporal bone for cochlear implantation. We focussed our investigation on two stages of this procedure that require very different drilling technique, namely mastoidectomy and posterior tympanotomy. Mastoidectomy is the initial stage and typically requires long sweeping strokes with a large burr, while posterior tympanotomy is carried out in a very tight space and requires short, often more circular strokes, with a small burr.

For each performance, we randomly selected a 10 second sub-trajectory from each stage and labelled it manually (example shown in figure 1). Table 1 summarizes the statistics of our dataset. The ratio of turning points to normal points for the two stages was approximately $1:10$ and $1:8$. We randomly split the 26 labelled performances into three sets: a training set of 18, a validation set of 4, and a test set of 4. The training set was used to train the model, the validation set was used for parameter optimisation, and the test set was used to validate segmentation performance.

In order to further test our segmentation models, we also manually labelled a random 10 second sub-trajectory from each stage of six cadaveric temporal bones. The details of the data collection procedure for cadaveric temporal bones can be found in [7].

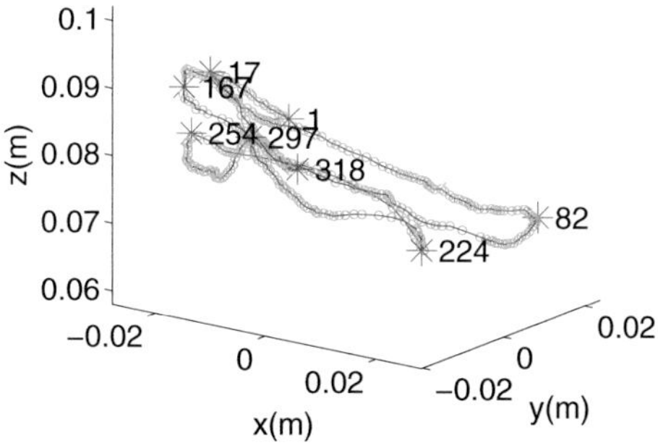

Fig. 1. Example of a manually segmented sub-trajectory from a mastoidectomy procedure containing 7 strokes. Units are in metres. Red crosses mark turning points and green dots mark normal points.

Table 1. Statistics of labelled trajectory dataset

dataset	task	# turning points	# normal points	# strokes
Simulator	mastoidectomy	786	7501	764
	posterior tympanotomy	936	7661	911
Cadaveric	mastoidectomy	7	211	6
	posterior tympanotomy	29	248	28

Proposed Method: Figure 2 provides an overview of the four steps that comprise the proposed automatic trajectory segmentation method. As a first step, noise and irrelevant points (such as non-drilling points) are filtered out of the trajectory, since these points do not reflect the true spatio-temporal characteristics of drilling technique. For the purposes of this paper, points separated by a Euclidean distance of less than 0.25 mm from their neighbours were considered noise, as they are more likely to be generated by limitations in the position sensing apparatus rather than intentional human motion.

The second step is to derive the spatio-temporal features of each point. The features of point p_i are denoted as $\phi(p_i)$. These features are derived from the current point p_i and two other points p_{i-k} and p_{i+k}, which are k points before and after p_i. We choose k equal to 3 in our experiment. Spatio-temporal features

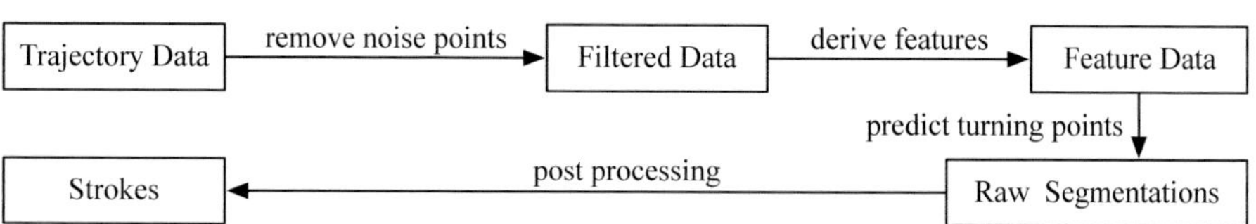

Fig. 2. Overview of trajectory segmentation steps

are expected to be fairly uniform during a stroke, but change significantly at its end points, when there is a change in direction. The features below were chosen for their ability to capture a variety of different strokes encountered in drilling, such as sharp turns and smooth, circular turns. We illustrate each feature using examples only in the X and Y axes for convenience, but all features were in fact derived using all three axes for our experiments.

- Speed [4]: the velocity (in x, y, z directions) and speed magnitude at point p_t. Turning points typically feature lower speeds than normal points.
- Direction: Figure 3a illustrates the angle $\alpha_x(t)$ between the line segment $\overline{p_{t-k}p_{t+k}}$ and the x-axis. Angle $\alpha_x(t)$ is smaller for turning points compared to normal points. The sine and cosine values of $\alpha_x(t)$ are derived as two features to capture the direction of p_t with respect to the x-axis. The sine and cosine values of $\alpha_y(t)$ and $\alpha_z(t)$ are also calculated with respect to the y-axis and z-axis respectively, using the same approach.
- Bow [6]: The bow of p_t is represented by the cosine of the angle $\beta(t)$ between the line segments $\overline{p_{t-k}p_t}$ and $\overline{p_tp_{t+k}}$, as shown in figure 3b. The cosine value of $\beta(t)$ is derived using vector inner product. The bow of a sharp turning point is usually larger than that of a normal point.
- Curvature: This value is defined as the ratio between the angle $\beta(t)$ and the sum of the lengths of its line segments: $\frac{\beta(t)}{|\overrightarrow{p_{t-k}p_t}|+|\overrightarrow{p_tp_{t+k}}|}$. This feature considers both the angle between the two line segments as well as their length to enable the capture of circular turning points, which usually have similar bow to normal points, but lower curvature.
- Vicinity aspect [9]: This feature captures the incremental change in position between points p_{t-k} and p_{t+k} over two axes, as shown in Figure 3c. Vicinity aspect is the ratio of the change in position across the x-axis and y-axis, defined as $VA(X,Y) = \frac{\Delta X(t)-\Delta Y(t)}{\Delta X(t)+\Delta Y(t)}$. $VA(X,Z)$ and $VA(Y,Z)$ are calculated using the same method. Vicinity aspect remains fairly constant for normal points, while it increases or decreases for turning points, depending on symmetry and turn direction.

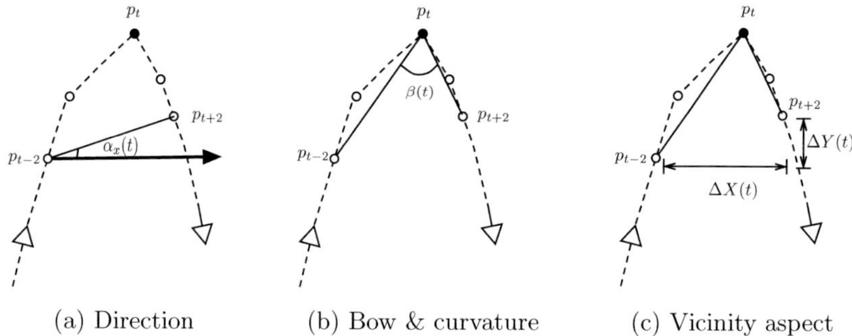

(a) Direction (b) Bow & curvature (c) Vicinity aspect

Fig. 3. Extracted features for a trajectory using $k = 2$

The third step of our approach uses the above features as input to derive a trajectory segmentation model. Most previous frameworks carry out this task using a variety of predefined thresholds for spatio-temporal criteria [2,6]. They pick a start time t_i and examine the subsequent data points until they find the longest sub-trajectory $\tau[t_i, t_j]$ that satisfies the predefined criteria. Then the end point of the stroke is regarded as the start point of the next stroke and the above process is repeated to the end of the trajectory. However, it is difficult to derive pre-defined criteria that will detect all types of strokes encountered during surgery. For example, in temporal bone surgery, surgeons tend to start with long fast strokes to efficiently remove bone that is far from sensitive anatomical structures, but switch to a more cautious technique as they approach structures such as the facial nerve. Predefined criteria are unlikely to be equally effective at detecting both types of stroke. Our approach treats trajectory segmentation as a supervised learning problem, whereby a functional mapping is derived from the value of the features $\phi(p_i)$ to two labels: a turning point and a normal point. This process is described in detail later in this section.

Once points are labelled, stroke start and end points are derived automatically from the labels. Since there are far more normal points than turning points in a typical trajectory, it is very unlikely that a set of consecutive points are all turning points. Hence, the fourth step of the process smooths stroke prediction by examining consecutive turning points, identifying the point with the maximum probability of being a turning point, and changing the other consecutive turning points to normal points. The proposed classification approach was compared to an existing method; both are described below.

Baseline: Previous work used bow to detect turning points based on the knowledge that the bow of points inside a stroke is typically different to that of turning points [10]. However, the threshold of bow that denotes a turning point is unpredictable, due to the great variety of stroke techniques encountered during bone drilling. This implementation assumed that bow follows normal distribution, so a threshold $ST = \mu + i \times \sigma$ for each trajectory is derived, where $i \in 1, 2$. The model computes the bow of a point p_i and compares it to ST. If the value is larger than ST, it is classified as a turning point, otherwise the point p_i is regarded as a normal point. If a list of consecutive turning points is encountered, the point with the minimum speed is chosen as the turning point.

Classification-Based Segmentation: Instead of using bow alone, supervised learning uses several features to perform turning point prediction. A point's label is not only dependent upon its own feature values, but those of its neighbouring points as well. Hence, we concatenate the features $\phi(p_i)$ of point p_i with those of the l nearest neighbour points. We formally define this operation as $concatenate(\phi(p_i), l) = [\phi(p_{i-l}), ..., \phi(p_i), ..., \phi(p_{i+l})]$. The length of concatenated features is $(2 \times l + 1) \times \#\phi(p_i)$, where $\#\phi(p_i)$ is the number of features for point p_i. l is usually a small number, since the concatenation operation increases feature size significantly. For the purposes of this work, we used $l = 3$ and $\#\phi(p_i) = 18$, which resulted in 126 features after concatenation.

The next task was to choose an appropriate classifier. Upon examination of the dataset (table 1), it was evident that the turning point class is a minor class (having a smaller number of instances than the other class), therefore the choice of classifier had to take into account the imbalance of the dataset. Since most tree-based classifiers are biased towards the major classes (which have a larger number of instances), we tried only Nearest Neighbour(NN), Linear Discriminant Analysis (LDA) and Naive Bayes(NB) classifiers. Preliminary results showed that LDA achieved acceptable turning point prediction accuracy, while other classifiers tended to ignore the turning point class. In addition, we experimented with kernel-based discriminant analysis (KDA) [3], which performed slightly better than LDA. However, parameter optimisation for KDA is far more time consuming than LDA. Therefore, we chose LDA as our classifier.

LDA estimates the prior probability of each class (i.e. $P(turning) = \frac{\#turning}{\#total}$) based on its frequency in the dataset. For an imbalanced dataset, this estimation skews the prediction towards the majority class. Since missing a turning point is a major error in trajectory segmentation, we treated this prior probability as a parameter and varied it to maximise the recall of turning point class prediction. However, high recall may be a result of more false positive predictions. Usually, a point is regarded as a turning point if the posterior probability of a point belonging to the turning class is larger than 50%. Since the prior probability affects the posterior probability, we treated the threshold of posterior probability as another parameter. These two parameters were tuned to achieve optimal balance between high recall and low false positive predictions, therefore providing the most accurate classification.

3 Experiment Results

Evaluation Measures: Precision and recall are often used as measures of classification performance on imbalanced data sets [5]. The precision and recall of turning points was computed as $Precision = \frac{TP}{TP+FP}$ and $Recall = \frac{TP}{TP+FN}$ where TP, FP, and FN represent the number of true positives, false positives, and false negatives respectively. However, these measures do not completely capture our goal of segmenting the trajectory such that the detected strokes are as similar to the ground truth as possible. Figure 4 illustrates the reason. Both cases have the same recall and precision, but figure 4a is obviously a better result.

To address this limitation, we define a new performance measure to capture the matching percentage between a ground truth stroke s_i and a classified stroke s_j as $match(s_i, s_j) = \frac{|\cap(s_i,s_j)|}{max(|s_i|,|s_j|)}$, where $|s_*|$ denotes the number of points in each stroke and $\cap$ denotes the overlapping part of the two strokes. For each classified stroke, we used the Kuhn-Munkres algorithm to find the best corresponding ground truth stroke, such that the average match rate for each surgical performance is maximized.

Segmentation Results: Table 2 shows the performance achieved by LDA models compared to the baseline. The match rate of the LDA approach was significantly better than the baseline for both surgical tasks. For simulation data, LDA

(a) Minor error: predicted turning point is 1 point away from ground truth

(b) Major error: predicted turning point is 4 points away from ground truth

Fig. 4. Example of two classifications representing a minor error and a major error. Filled black dots represent predicted turning points, white squares represent ground truth turning points and empty white dots represent normal points. Precision and recall are zero in both cases.

Table 2. Segmentation performance

		mastoidectomy			posterior tympanotomy		
dataset	**approach**	**precision**	**recall**	**match rate**	**precision**	**recall**	**match rate**
Simulator	Baseline	0.58	0.64	62.25%	0.17	0.13	57.24%
	LDA	0.66	0.62	79.44%	0.51	0.57	67.93%
Cadaveric	Baseline	0.5	0.42	20.7%	0.57	0.37	34.77%
	LDA	1	0.28	82.95%	0.33	0.34	51.35%

achieved an improvement of 17.2% for mastoidectomy and 10.7% for posterior tympanotomy. The improvement in match rate was greater in mastoidectomy than posterior tympanotomy, but LDA achieved dramatically better precision and recall in the latter, while these measures remained similar in mastoidectomy. For cadaveric data, LDA achieved an improvement of 62.25% for mastoidectomy and 16.58% for posterior tympanotomy in match rate. LDA also achieved dramatically better precision in mastoidectomy.

Since match rate is a better indicator of accuracy, we will focus on that measure. The higher match rate observed in mastoidectomy indicates that the longer strokes with sharper turning points were classified more precisely, which is to be expected. When the change in direction is small (as in the case of the circular strokes used during posterior tympanotomy), LDA models may produce false negatives. Posterior tympanotomy also includes more short, jittery movements, and it is not always clear whether these represent genuine surgical motion or noise. In this case, the LDA classifier may produce false positives. Many strokes in the posterior tympanotomy stage do not have clearly defined turning points, which makes even manual segmentation challenging and subjective. Therefore, the difference in match rate between the two stages may be a result of genuine ambiguity.

4 Discussion and Conclusion

We have presented an automated method for segmenting drilling-based surgical motion into its component drill strokes. This technique was validated on two temporal bone surgery tasks and shown to achieve acceptable accuracy despite encountering a great variety of surgical strokes. In the future, we may investigate the use of semi-supervised learning or Hidden Markov Models to further improve classification accuracy.

The ability to accurately segment a long surgical tool trajectory into smaller motions that are surgically meaningful is highly beneficial in facilitating the analysis of surgical technique in a variety of situations, ranging from simulation-based training to the operating theatre. The detailed characteristics of good surgical technique can be objectively quantified, and this understanding can be built into intelligent surgical training and guidance systems that guide surgeons towards optimal performance.

References

1. Bengio, Y., LeCun, Y., Nohl, C.R., Burges, C.J.C.: Lerec: a nn/hmm hybrid for on-line handwriting recognition. Neural Computation 7(6), 1289–1303 (1995)
2. Buchin, M., Driemel, A., van Kreveld, M., Sacristán, V.: An algorithmic framework for segmenting trajectories based on spatio-temporal criteria. In: Advances in Geographic Information Systems, pp. 202–211. ACM (2010)
3. Cai, D., He, X., Han, J.: Speed up kernel discriminant analysis. The VLDB Journal 20(1), 21–33 (2011)
4. Forestier, G., Lalys, F., Riffaud, L., Trelhu, B., Jannin, P.: Classification of surgical processes using dynamic time warping. J. Biomed. Inform. 45(2), 255–264 (2012)
5. Gu, Q., Zhu, L., Cai, Z.: Evaluation measures of the classification performance of imbalanced data sets. In: Cai, Z., Li, Z., Kang, Z., Liu, Y. (eds.) ISICA 2009. CCIS, vol. 51, pp. 461–471. Springer, Heidelberg (2009)
6. Hall, R., Rathod, H., Maiorca, M., Ioannou, I., Kazmierczak, E., O'Leary, S., Harris, P.: Towards haptic performance analysis using K-metrics. In: Pirhonen, A., Brewster, S. (eds.) HAID 2008. LNCS, vol. 5270, pp. 50–59. Springer, Heidelberg (2008)
7. Ioannou, I., Avery, A., Zhou, Y., Szudek, J., Kennedy, G., O'Leary, S.: The effect of fidelity: How expert behavior changes in a virtual reality environment. The Laryngoscope 124(9), 2144–2150 (2014)
8. Izadi, S., Haji, M., Suen, C.Y.: A new segmentation algorithm for online handwritten word recognition in persian script. In: Frontiers in Handwriting Recognition, pp. 598–603 (2008)
9. Sanna, M., Khrais, T.: Temporal Bone: A Manual for Dissection and Surgical Approaches. Thieme (2011)
10. Wijewickrema, S., Ioannou, I., Zhou, Y., Piromchai, P., Bailey, J., Kennedy, G., O'Leary, S.: A temporal bone surgery simulator with real-time feedback for surgical training. NextMed/MMVR21 196, 462 (2014)

Vision-Based Intraoperative Cone-Beam CT Stitching for Non-overlapping Volumes

Bernhard Fuerst[1,2], Javad Fotouhi[1], and Nassir Navab[1,2]

[1] Computer Aided Medical Procedures, Johns Hopkins University, Baltimore, MD
[2] Computer Aided Medical Procedures, Technische Universität München, Germany

Abstract. Cone-Beam Computed Tomography (CBCT) is one of the primary imaging modalities in radiation therapy, dentistry, and orthopedic interventions. While providing crucial intraoperative imaging, CBCT is bounded by its limited imaging volume, motivating the use of image stitching techniques. Current methods rely on overlapping volumes, leading to an excessive amount of radiation exposure, or on external tracking hardware, which may increase the setup complexity. We attach an optical camera to a CBCT enabled C-arm, and co-register the video and X-ray views. Our novel algorithm recovers the spatial alignment of non-overlapping CBCT volumes based on the observed optical views, as well as the laser projection provided by the X-ray system. First, we estimate the transformation between two volumes by automatic detection and matching of natural surface features during the patient motion. Then, we recover 3D information by reconstructing the projection of the positioning-laser onto an unknown curved surface, which enables the estimation of the unknown scale. We present a full evaluation of the methodology, by comparing vision- and registration-based stitching.

1 Introduction

Cone-Beam Computed Tomography (CBCT) enables intraoperative 3D imaging for various applications, for instance orthopedics [3], dentistry [13] or radiation therapy [4]. Consequently, CBCT is aimed at improving localization, structure identification, visualization, and patient positioning. However, the effectiveness of CBCT in orthopedic surgeries is bounded by its limited field of view, resulting in small volumes. Intraoperative surgical planning and verification could benefit of an extended field of view. Long bone fracture surgeries could be facilitated by 3D absolute measurements and multi-axis alignment in the presence of large volumes, assisting the surgeon's mental alignment.

The value of stitched fluoroscopy images for orthopedic surgery was investigated in [8]. Radio-opaque referencing markers attached to the tool were used to perform the stitching. Trajectory visualization and total length measurement were the most frequent features used by the surgeons in the stitched view. The outcome was overall promising for future development, and the usability was counted as good. Similarly, [5, 10] employed X-ray translucent references positioned under the bone for 2D X-ray mosaicing. In [15, 16], optical features

N. Navab et al. (Eds.): MICCAI 2015, Part I, LNCS 9349, pp. 387–395, 2015.
DOI: 10.1007/978-3-319-24553-9_48

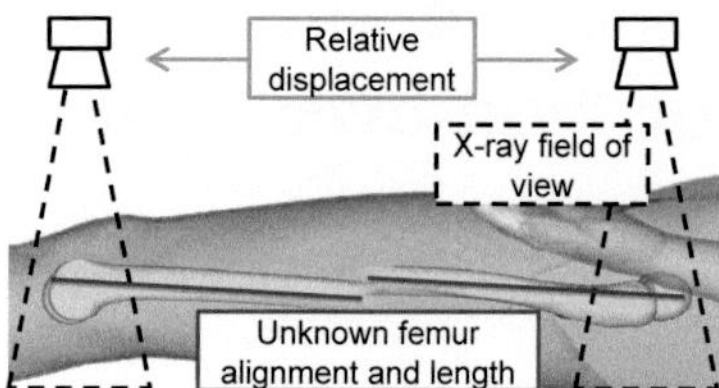

Fig. 1. The 3D misalignment of bones (red lines) may be difficult to quantify using 2D images. CBCT contributes as a valuable tool for interventions in which the 3D alignment is of importance, for instance in acute fracture treatment or joint replacement. Background image courtesy of BodyParts3D, Center for Life Science, Japan.

acquired from an adjacent camera were used to recover the transformation. The aforementioned methods all benefit from external features for 2D mosaicing, thus do not require large overlaps. However, it remains a challenge to generalize these approaches to perform 3D volume stitching, as illustrated in Fig. 1.

A validation study on using 3D rotational X-ray over conventional 2D X-rays was conducted for intra-articular fractures of the foot, wrist, elbow, and shoulder [3]. The outcome reported a reduction of indications for revision surgery. A panoramic CBCT is proposed in [4] by stitching overlapping X-rays acquired from all the views around the interest organ. Reconstruction quality is ensured by introducing a sufficient amount of overlapping regions, which in return increases the X-ray dose. Moreover, the reconstructed volume is vulnerable to artifacts introduced by image stitching. An automatic 3D image stitching technique is proposed in [6]. Under the assumption that the orientational misalignment is negligible, and sub-volumes are only translated, the stitching is performed using phase correlation as a global similarity measure, and normalized cross correlation as the local cost. Sufficient overlaps are required to support this method. To reduce the X-ray exposure, [7, 9] incorporate prior knowledge from statistical shape models to perform a 3D reconstruction.

Previous approaches are either limited to the overlap size or the existing prior shape models. Providing large overlaps will significantly increase the exposure. On the other hand, the bone fractures cause large deformation, hence preoperative and postoperative structures of the region of interest are significantly different, and one cannot benefit from prior scans for alignment. Lastly, incorporating external trackers leads to an increase in surgical complexity and line of sight problem. In this work, we propose a novel stitching approach, using a co-registered X-ray source with an optical camera attached to the C-arm [11,12], and a patient positioning-laser to recover the depth scale. Therefore, the system is mobile, self-contained and independent of the OR, and the workflow remains intact. It could be deployed after a single factory calibration. The alignment transformation of volumes is computed based on the video frames, and prior models are not required. We target cases with large gaps between the volumes and focus our approach on spatial alignment of separated regions of interest.

Image quality will remain intact, and the radiation dose will be linearly proportional to the size of the individual non-overlapping sub-volumes of interest.

2 Materials and Methods

2.1 System Setup and Calibration

The CBCT-enabled motorized C-arm is positioned relative to the patient by utilizing the positioning-lasers, which are built into the image intensifier and C-arm base. To enable the stitching of multiple sub-volumes, the transformation of the patient relative to the C-arm center must be recovered. In contrast to existing techniques we do not require additional hardware setup around the C-arm, but we attach a camera to the C-arm in such manner that it does not obstruct the surgeons access to the patient. By using one mirror, the camera and the X-ray source centers are optically identical. The system setup is outlined in Fig. 2.

Our system is composed of a mobile C-arm, ARCADIS Orbic 3D, from Siemens Medical Solutions and an optical video camera, Manta G-125C, from Allied Vision Technologies. The C-arm and the camera are both connected via ethernet to the computer with custom software to store the CBCT volumes and video. The X-ray and optical images are calibrated in an offline phase [11,12].

The positioning-laser in the base of the C-arm spans a plane, which intersects with the unknown patient surface, and can be observed as a curve in the camera image. To determine the exact position of the laser relative to the camera, we perform a camera-to-plane calibration. Multiple checkerboard poses (n) are recorded for which the projection of the positioning-laser intersects with the

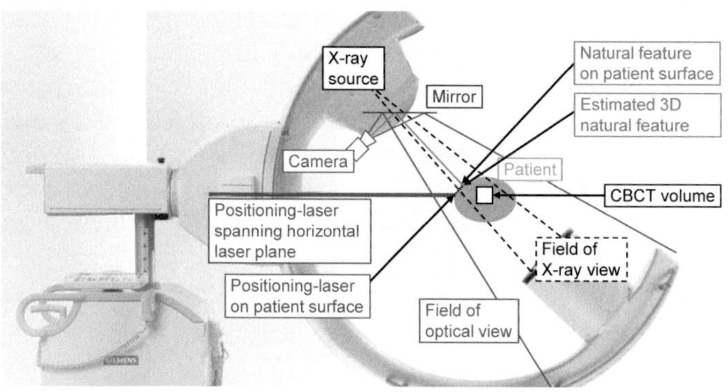

Fig. 2. A mobile C-arm, the positioning-laser (red), and an optical camera (blue) are illustrated. The mirror (purple) aligns the optical camera and X-ray source centers. The patient motion relative to the C-arm is estimated by observing both the positioning-laser and natural features (green) on the patient's surface. The 3D positions of the features are estimated using the depth of the nearest positioning-laser on the patient (black dotted line intersecting green line), of which the depth is based on calibration.

origin of the checkerboard. Once the camera intrinsics are estimated, the camera-centric 3D checkerboard poses are computed. Under the assumption that the 3D homogeneous checkerboard origins, $\mathbf{x}^{(3)} = \{\mathrm{x}_i \,|\, \mathrm{x}_i = [x, y, z, 1]^\top\}_{i=0}^{n}$ (see footnote [1] for notation), lay on the laser plane, the plane coefficients $A = [a, b, c, d]$ are determined by performing RANdom SAmple Consensus (RANSAC) based plane fitting to the observed checkerboard origins, which attempts to satisfy:

$$\arg\min_{A} \sum_{x_j \in \Omega} |Ax_j|, \tag{1}$$

where Ω is subset of checkerboard origins, which are inliers to the plane fitting.

2.2 CBCT Volume and Video Acquisition

To acquire a CBCT volume, the patient is positioned under guidance of the lasers. Then, the motorized C-arm orbits 190° around the center visualized by the laser lines, and automatically acquires a total of 100 2D X-ray images. The reconstruction is performed using the Feldkamp method, which utilizes filtered back-projection, resulting in a cubic volume with a 256 voxels along each axis and an isometric resolution of 0.5 mm. During the re-arrangement of C-arm and patient for the next CBCT acquisition, the positioning-laser is projected at the patient, and each video frame is recorded. For simplicity, we will assume that in the following the C-arm is static, while the patient is moving. However, as only the relative movement of patient to C-arm is recorded, there are no limitations on allowed motions.

2.3 Two-Dimensional Feature Detection and Matching

The transformation describing the relative patient motion observed between two video frames is estimated by detecting and matching a set of natural surface features and the recovery of their scale. For each frame, we automatically detect Speeded Up Robust Features (SURF) as described in [2], which are well suited to track natural shapes and blob-like structures. To match the features in frame k to the features in frame $k + 1$, we find the nearest neighbor by exhaustively comparing the features, and removing weak or ambiguous matches. Outliers are removed by estimating the Fundamental Matrix, $\mathbf{F}_k$, using a least trimmed squares formulation and rejecting up to 50% of the features, resulting in a set of n_k features $\mathbf{f}_k^{(2)} = \{\mathrm{f}_{k,j} \,|\, \mathrm{f}_{k,j} = [x, y, 1]^\top\}_{j=1}^{n_k}$ in frame k (see Fig. 3). To estimate the 3D transformation, the 3D coordinates of this set of features need to be estimated.

2.4 Recovering Three-Dimensional Coordinates

In each frame k, the laser is automatically detected. First the color channel corresponding to the laser's color is thresholded and noise is removed by analyzing connected components. To find the m_k 2D points, $\mathbf{p}_k^{(2)} = \{\mathrm{p}_{k,i} \,|\, \mathrm{p}_{k,i} = [x, y, 1]^\top\}_{i=1}^{m_k}$,

[1] Superscripts $^{(2)}$ and $^{(3)}$ denote 2D and 3D points; $^{(s)}$ denotes points up to a scale.

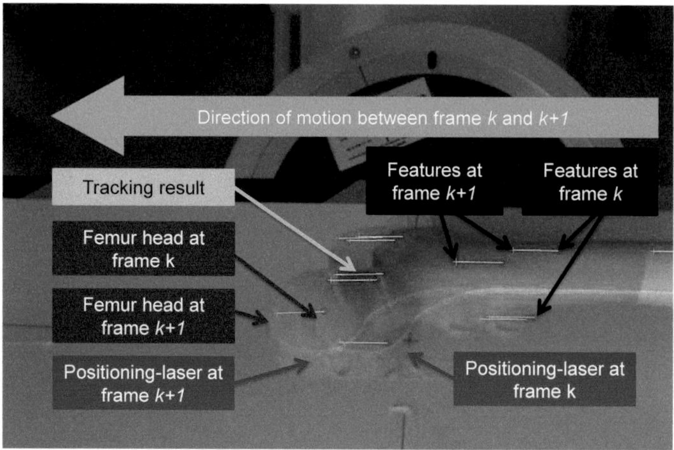

Fig. 3. The figure shows the overlay of two frames to illustrate the feature correspondences to estimate the movement of the patient. From both frames, the positioning-laser (red) and natural surface features are extracted. The tracking results of the matched features in frame k (+) and frame $k+1$ (○) are illustrated as yellow lines.

which are most likely on the plane, the resulting binary image is thinned [17]. Each 2D laser point $\mathrm{p}_{k,i}^{(2)}$ is projected back to a point up to a scale $\mathrm{p}_{k,i}^{(s)} = [x_{k,i}^{(s)}, y_{k,i}^{(s)}, 1, 1]^\top$ using the Moore-Penrose pseudo-inverse of the camera projection matrix, $\mathbf{P}$:

$$\mathrm{p}_{k,i}^{(3)} = s_{k,i}\mathrm{p}_{k,i}^{(s)} = s_{k,i}\mathbf{P}^{+}\mathrm{p}_{k,i}^{(2)}, \tag{2}$$

where the scale $s_{k,i}$ is recovered by intersecting the point up to a scale $\mathrm{p}_{k,i}^{(s)}$ with the plane:

$$s_{k,i} = \frac{-d}{ax_{k,i}^{(s)} + by_{k,i}^{(s)} + c}. \tag{3}$$

Once the 3D laser points are recovered, the scale for each feature, $\mathrm{f}_{k,j}^{(s)} = s_{k,j}\mathbf{P}^{+}\mathrm{f}_{k,j}^{(2)}$, can be estimated by interpolating the scales of the closest points $\mathrm{p}_{k,i}^{(3)}$.

2.5 Estimating 3D Transformation and CBCT Volume Stitching

After the estimation of the 3D coordinates of the matched features, the transformation for the frames k and $k+1$ is computed by solving the least squares fitting for two sets of 3D points [1], obtaining the transformation matrix T_k. Note that, only features in a small neighborhood of the laser line, < 1 cm, are used. Hence, features on other body parts, e.g. the opposite leg, are discarded. To verify the estimated transformation, the Iterative Closest Point (ICP) algorithm is used to perform a redundancy test using the laser points. In other words, ICP is applied after transforming the laser points $\mathrm{p}_i^{(3)}$ from frame k to the next $k+1$ only for verification. Consequently, for long bones, translation along the laser line is not

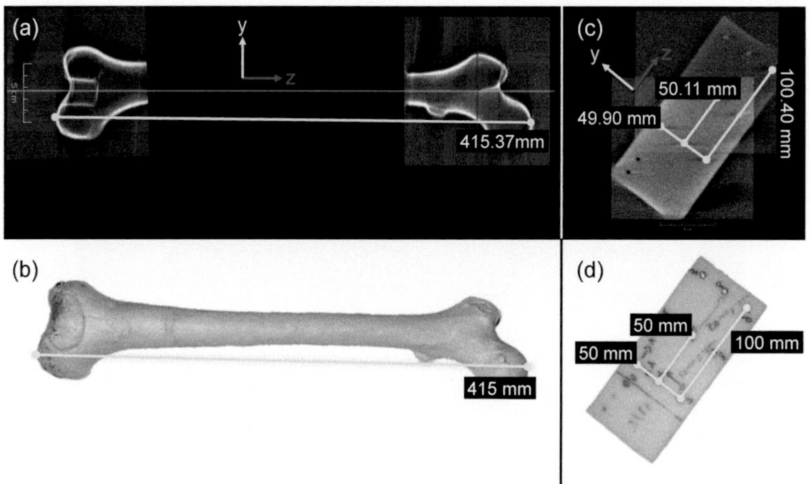

Fig. 4. Absolute distance of the aligned sub-volumes in (a) is measured (415.37 mm), and compared to the real world measurements (415 mm) of the femur phantom in (b). Similarly, a fiducial phantom was scanned and the vision-based stitching (c) compared to the real world object (d). For visualization purposes and volumetric appearance in (a) and (c), multiple parallel slices are averaged.

lost. This results in a transformation $\hat{\mathrm{T}}_k$. If $\hat{\mathrm{T}}_k$ is not nearly identity, the frame $k+1$ is rejected and the frames k and $k+2$ are used to compute $\hat{\mathrm{T}}_k$. To obtain the overall transformation $\mathrm{T}_{\mathrm{CBCT}}$, all transformations $\mathrm{T}_k \in \Gamma$ are accumulated, where Γ is the domain of all valid transformations:

$$\mathrm{T}_{\mathrm{CBCT}} = {}^{\mathrm{CBCT}}\,\mathrm{T}_{\mathrm{camera}} \prod_{\mathrm{T}_k \in \Gamma} \mathrm{T}_k, \tag{4}$$

where ${}^{\mathrm{CBCT}}\mathrm{T}_{\mathrm{camera}}$ is the transformation from camera coordinate system to the CBCT coordinate system obtained during calibration.

3 Experiments and Results

The novel laser-guided stitching method is evaluated in two different, but realistic scenarios. For each phantom, we performed vision-based stitching and evaluated the quality by measuring 3D distances in the stitched volumes and real object. In addition, the stitching quality was compared to intensity-based mosaicing using overlapping CBCT volumes, indicating the accuracy of the overall 3D transformation $\mathrm{T}_{\mathrm{CBCT}}$.

The result of vision-based stitching is illustrated in Fig. 4 (a) on the long bone phantom in the absence of overlaps, and in Fig. 4 (c) on the fiducial phantom with overlaps. The absolute distances are compared to real world measurements which are illustrated in Fig. 4 (b) and (d). Detailed results are reported in table 1, which shows the differences of measurements of the vision-based stitched CBCT volumes and real objects. The errors are apportioned according to the coordinate frames illustrated in Fig. 4, while the *norm* reflects the overall error. In addition, the *absolute distance error* reports the percentage of error with respect to the absolute distances measured. Average errors are in the range of 0.65 ± 0.28 mm and 0.15 ± 0.11 mm for long bone and fiducial phantom stitching, respectively. Lastly, for overlapping volumes, we have compared the vision- and intensity-based stitching by performing rigid registration using normalized cross correlation as similarity measure. The intensity-based stitching deviated from the vision-based stitching by 0.23 mm, indicating an overall good alignment.

Table 1. Errors are computed by comparing the vision-based stitched CBCT to the real objects. The final row presents the difference to the intensity-based stitching.

Error	X	Y	Z	Norm
Long Bone (Femur) Phantom				
Alignment error (mm)	0.75	0.83	0.37	1.18
Absolute distance error (%)	1.30	1.11	0.10	n/a
Fiducial Phantom				
Alignment error (mm)	0.08	0.10	0.26	0.29
Absolute distance error (%)	0.52	2.00	2.60	n/a
Vision- vs. intensity-based (mm)	0.11	0.08	0.18	0.23

4 Discussion and Conclusion

The proposed technique is an overlap-independent, low dose, and accurate stitching method for CBCT sub-volumes with minimal increase of workflow complexity. We attached an optical camera to a mobile C-arm, and used the positioning-laser to recover the 3D depth scales, and consequently aligned the sub-volumes. As a result of this method, the stitching is performed with low dose radiation, linearly proportional to the size of non-overlapping sub-volumes. We expect this to be applicable to intraoperative planning and validation for long bone fracture or joint replacement interventions, where multi-axis alignment and absolute distances are difficult to visualize and measure from the 2D X-ray views.

Our approach does not limit the working space, nor does it require any additional hardware besides a simple camera. The C-arm remains mobile and independent of the OR. One requirement is that the C-arm does not move during the CBCT acquisition, but we believe that the use of external markers could solve this problem and may yield a higher accuracy. However, in our scenario we intentionally did not rely on markers, as they would increase complexity and alter the surgical workflow. Our approach uses frame-to-frame tracking, which can cause drift. In fact, the ICP verification helps us to detect such drifts as it is based on points which were not used for motion estimation. Therefore, if the estimated motion from ICP increases over time, we can detect the drift and use

ICP to correct if necessary. Alternatively, the transformations could be refined using bundle adjustments [14]. Further studies on the effectiveness during interventions are underway. Also, the reconstruction of the patient surface during the CBCT acquisition may assist during the tracking of the patient motion.

References

1. Arun, K.S., Huang, T.S., Blostein, S.D.: Least-squares fitting of two 3-D point sets. IEEE Transactions on PAMI (5), 698–700 (1987)
2. Bay, H., Tuytelaars, T., Van Gool, L.: SURF: Speeded Up Robust Features. In: Leonardis, A., Bischof, H., Pinz, A. (eds.) ECCV 2006, Part I. LNCS, vol. 3951, pp. 404–417. Springer, Heidelberg (2006)
3. Carelsen, B., Haverlag, R., Ubbink, D., Luitse, J., Goslings, J.: Does intraoperative fluoroscopic 3D imaging provide extra information for fracture surgery? Archives of Orthopaedic and Trauma Surgery 128(12), 1419–1424 (2008)
4. Chang, J., Zhou, L., Wang, S., Clifford Chao, K.S.: Panoramic cone beam computed tomography. Medical Physics 39(5) (2012)
5. Chen, C., Kojcev, R., Haschtmann, D., Fekete, T., Nolte, L., Zheng, G.: Ruler Based Automatic C-Arm Image Stitching Without Overlapping Constraint. Journal of Digital Imaging, 1–7 (2015)
6. Emmenlauer, M., Ronneberger, O., Ponti, A., Schwarb, P., Griffa, A., Filippi, A., Nitschke, R., Driever, W., Burkhardt, H.: XuvTools: free, fast and reliable stitching of large 3D datasets. Journal of Microscopy 233(1), 42–60 (2009)
7. Fleute, M., Lavallée, S.: Nonrigid 3-D/2-D registration of images using statistical models. In: Taylor, C., Colchester, A. (eds.) MICCAI 1999. LNCS, vol. 1679, pp. 138–147. Springer, Heidelberg (1999)
8. Kraus, M.: von dem Berge, S., Schoell, H., Krischak, G., Gebhard, F.: Integration of fluoroscopy-based guidance in orthopaedic trauma surgery - a prospective cohort study. Injury 44(11), 1486–1492 (2013)
9. Lamecker, H., Wenckebach, T., Hege, H.C.: Atlas-based 3D-Shape Reconstruction from X-Ray Images. In: 18th International Conference on Pattern Recognition, ICPR 2006, vol. 1, pp. 371–374 (2006)
10. Messmer, P., Matthews, F., Wullschleger, C., Hgli, R., Regazzoni, P., Jacob, A.: Image Fusion for Intraoperative Control of Axis in Long Bone Fracture Treatment. European Journal of Trauma 32(6), 555–561 (2006)
11. Navab, N., Heining, S.M., Traub, J.: Camera Augmented Mobile C-Arm (CAMC): Calibration, Accuracy Study, and Clinical Applications. IEEE Transactions on Medical Imaging 29(7), 1412–1423 (2010)
12. Nicolau, S., Lee, P., Wu, H., Huang, M., Lukang, R., Soler, L., Marescaux, J.: Fusion of C-arm X-ray image on video view to reduce radiation exposure and improve orthopedic surgery planning: first in-vivo evaluation. Proceedings of Computer Assisted Radiology and Surgery 6, 115–116 (2011)
13. Pauwels, R., Araki, K., Siewerdsen, J., Thongvigitmanee, S.S.: Technical aspects of dental CBCT: state of the art. Dentomaxillofacial Radiology 44(1) (2014)
14. Triggs, B., McLauchlan, P.F., Hartley, R.I., Fitzgibbon, A.W.: Bundle adjustment – a modern synthesis. In: Triggs, B., Zisserman, A., Szeliski, R. (eds.) ICCV-WS 1999. LNCS, vol. 1883, pp. 298–372. Springer, Heidelberg (2000)

15. Wang, L., Traub, J., Heining, S.M., Benhimane, S., Euler, E., Graumann, R., Navab, N.: Long bone X-Ray image stitching using camera augmented mobile C-arm. In: Metaxas, D., Axel, L., Fichtinger, G., Székely, G. (eds.) MICCAI 2008, Part II. LNCS, vol. 5242, pp. 578–586. Springer, Heidelberg (2008)
16. Wang, L., Traub, J., Weidert, S., Heining, S.M., Euler, E., Navab, N.: Parallax-free intra-operative X-ray image stitching. Medical Image Analysis 14(5)
17. Zhang, T., Suen, C.Y.: A fast parallel algorithm for thinning digital patterns. Communications of the ACM 27(3), 236–239 (1984)

Visibility Map: A New Method in Evaluation Quality of Optical Colonoscopy

Mohammad Ali Armin[1,2], Hans De Visser[2], Girija Chetty[1], Cedric Dumas[2], David Conlan[2], Florian Grimpen[3], and Olivier Salvado[2]

[1] Department of Computer Science, University of Canberra, Australia
m.a.armin@gmail.com
[2] CSIRO Digital Productivity Flagship, Australia
Olivier.Salvado@csiro.au
[3] Department of Gastroenterology and Hepatology, Royal Brisbane and Women's Hospital

Abstract. Optical colonoscopy is performed by insertion of a long flexible endoscope into the colon. Inspecting the whole colonic surface for abnormalities has been a main concern in estimating quality of a colonoscopy procedure. In this paper we aim to estimate areas that have not been inspected thoroughly as a quality metric by generating a visibility map of the colon surface. The colon was modeled as a cylinder. By estimating the camera motion parameters between each consecutive frame, circumferential bands from the cylinder of the colon surface were extracted. Registering these extracted band images from adjacent video frames provide a visibility map, which could reveal uncovered areas by clinicians from colonoscopy videos. The method was validated using a set of realistic videos generated using a colonoscopy simulator for which the ground truth was known, and by analyzing results from processing actual colonoscopy videos by a clinical expert. Our method was able to identify 100% of uncovered areas on simulated data and achieved with sensitivity of 96% and precision of 74% on real videos. The results suggest that visibility map can increase clinicians' awareness of uncovered areas, and would reduce the chance of missed polyps.

Keywords: Optical colonoscopy, Visibility map, Colonoscopy Quality, Uncovered area, Camera motion parameters.

1 Introduction

Colorectal or Bowel cancer is the second cause of cancer related death after lung cancer, in Australia and the Western world [1]. Early diagnosis of bowel cancer can increase the chance of survival for patients by up to 90%. Colonoscopy is the gold standard method for detection and removal of colonic polyps. The efficiency of a colonoscopy procedure is influenced by many factors, including the amount of the colon surface that is inspected for the presence of polyps by the clinician. Studies have reported that even experienced gastroenterologists can still miss up to 33% of polyps [2, 3]. This is in part due to polyps, in particular flat lesions such as sessile serrated adenomas, not being recognized even though they are in view, but also due to polyps not being viewed because they were never inspected by the camera.

N. Navab et al. (Eds.): MICCAI 2015, Part I, LNCS 9349, pp. 396–404, 2015.
DOI: 10.1007/978-3-319-24553-9_49

One way to address this problem is to increase clinicians' skills through training; another way is to provide assistance to clinicians during the intervention by developing assistive technologies. There are several techniques which can measure the quality of a colonoscopy inspection by metrics such as withdrawal time [4], number of informative frames [5], and uncovered areas [6]. Hoang et al. proposed a method to identify colon folds to reconstruct individual 3D colon segments for every frame and determine their visible areas, without providing a combined feedback [6]. We aim to develop a technology that estimates uncovered areas by generating a visibility map of the flattened colon surface. To do this, we modeled the colon as a cylinder, and we hypothesized that circumferential bands of the colon surface could be extracted by projecting a 3D cylinder onto each frame. To know where on a frame to project the 3D cylinder, camera motion parameters between successive frames were estimated through epipolar geometry analysis [7], which has demonstrated high accuracy in endoscope camera pose estimation [8, 9]. Others have used a combination of different techniques to increase the robustness of camera motion estimation [10] but at the cost of extra computation time. Finally, each extracted band was registered to the one from the previous frame, and rastered to build a visibility map of the colon internal surface. A diagram of our method is shown in Fig. 1 and described in the next section.

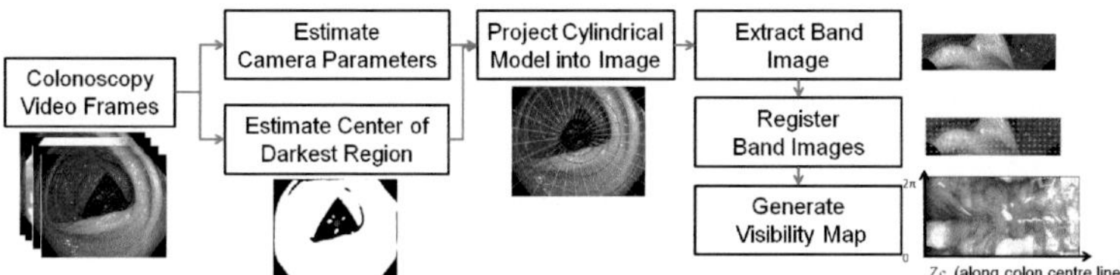

Fig. 1. Main processing steps of our proposed method

2 Method

2.1 Camera Motion Estimation

In this section, first we briefly describe the mathematical model for a colonoscope camera, then explain in detail the epipolar geometry based algorithm [7] to obtain the camera location and orientation relative to the colon lumen.

Colonoscope Camera Model. The camera of the colonoscope used in our setup had a fisheye lens (190HD Olympus endoscope), introducing image deformation. We used a mathematical model proposed by Scaramuzza et al. [11] to model fisheye lens camera projection. Using this model a 3D point (X,Y,Z) can be projected into image point (u,v) through the following equation:

$$\lambda \begin{bmatrix} u \\ v \\ a_0 + a_1\rho + \cdots + a_{n-1}\rho^{n-1} \end{bmatrix} = R.\begin{bmatrix} X \\ Y \\ Z \end{bmatrix} + T \tag{1}$$

where λ is scaling factor, $\rho = \sqrt{(u-u_0)^2 + (v-v_0)^2}$ indicates distance from image center (u_0, v_0) and $a_0, a_1, \ldots, a_n$ are intrinsic parameters used to correct the deformation in the colonoscopy images. R and T represent extrinsic camera parameters (rotation and translation).

Since the colonoscopy camera motion is parallax in most of the scene (each consecutive frame pair can be assumed as a stereo pair), an epipolar geometry based algorithm was employed to estimate the camera motion as follows:

Camera Calibration and Distortion Correction. An offline calibration specific to each colonoscope was performed using a fisheye model described in [11] to obtain the intrinsic camera parameters and correct image deformation. To reduce the computing time, only features' positions on the image were corrected for distortion.

Feature Detection and Uninformative Frame Removal. A set of feature points was automatically extracted and matched between each pair of consecutive frames using the Kanade-Lucas-Tomasi (KLT) algorithm [12]. Features consisted mostly of blood vessel patterns and soft tissue structures. Frames with no features (e.g. blurry frames) were excluded from further computation and assumed to be uninformative.

The RANdom Sample Consensus (RANSAC) [13] and deviation of distances between the corresponding points were employed to remove unreliable matches (outliers) and increase robustness of the motion estimation algorithm.

Extrinsic Camera Parameters Estimation. A combination of five and eight point algorithms explained in [7, 14] were used to calculate extrinsic camera parameters.

The 3D positions of tracked features were calculated using triangulation and extrinsic camera parameters. The distance between the coordinate of 3D points projected into the image plane and the feature points defined a reprojection error obtained by

$$E = \sum_{i=1}^{M} \sum_{l=1}^{N} \left|\left| p_{il} - \acute{p}_i \right|\right|^2 \quad (2)$$

where N is the number of features on M images and $\acute{p}_i$ is the projection of a 3D point P_i estimated through triangulation and camera parameters to the image plane, and p_{il} is the correspondence tracked feature on the image.

First we estimated the reprojection error of camera parameters computed by five and eight point algorithms, then the camera parameters with a lower reprojection error were optimized using a Levenberg-Marquardt technique [15] by minimizing the cost function defined in Eqn. (2). The optimized extrinsic camera parameters (camera pose) inferred from consecutive frames was then concatenated to estimate camera position [16].

Kalman Filtering. To predict the camera pose in presence of uninformative frames, it is assumed that acceleration was constant, and the standard Kalman filter (Eqn. (3)) was used to predict each camera pose x_k from previous optimized camera pose x_{k-1}

$$x_k = Ax_{k-1} + Gw_{k-1}, \qquad z_{k-1} = Hx_{k-1} + \mathrm{v}_{k-1} \quad (3)$$

with A the state matrix similar to [17], z_{k-1} the observation at time k, $G = (I_6\, I_6\, I_6)$ and $H = (I_6\, 0_6\, 0_6)$ the driving and measurement matrices, where 0_6 and I_6 are

6×6 zero and identity matrices. w_{k-1} and v_{k-1} are process and Gaussian noise (1e-4 and 0.06 determined experimentally for best qualitative results).

2.2 Generating Visibility Map

In this section we describe how circumferential bands of the colon surface (band image) were extracted from a video frame (area between green and red circle in Fig. 2) and merged to build a visibility map of a colon segment.

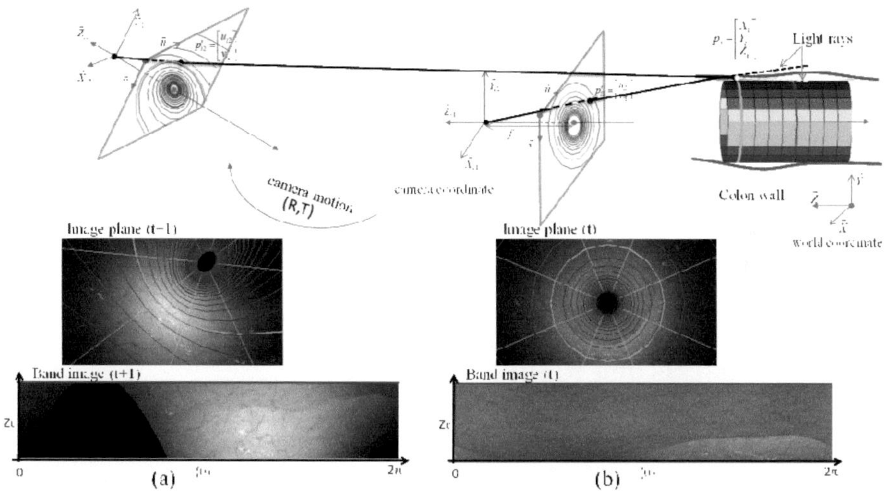

Fig. 2. Projection of cylinder into video frames and extracted band images (area between green and red perimeters), when camera moving backward from time (t) to (t+1); camera looking toward center of colon (b), the camera location and orientation change (a).

Cylindrical Model. We assumed that a colon can be modeled as a cylinder. Fig. 2 represents the cylindrical model; this cylinder was made of concentric 3D circles. Every point $P_i = (X_i, Y_i, Z_i)$ on a 3D circle was calculated by:

$$X_i = r.cos(\theta_i), \quad Y_i = r.sin(\theta_i), \quad Z_i = Z_{ci} + \Delta Z \tag{4}$$

where r is the radius of cylinder. We assumed an average colon diameter of 4cm (anatomical average), and we found that values from 3cm to 5cm did not change substantially the results. Z_{ci} is distance of cylinder from camera, ΔZ is the distance between each two circle on the cylinder, θ_i is the radian in a 3D circle. θ_i ranged from 0 to 2π with a step size $\Delta\theta$ related to the number of points (NP) on a 3D circle calculated by ($2\pi/NP$).

Cylindrical Model Projection and Band Image Extraction. From the camera parameters (intrinsic and pose), the 3D cylinder was projected into the image plane, using the camera model defined by Equation 1.

The orientation of the camera was updated by forcing its line of sight to go through the center of dark region (deepest area) of each frame, which was computed as barycenter of the darkest class of a two class segmentation using Otsu thresholding similar to [18].

The cylinder model had two perimeters, defined between Z_{ci}+1 cm and Z_{ci}+3 cm, from the camera defining a band on the cylinder circumference. We chose those values based on testing using the simulator and feedback from clinicians as to where the image quality is best and the lighting optimal. These perimeters defined a circumferential band that was moved at each frame depending on the camera pose. For example, when the camera was facing the wall, the perimeters could be seen on each side of the camera field of view. The image segment defined by that band was unwrapped and formed a rectangular patch (band image). The part of the band image outside the field of view was rastered in black.

Visibility Map Generation. Each extracted band image was assumed to overlap with the one from the previous frame, and two consecutive band images were registered by Local Weight Mean (LWM) registration algorithm [19] and merged on a plan corresponding to the internal colon surface that we call the visibility map. Fig. 4 shows an example of a visibility map.

3 Experiments and Results

3.1 Simulated Video

First we validated our algorithm on videos generated by a colonoscopy simulator. The simulator consists of a computer simulation of the colon model and a haptic device that allows insertion of an instrumented colonoscope to drive the simulation [20]. The colon model designed for this simulator has a parametric mathematical model of the colon allowing the generation of realistic human colon geometry. The simulator could also generate the ground truth camera poses and uncovered areas that were used for validation. We validated our method on ten different realistic videos from different parts of the colon generated by the simulator (each video on average covered 20cm of a colon length). Errors of the extrinsic camera parameters (orientation and translation) were computed between the ones estimated from the videos and those used by the simulator. Errors were averaged over each of the ten videos resulting in 10 errors for each parameter shown as boxplot in Fig. 3.

Translation errors between consecutive frames were less than 2 mm and rotation errors were less than 0.6 degrees. This corresponded to scenario without lens or colon obstructions, and in simulated videos using constant acceleration. It is expected that in real conditions, those errors might be higher.

3.2 Extracted Visibility Map from Simulated Videos

One example of implementation of our method is shown in Fig. 4, where dark spots represent uncovered areas. During any given actual colonoscopy the physician continuously moves the colonoscope back and forth, naturally resulting in bands overlapping each other with different views (e.g. some might be darker/brighter due to lighting differences). Fig. 5 shows a case when the camera was moving forward and facing one side of the colon, and then moving backward while facing another side of the colon. The final composite image correctly filled in the internal surface, which Zc is the traveled distance along colon center line.

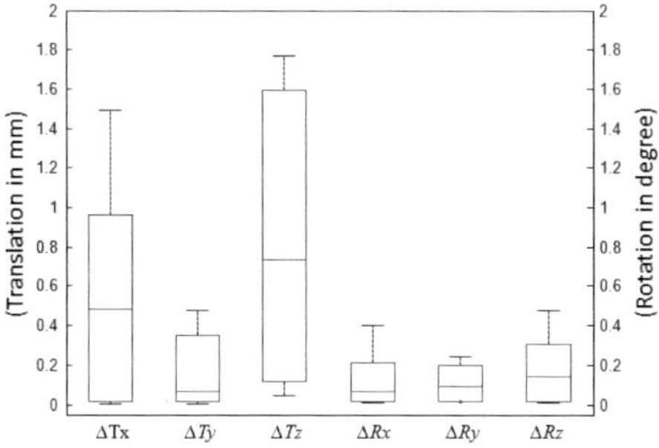

Fig. 3. The root mean square (RMS) error of camera motion parameters estimated on realistic videos generated by the simulator.

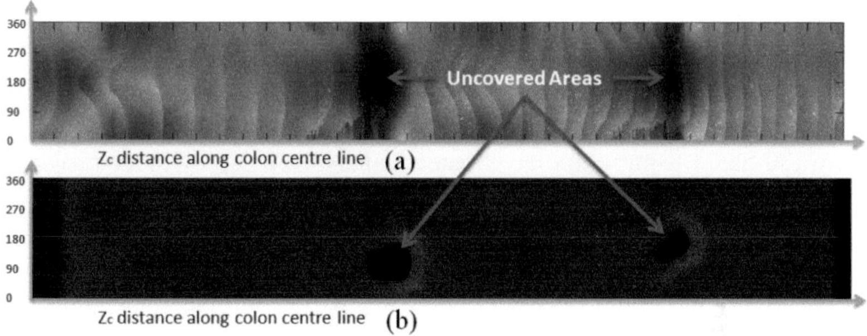

Fig. 4. Visibility map from a simulated colonoscopy video by our method (a), and its ground truth generated by the simulator (b), the black areas indicate uncovered areas.

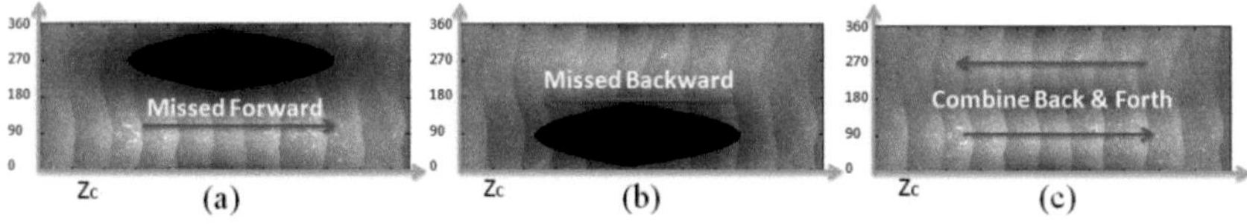

Fig. 5. Visibility map generated from a segment of the simulated colon: Parts of the colon are missed in forward motion (a), and backward motion in same place (b). Combination of two maps by max of pixel value shows the final coverage area (c).

3.3 Application to Actual Colonoscopy Video

We implemented our algorithm on nine segments of around 20 cm were inspected from five different videos of a 190HD Olympus endoscope, with 50 frame/sec and each frame sized 1856×1044 pixels. Two experiments were conducted. First, the expert noted the uncovered areas from the video extracts. Second, the expert noted again the uncovered areas while seeing the visibility maps when the videos were shown. In the first case he identified nineteen uncovered areas, whereas in the second experi ment he noted twenty-four uncovered areas. The latter was used as the ground truth to validate our automated method by computing sensitivity and precision [21]. The sensitivity was 96% and precision was 74%. Fig. 6 represents the visibility map of a segment of a colon. Mean typical processing time was 1.5 min per frame using a standard PC, Matlab, and non-optimized scripts.

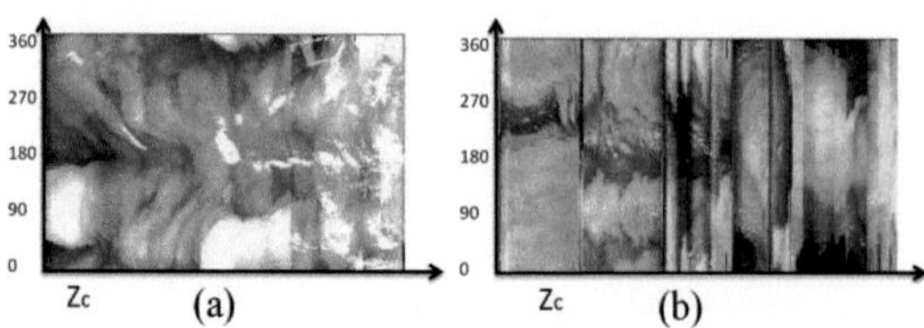

Fig. 6. Visibility map generated from a segment of a real colon, which is fully covered (a), and a map from another part of colon with some dark spot as uncovered areas (b).

4 Discussion and Conclusion

In this paper, we present a new method to estimate uncovered areas during optical colonoscopy. To achieve this, we modeled the colon as a cylinder, the camera parameters were estimated using epipolar geometry analysis, a 3D cylinder projected into colonoscopy image. The band image that could be extracted was then rastered on a visibility map showing the internal colon wall.

Estimating camera parameters from a colonoscopy video is challenging because of the non-rigidity of the colon anatomy, the presence of uninformative frames (e.g. a dirty lens), and low feature content of some tissue. Those issues were addressed in our technique by use of epipolar geometry to estimate camera pose, and a Kalman filter to estimate the camera parameters in the presence of uninformative frames.

On the visibility map of the colon surface, uncovered areas, or areas with lack of focus (removed uninformative frames) showed up as black areas. However, errors in the camera parameters translated into error of the position of the band images on the visibility map. This was reduced by registering successive band images, but could be improved by correcting the camera parameters with the registration results, thereby reducing drift in estimating the camera position, for example. This will be part of our future work, which will also include the identification and characterization of haustral folds to detect suspicious folds where potential polyps could be hidden.

Another challenge while extracting band images is the structure of colon that might depart from the cylinder model that we used. In our test this created problems at the flexure (high curvature). In future work, we will model the colon as a generalized cylinder around the center line defined by the camera trajectory.

By making the clinicians aware of uncovered areas post-procedurally, awareness of challenging areas as well as automated reports could lead to improved inspection efficacy and reduce the chance of missing polyps. This was already seen during our tests when the expert changed his opinion after seeing the visibility map and added uncovered areas that he thought he had missed before. The processing time of the proposed method is still too slow to achieve real-time assistance, however code optimization was not the focus of our research, and processing time could be significantly accelerated by using compiled code, particularly for graphical processing unit (GPU). Real-time computation would allow providing feedback during the procedure.

References

1. Australian Institute of Health and Welfare. http://www.aihw.gov.au/
2. Pickhardt, P.J., et al.: Location of adenomas missed by optical colonoscopy. Ann. Intern. Med. 141, 352–359 (2004)
3. Rex, D.K.: Who is the best colonoscopist? Gastrointest. Endosc. 65, 145–150 (2007)
4. Nawarathna, R., Oh, J., Muthukudage, J., Tavanapong, W., Wong, J., de Groen, P.C.: Real-time phase boundary detection for colonoscopy videos using motion vector templates. In: Yoshida, H., Hawkes, D., Vannier, M.W., et al. (eds.) Abdominal Imaging 2012. LNCS, vol. 7601, pp. 116–125. Springer, Heidelberg (2012)
5. Arnold, M., et al.: Indistinct frame detection in colonoscopy videos. In: MVIPC, pp. 47–52 (2009)
6. Hong, D., et al.: 3D Reconstruction of Virtual Colon Structures from Colonoscopy Images. Comput. Med. Imaging Graph. 38, 22–33 (2013)
7. Hartley, R., et al.: Multiple view geometry in computer vision. Cambridge University Press, Cambridge (2003)
8. Wang, H., et al.: Robust motion estimation and structure recovery from endoscopic image sequences with an adaptive scale kernel consensus estimator. In: CVPR, pp. 1–7 (2008)
9. Puerto-Souza, G.A., Staranowicz, A.N., Bell, C.S., Valdastri, P., Mariottini, G.-L.: A comparative study of ego-motion estimation algorithms for teleoperated robotic endoscopes. In: Luo, X., Reich, T., Mirota, D., Soper, T., et al. (eds.) CARE 2014. LNCS, vol. 8899, pp. 64–76. Springer, Heidelberg (2014)
10. Liu, J., et al.: A robust method to track colonoscopy videos with non-informative images. Int. J. Comput. Assist. Radiol. Surg. 8, 575–592 (2013)
11. Scaramuzza, D., et al.: A flexible technique for accurate omnidirectional camera calibration and structure from motion. In: ICVS, pp. 45–45 (2006)
12. Shi, J., et al.: Good features to track. In: CVPR, pp. 593–600 (1994)
13. Fischler, M.A., et al.: Random sample consensus: a paradigm for model fitting with applications to image analysis and automated cartography. CACM 24, 381–395 (1981)
14. Nister, D.: An efficient solution to the five-point relative pose problem. IEEE Trans. Pattern Anal. Mach. Intell. 26, 756–770 (2004)
15. More, J.: The Levenberg-marquardt algorithm: implementation and theory. In: Cleaveland, W.R. (ed.) CONCUR 1992. LNCS, vol. 630, pp. 105–116. Springer, Heidelberg (1992)
16. Scaramuzza, D., et al.: Visual Odometry. IEEE Robot. Autom. Mag. 18, 80–92 (2011)

17. Nagao, J., et al.: Fast and accurate bronchoscope tracking using image registration and motion prediction. In: Barillot, C., Haynor, D.R., Hellier, P., et al. (eds.) MICCAI 2004. LNCS, vol. 3217, pp. 551–558. Springer, Heidelberg (2004)
18. Zhen, Z., et al.: An Intelligent Endoscopic Navigation System, MA, pp. 1653–1657 (2006)
19. Goshtasby, A.: Image registration by local approximation methods. J. IVC. 6, 255–261 (1988)
20. De Visser, H., et al.: Developing A Next Generation Colonoscopy Simulator. Int. J. Image Graph. 10, 203–217 (2010)
21. Han, J.: Data mining: concepts and techniques. Elsevier Morgan Kaufmann, Amsterdam, Boston (2006)

Tissue Surface Reconstruction Aided by Local Normal Information Using a Self-calibrated Endoscopic Structured Light System

Jianyu Lin[1,2], Neil T. Clancy[1,3], Danail Stoyanov[4,5], and Daniel S. Elson[1,3]

[1] Hamlyn Centre for Robotic Surgery, Imperial College London, UK
[2] Department of Computing, Imperial College London, UK
[3] Department of Surgery and Cancer, Imperial College London, UK
[4] Centre for Medical Image Computing, University College London, UK
[5] Department of Computer Science, University College London, UK

Abstract. The tissue surface shape provides important information for both tissue pathology detection and augmented reality. Previously a miniaturised structured light (SL) illumination probe (1.9 mm diameter) has been developed to generate sparsely reconstructed tissue surfaces in minimally invasive surgery (MIS). The probe is inserted through the biopsy channel of a standard endoscope and projects a pattern of spots with unique spectra onto the target tissue. The tissue surface can be recovered by light pattern decoding and using parallax. This paper introduces further algorithmic developments and analytical work to allow free-hand manipulation of the SL probe, to improve the light pattern decoding result and to increase the reconstruction accuracy. Firstly the "normalized cut" algorithm was applied to segment the light pattern. Then an iterative procedure was investigated to update both the pattern decoding and the relative position between the camera and the probe simultaneously. Based on planar homography computation, the orientations of local areas where the spots are located in 3D space were estimated. The acquired surface normal information was incorporated with the sparse spot correspondences to constrain the fitting of a thin-plate spline during surface reconstruction. This SL system was tested in phantom, *ex vivo*, and *in vivo* experiments, and the potential of applying this system in surgical environments was demonstrated.

Keywords: Structured light, Endoscopy, Light pattern decoding, Self-calibration, Normal, Reconstruction.

1 Introduction

The measurement of tissue surface shape is important in medical applications since it may indicate tissue pathology and facilitate navigation in MIS. For instance, colonic polyp detection is aided by their morphological appearance [1]. Furthermore, intra-operative information, which can be acquired by optical techniques for surface detection, may be combined with pre-operative information provided by imaging modalities such as MRI and CT, facilitating augmented reality for surgical guidance [2, 3].

N. Navab et al. (Eds.): MICCAI 2015, Part I, LNCS 9349, pp. 405–412, 2015.
DOI: 10.1007/978-3-319-24553-9_50

SL has demonstrated potential in challenging surgical environments due to its non-reliance on salient features [3-5]. In SL a setup is designed to generate a pattern of light and project it through a probe onto the target object. According to the location of the projected light pattern recorded by a single camera, the object surface is estimated. Similar to stereoscopy a geometrical calibration should be applied to establish the spatial relationship between the projector and camera prior to 3D reconstruction.

A unique system has been developed [6] using a 4W supercontinuum laser (420-750 nm) dispersed by an SF-11 prism and focused onto a linear array of fibres. Those fibres, each carrying light of a unique narrowband spectrum, are converted into a random 1.9 mm diameter circular distribution at the distal tip, which is then imaged onto the tissue using a gradient refractive index (GRIN) lens. The system has many advantages, including the use of a narrow diameter flexible probe compatible with instrument ports, unique spectra for each fibre and high pattern brightness due to the use of a coherent laser source that can be focused into the 50 micron core diameters of the fibre array. The system schematic and the projected pattern are shown in Fig. 1(a). Despite its advantages SL systems have limitations, for instance, the calibration needs to be applied every time the flexible probe pose changes. Furthermore, SL systems do not generally provide a reconstruction result denser than the inter-spot spacing.

A system specific software platform has been established previously for surface recovery by conventional calibration and pattern decoding methods [7]. New algorithmic developments and analytical work is proposed to make full use of SL, emphasising two aspects: on-the-fly self-calibration which enables a free-hand manipulation of the probe; incorporation of local normal information in surface reconstruction. Both of these are general techniques that can also be applied to other SL systems. Self-calibration can be used whenever the relative positions of projector and camera are changed, and local normal incorporation can be used whenever light patterns with specific known shapes or sub-patterns are used.

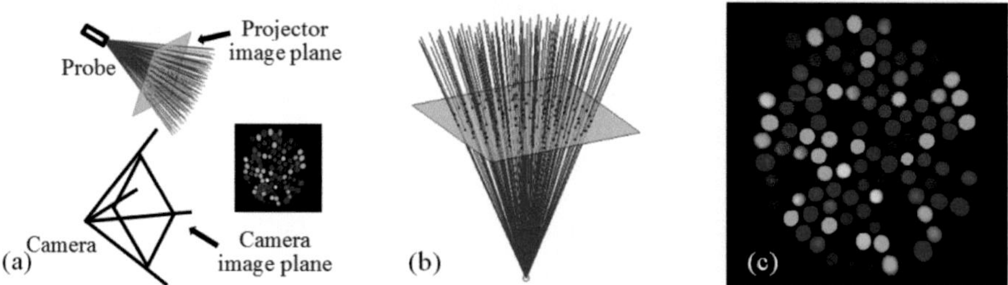

Fig. 1. (a). SL system schematic. (b). The projector model with probe centre (red circle), rays (blue lines), image plane (green), and features (red dots). (c). Virtual projector image plane.

2 Methods

Pre-calibration. Pre-calibration to estimate the intrinsic parameters of the SL system is applied prior to the experiment (Fig. 1 (b)) [7]. However, a virtual projector image plane, which provides a pixel-level description of the ellipse shapes, is also useful as it allows 3D plane orientation estimation and denser reconstruction. A white planar target is used to generate the projector image plane. The probe projects light onto the target and the SL image is captured by the camera. Induced by a plane at a general position in 3D space, a homography matrix estimated according to the spot centroid correspondences links the projector and camera image planes. The pixels of each spot in the camera image plane are mapped to the projector image plane using this homography and, after interpolation, a virtual projector image plane is generated (Fig. 1 (c)).

Pre-processing. Colour is the most important feature for light pattern decoding using this SL system. A colour vector, defined by the normalised magnitude of each colour component (red, blue and green), is used to represent pixel colour. The colour difference between two pixels can be quantified by the angle between their colour vectors. Due to strong light-tissue interaction pre-processing of SL images is required prior to light pattern decoding. This begins with specular highlight removal and includes high intensity and low saturation area detection, morphological transformation, and interpolation. Colour vectors for all pixels are calculated after Gaussian smoothing.

Light Pattern Decoding. SL images acquired during surgery have a number of challenges. For instance inter-spot distances are small and, due to lateral diffusion at longer wavelengths, may overlap, causing "contamination". In this work we use "normalized cut", which formulates the segmentation problem as spectral clustering [8]. Prior to segmentation, a mask is firstly generated based on regional maxima detection and morphological transformation to cover the spots (foreground). Then spectral clustering is applied to the pixels inside this mask to cluster them into different spots.

Spots on the SL image should be identified to find the correspondences between the projector image plane and camera image plane. In this work, by comparing the projector image with the captured SL image, unique labels are assigned to the spots. Firstly, neighbours for all the spots in both the projector and SL images are detected based on Delaunay triangulation. Then their colour vectors are computed and stacked in a clockwise sequence allowing some unique correspondences to be built. Next, the spot matching procedure is propagated to their neighbourhood from these initial matches until no more correspondences can be found and the projected spots are labelled.

On-the-fly Calibration. Calibration is required whenever the relative position between the probe and the camera changes. We propose on-the-fly self-calibration to estimate the relative positions, enabling free-hand manipulation during surgery.

In this SL system, the image plane of the projector can be regarded as the image plane of the second camera in a normal passive stereo system. The coordinates for all spot centroids X_p on the image plane are calculated in the pre-calibration procedure. On the camera image plane the image coordinates of corresponding spots X_c, after distortion correction and normalisation by the camera matrix, are also available after pre-calibration. Assuming that X_p and X_c correspond to X in 3D space the projective matrices of the projector P_p and the camera P_c, which satisfy $X_p = P_pX$ and $X_c = P_cX$, can be defined as $P_p = [R|t]$, $P_c = [I|0]$. Here R stands for the rotation matrix of the projector, and $t = -Rc$, where c is the position of the probe. The fundamental matrix F indicating the correspondences between these two image planes can be defined as

$$X_p{}^T F X_c = 0. \tag{1}$$

Together with the constraint that $\det F = 0$, F can be derived using the Maximum Likelihood (ML) estimation which minimizes the reprojection error [9]. In practice during the experiment, RANSAC [10] is applied to exclude wrong correspondences (outliers), and only those reliable correspondences are used to estimate F. The essential matrix E, which describes the relative position, is defined as $E = [t]_\times R$. E can be estimated from F based on the SVD and the geometrical interpretation of four possible solutions. In this way, both the probe orientation R and position c can be acquired, and the 3D position of spot centres can be estimated up to scale.

Feature Matching Refinement Using the Epipolar Constraint. Occasionally, due to strong optical scattering or absorption, the spot identification method fails to provide a perfect feature matching result. Therefore, the following iterative procedure is applied to refine both the epipolar geometry and spot identification: In each iteration, the fundamental matrix F is estimated with RANSAC outlier rejection and F optimisation. We then search for more correspondences using F as a constraint. A tolerance is set as the stopping criterion. Then F and correspondences are both updated.

Incorporation of Local Normal Information in 3D Reconstruction. In two view geometry, points on one plane can be related to corresponding points on another plane by a homography uniquely induced by a plane at a general position in 3D space [9]. Given the projective matrices P_p and P_c, and a plane defined by $N^T X = 0$ with $N = (n^T, 1)^T$ in 3D space, a point X on the plane is projected as X_p and X_c on the projector and camera planes, respectively. Then $X_p = HX_c$, where

$$H = R - t * n^T. \tag{2}$$

Normally, H can be estimated according to at least four 2D to 2D point correspondences. If H is known and R and t are calibrated beforehand, the normal of the plane n can be estimated. Based on this, we propose a method to estimate the orientation of the object surface at the reconstructed spot centres. Given that the individual spots are very small in 3D space, we assume that all the pixels inside spot S_i are located on one plane defined by $N_i{}^T X = 0$, with $N_i = (n_i{}^T, 1)^T$, then the image coordinates of those pixels on two image planes can be linked by a homography H_i. However, since pixelwise correspondences cannot be built between the two image planes in our SL system, another method is adopted to estimate H_i. It is noticeable that the shapes of spots on the projector image plane, which represents the intersection between the cone-like rays and the image plane, are all ellipses. It can also be observed that the shapes of most spots on the camera image plane are similar to ellipses, showing the feasibility of the assumption, since a conic can be transformed into another conic by a given homography. An ellipse on a 2D plane can be represented as

$$Ax^2 + 2Bxy + Dy^2 + 2Ex + 2Fy + G = 0. \tag{3}$$

Eq. (3) can be written as $X^T C X = 0$, where $X = [x, y, 1]^T$, and

$$C = \begin{bmatrix} A & B & E \\ B & D & F \\ E & F & G \end{bmatrix}. \tag{4}$$

In our SL system, if a pair of corresponding conics C_p and C_c on two image planes are known, they can be related by a homography H [9]:

$$C_c \sim H^T C_p H. \tag{5}$$

Combining eq. (2) and eq. (5),

$$C_{ci} \sim (R - t * n^T)^T C_{pi} (R - t * n^T), \tag{6}$$

Since eq. (6) defines an overdetermined system, n^T can be estimated through optimisation as long as the conics are non-degenerate. Based on the assumption that each pair of projected spots are located on one single plane in 3D space, corresponding spots in the two image planes of the SL system can be seen as pairs of corresponding conics C_p and C_c. Therefore, we start with ellipse fitting for all the spots to acquire the conic coefficient matrices, using the method proposed by Fitzgibbon et al. [11]. Based on the fitting cost, some spots are excluded since either they are not accurately delineated or they are not located in single planes, hence do not affect the reconstruction. Because all the fitted ellipses are non-degenerate, the local normal n where the spot is located can always be estimated by optimising eq. (6). The optimisation procedure is applied with the constraint that the estimated plane should always go through the 3D location of the spot centre, which is acquired in the previous self-calibration step. The initial guess of a local normal can be estimated from the normal of plane determined by the three surrounding spot locations in 3D space. After optimisation, the estimated normals are filtered using the cost of the optimised objective function. Given the 3D locations of spot centres, the object surface is reconstructed using a thin-plate spline (TPS) [12]. A simple but effective method is used to constrain the surface orientation: for one point with estimated orientation, six new neighbouring points close to it on the estimated plane are added. All the points including both the original and the newly added ones are used to fit the TPS model. In this way, those newly added neighbouring points constrain the local surface direction when TPS fitting takes place.

3 Experiments and Results

In order to evaluate the feasibility of the software platform, experiments on different objects have been carried out. Previous studies with this system have shown that, due to the narrowband spectra of the spots, pattern decoding is robust to changes in background hue and albedo [6]. Additional experiments have been carried out to measure the hue difference for the projected patterns on paper with different colours, finding an RMS difference of approx. 0.01. The accuracy of reconstruction and normal estimation depend on pattern decoding results, which has been demonstrated in previous work on tissue of varying albedos and hues *ex vivo* and *in vivo* [7]. The following section is divided into two parts: evaluation of self-calibrated reconstruction accuracy through comparison with corresponding manually calibrated results; observation of changes in 3D reconstruction brought by incorporating local normal information.

Reconstruction Results Using Self-calibration. The accuracy of reconstruction with manual calibration has been demonstrated in previous work (0.65 mm error at ~100 mm working distance) [7] and it was used to evaluate the self-calibration result. A silicon heart phantom was imaged as well as *ex vivo* porcine liver, kidney, heart, and *in vivo* porcine large bowel. In total 49 SL images were used and the result was evaluated by registering surfaces from manual and self-calibration. Since the surfaces are reconstructed up to scale, the scaling factor along line-of-sight rays is the only variable used in registration. The average and maximum distances between the two surfaces in percentages are used as indicators of reconstruction error (Fig. 2) (Table 1).

Table 1. Reconstruction errors using the self-calibration technique on benchmark data

Object	Mean distance	Median of mean distance	Max. distance	Median of Max. distance
Heart phantom	0.32% ± 0.13%	0.28%	1.03% ± 0.51%	0.88%
Liver	2.36% ± 5.26%	0.80%	3.84% ± 2.54%	2.68%
Kidney	0.40% ± 0.37%	0.20%	1.76% ± 1.70%	0.88%
Heart	0.81% ± 0.68%	0.44%	2.93% ± 2.39%	1.43%
Large Bowel	3.58% ± 4.38%	2.07%	16.70% ± 23.29%	7.55%

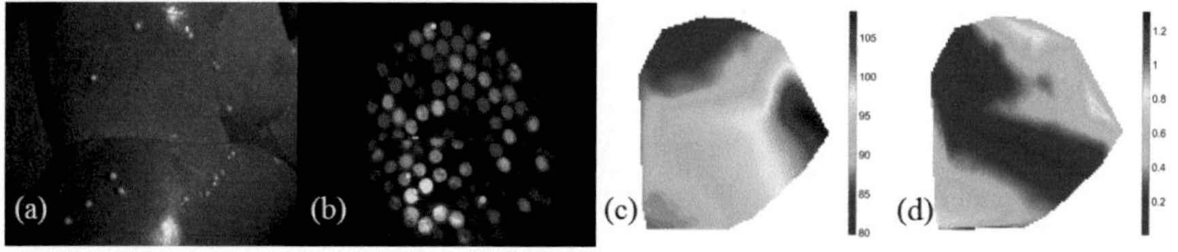

Fig. 2. (a). Liver under white light. (b). Liver under SL. (c). Reconstructed surface using self-calibration where colour indicates the surface depth (in mm). (d). Relative error map on the reconstructed surface using self-calibration where colour indicates the reconstruction error (%).

The mean and median values of both the average and maximum distance show promise for tissue reconstruction using the self-calibration technique. But it is noticeable that according to the maximum distance, despite generally good performance for the case of porcine large bowel, large errors still occur in some areas. This phenomenon was caused by the poor light pattern imaging due to strong scattering of light at long wavelengths and absorption of light at short wavelengths. But the performance does show the potential of the self-calibration technique in surgical environments.

Incorporation of Local Normal Information. The estimated local normals provide additional surface detail. The TPS interpolation is able to provide a reconstruction with high quality for objects with smooth surfaces. However, adding normal information helps to improve the surface detail when the object surface is more complex.

We tested the normal estimation algorithm on a rectangular box, a cylinder, and a liver phantom. Fig. 3 (b), (d), (f) demonstrate the reconstruction of an area around one edge of a rectangular box, a cylinder, and the liver phantom, respectively. The local normals (red arrows) are well estimated using the proposed method.

Since local normals do not benefit the reconstruction much on relatively smooth surfaces, a small object consisting of two steps was used to intuitively show the improvement of surface reconstruction after incorporating normal information. Light patterns were projected onto the object, and Fig. 3 (g) and (h) show the reconstructed surfaces before and after addition of local normal information. The step shape is only accurately defined when incorporating normal information, demonstrating that this method could improve the reconstruction when a sparse light pattern is projected on a non-smooth object surface. Images were acquired using 33 ms exposure times and it took ~50 s to process a single frame using Matlab (Intel i7-3770, 8 GB RAM).

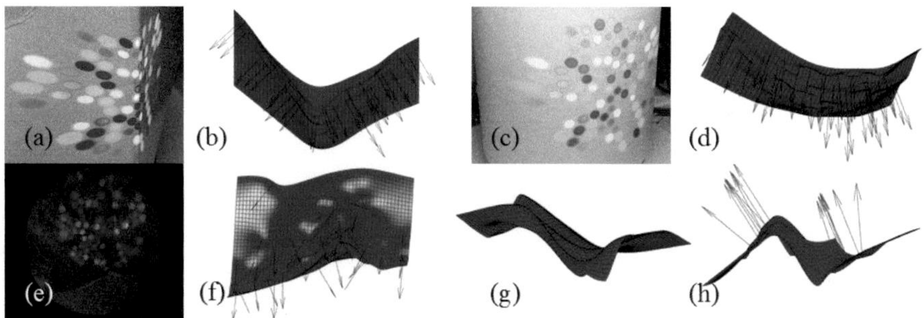

Fig. 3. (a). Rectangular box edge under white light and SL. (b). Reconstructed rectangular box edge (blue) aided by normals (red). (c). cylinder under white light and SL. (d). Reconstructed cylinder (blue) aided by normals (red). (e). Liver phantom under white light and SL. (f). Reconstructed liver phantom (blue) aided by normals (red). (g). Reconstructed step surface (blue) without normal information. (h). Reconstructed step surface (blue) aided by normals (red).

4 Discussion and Conclusion

In this paper we have developed an SL system that is capable of estimating 3D depth as well as inferring information about the surface normal at each SL point. We propose an on-the-fly self-calibration technique along with an iterative algorithm to update both the epipolar geometry and feature matching to enhance SL inference of 3D structural information. Comparison between the resulting reconstruction and that from manual calibration exposes the feasibility and robustness of this technique in object surface reconstruction. But further studies are needed to localise depth in metric space. This method is appropriate for fibre-based SL systems that rely on point projection. Based on the assumption that some projected spots are located on one plane in 3D space, local normal information is estimated according to the homography between two corresponding ellipses. Our experiments show that the improvement of incorporating normal information is notable and that this technique can also be adapted in other SL systems using light patterns with specific known shapes. Future work will focus on further hardware improvements to reduce ambiguities in pattern decoding and development of implementations where real-time robust and dense tissue surface reconstruction is possible through algorithm design and parallelisation architectures. This would allow dynamic tissue imaging on a per-frame basis.

Acknowledgements. This work is funded by ERC 242991 and an Imperial College Confidence in Concept award. NC is supported by an Imperial College Junior Research Fellowship. The authors thank Northwick Park Institute for Medical Research for surgical arrangements.

References

1. Schwartz, J.J., Lichtenstein, G.R.: Magnification endoscopy, chromoendoscopy and other novel techniques in evaluation of patients with IBD. Techniques in Gastrointestinal Endoscopy 6, 182–188 (2004)
2. King, A.P., Edwards, P.J., Maurer, C.R., Cunha, D.A.D., Gaston, R.P., Clarkson, M., Hill, D.L.G., Hawkes, D.J., Fenlon, M.R., Strong, A.J., Cox, T.C.S., Gleeson, M.J.: Stereo Augmented Reality in the Surgical Microscope. Presence: Teleoper. Virtual Environ. 9, 360–368 (2000)
3. Maier-Hein, L., Mountney, P., Bartoli, A., Elhawary, H., Elson, D., Groch, A., Kolb, A., Rodrigues, M., Sorger, J., Speidel, S., Stoyanov, D.: Optical techniques for 3D surface reconstruction in computer-assisted laparoscopic surgery. Medical Image Analysis 17, 974–996 (2013)
4. Maier-Hein, L., Groch, A., Bartoli, A., Bodenstedt, S., Boissonnat, G., Chang, P.L., Clancy, N.T., Elson, D.S., Haase, S., Heim, E., Hornegger, J., Jannin, P., Kenngott, H., Kilgus, T., Muller-Stich, B., Oladokun, D., Rohl, S., dos Santos, T.R., Schlemmer, H.P., Seitel, A., Speidel, S., Wagner, M., Stoyanov, D.: Comparative Validation of Single-Shot Optical Techniques for Laparoscopic 3-D Surface Reconstruction. IEEE Transactions on Medical Imaging 33, 1913–1930 (2014)
5. Schmalz, C., Forster, F., Schick, A., Angelopoulou, E.: An endoscopic 3D scanner based on structured light. Medical Image Analysis 16, 1063–1072 (2012)
6. Clancy, N.T., Stoyanov, D., Maier-Hein, L., Groch, A., Yang, G.-Z., Elson, D.S.: Spectrally encoded fiber-based structured lighting probe for intraoperative 3D imaging. Biomedical Optics Express 2, 3119–3128 (2011)
7. Lin, J., Clancy, N.T., Elson, D.S.: An endoscopic structured light system using multispectral detection. In: International Journal of Computer Assisted Radiology and Surgery (2015) ISSN:1861-6410
8. Shi, J., Malik, J.: Normalized cuts and image segmentation. IEEE Transactions on Pattern Analysis and Machine Intelligence 22, 888–905 (2000)
9. Hartley, R., Zisserman, A.: Multiple View Geometry in Computer Vision. Cambridge University Press (2004). ISBN: 0521540518
10. Fischler, M.A., Bolles, R.C.: Random sample consensus: a paradigm for model fitting with applications to image analysis and automated cartography. Commun. ACM 24, 381–395 (1981)
11. Fitzgibbon, A., Pilu, M., Fisher, R.B.: Direct least square fitting of ellipses. IEEE Transactions on Pattern Analysis and Machine Intelligence 21, 476–480 (1999)
12. Franke, R.: Smooth interpolation of scattered data by local thin plate splines. Computers & Mathematics with Applications 8, 273–281 (1982)

Surgical Augmented Reality with Topological Changes

Christoph J. Paulus[1,2], Nazim Haouchine[1,2], David Cazier[2], and Stéphane Cotin[1,2]

[1] Inria Nancy Grand Est, Villers-les-Nancy, France
[2] Université de Strasbourg, ICube Lab, CNRS, Illkirch, France

Abstract. The visualization of internal structures of organs in minimally invasive surgery is an important avenue for improving the perception of the surgeon, or for supporting planning and decision systems. However, current methods dealing with non-rigid augmented reality only provide augmentation when the topology of the organ is not modified. In this paper we solve this shortcoming by introducing a method for physics-based non-rigid augmented reality. Singularities caused by topological changes are detected and propagated to the pre-operative model. This significantly improves the coherence between the actual laparascopic view and the model, and provides added value in terms of navigation and decision making. Our real time augmentation algorithm is assessed on a video showing the cut of a porcine liver's lobe in minimal invasive surgery.

1 Introduction

In recent decades, considerable advances in the introduction of augmented reality during surgery have been achieved [1]. More particularly, the scientific community and clinicians have been focusing on minimally invasive surgery (MIS). This kind of surgery has gained popularity and become a well-established procedure thanks to its benefits for the patients in term of haemorrhaging risk reduction and shortened recovery time. However, it remains complex from a surgical point of view, mainly because of the reduced field of view which considerably impacts depth perception and surgical navigation.

Recently, there has been a great deal of ongoing research efforts towards automatic registration between pre- and intra-operative data in MIS considering the elastic organ behavior. Patient-specific biomechanical models have demonstrated their relevance for volume deformation, as they allow to account for anisotropic and elastic properties of the shape and to infer in-depth structure motion [2], [3]. In [4], a 4D scan of the heart is jointly used with a biomechanical model to couple the surface motion with external forces derived from camera data. This method uses the cyclic pattern of the heart deformations to improve the registration. A local tuning of the deformation is used to propagate the surface deformation to in-depth invisible structures. In the context of augmented reality for liver surgery, [3] used a heterogeneous model that takes into account

N. Navab et al. (Eds.): MICCAI 2015, Part I, LNCS 9349, pp. 413–420, 2015.
DOI: 10.1007/978-3-319-24553-9_51

the vascular network to improve the soft tissue behavior while real-time performance is obtained using adequate mesh resolution and pre-computed solvers. In [2], a physics-based shape matching approach is proposed. Non-rigid registration between the pre-operative elastic model and the intra-operative organ shape is modeled as an electrostatic-elastic problem. The elastic model is electrically charged to slide into an oppositely charged organ shape representation.

Despite such recent improvements in the field of surgical augmented reality, no study has yet investigated the impact of cutting or resection actions performed during the operation. Given that these are essential steps of any surgical procedure, it is obvious that if the meshes of the underlying mechanical model are not correctly modified, significant errors are generated in the registration and consequently in the estimation of internal structures or tumor localization. In the context of image-guided neurosurgery, Ferrant *et al.* [5] proposed to handle registration issues induced by tumor resection by updating a biomechanical brain model accordingly with topological changes. These changes consist of removing the elements of the brain model that contains the resected tumor and surrounded area.

In the computer graphics domain, there is ongoing work on methods that take account of the mesh updates induced by cutting, fracture or tearing. A comprehensive overview of cuts in soft tissue simulation is provided in [6]. The simulation of surgical cuts raises specific questions. Elastic and in some cases plastic deformations are required for accurate simulations. The surgeon's manipulations may include cuts, cauterization or tearing of the organs. The computations must therefore handle topological changes or updates in the connectivity of the underlying mesh. Handling such mechanical models and mesh operations implies elevated computational costs and makes it challenging to maintain real-time performance, that is required by augmented reality applications. The approach presented in [7] addresses these issues. The method is based on the composite finite element method, that embeds a fine grid into a coarse uniform hexahedral grid. The fine mesh is used for the visualization and collision and the simulation uses the coarse one, reducing the computation time. Cuts are performed on the fine level grid that stores the separation information. As soon as a complete separation of the fine grid occurs in a coarse element, it is duplicated to represent the cut. Visually pleasing results are obtained in real-time. However, as the elements of the coarse mesh can only be completely cut, the simulation does not react instantly on partial cuts.

The main contributions of this paper are 1) a method to detect a cut in three-dimensional soft structures by analyzing the motion of tracked surface points and 2) an algorithm for applying the detected topological changes to the preoperative model in real-time. This leads to an improved coherence between the actual surgical situation and the (updated) pre-operative data, therefore positively impacting the accuracy of the navigation.

2 Method

In this section we give a short overview of our method. We process the information from a monocular video stream similar to that provided by endoscopic cameras. This video captures the manipulations of a surgeon on the targeted organ on which deformations and cuts are performed with a scissor-grasper or any similar surgical tool. We suppose that a virtual 3D model of the organ is provided and initially registrated to the first frame of the video. Such model is usually obtained during pre-operative diagnostic operations from some medical imaging techniques. The biomechanical behavior of the virtual organ is modeled using a non-linear elastic deformation law computed using a finite element method (FEM). The real organ, through feature points captured on the video, and the virtual organ are coupled in a way that the motions in the videos are reproduced by the virtual organ. After a surgical cut, differences between the motions of the real and virtual organs appear. We detect and analyze those differences to predict the occurrence of a cut. Detected cuts are then reproduced on the virtual organ thus improving the following registration steps.

2.1 Coupling Real and Virtual Organs

We rely on the tracking and spatiotemporal registration as described in [8] where feature points acquired from a camera constrain a non-linear elastic model. The visual tracking yields a set of features $\mathcal{F} = \{f_i \in \mathbb{R}^2\}$ chosen in the video stream. The virtual organ is represented by a 3D mesh with vertices in the set $\mathcal{V} = \{v_m \in \mathbb{R}^3\}$. Each feature point f_i is associated with a virtual feature point $f_i^v \in \mathbb{R}^3$ lying on the boundary surface of $\mathcal{V}$. The points f_i^v are initialized with the first frame of the video as the intersection of the line of sight – from the camera's position to f_i – with the boundary of $\mathcal{V}$. Each virtual feature is registered in an element of the FEM mesh and expressed as barycentric coordinates of the element's vertices.

In order to compare the positions of the features f_i and the corresponding virtual features f_i^v, the points f_i^v are projected onto the plane of the f_i, i.e. the 2D plane of the video in the 3D scene. In the following, we use $\overline{f_i^v} = P(f_i^v)$ to denote those projections, with the projection matrix P of the camera. As the features move in the video, they introduce a stretching energy $W_S(\mathcal{F}, \mathcal{V})$ between each feature f_i and its projected virtual feature $\overline{f_i^v}$:

$$W_S(\mathcal{F}, \mathcal{V}) = \sum_i \frac{1}{2} k_i \| f_i - \overline{f_i^v} \|^2$$

The parameters k_i are experimentally chosen and are in the same order of magnitude as the Young's modulus of the organ. In addition, the biomechanical object is constrained by fixing nodes at predefined positions: $v_m = v_m^D, m \in B$. The internal elastic energy of the virtual organ is $W_I(\mathcal{V}) = \sum_e W_e$, accumulating the strain energy W_e of the elements related to a Saint Venant-Kirchhoff material. Finally, the deformation of the virtual organ is expressed as a minimization problem between internal elastic energy and stretching energy $W_I(\mathcal{V})+W_S(\mathcal{F},\mathcal{V})$ with the constraint that $v_m = v_m^D$, for all $m \in B$. The solution of the problem is the updated set of vertices $\mathcal{V}$. The positions of the virtual features f_i^v are updated using the stored barycentric coordinates and the updated $\mathcal{V}$.

The stretching energy links the virtual features f_i^v to the real ones f_i. When the virtual organ correctly follows the motion of the real one, the vector $d_i = f_i - \overline{f_i^v}$ changes continuously in the neighborhood of f_i. This vector encodes simultaneously the Euclidean distance between f_i and $\overline{f_i^v}$ and direction of the relative motion of the organ and its virtual representation. In the next section, the vector d_i is used to detect potential cuts in the real organ.

2.2 Detecting Discontinuities in Motion

With a continuous deformation of the manipulated organ, the projections of the virtual features $\overline{f_i^v}$ smoothly follow the tracked points f_i. When a cut occurs, the motion of $\overline{f_i^v}$ and f_i starts to diverge, because the cut is not represented in the virtual organ. To detect such divergent motions, we analyze the vectors d_i of neighboring virtual features. We define the set $N = \{(i,j)\}$ of neighbor pairs of virtual features such that the Euclidean distance $\|\overline{f_i^v} - \overline{f^v}_j\|$ is lower than a given radius r that depends on the detected features. The neighborhood $\mathcal{N}$ is initialized based on the features obtained in the first frame of the video. These notions are illustrated in figure 1.

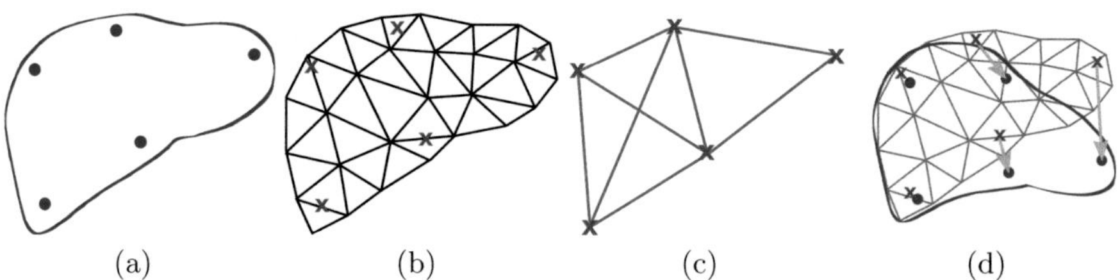

Fig. 1. (a) Real object with features f_i (blue disks); (b) Mesh with the virtual features $\overline{f_i^v}$ (red crosses); (c) Set $\mathcal{N}$ of neighboring virtual features (neighborhood relations in green); (d) Differences d_i between f_i and $\overline{f_i^v}$ (orange vectors)

To evaluate whether a discontinuity occurs in the way d_i evolves, we introduce the measure $\mu_{ij} = \|d_i - d_j\|$. We calculate the average distance $\bar{\mu}$ of the measures μ_{ij} over the set $\mathcal{N}$. Discontinuities between two features f_i and f_j are detected by finding the outliers $\mu_{ij} > \bar{\mu}\epsilon$, with a threshold ϵ dependent on the scenario. For the moment the monocular camera fixes the tracked features to the plane of the video, thus discontinuities in the motion along the z-axis can not be detected. Intuitively, the outliers correspond to pairs of features f_i, f_j whose difference vectors d_i, d_j differ too much – either in length or direction (figure 2(a)).

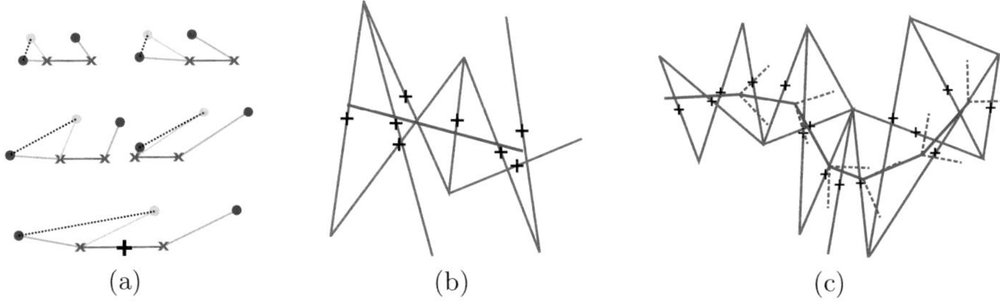

Fig. 2. (a) Neighbor configurations: dotted lines illustrate computation of measure μ_{ij}, the last configuration introduces a separation point (black cross); (b) Initialization of the cut (red line) averaging the separation points (black crosses) (c) Progression of the cut, with the angular restriction (dashed red lines)

The computed outliers define a region where a cut is likely to occur. To capture the location of this cut, we insert separation points between diverging features near their barycenters. The simulated cut is thus initialized as a line minimizing the Euclidean distance to a fixed number of separation points (figure 2(b)). We assume that the cutting process is continuous, i.e. that the separation path can advance in two directions, starting from the extremities of the initial separation line. Thus, we represent the separation as two lines l_1 and l_2, that can move independently from the first initialization line. This sequence of lines defines a separation polygon for each time step (figure 2(c)). The separation polygon is finally extruded along a depth vector to define a separation surface. This vector is either the direction of the camera or a predefined direction.

2.3 Robust Processing of the Cut

To ensure a trustworthy and robust detection of cuts, unrealistically tracked features that jump or slide in improbable directions need to be filtered out. The underlying mechanical model used to deform the virtual organ has the desirable property of regularizing and smoothing the movements of the points $\overline{f_i^v}$.

Again, we use the difference vector between the positions of neighbors to determine outliers, but this time comparing along the combination of the resolution of time and space. Precisely, we consider the evolution of d_i during a time step using the measure $E_i = \|d_i(t+\Delta t) - d_i(t)\|$ and we determine outliers comparing to the average of this measure. If a feature f_i has been identified as an outlier, then it is not used for the detection of the cut.

In addition, the propagation of the cut can be restricted in order to react on noisy data. First, an angular restriction α constrains the lines to only move in the desired direction. Secondly, the length of each line can be adapted, introducing a minimal and a maximal progression for each cut line. Thirdly, new cut lines are only inserted when a sufficient number of separation points have been inserted. Those constraints present two advantages: (i) it reduces the wrong detections due to too large motions and (ii) the detail of the separation polygon can be controlled.

The separation is incorporated into the volumetric mesh combining a remeshing approach with a simple snapping of the volumetric vertices to the cut [11]. However, the detection method we propose is independent of the separation algorithm, other efficient algorithms like [7] could be used as well.

3 Experimental Results

In this section, we demonstrate the potential of our approach to detect a surgical cut from the motion of features f_i extracted from a video stream and to replicate the corresponding topological changes on a virtual model $\mathcal{V}$ augmenting the view.

Our algorithm was applied on two scenarios involving highly elastic silicone bands which are cut and then video recorded while being manipulated to induce deformations. The feature tracking, deformable model update, cut detection and topological changes are performed in real-time. The final positions show the advantage of our method over an uncut mesh (see figure 3). This is quantitatively evaluated using a classical dice coefficient on the two dimensional domain of the video data. The results for the first case scenario (object cut on the side) are 0.815 when not accounting for topological changes, and 0.952 when using our algorithm. Results for the second case scenario (object cut in the middle) are 0.900 for the uncut mesh, and 0.964 when applying our method.

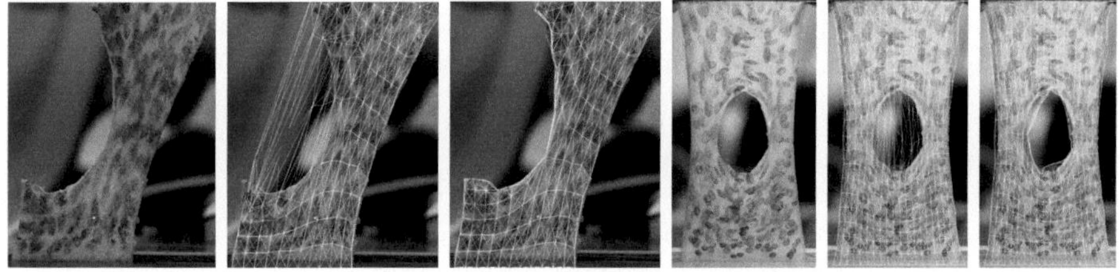

Fig. 3. Examples of a detected cut in silicone, augmented with an uncut/cut model

We then evaluated our approach on a video clip involving a cut being performed on a porcine liver lobe. The initial and the final frames are shown in figures 4(a) and 4(d). In this example, the algorithm extracts 438 features f_i from the video stream (figure 4(a)), 32 are identified to be outliers in the advancement of the video. The features deform a volumetric mesh, using the spring energy $W_S(\mathcal{F}, \mathcal{V})$. Figure 4(b) illustrates the initial configuration of the vertices $\mathcal{V}$. We calculate the measure μ on 18503 pairs of features and lose 1478 of these pairs in the course of the simulation due to identified outliers – the initial neighborhood information $\mathcal{N}$ is displayed in figure 4(c).

When applying our method, the measure μ_{ij} is calculated on the neighboring pairs of features in $\mathcal{N}$ and a pair of features is identified to be cut using a

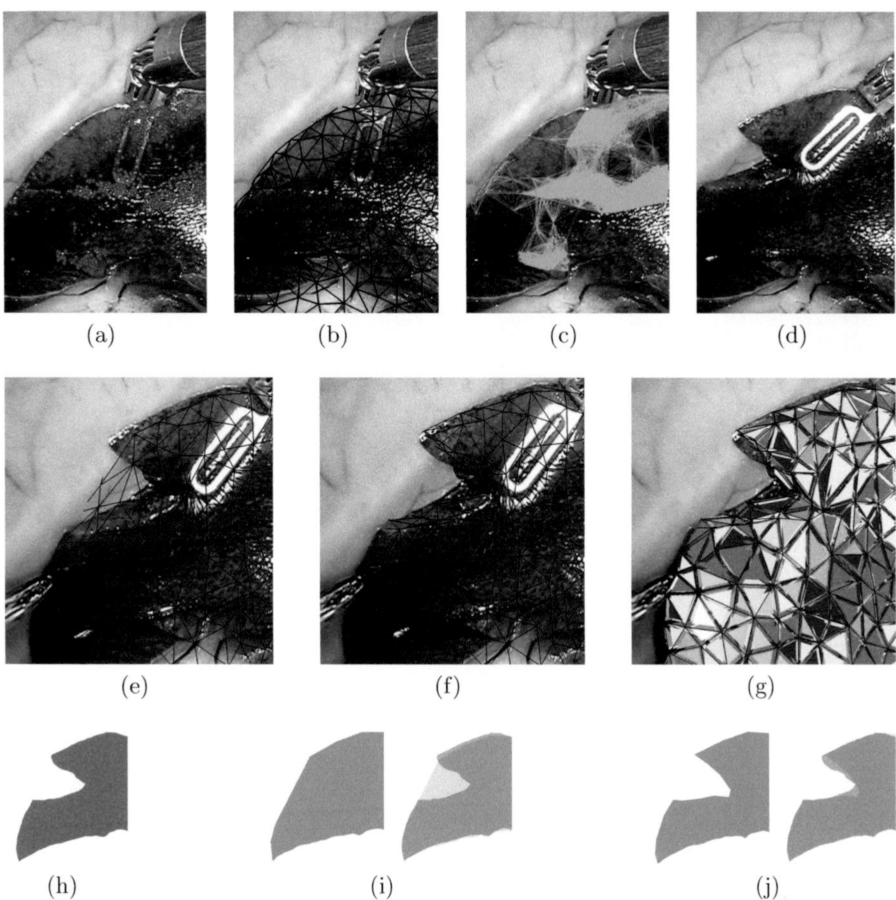

Fig. 4. (a) Detected features f_i; (b) FEM mesh of the virtual organ; (c) Computed neighborhood $\mathcal{N}$; (d) Organ manipulation after a cut; Augmented reality on cut and deformed liver without cut in the virtual organ (e) and with our method applying the cut to the virtual organ (f), (g); Surface areas of the real cut surface (h), models without/with cutting (i)/(j)

threshold $\epsilon = 7.0$. The resulting three-dimensional representation of the liver, as illustrated in figures 4(f) and (g), is very similar to the actual organ shape.

To analyze our results, we compute the dice measure comparing the surfaces of the uncut pre-operative mesh and the cut mesh obtained with our method. The dice coefficient associated with our result is 0.963, whereas it was 0.906 for the uncut object, confirming the benefits of the proposed method.

4 Conclusion and Discussion

This work addresses the important and little studied problem of cutting during surgical augmented reality. The proposed method is able to detect a surgical cut applied on soft deformable structures, by analyzing the discontinuities in the motion of feature points obtained by visual tracking. The cut is applied on the preoperative model in real-time using an efficient combination of re-meshing and snapping techniques, to maintain a realistic augmentation after a performed cut. Convincing preliminary results are demonstrated for both *in vitro* and *in vivo* examples. Let us point out that cuts can be detected even if the tracked features relatively far around the cut region, but with a deteriorated accuracy. More validation is obviously required though it is worth mentioning that validation implying actual organs are seldom reported in previous works. The current method is restricted to precut objects, the next steps in the context of this research will be an expansion to live cutting, tearing and fracture. For this step it is important to use less parameters or to automatically tune parameters to a specific scene. Beyond that – as our method does not address the depth of the cut – it would be specifically interesting to investigate into organs partially cut in the direction of the camera.

References

1. Nicolau, S., Soler, L., Mutter, D., Marescaux, J.: Augmented reality in laparoscopic surgical oncology. Surgical Oncology 20(3) (2011)
2. Suwelack, S., et al.: Physics-based shape matching for intraoperative image guidance. Medical Physics 41(11) (2014)
3. Haouchine, N., Dequidt, J., Peterlik, I., Kerrien, E., Berger, M.O., Cotin, S.: Image-guided simulation of heterogeneous tissue deformation for augmented reality during hepatic surgery. In: International Symposium on Mixed and Augmented Reality (ISMAR) (2013)
4. Pratt, P., Stoyanov, D., Visentini-Scarzanella, M., Yang, G.-Z.: Dynamic guidance for robotic surgery using image-constrained biomechanical models. In: Jiang, T., Navab, N., Pluim, J.P.W., Viergever, M.A. (eds.) MICCAI 2010, Part I. LNCS, vol. 6361, pp. 77–85. Springer, Heidelberg (2010)
5. Ferrant, M., Nabavi, A., Macq, B., Black, P., Jolesz, F., Kikinis, R., Warfield, S.: Serial registration of intraoperative mr images of the brain. Medical Image Analysis 6 (2001)
6. Wu, J., Westermann, R., Dick, C.: Physically-based simulation of cuts in deformable bodies: A survey. In: Eurographics 2014 State-of-the-Art Report (2014)
7. Dick, C., Georgii, J., Westermann, R.: A hexahedral multigrid approach for simulating cuts in deformable objects. IEEE Transactions on Visualization and Computer Graphics 17(11) (2011)
8. Haouchine, N., Dequidt, J., Berger, M.O., Cotin, S.: Single view augmentation of 3D elastic objects. In: ISMAR (2014)
9. Koschier, D., Lipponer, S., Bender, J.: Adaptive tetrahedral meshes for brittle fracture simulation. In: Proceedings of the 2014 ACM SIGGRAPH/Eurographics Symposium on Computer Animation (2014)
10. Nienhuys, H.-W., van der Stappen, A.F.: A surgery simulation supporting cuts and finite element deformation. In: Niessen, W.J., Viergever, M.A. (eds.) MICCAI 2001. LNCS, vol. 2208, pp. 145–152. Springer, Heidelberg (2001)
11. Paulus, C.J., Untereiner, L., Courtecuisse, H., Cotin, S., Cazier, D.: Virtual cutting of deformable objects based on efficient topological operations. The Visual Computer 31(6-8), 831–841 (2015)

Towards an Efficient Computational Framework for Guiding Surgical Resection through Intra-operative Endo-microscopic Pathology

Shaohua Wan[1,⋆], Shanhui Sun[1], Subhabrata Bhattacharya[1], Stefan Kluckner[1], Alexander Gigler[2], Elfriede Simon[2], Maximilian Fleischer[2], Patra Charalampaki[3], Terrence Chen[1], and Ali Kamen[1]

[1] Siemens Corporation, Corporate Technology, Princeton, NJ, USA
[2] Siemens AG, Corporate Technology, Munich, Germany
[3] Department of Neurosurgery, Hospital Merheim, Cologne Medical Center, Germany

Abstract. Precise detection and surgical resection of the tumors during an operation greatly increases the chance of the overall procedure efficacy. Emerging experimental in-vivo imaging technologies such as Confocal Laser Endomicroscopy (CLE), could potentially assist surgeons to examine brain tissues on histological scale in real-time during the operation. However, it is a challenging task for neurosurgeons to interpret these images in real-time, primarily due to the low signal to noise ratio and variability in the patterns expressed within these images by various examined tissue types. In this paper, we present a comprehensive computational framework capable of automatic brain tumor classification in real-time. Specifically, our contributions include: (a) an end-to-end computational pipeline where a variety of the feature extraction methods, encoding schemes, and classification algorithms can be readily deployed, (b) thorough evaluation of state-of-the-art low-level image features and popular encoding techniques in context of CLE imagery, and finally, (c) A highly optimized feature pooling method based on codeword proximity. The proposed system can effectively classify two types of commonly diagnosed brain tumors in CLE sequences captured in real-time with close to 90% accuracy. Extensive experiments on a dataset of 117 videos demonstrate the efficacy of our system.

1 Introduction

Glioblastoma is the most predominant and most aggressive malignant brain tumor in humans that accounts for 52% of all brain tumor cases and 20% of all intracranial tumors [1]. Meningioma, on the other hand, although benign, accounts for more than 35% of primary brain tumors in the US, and occurs in approximately 7 of every 100,000 people [2, 3], with an approximate 5 year survival time-line of the diagnosed patient. Optimal surgical resection is primarily based on accurate detection of tumor tissue during the surgical resection.

Recently, Confocal Laser Endomicroscopy (CLE) [4] has emerged as a promising in-vivo imaging technology that allows real-time examination of body tissues on a scale

⋆ Shaohua Wan (from University of Texas at Austin, Austin, TX, US) contributed to this work during his internship at Siemens Corporation, Corporate Technology, Princeton, NJ, USA.

N. Navab et al. (Eds.): MICCAI 2015, Part I, LNCS 9349, pp. 421–429, 2015.
DOI: 10.1007/978-3-319-24553-9_52

that was previously only possible on histologic slices. Neurosurgeons could now use CLE as a surgical guidance tool for brain tumors. However, as a manual examination task, this can be highly time-consuming and error-prone. Thus, there has been an increasing demand in employing computer vision techniques for brain tumor tissue typing and pathology in the CLE probing process.

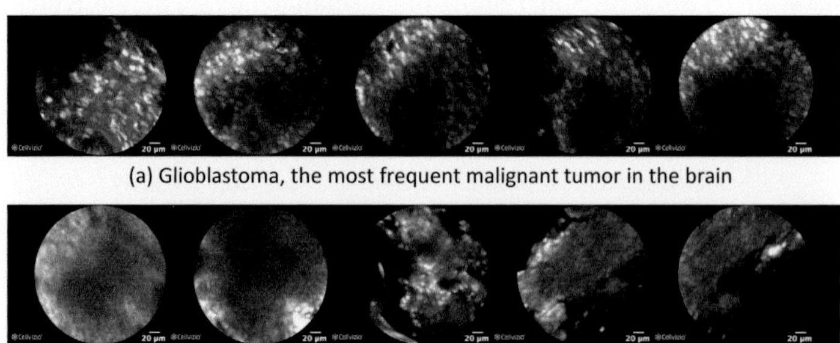

(a) Glioblastoma, the most frequent malignant tumor in the brain

(b) Meningioma, the most frequent benign tumor in the brain

Fig. 1. Top row shows representative frames from Glioblastoma and bottom row from Meningioma cases, captured using CLE imagery. Note how the former is characterized by sharp granular patterns while the latter by smooth homogeneous patterns.

Tissues affected by Glioblastoma and Meningioma, are usually characterized by sharp granular and smooth homogeneous patterns [1], respectively. However, the low resolution of current CLE imaging systems, coupled with the presence of both kind of patterns in the probing area, makes it extremely challenging for common image classification algorithms. As seen in Figure 1, besides the great variability between images from the same tumor class, the differences between the two classes of tumors are not clearly evident when both granular and homogeneous patterns are present in the image.

However, CLE technology still being at an inchoate state, there have been only a few notable earlier endeavors that address automatic analysis of CLE images [5,6]. To this end, André *et al.* introduce a Bag-of-visual Words (BoW) based framework [7] to perform endoscopic image retrieval [5]. On a different note, Bauer *et al.* [8] introduce a conditional random field based segmentation approach to localize tumor affected brain tissues. Inspired by the success of [5], the authors of [9] employ an improved feature descriptor based on Radial Gradients descriptors on a similar BoW based computational framework. Recently, the authors of [10] find applications for BoW based CLE video representation for retrieval purpose.

BoW based approaches and their variants have caught immense attention in generic image recognition tasks, and they still continue to be the natural choice for practitioners due to their simplicity in implementation. As part of this work, we adapt an efficient, yet accurate encoding that exploits spatial locality of visual features that outperforms conventional BoW based methods as well as three other popular encoding methods [11–13]. Our intuition behind using this encoding scheme is driven by the spatial proximity of the granular patterns in Glioblastoma affected tissues. The proposed locality constrained coding scheme, thus will be able to create a highly discriminative representation for the different kind of texture patterns as observed in Fig. 1.

Additionally, we investigate the efficacy of some of the state-of-the-art feature descriptor algorithms [14–17]. We organize our paper as follows: In Section 2 we describe our computational methodology. This is followed by Section 3 where we discuss our experimental setup, results on a challenging dataset, and compare quantitatively with the state-of-the-art. Finally we conclude our observations in Section 5.

2 Computational Pipeline

Our task of automatic brain tumor classification, like all supervised learning tasks, requires a training phase which is performed off-line. The training phase consists of extracting low-level features from frames from CLE video sequences. The implementation specific details of this step is provided in Section 3. Extracted features are typically pooled using an encoding strategy (Fig. 2). We briefly explain the pooling strategies employed in BoW, to set up the context for the various encoding strategies [11–13, 18] we evaluate in this work.

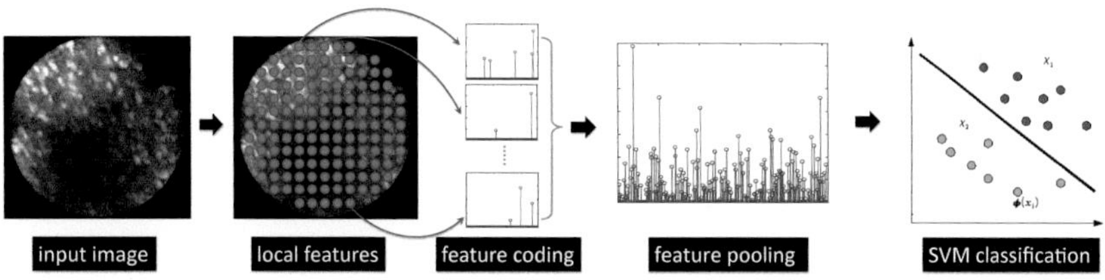

Fig. 2. Schematic diagram of the computational pipeline.

Let $\boldsymbol{X}$ be a set of d-dimensional local descriptors extracted from an image, i.e., $\boldsymbol{X} = [\boldsymbol{x}_1, \cdots, \boldsymbol{x}_n] \in \mathcal{R}^{d \times n}$. Representative descriptors from a reasonably large image set can be extracted using clustering or vocabulary tree [19] based indexing scheme. The objective of constructing a vocabulary from these local descriptors is to obtain a compact global representation for any given image.

Thus, given a vocabulary with m entries, $\boldsymbol{B} = [\boldsymbol{b}_1, \cdots, \boldsymbol{b}_n] \in \mathcal{R}^{d \times m}$, each descriptor from an image, is converted into an m-dimensional code $\boldsymbol{c}_i = [c_{i1}, \cdots, c_{im}]^T \in \mathcal{R}^m$, depending on the encoding scheme. Traditional BoW employs hard quantization, wherein for a local feature $\boldsymbol{x}_i$, there is only one non-zero coding coefficient, corresponding to the nearest visual word subject to a predefined distance threshold. Thus, the code $\boldsymbol{c}_i$ is calculated as:

$$c_{ij} = \begin{cases} 1 & \text{if } j = \arg\min_{j=1,\cdots,n} \|\boldsymbol{x}_i - \boldsymbol{b}_j\|_2^2 \\ 0 & \text{otherwise} \end{cases} \tag{1}$$

The encoding strategy as described in Eqn. 1, although straight-forward, often shown to suffer from quantization errors [12, 13]. A notable improvisation in this direction includes the use of Gaussian Mixture Models based clustering followed by soft- assignment of each descriptor to the mixtures [12], popularly known as Fisher Kernel based encoding. This technique although, results in relatively denser and higher-dimensional image representations than BoW, becomes computationally intractable for real-time classification applications. Based on a similar yet simplified theoretical foundation, Vector of Large Aggregated Descriptors (VLAD [13]) has been recently made popular, which jointly optimizes dimensionality reduction and the descriptor search space, while preserving the quality of vector comparison. We integrate both of these techniques in our evaluation framework to perform an in-depth analysis of the effect of encoding on classification.

Since typical vocabulary based representations (BoW) are sparse, encoding methods that exploit sparsity [11], are being increasingly used. Under the sparsity assumption, a local feature $\boldsymbol{x}_i$ is represented as a linear combination of a sparse set of basis vectors in the vocabulary. The coefficient vector $\boldsymbol{c}_i$ is obtained by solving an l_1-norm regularized problem:

$$\boldsymbol{c}_i = \arg\min \|\boldsymbol{x}_i - \boldsymbol{B}\boldsymbol{c}_i\|_2^2 + \lambda\|\boldsymbol{c}_i\|_1 \quad \text{s.t.} \quad \mathbf{1}^T\boldsymbol{c}_i = 1, \forall i \tag{2}$$

where $\|\cdot\|_1$ denotes the l_1-norm of a vector. This vector, in turn can be used as a compact code to represent an image and is suitable for discriminative classification.

In order to capture higher order texture patterns in CLE sequences, we enforce a locality constraint, originally proposed in [18], during the encoding process. The Linear Locality Constraint (LLC) based coding is incorporated into Eqn. 2 as follows:

$$\boldsymbol{c}_i = \arg\min \|\boldsymbol{x}_i - \boldsymbol{B}\boldsymbol{c}_i\|_2^2 + \lambda\|\boldsymbol{d}_i \odot \boldsymbol{c}_i\|_2^2 \quad \text{s.t.} \quad \mathbf{1}^T\boldsymbol{c}_i = 1, \forall i \tag{3}$$

where $\odot$ denotes the element-wise multiplication, and $\boldsymbol{d}_i \in \mathcal{R}^m$ is the locality adapter (Euclidean distance between basis vectors, $\boldsymbol{B}$ and input descriptor $\boldsymbol{x}_i$). Similar to the original sparse coding formulation, the coefficients $\boldsymbol{c}_i$ represent each image and can be used for discriminative classification.

3 Experiments

The global representation of a given frame as achieved using the encoding strategies proposed in Eqns. 1- 3, or [12, 13] is used as input to SVM classifiers.

Data Collection: We use a commercially available clinical endo-microscope on the market called Cellvizio (Mauna Kea Technologies, Paris, France). Cellvizio is a probe-based CLE system. It consists of a laser scanning unit, proprietary software, a flat-panel display and fiber optic probes providing a circular field of view with a diameter of $160\mu m$. The device is intended for imaging the internal microstructure of tissues in the anatomical tract that are accessed by an endoscope. The system is clinically used during an endoscopic procedure for analysis of sub-surface structures of suspicious lesion, which is primarily referred to as optical biopsy [20]. In a surgical resection application, a neurosurgeon inserts a handheld proof into a surgical bed to examine the remainder of the tumor tissue to be resected.

The equipment is used to collect 86 short videos, each from a unique patient suffering from Glioblastoma and 29 relatively longer videos from patients with Meningioma. All videos are captured at 24 frames per second, under a resolution of 464×336. The collection of videos are hereafter being referred to as the Brain Tumor Dataset. Some sample frames are shown in Fig. 1.

Pre-processing: Due to the limited imaging capability of CLE devices or intrinsic properties of brain tumor tissues, the resultant images often contain little categorical information and are not useful for recognition algorithms. Image entropy has been constantly used in the past [21] to quantitatively determine the information content of an image. Specifically, low-entropy images have very little contrast and large runs of pixels with the same or similar values.

Uninformative video frames are discarded using entropy based thresholding. The threshold is determined to be 4.05 after computing gray-level entropies of $34,443$ frames in our dataset. This simple thresholding scheme allows us to select $16,939$ frames containing Glioblastoma and $10,892$ frames containing Meningioma cases, respectively. We select 80% of these, evenly distributed over either classes, for training and the remaining 20% for testing. All experiments report average classification accuracy on 5 such training/ testing splits, ensuring no frame from a training video ending up on the validation split.

Feature Extraction: Low-level feature representation being a decisive factor in almost all automatic image recognition tasks, we systematically evaluate the performance of our encoding method across 4 different feature representations. We employ a dense sampling strategy during the feature extraction phase to ensure a fair comparison across all feature descriptors. From each frame, 500 keypoints are uniformly sampled after applying a circular region of interest (approximately of the same radius as the endoscopic lens). Each keypoint is then described using the following descriptor types: Scale Invariant Feature Transform (SIFT [15]), Oriented FAST and Rotated BRIEF (ORB [16]), Fast Retina Keypoint (FREAK [17]) and finally, Local Binary Patterns (LBP [14]). SIFT captures Spatial Gradient Orientation and encodes these into a histogram which can be represented using a 128 dimensional feature vector. The ORB descriptor smartly samples intensities in a region and encodes their differences in a binary string which is represented using a 32 dimensional feature vector. The FREAK descriptor uses retinal sampling while describing neighboring regions into 64 dimensional feature vector. LBP quantizes intensity differences in a circular neighborhood, accounting for commonly occurring patterns. The resultant feature vector is a 59 dimensional histogram of pattern codes.

In our computational framework, we use freely available implementations of SIFT [15]and LBP [14]from the VLFeat library [1]. We use OpenCV based C++ implementations [2] of the remaining two feature descriptor algorithms.

Baseline:A baseline recognition pipeline, similar to the Bag-of-Words based method proposed in [9], is implemented for a given feature modality as follows: We randomly select 10% of descriptors from the training split and perform k-means ($k = 512$ is empirically determined from one of the training testing split) clustering to construct 4 different vocabularies. Features from each frame are then quantized using these different sets of vocabularies. This baseline is hereafter being referred to as BoW.

[1] `http://www.vlfeat.org/download/vlfeat-0.9.20-bin.tar.gz`

[2] `http://opencv.org/`

In conjunction to the above baseline, we evaluate our method against two independent state-of-the-art feature encoding methods: Super-vector coding (VLAD [13]) and Fisher Kernel (F-K [12]). All frame level representations are used separately to train a two class Support Vector Machine (SVM) [22] with RBF kernel. The optimal parameters of the SVM classifier ($c = 0.81, \gamma = 0.0025$) are selected using coarse-grid search.

4 Results and Discussions

In this section, we present our evaluation in detail. Fig. 3 provides a comprehensive summary of the average accuracy achieved using 5 encoding schemes on 4 stated feature description algorithms. Error bars indicate the variance of accuracy obtained using each approach. Clearly, the proposed locality constraint based encoding method outperforms all other encoding methods, under 3 out of 4 low-level feature description strategies. This empirically argues in favor of our hypothesis that LLC is capable of efficiently capturing the spatial distribution of local texture, which provides vital cues for the tumor classifier.

Among all the encoding strategies evaluated, Fisher Kernel (F-K) based representation is least informative. Also, it is interesting to note how the FAST Oriented and Rotated Brief descriptor, when used in conjunction with LLC, achieves above 90% classification accuracy. This is primarily because the information captured using this descriptor /encoding combination is complementary in nature. While the ORB descriptor captures patch level local gradients efficiently, capturing the spatial proximity between different patches is a highly discriminative cue to identify the nature of either tumors visually.

In Fig. 4 we plot the sensitivity (true positive rate) versus specificity (1-false positive rate) of the algorithms under evaluation. It is evident that, even at a low false alarm rate ($\sim 5\%$) LLC based encoding performs the best with ORB based low-level feature description. This clearly argues in favor of ORB as the feature description, and LLC as the encoding method of choice.

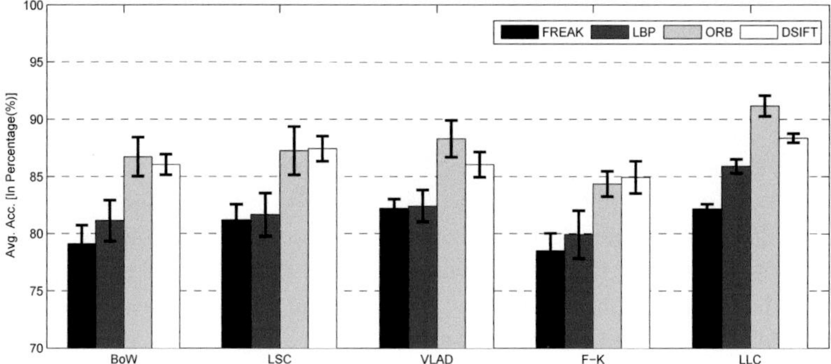

Fig. 3. Average accuracy of various combinations of feature descriptors and encoding strategies. Each group of four bars indicate an encoding strategy, while the individual bar indicates the feature description algorithm used.

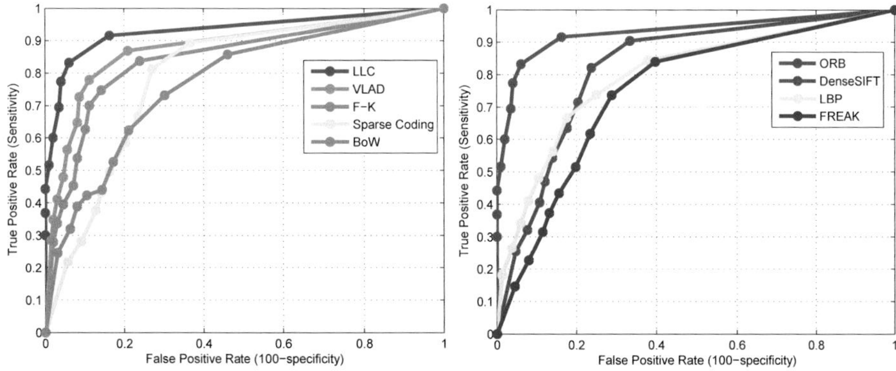

Fig. 4. Receiver operating characteristic curves: The group of curves on the left indicate the recognition performance of different encoding strategies, keeping feature description method [16] constant. On the right, we show the performance of our proposed encoding scheme (LLC) over the different feature description algorithms.

Table 1. Computational speed (in frames per second) of the various feature extraction and representation methods used in our experiments.

Encoding Schemes	Feature Descriptor			
	SIFT [15]	ORB [16]	FREAK [17]	LBP [14]
BoW [9]	19.87	23.1	19.14	20.10
VLAD [13]	11.21	22.2	18.80	21.43
F-K [12]	11.86	22.34	19.21	18.43
LSC	0.15	0.12	0.34	0.23
LLC	15.01	17.71	16.13	18.11

Table 1 gives a coarse estimate of the computational time of the each combination of methods. The numbers indicate processing speed in frames per second as observed in a Intel Quad Core workstation (3.2GHz with 4GB physical memory). Although LLC encoding is not certainly the fastest, it is comparable in terms of speed with the faster encoding methods. The sparse coding scheme without any proximity constraint (LSC), being the slowest of all, is not suited for real-time classification purposes.

5 Conclusion

We presented a comprehensive computational framework capable of performing automatic brain tumor classification in real-time. To this end, we thoroughly evaluated 4 state-of-the-art low-level image features and 4 popular encoding techniques in context of CLE imagery. Additionally, we presented a highly optimized feature pooling method based on codeword proximity. Our proposed system can effectively classify two types of commonly diagnosed brain tumors in CLE sequences captured in real-time with close to 90% accuracy. As part of future work, we intend to investigate better classifier fusion strategies in the existing computational framework.

References

1. Bleeker, F.E., et al.: Recent advances in the molecular understanding of glioblastoma. Journal of Neuro-Oncology 108(1), 11–27 (2012)
2. Lee, J.H., Sade, B.: Meningiomas of the central neuraxis: unique tumors. In: Meningiomas, pp. 157–162 (2009)
3. Lee, E.J., et al.: Two primary brain tumors, meningioma and glioblastoma multiforme, in opposite hemispheres of the same patient. Journal of Clinical Neuroscience 9(5), 589–591 (2002)
4. Paull, P.E., et al.: Confocal laser endomicroscopy: a primer for pathologists. Arch. Pathol. Lab. Med. 135(10), 1343–1348 (2011)
5. André, B., Vercauteren, T., Perchant, A., Buchner, A.M., Wallace, M.B., Ayache, N.: Introducing space and time in local feature-based endomicroscopic image retrieval. In: Caputo, B., Müller, H., Syeda-Mahmood, T., Duncan, J.S., Wang, F., Kalpathy-Cramer, J. (eds.) MCBR-CDS 2009. LNCS, vol. 5853, pp. 18–30. Springer, Heidelberg (2010)
6. Andre, B., et al.: A smart atlas for endomicroscopy using automated video retrieval. Med. Image. Anal. 15(4), 460–476 (2011)
7. Csurka, G., Bray, C., Dance, C., Fan, L.: Visual categorization with bags of keypoints. In: Workshop ECCV, pp. 1–22 (2004)
8. Bauer, S., Nolte, L.-P., Reyes, M.: Fully automatic segmentation of brain tumor images using support vector machine classification in combination with hierarchical conditional random field regularization. In: Fichtinger, G., Martel, A., Peters, T. (eds.) MICCAI 2011, Part III. LNCS, vol. 6893, pp. 354–361. Springer, Heidelberg (2011)
9. Couceiro, S., Barreto, J.P., Freire, P., Figueiredo, P.: Description and classification of confocal endomicroscopic images for the automatic diagnosis of inflammatory bowel disease. In: Wang, F., Shen, D., Yan, P., Suzuki, K. (eds.) MLMI 2012. LNCS, vol. 7588, pp. 144–151. Springer, Heidelberg (2012)
10. Kohandani Tafresh, M., Linard, N., André, B., Ayache, N., Vercauteren, T.: Semi-automated query construction for content-based endomicroscopy video retrieval. In: Golland, P., Hata, N., Barillot, C., Hornegger, J., Howe, R. (eds.) MICCAI 2014, Part I. LNCS, vol. 8673, pp. 89–96. Springer, Heidelberg (2014)
11. Yang, J., Yu, K., Gong, Y., Huang, T.S.: Linear spatial pyramid matching using sparse coding for image classification. In: IEEE CVPR, pp. 1794–1801 (2009)
12. F., Perronnin, Y.L., Sanchez, J., Poirier, H.: Large-scale image retrieval with compressed fisher vectors. In: IEEE VPR, pp. 3384–3391, June 2010
13. Arandjelović, R., Zisserman, A.: All about VLAD. In: IEEE CVPR (2013)
14. Ojala, T., et al.: Multiresolution gray-scale and rotation invariant texture classification with local binary patterns. IEEE TPAMI 24(7), 971–987 (2002)
15. Lowe, D.G.: Distinctive image features from scale-invariant keypoints. IJCV 60(2), 91–110 (2004)

16. Rublee, E., Rabaud, V., Konolige, K., Bradski, G.: Orb: An efficient alternative to sift or surf. In: ICCV, pp. 2564–2571, November 2011
17. Ortiz, R.: Freak: Fast retina keypoint. In: IEEE CVPR, pp. 510–517 (2012)
18. Wang, J., et al.: Locality-constrained linear coding for image classification. In: IEEE CVPR (2010)
19. Nister, D., Stewenius, H.: Scalable recognition with a vocabulary tree. In: IEEE CVPR, pp. 2161–2168 (2006)
20. Hoffman, A., et al.: Confocal laser endomicroscopy: technical status and current indications. Endoscopy 38, 1275–1283 (2006)
21. Gonzalez, R.C., Woods, R.E.: Digital Image Processing. Prentice-Hall, Inc., Upper Saddle River (2008)
22. Chang, C.-C., Lin, C.-J.: LIBSVM: A library for support vector machines. ACM Trans. on Intel. Sys. and Tech. 2, 27:1–27:27 (2011)

Automated Assessment of Surgical Skills Using Frequency Analysis

Aneeq Zia[1], Yachna Sharma[1], Vinay Bettadapura[1], Eric L. Sarin[2], Mark A. Clements[1], and Irfan Essa[1]

[1] Georgia Institute of Technology, Atlanta, GA, USA
[2] Emory University, Atlanta, GA, USA

Abstract. We present an automated framework for visual assessment of the expertise level of surgeons using the OSATS (Objective Structured Assessment of Technical Skills) criteria. Video analysis techniques for extracting motion quality via frequency coefficients are introduced. The framework is tested on videos of medical students with different expertise levels performing basic surgical tasks in a surgical training lab setting. We demonstrate that transforming the sequential time data into frequency components effectively extracts the useful information differentiating between different skill levels of the surgeons. The results show significant performance improvements using DFT and DCT coefficients over known state-of-the-art techniques.

1 Introduction

Timely evaluation and feedback is essential in surgical training. In medical schools, surgical skills are traditionally assessed manually by a supervising surgeon who observes a trainee surgeon performing a procedure. Although, supervision is necessary for resident training, manual evaluation and observing each individual trainee is time consuming and subjective, with known complications [1]. Structured manual grading systems, such as the Objective Structured Assessment of Technical Skills (OSATS) [2] are used in medical schools to alleviate the problem of subjectivity in manual assessments. OSATS covers several assessment criteria such as respect for tissue (RT), time and motion (TM), instrument handling (IH), suture handling (SH), flow of operation (FO), knowledge of procedure (KP) and overall performance (OP). However, manual assessment of each trainee surgeon on a variety of OSATS criteria is still time consuming besides being inherently subjective due to the manual nature of the assessment.

Overall, surgery is a complex task, including, basic surgical skills such as suturing and knot tying that involve hand movements in a repetitive manner. Every surgical resident masters these basic skills before moving on to complicated procedures. Considering the volume of trainees that need to go through basic surgical skills training along with the time consuming and subjective nature of manual OSATS evaluations, automated assessment of these basic surgical skills can be of a huge benefit to medical schools and teaching hospitals.

In this work, we propose a frequency based video analysis system for OSATS assessment of basic surgical skills such as suturing and knot tying. First, we

N. Navab et al. (Eds.): MICCAI 2015, Part I, LNCS 9349, pp. 430–438, 2015.
DOI: 10.1007/978-3-319-24553-9_53

compute motion features from video data of surgeons performing basic surgical tasks to obtain multi-dimensional time series representation of their motions. Then, frequency coefficients of the time series are calculated and used to predict the proficiency level of the surgeon. Our system requires minimal setup, is inexpensive, and is portable for ubiquitous data collection and analysis.

Our contributions are: (1) A novel analysis method of surgical motion without any a priori (and manual) segmentation of the movements; (2) A framework that leverages simple inexpensive equipment with potential for ubiquitous surgical assessment, with easy setup, relieving the time and resource requirements for surgical training in medical schools and; (3) A frequency based analysis method applied to video motion data, which provides better OSATS skill assessment as compared to state-of-the-art techniques.

2 Background

Automated analysis of surgical motion has received attention in recent years [3,4,5,6,7]. The pioneering works addressed skill assessment in robotic minimally invasive surgery (RMIS) [3,4] and proposed techniques for automatic detection and segmentation of robot-assisted surgical motions. The techniques described in these works are specifically for RMIS and laparoscopic surgeries and have not, to our knowledge, addressed the traditional OSATS based trainee evaluation.

Several RMIS works have used Hidden Markov Modeling (HMM) to represent the surgical motion flow. The motivation for HMMs and gesture based analysis is derived from speech recognition techniques and the goal is to develop *a language of surgery* where a surgical task can be modeled as a sequence of predefined gestures (also known as *surgemes* analogous to phonemes in speech recognition). Some recent works such as [3,4] have also used linear dynamical systems (LDS) and bag-of-features (BoF) (or Bag-of-Words (BoW)) for surgical gesture classification.These RMIS works provide background and motivation for our work on surgical skill assessment. However, in this work our focus is on OSATS based skill assessment in traditional setting with trainee surgeons practicing basic surgical skills such as suturing and knot tying.

Our goal is to develop an automated, portable and cost effective assessment system that replicates the traditional OSATS assessment without any manual intervention. Some works based on automated assessment of the OSATS criteria for general surgical training have been proposed recently. In [5], the authors introduced Augmented BoW (A-BoW), in which time and motion are modeled as short sequences of events and the underlying local and global structural information is automatically discovered and encoded into BoW models. They classified surgeons into different skill levels based on the holistic analysis of time series data. In [6], the authors proposed Motion Texture (MT) analysis technique in which each video is represented as a multi-dimensional sequence of motion class counts to obtain a frame kernel matrix. The textural features derived from the frame kernel matrix are used for prediction of OSATS criteria. Although, MT technique provided good OSATS prediction, it is computationally intensive

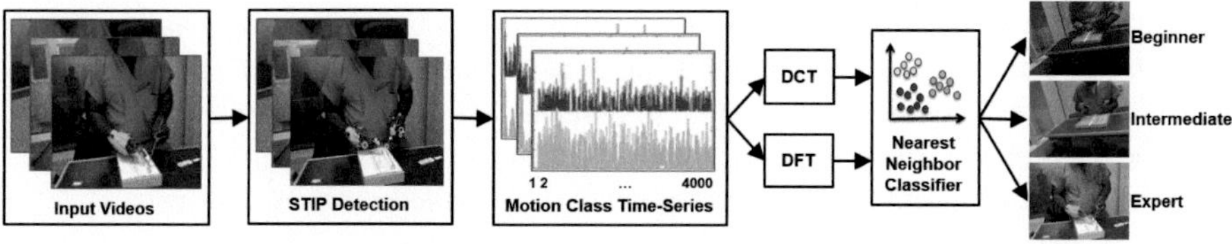

Fig. 1. An overview of our OSATS skill assessment system for suturing and knot tying.

($N \times N$ sized frame kernel matrix for a video with N frames) and does not account for the sequential motion aspects in surgical tasks. A variant of MT, called Sequential Motion Texture (SMT) [7], encoded both the qualitative and sequential motion aspects.

However, none of these past works represent periodic motion elements inherent in basic surgical tasks such as suturing and knot tying. This limitation is addressed in our representation and we show that our proposed method outperforms both traditional techniques like HMMs and the more modern techniques like BoW, A-BoW, MT and SMT.

Some recent skill assessment works in other domains such as competitive sports [8] have used frequency analysis techniques such as Discrete Fourier Transform (DFT) and Discrete Cosine Transform (DCT) to assess the quality of sporting actions. We hypothesize that frequency analysis via DFT and DCT could provide similar results in the assessment of basic surgical skills such as suturing and knot tying due to inherent repetitive motion involved in these tasks.

3 Framework for Skill Assessment

The sequential and repetitive nature of basic surgical tasks such as suturing and knot tying results in an inherent dependency on consecutive time series samples. To reveal this time dependency and repetitiveness, we encode the video motion information into a time series, which is then analyzed by using two different frequency analysis methods (DCT and DFT). Our technique involves the following steps: (1) Computing motion features from video data; (2) Generating a time-series from motion features; (3) Computing frequency coefficients of the extracted time series; (4) Selecting the optimum frequencies distinguishing the three skill levels and classifying the skill level of the surgeon. Figure 1 shows the flow diagram of our system. We describe each of these steps in detail:

Step 1: Extraction of motion information from video data: We use computer vision based local features such as Spatio-Temporal Interest Points (STIPs) that have been shown to work well in action classification [9,10] tasks. Let V be the set containing all videos in our dataset. For all $v \in V$, we use a Harris3D detector to compute the spatio-temporal second-moment matrix μ at each video point (using independent spatial and temporal scales, a separable Gaussian smoothing function and space-time gradients). The final location of the STIPs are given by the local maxima of $H = \det(\mu)$ - $k\text{trace}^3(\mu)$ with a standard parameter setting of $k = 0.0005$ as per the original implementation [10]. Then we compute 162-element HoG-HoF (histogram of oriented gradients-histogram of optical flow) descriptors $\forall v \in V$ as described in [10].

Step 2: Transformation of motion data into time-series: We use two expert videos for motion class learning (via K-means clustering) since expert motions provide exemplary templates of the surgical task to be evaluated. The learned clusters essentially represent the different moving parts in the video which include arms and tool of the surgeon. For each remaining video, we assign its STIPs to one of the K motion classes learnt by clustering expert videos using minimum Mahalanobis distance. This gives a time series $S \in \Re^{K \times N}$, where N is the number of frames in the video and each element $S(k, n)$ represents the number of STIPs belonging to the nth frame and the kth cluster.

Step 3: Frequency analysis: Recent works such as [8] have used frequency coefficients in assessing the quality of competitive sports, like diving and ice-skating. Since the basic surgical tasks of suturing and knot tying are inherently repetitive in nature, the use of frequency coefficients would essentially be effective in extracting the useful information differentiating between the different skill levels of the surgeons. We use DCT and DFT to obtain frequency coefficients as follows: Let $s_k \in \Re^N$ be the kth dimension of the time series S. We calculate the frequency coefficient vector $\Theta_k \in \Re^N$ by evaluating the expression $\Theta_k = (F s_k^T)^T$ for $k \in [1, 2, \ldots, K]$, where $F \in \Re^{N \times N}$ representing the discrete Cosine/Fourier transformation matrix. For DFT, each element of the transformation matrix is given by $F(m, n) = e^{-j2\pi \frac{mn}{N}}$ for $m \in [0, 1, \ldots, N-1]$ whereas, for DCT, $F(0, n) = \sqrt{\frac{1}{N}}$ and $F(m, n) = \sqrt{\frac{2}{N}} cos(\frac{\pi(2n+1)m}{2N})$ for $m \in [1, 2, \ldots, N-1]$. All the Θ_k's are then concatenated vertically to produce a feature matrix $\Theta \in \Re^{K \times N}$, where each entry in the matrix $\Theta(k, n)$ represents the nth frequency coefficient of the kth dimension of the time series S. Since higher frequencies are likely a result of noisy or abrupt movements, we use the lowest D frequencies producing a reduced sized feature matrix $\bar{\Theta} \in \Re^{K \times D}$. The value of D was then selected empirically depending on the classification accuracy and computation time. The rows of the reduced feature matrix $\bar{\Theta}$ were then concatenated horizontally giving a feature vector $\phi \in \Re^{KD}$ representing the video.

Step 4: Feature selection and skill classification: Since all DCT and DFT frequency coefficients may not be relevant for skill assessment, we perform feature selection to determine a subset of skill defining frequency coefficients. We use Sequential Forward Feature Selection (SFFS) [11] to select a subset of relevant features for each OSATS criteria giving a final feature vector $\hat{\phi} \in \Re^P$, where P is the number of features selected by SFFS. We use a Nearest-Neighbor (NN) classifier with cosine distance metric as a wrapper function for SFFS and select a subset of features with minimum classification error in leave-one-out cross-validation (LOOCV) as reported in [5,7,6].

4 Experimental Evaluation

Data Acquisition: We recruited 18 participants (surgical residents and nurse practitioners) to collect data for skill evaluation using a standard off-the-shelf

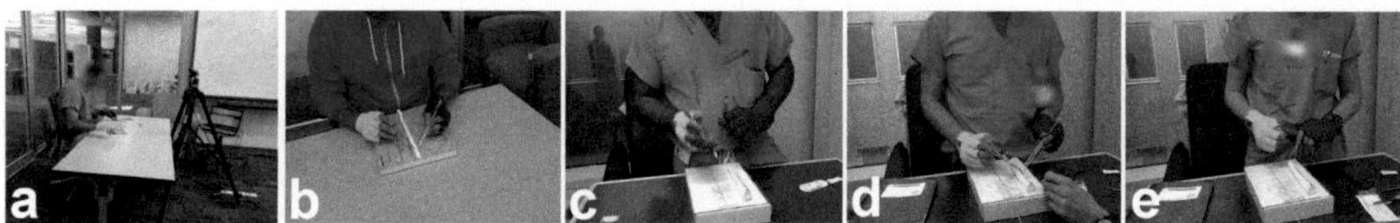

Fig. 2. (a) Setup for data acquisition, (b-e) Sample frames for suturing and knot tying

camera. The camera was mounted on a tripod and the participants performed the surgical task wearing colored finger-less gloves. Figure 2 shows the set up for data acquisition along with a few sample frames with participants performing the two surgical tasks. The videos were acquired at 30 frames per second.

We collected two instances for the suturing and knot tying task from each participant, resulting in 36 videos for knot tying and 35 videos for suturing (one video discarded due to data corruption). The number of frames for each video was 4000 for suturing and 1000 for knot tying with the RGB resolution of 640×480 pixels. The videos were captured with varying camera positions and in different rooms to make the dataset invariant to view and illumination changes.

The videos were viewed by an expert (Professor and MD of Surgery and Surgical Translational Studies) who provided the ground-truth OSATS scores. A beginner was given a score of 1, an intermediate was given a score of 2 and an expert was given a score of 3. The distribution of the different skill levels for each OSATS criteria is given in Table 1.

Comparison with State-of-the-Art: All the experiments were performed using leave-one-out cross-validation (LOOCV). We evaluated our proposed technique against five previously published methods: traditional Hidden Markov Models (HMM) and more modern approaches such as Bag of Words (BoW), Augmented-BoW (A-BoW), Motion Textures (MT) and Sequential Motion Texture (SMT).

HMM: Our HMM employed semi-continuous modeling with Gaussian mixture models (GMM) as feature space representations. The $K \times N$ time series was converted into a vector of discrete symbols using k-means with $k \in [3, \ldots, 10]$ and the GMMs were derived by means of an unsupervised density learning procedure.The HMM model is based on linear left-right topologies and are trained

Table 1. Distribution of skill levels for different OSATS criteria (Suturing|Knot Tying). NA corresponds to either samples not available or the respective OSATS criteria being not applicable for the task (explained in results section)

	RT	TM	IH	SH	FO	OP
Beginner	5 | NA	13 | 6	13 | NA	14 | 5	12 | 2	NA | 2
Intermediate	20 | NA	11 | 12	10 | NA	13 | 17	14 | 19	NA | 17
Expert	10 | NA	11 | 18	12 | NA	8 | 14	9 | 15	NA | 17

Abbreviations: RT: Respect for Tissue, TM: Time and Motion, IH: Instrument Handling, SH: Suture Handling, FO: Flow of Operation, OP: Overall Performance.

using classical Baum-Welch training. Classification is pursued using Viterbi-decoding. HMMs with 4, 8, 10, 12 and 14 states were trained and used in the experiments. Classification results were obtained for all possible combinations of states and symbols. A final model with 4 states and 7 symbols was empirically selected. We use a discrete HMM instead of a continuous one in order to have a fair comparison with some of the state-of-the-art methods used in surgical skill evaluation. However, a continuous HMM could also be used in which the observation sequence would simply be the $K \times N$ time series matrix.

BoW/A-BoW: While BoW approaches are good at building powerful and sparser representations of the data, they ignore the ordering information of the particular words and disregard the underlying temporal information. The A-BoW approach [5] attempts to solve this by quantizing time into N bins and encoding them into bag-of-words models using n-grams. We used the BoW and A-BoW code publicly available using the values of $n = 3$ and $N = 5$.

MT/SMT: Motion Texture [6] and Sequential Motion Texture [7] were implemented as proposed in the original papers. As described for OSATS assessment and for computational simplicity, Gray Level Co-Occurrence Matrices (GLCM) texture features with 8 gray levels were used for both MT and SMT. For SMT, the number of windows was set to 10 (determined empirically).

DCT/DFT: We use the DCT coefficients in their original form. However, since the DFT coefficients are complex numbers, we only use their magnitudes in the feature matrix. Once the feature matrix $\Theta \in \Re^{K \times N}$ of the frequency coefficients is obtained, we reduce the number of features by using only the lowest 50 frequency coefficients ($D = 50$) in each dimension of the time series giving the $50K$-dimensional feature vector. Due to a relatively small dataset and to avoid over-fitting, we further reduce the number of features using SFFS feature selection. The number of selected features was empirically set to 30. It was observed that including frequency coefficients greater than 50 (for each dimension) and number of final features greater than 30 did not result in any substantial improvement in the classification accuracy.

5 Results and Discussion

We report the skill classification accuracies of surgeons performing basic surgical tasks of suturing and knot tying for the OSATS criteria applicable and used for each task, except Knowledge of Procedure (KP). KP was excluded since suturing and knot tying are both repetitive tasks and are not procedures with technical progression. Hence, there really is no knowledge component to assess in these tasks. Figure 3 shows the heat maps generated for the classification accuracies for different OSATS criteria using all 7 techniques described and for all the values of K in the motion count time-series. We can see a clear improvement when moving from left to right (HMM to DCT) for all the OSATS criteria and for both the surgical tasks. But overall, all the techniques seem to work well for $K = 6$ and hence those results are presented in Table 2.

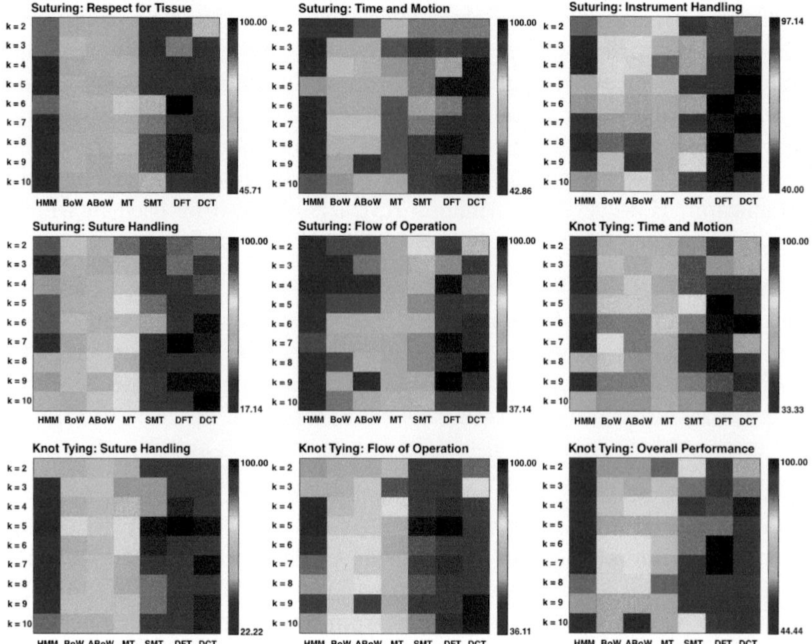

Fig. 3. Heatmaps showing the classification accuracies for the different OSATS criterion for Suturing and Knot Tying. The columns show the proposed DFT and DCT methods and the 5 other method that they are compared against (for the various K in the motion count time-series). We can see a clear improvement in accuracies from left to right (from HMM to DCT).

In Table 2, the first number corresponds to suturing and the second to knot tying. Some OSATS are not applicable to the knot tying tasks (shown as NA in Table 2) e.g. IH (third column) since there was no instrument used. Suturing scores for OP were not available. For almost all the OSATS criteria, the use of DCT and DFT significantly improves the classification accuracy for both the surgical tasks as compared to the state-of-the-art methods.

The basic surgical tasks of suturing and knot tying are both sequential periodic activities. An expert surgeon seems to do much more of a task in a given time as compared to a beginner. Thinking in terms of a signal, the expert 'signal' will have a different frequency as compared to a beginner or intermediate. Our technique exploits the periodicity of the two surgical tasks and successfully extracts the frequency coefficients to distinguish the three skill levels of the surgeons. Our technique is also computationally less expensive as compared to SMT which gives reasonably good results too. SMT divides the time series into windows and uses texture analysis on a self-similarity matrix which is computationally expensive. Our technique does not require complex texture analysis and dividing the time-series into windows. One should note that our method is designed for basic repetitive type of surgical motions. For other non-repetitive

Table 2. Percentage of correctly classified subjects (suturing | knot tying) for $K = 6$

Method	RT	TM	IH	SH	FO	OP
HMM	60.0 | NA	48.5 | 36.1	57.1 | NA	37.1 | 36.1	48.5 | 47.2	NA | 44.4
BoW	65.7 | NA	62.8 | 83.3	71.4 | NA	60.0 | 58.3	60.0 | 75.0	NA | 80.5
A-BoW	65.7 | NA	62.8 | 83.3	65.7 | NA	57.1 | 61.1	60.0 | 75.0	NA | 80.5
MT	77.1 | NA	57.1 | 77.7	60.0 | NA	60.0 | 69.4	60.0 | 63.8	NA | 75.0
SMT	82.8 | NA	82.8 | 83.3	80.0 | NA	74.2 | **94.4**	68.5 | 86.1	NA | 86.1
DFT	**100** | NA	85.7 | 97.2	**97.1** | NA	88.5 | 91.6	91.4 | 88.8	NA | **100**
DCT	91.4 | NA	**94.2** | **100**	94.2 | NA	**97.1** | 91.4	**94.2** | **91.4**	NA | 91.4

Abbreviations: RT: Respect for Tissue, TM: Time and Motion, IH: Instrument Handling, SH: Suture Handling, FO: Flow of Operation, OP: Overall Performance.

tasks, frequency based features could be used along with other feature types that are not dependent upon periodicity of the task.

In Summary, we present an automated framework for surgical skill assessment. Using our technique, we classified surgical residents and nurse practitioners into different OSATS skill groups. Our method enables skill assessment without using time windowing, texture analysis or manually defined surgical gestures. The proposed system is simple, easy to setup and is cost effective to deploy.

References

1. Dennis, B.M., Long, E.L., Zamperini, K.M., Nakayama, D.K.: The effect of the 16-hour intern workday restriction on surgical residents' in-hospital activities. Journal of Surgical Education 70(6), 800–805 (2013)
2. Martin, J., Regehr, G., Reznick, R., MacRae, H., Murnaghan, J., Hutchison, C., Brown, M.: Objective structured assessment of technical skill (osats) for surgical residents. British Journal of Surgery 84(2), 273–278 (1997)
3. Béjar Haro, B., Zappella, L., Vidal, R.: Surgical gesture classification from video data. In: Ayache, N., Delingette, H., Golland, P., Mori, K. (eds.) MICCAI 2012, Part I. LNCS, vol. 7510, pp. 34–41. Springer, Heidelberg (2012)
4. Zappella, L., Béjar, B., Hager, G., Vidal, R.: Surgical gesture classification from video and kinematic data. Medical Image Analysis 17(7), 732–745 (2013)
5. Bettadapura, V., Schindler, G., Plötz, T., Essa, I.: Augmenting bag-of-words: Data-driven discovery of temporal and structural information for activity recognition. In: IEEE VPR (2013)
6. Sharma, Y., Plötz, T., Hammerla, N., Mellor, S., Roisin, M., Olivier, P., Deshmukh, S., McCaskie, A., Essa, I.: Automated surgical OSATS prediction from videos. In: IEEE ISBI (2014)
7. Sharma, Y., Bettadapura, V., Plötz, T., Hammerla, N., Mellor, S., McNaney, R., Olivier, P., Deshmukh, S., McCaskie, A., Essa, I.: Video based assessment of OSATS using sequential motion textures. In: International Workshop on Modeling and Monitoring of Computer Assisted Interventions (M2CAI)-Workshop (2014)

8. Pirsiavash, H., Vondrick, C., Torralba, A.: Assessing the quality of actions. In: Fleet, D., Pajdla, T., Schiele, B., Tuytelaars, T. (eds.) ECCV 2014, Part VI. LNCS, vol. 8694, pp. 556–571. Springer, Heidelberg (2014)
9. Laptev, I., Marszalek, M., Schmid, C., Rozenfeld, B.: Learning realistic human actions from movies. In: IEEE CVPR, pp. 1–8 (2008)
10. Wang, H., Ullah, M.M., Kläser, A., Laptev, I., Schmid, C.: Evaluation of local spatio-temporal features for action recognition. In: BMVC (2009)
11. Pudil, P., Novovičová, J., Kittler, J.: Floating search methods in feature selection. Pattern Recognition Letters 15(11), 1119–1125 (1994)

Robust Live Tracking of Mitral Valve Annulus for Minimally-Invasive Intervention Guidance

Ingmar Voigt[1], Mihai Scutaru[2], Tommaso Mansi[3], Bogdan Georgescu[3], Noha El-Zehiry[3], Helene Houle[4], and Dorin Comaniciu[3]

[1] Imaging and Computer Vision, Siemens Corporate Technology, Erlangen, Germany
[2] Imaging and Computer Vision, Siemens Corporate Technology, Brasov, Romania
[3] Imaging and Computer Vision, Siemens Corporate Technology, Princeton, NJ
[4] Siemens Corporation, Healthcare Clinical Products, Ultrasound

Abstract. Mitral valve (MV) regurgitation is an important cardiac disorder that affects 2-3% of the Western population. While valve repair is commonly performed under open-heart surgery, an increasing number of transcatheter MV repair (TMVR) strategies are being developed. To be successful, TMVR requires extensive image guidance due to the complexity of MV physiology and of the therapies, in particular during device deployment. New trans-esophageal echocardiography (TEE) enable real-time, full-volume imaging of the valve including 3D anatomy and 3D color-Doppler flow. Such new transducers open a large range of applications for TMVR guidance, like the 3D assessment of the impact of a therapy on the MV function. In this manuscript we propose an algorithm towards the goal of live quantification of the MV anatomy. Leveraging the recent advances in ultrasound hardware, and combining machine learning approaches, predictive search strategies and efficient image-based tracking algorithms, we propose a novel method to automatically detect and track the MV annulus over very long image sequences. The method was tested on 12 4D TEE annotated sequences acquired in patients suffering from a large variety of disease. These sequences have been rigidly transformed to simulate probe motion. Obtained results showed a tracking accuracy of 4.04mm mean error, while demonstrating robustness when compared to purely image based methods. Our approach therefore paves the way towards quantitative guidance of TMVR through live 3D valve modeling.

1 Introduction

The mitral valve (MV), which ensures the unidirectional flow from the left atrium (LA) to the left ventricle (LV), is often affected by heart failure or degenerative diseases [5]. One particular MV pathology is MV regurgitation, where the valve does not close properly and blood can flow back to the LA. Following the success of transcatheter aortic valve repair, transcatheter mitral valve repair (TMVR) strategies are being explored by the medical industry. MitraClip™ is today an established treatment, but approaches for minimally-invasive annuloplasty or

N. Navab et al. (Eds.): MICCAI 2015, Part I, LNCS 9349, pp. 439–446, 2015.
DOI: 10.1007/978-3-319-24553-9_54

complete valve repair are being developed [1]. The MV physiology brings important challenges to solve: MV anatomy is more complex than the aortic valve, including papillaries, chordae, complex leaflets geometry and non-symmetrical annulus. The pathologies are also more heterogeneous. For these reasons, advanced, quantitative 3D imaging is required during TMVR.

So far TMVR imaging guidance is mostly performed under 2D trans-esophageal echocardiography (TEE), since high-temporal resolution and color flow quantification are required for a complete monitoring of device deployment and its impact on MV function. Recent breakthroughs in ultrasound hardware have made possible to acquire non-stitched, full-volume 3D images at high frame-rates while combining both anatomical images (B-mode) and color-flow Doppler [5]. Such new probes pave the way to 3D TMVR guidance through MV physiology imaging, which would make the current therapies easier to perform, but also opening new therapeutic possibilities. One requirement is to have live and continuous 3D MV modeling, quantification and tracking within the interventional setup.

Several approaches for MV modeling from 3D TEE have been proposed in the past [4,8,10]. Yet, all of them still require from seconds to minutes to process a single frame and are therefore not adapted for continuous, live 3D valve modeling. At the same time, very efficient object tracking methods have been developed in other fields. In [3] for instance, a graph-based approach was proposed to track devices in 2D X-ray images. In [6], the authors propose a real-time tracking of four MV annulus landmarks from 2D TEE. To the best of our knowledge, no solution is able to track and model the complete MV annulus continuously in live 3D TEE images.

This paper proposes an approach towards live, continuous 3D MV annulus modeling from 3D TEE to support TMVR. Tracking a structure in live images requires a fast but accurate algorithm (10-15 or more frame per seconds) that does not drift over time. To cope with potentially large deformations due to probe motion, a combination of machine-learning based detection algorithm and fast optical flow tracking method is employed, which both leverage non-stitch, full-volume 3D TEE imaging (Sec. 2). The method was tested on 12 synthetic sequences (up to 46s-long) obtained by concatenating fully annotated 3D TEE data acquired in patients, which are continuously deformed according to random rigid deformations that mimicked probe motion (Sec. 3). Our approach achieved a point-to-mesh accuracy of 4.04mm (3978 frames in total) at a frame-rate of 12.5fps. Sec. 4 concludes the manuscript.

2 Methods

The proposed approach combines two components that complement each other in robustness and speed (Fig. 1): 1) a **learning-based detector** of MV location, pose and size as well as landmarks and annulus, which is robust to image alterations from transducer motion (image translation and rotation from probe flexing) and artifacts; and 2) an **optical-flow tracker**, which is capable of running at high frame rates, implements a key-frame approach for drift control while obtaining smooth and temporally-consistent motion estimates.

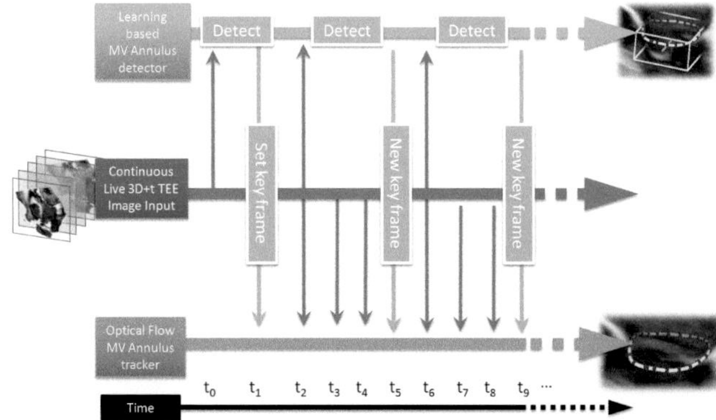

Fig. 1. System Overview. A continuous stream of images (**blue**) is being processed by two system components in parallel: a high frame rate optical flow tracker (**orange**), which is periodically re-initialized by a robust learning-based annulus detector (**green**).

The two components, described in details in the following sections, are run in parallel. On system initialization, the detector component starts and determines valve presence in the ultrasound image. If the valve is found, the detector estimates the MV annulus curve, which is transfered to the flow tracker component for high frame-rate anatomy tracking. Subsequent images are being processed in parallel, i.e. the optical flow tracker processes each new image, while the detector runs in a separate thread to periodically re-detect valve presence and annulus, which is then fed back into the tracker to achieve robustness to large motion and ensure continuous control of tracking drift.

2.1 Mitral Valve Annulus Detector

The MV annulus detector is composed of a series of learning-based elements, as illustrated in Fig. 2. Learning-based detectors D_{rigid} of MV presence, location, orientation and size, as well as detectors of annulus landmarks and curve $D_{annulus}$, estimate model parameters $\phi_{rigid}(t)$ and $\phi_{annulus}(t)$ for an image $I(t)$ by maximizing the posterior probability p modeled by probabilistic boosting tree (PBT) [9] classifiers, $\phi(t) = argmax_{\phi} p(\phi|I(t))$. PBT classifiers are trained with Haar-like and steerable features from a manually generated database of ground truth locations of MV annulus and landmarks.

On system initialization, D_{rigid} is evaluated on the entire volume $I(t_0)$ using efficient search along increasing dimensionality of the parameter space employing the framework of marginal space learning (MSL) [11]. The search on the complete volume is repeated for subsequent images $I(t_1...t_n)$ until the MV is detected with high confidence ($p(\phi_{rigid}(t)) \geq 0.85$) on at least three consecutive images. Then the MV is assumed to be present within the volume and a region of interest (ROI) $\Phi_{rigid}(t)$ is computed from the three last estimates to reduce the computational demand for estimating valve location. For subsequent detector invocations $t >$

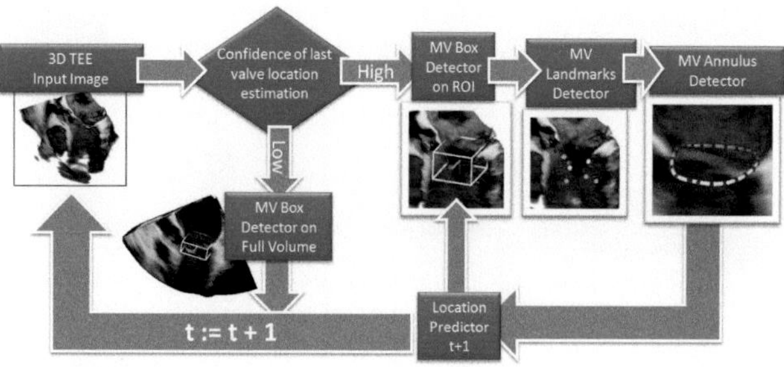

Fig. 2. Learning based hierarchical detector pipeline: on initialization the detector of MV presence, location, orientation and scale (box detector) runs on the full volume until at least three consecutive iterations were detected with high confidence estimates. Assuming MV presence, an ROI is computed and used for reducing the computational load. The ROI is updated at each iteration to account for probe motion.

t_n, D_{rigid} is estimated by searching only within that ROI until the estimator confidence drops, i.e. $p(\phi_{rigid}(t)) < 0.85$, where the process is automatically reinitialized, i.e. runs again on the full volume.

To be robust to potential transducer motion, at each detector invocation a predictor P_{rigid} estimates the valve location for the next time the detector is invoked and updates the ROI center accordingly. In this work, P_{rigid} is empirically defined as the average trajectory over the last six iterations:

$$\Phi_{rigid}(t+1) = P_{rigid}(\phi_{rigid}) = \sum_{t-6}^{t} (\phi_{rigid}(t) - \phi_{rigid}(t-1)) \tag{1}$$

Following the estimation of the rigid paramaters ϕ_{rigid}, $D_{annulus}$ detects anatomically defined landmarks – namely the left and right trigones as well as the postero-annular midpoint – by scanning respective classifiers over search ranges within ϕ_{rigid}. Finally the annulus is initialized as a closed curve by fitting a mean annulus shape composed of 58 points to the previously detected landmarks using thin plate splines (TPS). Specially trained PBT classifiers are evaluated by sampling the volume along planes that are transversal to the annulus curve at each curve point. The resulting curve $\phi_{annulus}(t)$ is spatially constrained using a point distribution shape model [2].

2.2 Optical Flow Key Frame Tracker

The optical flow key-frame tracker is a composite of two ordinary Lukas Kanade optical flow trackers [7]: a sequential tracker T_{seq}, which tracks landmarks from $I(t-1)$ to $I(t)$ and a second non-sequential key-frame tracker T_{key}, which registers the landmark defined on a past key frame $I(t_k < t)$ to the current frame $I(t)$. The estimation results of both trackers are averaged to obtain the final estimate. In this way the tracker obtains smooth motion (via the frame by frame

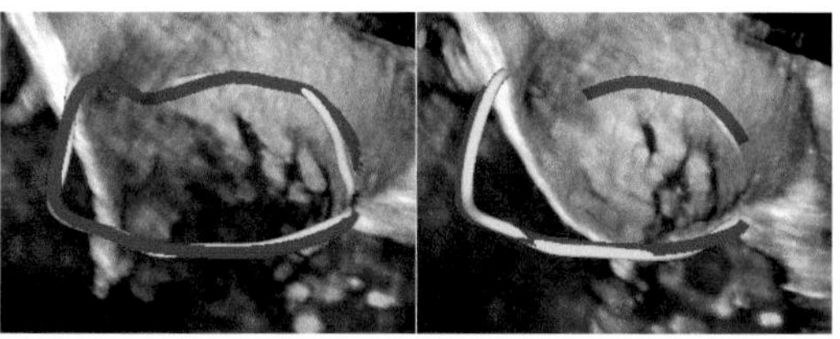

Fig. 3. Detection results for Mitral Valve annulus with 1.25mm mean error; yellow - ground truth, red: detector output

component T_{seq}) while reducing drift across cardiac cycles (via the key frame component T_{key}). The tracker estimates higher order terms iteratively by creating a warped image $I^1(t-1)$ out of the template image $I^0(t-1) = I(t-1)$ by applying the previously estimated motion vector field u^0 at locations x

$$\begin{aligned} I^1(x, t-1) &= I^0(x + u^0, t-1) \\ \mathbf{M^1} u^1 &= b^1 \\ u^0 &:= u^0 + u^1 \end{aligned}$$

with $\mathbf{M^1}$ and b^1 computed from derivatives over space and time [7]. The scheme is repeated over six iterations, which was experimentally determined as point of convergence. In order to achieve high frame rates, the tracker runs directly on the spherical coordinate representation of the ultrasound image (acoustic space). Although the error is expected to increase with the distance to the transducer array due to the anisotropic image sampling, that limitation does not hinder our application as the mitral valve is typically located 50-70mm away from the transducer array, where the voxel distance is typically 1.2mm in the spherical coordinates representation of the image (assuming a typical angular resolution of about 1.3 degrees).

As the runtime of the detectors D (0.18 sec) exceeds the processing time of the optical flow trackers T (0.08 sec), both are run in parallel. The trackers are reinitialized each time the detector completes processing, by setting the respective annulus detection result $\phi_{annulus}(t_{key})$ and corresponding image $I(t_{key})$ as key frame for T_{key}, while T_{seq} restarts sequential tracking from the frame that D has finished at. For instance, following Fig. 1, let D start processing at time t_2 and complete at time t_5. The new key frame is set $t_{key} = t_2$ and T_{seq} restarts tracking by computing optical flow using $I(t_2)$, $I(t_6)$ and $\phi_{annulus}(t_2)$. While this means cardiac motion occurs in between t_2 and t_5, we observed that the annulus motion within 0.18s is typically small.

3 Experiments and Results

For our experiments, the detectors were implemented using CUDA version 3.2 and executed on a test machine using an nVidia Quadro K2100M graphics card, an Intel Core i7-4800MQ 2.70GHz processor and 16GB of RAM.

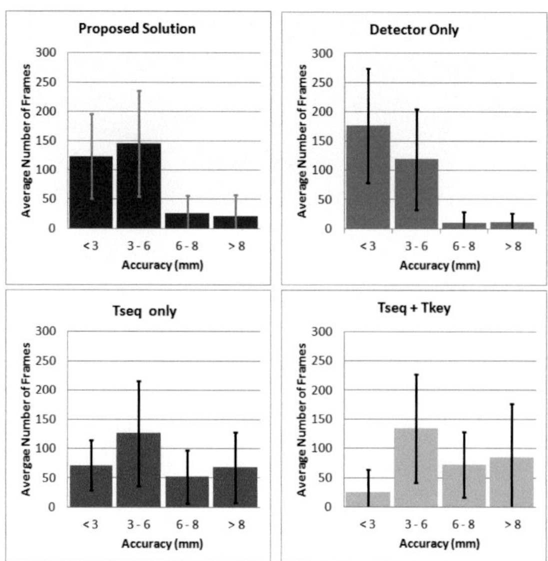

Fig. 4. Average error distributions over the testing set illustrated by error histograms for the proposed approach as well as isolated components. While the detector component operates with bounded error, the tracker components T_{seq} and T_{key} are subject to drift as can be seen by the higher number of error samples in histogram bins above 6mm error. Through the combination of all techniques, the proposed approach obtains the similar robustness as the detector while achieving the same frame rates an optical flow tracker

3.1 Dataset

The detector components were trained on 800 3D+t TEE volume sequences. To allow quantitative and thorough evaluation, the algorithm was fed with ever-looping recorded data from a separate set of 12 3D+t TEE volume sequences. The sets were manually annotated by an expert by manually fitting MV annulus ground truth models into the image data.

To test the method in operating room (OR) like conditions, the data were manipulated with rigid transformations that simulated probe motion based on the degrees of freedom that are typically observed during a clinical exam, i.e. transducer rotation along roll and yaw angles by 15 degrees (rotating and flexing) as well as shifts of 60mm collinear with the probe shaft (displacement along esophagus). The resulting sequences, obtained by looping, altering and concatenating an original sequence 26 times, ranged between 182 and 728 frames with frame rate between 5 to 32 fps, covering a total duration of 33 to 46 seconds. The volumes covered fields of view between $83° \times 81° \times 77$mm to $91° \times 90° \times 141$mm, typically covering both valves or mitral valve as well left and right ventricles. In total the resulting testing set comprised 3978 annotated 3D frames.

Table 1. Overall MV Annulus estimation accuracy reported in terms of mean ± std dev over the complete testing set.

Proposed approach	Detector only	$T_{seq} + T_{key}$	T_{seq} only
4.04±1.06 mm	3.37±0.69 mm	6.57±2.04 mm	5.28±1.19 mm

3.2 Quantitative Evaluation

For a quantitative analysis of the method, we evaluated the overall accuracy as well as tracking drift over time. Fig. 3 shows an example of ground truth annulus curve and obtained estimation result. As an accuracy metric the distance was computed from each point of the estimated MV annulus curve to the respective ground truth curve and vice versa, and finally averaged over the curve. Table 1 reports the overall accuracy of the proposed approach as well as detector and tracker components independently. The accuracy of the proposed approach ranges within the accuracy of the detector, the tracking components are subject to higher errors, due to drift. While the detector components ran with constant error and followed the probe motion, the trackers were subject to error accumulation over time, particularly in the presence of probe motion. This fact is particularly highlighted in Fig. 4, where the error distribution for the same categories showed significant amounts of outliers for the tracker only based approaches as a consequence of drift and changes in image appearance over time. On the other hand the detector ran at an average frame rate of 5.5fps, hence was not able to keep up with the imaging capabilities of state-of-the-art 4D imaging hardware. In contrast the tracker components operated at an average frame rate of 12.5fps, which is near interactive. Combining the two techniques, our approach was hence able to operate at high frame rates (12.5fps), while obtaining the same level of robustness as the detector, being robust to noise and probe motion.

Finally we evaluated the average accuracy of the acoustic space tracking vs. Cartesian space tracking (same algorithm, but on Cartesian grids), particularly knowing that the tracking error could increase with the distance to the transducer array due to the non-linear acoustic sampling space. Both techniques exhibited similar performances with average errors of 4.36±2.2mm (Cartesian space tracking) vs. 4.13±1.43 (acoustic space tracking).

4 Conclusion

This paper presented an approach for robust tracking of MV annulus from 3D+t TEE volumetric data at high frame rates. It combines robust machine learning methods with image based tracking, hence enabling for robust live tracking within an interventional setting, where ultrasound imaging is subject to constant changes of the field of view and motion. The approach was tested on a set of 3978 3D image frames generated out of 12 volume sequences of patient data, which included simulated probe motion to test the method in an operating room like setting. Reaching high frame rates and robustness, our approach enables real-time quantitative assessment of therapies and their impact on MV function, and could thus benefit emerging therapies such as TMVR.

Acknowledgement. This paper is supported by the Sectoral Operational Programme Human Resources Development (SOP HRD), ID134378 financed from the European Social Fund and by the Romanian Government.

References

1. Anyanwu, A.C., Adams, D.H.: Transcatheter mitral valve replacement: The next revolution? Journal of the American College of Cardiology 64(17), 1820–1824 (2014)
2. Cootes, T.F., Taylor, C.J., Cooper, D.H., Graham, J.: Active shape models—their training and application. Comput. Vis. Image Underst. 61(1), 38–59 (1995)
3. Heibel, H., Glocker, B., Groher, M., Pfister, M., Navab, N.: Interventional tool tracking using discrete optimization. IEEE Trans. Med. Imag.
4. Ionasec, R.I., Voigt, I., Georgescu, B., Wang, Y., Houle, H., Vega-Higuera, F., Navab, N., Comaniciu, D.: Patient-Specific Modeling and Quantification of the Aortic and Mitral Valves From 4-D Cardiac CT and TEE. IEEE Transactions on Medical Imaging 29(9), 1636–1651 (2010)
5. Lancellotti, P., Zamorano, J.-L., Vannan, M.A.: Imaging challenges in secondary mitral regurgitation unsolved issues and perspectives. Circulation: Cardiovascular Imaging 7(4), 735–746 (2014)
6. Li, F.P., Rajchl, M., Moore, J., Peters, T.M.: A mitral annulus tracking approach for navigation of off-pump beating heart mitral valve repair. Medical Physics 42 (2015)
7. Paragios, N., Chen, Y., Faugeras, O. (eds.): Mathematical Models in Computer Vision: The Handbook, chap. 15, pp. 239–258. Springer (2005)
8. Schneider, R.J., Perrin, D.P., Vasilyev, N.V., Marx, G.R., Pedro, J., Howe, R.D.: Mitral annulus segmentation from four-dimensional ultrasound using a valve state predictor and constrained optical flow. Medical Image Analysis 16(2), 497–504 (2012)
9. Tu, Z.: Probabilistic boosting-tree: Learning discriminative models for classification, recognition, and clustering. In: 10th IEEE International Conference on Computer Vision (ICCV 2005), Beijing, China, October 17–20, pp. 1589–1596 (2005). `http://doi.ieeecomputersociety.org/10.1109/ICCV.2005.194`
10. Weber, F.M., Stehle, T., Waechter-Stehle, I., Götz, M., Peters, J., Mollus, S., Balzer, J., Kelm, M., Weese, J.: Analysis of mitral valve motion in 4D transesophageal echocardiography for transcatheter aortic valve implantation. In: Camara, O., Mansi, T., Pop, M., Rhode, K., Sermesant, M., Young, A. (eds.) STACOM 2014. LNCS, vol. 8896, pp. 168–176. Springer, Heidelberg (2015)
11. Zheng, Y., Georgescu, B., Ling, H., Zhou, S.K., Scheuering, M., Comaniciu, D.: Constrained marginal space learning for efficient 3d anatomical structure detection in medical images. In: 2009 IEEE Computer Society Conference on Computer Vision and Pattern Recognition (CVPR 2009), Miami, Florida, USA, June 20–25, pp. 194–201 (2009). `http://dx.doi.org/10.1109/CVPRW.2009.5206807`

Motion-Aware Mosaicing for Confocal Laser Endomicroscopy

Jessie Mahé[1,*], Nicolas Linard[1*], Marzieh Kohandani Tafreshi[1,2], Tom Vercauteren[3], Nicholas Ayache[2], Francois Lacombe[1], and Remi Cuingnet[1]

[1] Mauna Kea Technologies, Paris, France
[2] Inria Asclepios Project-Team, Sophia Antipolis, France
[3] Translational Imaging Group, University College London, London, UK

Abstract. Probe-based Confocal Laser Endomicroscopy (pCLE) provides physicians with real-time access to histological information during standard endoscopy procedures, through high-resolution cellular imaging of internal tissues. Earlier work on mosaicing has enhanced the potential of this imaging modality by meeting the need to get a complete representation of the imaged region. However, with approaches, the dynamic information, which may be of clinical interest, is lost. In this study, we propose a new mosaic construction algorithm for pCLE sequences based on a min-cut optimization and gradient-domain composition. Its main advantage is that the motion of some structures within the tissue such as blood cells in capillaries, is taken into account. This allows physicians to get both a sharper static representation and a dynamic representation of the imaged tissue. Results on 16 sequences acquired *in vivo* on six different organs demonstrate the clinical relevance of our approach.

Introduction

Probe-based Confocal Laser Endomicroscopy (pCLE) [10] is a recent modality for *in situ* and *in vivo* imaging in the context of endoscopy. Basically, the objective of a confocal microscope is replaced by a flexible optical probe of length and diameter compatible with the working channel ($\varnothing \sim$ a few mm) of an endoscope in order to be able to perform *in situ* and *in vivo* imaging. Thus, pCLE provides physicians with real-time access to histological information during standard endoscopy procedures, through high-resolution cellular imaging of internal tissues, which is of particular interest for early detection of cancer (e.g. [2]).

Since pCLE is a contact real-time imaging modality, there is an inevitable hardware trade-off between invasiveness, frame rate, resolution and field-of-view. A typical pCLE acquisition system images, with a micrometrical resolution at 12 frames per second, a 600×600 μm optical section parallel to the tissue surface. Since most pCLE videos interpretations are based on the morphological characteristics of micro-cellular architecture in deep layers of the epithelium with structures' sizes ranging from one to a few hundred microns (e.g. ~ 200 μm for

[*] Authors have contributed equally to the paper.

N. Navab et al. (Eds.): MICCAI 2015, Part I, LNCS 9349, pp. 447–454, 2015.
DOI: 10.1007/978-3-319-24553-9_55

a colonic crypt in a healthy tissue), an increase of the field of view helps the clinicians in analyzing pCLE videos. Therefore, earlier work on mosaicing [12,16,19] has enhanced the potential of this imaging modality by meeting the need to get a complete representation of the imaged region. However, with such approaches, the dynamic information, which may be of clinical interest, is lost. For some organs such as the pancreas, dynamic information is required to draw a proper diagnosis. For instance, it helps distinguishing vessels from other structures by visualizing cells circulating in the blood stream.

In this study, we propose a new mosaicing construction algorithm to enlarge the field of view of pCLE sequences while preserving their motion information. It is based on a min-cut optimization and gradient domain composition. Our work has been inspired by the works of Agarwala et al., Ravi-Acha et al. and Joshi et al. on *panoramic video texture* (PVT) [1], *dynamosaicing* [15] and *cliplets* [7] respectively for manual video editing. The main advantage of our approach over previous works [12,16,19] is that the motion of some structures within the tissue, such as blood cells in capillaries, is taken into account. This allows physicians to get a dynamic representation of the imaged tissue whose field of view is no longer defined by the imaging system but by the size of the imaged region.

1 Dynamic Mosaicing

1.1 Problem Statement and Related Work

The goal of our method is to enlarge the field of view of a pCLE sequence while preserving its motion information. To that end, we begin by assuming that all the images have been spatially registered into a single coordinate system [19] and have an isotropic resolution. Thus, the registered pCLE sequence can be represented by a real value function I defined on $\mathcal{D} = \bigcup_{t\in[0,T]} \Omega_t \times \{t\}$ where T is the video duration and Ω_t is the imaged region at time t. We would like to create from I a new function $\tilde{I}$ defined on $\Omega \times [0,T]$ where $\Omega = \bigcup_{t\in[0,T]} \Omega_t$ is the whole imaged region. Since we visualize a 2D optical section at 12 Hz, motion quantification cannot be directly obtained from the pCLE sequence. Indeed, estimating out-of-plane motions is an ill-posed problem. Furthermore, the Nyquist-Shannon sampling theorem shows that the motion of blood cells cannot always be properly estimated. Motion information is mainly used to distinguish vessels from other structures by vizualising moving blood cells.

One way to deal with this problem would have been to consider it as an inpainting or video completion problem and search $\tilde{I}$ among functions extending I. This is the solution chosen by Matsushita et al. [13]. However, their method based on motion inpainting cannot be applied to our problem since motion estimation in a 2D section is an ill-posed problem. Rav-Acha et al. [15] tackled this problem differently by considering $\tilde{I} = I \circ \phi$ where ϕ is a deformation field. ϕ is chosen as a trade-of between a user defined deformation field ϕ_0 and a image regularization term chosen to reduce stitching artifacts. While their method is well adapted for manual video editing, it has several limitations for dynamic mosaicing of pCLE sequences. First, chosing a suitable ϕ_0 is not obvious. Moreover, it does not have the ability to have discrete jumps in time, which is more adapted to repetitive stochastic textures, neither has it the ability to generate infinite dynamics. Agarwala et al. [1] proposed a very similar approach that does not have all these limitations: the *panoramic video textures* (PVT).

1.2 Markov Random Field Formulation

Agarwala et al. [1] considered $\tilde{I} = I \circ \phi$ with $\phi : (\mathbf{x}, t) \mapsto (\mathbf{x}, t + \Delta(t) \bmod T_{\max})$ where Δ is a time-offset function and $T_{\max}$ is the ouput video duration. In the following, we drop the modulo notation for clarity sake. In a nutshell, ϕ is obtained by solving a 3D Markov random field (MRF) problem where $\Omega \times [0, T_{\max}]$ is the domain and Δ are the free variables taking values in $\{0, 1, \cdots, T\}$. The unitary potential function U^{PVT}, defined as $U_i^{\mathrm{PVT}}(\Delta) := 0$ if $(\mathbf{x}_i, t_i + \Delta(\mathbf{x}_i)) \in \mathcal{D}$ and $U_i^{\mathrm{PVT}}(\Delta) := +\infty$ otherwise, ensures that all the pixels of the output video are defined. Agarwala et al. [1] defined the pairwise potential function as

$$V_{(i,j)}^{\mathrm{PVT}}(\Delta_i, \Delta_j) := \sum_{k=i,j} \|I(\mathbf{x}_k, t_k + \Delta_i) - I(\mathbf{x}_k, t_k + \Delta_j)\|^n \tag{1}$$

for every adjacent points (i, j) in the spatio-temporal volume (6-connectivity) where I is defined and $V_{(i,j)}^{\mathrm{PVT}}(\Delta_i, \Delta_j) = +\infty$ otherwise.

When applied to pCLE sequences, solving PVT energy function may yield either rather static videos or oscillation and jitter motions. In [1], the rationale behind the temporal pairwise potential is to consider a transition to be correct provided a similar one exists at the same position in the original (registered) video. As a matter of fact, with such regularization term, only temporal transitions that are similar to existing ones are considered, even if it means only keeping a small proportion of existing transitions. In [1], removing motion information is less critical than adding temporal artifacts. Since we rather avoid removing motion information, our temporal regularization penalizes label changes without regard to the pixel intensity. We therefore modify the energy pairwise potential to enforce temporal consistency with the original video.

To do so, we do not make any assumptions on the intensity evolution. Instead, we consider that a temporal intensity change of a given pixel is plausible if and only if it exists in the original video for the same pixel. Hence, in our approach, the pairwise potential function V is defined, for two adjacent points $i = (\mathbf{x}_i, t_i)$ and $j = (\mathbf{x}_j, t_j)$ in the spatio-temporal volume (6-connectivity), as

$$V_{(i,j)}(\Delta_i, \Delta_j) := \begin{cases} C & \text{if } \Delta_i \neq \Delta_j \text{ and } \mathbf{x}_i = \mathbf{x}_j \text{ (temporal)} \\ V_{(i,j)}^{\mathrm{PVT}}(\Delta_i, \Delta_j) & \text{otherwise} \qquad\qquad\qquad \text{(spatial)} \end{cases} \tag{2}$$

where C is a positive constant. The unitary potential function is $U = U^{\mathrm{PVT}}$.

Since the pairwise potential V is a metric, we solve this MRF energy's optimization problem by α-expansion [4,8]. The time-offset function Δ is initialized to 0, which is equivalent to consider the original mosaic video as initialization.

1.3 Hierachical Optimization

Basically, the α-expansion algorithm [4] is a sequence of min-cut / max-flow optimization problems. To solve a min cut optimization problem, algorithms such as the the *relabel-to-front* algorithm are running in $O(|v|^3)$ where $|v|$ is the number of nodes of the optimization graph. When applied to our problem, each node represent one pixel in the reconstructed video. Thus, the number of nodes is $|v| = |\Omega \times [0, T_{\max}]|$.

For typical pCLE sequences, Ω ranges from 500×500 to 1000×1000 pixels and T from 30 to 200 frames. Therefore, to lessen the computational burden, hierachichal min-cut optimizations were performed (e.g. [1, 11]). The heuristic we followed is based on the assumption that the computed seams at the finer resolution are roughly similar to the ones at a coarser resolution. Hence, the problem is first solved at a coarse resolution. At finer resolution, the optimization is then only performed within the neighborhood of the seams.

1.4 Gradient-Domain Composition

In the reconstructed video, the computed seams may remain visible after optimization. This is mainly due to intensity variation resulting from the photobleaching of optical probe's doping fluorophore as well as an evolution of the fluorophore concentration in the tissue. Residual errors in the registration process may also yield similar visual artifacts. To reduce them, a gradient-domain composition [14,21] with mixed Neuman and Dirichlet boundary conditions was performed to create the final video. For sake of efficiency, we solve the Poisson equation frame by frame instead of considering the whole 3D volume. To avoid bleaching artifacts, we used a still mosaic reconstruction to define the same Dirichlet boundary condition for all the pixels lying on still regions along the boundary of the entire imaged region.

1.5 Looping Mosaic

The time required to analyze a dynamic mosaic might be longer than its duration $T_{\max}$. Therefore, generating infinite dynamics is of interest. A first approach would be to post-process the constructed video $\tilde{I}$ with the *video texture* algorithm [18]. Note that the frame transition obtained in [18] cannot be directly used in the MRF formulation since they are not symmetric. As for the PVT method, Agarwala et al. [1] proposed to generate infinite dynamics by merely playing the video in an infinite loop mode. An optimal duration $T_{\max}$ of the video is then chosen to reduce temporal artifacts.

In our algorithm, the output video duration ($T_{\max}$) is defined by the user. We create a looping mosaic by slighlty changing the MRF graph. Every point $(\mathbf{x}, T_{\max})$ of the last frame is then connected to the point $(\mathbf{x}, 0)$ of the first frame. Thus, the infinite dynamics directly results from the temporal consistency constraints. Our approach is rather simple and yet gives good results.

2 Combining Static and Dynamic Mosaics

Acquired pCLE videos are rarely solely composed of dynamic regions. Hence, solving the MRF optimization problem described in section 1.2 on the whole input image unnecessarily increases the computational burden. Besides, residual registration errors on static region may result in flickering artifacts when considered as dynamic. Therefore, we combine still and dynamic mosaic [1,7].

2.1 Texture Preserving Static Mosaicing

Reconstruction used in standard mosaicing algorithm [12,16,19] is an average of registered frames. This can bring superresolution or increase the signal-to-noise ratio provided there is no residual registration error. However, this in not always the case when observing *in vivo* tissues. Moving structures such as blood cells in capillaries appear blurred. Besides, texture information, which may be used for diagnosis in some organs (e.g. eosophagus), is lost when averaging. Several methods for mosaicing non rigid dynamical scenes have been proposed in the literature (e.g. [6,15,20]). In this study, we simply notice that using the MRF formulation (section 1.2) with $T_{\max} = 0$ results in a static mosaic obtained by stitching. This optimization is similar to texture synthesis [9] with the *image quilting*'s pairwise potential function [5]. This constructs a static mosaic that preserves texture information. Besides, it does not blur moving structures neither regions with residual registration error. Note that we do not use the pairwise potential described in [9], for it is a semi-metric and not a metric. Hence, α-expansion does not apply [4]. The α-β-swap algorithm [4] could be used instead but there is no guarantee to converge to a solution close to the global minimum.

2.2 Static Background Detection

Combining still and dynamic mosaicing requires a partition of imaged tissue into static and dynamic regions. In [1], this partition required user inputs. To do it automatically we focused on background substraction and motion detection algorithms. There is an extended literature on this subject [3]. To the best of our knowledge, these methods based on motion estimations or density estimations are not adapted to our problem for the reasons described in section 1.2. Therefore, our approach consists in thresholding the temporal variance computed on locally normalized frames (zero mean and unit variance).

2.3 Combining Still Images and Video Segments

To combine still images and video segments, Joshi et al. [7] used feathering and Laplacian blending. Agarwala at al. [1] adapt the unitary potential function on the boundary to stitch the video segments to a static mosaic. Using either of these approaches on thin structures such as vessels results in rather static videos. To solve this problem, we drop the stitching constraint in the MRF and we use a Dirichet boundary condition on the frontier between static and dynamic region for the gradient domain composition.

Table 1. Consistency of visual summaries with the original video rated by four experts with a five-level Likert scale (SD: strongly disagree; D: disagree; NAND: neither agree nor disagree; A: agree; SA: strongly agree).

Expert	SD	D	NAND	A	SA
1	13%	19%	31%	31%	06%
2	13%	69%	00%	19%	00%
3	06%	00%	44%	50%	00%
4	00%	13%	00%	56%	31%

Averaging Mosaicing

Expert	SD	D	NAND	A	SA
1	00%	00%	06%	31%	63%
2	00%	31%	00%	44%	25%
3	00%	00%	00%	13%	87%
4	00%	00%	13%	06%	81%

Stitching Mosaicing

Expert	SD	D	NAND	A	SA
1	06%	00%	00%	06%	88%
2	00%	00%	00%	25%	75%
3	00%	00%	00%	13%	87%
4	00%	06%	00%	13%	81%

Dynamic Mosaicing

3 Experiments and Results

3.1 Materials

The validation of our method was performed by four experts on a dataset composed of 16 sequences coming from six organs (oesophagus, stomach, pancreas, bladder, biliary duct and colon) with various conditions. Sequences have been acquired and preprocessed following [10,17]. To register all the input video frames we used the deformation fields obtained with the algorithm proposed by Vercauteren et al. [19]. In our experiments, we chose $T_{\max} = T$ and $n = 2$ (note that we also tried $n = 1$ and $n = 8$ and obtained similar results). As for the trade-off parameter C, we set it relatively to the dynamic of the image intensity. Parameter C was set proportionally to the median of $\max_{\Delta_i,\Delta_j} V_{(i,j)}(\Delta_i, \Delta_j)$ over all couples (i, j) of spatially adjacent points. The proportion parameter was set to 10, which we found to be a good trade-off between the spatial and temporal coherency constraints. Examples of reconstructed videos are available as supplementary materials (`https://sites.google.com/site/motionawaremosaicingpcle/`).

3.2 Consistency of the Visual Summary

To validate the clinical relevance of our mosaicing method, we asked four experts to assess the clinical consistency of the constructed mosaics with the original pCLE videos. Each expert rated, with a five-level Likert scale, a static mosaic reconstructed by weighting average as well as both a static and a dynamic mosaic constructed using our method. Results are presented in Table 1.

We also asked each expert to rank static mosaics obtained by averaging and by stitching. Our method was considered to give significantly better results (p-value < 0.05 with a Wilcoxon signed rank test). Stitched mosaics were preferred 97% of the time. We carried out the same experiment between the dynamic mosaics and the best static mosaics. Dynamic mosaicing was considering to give

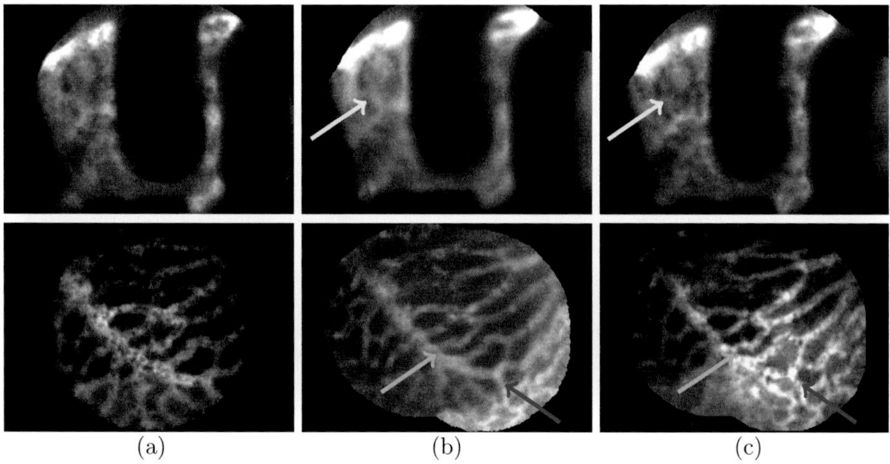

Fig. 1. (a) frame from a pCLE sequence; (b) static mosaic reconstructed by averaging; (c) static mosaic reconstructed with our method; it yields sharper images (yellow), preserves moving cells (green) in vessels and removes intensity change artifacts (red).

a significantly more consistent summary (p-value < 0.05). Dynamic mosaics were preferred 78% of the time over static mosaics.

We also show visually the benefits of our algorithm over the averaging reconstruction methods in Figure 1. Compared to the averaging approach, the stitching method better preserves texture information and does not blur moving structures such as blood cells. Besides, the gradient domain composition removes bleaching artifacts.

4 Discussion

By introducing time information in the mosaicing construction algorithm, we manage to have a dynamic mosaic reconstruction that preserves texture information and maintains motion appearance. Such mosaics help clinicians to distinguish specific structures such as capillaries by visualizing moving cells in the blood stream. We also derived a method to get a static and a dynamic mosaic. Both mosaics have sharper reconstructed images by reducing blur induced by residual registation error.

The clinical relevance of our methods was assessed by four expert users on 16 pCLE sequences aquired *in vivo* and *in situ* on six different organs. Results showed that our methods yield more consistent visual summaries of the original videos.

References

1. Agarwala, A., Zheng, K.C., Pal, C., Agrawala, M., Cohen, M., Curless, B., Salesin, D., Szeliski, R.: Panoramic video textures. In: TOG, SIGGRAPH, vol. 24, pp. 821–827. ACM (2005)

2. Becker, V., Vercauteren, T., von Weyhern, C.H., Prinz, C., Schmid, R.M., Meining, A.: High-resolution miniprobe-based confocal microscopy in combination with video mosaicing (with video). Gastrointest Endosc. 66(5), 1001–1007 (2007)
3. Benezeth, Y., Jodoin, P.-M., Emile, B., Laurent, H., Rosenberger, C.: Comparative study of background subtraction algorithms. J. Electron. Imaging 19(3) (2010)
4. Boykov, Y., Veksler, O., Zabih, R.: Fast approximate energy minimization via graph cuts. TPAMI 23(11), 1222–1239 (2001)
5. Efros, A.A., Freeman, W.T.: Image quilting for texture synthesis and transfer. In: Proc. SIGGRAPH, pp. 341–346. ACM (2001)
6. Fitzgibbon, A.W.: Stochastic rigidity: Image registration for nowhere-static scenes. In: Proc. ICCV, vol. 1, pp. 662–669. IEEE (2001)
7. Joshi, N., Mehta, S., Drucker, S., Stollnitz, E., Hoppe, H., Uyttendaele, M., Cohen, M.: Cliplets: juxtaposing still and dynamic imagery. In: Proc. 25th Annual ACM Symposium on User Interface Software and Technology, pp. 251–260. ACM (2012)
8. Kolmogorov, V., Zabin, R.: What energy functions can be minimized via graph cuts? TPAMI 26(2), 147–159 (2004)
9. Kwatra, V., Schödl, A., Essa, I., Turk, G., Bobick, A.: Graphcut textures: image and video synthesis using graph cuts. In: ACM Transactions on Graphics (ToG), vol. 22, pp. 277–286 (2003)
10. Le Goualher, G., Perchant, A., Genet, M., Cavé, C., Viellerobe, B., Berier, F., Abrat, B., Ayache, N.: Towards optical biopsies with an integrated fibered confocal fluorescence microscope. In: Barillot, C., Haynor, D.R., Hellier, P. (eds.) MICCAI 2004. LNCS, vol. 3217, pp. 761–768. Springer, Heidelberg (2004)
11. Lombaert, H., Sun, Y., Grady, L., Xu, C.: A multilevel banded graph cuts method for fast image segmentation. In: Tenth IEEE International Conference on Computer Vision, ICCV 2005, vol. 1, pp. 259–265. IEEE (2005)
12. Mahé, J., Vercauteren, T., Rosa, B., Dauguet, J.: A viterbi approach to topology inference for large scale endomicroscopy video mosaicing. In: Mori, K., Sakuma, I., Sato, Y., Barillot, C., Navab, N. (eds.) MICCAI 2013, Part I. LNCS, vol. 8149, pp. 404–411. Springer, Heidelberg (2013)
13. Matsushita, Y., Ofek, E., Ge, W., Tang, X., Shum, H.-Y.: Full-frame video stabilization with motion inpainting. TPAMI 28(7), 1150–1163 (2006)
14. Pérez, P., Gangnet, M., Blake, A.: Poisson image editing. In: TOG, vol. 22, pp. 313–318. ACM (2003)
15. Rav-Acha, A., Pritch, Y., Lischinski, D., Peleg, S.: Dynamosaicing: Mosaicing of dynamic scenes. TPAMI 29(10), 1789–1801 (2007)
16. Rosa, B., Erden, M.S., Vercauteren, T., Herman, B., Szewczyk, J., Morel, G.: Building large mosaics of confocal edomicroscopic images using visual servoing. IEEE Transactions on Biomedical Engineering 60(4), 1041–1049 (2013)
17. Savoire, N., André, B., Vercauteren, T.: Online blind calibration of non-uniform photodetectors: Application to endomicroscopy. In: Ayache, N., Delingette, H., Golland, P., Mori, K. (eds.) MICCAI 2012, Part III. LNCS, vol. 7512, pp. 639–646. Springer, Heidelberg (2012)
18. Schödl, A., Szeliski, R., Salesin, D.H., Essa, I.: Video textures. In: Proc. SIGGRAPH, pp. 489–498. ACM (2000)
19. Vercauteren, T., Perchant, A., Malandain, G., Pennec, X., Ayache, N.: Robust mosaicing with correction of motion distortions and tissue deformations for in vivo fibered microscopy. Medical Image Analysis 10(5), 673–692 (2006)
20. Vidal, R., Ravichandran, A.: Optical flow estimation & segmentation of multiple moving dynamic textures. In: Proc. CVPR, vol. 2, pp. 516–521. IEEE (2005)
21. Wang, H., Raskar, R., Ahuja, N.: Seamless video editing. In: Pattern Recognition, vol. 3, pp. 858–861. IEEE (2004)

A Registration Approach to Endoscopic Laser Speckle Contrast Imaging for Intrauterine Visualisation of Placental Vessels

Gustavo Sato dos Santos[1,2], Efthymios Maneas[1,2], Daniil Nikitichev[2], Anamaria Barburas[2], Anna L. David[3], Jan Deprest[4], Adrien Desjardins[2], Tom Vercauteren[1,2], and Sebastien Ourselin[1,2]

[1] Translational Imaging Group, CMIC, University College London, NW1 2HE, UK
[2] Dept. Med. Phys. and Biomed. Eng., University College London, WC1E 6BT, UK
[3] Institute for Women's Health, University College London, WC1E 6HX, UK
[4] Dept. of Obstetrics, University Hospitals KU Leuven, Belgium

Abstract. Intrauterine interventions such as twin-to-twin transfusion syndrome procedure require accurate mapping of the fetal placental vasculature to ensure complete photocoagulation of vascular anastomoses. However, surgeons are currently limited to fetoscopy and external ultrasound imaging, which are unable to accurately identify all vessels especially those that are narrow and at the periphery. Laser speckle contrast imaging (LSCI) is an optical method for imaging blood flow that is emerging as an intraoperative tool for neurosurgery. Here we explore the application of LSCI to minimally invasive fetal surgery, with an endoscopic LSCI system based on a 2.7-mm-diameter fetoscope. We establish using an optical phantom that it can image flow in 1-mm-diameter vessels as far as 4 mm below the surface. We demonstrate that a spatiotemporal algorithm produces the clearest images of vessels within 200 ms, and that speckle contrast images can be accurately registered using groupwise registration to correct for significant motion of target or probe. When tested on a perfused term *ex vivo* human placenta, our endoscopic LSCI system revealed small capillaries not evident in the fetoscopic images.

1 Introduction

An augmented view of vasculature and blood flow is required for surgical procedures that rely on accurate identification of the vessels. Laser speckle contrast imaging (LSCI) is emerging as an intraoperative tool for monitoring tissue perfusion and blood flow, particularly in neurosurgery where its clinical potential has been recently demonstrated [1]. Despite its potential for imaging perfusion and blood flow in minimally invasive procedures, relatively few applications of LSCI for endoscopic surgery have been described [2]. The present study proposes a novel application for endoscopic LSCI for intrauterine fetal surgery.

In twin-to-twin transfusion syndrome (TTTS) therapy, the surgeon aims to photocoagulate anastomosing placental vessels that cause a net transfusion of

N. Navab et al. (Eds.): MICCAI 2015, Part I, LNCS 9349, pp. 455–462, 2015.
DOI: 10.1007/978-3-319-24553-9_56

blood between identical twins sharing a placenta [3]. Success depends on the degree of remaining anastomoses, since perinatal morbidity and mortality is highest in cases where anastomoses are not identified or completely photocoagulated [4]. Narrow vessels (<2mm) are most likely to be missed or incompletely photocoagulated. Endoscopic LSCI can potentially help the surgeon identify smaller and less accessible vessels that are difficult to see in standard fetoscopy images.

Due to its nature, LSCI is highly sensitive to motion of the camera relative to tissue. This sensitivity is of particular concern in endoscopic surgeries when the camera is often handheld and the tissue can also move substantially. We aim to address this issue in two complementary ways: (1) by generating the clearest images within a short acquisition interval; and (2) by compensating for motion over longer intervals. For the first way, we evaluate three methods for estimating speckle statistics from data acquired in 200 ms to determine which yields the largest contrast between vasculature and background. And for the second way we evaluate two approaches for registering speckle contrast images in the presence of motion between the endoscope and the anatomy, and demonstrate that groupwise registration is preferable to a previously proposed method [5,6]. We tested our approach on an optical phantom and also on a perfused *ex vivo* human placenta, and in both cases tested the method's robustness to motion.

2 Methods

Endoscopic LSCI. A typical LSCI paradigm involves illumination of tissue with a spatially and temporally coherent laser source and reception of light with a camera. Our approach for endoscopic LSCI comprised a high-resolution sCMOS camera (ORCA-Flash4.0v2, Hamamatsu, Japan; pixel size: 6.5 μm) with high-magnification zoom lens (MVL6X12Z, Thorlabs, Germany), a 2.7-mm diameter fetoscope (Hopkins II, Karl Storz, Germany), and a 785 nm, 450 mW fibre-coupled laser (BWF1, B&W Tek, USA). The fibre-coupled laser was positioned to create a specular illumination on the target area, and images were acquired using the sCMOS camera placed at the proximal end of the fetoscope (Fig. 1(a)). In all experiments, the sCMOS sensor's exposure time was set to 5 ms and frames were acquired at 100 fps and at full resolution (2048x2048).

Speckle Contrast Estimation. When coherent light reflects off an irregular surface such as tissue, it forms a speckle pattern due to random interference. LSCI is based on the principle that the rate of change of speckle intensity is a function of the average velocity of the tissue particles that reflect light [7]. Speckles depend on the movement of scatterers and the sensor exposure time; by measuring the statistics of speckle intensities, it is possible to obtain high-resolution images of the vasculature and also relative estimates of blood flow [1]. Speckle contrast images are computed from raw images by taking the ratio of the standard deviation to the mean pixel intensity: $K = \sigma/\mu$. There are three algorithms for estimating speckle contrast: (1) temporal, by computing the statistics of each pixel across time; (2) spatial, by computing the statistics within a square window around each pixel; and (3) spatiotemporal, by computing the statistics in a spatiotemporal cube window around each pixel. To evaluate these algorithms, we generate speckle contrast images from stacks of 20 raw images using each algorithm and compare the resulting images. For the spatial algorithm, we use a 14x14 kernel (typical kernel size: 0.2 mm) to compute the spatial statistics and take the average of the 20 spatial contrast images to obtain a single image. A 14x14x20 kernel is used for the spatiotemporal algorithm.

Registration of Speckle Contrast Images. We compared two strategies for registering speckle contrast images to compensate for motion during image acquisition. The first one was proposed in [5,6], and uses the image at the start of acquisition as a fixed reference for the registration of all other images. We propose an alternative strategy: to use groupwise registration and register all images to their average image, which is iteratively refined after each round of registrations. This approach was adapted from [8], except that affine transformations are applied on 2D images. Groupwise registration starts by taking the average of all unregistered images and using it as the initial fixed image; after registering all images relative to it, the fixed image is recomputed as the average of the registered images, and this procedure is repeated. We used a total of 5 iterations to register 20 images in the moving phantom experiments, and 10 iterations to register 100 images in the placenta experiment. Both registration strategies described above used the same spatial speckle contrast images and the same number of iterations. We used Elastix to perform the registrations [9], and in all cases used the same set of registration parameters: affine transform as the transformation type, mutual information as the similarity measure, and adaptive stochastic gradient descent as the optimisation procedure.

Experimental Setup. An optical phantom was used to evaluate the ability to image flow at different depths using our endoscopic LSCI approach. The phantom was made using a 3D-printed mould comprising two parts: a 13x26 mm rectangular chamber with 1mm holes on the side, and a plate with 1-mm diameter rods spaced 2 mm horizontally and 1 mm vertically (Fig. 2(a)). The mould was filled with 5.5% agar solution mixed with 0.5% intralipid (Sigma-Aldrich, USA), and the rods were removed after the agar had set to create wall-less vessels (i.e., grooves in the agar). Speckle images were acquired as the phantom vessels were perfused with 1% intralipid at a constant rate (60 mL/h) using a syringe driver (Alaris, CareFusion, USA). Intralipid has similar optical properties as biological tissue and, at 1% concentration, it has been used as blood phantom in LSCI studies. For the moving phantom experiments, the phantom was mounted on a motorised linear stage (MT1-Z8, Thorlabs, Germany) and moved at a constant speed of 4mm/s or 2mm/s longitudinally to the imaging plane. The working distance between fetoscope tip and phantom was 1.3 cm or 2.5 cm. Constant intralipid flow was maintained in the 2-mm-deep vessel.

Speckle contrast images were evaluated by computing the average signal-to-noise ratio (SNR) of the pixel contrast values in the perfused vessel region. ROI and background region were defined for each vessel (Fig. 2(b)), and the SNR was computed as: $SNR = |\mu_{ROI} - \mu_{bg}|/\sigma_{bg}$, where μ_{ROI} is the average contrast value in the ROI, and μ_{bg} and σ_{bg} are the average and standard deviation of the contrast values in the background, respectively. Different selections for the background region were tested, with similar results.

For testing on *ex vivo* placenta, a term placenta was collected at UCLH following a C-section delivery and after obtaining a written informed consent from the mother (all procedures were approved by UCLH Ethics Committee). The placenta was placed on a flat surface and one of its surface vessels was perfused with 1% intralipid at 30 mL/h. The perfused vessel was imaged downstream from the cannula with our endoscopic LSCI system (Fig. 1(b)). To simulate handheld movement of the fetoscope, the distal end of the fetoscope was tapped and made to wobble by <1 cm over 1 s during image acquisition.

3 Experiments and Results

Endoscopic LSCI of a Perfused Placenta. The endoscopic LSCI system was initially tested on a perfused *ex vivo* placenta (Fig.1(b)). A 1-mm-diameter placental vessel was cannulated and continuously perfused with 1% intralipid solution, and the fetoscope was positioned to image the perfused vessel (Fig. 1(c)). 100 raw speckle images were acquired, and the estimated spatiotemporal

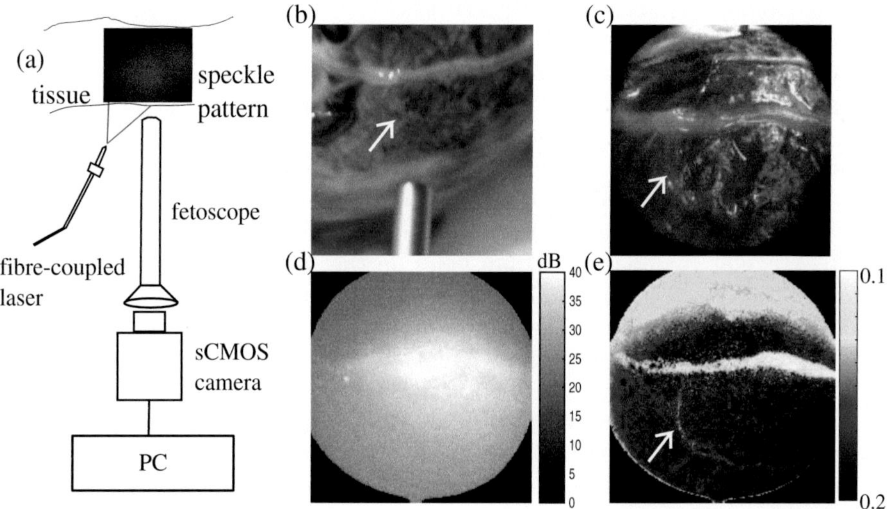

Fig. 1. **(a)** Diagram of the endoscopic LSCI system. **(b)** A photograph showing the tip of the fetoscope and the area on the placenta being imaged. The vessel at the image top is 1 mm in diameter and was continuously perfused with 1% intralipid. **(c)** Fetoscopic image acquired under white light illumination. **(d)** Raw fetoscopic speckle image acquired using laser illumination. **(e)** Speckle contrast image showing perfused vessel and a branching capillary; lower contrast values (warmer colours) indicate flow. The white arrows in (b), (c) and (e) indicate the capillary's location in each image.

speckle contrast image revealed the perfused vessel in high contrast relative to background (average pixel SNR = 3.28; Fig. 1(e)). Furthermore, a branching capillary was clearly visible in the speckle contrast image (Fig. 1(e)), but was not as evident under white light illumination (Fig. 1(b) and Fig. 1(c)).

Evaluation of Registration-Free Speckle Contrast Estimation Methods in the Absence of Confounding Motion. Three algorithms for estimating speckle contrast were tested on a perfused optical phantom (Fig.2(a) and Fig. 2(b)). Vessels at 1, 2, 3 and 4mm depth were perfused one at a time, and the phantom was placed at 1 or 2 cm from the fetoscope in air, or 1 cm in wa-

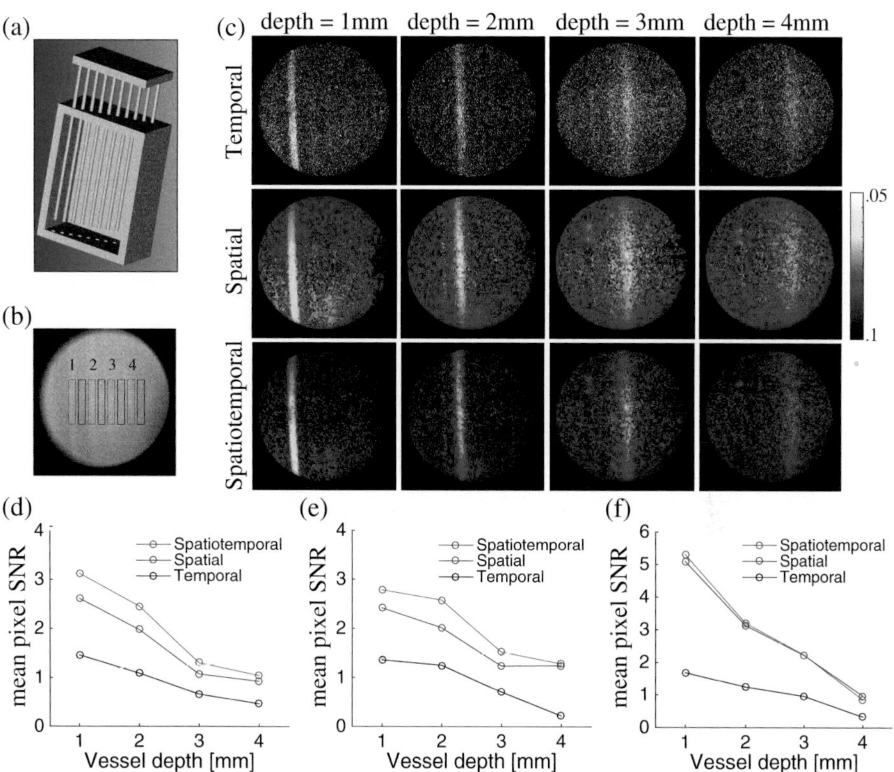

Fig. 2. **(a)** 3D-printed mould used for manufacturing the agar-based optical phantom. **(b)** Fetoscopic view of the phantom placed 1 cm from the fetoscope tip under white light illumination; vessels are filled with 1% intralipid. Numbers indicate the location and depth (in mm) of the vessels, and red and black rectangles show the ROI and background region for each vessel. **(c)** Speckle contrast images of intralipid flow at variable vessel depths (columns) and obtained with different estimation algorithms (rows), with the same phantom position as in (b). **(d-f)** Signal to noise (SNR) analysis of contrast estimation algorithms in different setups: (d) phantom placed at 1 cm distance or (e) 2 cm distance; and (f) imaging in water with phantom at 1 cm distance.

ter. Intralipid flow could be reliably imaged down to 4 mm depth in air, or 3 mm depth in water (Fig. 2(c) and Fig. 2(d)). SNR analysis indicated that the spatiotemporal method consistently produced the highest contrast for intralipid flow.

Evaluation of Registration Algorithms on a Moving Phantom. The phantom was placed on a linear stage and moved at 4 mm/s or 2 mm/s longitudinally to the image plane (Fig. 3(a)) with the fetoscope at a fixed position and orientation. 20 frames of raw speckle image were acquired during movement, and the resulting 20 spatial speckle contrast images were registered, or spatially normalised, to estimate motion. Groupwise registration recovered the linear translation in the X direction with the phantom at 1.3 cm or 2.5 cm dis-

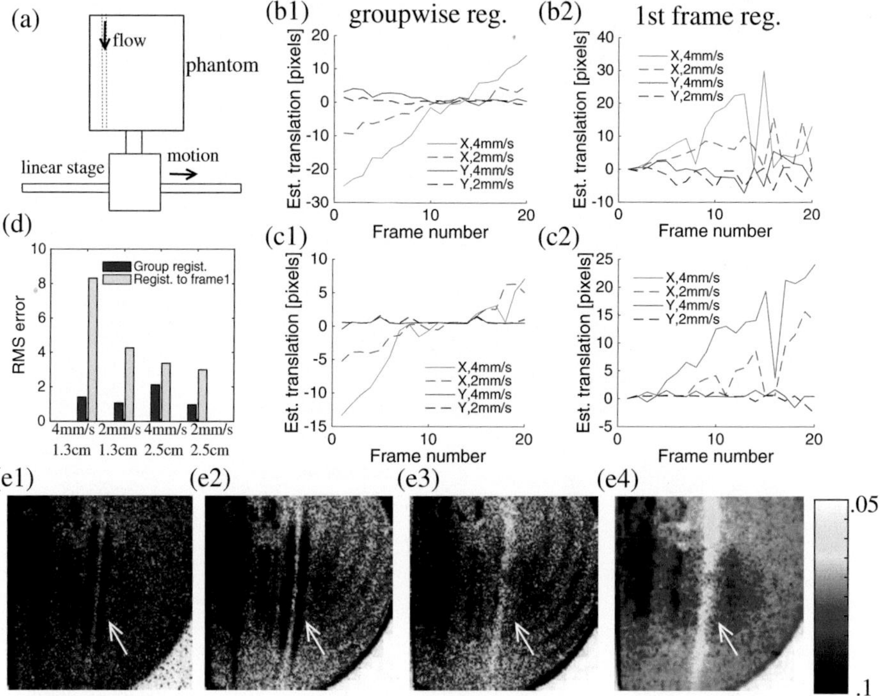

Fig. 3. **(a)** Setup for testing speckle contrast image registration. **(b)** Estimated X-Y translations for each frame using (b1) groupwise registration or (b2) registration to the 1st frame. Phantom was 1.3 cm away from fetoscope tip. **(c)** Same as in (b), but with phantom placed at 2.5 cm distance. **(d)** RMS error of estimated X displacements with respect to linear fits. **(e)** Speckle contrast images of vessel region (phantom distance: 1.3 cm, speed: 4 mm/s) using different combinations of contrast estimation and registration algorithms: (e1) no registration, temporal estimation; (e2) registration to 1st frame, temporal estimation; (e3) groupwise registration, temporal estimation; and (e4) groupwise registration, spatiotemporal estimation. Arrow: perfused vessel.

tance, whereas registering to the first frame failed in both accounts (Fig. 3(b), Fig. 3(c)). Speckle contrast images were clearest with a combination of groupwise registration and spatiotemporal contrast estimation (Fig. 3(e)).

Evaluation of Groupwise Registration on Perfused Placenta. While imaging the same region of the placenta as in Fig. 1 the tip of the fetoscope was tapped, making it wobble vertically. The spatiotemporal contrast image of the data acquired during motion contains dark artefacts in the background (Fig. 4(a)) - these are areas with higher speckle contrast, in some cases caused by specular reflection due to accumulation of water. Applying groupwise registration reduced the artefacts in the contrast image (Fig. 4(b)) and improved flow contrast (SNR: 2.88 without registration vs. 2.97 with registration).

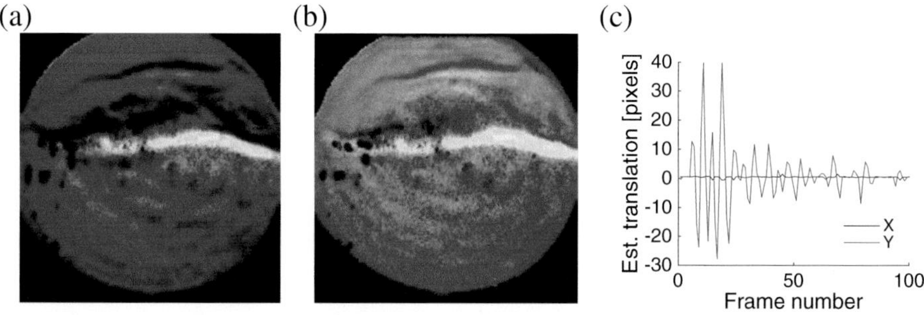

Fig. 4. Imaging placenta perfusion with motion. (a) Spatiotemporal contrast image of unregistered data (100 frames). (b) Spatiotemporal contrast estimation after groupwise registration, with fewer irregularities in background. (c) Estimated X-Y translation.

4 Discussion

Our results demonstrate the potential of endoscopic LSCI for imaging the fetal placental vasculature during intrauterine procedures. Our approach revealed the perfused vessels in high contrast relative to background both in the optical phantom and in the *ex vivo* human placenta, in air or under water, and in the presence of motion. Intralipid flow could be imaged down to a depth of 4 mm in the static phantom, 3 mm in the phantom under water, and 2 mm in the moving phantom. In the placenta, small branching capillaries could be clearly identified in the speckle contrast images but not as easily under white light illumination.

Groupwise registration significantly improved the ability to correct for motion during image acquisition. Registering to the first frame, as proposed in [5,6], may be adequate for near static conditions such as in neurosurgery, but may not be sufficiently robust for endoscopic LSCI. Our results showed that registration to the first frame failed to converge in several cases (Fig. 3), whereas groupwise registration had converged within the same number of iterations and using the same parameters. The next stage that we started implementing is to develop a real-time endoscopic LSCI system using a fast registration algorithm running on GPUs. Speckle contrast image registration can potentially be improved further by performing it simultaneously to endoscopic video registration, taking advantage of the richer texture information in the video images. Additionally, camera stabilisation using robotic surgical systems may help LSCI.

Endoscopic LSCI lends itself well to integration into current clinical workflow, as fibre-coupled lasers are already used in conjunction with imaging. Ultimately, we envisage that the same laser fibre could be used for two purposes. For instance, with a double-clad fibre, the single-mode core could deliver light for speckle imaging while the outer multi-mode cladding could deliver light for photocoagulation. Together with suitable spectral filters, this type of system could potentially be used to monitor photocoagulation in real-time. An integrated photocoagulation and endoscopic LSCI system would have great potential for use in intrauterine procedures, particularly for the TTTS procedure. Future work will focus on the development of this integrated system.

Acknowledgements. This work was supported through an Innovative Engineering for Health award by the Wellcome Trust [WT101957]; Engineering and Physical Sciences Research Council (EPSRC) [NS/A000027/1] and an NIHR BRC UCLH/UCL High Impact Initiative.

References

1. Hecht, N., Woitzik, J., König, S., Horn, P., Vajkoczy, P.: Laser speckle imaging allows real-time intraoperative blood flow assessment during neurosurgical procedures. Journal of Cerebral Blood Flow and Metabolism 33, 1000–1007 (2013)
2. Bray, R.C., Forrester, K.R., Reed, J., Leonard, C., Tulip, J.: Endoscopic laser speckle imaging of tissue blood flow: Applications in the human knee. Journal of Orthopaedic Research 24, 1650–1659 (2006)
3. Senat, M.V., Deprest, J., Boulvain, M., Paupe, A., Winer, N., Ville, Y.: Endoscopic laser surgery versus serial amnioreduction for severe twin-to-twin transfusion syndrome. New England Journal of Medicine 351(2), 136–144 (2004)
4. Slaghekke, L.L., Middeldorp, J.M., Weingertner, A.S., Klumper, F.J., Dekoninck, P., Devlieger, R., Lanna, M.M., Deprest, J., Favre, R., Oepkes, D., Lopriore, E.: Residual anastomoses in twin-twin transfusion syndrome after laser: the Solomon randomized trial. American Journal of Obstetrics and Gyn. 211(3), 285–e1 (2014)
5. Miao, P., Rege, A., Li, N., Thakor, N.V., Tong, S.: High resolution cerebral blood flow imaging by registered laser speckle contrast analysis. IEEE Transactions on Biomedical Engineering 57, 1152–1157 (2010)
6. Richards, L.M., Towle, E.L., Fox, J.D.J., Dunn, A.K.: Intraoperative laser speckle contrast imaging with retrospective motion correction for quantitative assessment of cerebral blood flow. Neurophotonics 1(1), 15006 (2014)
7. Boas, D.A., Dunn, A.K.: Laser speckle contrast imaging in biomedical optics (2010)
8. Guimond, A., Meunier, J., Thirion, J.P.: Average brain models: A convergence study. Computer Vision and Image Understanding 77(2), 192–210 (2000)
9. Klein, S., Staring, M., Murphy, K., Viergever, M.A., Pluim, J.P.: Elastix: a toolbox for intensity-based medical image registration. IEEE Transactions on Medical Imaging 29(1), 196–205 (2010)

Marker-Less AR in the Hybrid Room Using Equipment Detection for Camera Relocalization

Nicolas Loy Rodas, Fernando Barrera, and Nicolas Padoy

ICube, University of Strasbourg, CNRS, IHU Strasbourg, France
{nloyrodas,barreracampo,npadoy}@unistra.fr

Abstract. Augmented reality (AR) permits clinicians to visualize directly in their field of view key information related to the performance of a surgery. To track the user's viewpoint, current systems often use markers or register a reconstructed mesh with an a priori model of the scene. This only allows for a limited set of viewpoints and positions near the patient. Indeed, markers can be intrusive and interfere with the procedure. Furthermore, changes in the positions of equipment or clinicians can invalidate a priori models. Instead, we propose a marker-free mobile AR system based on a KinectFusion-like approach for camera tracking and equipment detection for camera relocalization. Our approach relies on the use of multiple RGBD cameras: one camera is rigidly attached to a hand-held screen where the AR visualization is displayed, while two others are rigidly fixed to the ceiling. The inclusion of two static cameras enables us to dynamically recompute the 3D model of the room, as required for relocalization when changes occur in the scene. Fast relocalization can be performed by looking at an equipment that is not required to remain static. This is particularly of advantage during hybrid surgeries, where an obvious choice for such an equipment is the intraoperative imaging device, which is large, can be seen in all views, but can also move. We propose to detect the equipment using a template based approach and further make use of the static cameras to speed-up the detection in the moving view by dynamically adapting the subset of tested templates according to the actual room layout. The approach is illustrated in a hybrid room through a radiation monitoring application where a virtual representation of the radiation cone beam, main X-ray scattering direction and dose distribution deposited on the surface of the patient are displayed on the hand-held screen.

Keywords: Augmented reality, RGBD cameras, Equipment detection, Camera relocalization, Radiation safety monitoring.

1 Introduction

This paper presents the development of a marker-free approach to perform mobile augmented reality (AR) in the operating theatre during hybrid surgery. By mobile AR, we refer to the display of information directly in the user's view by using a mobile screen or a head-mounted display (HMD). The targeted application is the display of 3D information related to radiation safety during X-ray

N. Navab et al. (Eds.): MICCAI 2015, Part I, LNCS 9349, pp. 463–470, 2015.
DOI: 10.1007/978-3-319-24553-9_57

guided procedures or during training sessions for such procedures. Consequently, the approach should allow a user, such as the clinician or the radio-manipulator, who can be located at different distances and positions around the patient table, to look anywhere around the table and benefit from the AR overlay. This application is subject to several constraints, such as the presence of motion in the scene, for instance the rotation and translation of the X-ray device, and the impracticability of having multiple markers visible from all interesting viewpoints. It is however important to note that precision requirements are less stringent here than in traditional image guided applications designed to guide precise gestures, for instance for tumor resection or screw placement.

The last decades have seen the development of several medical AR visualization solutions that overlay pre-operative or intra-operative patient images directly in the view of the clinician. Due to limited space, we refer the reader to [10,4] for a detailed review of these approaches and also for a description of other available visualization methods. These systems rely either on markers to locate the viewing device or on registration between a reconstructed surface and a model of the patient. For instance, the RAMP system [9] uses an inside-out approach, where a pattern of markers located near the patient is tracked with a camera placed on the HMD. In [6], an iterative closest point (ICP) matching approach is applied to register a pre-operative patient model to the view of a time-of-flight camera fixed on a mobile display. Such approaches are designed to display information related to the anatomy of the patient. In contrast, we are interested in displaying information concerning the surroundings of the patient and of the operating table, such as the skin dose and the scattered radiation map. A modeling of the scene beyond the patient is therefore required.

Several studies on radiation safety during X-ray guided procedures [11] have pointed out that clinicians and patients can be overexposed to radiation due to improper positioning of the X-ray device. Small changes in the angulation of the device can multiply the dose received by the patient or clinician by several factors. Similarly, overexposure can occur if the clinician or the lead protection devices are incorrectly positioned. In such situations, appropriate feedback could strongly reduce the received doses. To increase the awareness of clinicians w.r.t. radiation safety, [12] proposes a software that shows the radiation scattering in a virtual OR during training sessions. [3,5] propose to increase awareness by showing the dose received by the clinicians using radiation simulation and 3D person tracking. The risk is shown on a screen that overlays the radiation map over a 3D model of the room. This paper proposes a new approach to provide feedback to clinicians and staff when the X-ray device is used. It relies on mobile AR to display directly in the view of the staff key information about an upcoming X-ray image, such as the radiation beam, the main scattering direction, the radiation exposure of the patient and the current device parameters.

The AR approach that we propose uses one RGBD camera fixed on a mobile display and two static RGBD cameras fixed on the ceiling. Tracking of the moving camera is performed using an approach similar to KinectFusion [7], referred to as KinFu in the rest of this paper. One inconvenience of KinFu is the loss of tracking when motions occur in the scene or when the view changes abruptly. The static cameras are therefore a key element in the system to enable fast and convenient relocalization by keeping an up-to-date picture of the scene. We perform relocalization by detecting the same equipment simultaneously in the moving view and in at least one static view. Motivated by our clinical application, we detect the C-arm, which is large and can be partially seen in all views. We use an extended template-based detection approach based on [2]. It detects equipment *parts* for robustness and integrates natural constraints on the mobile camera location by dynamically adapting the set of tested templates according to the equipment configuration detected in the static views. This approach allows for fast relocalization in the presence of changes in the scene, as opposed to approaches like [1,8], which use a single camera and are designed for static scenes.

The contributions of this paper are as follows: we propose a KinFu based approach for mobile AR in the hybrid room using multiple RGBD cameras and equipment detection for relocalization. We also introduce a dynamic template-based approach for detection in the mobile view to fully integrate the information provided by the static cameras. To the best of the authors' knowledge, this is the first time that equipment detection is attempted in the OR using vision. Finally, we suggest a new application for mobile AR in the OR, namely the monitoring of patient dose and main direction of scatter during X-ray guided procedures.

2 Methods

The setup is composed of three synchronized and calibrated RGBD cameras (Asus Xtion Pro): two are rigidly mounted to the ceiling of the operating room and a third one is attached to the tracked hand-held display.

2.1 System Setup

Fig. 1 presents the proposed system setup and the different transformations involved. In the calibration procedure, the transformations $T_{C_i}^{R}$ between each static camera ($\mathbf{C}_i$) and the room ($\mathbf{R}$) are obtained using the procedure presented in [5]; these remain constant for each setup.

The mobile device ($\mathbf{M}$) is tracked using KinFu, yielding at each time step t a relative pose ${}^{t}T_{M}^{K}$ with respect to the virtual KinFu volume ($\mathbf{K}$) generated during tracking. The simultaneous detections at t_0 of a piece of equipment $\mathbf{E}$ in at least one static camera ($\mathbf{C_1}$ in Fig. 1a) and in the moving view, provide object-to-camera transformations used for computing an initial registration ${}^{t_0}T_{M}^{R}$ of the hand-held device with respect to the room coordinate system $\mathbf{R}$ in the following manner:

$$ {}^{t_0}T_{M}^{R} = {}^{t_0}T_{M}^{E}\, ({}^{t_0}T_{C_1}^{E})^{-1}\, T_{C_1}^{R}. \tag{1} $$

During tracking, ${}^{t_0}T_{M}^{R}$ is applied to the current relative transformation ${}^{t}T_{M}^{K}$ to obtain at each time step the pose of the moving device with respect to the room:

$$ {}^{t}T_{M}^{R} = {}^{t}T_{M}^{K}\, (T_{M}^{K})^{-1}\, {}^{t_0}T_{M}^{R}, \tag{2} $$

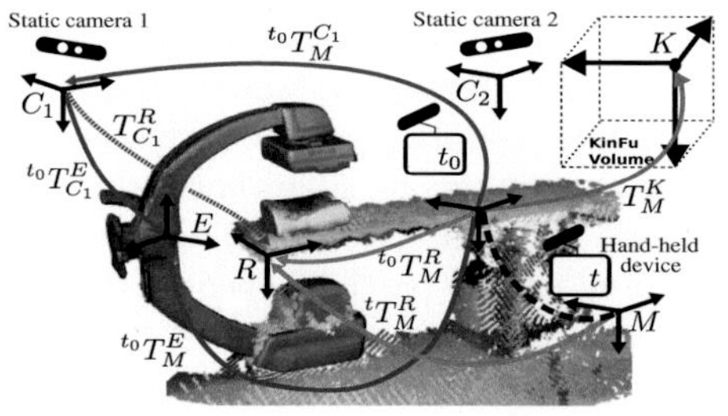

(a) Setup and corresponding transformations.

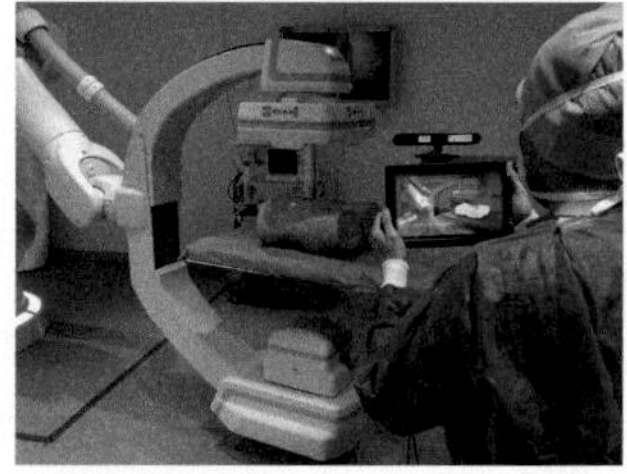

(b) Hand-held device displaying the AR visualization.

Fig. 1. System setup.

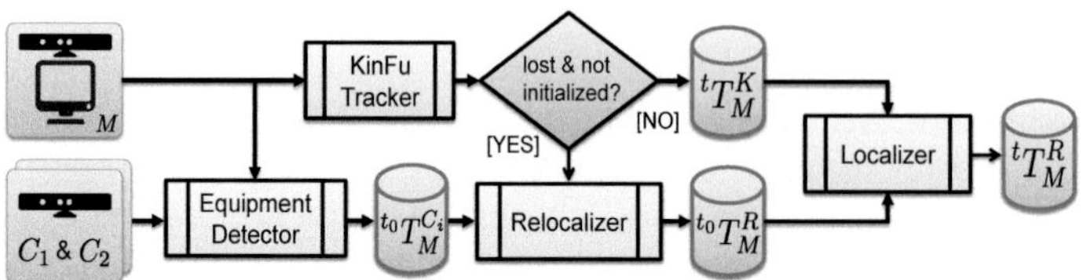

Fig. 2. Tracking pipeline.

where T_M^K is a constant transformation in the system. When tracking is lost, camera relocalization is achieved by recomputing ${}^{t_0}T_M^R$ using new simultaneous equipment detections in both views.

2.2 Tracking Pipeline

An overview of the tracking pipeline is shown in Fig. 2. All processes are executed concurrently in different threads.

KinFu Tracker: This process makes use of an open-source implementation of KinectFusion [7] to track the motion of **M**. It uses the GPU to simultaneously construct a 3D map of the environment and to estimate with ICP the transformation relating **M** to **K**. At each time step, the ICP error is compared to a threshold in order to detect any tracking failure.

Equipment Detector: This process performs equipment detection in each view and is further described in Sec. 2.3. Detecting an object in the moving view alone is not sufficient for camera relocalization due to the possible ambiguities caused by the fact that the object can also be moving.

Relocalizer: This process corresponds to the equipment-based relocalization algorithm. It uses simultaneous equipment detections to compute ${}^{t_0}T_M^R$ at initialization or to recompute it when **M** is lost. The transformation from Eq. 1 is refined by applying ICP between the point cloud of the moving camera and the merged point cloud from the static cameras, restricted to a large area around the object.

Localizer: This process applies ${}^{t}T_{M}^{K}$ and ${}^{t_0}T_{M}^{R}$ to compute the pose ${}^{t}T_{M}^{R}$ of the mobile camera w.r.t. the room using Eq. 2 for the AR visualization.

2.3 Equipment Detection

We apply a multimodal template matching approach inspired by [2] for detecting equipment in each of the views and estimating the cameras' relative poses w.r.t. the detected equipment. The templates sample the possible appearances of an object and are built from densely sampled color gradients and depth map normals. Because each template is labeled with the corresponding relative camera-object transformation, when a template is found at test time, a coarse estimation of the object's pose is also provided. This pose is further refined using ICP.

Template Generation: Since CAD models of the equipment from an operating room are not easily available, we first generate a 3D model by scanning the object with a RGBD camera. Then, as in [2], we equally sample a set of viewpoints with respect to the coordinate center of the model by recursively dividing the space into a polyhedron. Each obtained vertex is considered as a camera viewpoint from where virtual color and depth images are generated and used for computing the templates. This is repeated for polyhedrons with different sizes to generate images at different scales. In [2], the assumption is made that the objects to detect are placed over a planar surface. Therefore, viewpoints are only sampled from the upper hemisphere of the model. They are also only sampled using a camera parallel to the horizon and looking at the object's center. In our case, the cameras are not necessarily horizontal and have very different viewpoints. Furthermore, the C-arm has a large set of possible orientations. To generate templates for all possible situations, virtual images are first generated from views sampled from a sphere around the object (Fig. 3a) using a horizontal camera pointing towards the object's centre. The same procedure is then repeated for a discrete set of n 3D orientations of the object $\Theta = \{\theta_1, \ldots, \theta_n\}$. Since objects are not constantly moving in an OR, the slower detection speed caused by the larger set of templates is not a limitation for detection in the static views. However, faster detection is required in the moving view for a comfortable user experience. We therefore dynamically adapt the set of templates tested in the moving camera based on the object pose detected in the static views, as described below.

Dynamic Template Subset Selection: We make use of the detected 3D object position in the static cameras to gain information about the object poses that the moving camera should expect. We include the additional assumption that the moving device is constrained to move within a certain part of the room and between pre-defined heights. The set of relevant templates is thereby drastically reduced. In practice, we precompute for each 3D orientation $\theta \in \Theta$ the subset S_θ of potentially visible templates (Fig. 3a). At test time, the static cameras detect the current object orientation and the system dynamically loads the corresponding template subset to be used by the moving camera detector. This procedure reduces the number of computations per frame and accelerates the tracking initialization and relocalization procedures.

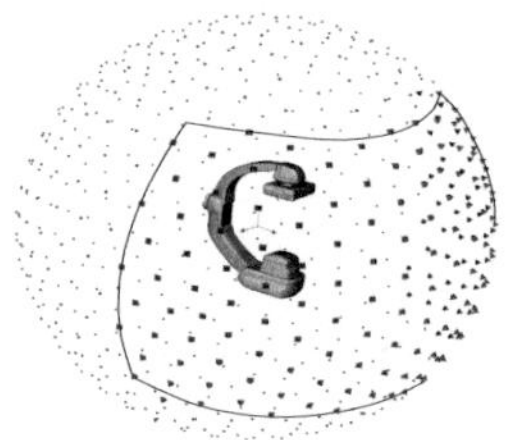

(a) Sampling procedure. Red poses form a template subset.

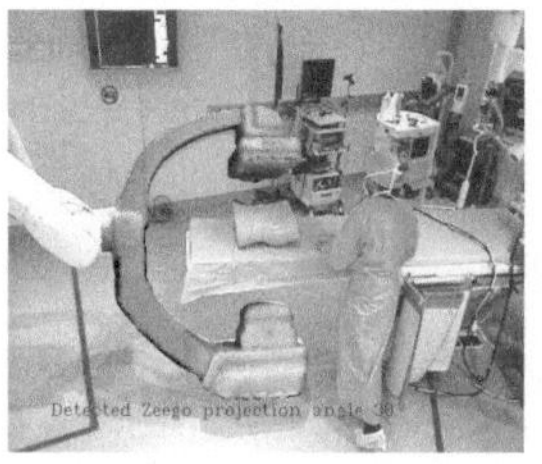

(b) Detected equipment overlaid in static view.

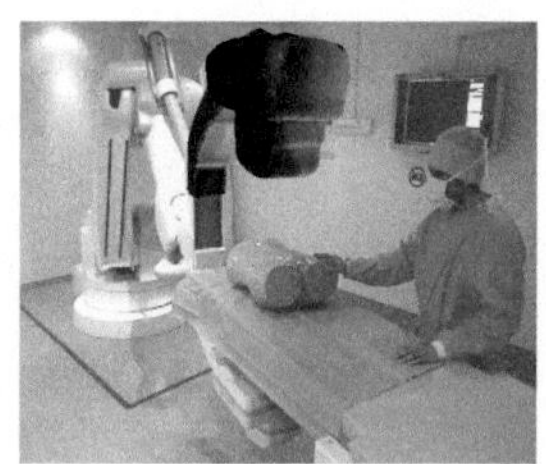

(c) Part detected and overlaid in moving view.

Fig. 3. Equipment detection: template generation and result examples.

Part-Based Detection: A known drawback of template matching approaches is the fact that the complete template must be visible in the image for it to be detected. This can become an issue when dealing with large objects or close views of the object. We use a part-based detection approach that copes with these limitations by looking for separate parts of the same object in the images. First, we divide the object's model into a finite number of parts to obtain separate models sharing the same reference coordinate system. Then, templates are generated for each part using the procedure described above. Detection is performed separately per part for finding the complete object even when this one is partially occluded or not fully visible. Making the assumption that the parts located higher than the table are the most visible, the parts are tested by decreasing order of heights, making use of the equipment pose estimated by the static cameras.

Mobile AR Visualization: The estimation of ${}^{t}T_{M}^{R}$ allows us to overlay virtual elements directly into the user's point of view. We do so by back-projecting the virtual objects directly into the RGB image, shown on the moving screen. We make use of the depth map from the moving camera to detect when the virtual object is occluded and display only its parts visible in the current view.

3 Results

To validate our system, we recorded several sequences illustrating its typical use and several challenges that can occur, such as C-arm rotation, abrupt changes of viewpoint orientation, large changes in the position of the user around the table, clinicians walking in the view and other types of occlusions. The medical imaging system used in the room is a Siemens Zeego. Note, however, that the kinematic information was not available. Some of the results are described below. They are more comprehensively presented in the supplementary video[1], which also includes live recordings, since video material is better suited for evaluation.

The approach is tested using a computer equipped with an i7-3930K 6-core processor along with a GeForce GTX Titan GPU. Parallelization occurs through

[1] Supplementary video can be found at: `http://camma.u-strasbg.fr/videos/`

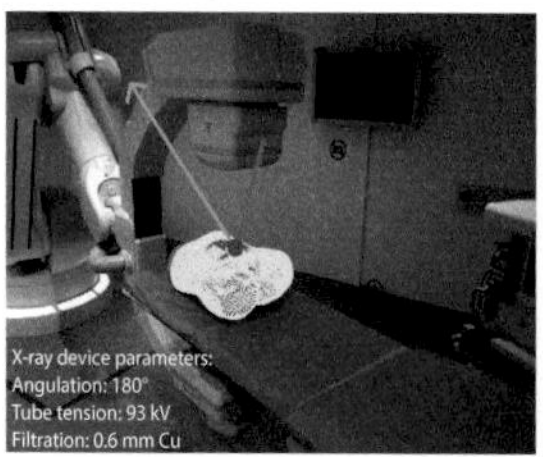

(a) AR visualization showing the main direction of scatter (orange), patient exposure and current device angulation.

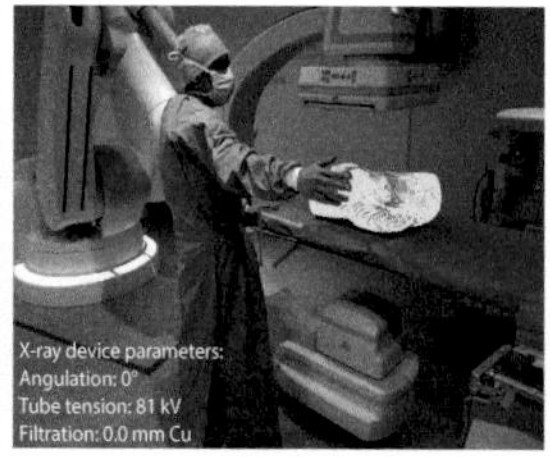

(b) AR visualization in the moving view where depth is used for consistent display in case of occlusion.

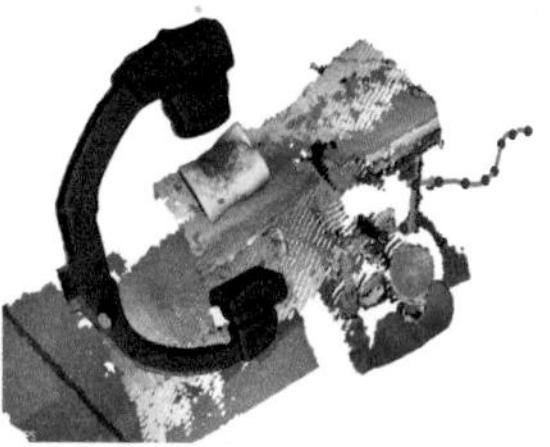

(c) Hand-held device trajectory displayed in the fused point cloud obtained from the static cameras.

Fig. 4. Illustration of the AR and tracking results for our clinical application.

multi-threading as described in Sec. 2.2 and through the use of the GPU for KinFu. In these experiments, the radiation maps are pre-computed offline using the approach presented in [5]. The patient is represented by an anatomical phantom, whose 3D shape has been scanned. Its exposure to radiation is displayed by texturing the phantom's surface according to the dose value at each 3D location for the current device configuration. Radiation scattering is caused by the interactions of the radiation with the surface of the patient. The main direction of scatter is computed from the position and orientation of the X-ray tube provided by the equipment detection.

Fig. 3 shows examples of object detections in the moving and static views. The 3D models are overlaid over the original images. In Fig. 3c, only the top part of the C-arm was detected. With the parameters used in our experiments, the dynamic template selection permits to divide the number of tested templates in the moving view by a factor of 10. Two examples of visualizations seen by the user are shown in Fig. 4 for different layouts of the room and positions. They illustrate the robustness of the system to occlusions and also the benefits of using the depth for consistent display of the virtual information in such situations. The overall system, including the visualization, runs at a framerate of 27 fps. The tracked path of the moving camera is shown in Fig. 4c inside the merged point clouds from the static cameras.

4 Conclusion

We have presented a mobile augmented reality approach for radiation awareness in the hybrid room. It relies on KinFu for camera tracking and on equipment detection for relocalization. By using three RGBD cameras, it has the advantage of being flexible and non-intrusive. The system is a proof-of-concept demonstrated on an important medical use-case. It is currently limited by the fact that the computation of the radiation risk map is not real-time and that the patient is not tracked. Future work will need to address these limitations. This system is however useful in its current form for radiation awareness training and can also be employed for other AR applications.

Acknowledgements. This work was supported by French state funds managed by the ANR within the Investissements d'Avenir program under references ANR-11-LABX-0004 (Labex CAMI), ANR-10-IDEX-0002-02 (IdEx Unistra) and ANR-10-IAHU-02 (IHU Strasbourg).

References

1. Glocker, B., Izadi, S., Shotton, J., Criminisi, A.: Real-time rgb-d camera relocalization. In: ISMAR, pp. 173–179 (2013)
2. Hinterstoisser, S., Lepetit, V., Ilic, S., Holzer, S., Bradski, G., Konolige, K., Navab, N.: Model based training, detection and pose estimation of texture-less 3D objects in heavily cluttered scenes. In: Lee, K.M., Matsushita, Y., Rehg, J.M., Hu, Z. (eds.) ACCV 2012, Part I. LNCS, vol. 7724, pp. 548–562. Springer, Heidelberg (2013)
3. Ladikos, A., Cagniart, C., Ghotbi, R., Reiser, M., Navab, N.: Estimating radiation exposure in interventional environments. In: Jiang, T., Navab, N., Pluim, J.P.W., Viergever, M.A. (eds.) MICCAI 2010, Part III. LNCS, vol. 6363, pp. 237–244. Springer, Heidelberg (2010)
4. Linte, C., Davenport, K., Cleary, K., Peters, C., Vosburgh, K., Navab, N., Edwards, P., Jannin, P., Peters, T., Holmes, D., Robb, R.: On mixed reality environments for minimally invasive therapy guidance: Systems architecture, successes and challenges in their implementation from laboratory to clinic. Comput. Med. Imaging Graph. 37(2), 83–97 (2013)
5. Loy Rodas, N., Padoy, N.: Seeing is believing: increasing intraoperative awareness to scattered radiation in interventional procedures by combining augmented reality, monte carlo simulations and wireless dosimeters. International Journal of Computer Assisted Radiology and Surgery (2015)
6. Maier-Hein, L., Franz, A., Fangerau, M., Schmidt, M., Seitel, A., Mersmann, S., Kilgus, T., Groch, A., Yung, K., dos Santos, T., Meinzer, H.P.: Towards mobile augmented reality for on-patient visualization of medical images. In: Bildverarbeitung für die Medizin, pp. 389–393. Springer (2011)
7. Newcombe, R.A., Izadi, S., Hilliges, O., Molyneaux, D., Kim, D., Davison, A.J., Kohli, P., Shotton, J., Hodges, S., Fitzgibbon, A.W.: Kinectfusion: Real-time dense surface mapping and tracking. In: ISMAR, pp. 127–136 (2011)
8. Salas-Moreno, R.F., Newcombe, R.A., Strasdat, H., Kelly, P.H.J., Davison, A.J.: SLAM++: simultaneous localisation and mapping at the level of objects. In: CVPR, pp. 1352–1359 (2013)
9. Sauer, F., Khamene, A., Bascle, B., Rubino, G.J.: A head-mounted display system for augmented reality image guidance: Towards clinical evaluation for imri-guided neurosurgery. In: Niessen, W.J., Viergever, M.A. (eds.) MICCAI 2001. LNCS, vol. 2208, pp. 707–716. Springer, Heidelberg (2001)
10. Sielhorst, T., Feuerstein, M., Navab, N.: Advanced medical displays: A literature review of augmented reality. Journal of Display Technology 4(4), 451–467 (2008)
11. Vanhavere, F., Carinou, E., Gualdrini, G., Clairand, I., Merce, M., Ginjaume, M.: The oramed project: Optimisation of radiation protection for medical staff. IFMBE Proceedings, vol. 25/3, pp. 470–473 (2009)
12. Wagner, M., Dresing, K., Wolfram, L., Ahrens, C.A., Bott, O.J.: Siscar-gpu: fast simulation and visualization of intraoperative scattered radiation to support radiation protection training. MIE 180, 968–972 (2012)

Hybrid Retargeting for High-Speed Targeted Optical Biopsies

André Mouton[1], Menglong Ye[1], François Lacombe[2], and Guang-Zhong Yang[1]

[1] The Hamlyn Centre for Robotic Surgery, Imperial College London, UK
[2] Mauna Kea Technologies, Paris, France
{a.mouton,menglong.ye11}@imperial.ac.uk

Abstract. With the increasing maturity of optical biopsy techniques, routine clinical use has become more widespread. This wider adoption of the technique demands effective tracking and retargeting of the biopsy sites, as no visible markers are left following examination. This study presents a high-speed framework for intra-procedural retargeting of probe-based optical biopsies in gastrointestinal endoscopy. A probe tip localisation method using active shape models and geometric heuristics, which eliminates the traditional dependency on shaft visibility, is proposed for automated initialisation. Partial occlusion and tissue deformation are addressed by exploiting the benefits of indirect and direct tracking through a novel combination of geometric association and online learning. Robustness to rapid endoscope motion and improvements in computational efficiency are achieved by restricting processing to the automatically detected video content area and through a feature-based rejection of non-informative frames. Performance evaluation in phantom and *in-vivo* environments demonstrates accurate biopsy site initialisation, robust retargeting and significant improvements over the state-of-the-art in processing time and memory usage.

1 Introduction

Gastrointestinal (GI) endoscopy together with histopathological tissue examination is the gold-standard for the diagnoses of pathologies in the digestive tract. Endoscopy-guided probe-based optical biopsies, however, allow for *in-vivo* visualisation of tissues at a cellular level, forgoing the need for tissue excision. Macroscopic retargeting of previously examined sites in this context is challenging due to the absence of physical scars at the biopsy sites [1]. Traditional retargeting, performed by tattooing the examined tissue with ink or Argon Plasma Coagulation (APC), is limited as the ink tends to diffuse and APC causes tissue damage. This study proposes a non-invasive alternative for automated intra-procedural retargeting using purely vision-based techniques, seeking high-speed performance and robustness to rapid endoscope movements, natural tissue deformation and partial site occlusion.

Mountney *et al.* [6] perform intra-procedural retargeting using a visual SLAM-based approach (assuming large-scale rigidity) to generate a 3D model of the

N. Navab et al. (Eds.): MICCAI 2015, Part I, LNCS 9349, pp. 471–479, 2015.
DOI: 10.1007/978-3-319-24553-9_58

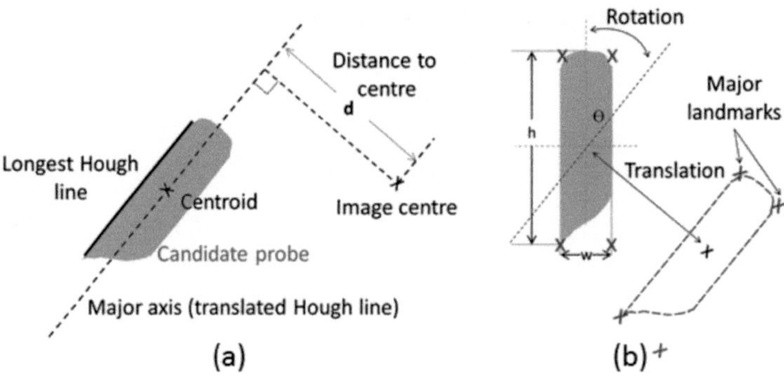

Fig. 1. Tip localisation: (a) Orientation constraint. (b) Major landmarks computation.

tissue surface. Initialisation is automated by a probe detection technique which exploits the achromatic properties of the probe shaft. Atasoy *et al.* [2] address tissue deformation using a geometrically-constrained MRF model, while Allain *et al.* [1] propose retargeting based on epipolar lines, derived from multiple views of a given biopsy site. Ye *et al.* [9] model tissue deformation as locally affine and perform indirect retargeting by geometric association and online-learning. Partial occlusion is addressed by reinitialising the associated sites when the optical probe exits the field of view (determined by simple blob detection).

This work expands upon these prior studies, each of which addresses only part of the retargeting problem, through the development of a novel, end-to-end framework for high-speed, automated and robust retargeting. The principal contributions include: real-time detection of non-informative frames; geometry-independent content area detection; shape-based probe tip localisation for automated initialisation and hybrid retargeting for improved performance under partial occlusion and tissue deformation.

2 Methods

An automated, high-speed solution for targeted optical biopsies in GI endoscopy, comprised of the following five components, is proposed: **1)** non-informative frame rejection; **2)** video content area detection; **3)** probe tip localisation; **4)** retargeting under partial occlusion and **5)** retargeting without occlusion.

Frame Rejection: Redundant processing is mitigated by discarding clinically non-informative frames using a novel quantification of image saliency based on the number of FAST keypoints detected [8] (Fig. 2). In particular, frames are rejected by placing a lower bound, τ_σ, on the number of detected keypoints. High frame rates in endoscopic sequences ($\geq$ 25fps) result in significant information overlap between a certain number of consecutive frames, making the selection of τ_σ non-critical as information lost in incorrectly discarded frames is likely to be recaptured in subsequent frames.

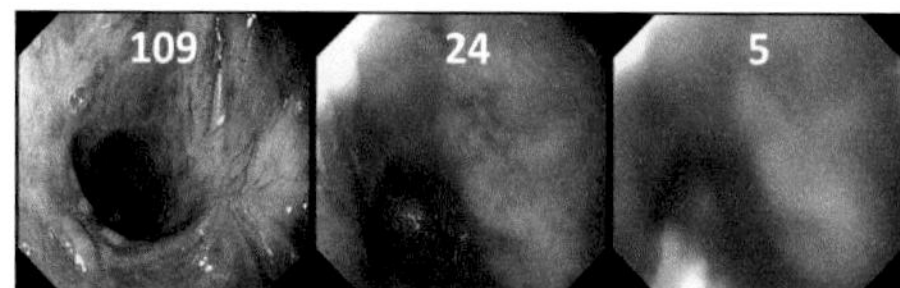

Fig. 2. Number of FAST keypoints detected.

Content Detection: Subsequent processing is restricted to the automatically-detected central content area (Fig. 3). While Munzer *et al.* [7] proposed a method to automatically detect circular content regions, here a technique for annotating the content area of all endoscopic sequences, regardless of the FoV geometry, is presented. Binary thresholding is applied to a greyscale input image to eliminate low-intensity noise in the background regions. The largest connected component in the binary image is then found and refined via morphological opening, which reduces unwanted spurious details.

Probe Tip Localisation: The initial biopsy site is assumed to be located at the tip of the optical probe and is found via probe detection and tip localisation. A limitation of prior work in vision-based endoscopic instrument detection is the reliance on the visibility of the achromatic instrument shaft [6]. This limitation is addressed via a markerless probe detection approach that combines colour-based segmentation with active shape modelling and geometric heuristics. The technique focusses directly on the detection of the probe tip, ignoring the instrument shaft and thereby compensating for scenarios where the shaft is not visible. Candidate segmentations are obtained by thresholding and connected component analysis in a *texture-reduced* image, obtained by greyscale morphological closing. Closing attenuates darker features in the image, reducing the characteristic mucosal and vascular patterns (i.e. reducing the texture) without impacting the appearance of the comparatively homogeneous probe tip and thereby simplifies the segmentation task. The candidate set is refined by applying two geometric constraints based on *a priori* knowledge of probe size and orientation. All components falling outside of a predefined size range are eliminated, while the orientation constraint is formulated based on the knowledge that the optical probe is inserted through the operating channel of the endoscope and is thus radially orientated. The constraint is enforced by placing a threshold on the distance between the extended major axis of the component and the image centre. The major axis is found by computing the longest straight line segment in the component using the Hough transform. This line (which is expected to represent one of the two longitudinal edges of the probe) is translated to pass through the centroid of the component, yielding the major axis (Fig. 1). The final coarse segmentation is that component with the longest straight line segment satisfying these constraints.

The texture-reduced image is searched using an Active Shape Model (ASM) [3] of the probe tip, the accuracy of which is optimised by initialising the search with the coarse segmentation. This is achieved by defining four *major* landmarks in the ASM located at the end-points of the longitudinal edges of the probe. The corresponding points in the coarse segmentation are estimated by centring the probe at the origin (by translation) and rotating it according to the orientation of its longest line segment (Fig. 1). The height and width of the probe are estimated as the maximum differences in the (x, y) components of any two points in the probe. The landmarks are then approximated as the corresponding offsets from the probe centroid, translated and rotated back to the initial pose. A linear transformation that minimises the Procrustes distance between the major landmarks in the mean and initial shapes is used to align the ASM with the coarse segmentation. This approach significantly improves segmentation accuracy, compared to the traditional approach of initialising the search with the mean shape and a fixed pose.

Pathological Site Retargeting (PSR): A hybrid retargeting approach is proposed, whereby the underlying methodology is based on the degree of partial site occlusion. A site is considered occluded if the overlap O between its bounding box (defined by the set of pixels A) and the optical probe (defined by the set B) exceeds a predefined threshold where $O = \frac{|A \cap B|}{|A|}$.

PSR with Partial Occlusion is performed by geometric association (Fig. 3). Similarly to [9], the associated sites are defined as the vertices of a set of n concentric, fixed radius pentagons. The set is constructed by incremental rotation of an initial pentagon by $\{0, \theta, 2\theta, \ldots, (n-1)\theta\}$ such that $n\theta = 72$. Based on the assumption that tissue deformation is locally affine [9], the biopsy site location is computed using the perspective transformation that minimises the reprojection error between the associated sites in the previous and current frames. The critical difference to [9], where each associated site is retargeted independently using TLD [5], is that the sites are tracked directly using Lucas-Kanade optical flow, which significantly reduces computational overhead. This approach is motivated by the fact that initial tracking of the site, while the probe is visible, does not generally involve endoscope motion and is thus unlikely to require site re-detection. This makes a short-term tracking solution more suitable in terms of computational overhead.

PSR without Partial Occlusion: The retargeting methodology switches to TLD when the overlap between the optical probe and the local neighbourhood of the biopsy site falls below a threshold (Fig. 3). TLD is an established long-term tracking method that integrates a median flow tracker, a cascaded classifier and online learning. In [9] tissue deformation is addressed by modelling the local neighbourhood with 180 separate bounding boxes. Here it is proposed that the same local information is captured by initialising TLD with a single, suitably-sized bounding box centred on the biopsy site. Since TLD is robust to affine transformations, the tracking of this bounding box is not affected by affine tissue deformation. This direct retargeting approach offers a significant reduction in computational overhead (1 site vs. 180 sites). In order to avoid corrupting the positive training samples of the cascaded classifier (generated online), the

Table 1. Probe tip localisation results.

Method	P	R	FPR	ALE (pixels)	FPS
TipLoc	0.91	0.89	0.05	3.84 ± 1.80	10
Mount [6]	0.09	0.05	0.41	43.26 ± 49.30	25

retargeting methodology reverts back to geometric association at any stage that the probe re-enters the local neighbourhood of the site.

3 Results

Performance was evaluated using both phantom and *in-vivo* gastrointestinal data, captured with an Olympus Narrow Band Imaging (NBI) endoscope. Two phantoms (modelling the textural mucosal and vascular characteristics of the human oesophagus) were used. Ground-truth annotations were performed by an experienced observer. Since probe-based optical biopsies are not currently practised in GI endoscopy in the UK, the procedure was simulated in the phantom environment using a Cellvizio optical probe manufactured by Mauna Kea Technologies. Tissue deformation was simulated by manually applying an external force to the phantom. All components of the proposed methodology related to probe tip localisation were evaluated in this environment.

Probe Tip Localisation: The ASM model was built using 50 training images and the number of search iterations was restricted to 10, such that overall processing times were not significantly compromised. Accuracy was measured as the Average Localisation Error (ALE) in pixels between the computed and ground-truth probe tip positions. Performance was quantified further according to the recall rate (R), False Positive Rate (FPR), and precision (P). Localisation errors of less than 10 pixels were considered true positives. Performance of the proposed method (denoted *TipLoc*) was compared to [6] (denoted *Mount*) - chosen as its methodology is representative of the majority of the related vision-based methods that rely on the visibility of the achromatic instrument shaft. With reference to Tab. 1, the proposed technique significantly outperformed [6] in terms of both tip localisation and detection accuracy. The poor performance of [6] is attributed to the failed initial segmentations and not to inaccurate tip localisations, as the current dataset consists predominantly of images where the shaft is not visible. Despite the lower average frame rate, Tab. 1 highlights the advantages of the proposed technique over the popular shaft-based segmentation approaches.

Retargeting: Performance was evaluated using three phantom and three *in-vivo* sequences and quantified using precision, recall and the ALE between the centres of the ground-truth and predicted bounding boxes. In particular, an object-based evaluation (c.f. pixel-based) was considered, whereby a true positive instance is defined as an overlap $\sigma_i = \frac{B_i^G \cap B_i^T}{B_i^G \cup B_i^T}$ of greater than a threshold τ_σ between the ground-truth and predicted bounding boxes (B^G, B^T respectively).

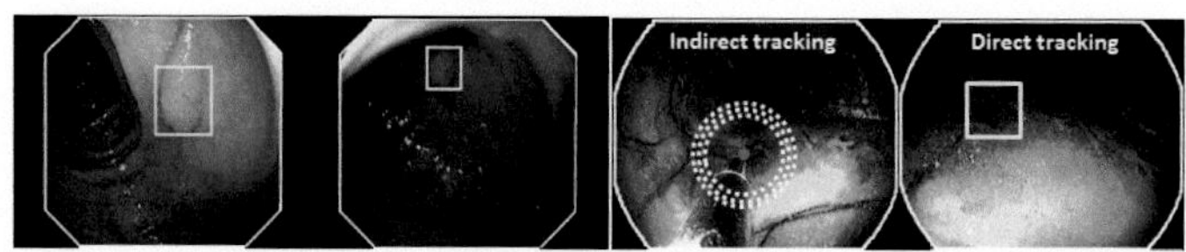

Fig. 3. Sample *in-vivo* (left) and phantom (right) PSR results. Content areas in white.

It is worth noting that ALE is not scale-invariant [??] and that it is thus not generally possible to perform ROC analysis using object-based metrics (as the false-positive rate cannot be computed) [4]. Therefore, in accordance with [4,5,??], the scalar-valued $F1$-measure ($F1 = 2\left(\frac{P \cdot R}{P+R}\right)$) was computed in addition to P, R and ALE, to provide an objective overall performance measure. The *in-vivo* performance of the proposed methodology (denoted *PSR*) was compared to the baseline intra-procedural approach of Ye *et al.* [9] (denoted *PSR_Ye*). A direct comparison was not possible in the phantom environment as PSR_Ye does not consider probe detection, thus requiring manual initialisation. Optimal parameter values were determined empirically, based on performance in a single sequence (not included in the results). The chosen parameter set was used for all tests (*in-vivo* and phantom).

PSR performed well in the phantom environment (Tab. 2), with perfect precision and a worst-case F1 of 0.91. Retargeting localisation accuracy was high for all three sequences (9.75-13.72 pixels). Performance is comparable to the state-of-the-art [9] (achieved in a similar phantom environment). PSR maintained high precision (0.91-0.96), recall (0.80-0.94) and F1 (0.85-0.94) scores *in-vivo* (Tab. 2). In contrast, PSR_Ye performed poorly, particularly with regard to recall (0.12-0.44), resulting in considerably lower F1 scores (0.23-0.61). In all three cases, PSR_Ye lost track of the biopsy site before it had exited the FoV and was not able to re-detect it in subsequent frames. As noted in [9], a decrease in textural saliency and an increase in the number of out-of-focus frames relative to the phantom data (due to rapid endoscope motion) negatively affects the feature-based classification in TLD. PSR_Ye, which relies on multi-site TLD and does not discard non-informative frames, is thus affected more significantly by these factors than PSR. The relative decline in performance of PSR *in-vivo* may be further attributed to the absence of partial probe occlusion, which biases overall phantom performance due to the relative ease of short-term tracking in partially occluded frames. The *in-vivo* and phantom results suggest that direct tracking is favourable to geometric association in non-occluded scenarios.

Content detection used in conjunction with frame rejection was found to yield optimal performance, when considering F1 scores in conjunction with processing times (Tab. 3). Although a negligible drop in recall was caused by the inevitable rejection of a small number of informative frames, frame-rejection crucially improved precision by reducing the number of false-positive containing frames and significantly decreased processing times by eliminating redundant sliding window searches.

Computational Performance: The improvements in computational efficiency of PSR relative to PSR_Ye were evaluated according to CPU usage, memory

Table 2. Phantom and *in-vivo* performance.

Name	Method	P	R	F1	ALE (pixels)
Phantom 1	PSR	1.00	0.98	0.99	13.72
Phantom 2	PSR	1.00	0.96	0.98	13.06
Phantom 3	PSR	1.00	0.91	0.95	9.75
***In-vivo* 1**	PSR	0.96	0.81	0.88	10.94
	PSR_Ye	1.00	0.27	0.43	4.60
***In-vivo* 2**	PSR	0.94	0.94	0.94	15.89
	PSR_Ye	1.00	0.44	0.61	3.40
***In-vivo* 3**	PSR	0.91	0.80	0.85	12.24
	PSR_Ye	1.00	0.13	0.23	14.19

Table 3. Impact of content detection (CD) and frame rejection (FR). Optimal results in bold.

Name	CD	FR (discarded)	P	R	F1	Time (s)
	no	no	0.79	0.37	0.50	131.87
***In-vivo* 1**	yes	no	0.94	0.83	0.88	120.73
	no	yes (275)	0.77	0.87	0.82	101.00
	yes	**yes (325)**	**0.96**	**0.81**	**0.88**	**91.12**
	no	no	0.94	0.67	0.78	46.73
***In-vivo* 3**	yes	no	0.87	0.80	0.83	41.18
	no	yes (6)	0.63	0.69	0.66	41.47
	yes	**yes (15)**	**0.91**	**0.80**	**0.85**	**39.00**

usage and processing time for single-site retargeting in a 419-frame *in-vivo* sequence. Additionally, the feasibility of multi-site PSR was evaluated by measuring computational performance for one, two, three and five sites. Multi-site PSR was implemented by brute-force, whereby each site was retargeted independently (resource sharing and/or parallelisation were not considered). Processing was performed on an Intel® Core™ i7, 3.4GHz quad-core CPU with 16GB of RAM. PSR outperformed PSR_Ye in every aspect of computational performance for single-site retargeting with reductions of approximately 50% in mean CPU usage and 90% in mean memory usage (Fig. 4a-c). Most significantly (with regard to clinical feasibility), PSR gave an improvement of two orders of magnitude in frame rate over PSR_Ye (10-30fps vs. ≈ 0.5fps). These are significant improvements in computational efficiency and highlight the benefits of the proposed hybrid retargeting approach. Fig. 4d shows the results of regression analyses for each metric (averaged over the entire sequence) for multi-site PSR. Memory usage and CPU usage exhibited quadratic and linear relationships with the number of retargeted sites respectively, while frame rate decreased exponentially. While this is not encouraging for clinical feasibility (where approximately 10-20 sites would need to be retargeted), it is proposed that parallelisation and resource sharing would improve performance significantly. This claim is substantiated by the results for single-site PSR_Ye (Fig. 4a-c). PSR_Ye, which has been parallelised, simultaneously retargets 180 associated sites for a single biopsy site, yet operates with manageable computational overhead and maintains a frame rate of approximately 0.5fps.

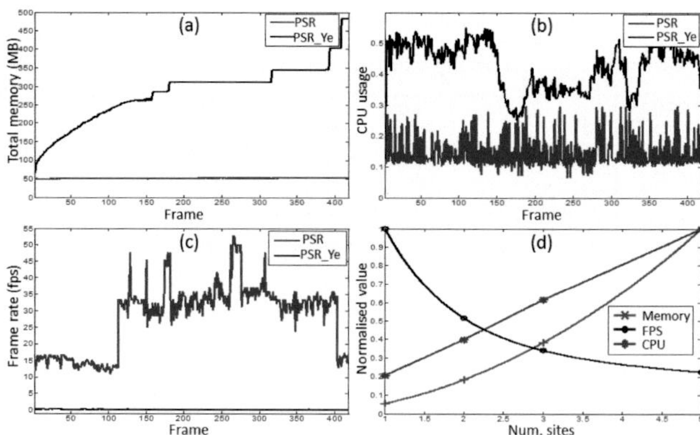

Fig. 4. Computational performance: (a) Single-site memory usage. (b) Single-site CPU usage. (c) Single-site frame rates. (d) Multi-site regression analyses.

4 Conclusion

This study has presented a high-speed, automated solution for targeted optical biopsies in GI endoscopy. Initialisation is performed via a novel probe tip localisation method using active shape modelling and geometric heuristics. Partial occlusion and tissue deformation have been addressed by adopting a hybrid retargeting approach which combines indirect tracking by geometric association and direct tracking by online learning. Additionally, a method for the detection of non-informative frames using the FAST feature detector has been presented, improving robustness to rapid endoscope motion and facilitating high-speed implementation. Computational efficiency has been optimised further by restricting processing to the automatically-detected video content area. State-of-the-art probe tip localisation accuracy has been presented with an average error of 3.84 pixels and consistently high recall (0.89) and precision (0.91) rates. Crucially, the traditional dependency on the visibility of the probe shaft has been eliminated. Retargeting is achieved with consistently high F1 scores (0.85-0.99) for both phantom and *in-vivo* data. Together with an improvement of two orders of magnitude in processing time, this corresponds to a significant improvement over the state-of-the-art [9]. Future work will seek to further improve computational efficiency to facilitate the implementation of multi-site retargeting.

References

1. Allain, B., Hu, M., Lovat, L.B., Cook, R.J., Vercauteren, T., Ourselin, S., Hawkes, D.J.: A system for biopsy site re-targeting with uncertainty in gastroenterology and oropharyngeal examinations. In: Jiang, T., Navab, N., Pluim, J.P.W., Viergever, M.A. (eds.) MICCAI 2010, Part II. LNCS, vol. 6362, pp. 514–521. Springer, Heidelberg (2010)

2. Atasoy, S., Glocker, B., Giannarou, S., Mateus, D., Meining, A., Yang, G.-Z., Navab, N.: Probabilistic region matching in narrow-band endoscopy for targeted optical biopsy. In: Yang, G.-Z., Hawkes, D., Rueckert, D., Noble, A., Taylor, C. (eds.) MICCAI 2009, Part I. LNCS, vol. 5761, pp. 499–506. Springer, Heidelberg (2009)
3. Cootes, T.F., Taylor, C.J., Cooper, D.H., Graham, J.: Active shape models-their training and application. CVIU 61(1), 38–59 (1995)
4. Hua, Y., Alahari, K., Schmid, C.: Occlusion and motion reasoning for long-term tracking. In: Fleet, D., Pajdla, T., Schiele, B., Tuytelaars, T. (eds.) ECCV 2014, Part VI. LNCS, vol. 8694, pp. 172–187. Springer, Heidelberg (2014)
5. Kalal, Z., Mikolajczyk, K., Matas, J.: Tracking-learning-detection. IEEE TPAMI 34(7), 1409–1422 (2012)
6. Mountney, P., Giannarou, S., Elson, D., Yang, G.-Z.: Optical biopsy mapping for minimally invasive cancer screening. In: Yang, G.-Z., Hawkes, D., Rueckert, D., Noble, A., Taylor, C. (eds.) MICCAI 2009, Part I. LNCS, vol. 5761, pp. 483–490. Springer, Heidelberg (2009)
7. Munzer, B., Schoeffmann, K., Boszormenyi, L.: Detection of circular content area in endoscopic videos. In: IEEE Inter. Symp. on Computer-Based Medical Systems, pp. 534–536 (2013)
8. Rosten, E., Drummond, T.W.: Machine learning for high-speed corner detection. In: Leonardis, A., Bischof, H., Pinz, A. (eds.) ECCV 2006, Part I. LNCS, vol. 3951, pp. 430–443. Springer, Heidelberg (2006)
9. Ye, M., Giannarou, S., Patel, N., Teare, J., Yang, G.-Z.: Pathological site retargeting under tissue deformation using geometrical association and tracking. In: Mori, K., Sakuma, I., Sato, Y., Barillot, C., Navab, N. (eds.) MICCAI 2013, Part II. LNCS, vol. 8150, pp. 67–74. Springer, Heidelberg (2013)

Visual Force Feedback for Hand-Held Microsurgical Instruments

Gauthier Gras, Hani J. Marcus, Christopher J. Payne, Philip Pratt, and Guang-Zhong Yang

The Hamlyn Centre for Robotic Surgery, Imperial College London, SW7 2AZ, London, UK
gauthier.gras12@imperial.ac.uk

Abstract. Microsurgery is technically challenging, demanding both rigorous precision under the operating microscope and great care when handling tissue. Applying excessive force can result in irreversible tissue injury, but sufficient force must be exerted to carry out manoeuvres in an efficient manner. Technological advances in hand-held instruments have allowed the integration of force sensing capabilities into surgical tools, resulting in the possibility of force feedback during an operation. This paper presents a novel method of graduated online visual force-feedback for hand-held microsurgical instruments. Unlike existing visual force-feedback techniques, the force information is integrated into the surgical scene by highlighting the area around the point of contact while preserving salient anatomical features. We demonstrate that the proposed technique can be integrated seamlessly with image guidance techniques. Critical anatomy beyond the exposed tissue surface is revealed using an augmented reality overlay when the user is exerting large forces within their proximity. The force information is further used to improve the quality of the augmented reality by displacing the overlay based on the forces exerted. Detailed user studies were performed to assess the efficacy of the proposed method.

1 Introduction

Delicate neurovascular tissue requires the performance of microsurgical procedures with high dexterity and accuracy. Technological advances of the past decade have facilitated the integration of force-sensing with new surgical devices. Robotic platforms such as the NeuroArm and the Steady-Hand Robot have incorporated force limiting, scaling, and feedback capabilities. Hand-held microinstruments have also benefited from increased force-sensing capabilities. These instruments represent simple, low cost, yet intrinsically robust alternatives to conventional master-slave and co-operative control platforms.

Various modes of force-feedback have been used in both hand-held and robotic devices including tactile, auditory, and visual cues [1,2]. Previous work has suggested that all of these forms of feedback have a comparable influence on surgical performance [3]. However, these modes differ considerably in the nature in which

N. Navab et al. (Eds.): MICCAI 2015, Part I, LNCS 9349, pp. 480–487, 2015.
DOI: 10.1007/978-3-319-24553-9_59

they may be integrated into the operative workflow. Tactile feedback may represent the most intuitive method to indicate when a force threshold is breached, but is best suited to conveying binary rather than graduated information. Auditory feedback does allow for more granular feedback, but may not be recognised above the ambient noise of a busy operating room. Visual feedback can provide detailed information in an unambiguous fashion, but it risks inattention blindness - cues located away from the operating site may distract the surgeon, and cues overlying the operating site may obstruct the surgical scene.

In this paper, we propose a new way of visual force-feedback for hand-held microsurgical instruments that allows graduated force feedback to be presented over the operating site, while preserving the salient anatomical features. The preservation of anatomical information in the image is achieved by using a Non-Photorealistic Rendering (NPR) scheme. As shown in [4], this method is particularly effective in augmented reality applications with high-fidelity depth perception. The proposed technique makes use of this feature for seamless integration with image guidance techniques. By detecting the proximity of the surgeon's instrument to critical anatomical structures beyond the exposed tissue surface, the proposed technique is used to reveal these structures when exerted forces are deemed too high. Finite element modelling is performed to ensure physically accurate deformation rendering. The efficacy of the method is assessed by detailed user studies involving a retraction and dissection study to quantify the forces exerted with and without the visual force-feedback; and a depth study to quantify the effect of the movement of the overlaid structure on depth perception.

2 Materials and Methods

2.1 System Overview

A blunt surgical dissector (Yasargil FD304R, Braun Aesculap) was axially affixed to a force-torque (F/T) sensor (ATI Nano17, ATI Industrial Automation, Inc) that can sense both lateral and axial forces that are applied to the dissector tip. This dissector and F/T sensor assembly were integrated into a hand-held casing that incorporated optical tracking markers, as shown in Figure 1. The force signal was acquired by a realtime linux computer through a PCI interface. Images from the Leica M525 OH4 (Leica Microsystems Ltd., UK) surgical microscope were acquired with an AJA HA5-Plus HDMI to SDI converter (AJA Video Systems Inc., California, USA) linking to an AJA Kona 4 PCIe card. A Polaris Vicra optical tracking system by NDI (Waterloo, Ontario, Canada) served to track the microscope, the hand-held tool, and register the virtual scene.

2.2 Visual Force-Feedback

The principal purpose of NPR is to render the surface tissue as a translucent layer, while keeping salient anatomical features distinct enough to provide navigation and depth cues [4]. To accomplish this NPR computes p-q values representing a measure of the local surface slope of the tissue. In force feedback

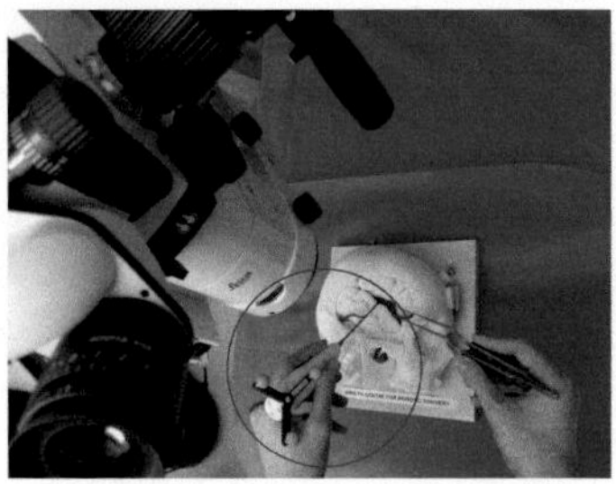

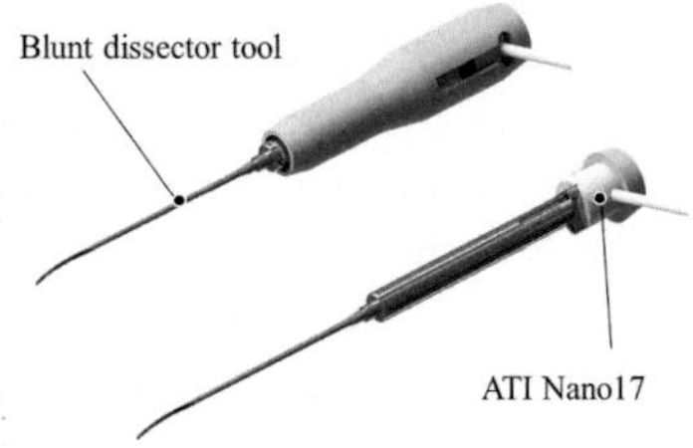

Fig. 1. Left: surgical setup under a microscope with a blunt dissector with force feedback (left hand), and forceps (right hand) Right: design of the blunt dissector

these values are multiplied by a scaling factor proportional to the force exerted, to increase the level of details in the highlighted features when higher forces are applied. The output of the rendering is a texture referred to as the inverse realism texture (IR texture), of width W_{ir} and height H_{ir}, and centred around a point $P_c(x_c, y_c)$.

Smooth surfaces are represented as uniform dark blue patches, and high surface gradients are brightened proportionally to their gradient value. Furthermore, pixels shift from the IR texture values to the original image values proportionally to their distance from the texture centre. For NPR to be useful for visual force-feedback, these properties must be modulated by the forces detected. The parameters used to modulate the IR texture are:

- The detail level of features during the pq value generation.
- The radius R_{ir} of the circular texture, when $W_{ir} = H_{ir} = R_{ir}$.
- The blending between the input image and the IR texutre, G_{ir}.
- The colour palette of the IR texture.

Let A be the output pixel, B the input pixel, and C the IR texture pixel at the point $P(x, y)$. Let G_{ir} be the blending coefficient between B and C. The blending is modulated by:

$$A = S_{ir} \times B + (1 - S_{ir}) \times C, \tag{1}$$

with

$$S_{ir} = \left(\frac{(x - x_c)^2}{W_{ir}} + \frac{(y - y_c)^2}{H_{ir}} \right)^{G_{ir}}. \tag{2}$$

And so:

$$A = C + (B - C) \times \left(\frac{(x - x_c)^2}{W_{ir}} + \frac{(y - y_c)^2}{H_{ir}} \right)^{G_{ir}} \tag{3}$$

2.3 Augmented Reality Integration

Recent studies have demonstrated that the use of inverse realism techniques using NPR improve depth perception [5]. The proposed method makes use of this property to combine visual force feedback with image guidance techniques. When exerting excessive force near critical pathology, the proposed method reveals anatomical structures hidden under the tissue surface, alerting the surgeon to their presence. A virtual surgical scene containing triangle meshes of the structures of interest is registered to the real-world operating scene, allowing correct overlaying of the virtual elements on the operative images. The resulting combination of the IR texture modulation with the augmented reality is shown in Figure 2.

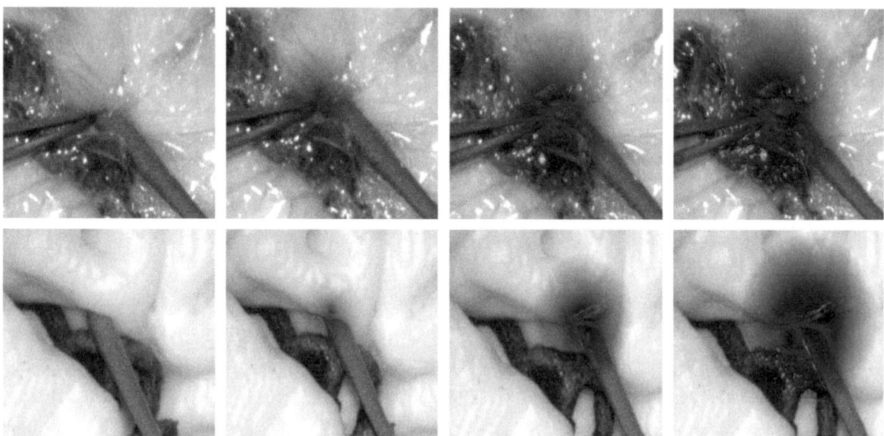

Fig. 2. From left to right: gradual increase in forces exerted, Top: with plastic membrane to simulate the dura, Bottom: without the plastic membrane

2.4 Force-Based Displacement

While the IR texture allows the augmented reality overlay to appear embedded below the tissue surface, it does not provide any motion cues. Unless the registered microscope or skull are moved, the overlaid structure will appear static regardless of the deformation of the surface tissue. The force information from the hand-held instrument can be used to simulate this motion, by displacing the overlaid structure relative to the forces exerted.

Preliminary work with a linear displacement model suggested that the model did not have to be highly accurate in order to be compelling, due to the visual nature of the application. In order to strike a balance between simplicity and accuracy, a finite element model (FEM) simulation was conducted. A professional neurosurgical phantom (Kezlex, Tokyo, Japan) was scanned and a tetrahedral mesh of 1483 nodes obtained. A downwards force exerted from the top of the brain tissue simulated the push of a blunt dissector, and the boundary conditions were set by areas of the skull consistent with a microscopic operation. An implementation of the total Lagrangian explicit dynamics (TLED) algorithm was used to model tissue deformation, employing a constant lumped mass matrix and a

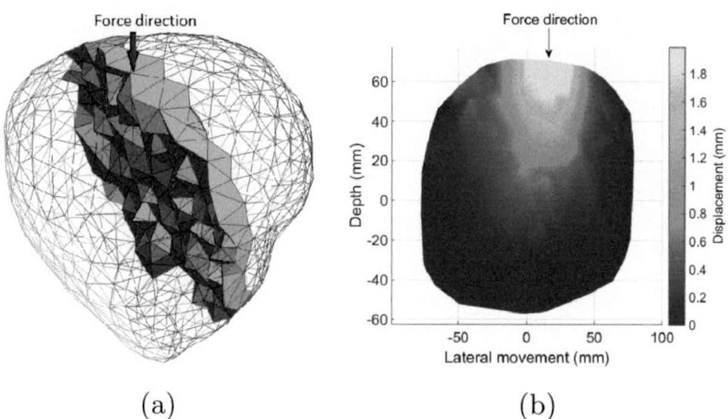

Fig. 3. Propagation of displacements in the brain for a surface deformation of 2mm. (a) section of the model, (b) map of displacements in the section

proportional damping matrix with Rayleigh damping coefficient $\alpha = 7.5E+01$. The constitutive law followed that of a compressible neo-Hookean material, with Young's modulus $E = 3240$ Pa and Poisson's ratio $\eta = 0.499$ [6]. The results of the simulation were studied for different sections of the model, as shown in Figure 3. For each of five simulations chosen to cover the range of forces typically applied in neurosurgery, displacement data of the tissue at different depths was recorded. Polynomials of up to degree 6 were fitted to the data. Degree 4 polynomials were chosen as they presented the best global fitting while retaining a monotonic behaviour which matched the original data over the interval of interest, as shown in Figure 4a. Results from the literature [6] are used to convert force values from the sensor to surface displacements. Finally a generalized model was developed, describing the displacement $D(x)$ at a depth x for a surface displacement D_0:

$$D(x) = \frac{D_0}{n}\left(\sum_{i=1}^{n} \frac{a_i \times x^4 + b_i \times x^3 + c_i \times x^2 + d_i \times x + e_i}{D_{0_i}}\right), \tag{4}$$

where n is the number simulations (5 in this paper), D_{0_i} is the surface displacement for the ith simulation, and a_i, b_i, c_i, d_i, and e_i the coefficients of the fitted polynomial for the ith simulation. The generalized model is compared to the polynomials of the individual simulations in Figure 4b.

The model described in 4 can be derived by normalizing the results from the different simulations. This is achieved by dividing all the displacement values obtained in a simulation i by the surface displacement for that simulation D_{0_i} (i.e the maximum displacement). In so doing all the displacement values are normalized to a $[0;1]$ range, and the resulting normalized polynomials of each simulation can be averaged to a polynomial P_{norm}. The displacement $D(x)$ at a depth x for a surface displacement D_0 can then be derived as follows:

$$D(x) = D_0 \times P_{norm}(x) \tag{5}$$

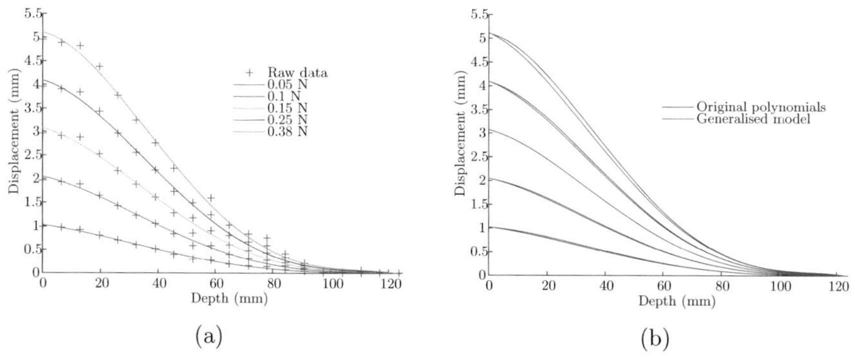

Fig. 4. Displacements relative to depth (a) Raw data (1 out of 5 points) and polynomial fitting (b) Comparison between the generalised model and the polynomial fitting

3 Experimental Setup and Results

In the studies below, the live input video stream used was obtained from a Leica M525 OH4 surgical microscope. The output HD video stream was displayed on a screen with stereo capabilities.

3.1 Retraction Study

Tissue retraction is among the most common manoeuvres performed in surgery. Eight participants were asked to use the blunt dissector in their non-dominant hand to provide retraction, and use the forceps in their dominant hand to simultaneously perform a peg transfer task. The forces exerted on through the instrument were recorded, and a coloured display used to indicate when a minimum effective force of 0.2 N was applied (red for forces under 0.2 N, grey otherwise). Each participant was asked to apply an increasing retraction force with the dissector, until the colour became grey. Participants were then asked to keep the indicator grey by maintaining this minimum force of 0.2 N for 60 s. A force threshold of 0.3 N was selected as indicative of excessive force. Participants performed the experiment 6 times, 3 times with visual force-feedback and 3 times without in a randomized manner. The primary outcomes of the study were the median forces exerted (N), the maximum forces exerted (N), the time exerting forces under 0.2N, and the time exerting forces more than 0.3N. These results are shown in Figure 5.

3.2 Dissection Study

Tissue dissection is also commonly performed in surgery, but represents a more complex manoeuvre than retraction. A surgical resident was recruited from a university hospital, and performed a dissection alternating at 2 min intervals between no force-feedback, and NPR visual force-feedback. The participant was

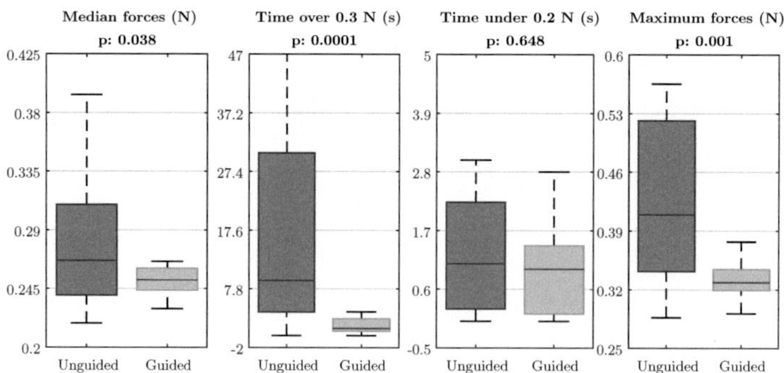

Fig. 5. Primary outcomes of the retraction study

asked to use the blunt dissector in their right hand to perform dissection, and use a sucker in their left hand to simultaneously provide counter-traction. A model brain was used to simulate dissection (Kezlex, Tokyo, Japan). The participant was asked to perform blunt arachnoid dissection of the Sylvian fissure on the model brain. A force threshold of 0.3 N was selected as indicative of excessive force. The study showed the use of NPR visual force-feedback resulted in a 31% decrease of median forces, as well as a 48% decrease in the overall time spent above 0.3 N. The maximum forces exerted also decreased by 51%.

3.3 Depth Perception Study

The application of inverse realism overlay to microsurgery represents a unique challenge, because image injection on commercial operating microscopes is 2D. To mitigate for the loss of binocular depth cues, we developed and evaluated a modified image guidance platform that incorporates force data to displace the virtual embedded object. Six participants were asked to use the blunt dissector in their right hand to interact with a series of scenes, each containing two virtual spheres located within the brain phantom used for the FEM simulation. One sphere was 50% larger than the other, but both were placed at different depths under the brain tissue so that size alone could not be a sufficient depth indicator. Each participant was asked to contact both virtual sphere three times with the dissector, and then select which was deeper. Participants performed the experiment 24 times, 12 times with displacement feedback and 12 times without in a randomized manner.

Without force feedback (unguided), the average success rate was 50% in 2D (random), and 70.8% in 3D. With force feedback (guided), the average success rate rose to 91.7% in 2D, and 97.2% in 3D. The differences between guided and unguided were statistically significant in both 2D and 3D ($p < 0.01$). Guided 2D also showed statistically significant improvements over unguided 3D.

4 Discussion and Conclusion

In this paper, we have presented a new visual force feedback scheme for hand-held microsurgical instruments. Results from the retraction and dissection studies show a clear improvement of the median forces exerted, maximum forces exerted, and time spent over the force threshold. The retraction study does not display significant results for the time spent under the minimum force. This is due to the fact that both study cases had visual feedback of that limit through the red indicator. The visual force feedback seemed particularly apt at preventing drift over time of the forces exerted.

The results show significant improvement between the cases with and without force feedback, both in 2D and in 3D. The results of the experiment in 2D without force feedback show nearly 50% correct answers, which was expected as participants did not have any valid cues to judge the depth. The addition of 3D shows a statistically significant improvement for the unguided case. While the improvement in the percentage of correct answers is not statistically significant between guided 2D and 3D, the success rate for both is significantly higher than unguided. From these results it can be concluded that the force displacement is essential for estimating the relative depth of objects in a neurosurgical scene, at least equivalent to stereo alone. Furthermore the results suggest that the force displacement enhances the effect of a stereo display, due to added 3D motion cues.

References

1. Payne, C.J., Yang, G.Z.: Hand-held medical robots. Annals of Biomedical Engineering 42(8), 1594–1605 (2014)
2. Akinbiyi, T., Reiley, C.E., Saha, S., Burschka, D., Hasser, C.J., Yuh, D.D., Okamura, A.M.: Dynamic augmented reality for sensory substitution in robot-assisted surgical systems. In: Conf. Proc. IEEE Eng. Med. Biol. Soc. pp. 315–333 (2006)
3. Kitagawa, M., Dokko, D., Okamura, A.M., Yuh, D.D.: Effect of sensory substitution on suture-manipulation forces for robotic surgical systems. J. of Thorac. and Cardiovas. Surg. 129(1), 151–158 (2005)
4. Lerotic, M., Chung, A.J., Mylonas, G.P., Yang, G.Z.: *pq*-space based non-photorealistic rendering for augmented reality. In: Ayache, N., Ourselin, S., Maeder, A. (eds.) MICCAI 2007, Part II. LNCS, vol. 4792, pp. 102–109. Springer, Heidelberg (2007)
5. Marcus, H.J., Pratt, P., Hughes-Hallett, A., Cundy, T.P., Marcus, A.P., Yang, G.Z., Darzi, A., Nandi, D.: Comparative effectiveness and safety of image guidance systems in neurosurgery: a preclinical randomized study. J. of Neurosur. (2015)
6. Miller, K., Chinzei, K., Orssengo, G., Bednarz, P.: Mechanical properties of brain tissue in-vivo: Experiment and computer simulation. J. of Biomechanics 33(11), 1369–1376 (2000)

Automated Three-Piece Digital Dental Articulation

Jianfu Li[1], Flavio Ferraz[1], Shunyao Shen[1], Yi-Fang Lo[1], Xiaoyan Zhang[1], Peng Yuan[1], Zhen Tang[1], Ken-Chung Chen[1], Jaime Gateno[1,2], Xiaobo Zhou[3], and James J. Xia[1,2]

[1] Department of Oral & Maxillofacial Surgery, Houston Methodist Research Institute, TX, USA
[2] Department of Surgery, Weill Medical College, Cornell University, New York, NY, USA
[3] Department of Radiology, Wake Forest School of Medicine, Winston-Salem, NC, USA

Abstract. In craniomaxillofacial (CMF) surgery, a critical step is to reestablish dental occlusion. Digitally establishing new dental occlusion is extremely difficult. It is especially true when the maxilla is segmentalized into 3 pieces, a common procedure in CMF surgery. In this paper, we present a novel midline-guided occlusal optimization (MGO) approach to automatically and efficiently reestablish dental occlusion for 3-piece maxillary surgery. Our MGO approach consists of 2 main steps. The anterior segment of the maxilla is first aligned to the intact mandible using our ergodic midline-match algorithm. The right and left posterior segments are then aligned to the mandible in sequence using an improved iterative surface-based minimum distance mapping algorithm. Our method has been validated using 15 sets of digital dental models. The results showed our algorithm-generated 3-piece articulation is more efficient and effective than the current standard of care method. The results demonstrated our approach's significant clinical impact and technical contributions.

1 Introduction

Craniomaxillofacial (CMF) surgery involves surgical correction of congenital or acquired deformities of the skull and face. Throughout the world, many patients suffering from CMF deformity require surgical correction. In the CMF surgery, one of the critical steps is to reestablish a good dental occlusion (the relationship between the upper and the lower teeth). Current standard of care to reestablish occlusion (called *stone dental cast surgery*) is very convoluted and time-consuming. When a doctor uses upper and lower stone dental casts to establish the occlusion (called *dental articulation*), the physical action of articulating upper and lower models into a maximal contact (called *maximum intercuspation (MI)*) is relatively easy and accurate. It becomes more difficult when the maxilla is segmentalized into 3 individual segments, 1 anterior and 2 posteriors (usually takes 4-6 hours manually). Each individual piece has its own 6-degree of freedom and lesser geometric features that can be extracted for dental articulation. The process of articulating the 3 upper segments to the lower teeth is a common procedure in CMF surgery (called *3-piece articulation*). In this procedure, lower dental arch usually remains intact. The dental articulation becomes even more difficult in virtual world, where the digital dental models are represented by three-dimensional (3D) images that lack collision constraints [1].

N. Navab et al. (Eds.): MICCAI 2015, Part I, LNCS 9349, pp. 488–496, 2015.
DOI: 10.1007/978-3-319-24553-9_60

Generally, the following rules are applied to the dental articulation: the upper and lower teeth should be maintained in MI; and both upper and lower central dental midlines should be aligned straight in the middle. Additional rules are applied to the 3-piece dental articulation: the anterior and the two posterior segments should maintain an appropriate smoothly curved relationship in the new upper dental arch, and to their corresponding lower dental arch; the upper and lower incisors should maintain appropriate overbite and overjet (vertical and horizontal distances between the upper and lower incisors); and the new upper dental arch should maintain appropriate Curve of Wilson (a U-shape curve in front view) between the posterior segments.

Currently, there is no report on establishing the 3-piece dental articulation digitally. Only the research works on 1-piece articulation were reported. Hiew et al. [2] described a technique in which plaster orthodontic study models with their distinctive heptagonal bases were created for a corresponding set of upper and lower dental models. DeLong et al. [3] proposed to align a set of digital dental models into MI based on three-point alignment. Zhang et al. [4] developed a two-stage occlusal analysis algorithm to manually align the models in the computer. However, none of above approach can be actually used in real clinical practice. More recently, Chang et al. [1] developed an approach to achieve single-piece dental articulation using an Iterative Surface-based Minimum Distance Mapping with collision constraints (ISMDM). Although this approach was validated clinically, it could be only used for 1-piece dental articulation, but not for 3-piece articulation.

In this article, we present a novel and effective midline-guided occlusal optimization (MGO) approach to automatically reestablish dental occlusion for 3-piece maxillary osteotomy (within 30 minutes using MATLAB codes on a regular office PC). Our MGO approach includes two main steps. The first step is to align the maxillary anterior segment to the intact mandible based on a robust ergodic midline-match algorithm. The second step is to align the right and left posterior segments to the mandible in sequence using an improved ISMDM optimization algorithm combined with occlusal plane transformation, new constraints for deviations among the 3 pieces, and adaptive constraints parameter adjustment. Finally, our method is validated using 15 sets of dental models that are required for 3-piece dental articulation. The clinical contribution of this project is significant. It allows clinicians to plan CMF surgery completely in the computer, including the most challenging 3-piece digital dental articulation. This has never been achieved before. The plan can then be transferred to the patient at the time of the surgery using surgical templates [5]. The technical contribution is that our novel ergodic midline-match algorithm can ensure the upper and lower dental midlines are ideally aligned to each other, and the arc of the anterior segment is aligned to the lower dental arch with their incisors maintaining appropriate overjet, overbite and inclination. Additionally, guided by the midline-matched anterior segments, our MGO approach further applies an improved ISMDM aligning the two posterior segments of the upper model to the lower model to ensure they are in MI.

2 Algorithm for Automatic 3-Piece Dental Articulation

The 3 pieces of the upper digital dental model and the intact lower dental model are represented by closed mesh surfaces. For 3-piece dental articulation, we need to align not only the occlusal surfaces between the upper and lower teeth, but also the cutting surfaces among the anterior and the two posterior segments of the upper model. In our algorithm, we first extract dental features for both the occlusal and cutting surfaces.

The occlusal surfaces feature points are extracted based on the work in [1]. For cutting surface feature points, a kd-tree [6] is constructed for mesh vertices on the anterior segment of maxilla. The nearest neighbor search (NN) algorithm is then applied to find the closest points between the posterior and anterior segments of maxilla. Finally, the cutting surface feature points are constructed from the closest points. Fig. 1 shows the feature points of the occlusal and cutting surfaces for the 3-piece upper models, and the occlusal feature points for the lower model. These feature points are used for the alignment of the anterior and two posterior segments. They are described below in details.

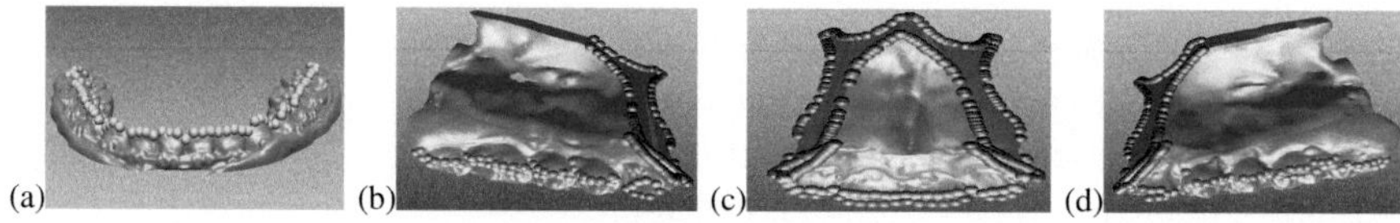

Fig. 1. Feature points for occlusal and cutting surfaces. (a) lower model; (b) right posterior segment of upper model; (c) anterior segment of upper model; (d) left posterior segment of upper model. Light yellow and Gray represent occlusal surface feature points. Dark yellow represents cutting surface feature points.

2.1 Anterior Segment Alignment

Anterior alignment plays an important role in dental occlusion. In our 3-piece MGO approach, we first align the anterior segment to an ideal position based on a group of clinical rules, followed by right and left posterior segment alignment. We develop an ergodic midline-match algorithm to solve the anterior segment alignment problem.

The midline-match algorithm is to align the dental midlines of the upper anterior segment and the lower teeth, and to set an appropriate overjet and overbite. For a given target overjet and overbite with a resulted upper and lower incisal inclination (calculated based on overjet and overbite), we can estimate a new position of upper midline plane (black intersectional lines in Fig. 2(a)) based on lower midline plane (green intersectional lines in Fig. 2(a)). Each central incisal midline plane is determined by manually digitizing 2 midpoints of right and left incisal edges, and a midpoint between the 2 roots (the circles in Fig.2). A transform matrix is then calculated by matching the original (red in Fig. 2(a)) and estimated upper midline planes. During the alignment, the upper and lower dental midlines are perfectly aligned to each other with appropriate overjet and overbite. The arc of the anterior segment is also aligned to the arc of the lower dental arch (blue in Fig. 2(a)).

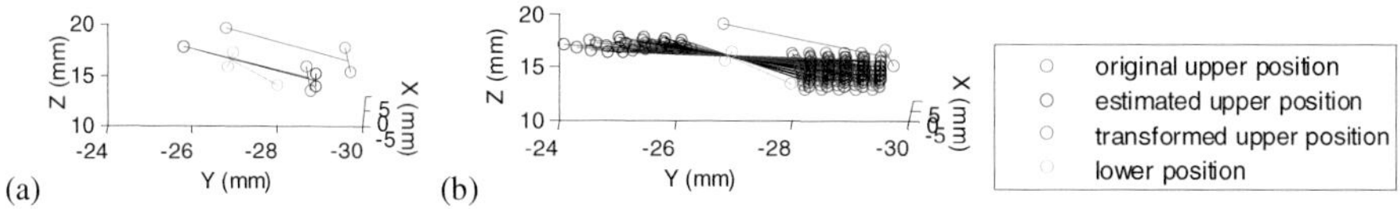

Fig. 2. Schema of ergodic midline-match transform; (a) a given transform; (b) ergodic transforms.

In order to eliminate any possible penetration between the anterior segment of upper teeth and lower teeth, a penetration-adjustment procedure is applied to the initial midline-matched upper and lower models. The penetrations are detected by finding the intersection of the lower teeth surface and the transformed upper anterior segment surface. The penetrations are eliminated by performing a pitch rotation (rotating around the mediolateral axis) of the upper anterior segment. The pitch rotational angle is computed based on the penetrated points between lower and upper surfaces.

It is challenge to determine a definitive combination of overjet, overbite and the inclination of the upper and lower incisors, since the clinical normative value of each measurement has a mean and a standard deviation. Therefore, in our algorithm, we generate a series of anterior segment midline-match transformations in a range of overjet, overbite and inclination between the upper and lower incisors using clinical norms (Fig. 2 (b)). Overjet is set in a range of 1.4 - 2.6mm (0.3mm per step) while overbite is set in a range of 0.5-2.5mm (0.4mm per step) [7]. The algorithm generates a total of 30 positions for midline-matched upper models. All the midline-matched upper models are then ranked based on clinical criteria (the balance among overjet, overbite and the resulted inclination of the upper and lower incisors (normal value: 131±11° for male and 136±11° for female [7])). At this stage, both the right and left posterior segments are transformed together with the anterior segment without breaking their original relationship. Finally, top 5 optimal positions of the anterior segment are automatically determined based on normal values and saved for the next step.

2.2 Right and Left Posterior Segments Alignment

After the anterior segment of the upper dental model is aligned to the lower dental model, the right and left posterior segments are individually articulated to the mandible. We develop an improved ISMDM algorithm to achieve the posterior segment alignment. The original ISMDM algorithm [1] iteratively minimizes the distance of 1-piece upper and lower occlusal surfaces to acquire an MI using small-angle approximation and quadratic optimization. It requires an initial alignment of the upper model to the lower model by matching the whole occlusal surfaces feature points. However, in 3-piece dental alignment, the use of the full occlusal surfaces feature points matching cannot achieve a rough alignment of the 3 pieces of upper model to the lower model. Three-piece articulation requires more constraints for the relationships between the anterior and posterior segments. To solve these problems and ensure that the optimization is feasible and convergent, we improve the ISMDM by developing an occlusal plane transform method to align the upper posterior segments to the lower model with extra constraints in the framework of ISMDM. The constraint parameters are adjusted adaptively during the iterative optimization process.

In the occlusal plane transformation, three distinct feature points (canine cusp *P1*, the 1st molar mesiobuccal cusp *P2*, and 1st molar mesiopalatal cusp *P3*) on the posterior segment are used to guide the transformation. Clinically, we have a definition on where each cusp of the upper teeth should be around the corresponding lower teeth. Using these clinical rules, we can automatically estimate initial positions of these feature points (*P1'*, *P2'*, *P3'*). A rigid transformation is thus calculated and applied to the posterior segment to roughly align it to the lower model.

Based on the initial alignment, the optimal alignment is achieved by minimizing the distance of the two pairs of feature points (shown in Fig. 1) on posterior occlusal surfaces:

$$d_S^2(R,t) = \frac{1}{N}\sum_{j=0}^{N-1}\left\|u_{i_j} - v_j'(R,t)\right\|^2 \quad (1)$$

where, v_j' is the transformed feature point of v_j on the posterior segment, u_{i_j} is the matched feature point of v_j on the mandible, N is the number of feature points on the posterior segment, R is the rotation matrix and t is the translation vector. In addition, the posterior segment should maintain an appropriate smoothly curved relationship with the anterior segment. Therefore, we add a deviation constraint to limit the distance (within a range of 0-2mm) of a cutting surface feature point a_j on the posterior segment, and the corresponding cutting surface feature point b_j on the anterior segment. The constraint is $\left\|a_j - b_j\right\|^2 < h_1$, where h_1 is the threshold distance (2mm) [8]. We also use a deviation constraint between upper canine p_1 and lower interstices between canine and 1st premolar p_2, $\|p_1 - p_2\|^2 < h_2$ (h_2 is a threshold distance, also 2mm). This constraint is to achieve a correct canine intercuspation.

By only using small-angle approximation with the two extra constraints, the iterative quadratic optimization may be infeasible. Therefore, we adjusted the constraint parameters h_1 and h_2 adaptively during the iterative optimization process. Large parameter values are used first to start the iterative optimization process. Once the iteration became feasible, the parameters are then gradually adjusted to a strict level until the optimization converged.

3 Experiments and Results

3.1 Dental Models and Digital Dental Articulation

Patient Digital Dental Models. A total of 15 sets of patient digital dental models were randomly selected from our digital archives [IRB(2)#1011-0187x]. Each patient dataset included a set of hand-articulated 3-piece upper and 1-piece corresponding lower dental models, and an unarticulated original uncut upper model. The digital dental models (in .STL format) were generated using a high-resolute laser scanner. The hand articulated 3-piece upper and lower dental models were achieved using a current standard of care method [9], scanned together, and used in the actual surgery.

They served as reference models (controls). In the computer, the stand-alone uncut upper dental casts were manually segmentalized into 3 pieces between lateral incisors and canines without disturbing the relationship among the 3 pieces. The stand-alone 3-piece upper digital models served as an experimental group.

Three-Piece Digital Dental Articulation. In order to compare our algorithm-articulated 3-piece models to the reference models, we used the reference lower dental model as the target. The 3-piece segments of each experimental model were automatically articulated to the reference lower model using our MGO approach within 30 minutes. All codes were written in MATLAB and run on a regular office PC. A total of 5 articulated 3-piece upper models for each patient were generated. They were evaluated together with the reference models qualitatively and quantitatively.

3.2 Qualitative Validation and Results

In order to qualitatively validate our method, 3 experienced evaluators (2 oral surgeons and 1 orthodontist) were asked independently to evaluate our results. The evaluation was conducted in two steps. The first step was to rank the blinded 6 sets of 3-piece articulated models (1 reference and 5 algorithm-generated models) for each patient, while the second step was to evaluate whether the best ranked algorithm-articulated model in each patient was ready for the surgery by comparing it to the unblind reference model.

In the first step of the evaluation, the 6 sets of models for each patient were shown as a group to the evaluators. The order of them was randomly generated and the evaluators were blind to the nature of the models. The evaluators were asked to give a rank to each of the 6 models based on the clinical criteria, i.e., upper and lower midlines, arcs of the upper and lower dental arch alignment, appropriate overjet, overbite and inclination, MI, and appropriate Curve of Wilson. A rank of "6" indicated the best articulated models while a score of "1" indicated the worst.

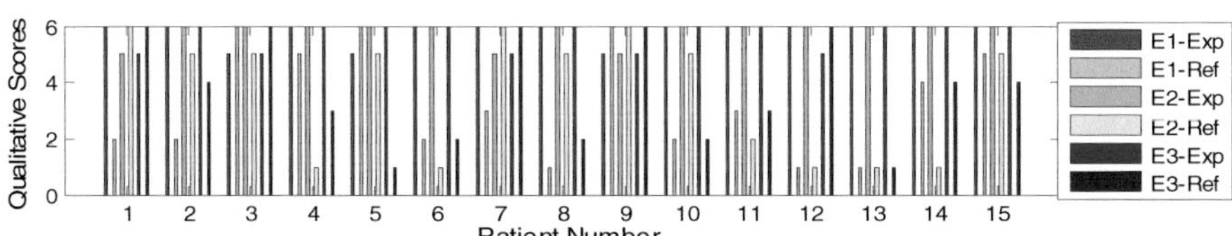

Fig. 3. Comparisons between the best rank of the algorithm-articulated model and the rank of reference model when were blended together. E1-, E2- and E3-Exp: 3 evaluators' the best ranked algorithm-articulated models; E1-, E2- and E3-Ref: 3 evaluators' ranks for reference models.

The results of the blind evaluation were shown in Fig. 3. For each patient, only the best rank of the algorithm-articulated models and the rank of the reference model were shown (due to the page limit). While all 3 evaluators agreed that 9 algorithm-articulated models (#2, 4, 6, 8, 10, 11, and 13-15) were superior than the reference models, all also agreed that the model (# 9) was inferior.

In the second step of the evaluation, the blind was broken. The evaluators were asked to evaluate whether the best ranked algorithm-articulated model was ready for the surgery based on the clinical criteria and by comparing it to the reference model (which was used for the surgery). The results of unblinded evaluation showed that all 3 evaluators agreed that 12 algorithm-articulated models (#2, 4-8, and 10-15) were clinical acceptable and ready for the surgery. In addition, 2 evaluators agreed that 2 of the rest algorithm-generated models (#1 and 3) were ready for surgery, while the other only agreed the model (#3) was ready. Finally, all 3 evaluators agreed that 1 algorithm-generated model (#9) was not ready for the surgery. The problem of the model #9 was mainly due to a significant step between the anterior and right posterior segments which resulted in a right posterior open-bite (upper and lower posterior teeth did not bite together tightly). Fig. 4 showed an example of well algorithm-articulated model (#8) and the unacceptable model #9.

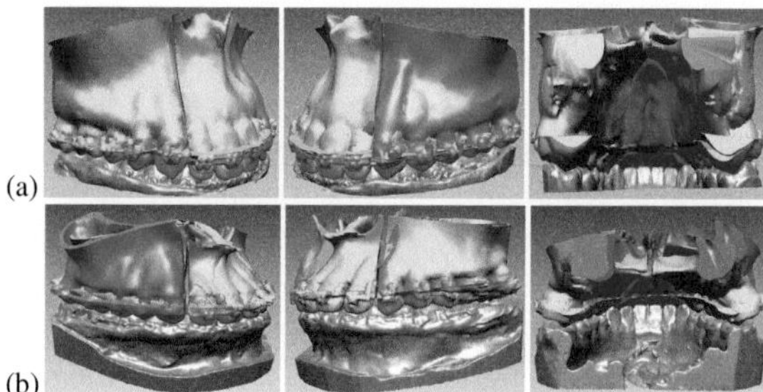
(a)
(b)

Fig. 4. Examples of algorithm-generated 3-piece articulation. Yellow: reference model; Blue: experimental model. From left to right: right oblique, left oblique and posterior views. (a) Model #8 - an algorithm-generated 3-piece articulation that is better than the reference model. (b) Model #9 – a clinical unacceptable articulation (the right posterior segment flares out significantly and has a significant posterior open-bite).

3.3 Quantitative Validation

To quantitatively validate our method, we computed overjets, overbites, and upper canines deviations (calculated between the upper canines tips and the corresponding lower interstices between the canines and the first premolars). The computations were completed based on the coordinates of the manually digitized two pairs of 4 landmarks on upper and lower models for reference and experimental groups (Fig. 5).

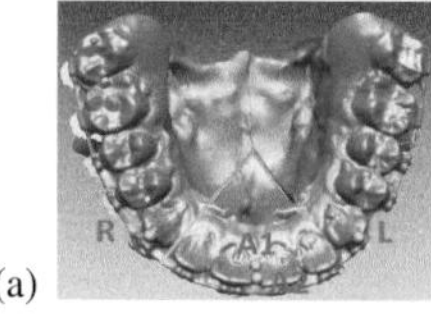
(a)

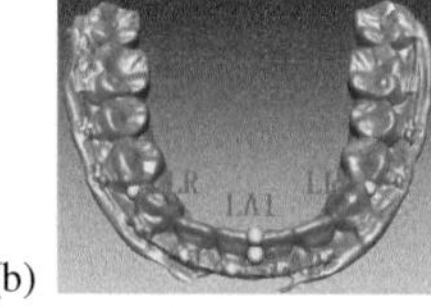
(b)

Fig. 5. Four sets of corresponding landmarks were digitized on the reference upper and lower models. The landmarks on experimental models used the same definition. (a) upper; (b) lower.

The overjets and overbites were computed using the landmark pairs of the upper and lower central dental midlines (A1-A2 and LA1-LA2 for reference; A1'-A2' and LA1'-LA2' for experimental). The deviations for canines were computed using the landmark pairs of the upper canines and the corresponding lower interstices (R-LR and L-LL for reference, and R'-LR' and L'-LL' for experimental). Because our algorithm enforced the perfect alignment of the upper and lower central dental midlines, the midline deviations were therefore not calculated. Means and standard deviations (SD) of these measurements were computed for both reference and the best ranked algorithm-articulated models. The results of the means and SDs are shown in Fig. 6. All of them were clinically acceptable even with the model #9 that was considered clinically not acceptable for surgery. This was because our quantitative evaluation was designed to evaluate overjets and overbites for the anterior segments, and upper canines deviations for the front part of the posterior segments.

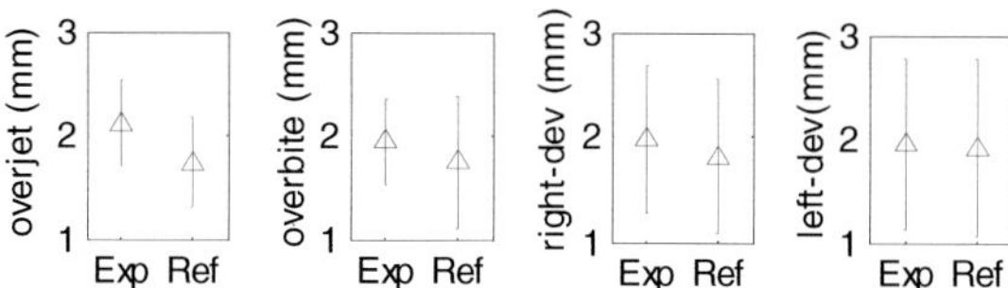

Fig. 6. Mean and SD error bars of overjets, overbites, and deviations for canines for reference (Ref) and experimental (Exp) models. From left to right: overjet, overbite, deviation for right canine, and deviation for left canine.

4 Discussion and Future Work

Unlike 1-piece dental articulation, it is difficult to reestablish 3-piece articulation even with stone dental casts. Although there are some clinical rules to guide 3-piece articulation, different doctors may have different opinions and habits. Even though each segment is segmentalized at the same location, no articulated 3 pieces of the same patient are the same if they are established by different doctors even with the same clinical rules applied. It becomes even more difficult, if not impossible, to automatically articulate the 3-piece segments in computer. Therefore, it is the authors' believe that the clinical qualitative evaluation is a vital part to the success of the study.

In order to solve above (different opinions among doctors) problems and make the automated 3-piece dental articulation clinically useful, we use a combination of different parameters to articulate the 3 pieces in our MGO approach. Our robust ergodic midline-match algorithm automatically articulates, ranks, and fetches the top 5 optimal positions of the anterior piece. The right and left posterior segments are then aligned to the anterior segment based on its position, and further aligned to the lower teeth using our improved ISMDM algorithm. The results of the validations show an exceptional agreement among the 3 experienced doctors. To our knowledge, this will be the first publication on automatic 3-piece dental articulation.

Currently we are working on optimizing our algorithms for both anterior and posterior alignments. We are also transferring our MATLAB codes into C/CPP. Our goal is to complete the entire 3-piece articulation within a couple of minutes on a regular office PC. In addition, artificial intelligence will be used to summarize and incorporate different doctor's preferences into the algorithm. Furthermore, although we believe our qualitative evaluation is well designed and clinically relevant, we will improve our quantitative evaluation by adding the measurements to detect the maximal intercuspation for the posterior segments. Finally, we will validate our algorithm using partially edentulous models, in which some teeth are missing.

References

1. Chang, Y.B., et al.: An automatic and robust algorithm of reestablishment of digital dental occlusion. IEEE Transactions on Medical Imaging 29(9), 1652–1663 (2010)
2. Hiew, L.T., et al.: Optimal occlusion of teeth. In: 9th International Conference on Control, Automation, Robotics and Vision, pp. 1–5 (2006)
3. DeLong, R., et al.: Comparing maximum intercuspal contacts of virtual dental patients and mounted dental casts. J. Prosth. Dent. 88, 622–630 (2002)
4. Zhang, C., Chen, L., Zhang, F., Zhang, H., Feng, H., Dai, G.: A new virtual dynamic dentomaxillofacial system for analyzing mandibular movement, occlusal contact, and TMJ condition. In: Duffy, V.G. (ed.) Digital Human Modeling, HCII 2007. LNCS, vol. 4561, pp. 747–756. Springer, Heidelberg (2007)
5. Xia, J.J., et al.: New clinical protocol to evaluate craniomaxillofacial deformity and plan surgical correction. J. Oral Maxillofacial Surg. 67(10), 2093–2106 (2009)
6. DeBerg, M., et al.: Computational geometry: algorithms and applications. Springer (2000)
7. Bhatia, S.N.: A manual of facial growth: a computer analysis of longitudinal cephalometric growth data. Oxford University Press, Oxford (1993)
8. Hsu, S., et al.: Accuracy of a computer-aided surgical simulation protocol for orthognathic surgery: a prospective multicenter study. J. Oral Maxillofac. Surg. 71(1), 128–142 (2013)
9. Bell, W.H., et al.: Modern practice in orthognathic and reconstructive surgery, vol. 1. W B Saunders Co. (1992)

A System for MR-Ultrasound Guidance during Robot-Assisted Laparoscopic Radical Prostatectomy

Omid Mohareri[1,2], Guy Nir[1], Julio Lobo[1], Richard Savdie[3], Peter Black[3], and Septimiu Salcudean[1]

[1] Department of Electrical and Computer Engineering, University of British Columbia, Vancouver, BC, Canada
{tims,omidm}@ece.ubc.ca

[2] Intuitive Surgical Inc., Sunnyvale, CA

[3] Department of Urological Sciences, University of British Columbia, Vancouver, BC, Canada

Abstract. We describe a new ultrasound and magnetic resonance image guidance system for robot assisted radical prostatectomy and its first use in patients. This system integrates previously developed and new components and presents to the surgeon preoperative magnetic resonance images (MRI) registered to real-time 2D ultrasound to inform the surgeon of anatomy and cancer location. At the start of surgery, a trans-rectal ultrasound (TRUS) is manually positioned for prostate imaging using a standard brachytherapy stepper. When the anterior prostate surface is exposed, the TRUS, which can be rotated under computer control, is registered to one of the da Vinci patient-side manipulators by recognizing the tip of the da Vinci instrument at multiple locations on the tissue surface. A 3D TRUS volume is then taken, which is segmented semi-automatically. A segmentation-based, biomechanically regularized deformable registration algorithm is used to register the 3D TRUS image to preoperatively acquired and annotated T2-weighted images, which are deformed to the patient. MRI and TRUS images can then be pointed at and examined by the surgeon at the da Vinci console. We outline the approaches used and present our experience with the system in the first two patients. While this work is preliminary, the feasibility of fused MRI and TRUS during radical prostatectomy has not been demonstrated before. Given the significant rates of positive surgical margins still reported in the literature, such a system has potentially significant clinical benefits.

1 Introduction

A standard treatment of prostate cancer is radical prostatectomy (RP), or the surgical removal of the prostate gland, via open, laparoscopic or robot assisted surgery. Studies seem to indicate that robot-assisted laparoscopic RP (RALRP) has the best outcomes, yet the rates of positive surgical margins (cancer left behind after surgery) still range between 9% and 30%, depending on the center

N. Navab et al. (Eds.): MICCAI 2015, Part I, LNCS 9349, pp. 497–504, 2015.
DOI: 10.1007/978-3-319-24553-9_61

[1]. The goal of the surgery is to remove the entire prostate and the cancer within it and extending from it, while attempting to spare as much as possible the adjacent critical structures responsible for continence (sphincter muscle) and potency (neurovascular bundles (NVB) and the cavernosal nerves). The main reason why the best trade-off between achieving oncological success (cancer removal) and functional success (continence and potency) cannot be achieved is the inability to localize, intra-opratively, the location and extent of cancer. Advances in MRI may provide spatially localized information to fill this void and aid surgical planning [2]. The combination of conventional anatomical MRI with functional (diffusion-weighted (DW) and dynamic contrast-enhanced (DCE)) MRI, known as multi-parametric MRI (mp-MRI), is emerging as an accurate tool for identifying clinically relevant tumors [3]. mp-MRI is becoming an integral diagnostic tool in preoperative planning of RALRP, specifically for prediction of pathologic stage in extracapsular extension (ECE) and NVB invasion. This capability of mp-MRI to generate the most accurate characterization of prostate cancer [4], has led to the development of methods for MRI-guided treatments, mainly biopsy and brachytherapy [5].

Direct MRI-guided methods have been reported for prostate biopsy and brachytherapy, but intraoperative MRI is still cumbersome, time consuming and resource costly. Cognitive fusion, in which the clinician estimates the lesion's location in the intraoperative TRUS based on a preoperative MRI, varies greatly with expertise. A more feasible approach to allow integration of MRI data in the operating room involves registration of the preoperative MRI to the intraoperative TRUS, and visualization of the corresponding images to assist the clinician during treatment. Previously, such an approach was successfully demonstrated for prostate biopsy [6,7], and for prostate brachytherapy [8]. However, there exists no report on integration of such an approach for real-time surgical guidance using the da Vinci surgical system which is currently being used to perform more than 80% of RPs in North America.

In this work, we present a novel MR-guidance system for the da Vinci which involves an intraoperative segmentation-based MR-TRUS registration method that is integrated into a clinically used robotic TRUS imaging system, which in turn can be registered to the da Vinci system's coordinate frame. In this way a 3D MR volume and the preoperative surgical plan can be mapped to the da Vinci coordinate frame. The surgical instrument can then be visualized, in real-time, with respect to the preoperative MR volume. In addition, since the TRUS imaging system is robotic, it can track the tip of a da Vinci surgical instrument automatically, and is registered to the preoperative MR volume, the surgical instrument itself can be used as an intuitive and easy to use control device for the surgeon to manipulate both MR and TRUS images in real-time during the procedure. The system was initially tested and validated on a prostate phantom and a data-set of six patients offline. Next, it was used with a clinical da Vinci surgical system inside a robotic operating room and tested on two patients undergoing RALRP.

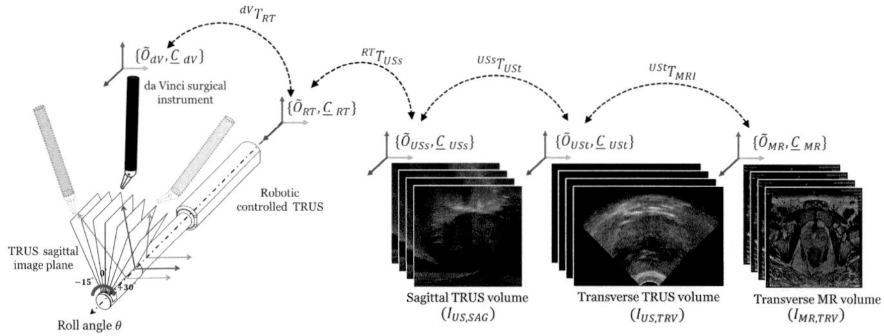

Fig. 1. A schematic of the system. da Vinci $\{O_{dV}, \underline{C}_{dV}\}$ and Robotic-TRUS $\{O_{RT}, \underline{C}_{RT}\}$ coordinate frames are registered in order to enable automatic tracking of the instrument with ultrasound. Images are then converted from cylindrical coordinates to cartesian spatial coordinates for MR-TRUS registration.

2 Materials and Methods

The components of our image-guided system are illustrated in Figure 1 and Figure 3. The system comprises: (i) an ultrasound system with a motorized TRUS transducer mounted on a brachytherapy setup, (ii) an external PC for image registration and display on the da Vinci console, and (iii) registration and tracking software. These components will be described next.

2.1 TRUS Imaging System

A previously designed and clinically used robotic TRUS manipulator was used for automatic and remote rotation (angle range ±45 degrees) of the TRUS transducer during the procedure [9]. The sagittal TRUS imaging plane is automatically repositioned using the robot, so that the 2D ultrasound image continuously contains the tip of a specified da Vinci surgical manipulator. Automatic instrument tracking is achieved by means of a rapid and clinically feasible intraoperative registration technique that solves for the rigid homogeneous transformation between the da Vinci and the TRUS robot coordinate systems (Figure 1). The registration involves defining points on tissue surface using the da Vinci instrument tip and accurate and automatic localization of the points in both da Vinci and Robotic TRUS coordinate frames [10]. This tracking method allows the surgeon at the console to control the TRUS imaging plane automatically with the tip of a da Vinci surgical instrument with an accuracy of less than 2 mm [9]. A BK ultrasound machine (BK Medical, Herlev, Denmark) with a 8848 4-12 MHz biplane transducer was used for imaging the prostate. Raw in phase quadrature (IQ) data was captured at 43.07 Hz sampling rate and saved into an external PC through a DALSA Xcelera-CL PX4 Full frame grabber card (Teledyne DALSA, Waterloo, ON). The TRUS robot was used for 3D TRUS volume acquisition by automatically controlling the rotation angle of the TRUS transducer and saving the location information of each image. All TRUS volumes were captured using the 214-element 6 cm long sagittal array with a transmit frequency of 9 MHz and an imaging depth of 5.6 cm. Volumes were obtained using a 90-degree rotary sweep about the probe axis with images acquired at increments of 0.2 degrees. The image capture time was 45 seconds per volume.

2.2 TRUS-MR Registration

The prostate gland on each transverse slice in the preoperative T2-weighted MR volume is segmented manually by a radiologist before surgery. After interpolating the intraoperative TRUS B-mode images into a 3D grid in order to obtain transverse slices from the sagittal volume, we employed a real-time semi-automatic algorithm for 3-D segmentation of the prostate in the ultrasound volume. This algorithm, described in [11], has been routinely employed during brachytherapy, and found to be a fast, consistent and accurate tool for the delineation of the prostate gland in 3D TRUS.

Based on the segmented surfaces of the prostate in the TRUS and MR volumes, we construct binary volumes. The two binary volumes can then be registered to each other in order to obtain a displacement map which can be applied to the MR volume. First, the MR binary volume is rigidly aligned (and scaled) to the TRUS binary volume using the principal axes transformation. Next, we deform the aligned MR volume to match the TRUS volume. The registration algorithm, based on the variational framework presented in [12], minimizes the

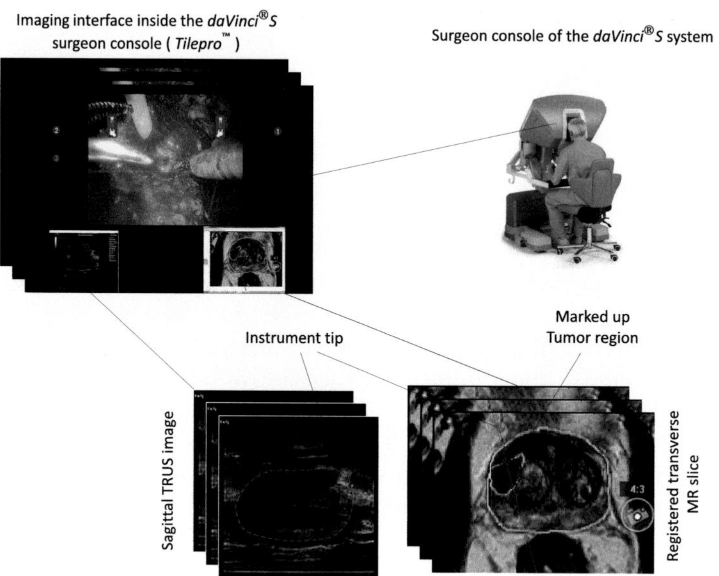

Fig. 2. Real-time imaging system interface using the da Vinci Si TilePro™ feature.

sum of squared differences between the two binary volumes with an elastic regularization of the displacement map. The proposed method was tested offline on $n = 6$ data sets of RP patients who underwent preoperative MR and intraoperative US. The MR volumes were acquired by a 3-Tesla system (Achieva 3.0T, Philips, The Netherlands) using a standard 6-channel cardiac coil with acceleration factor (SENSE) 2. In order to maintain consistent processing times, we ran the deformable registration algorithm a fixed number of 30 iterations that takes less than 60 seconds. Including the times for the semi-automated segmentation ($46 \pm 15sec$), the total run-time of the entire segmentation-based registration process is about 100 seconds. We evaluated the registration performance using the volume overlap (VO), in the sense of Dice's coefficient between the MR and the TRUS volumes after rigid and deformable registrations. The mean distance between splines on both modalities that were fitted through the center points of the urethra was also measured for the rigid and deformable registered volumes. The mean volume overlap (VO) between the registered MR and the TRUS volumes was $97.7 \pm 0.3\%$, and the mean distance between splines fitted to the segmented urethra in the two volumes was $1.44 \pm 0.42mm$.

2.3 *in-vivo* Patient Studies and Results

To date, two patients (ages 55 and 72; prostate specific antigen 13.5 and 28.5 ng/ml) with clinically organ confined prostate cancer undergoing RALRP agreed to participate in this institutional review board approved study. The main components and configuration of the system during this clinical study inside the operating room are shown in Figure 3. Both patients underwent preoperative mp-MR and a radiologist was asked to examine their MR volume and segment the prostate and the lesions. The lesions were identified in DCE-MR images and then marked on T2-weighted images.

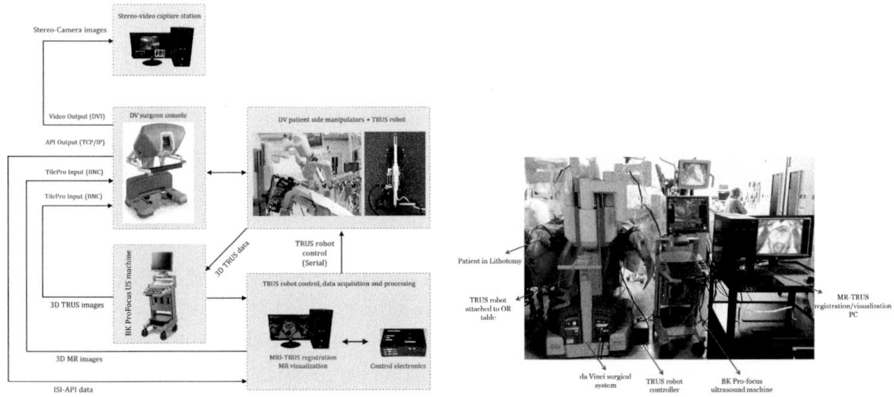

Fig. 3. The guidance system components and configuration in a da Vinci operating room is shown on the left and the operating room scenario is shown on the right.

Table 1. Table of patient study results. T_{reg} is the duration of each registration process, N_r is the number of times registration was repeated for that patient, N_f is the number of fiducial points selected for instrument registration, and $T_{TilePro}$ is the total duration of TilePro usage during each case.

	MR-TRUS reg.				TRUS-dV reg.		$T_{TilePro}$ (min)
	VO (%)	e_{reg} (mm)	T_{reg} (s)	N_r	N_f	T_{reg} (s)	
Patient 1	91.1 ± 0.1	2.1 ± 0.3	100	4	4	96	16
patient 2	93.0 ± 0.3	2.5 ± 0.1	100	5	4	110	28

Once the patient is placed on the operating table and before docking the da Vinci robot, we attached the Robotic-TRUS system to the foot of the operating table and placed the TRUS transducer to provide optimal transverse/sagittal images of the patient's prostate as performed in standard brachytherapy volume studies. After docking the da Vinci system and start of the procedure, once the anterior surface of the prostate is visible to the surgeon, we performed the TRUS to da Vinci calibration to enable automatic tracking of the surgical instrument with ultrasound. The calibration process was performed after incision of the endopelvic fascia with 4 instrument tip locations spread across both sides of the dorsal prostate and could be completed in approximately 2 minutes. Before activating the automatic instrument tracking control mode, we acquired 3D TRUS volumes (45 seconds each) to be used by the MR-TRUS registration algorithm. The TRUS volume used for the registration was acquired immediately before the part of the procedure when the surgeon wanted to use MR images to localize tumors. This was done to ensure that the MR volume was deformed to the most current patient anatomy making the display as intuitive as possible.

After the tracking was activated, the surgeon could examine the prostate anatomy and tumor locations by moving the registered surgical instrument around, placing it on the tissue surface in the area of interest and localizing the instrument tip with respect to anatomy seen in real-time sagittal TRUS images. The corresponding transverse MR slice is also displayed based on the position of the tool tip. As it is shown in Figure 2, both real-time TRUS and the corresponding MR images are sent to the da Vinci console and displayed to the surgeon using the TilePro^{TM}feature of the da Vinci system. The surgical view is divided into three tiles with adjustable sizes, one for the endoscopic view, one for the real-time TRUS and one for the corresponding deformed MR slice. Our graphical user interface for MR imaging display (shown in Figure 2) shows instrument tip location in the cylindrical coordinates of the TRUS system (roll angle) with a superimposed red cursor line on the 2D deformed MR slice. This cursor line was used by the surgeon for localization of the registered surgical instrument with respect to the segmented and annotated lesions displayed in MR images. Snapshots of the surgeon console images at the stages when the MR-guidance system was being used to localize tumors are shown in Figure 4. A summary of the registration results for both patients is listed in Table 1.

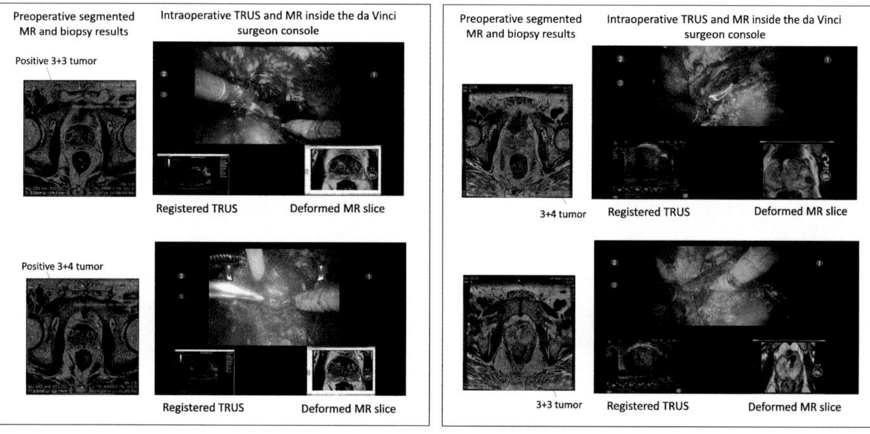

Fig. 4. Clinical study results. Both deformed MR and real-time TRUS are shown to the surgeon at the console along with the surgical endoscopic imaging for both cases.

3 Discussions and Conclusions

The performed surgical procedures were the first in which a surgeon was able to see registered MR images intraoperatively, and to refine the surgical planes accordingly for achieving a better surgical margin and functional outcome. During the first case, a lesion on the right side, stretching from the mid-gland anteriorly and superiorly was seen on the MR imaging system (shown in Figure 4). Based on this information, the surgeon attempted to leave as much of the NVB intact on the left "high" or more anterior dissection approach in order to get closer to the prostate. On the right, the surgeon attempted to get close to the prostate only posteriorly. The surgeon decided to perform a bilateral nerve sparing but more conservatively because of the anterior lesion on the right seen in MR images. If the lesion was posterior, then he would not have done nerve sparing on that side. During the second case, a lesion on the left posterior side was seen on the MR images and the surgeon avoided sparing the nerve on that side. The intraoperative MR imaging allows surgeons to fine tune the procedure based on the anatomy. Without MRI, they would just have a certain number and proportion of cores involved on one side or the other, but no other information on location - hence, relying mainly on intuition. Given the controversy on the "best" surgical approach in RP, as reflected in the literature, this MR-guidance could be a powerful tool to trade off positive surgical margins against potency.

Intraoperative TRUS-da Vinci and TRUS-MR registrations were performed successfully in two patients. The imaging was examined at the anterior surface of the prostate after the surgeon placed the dorsal venus complex (DVC) suture at the prostate apex, before bladder-neck dissection for localization of the tumor, and for finding the best surgical plane to achieve both better oncological and functional outcomes before performing NVB release. TRUS volume acquisition and MR-TRUS registration processes were redone (145 seconds acquisition and processing time) before any stage of the surgery when the surgeon wanted to use the system. An updated TRUS volume should be acquired as necessary to deform the preoperative MR images based on the current state of the prostate.

It is important for the surgeon to have intuitive control over the intraoperative imaging system in the surgical robot coordinate space. Previous work showed that surgeon-assistant coordination is inefficient. Other methods to interact with the imaging system would be adding control devices to the da Vinci console, such as another foot-pedal or hand controller or using the da Vinci masters as pointing devices [13]. A major advantage of our system is that the surgeon can seamlessly use the native da Vinci input controls to move through the 3D volume of both TRUS and MRI and manipulate the 3D data.

References

1. Ficarraa, V., et al.: Systematic review of methods for reporting combined outcomes after radical prostatectomy and proposal of a novel system: The survival, continence, and potency (scp) classification. European Urology 61(3), 541–548 (2012)
2. Tan, N., et al.: Radical prostatectomy: value of prostate MRI in surgical planning. Abdominal Imaging 37, 664–674 (2012)
3. Johnson, L.M., et al.: Multiparametric MRI in prostate cancer management. Nature Reviews Clinical Oncology 11, 346–353 (2014)
4. Kozlowski, P., et al.: Combined prostate diffusion tensor imaging and dynamic contrast enhanced MRI at 3T–quantitative correlation with biopsy. Magnetic Resonance Imaging 28(5), 621–628 (2010)
5. Tempany, C., et al.: MR-guided prostate interventions. Magnetic Resonance Imaging 27(2), 356–367 (2008)
6. Hadaschik, B.A., et al.: A novel stereotactic prostate biopsy system integrating pre-interventional magnetic resonance imaging and live ultrasound fusion. Journal of Urology 186(6), 2214–2220 (2011)
7. Ukimura, O., et al.: 3D elastic registration system of prostate biopsy location by real-time 3D transrectal ultrasound guidance with MR/TRUS image fusion. The Journal of Urology 187(3), 1080–1086 (2012)
8. Reynier, C., et al.: MRI/TRUS data fusion for prostate brachytherapy: preliminary results. Medical Physics 31(6), 1568–1575 (2004)
9. Mohareri, O., et al.: Intraoperative registered transrectal ultrasound guidance for robot-assisted laparoscopic radical prostatectomy. The Journal of urology 193(1), 302–312 (2015)
10. Yip, M.C., Adebar, T.K., Rohling, R.N., Salcudean, S.E., Nguan, C.Y.: 3D ultrasound to stereoscopic camera registration through an air-tissue boundary. In: Jiang, T., Navab, N., Pluim, J.P.W., Viergever, M.A. (eds.) MICCAI 2010, Part II. LNCS, vol. 6362, pp. 626–634. Springer, Heidelberg (2010)
11. Mahdavi, S.S., et al.: Semi-automatic segmentation for prostate interventions. Medical Image Analysis 15(2), 226–237 (2011)
12. Modersitzki, J.: Numerical methods for image registration. Oxford University Press (2004)
13. Leven, J., et al.: DaVinci canvas: A telerobotic surgical system with integrated, robot-assisted, laparoscopic ultrasound capability. In: Duncan, J.S., Gerig, G. (eds.) MICCAI 2005. LNCS, vol. 3749, pp. 811–818. Springer, Heidelberg (2005)

Computer Aided Diagnosis I: Machine Learning

Automatic Fetal Ultrasound Standard Plane Detection Using Knowledge Transferred Recurrent Neural Networks

Hao Chen[1], Qi Dou[1], Dong Ni[2,⋆], Jie-Zhi Cheng[2], Jing Qin[2], Shengli Li[3], and Pheng-Ann Heng[1]

[1] Dept. of Computer Science and Engineering, The Chinese University of Hong Kong
[2] School of Medicine, Shenzhen University, China
[3] Shenzhen Maternal and Child Healthcare Hospital of Nanfang Medical University

Abstract. Accurate acquisition of fetal ultrasound (US) standard planes is one of the most crucial steps in obstetric diagnosis. The conventional way of standard plane acquisition requires a thorough knowledge of fetal anatomy and intensive manual labors. Hence, automatic approaches are highly demanded in clinical practice. However, automatic detection of standard planes containing key anatomical structures from US videos remains a challenging problem due to the high intra-class variations of standard planes. Unlike previous studies that developed specific methods for different anatomical standard planes respectively, we present a general framework to detect standard planes from US videos automatically. Instead of utilizing hand-crafted visual features, our framework explores spatio-temporal feature learning with a novel knowledge transferred recurrent neural network (T-RNN), which incorporates a deep hierarchical visual feature extractor and a temporal sequence learning model. In order to extract visual features effectively, we propose a joint learning framework with knowledge transfer across multi-tasks to address the insufficiency issue of limited training data. Extensive experiments on different US standard planes with hundreds of videos corroborate that our method can achieve promising results, which outperform state-of-the-art methods.

1 Introduction

Obstetric ultrasound (US) examination generally involves the procedures of image scanning, standard plane selection, biometric measurement and diagnosis. Accurate acquisition of US standard planes, e.g., fetal abdominal standard plane (FASP), fetal face axial standard plane (FFASP) and fetal four-chamber view standard plane (FFVSP) of heart, is one crucial step for the subsequent biometric measurement and obstetric diagnosis. Clinically, US standard plane is manually acquired by searching the view with concurrent presence of key anatomical structures (KASs) in the regions of interest (ROI) [1]. Fig. 1 illustrates the KASs for

⋆ Corresponding author.

N. Navab et al. (Eds.): MICCAI 2015, Part I, LNCS 9349, pp. 507–514, 2015.
DOI: 10.1007/978-3-319-24553-9_62

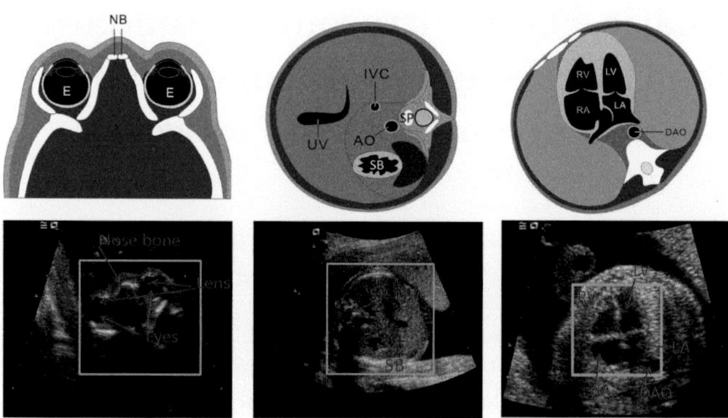

Fig. 1. Left: FFASP containing nose bone, eyes and lens; middle: FASP containing stomach bubble (SB), umbilical vein (UV) and spine (SP); right: FFVSP containing left atrium (LA), right atrium (RA), left ventricle (LV), right ventricle (RV) and descending aorta (DAO) (green rectangles denote the ROIs).

FFASP, FASP and FFVSP, respectively. The manual acquisition of standard planes heavily relies on clinical experience and is also very laborious. Hence, automatic detection methods are highly demanded to boost the examination efficiency [2]. However, this computerized detection task is quite challenging due to the high intra-class variations of US standard planes resulting from acoustic shadows, deformations of soft tissues and various transducer orientations [3].

Over the past few years, several methods have been proposed to address this challenging problem. Most of them either utilized hand-crafted features by observation [2,3,4] or incorporated component-based geometric constraints for a specific standard plane detection task, e.g., the radial component model and vessel probability map detection (RVD) method in [5]. However, these low level features may not accurately represent the complicated characteristics of standard planes. In addition, the insufficiency of training data in the medical domain usually leads to the overfitting problem in supervised learning based methods, and hence degrades the generalization performance. Chen *et al.* [6] compared the performance of randomly initialized convolutional neural network (R-CNN) and that of transferred convolutional neural network (T-CNN) on FASP detection. The method of T-CNN achieved a high accuracy by using deep learning based spatial feature representations with knowledge transfer from natural images. However, the cross-domain knowledge transfer may boost the detection performance with limited improvement due to the larger domain gap. Besides, only considering spatial features may not be the optimal solution, since temporal information of consecutive sequences in US videos could provide extra contextual clues for better discrimination.

Recently, the recurrent neural network (RNN), especially the long short-term memory (LSTM) model, has achieved success in sequence learning tasks, such as speech recognition [7] and video recognition [8]. In order to meet above challenges, we propose a knowledge transferred recurrent neural network (T-RNN) by exploring spatio-temporal feature learning. The major contributions of this paper are three-fold. First, to our best knowledge, this is the first work that considers spatio-temporal feature representations under the framework of deep learning for the detection of standard planes from US videos. Second, a joint learning model for effective spatial feature learning across multi-tasks is presented, which reduces the overfitting problem caused by the inadequacy of training data. Third, the proposed T-RNN is a general framework and can be easily extended to other US standard plane or anatomical structure detection problems. Extensive experiments on different US standard plane detection tasks with large scale datasets demonstrated the efficacy of our method.

2 Method

Fig. 2 (left) shows the architecture of the proposed T-RNN, which is a hybrid model integrating deep convolutional neural networks (CNN) and recurrent neural networks (LSTM model). A ROI classifier is first trained based on the joint learning of convolutional neural networks (J-CNN) across multi-tasks to locate the most discriminative regions for US standard plane detection. Then, the temporal information is explored via the LSTM model based on the features of ROIs in consecutive frames extracted from the J-CNN model. Finally, the score of each frame is obtained by averaging all predictions from the LSTM model and the frame is classified as the standard plane when the output score is larger than a threshold T_0.

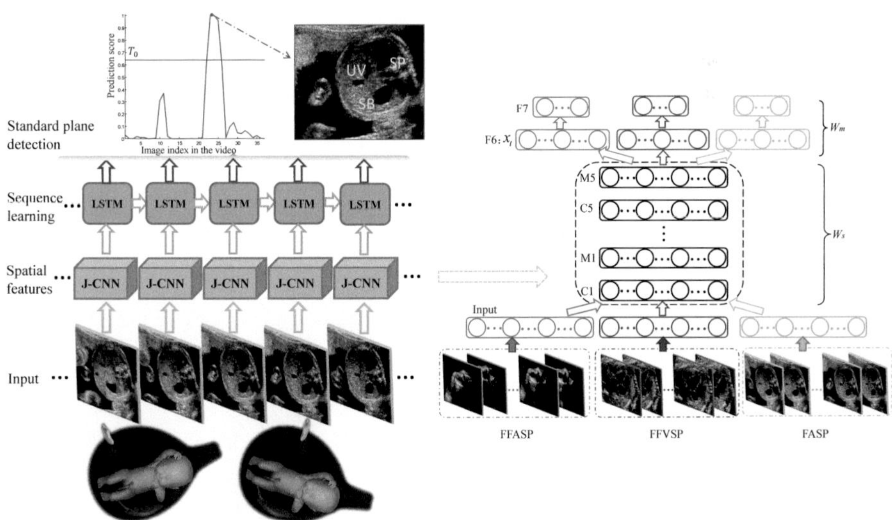

Fig. 2. Left: architecture of the proposed T-RNN; right: the proposed J-CNN.

2.1 Joint Learning with Knowledge Transfer across Multi-tasks

The basic structure of CNN includes several pairs of alternating convolutional (C) and max-pooling (M) layers, followed by fully-connected (F) layers. Previous studies have indicated that the knowledge learned from one domain or task via CNN could benefit the training for another domain or task with limited annotated data [6]. Inspired by these studies, it is reasonable to speculate that leveraging the transferred knowledge across similar US detection tasks can mitigate the challenge of insufficient training data for a specific task as well as improve the generalization performance of the learning. To the end, we propose a joint learning model with CNN across multiple detection tasks of US standard planes, as illustrated in Fig. 2 (right).

In the figure, the matrix W_s denoting the parameters of layers from C1 to M5 is trained from all training samples of the three detection tasks and shared among these tasks. The W_m ($m = 1, 2, 3$ represents the task of FFASP, FFVSP and FASP, respectively) denotes the parameters of F6 and F7 layers and is trained individually on each task for the discrimination of different standard planes. These parameters can be optimized by minimizing the following joint max-margin loss function $\mathcal{L}_1$:

$$\mathcal{L}_1 = \frac{\lambda}{2}(\sum_m ||W_m||_2^2 + ||W_s||_2^2) + \sum_m \sum_k max(0, 1 - y_{mk} F_m(f_{mk}^s; W_m))^2 \quad (1)$$

$$f_{mk}^s = F_s(I_{mk}; W_s) \quad (2)$$

where the first part of $\mathcal{L}_1$ is the regularization penalty term and the second part is the data loss term. The tradeoff between these two terms is controlled by the hyperparameter λ, which is determined by cross-validation in our experiments. The F_s denotes the shared feature extraction function while the F_m denotes the discriminant function for different US standard planes individually. The I_{mk} is the kth input frame of mth task and f_{mk}^s is the output of shared section (i.e., activations of M5 layer). The $y_{mk} \in \{-1, 1\}$ is the corresponding ground truth. The architecture of J-CNN model can be seen in Table 1 (padding and non-linear activation layers are not shown).

Table 1. Architecture of J-CNN

Layer	Feature maps	Kernel size	Stride
input	227x227x1	-	-
C1	55x55x24	11	4
M1	27x27x24	3	2
C2	14x14x24	5	2
M2	7x7x24	3	2
C3	7x7x24	3	1
C4	7x7x24	3	1
C5	7x7x24	3	1
M5	3x3x24	3	2
F6	100	-	-
F7	2	-	-

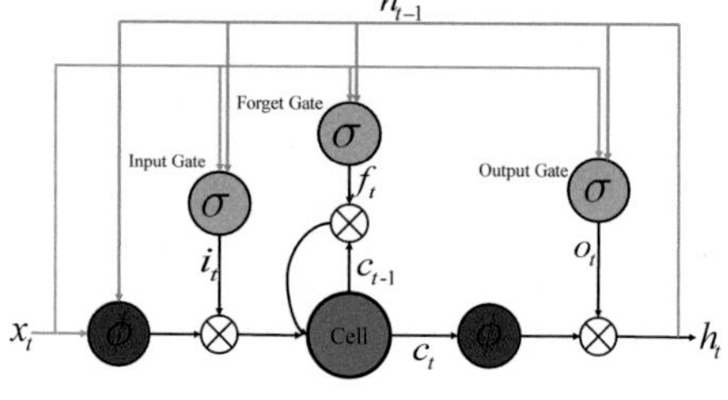

Fig. 3. LSTM model

2.2 US Standard Plane Detection via T-RNN

Temporal information in time-series videos could provide additional contextual clues for the improvement of detection performance. In our T-RNN model, spatio-temporal features in ROIs, which have been detected by the J-CNN model, are further explored by the LSTM. Given the input frame I_{mk}, the probability map of the ROI is computed by the J-CNN model in a sliding window way and the center of the ROI is located at the position with maximal value in the probability map. Features in the penultimate layer (i.e., activations of F6 layer) of the J-CNN model are then extracted from the ROI of each frame. Before inputting features into the LSTM, we manually clip each video into separated clips with the same number of T frames. Thus, each input video can be transformed into sequenced samples, where each sample is represented by a vector sequence $\mathbf{x} = \{x_1, ..., x_t, ..., x_T\}$ and $x_t \in \mathbb{R}^q$ ($q = 100$ in our experiments). The corresponding labelling vector is $\mathbf{y} = \{y_1, ..., y_t, ..., y_T\}$, where $y_t \in \{0, 1\}$.

In the traditional RNN, the back-propagation algorithm may result in vanishing or exploding gradients. The LSTM model tackles this problem by incorporating memory cells that allow the network to learn when to forget previous hidden states and when to update hidden states given the new input [7]. A simplified version of LSTM model is shown in Fig. 3. The element-wise nonlinear functions $\sigma(x) = \frac{1}{1+e^{-x}}$ and $\phi(x) = \frac{e^x - e^{-x}}{e^x + e^{-x}}$ squash their inputs into [0,1] and [-1,1], respectively. The gates serve to modulate the interactions between the memory cell c_t and its environment. The input gate i_t can allow incoming input x_t to alter the state of the memory cell or block it. The output gate o_t can allow the state of the memory cell to have an effect on hidden neurons or prevent it. The forget gate f_t can modulate the self-recurrent connection of the memory cell, allowing the cell to remember or forget its previous state c_{t-1}. All the gates and memory cells have the same vector size with hidden state $h_t \in \mathbb{R}^H$ (H is the number of hidden units). Specifically, they are updated with following equations:

$$
\begin{aligned}
i_t &= \sigma(W_{xi}x_t + W_{hi}h_{t-1} + b_i) \\
f_t &= \sigma(W_{xf}x_t + W_{hf}h_{t-1} + b_f) \\
o_t &= \sigma(W_{xo}x_t + W_{ho}h_{t-1} + b_o) \\
c_t &= f_t \odot c_{t-1} + i_t \odot \phi(W_{xc}x_t + W_{hc}h_{t-1} + b_c) \\
h_t &= o_t \odot \phi(c_t)
\end{aligned}
\tag{3}
$$

where $h_0 = 0$, W denotes the weight matrix (e.g., W_{xi} is the input-input gate matrix and W_{hi} is the hidden-input gate matrix), b is corresponding bias term, and $\odot$ denotes the element-wise multiplication. The predictions can be obtained by feeding h_t into a softmax classification layer. Thus, the parameters θ (including all W and b) of the model can be trained by minimizing the negative logarithm loss function with stochastic gradient descent method [9]:

$$
\mathcal{L}_2 = -\sum_{n=1}^{N}\sum_{t=1}^{T} \log p_n(y_t | x_t, h_{t-1}; \theta) \tag{4}
$$

where N is the total number of sequenced training samples after clipping.

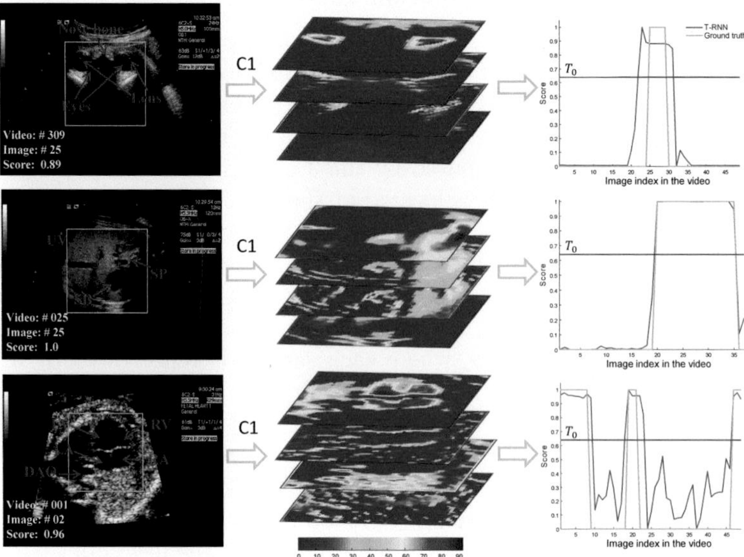

Fig. 4. Left: typical US standard plane detection results; middle: several feature maps of ROIs in C1 layer; right: sequenced predictions in the video.

3 Experiments and Results

Materials. Ultrasound videos were acquired by performing a conventional US sweep on the pregnant women (fetal gestational age from 18 to 40 weeks) in the supine position using a Siemens Acuson Sequoia 512 US scanner. Each video was acquired from one patient and contained 17-48 frames. They were manually annotated by an experienced obstetrician. For training the ROI classifier under the framework of J-CNN, training samples of FASP, FFASP and FFVSP were generated from 300 videos with a total of 11,942, 13,091 and 12,343 US images, respectively. In addition, 219 videos with 8718 US images of FASP, 52 videos with 2278 images of FFASP and 60 videos with 2252 images of FFVSP were used for the performance evaluation, respectively.

Qualitative Performance Evaluation. Fig. 4 (left) shows the typical detection results of three US standard planes. All the detected standard planes contained the KASs and the predicted scores were above the threshold T_0 (determined with cross validation). In addition, we input the ROIs of the detected standard planes into the J-CNN and visualized their feature maps in C1 layer in Fig. 4 (middle). It is observed that large responses of feature maps were excited in the regions of KASs, revealing the model captured the discriminative structures. Furthermore, as shown in Fig. 4 (right), the whole sequenced predictions of three videos by T-RNN demonstrated a good consistency with ground truth.

Table 2. Results of Standard Plane Detection

Method	FASP				FFASP				FFVSP			
	A	P	R	$F1$	A	P	R	$F1$	A	P	R	$F1$
T-RNN	**0.908**	**0.748**	**0.747**	**0.747**	**0.867**	**0.634**	**0.598**	**0.615**	**0.867**	**0.770**	**0.612**	**0.682**
J-CNN	0.902	0.729	0.739	0.734	0.854	0.605	0.513	0.555	0.835	0.718	0.611	0.660
T-CNN[6]	0.896	0.714	0.710	0.712	0.847	0.582	0.503	0.535	0.831	0.708	0.606	0.653
R-CNN[6]	0.857	0.594	0.681	0.635	0.831	0.530	0.443	0.482	0.826	0.688	0.608	0.651
RVD[5]	0.833	0.532	0.693	0.602	-	-	-	-	-	-	-	-

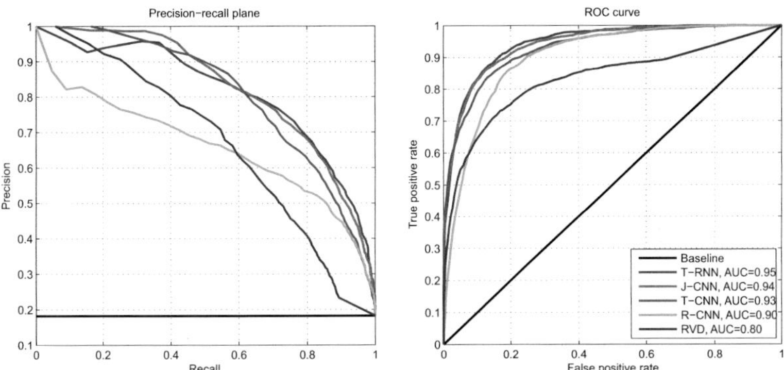

Fig. 5. The PR plane and ROC curves of different methods on FASP detection.

Comparison of Quantitative Performance. We compared our method with state-of-the-art methods [5,6] and the J-CNN that relies only on the spatial feature representations from three detection tasks. The evaluation measurements include *accuracy* (A), *precision* (P), *recall* (R), and $F1$ score. The results of different methods are shown in Table 2. The four deep learning based methods achieved better results than the method of RVD [5] on the FASP detection, which evidenced the efficacy of exploiting deep learning based feature representations. The detection results of J-CNN and T-CNN [6] outperformed those of R-CNN [6] on most measurements, demonstrating the advantages of the knowledge transfer strategy on reducing overfitting caused by the inadequacy of training data. In addition, the results of J-CNN were better than those of T-CNN, indicating that the knowledge transferred from images of the same domain reduced the gap between cross-domains (e.g., natural images used in the T-CNN). Compared with other methods, our T-RNN achieved the best performance on different measurements, which further highlighted the superiority of exploring spatio-temporal feature learning with knowledge transfer in standard plane detection from US videos. The precision-recall (PR) plane and receiver operating characteristic (ROC) curves of different methods on FASP detection are shown in Fig. 5, further demonstrating the advantages of the proposed T-RNN. The T-RNN method generally took less than 1 minute to detect the standard planes from a video containing 40 frames using a workstation equipped with a 2.50 GHz Intel(R) Xeon(R) E5-2609 CPU and a NVIDIA Titan GPU.

4 Conclusion

In this paper, we presented a knowledge transferred RNN to automatically detect fetal standard planes from US videos by exploring spatio-temporal feature learning. Experimental results on three US standard planes demonstrate the efficacy of our approach quantitatively on this challenging problem. Furthermore, our approach is a general framework and can be extended to the detection of other US standard planes or anatomical structures. In the future, we will accelerate the detection process and apply it in clinical practice.

Acknowledgements. The work described in this paper was supported in part by the Shenzhen Key Basic Research Project (No. JCYJ20140509172609164) and in part by the Shenzhen-Hong Kong Innovation Circle Funding Program (Nos. GHP/002/13SZ and SGLH20131010151755080). We also gratefully acknowledge the NVIDIA Corporation for the donated GPU used in this research.

References

1. Chen, H., Ni, D., Yang, X., Li, S., Heng, P.A.: Fetal abdominal standard plane localization through representation learning with knowledge transfer. In: Wu, G., Zhang, D., Zhou, L. (eds.) MLMI 2014. LNCS, vol. 8679, pp. 125–132. Springer, Heidelberg (2014)
2. Kwitt, R., Vasconcelos, N., Razzaque, S., Aylward, S.: Localizing target structures in ultrasound video–a phantom study. Medical Image Analysis 17(7), 712–722 (2013)
3. Maraci, M.A., Napolitano, R., Papageorghiou, A., Noble, J.A.: Searching for structures of interest in an ultrasound video sequence. In: Wu, G., Zhang, D., Zhou, L. (eds.) MLMI 2014. LNCS, vol. 8679, pp. 133–140. Springer, Heidelberg (2014)
4. Rahmatullah, B., Papageorghiou, A.T., Noble, J.A.: Integration of local and global features for anatomical object detection in ultrasound. In: Ayache, N., Delingette, H., Golland, P., Mori, K. (eds.) MICCAI 2012, Part III. LNCS, vol. 7512, pp. 402–409. Springer, Heidelberg (2012)
5. Ni, D., Yang, X., Chen, X., Chin, C.-T., Chen, S., Heng, P.A., Li, S., Qin, J., Wang, T.: Standard plane localization in ultrasound by radial component model and selective search. Ultrasound in Medicine & Biology 40(11), 2728–2742 (2014)
6. Chen, H., Ni, D., Qin, J., Li, S., Yang, X., Wang, T., Heng, P.: Standard plane localization in fetal ultrasound via domain transferred deep neural networks. IEEE Journal of Biomedical and Health Informatics (2015)
7. Graves, A.: Supervised Sequence Labell. with Recur. Neur. Networks. SCI, vol. 385, pp. 5–13. Springer, Heidelberg (2012)
8. Donahue, J., Hendricks, L.A., Guadarrama, S., Rohrbach, M., Venugopalan, S., Saenko, K., Darrell, T.: Long-term recurrent convolutional networks for visual recognition and description. arXiv preprint:1411.4389 (2014)
9. Williams, R.J., Zipser, D.: Gradient-based learning algorithms for recurrent networks and their computational complexity. In: Back-Propagation: Theory, Architectures and Applications, pp. 433–486 (1995)

Automatic Localization and Identification of Vertebrae in Spine CT via a Joint Learning Model with Deep Neural Networks

Hao Chen[1,⋆], Chiyao Shen[2,⋆], Jing Qin[3], Dong Ni[3], Lin Shi[4], Jack C.Y. Cheng[4], and Pheng-Ann Heng[1]

[1] Dept. of Computer Science and Engineering, The Chinese University of Hong Kong
[2] College of Computer Science and Technology, Zhejiang University, China
[3] School of Medicine, Shenzhen University, China
[4] Prince of Wales Hospital, The Chinese University of Hong Kong

Abstract. Accurate localization and identification of vertebrae in 3D spinal images is essential for many clinical tasks. However, automatic localization and identification of vertebrae remains challenging due to similar appearance of vertebrae, abnormal pathological curvatures and image artifacts induced by surgical implants. Traditional methods relying on hand-crafted low level features and/or a priori knowledge usually fail to overcome these challenges on arbitrary CT scans. We present a robust and efficient approach to automatically locating and identifying vertebrae in 3D CT volumes by exploiting high level feature representations with deep convolutional neural network (CNN). A novel joint learning model with CNN (J-CNN) is proposed by considering both the appearance of vertebrae and the pairwise conditional dependency of neighboring vertebrae. The J-CNN can effectively identify the type of vertebra and eliminate false detections based on a set of coarse vertebral centroids generated from a random forest classifier. Furthermore, the predicted centroids are refined by a shape regression model. Our approach was quantitatively evaluated on the dataset of MICCAI 2014 Computational Challenge on Vertebrae Localization and Identification. Compared with the state-of-the-art method [1], our approach achieved a large margin with 10.12% improvement of the identification rate and smaller localization errors.

1 Introduction

Vertebrae serve as the essential anatomical landmarks and provide an important prior structure of spinal shape. Accurate localization and identification of vertebrae in 3D images such as CT and MRI is significant for many subsequent tasks including pathological diagnosis, surgical planning and post-operative assessment. Moreover, it can benefit many other applications including vertebral body segmentation [2], idiopathic scoliosis diagnosis [3], and intervertebral disc labelling [4], to name a few.

⋆ Joint first authors.

N. Navab et al. (Eds.): MICCAI 2015, Part I, LNCS 9349, pp. 515–522, 2015.
DOI: 10.1007/978-3-319-24553-9_63

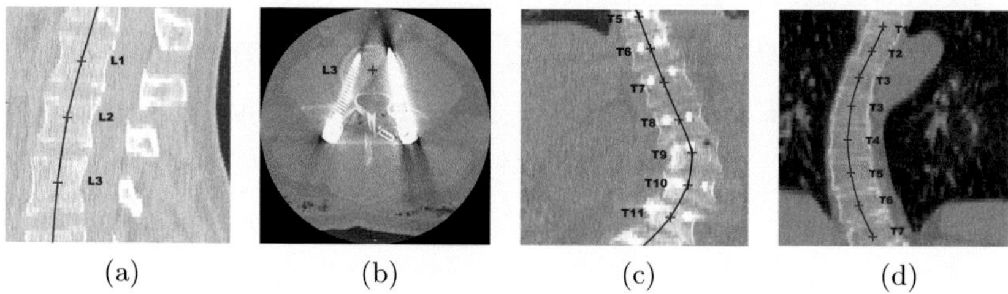

Fig. 1. Challenges of vertebrae localization and identification in 3D CT volume (vertebral centroids are marked as red crosses): (a) similar appearance of vertebrae; (b) image artifacts induced by the implanted pedicle screws; (c)(d) pathological cases of scoliosis.

In clinical practice, manual labelling of vertebrae is time consuming and subjective with limited reproducibility [5]. Therefore, an accurate and reliable automatic localization and identification method can greatly improve the examination efficiency and reliability. However, developing such a method faces several challenges. First, vertebrae often carry similar morphological appearance due to the repetitive nature of spine, which makes them difficult to be distinguished, as shown in Fig. 1 (a). Second, the existence of surgical metal implants, e.g., pedicle screws, induces severe image artifacts and reduces the contrast around bony boundary in the CT volume, as shown in Fig. 1 (b). Third, various pathological cases could cause different abnormalities in the vertebral shape and spinal curvature [6], as the examples shown in Fig. 1 (c) and (d). This task becomes more difficult when the CT scans are of limited field-of-view.

Over the past few years, several methods have been proposed to solve this challenging problem [4,5,7]. Most of them either concentrate on specific regions or make an assumption about the visible portion of spine. In addition, they achieved a high accuracy on normal cases but suffered from pathological cases. Glocker *et al.* [6] localized and identified vertebrae in arbitrary field-of-view CT scans with regression forests and hidden Markov model. They further proposed a new strategy by transforming the sparse centroid annotations into dense probabilistic labels for training the classifier [1]. This method achieved better results than previous methods in terms of identification rate on pathological cases. One limitation of above-mentioned methods was that they employed hand-crafted feature descriptors, such as histogram of oriented gradients (HOG), and/or a priori knowledge for identification of vertebrae. However, these feature descriptors cannot accurately represent the complicated characteristics of vertebrae when spinal pathologies or surgical implants exist. Besides, these methods did not consider structural information in a larger scale, such as the relationship of neighboring vertebrae, which may further improve the identification rate by circumventing the low discrimination of neighboring vertebrae.

Instead of employing low level hand-crafted features, deep neural networks with high level feature representations have made breakthroughs in various detection tasks [8]. Recently, Suzani [9] has employed a six-layer feed-forward neural network for vertebrae localization and identification. However, compared with convolutional neural network (CNN), feed-forward neural network cannot take full advantage of spatial information to better learn discriminative features. In this paper, we propose a novel joint learning model with deep convolutional neural network (J-CNN) to meet the challenges mentioned above. In our model, besides the high level feature representations learned from CNN, we also take the conditional dependency among neighboring vertebrae into consideration, as single vertebra without reference structures can impede the identification performance. In addition, a shape regression model is proposed to refine the predicted centroids of vertebrae. Our method achieves significant improvements compared with the state-of-the-art method [1] on the testing data of MICCAI 2014 Computational Challenge on Vertebrae Localization and Identification.

2 Method

The proposed method consists of three steps: coarse vertebra candidates localization, vertebrae identification and vertebral centroids refinement.

2.1 Coarse Vertebra Candidates Localization

Directly performing CNN on CT volumes is not computationally efficient. Thus, we employed an random forest (RF) classifier for fast localizing the vertebra candidates coarsely while preserving a high sensitivity. The RF is an effective ensemble learning method and has demonstrated good performance on the localization of anatomical structures in CT volumes [1]. We trained a binary RF classifier (i.e., vertebra and non-vertebra) based on HOG features from 3D training samples, which are extracted from ground truth and background (randomly selected). In the testing phase, the RF classifier retrieved the vertebra candidates coarsely by scanning the input CT volume in a sliding window way.

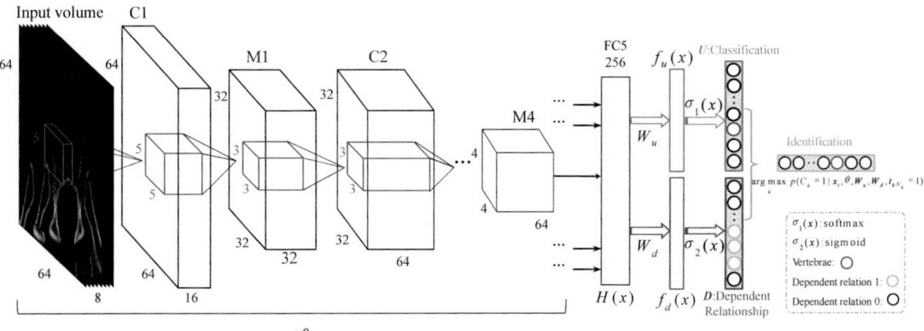

Fig. 2. The architecture of the proposed J-CNN model

2.2 J-CNN for Vertebrae Identification

We detail the J-CNN model after a brief introduction of CNN. The basic structure of CNN includes several pairs of altering convolutional and sub-sampling (e.g., average- or max-pooling) layers, followed by fully connected (FC) layers for classification [10]. The convolutional (C) layer takes local receptive field in the previous layer as input and extracts features while preserving the spatial position. The max-pooling (M) layer performs non-max suppression and down-samples the resolution of feature maps. The architecture of our J-CNN model (including four C layers, four M layers, two FC layers and two classification layers) is illustrated in Fig. 2.

Unary Appearance Posterior Term. Given an input training sample x_i, the softmax classification layer outputs the unary appearance posterior probability p_u for each class of vertebra. The p_u is defined as:

$$p_u(C_k = 1|x_i, \theta, W_u) = \frac{e^{f_u^k(x_i)}}{\sum_{j=1}^{K} e^{f_u^j(x_i)}}, k = 1, ..., K \tag{1}$$

$$f_u(x_i) = W_u H(x_i \otimes W_n + b) \tag{2}$$

where $f_u(x_i)$ is the output before softmax classification layer with weight W_u for inferring the probability of kth class $p_u(C_k = 1|x_i, \theta, W_u)$. The $H(\cdot)$ denotes the extracted features (i.e., activations of FC5 in Fig. 2) through the deep CNN. It is a highly non-convex compositional function with parameters $\theta = \{W_n, b\}$. We then define the unary appearance posterior term with cross-entropy loss as:

$$\mathcal{U}_i(x_i, y_i; \theta, W_u) = \sum_{k=1}^{K} y_i^k \log p_u(C_k = 1|x_i, \theta, W_u) \tag{3}$$

where $y_i \in \{0,1\}^K$ is the one-hot vector of label ($K = 27$ is number of classes including 26 types of vertebrae and the background) with the kth element as y_i^k.

Pairwise Conditional Dependency Term. The low inter-class difference among neighboring vertebrae can impose difficulties for vertebrae identification if only relying on the unary appearance posterior term via deep CNN. The neighboring vertebrae could provide more structural information for discrimination. The input volume, we argue that, could not only infer the type of vertebra but also the conditional relationship of neighboring vertebrae. The latter one incorporates the structure prior of spine, which acts as structural dependency constraints and contributes to vertebrae identification. Therefore, a novel conditional relationship probability p_d considering the pairwise inter-dependency with neighboring vertebrae is inferred with weight W_d. The p_d is defined as:

$$p_d(r_{kj} = 1|x_i, C_k = 1; \theta, W_d) = \frac{1}{1 + e^{-f_d^j(x_i)}}, j = 1, 2, ..., J \tag{4}$$

$$f_d(x_i) = W_d H(x_i \otimes W_n + b) \tag{5}$$

where J is the total number of relations r_{kj} between one particular vertebra k and the rest, $f_d^j(x_i)$ denotes the jth element in $f_d(x_i) \in \mathbb{R}^J$ ($J = 27$ in our experiments). Then the pairwise conditional dependency term is defined as:

$$\mathcal{D}_i(x_i, t_{kj}; \theta, W_d) = \sum_{j=1}^{J} t_{kj} \log p_d + (1 - t_{kj}) \log(1 - p_d) \tag{6}$$

where the binary dependent relationship t_{kj} is set as 1 for neighboring vertebrae set $\mathcal{N}_k$ with respect to the vertebra class k, otherwise 0. In our implementation, we consider the two adjacent vertebrae of a specified vertebra as its neighboring vertebrae. For the relationship of background, we regard all samples from background as neighbours.

Total Loss Function. Based on the above analysis, the total loss function, which aims at joint learning of the unary appearance and the pairwise dependency so as to improve the accuracy of vertebrae identification, is defined as:

$$\mathcal{L} = -\sum_{i=1}^{N} \mathcal{U}_i(x_i, y_i; \theta, W_u) + \lambda \mathcal{D}_i(x_i, t_{kj}; \theta, W_d) \tag{7}$$

where the hyperparameter λ controls the tradeoff between these two terms, and N is the number of training samples. Due to the non-convexity in Eq. 7, we employed stochastic gradient descent (SGD) method to solve it. Finally, the class of vertebra can be obtained by generating following maximum probability:

$$\begin{aligned} k^* &= \arg\max_k p(C_k = 1 | x_i; \theta, W_u, W_d, t_{k\mathcal{N}_k} = 1) \\ &= p(C_k = 1 | x_i; \theta, W_u) \prod_{j \in \mathcal{N}_k} p(t_{kj} = 1 | x_i; \theta, W_d) \end{aligned} \tag{8}$$

which considers both appearance of vertebra and dependency information among neighboring vertebrae jointly in order to achieve a better identification rate.

2.3 Localization Refinement with Shape Regression Modelling

The predicted vertebral centroids may have offsets with respect to the exact geometric centroids. This may arise from the coarse sliding window operation. Given the predicted centroids of vertebrae and ground truth, we observed that offsets mainly resulted from the deviation in vertical axis due to the low resolution in this direction. Hence we learned a shape regression model $g(d_s)$ to refine the coordinate in the vertical axis, denoted as v_s, with following energy function:

$$E = \sum_s (||g(d_s) - v_s||_2^2 + \gamma ||g(d_s) - \sum_{j \in \mathcal{N}_s} \beta_{js} g(d_j)||_2^2) \tag{9}$$

where d_s is the distance in vertical axis from the identified 1st vertebrae to the sth vertebrae, which is derived from the annotations of training data and acts as the spinal prior structure. As most of scans have a limited field-of-view, we set $g(d_s)$ as a quadratic polynomial curve. The first term $||g(d_s) - v_s||_2^2$ regresses the v_s of predicted centroids on d_s. The second term models the refined centroid among neighboring vertebrae $\mathcal{N}_s$ with weight β. The weight γ controls the balance of these two terms. In the test phase, the optimized parameters of $g(d_s)$ can be learned by minimizing the function E for each patient separately. Then the predicted vertebral centroids are refined by the learned shape regression model.

3 Experiments

The performance of our method was evaluated on the dataset of MICCAI 2014 Computational Challenge on Vertebrae Localization and Identification. It contains 302 annotated spine-focused CT volumes with various pathologies and numerous post-operative cases. For the training data (242 CT scans), manual annotations of vertebral centroids are provided, but the ground truth of testing data (60 CT scans) is held-out for evaluation. In the training, we augmented each extracted 3D volume by translation. Totally, we extracted 67,145 vertebrae samples and 7,260 background samples to train the RF classifier and J-CNN. The weights of network were initialized with Gaussian distribution and other hyperparameters were determined with cross validation.

We compared our results with the state-of-the-art method [1] and the general deep CNN without considering the conditional dependency term. We employed two evaluation metrics: *identification rate* and *localization error* defined same as in [1]. For the method of general CNN, we trained it on the same data with only unary appearance posterior term, and other steps were the same with the proposed J-CNN. The results were reported in Table 1. Our method outperformed the method of [1] and the general CNN with 10.12% and 7.03% improvement in term of identification rate for all vertebrae. The mean localization errors of our method were also smaller than those of other two methods. Note that in most cases, the results of general CNN were better than those of [1], demonstrating the high level features learned from CNN have better discriminative capability than hand-crafted features. The results of J-CNN further demonstrated the superiority of the joint learning model with neighboring dependency information.

Table 1. Comparison results of different methods

Method		Glocker [1]			CNN			J-CNN(Ours)		
Region	Counts	Id.Rate	Mean	Std	Id.Rate	Mean	Std	Id.Rate	Mean	Std
All	657	74.04%	13.20	17.83	77.13%	10.41	13.82	**84.16%**	**8.82**	13.04
Cervical	188	88.76%	6.81	10.02	84.00%	6.80	10.90	**91.84%**	**5.12**	8.22
Thoracic	324	61.75%	17.35	22.30	67.26%	13.06	16.29	**76.38%**	**11.39**	16.48
Lumbar	113	79.86%	13.05	12.45	85.21%	9.63	10.22	**88.11%**	**8.42**	8.62

Id.Rate: identification rate. Mean and Standard deviation (Std) errors (unit: mm).

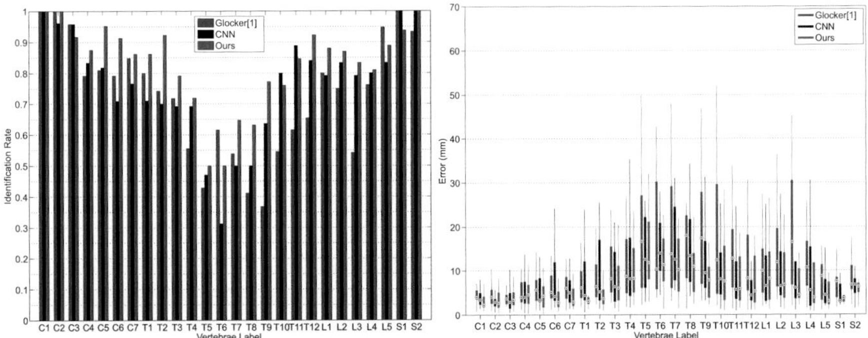

Fig. 3. (left) Identification rate on individual vertebra of testing data; (right) Error statistics for each type of vertebra

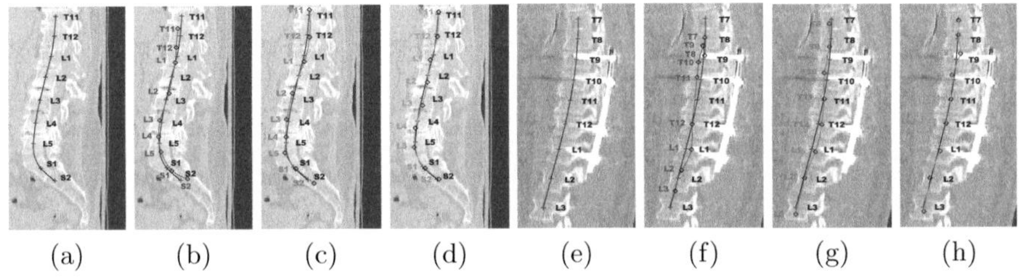

(a) (b) (c) (d) (e) (f) (g) (h)

Fig. 4. Two examples of results (localized and identified vertebral centroids are marked as brown diamonds): (a)(e): the ground truth of annotated centroids (both have 9 annotations marked as red crosses), (b)(f): the results of [1], (c)(g): the results of the general CNN, and (d)(h): the results of the proposed J-CNN.

Quantitative comparison of identification rate on each type of vertebra was reported in Fig. 3 (left). Our method achieved a higher identification rate on most of the vertebrae than other two methods. The localization error statistics for each type of vertebra were also evaluated for the three methods, as shown in Fig. 3 (right). In most cases, the proposed method achieved smaller mean errors than other two methods. We further evaluated the mean localization errors of all vertebrae for J-CNN with and without refinement step. The results were 8.82 ± 13.04 (mean $\pm$ std) mm and 9.99 ± 15.56 mm, respectively, demonstrating the efficacy of the shape regression model in localization refinement. Fig. 4 showed two typical examples of results. In both cases, our estimated vertebral centroids are more accurate compared with those of other two methods.

4 Discussion and Conclusion

We presented a novel automatic approach for vertebrae localization and identification in CT volumes. The proposed approach utilized the feature representations learned from CNN while taking neighboring dependency into consideration to improve the identification rate. Experimental results demonstrated the proposed method achieved better performance than the state-of-the-art method and the general CNN framework. Although the method is tailored for vertebrae detection here, it can be adapted to other similar anatomical structure detection tasks. Future investigations include integrating a statistical articulated model in the refinement step and testing the method on more datasets.

Acknowledgement. The work described in this paper was supported by a grant from the Research Grants Council of the Hong Kong Special Administrative Region (Project No. CUHK412513) and a GRF grant (No. CUHK 473012).

References

1. Glocker, B., Zikic, D., Konukoglu, E., Haynor, D.R., Criminisi, A.: Vertebrae localization in pathological spine CT via dense classification from sparse annotations. In: Mori, K., Sakuma, I., Sato, Y., Barillot, C., Navab, N. (eds.) MICCAI 2013, Part II. LNCS, vol. 8150, pp. 262–270. Springer, Heidelberg (2013)
2. Ben Ayed, I., Punithakumar, K., Minhas, R., Joshi, R., Garvin, G.J.: Vertebral body segmentation in MRI via convex relaxation and distribution matching. In: Ayache, N., Delingette, H., Golland, P., Mori, K. (eds.) MICCAI 2012, Part I. LNCS, vol. 7510, pp. 520–527. Springer, Heidelberg (2012)
3. Schlösser, T.P., van Stralen, M., Brink, R.C., Chu, W.C., Lam, T.P., Vincken, K.L., Castelein, R.M., Cheng, J.C.: Three-dimensional characterization of torsion and asymmetry of the intervertebral discs versus vertebral bodies in adolescent idiopathic scoliosis. Spine 39(19), E1159–E1166 (2014)
4. Oktay, A.B., Akgul, Y.S.: Localization of the lumbar discs using machine learning and exact probabilistic inference. In: Fichtinger, G., Martel, A., Peters, T. (eds.) MICCAI 2011, Part III. LNCS, vol. 6893, pp. 158–165. Springer, Heidelberg (2011)
5. Klinder, T., Ostermann, J., Ehm, M., Franz, A., Kneser, R., Lorenz, C.: Automated model-based vertebra detection, identification, and segmentation in CT images. Medical Image Analysis 13(3), 471–482 (2009)
6. Glocker, B., Feulner, J., Criminisi, A., Haynor, D.R., Konukoglu, E.: Automatic localization and identification of vertebrae in arbitrary field-of-view CT scans. In: Ayache, N., Delingette, H., Golland, P., Mori, K. (eds.) MICCAI 2012, Part III. LNCS, vol. 7512, pp. 590–598. Springer, Heidelberg (2012)
7. Kelm, B.M., Wels, M., Zhou, S.K., Seifert, S., Suehling, M., Zheng, Y., Comaniciu, D.: Spine detection in ct and mr using iterated marginal space learning. Medical Image Analysis 17(8), 1283–1292 (2013)
8. Bengio, Y., Courville, A., Vincent, P.: Representation learning: A review and new perspectives. IEEE Transactions on Pattern Analysis and Machine Intelligence 35(8), 1798–1828 (2013)
9. Suzani, A.: Automatic vertebrae localization, identification, and segmentation using deep learning and statistical models. In: thesis, Sharif University of Technology. University of British Columbia (2014)
10. LeCun, Y., Bottou, L., Bengio, Y., Haffner, P.: Gradient-based learning applied to document recognition. Proceedings of the IEEE 86(11), 2278–2324 (1998)

Identification of Cerebral Small Vessel Disease Using Multiple Instance Learning

Liang Chen[1], Tong Tong[1], Chin Pang Ho[1], Rajiv Patel[2], David Cohen[2], Angela C. Dawson[3], Omid Halse[3], Olivia Geraghty[1], Paul E.M. Rinne[1], Christopher J. White[1], Tagore Nakornchai[1], Paul Bentley[1], and Daniel Rueckert[1]

[1] Imperial College London, London, United Kingdom
[2] Northwick Park Hospital, London, United Kingdom
[3] Imperial College Healthcare NHS Trust, London, United Kingdom

Abstract. Cerebral small vessel disease (SVD) is a common cause of ageing-associated physical and cognitive impairment. Identifying SVD is important for both clinical and research purposes but is usually dependent on radiologists' evaluation of brain scans. Computer tomography (CT) is the most widely used brain imaging technique but for SVD it shows a low signal-to-noise ratio, and consequently poor inter-rater reliability. We therefore propose a novel framework based on multiple instance learning (MIL) to distinguish between absent/mild SVD and moderate/severe SVD. Intensity patches are extracted from regions with high probability of containing lesions. These are then used as instances in MIL for the identification of SVD. A large baseline CT dataset, consisting of 590 CT scans, was used for evaluation. We achieved approximately 75% accuracy in classifying two different types of SVD, which is high for this challenging problem. Our results outperform those obtained by either standard machine learning methods or current clinical practice.

1 Introduction

The World Health Organization (WHO) states that stroke is the second major cause of death in the world during 2000 and 2012. Stroke, which is a cerebrovascular accident, is the loss of brain function caused by the lack of blood supply [16]. It may lead to long-term disability. Ischemic stroke and hemorrhagic stroke are two different categories of strokes that require different treatments [6]. Ischemic stroke accounts for approximately 80% of all strokes [7]. Intravenous thrombolysis with recombinant tissue plasminogen activator (rt-PA) is the recommended therapy for acute ischemic stroke that reduces severe disability but causes deterioration due to symptomatic intracranial hemorrhage (SICH) in approximately 6% [18]. [4] demonstrates that cerebral SVD is associated with increased risk of ischemic stroke. Hypertensive SVD is the most common mechanism of hemorrhagic stroke [6]. In order to reduce the rate of SICH, which is associated with the worst outcome of stroke, management of SVD is pivotal. Cerebral SVD refers to a group of pathological aetiologies that affect the brain [12]. However, in this

N. Navab et al. (Eds.): MICCAI 2015, Part I, LNCS 9349, pp. 523–530, 2015.
DOI: 10.1007/978-3-319-24553-9_64

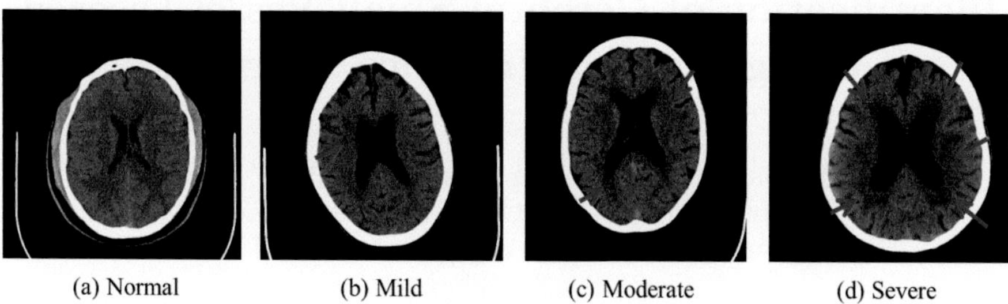

(a) Normal (b) Mild (c) Moderate (d) Severe

Fig. 1. Examples of CT images of the brain: (a) normal brain appearance, (b) brain with mild cerebral SVD, (c) brain with moderate SVD, and (d) cerebrum with severe SVD. The red arrows point out where the lesions are.

paper we will use the term to describe ischemic consequences of white matter (WM) lesions. Figure 1 presents examples of cerebrums with different kinds of SVD.

Advanced neuroimaging techniques have been widely used in the diagnosis of stroke. It is normally recommended that patients should undergo either magnetic resonance (MR) or CT imaging [19]. Diffusion-weighted imaging (DWI) and T2-fluid attenuated inversion recovery (FLAIR) should be included in the MR sequences, which are able to show any acute or chronic lesions. Although MR is the gold standard, CT is more frequently used in the acute phase of stroke treatment. This is due to the fact that there is typically no MR scanner access in emergency rooms in hospitals. For patients suffering from acute stroke it is therefore desirable to have reliable and automatic image analysis techniques for CT images.

There have been a large number of studies focusing on the automatic analysis of brain MR images. For instance, in Alzheimer's Disease (AD), machine learning techniques have been extensively used to classify controls and patients. However, there are very few works that focus on the classification of subjects suffering from stroke and even fewer which use CT images [5]. The cutting-edge studies on CT images, including [3], [17], and [9], are typically based on statistical values and threshold. These methods are fairly simple that it is difficult to apply to large datasets. To the best of our knowledge no machine learning approach has been proposed for the identification of SVD in a large dataset of CT images.

Fazekas et al. [8] proposed a standard approach for SVD grading. In this approach, SVD is divided into four categories according to the degree of the lesions: absent, mild, moderate, and severe. Generally, mild SVD is associated with normal brain ageing while moderate or severe SVD suggests potential risks for diseases such as stroke. One of the challenges for the grading of SVD is that the difference between absent/mild and moderate/severe SVD are often very subtle. In the context of similar challenging classification problems in medical images, semi-supervised machine learning approaches have been very successful. MIL is one example of such a semi-supervised learning method [21]. It solves the problem that standard approaches are difficult to distinguish lesions and normal tissues at a voxel or a patch.

In MIL, instances are contained in bags. A bag is positive if there is one positive instance in it; otherwise the bag is negative. Different bags may contain various numbers of instances. Compared to other standard supervised and unsupervised learning algorithms, there are many MIL methods that have been developed and applied, e.g. MIS-Boost [1], MIForest [11], and EM-Diverse Density [20]. In [1], the authors proposed a boosting based MIL, which outperforms a number of other similar algorithms on several benchmark datasets. This approach aims to learn a specific instance for each weak classifier, which is able to discriminate two categories of instances.

In this paper, we tackle the problem of automatic SVD identification. An MIL framework is formulated to classify SVD into normal (absent and mild) and abnormal (moderate and severe) groups, which is based on a large dataset of CT images. In Section 2, details of the MIS-Boost algorithm and our further optimization will be presented. Section 3 demonstrates how patches were extracted. We will show our imaging dataset, the pre-processing techniques, and our model based on MIS-Boost in Section 4. Comparisons between our model and other state-of-the-art algorithms will also be shown.

2 Methods

Given bags and their labels, MIL is recognized as a supervised learning method, which learns the mapping $\mathbf{X} \to \mathbf{Y}$, where $\mathbf{X}$ is a set of training data and $\mathbf{Y} = \{-1, +1\}$ is the set of corresponding labels. In this case, $\mathbf{X} = \{\mathbf{B}_1, \mathbf{B}_2, \dots, \mathbf{B}_N\}$ and for each bag $\mathbf{B}_i = \{\mathbf{I}_1, \mathbf{I}_2, \dots, \mathbf{I}_{n_i}\}$, where $\mathbf{I}_k \in \Re^r$ is the k-th instance in bag $\mathbf{B}_i$. N is the number of bags. n_i is the number of instances in the i-th bag. r is the size of a patch. The boosting-based MIL proposed in [1] aims to learn a 'bag-level' classifier

$$F(\mathbf{B}) = \text{sign}\left(\sum_{m=1}^{M} f_m(\mathbf{B})\right), \tag{1}$$

where $f_m(\cdot), m = 1, 2, \dots, M$, are weak classifiers defined as

$$f_m(\mathbf{B}) = \frac{2}{1 + e^{-(\beta_1 D(\mathbf{p}_m, \mathbf{B}) + \beta_0)}} - 1. \tag{2}$$

The task of each weak classifier is to find a patch $\mathbf{p}_m$, which serves as an instance, to discriminate different bags. In [1], the distance from an instance to a bag is defined as below

$$D(\mathbf{p}_m, \mathbf{B}) = \sum_{k=1}^{n} \pi_k d(\mathbf{p}_m, \mathbf{I}_k), \tag{3}$$

where $d(\mathbf{p}_m, \mathbf{I}_k) = \|\mathbf{p}_m - \mathbf{I}_k\|_2$ and $\pi_k = \frac{e^{-\alpha d(\mathbf{p}_m, \mathbf{I}_k)}}{\sum_{l=1}^{n} e^{-\alpha d(\mathbf{p}_m, \mathbf{I}_l)}}$. $d(\mathbf{p}_m, \mathbf{I}_k)$ is the distance between the specific instance and the k-th instance in the bag, which is the standard Euclidean distance and π_k is its weight. α is a constant. $D(\mathbf{p}_m, \mathbf{B})$ is the weighted average distance of $\mathbf{p}_m$ to each instance in the bag and $f_m(\cdot)$ maps the distance into the range $[-1, 1]$.

In order to learn $\mathbf{p}_m$, [1] defined an error function based on Gentle Adaboost. We obtained the parameters β_0, β_1, and $\mathbf{p}_m$ by minimizing the weighted error between the ground truth labels and the decision made by weak classifiers.

$$\min_{\mathbf{p}_m, \beta_0, \beta_1} \varepsilon_m = \sum_{i=1}^{N} w_i (y_i - f_m(\mathbf{B}_i))^2 \tag{4}$$

In [1] the optimization problem is solved via a coordinate descent algorithm. This uses a line-search method and therefore does not require the calculation of derivatives. However, each iteration is very time-consuming. In this work, we propose an optimization using a region-trust-reflective method [2] to allow a more efficient optimization that exploits the fact that the function above is differentiable. We formulated optimization of the objective function as a non-linear least square fitting problem.

For initialization, we performed k-means clustering for all instances in all the bags. The resulting K clustering centres were used as input for the initial $\mathbf{p}_m$ and we selected one leading to the minimum error ε_m among them. In order to decide on the number of weak classifiers M, we split the training dataset into sub-training and validation sets and pick up final M with minimum validation error.

3 Patch Extraction

In MIL, each bag contains a number of instances, which are patches in our case. Patches were extracted from original CT images since the slice thickness varies between different scans and resampling them to a constant voxel size will reduce the image quality. The extraction was guided by an atlas, which shows the regions with high probability of lesions. In order to construct such an atlas, we collected 277 MR images with SVD. For all MR images, clinical experts manually outlined regions of interests (ROIs) corresponding to the SVD lesions. They were then registered and normalized onto a standard space so that we are able to obtain the lesion atlas. The atlas constructed shows the probability for each voxel in the brain to be part of an SVD lesion. We excluded the regions with very low abnormal probability ($< 4\%$) in the atlas since they are likely to be outliers. Finally, the lesion atlas was mapped back to each individual CT image so that for each CT image a lesion atlas is available which shows regions with high probability of lesions. Figure 2 visualizes this processing pipeline.

4 Experiments and Results

4.1 Imaging Data and Pre-processing

In this study, all the data was collected from a local hospital. We collected 627 baseline CT brain images with stroke. For all patients, the imaging was carried

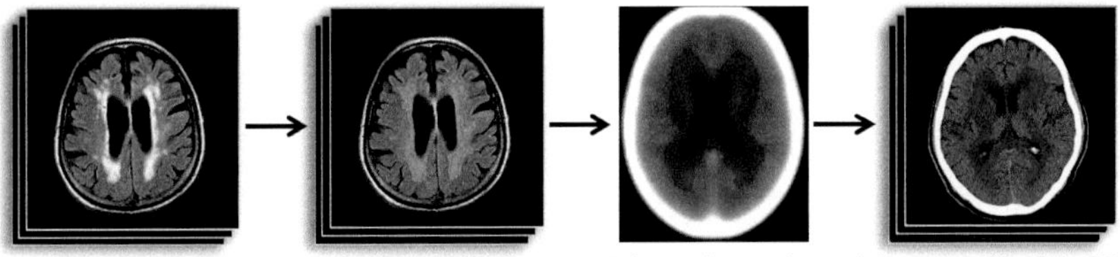

Raw MRI scans → Lesions outlined → Atlas on the template → Atlas mapped back to CT scans

Fig. 2. The process of atlas construction and mapping back. The red regions are the ROIs for patch extraction.

out within a short time window after stroke (4.5 hours). The average age of these subjects is 70.75 ± 10.83. There are 326 male and 301 female participants. The labels of these images were assessed by an expert according to [8] and there are inter-rater consistencies of about 75% between experts.

We developed a pipeline to normalize the images before analysis. All images were registered to a CT-based template and then resampled to a uniform voxel size. The template was developed by [14]. In order to reduce the radiation burden for patients, in some subjects the brains were scanned in two separate volumes including the cerebrum and the base using different voxel sizes. For the images scanned separately, the voxel sizes of cerebrum and base are approximately $0.45 \times 0.45 \times 7.2$ mm and $0.45 \times 0.45 \times 2.4$ mm; the voxel size of the whole-brain scans is approximately $0.38 \times 0.38 \times 3$ mm, while the template's voxel size is $2 \times 2 \times 2$ mm. We combined these sub-volumes into single volumes with constant voxel size. Subsequently we corrected the gantry tilt and rigidly co-registered all images to the template. Following this step, a non-rigid registration [15] was performed between all images and the template. Finally, all images were resampled onto the voxel grid of the template. The processing pipeline failed for 37 CT scans because of poor image quality and/or patient movement. These subjects were excluded and we used the remaining 590 scans in the following experiments, which consists of 350 with absent/mild SVD and 240 with moderate/severe SVD.

4.2 Patch-Based Identification of SVD

In order to have two SVD groups which are balanced in terms of number of subjects, we randomly sampled 240 subjects from the absent or mild group and performed leave-10%-out cross-validation. The random sampling was repeated for $T = 10$ times and the final results are average values of the T repeats. In this paper, abnormal bags and instances are regarded as positive.

In MIS-Boost, each subject is modelled as a bag, which can contain a number of patches as the instances. The patches were extracted from an ROI according to the atlas. The ROI is defined by those voxels in which the prior probability for lesions is not low. As different original CT scans have different numbers of slices and the size of the brain varies, different bags contain different numbers of instances. We obtain on average 2313 patches (SD: 762) in a bag. Given the

Table 1. Classification performance of different classifiers and features. Results of MIS-Boost and random forest are based on T times cross-validation.

Classifier	Feature	Accuracy(%)	Sensitivity(%)	Specificity(%)
MIS-Boost	Patch in ROI	**75.04**±1.37	**80.17**±1.65	69.92 ± 1.37
Random forest	Voxel in ROI	70.65 ± 0.03	69.63 ± 0.04	**71.67**±0.04
	Voxel in whole brain	65.25 ± 0.02	65.64 ± 0.04	64.96 ± 0.04
Threshold	t-Score	54.07	5.42	48.64

different slice thickness of the different scans, 2D patches were extracted with a patch size of 15 × 15. The performance is shown in Table 1.

In order to demonstrate the performance of our model, we compared the results to those obtained using alternative approaches. We compared our approach to random forests [10]. It is one of the most popular standard machine learning methods and has achieved a notable success in classification of AD patients and controls using imaging data [13]. As the CT images have been registered and normalized to the template, the voxels of processed images were selected as features for the random forests. Voxels were extracted from the whole brain and the ROI, respectively. We also compared the approach by [9] which has shown the ability for automated stroke lesion delineation using brain CT images. In this approach a t-score map is calculated, which when combined with a carefully selected threshold, can be used to delineate stroke lesions. Since acute stroke lesions are similar to SVD in terms of intensity and texture, this approach can be tested in terms of its performance for the evaluation of SVD. We collected 307 CT images without SVD to calculate the standard t-score map in template's space and mapped it back to each native image space. For each individual subject, we delineated the potential SVD lesions by applying the selected threshold to its t-score map and therefore obtained the volume of the lesions. We then sorted the volumes of all subjects and chose the median as the threshold to distinguish normal and abnormal subjects in terms of SVD.

According to Table 1, our implementation of patch-based MIS-Boost outperforms the other two methods. It is clear that a simple method based on thresholds is unreliable since its sensitivity is low. This means it cannot detect abnormal subjects. Compared with the threshold-based method, the random-forest-based method improves the accuracy by 10%. In addition, the random forest classifier is sufficiently robust as the gap between sensitivity and specificity is small. The use of voxels from the ROI defined by the atlas enhances the accuracy by 5% compared to using voxels from the whole brain. Furthermore, our proposed model boosts the classification accuracy by an additional 5%. Apart from the high accuracy of classification, the sensitivity of MIS-Boost is high.

5 Discussion and Conclusion

We have presented a framework in which boosting based MIL is used to learn patches for discrimination of normal or abnormal brain degeneration. A key feature of the proposed method is that it has been applied a large clinical CT dataset for automatic clinical identification of SVD. In addition, patches from original CT scans were employed, which avoids additional errors. To the best of our knowledge of this is the first such application of automated detection of SVD in such a large dataset. We have also shown that the classification results obtained using a state-of-the-art classification technique such as random forests is not as good as the proposed approach.

The proposed approach uses an atlas of SVD lesions derived from MR images. Compared with the low resolution of CT images, MR images are able to show brain lesions in detail. MR imaging is therefore regarded as the gold standard in the assessment of SVD. This provides prior knowledge where lesions occur frequently in the brain. The MR images used for the atlas construction are separate from the images that are used for training and/or testing.

The proposed method also showed its strength compared to standard clinical approaches, where basic statistical features are used. Since CT images show a low signal-to-noise ratio, small lesions like SVD are difficult to be identified at a voxel. In contrast, patch-based features decrease the effect of noise.

In the future, the proposed method will be applied to a larger dataset including data from different clinical centres so that the framework can be tested more widely in terms of robustness and accuracy. More importantly, our final goal is to predict the outcome of stroke - whether the stroke patients will hemorrhage or not. This will help to reduce the rate of SICH significantly, which will improve quality of patients' lives and reduce the pressure for the public health services.

References

[1] Akbas, E., Ghanem, B., Ahuja, N.: MIS-Boost: Multiple instance selection boosting. arXiv preprint:1109.2388 (2011)

[2] Byrd, R.H., Schnabel, R.B., Shultz, G.A.: Approximate solution of the trust region problem by minimization over two-dimensional subspaces. Mathematical Programming 40(1–3), 247–263 (1988)

[3] Chawla, M., Sharma, S., Sivaswamy, J., Kishore, L.: A method for automatic detection and classification of stroke from brain CT images. In: Annual International Conference of the IEEE Engineering in Medicine and Biology Society (EMBC), pp. 3581–3584. IEEE (2009)

[4] Conijn, M.M.A., Kloppenborg, R.P., Algra, A., Mali, W.P.T.M., Kappelle, L.J., Vincken, K.L., Van Der Graaf, Y., Geerlings, M.I.: Cerebral small vessel disease and risk of death, ischemic stroke, and cardiac complications in patients with atherosclerotic disease: The second manifestations of arterial disease-magnetic resonance (SMART-MR) study. Stroke 42, 3105–3109 (2011)

[5] Dalca, A.V., et al.: Segmentation of cerebrovascular pathologies in stroke patients with spatial and shape priors. In: Golland, P., Hata, N., Barillot, C., Hornegger, J., Howe, R. (eds.) MICCAI 2014, Part II. LNCS, vol. 8674, pp. 773–780. Springer, Heidelberg (2014)

[6] Donnan, G., Fisher, M., Macleod, M., Davis, S.M.: Stroke. The Lancet 371, 1612–1623 (2008)
[7] Durukan, A., Tatlisumak, T.: Acute ischemic stroke: Overview of major experimental rodent models, pathophysiology, and therapy of focal cerebral ischemia. Pharmacology Biochemistry and Behavior 87, 179–197 (2007)
[8] Fazekas, F., Chawluk, J.B., Alavi, A., Hurtig, H.I., Zimmerman, R.A.: MR signal abnormalities at 1.5 T in Alzheimer's dementia and normal aging. American Journal of Neuroradiology 8(3), 421–426 (1987)
[9] Gillebert, C.R., Humphreys, G.W., Mantini, D.: Automated delineation of stroke lesions using brain CT images. NeuroImage: Clinical 4, 540–548 (2014)
[10] Ho, T.K.: The random subspace method for constructing decision forests. IEEE Transactions on Pattern Analysis and Machine Intelligence 20(8), 832–844 (1998)
[11] Leistner, C., Saffari, A., Bischof, H.: MIForests: Multiple-instance learning with randomized trees. In: Daniilidis, K., Maragos, P., Paragios, N. (eds.) ECCV 2010, Part VI. LNCS, vol. 6316, pp. 29–42. Springer, Heidelberg (2010)
[12] Pantoni, L.: Cerebral small vessel disease: from pathogenesis and clinical characteristics to therapeutic challenges. The Lancet Neurology 9(7), 689–701 (2010)
[13] Ramírez, J., Górriz, J., Segovia, F., Chaves, R., Salas-Gonzalez, D., López, M., Álvarez, I., Padilla, P.: Computer aided diagnosis system for the Alzheimer's disease based on partial least squares and random forest SPECT image classification. Neuroscience Letters 472(2), 99–103 (2010)
[14] Rorden, C., Bonilha, L., Fridriksson, J., Bender, B., Karnath, H.O.: Age-specific CT and MRI templates for spatial normalization. NeuroImage 61, 957–965 (2012)
[15] Rueckert, D., Sonoda, L.I., Hayes, C., Hill, D.L., Leach, M.O., Hawkes, D.J.: Nonrigid registration using free-form deformations: application to breast MR images. IEEE Transactions on Medical Imaging 18(8), 712–721 (1999)
[16] Sims, N.R., Muyderman, H.: Mitochondria, oxidative metabolism and cell death in stroke. Biochimica et Biophysica Acta (BBA)-Molecular Basis of Disease 1802(1), 80–91 (2010)
[17] Takahashi, N., Tsai, D.Y., Lee, Y., Kinoshita, T., Ishii, K.: Z-score mapping method for extracting hypoattenuation areas of hyperacute stroke in unenhanced CT. Academic Radiology 17(1), 84–92 (2010)
[18] Wardlaw, J.M., Murray, V., Berge, E., Del Zoppo, G., Sandercock, P., Lindley, R.L., Cohen, G.: Recombinant tissue plasminogen activator for acute ischaemic stroke: An updated systematic review and meta-analysis. The Lancet 379, 2364–2372 (2012)
[19] Wintermark, M., Albers, G.W., Alexandrov, A.V., Alger, J.R., Bammer, R., Baron, J.C., Davis, S., Demaerschalk, B.M., Derdeyn, C.P., Donnan, G.A., et al.: Acute stroke imaging research roadmap. American Journal of Neuroradiology 29(5), e23–e30 (2008)
[20] Zhang, Q., Goldman, S.: EM-DD: An improved multiple-instance learning technique. In: Advances in Neural Information Processing Systems, pp. 1073–1080 (2001)
[21] Zhou, Z.H.: Multi-instance learning: a survey. Tech. rep., National Laboratory for Novel Software Technology, Nanjing (2004)

Why Does Synthesized Data Improve Multi-sequence Classification?

Gijs van Tulder[1] and Marleen de Bruijne[1,2]

[1] Biomedical Imaging Group Rotterdam
Erasmus MC University Medical Center, The Netherlands
[2] Department of Computer Science
University of Copenhagen, Denmark

Abstract. The classification and registration of incomplete multi-modal medical images, such as multi-sequence MRI with missing sequences, can sometimes be improved by replacing the missing modalities with synthetic data. This may seem counter-intuitive: synthetic data is derived from data that is already available, so it does not add new information. Why can it still improve performance? In this paper we discuss possible explanations. If the synthesis model is more flexible than the classifier, the synthesis model can provide features that the classifier could not have extracted from the original data. In addition, using synthetic information to complete incomplete samples increases the size of the training set.

We present experiments with two classifiers, linear support vector machines (SVMs) and random forests, together with two synthesis methods that can replace missing data in an image classification problem: neural networks and restricted Boltzmann machines (RBMs). We used data from the BRATS 2013 brain tumor segmentation challenge, which includes multi-modal MRI scans with T1, T1 post-contrast, T2 and FLAIR sequences. The linear SVMs appear to benefit from the complex transformations offered by the synthesis models, whereas the random forests mostly benefit from having more training data. Training on the hidden representation from the RBM brought the accuracy of the linear SVMs close to that of random forests.

1 Introduction

Multi-sequence data can be very informative in medical imaging, but using it may cause some practical problems. Training a classifier on multi-modal data, for instance, generally requires that all modalities are available for all samples. If some modalities are missing, there is a range of methods for handling or imputing the missing values in standard statistical analysis [1]. Specifically for image analysis, there are synthesis methods that predict missing modalities. Some methods model the physical properties of the imaging process, e.g., to derive intrinsic tissue parameters from MRI scans [2] or to derive pseudo-CT from MRI in radiotherapy applications [3,4]. But an explicit model of the imaging process is not even required, as image processing techniques can be sufficient: for example, pseudo-CT images have also been made with tissue segmentation [5,6], with Gaussian mixture models [7] or by registering and combining CT images [8,9].

N. Navab et al. (Eds.): MICCAI 2015, Part I, LNCS 9349, pp. 531–538, 2015.
DOI: 10.1007/978-3-319-24553-9_65

Interestingly, data synthesis can not only generate images but also helps as an intermediate step. For example, Iglesias et al. [10] found that synthetic data improved the registration of multi-sequence brain MRI. Roy et al. [11] showed that synthetic sequences can improve segmentation consistency in datasets with multiple MRI contrasts. Li et al. [12] predicted PET patches from MRI data with convolutional neural networks, and found that including this synthetic PET data could improve classification of Alzheimer's disease.

There is something paradoxical about these results: if the synthetic data is derived from the available data and does not add new information, how can it still improve the performance? If the data synthesis is more flexible than the existing model, the synthetic data could add a useful transformation that makes the data easier to analyze. Data synthesis may also help to use the training data more efficiently, by allowing samples with different missing modalities to be combined into a single, large training set. Finally, synthesis methods that use unlabeled data, such as those discussed here, are an elegant way to add unsupervised learning to supervised models. However, most studies with synthetic data do not feature mixed training data or extra unlabeled examples, which suggests that the extra modeling power of the synthesis method could be important.

We present experiments that compare simple and complex classifiers trained with synthetic data on multi-sequence MRI data from the BRATS brain tumor segmentation challenge [13]. We use neural networks and restricted Boltzmann machines (RBMs) to provide synthetic replacements for missing image sequences. These representation learning [14] methods aim to learn new, abstract representations from the data. We use these representations to train linear support vector machines (SVMs) and random forests. We compare the results of using data synthesis with those of simply replacing missing data with a constant value. The data synthesis models are non-linear, so we expect that they can improve the results of the linear SVM but have a smaller effect for the random forests.

2 Methods

Image Synthesis with Neural Networks. We use a neural network with three layers: an input layer with nodes v_i to represent the voxels from the 3D input patches, a hidden layer with nodes h_j, and a layer with nodes y_k representing the 3D patch to be predicted. In this feed-forward network the visible nodes v_i are connected with weights W_{ij} to the hidden nodes h_j, which are connected to the output nodes $\hat{y}_k$ with weights U_{jk}. The parameters b_j and c_k are biases. The activation of the nodes given input $\mathbf{v}$ is given by

$$h_j = \text{sigm}(\sum_i W_{ij} v_i + b_j) \quad \text{and} \quad \hat{y}_k = \sum_j U_{jk} h_j + c_k, \tag{1}$$

with $\text{sigm}\,(x) = \frac{1}{1+\exp(-x)}$. We use backpropagation to learn the weights that optimize the reconstruction error between the predicted $\hat{\mathbf{y}}$ and true values $\mathbf{y}$:

$$\text{err}\,(\mathbf{y}, \hat{\mathbf{y}}) = \sum_k |y_k - \hat{y_k}|\,. \tag{2}$$

Restricted Boltzmann Machines. A restricted Boltzmann machine (RBM) models the joint probability over a set of visible nodes $\mathbf{v}$ and hidden nodes $\mathbf{h}$, with an undirected connection with weight W_{ij} between each visible node v_i and hidden node h_j. Each visible node has a bias b_i, each hidden node a bias c_j. We use noisy rectified linear units in the hidden layer and real-valued nodes with a Gaussian distribution for the visible nodes [15]. The weights and biases define the energy function

$$E(\mathbf{v}, \mathbf{h}) = \sum_j \frac{(v_i - b_i)^2}{2\sigma_i^2} - \sum_{i,j} \frac{v_i}{\sigma_i} W_{ij} h_j - \sum_j c_j h_j \,, \tag{3}$$

where σ_i is the standard deviation of the Gaussian noise of visible node i. The joint distribution of the input $\mathbf{v}$ and hidden representation $\mathbf{h}$ is defined as

$$P(\mathbf{v}, \mathbf{h}) = \frac{\exp(-E(\mathbf{v}, \mathbf{h}))}{Z}, \tag{4}$$

where Z is a normalization constant. The conditional probabilities for the hidden nodes given the visible nodes and vice versa are

$$P(h_j | \mathbf{v}) = \max(0, \sum_i W_{ij} v_i + c_j + \mathcal{N}(0, \text{sigm}(\sum_i W_{ij} v_i + c_j))) \text{ and} \tag{5}$$

$$P(v_i | \mathbf{h}) = \mathcal{N}(\sum_j W_{ij} h_j + b_i,\ \sigma_i), \quad \text{with } \text{sigm}(x) = \frac{1}{1 + \exp(-x)}. \tag{6}$$

We use stochastic gradient descent with persistent contrastive divergence [15,16] to find weights $\mathbf{W}$ and biases $\mathbf{b}$ and $\mathbf{c}$ that give a high probability to samples from the training distribution.

Although the energy $E(\mathbf{v}, \mathbf{h})$ can be calculated with Eq. 3, the normalization constant Z prohibits computing the probability $P(\mathbf{v}, \mathbf{h})$ for non-trivial models. However, we can still sample from the distribution using Gibbs sampling and the conditional probabilities $P(h_j | \mathbf{v})$ and $P(v_i | \mathbf{h})$ (Eqs. 5 and 6).

The standard RBM has one set of visible nodes. To model the patches for multiple sequences we use a separate set of visible nodes $\mathbf{v}^s$ for each sequence s, connected to a shared set of hidden nodes $\mathbf{h}$. There are no direct connections between visible nodes, so the interactions between sequences are modeled through the hidden nodes. We train this RBM on training samples with the same patch in every sequence to learn the joint probability distribution of the four sequences.

Image Synthesis with RBMs. In theory we could calculate the probability of one sequence given the others, $P(\mathbf{v}^s | \mathbf{v} \backslash \mathbf{v}^s)$, to predict a missing sequence, but the normalization constant Z makes this impossible. We resort to Gibbs sampling to synthesize the missing sequence. We initialize the model with the available sequences and keep these values fixed. We set the visible nodes for the missing sequence to 0, the mean value for our normalized patches. During Gibbs sampling we alternate sampling from the visible and hidden layers. We use the final values of the visible nodes for the missing sequence as the synthesized patch.

3 Data and Implementation

We used data of 30 patients from the BRATS 2013 brain tumor segmentation challenge [13] with four MRI sequences per patient: T1, T1 post-contrast (T1c), T2 and FLAIR. The scans of each patient are rigidly registered to the T1c image, which has the highest resolution, and resampled to 1 mm isotropic resolution. The dataset includes brain masks and class labels for four tumor structures.

For each patient we extracted patches of $9 \times 9 \times 9$ voxels from the same location in each sequence. For feature learning we used 10 000 patches per scan, centered at random voxels in the brain mask. For classification we used the label data to create a balanced training set with approximately $\frac{1}{5}$th of the samples for each class (four tissue classes and the non-tumor background).

We normalized the data twice. First, each scan was normalized to zero mean and unit variance to remove large differences between scans. After extracting patches we calculated the mean intensity, standard deviation and the intensity of the center voxel for each patch, since these features may help to discriminate tissue classes. Finally, we normalized each patch before training the neural networks and RBMs, since this helps to learn the local image structures.

We trained the neural network and RBM on unlabeled patches, implemented with the Theano library [17] for Python. The neural networks had one hidden layer of 600 binary nodes; the RBMs had 600 noisy rectified linear units in the hidden layer. Using more nodes or layers did not improve the performance. We used stochastic gradient descent with a decreasing learning rate for both models, with persistent contrastive divergence to estimate the updates of the RBM.

After training the models, we synthesized missing sequences from three known sequences, using Eq. 1 for the neural network and Gibbs sampling (20 iterations) for the RBM. As a baseline method, we replaced missing sequences with all zeros, the mean value of the normalized patches.

We trained random forest and linear SVM classifiers from Scikit-learn [18] to classify the five tissue types. The feature vectors were composed of either the normalized intensity values of observed and synthesized patches, or the values of the hidden layer of the RBM. We also included the intensity of the center voxel and the mean intensity and standard deviation of the patch intensities.

We repeated our experiments for five train/validation/test splits, each with 20 training scans, 5 scans to validate the model parameters and 5 test scans. For each split, we used the validation set to optimize the number of trees (up to 200) in the random forest, the L2 regularization of the SVM, and the hyperparameters of the neural networks and RBMs. We report the mean accuracy on the test sets.

4 Experiments

We present two classification scenarios. In the first, all samples are missing the same sequence. As a baseline we use the classification accuracy without data synthesis, measured on the full dataset and on datasets where we removed one sequence from the training and test data. Next, we look at data synthesis to complete the missing sequences. We trained classifiers on complete samples and tested on samples with one synthetic sequence. We also give the accuracy of classifiers trained on samples with a synthetic sequence, because the synthetic data might have a different distribution than the real data. Training and testing a classifier on data with different distributions might reduce its performance. Finally, we trained classifiers on the hidden representation from the RBM directly.

The second scenario uses a mixed training set, in which every sample is still missing one sequence, but where every quarter of the training set is missing a different sequence to simulate a combination of heterogeneous datasets. Without data synthesis, a separate classifier is needed for each subset of samples with the same three sequences. We use this as a baseline for the synthesis experiments. The RBM can be trained on the mixed training set. The neural networks have a practical problem: with no training samples with four sequences, we cannot train a network that predicts one sequence from the other three. Instead, we trained networks with one (MLP 1–1) or two (MLP 2–1) input sequences to predict one output sequence. Each option yields three networks to predict one sequence for a sample with three available sequences; we used the average prediction. We used the synthesis methods to complete the training set and compare with replacing the missing values with zeros, the mean value of the normalized patches.

5 Results

Table 1 shows the results of removing one of the MRI sequences from the test set. When training without synthesis, removing T1c or FLAIR reduced the accuracy more than removing T1 or T2, suggesting that T1c and FLAIR provide information that is not in T1 or T2. (The T1c scans also had a higher resolution.)

Training and testing with one synthetic sequence gave an accuracy similar to that of training on the dataset without the sequence. Replacing the synthetic data with zeros also gave similar results. This fits with our hypothesis that the synthetic data might not add new information. Adding synthetic data did not make the results much worse, which is useful if the synthetic data is used to combine data from multiple datasets. Using RBM synthesis was slightly better than using a neural network or replacing the sequence with zeros. Training on synthetic data instead of on real data slightly improved the accuracy, most likely because classifiers were confused by the different distributions of the real and synthetic data. Training on the hidden representation from the RBM increased the accuracy of the linear SVM and brought it closer to that of the random forest. This suggests that although the RBM does not add new information, it can still transform the data in a way that helps the linear SVM. The RBM representation did not improve the accuracy of the more complex random forests.

Table 2 shows the results of training with a mixed training set with partially incomplete data. Training on subsets of complete samples (sharing the same three sequences, $\frac{1}{4}$th of the samples) gave a lower accuracy than training on the full set. Using the synthesis methods to complete the samples, we trained a classifier on all samples, which gave a higher accuracy than training on subsets. There

Table 1. Classification accuracy (linear SVM | random forest) for different synthesis methods, with test sets in which all samples are missing the same sequence. Results in bold are significantly different from the baseline results in the top row ($p < 0.05$).

		Missing sequence			
	Full set	T1	T1c	T2	FLAIR
Train and evaluate on voxel values, without synthesis					
	68.83|73.22	67.90|72.97	58.67|61.62	68.26|72.87	59.13|69.60
Train on complete samples, evaluate with synthesized data					
with zeros		67.32|72.61	54.26|59.77	**67.17**|**72.08**	58.10|**65.03**
by MLP		68.32|72.95	**56.21**|**60.00**	67.48|72.52	58.33|68.53
by RBM		68.42|73.06	**55.34**|**60.33**	67.35|**72.38**	59.66|**67.57**
Train and evaluate with synthesized data					
with zeros		**68.47**|**73.36**	57.88|61.75	67.90|72.73	**59.94**|**69.38**
by MLP		67.37|73.01	58.34|61.22	**66.59**|**72.89**	**60.19**|**69.90**
by RBM		69.25|73.24	**60.53**|**61.47**	68.17|72.55	**62.30**|**69.88**
Train and evaluate on values from the RBM hidden layer					
RBM	**72.89**|**74.16**	**72.18**|**73.47**	**61.68**|**61.51**	**70.78**|**72.93**	**66.33**|**69.52**

Table 2. Classification accuracy (linear SVM | random forest) with partially incomplete training data, in which every scan is missing a random sequence. Boldface indicates a significant difference with the baseline ($p < 0.05$). The results for the full test set are compared with the best performing baseline (missing T2).

		Missing sequence in evaluation			
	Full test set	T1	T1c	T2	FLAIR
Train on subsets with complete samples (three sequences, $\frac{1}{4}$th of the full set)					
		62.30|67.99	54.92|59.48	62.71|69.03	51.06|65.51
Train on the mixed training set, with missing sequences filled-in					
with zeros	**66.85**|**70.86**	63.64|**69.90**	58.21|**63.70**	62.90|70.55	54.03|67.63
by MLP 1–1	**66.99**|**71.44**	64.28|**69.99**	59.27|**63.95**	63.50|**71.17**	**55.82**|**68.73**
by MLP 2–1	**65.42**|**71.22**	65.03|**69.76**	59.15|**64.01**	63.88|**71.21**	55.84|68.38
by RBM	**57.81**|**70.26**	**54.56**|**69.25**	**51.94**|**63.23**	**56.12**|**70.65**	50.60|68.10
Train and evaluate on values from the RBM hidden layer (all samples)					
RBM	**70.17**|**70.79**	**69.80**|**69.60**	**59.72**|**59.78**	**68.57**|**70.30**	**62.90**|**65.90**

was little difference between the two neural network approaches and replacing the missing values by zeros. The RBM synthesis gave a lower accuracy, possibly because synthesizing the missing training sequences made it harder to optimize the model. Training directly on the hidden representation from the RBM gave the highest accuracy for the linear SVM, as in the first experiment. The results with random forests were comparable to those of training on synthesized data.

6 Discussion and Conclusion

Data synthesis methods can improve the classification accuracy of multi-modal image analysis by providing synthetic data for incomplete examples. We first explored the explanation that the synthesis models may offer data transformations that are useful to the classifier. In our experiments in which the same modality was missing for all samples, we found few significant improvements from using synthetic T1, T1c or T2. We suspect that these modalities are too similar to produce useful transformations. Synthesized FLAIR did give a small improvement. Moreover, training on the RBM hidden layer significantly improved the accuracy for both classifiers and brought the SVMs close to the random forests. This suggests that the RBM extracts features that are new to the linear SVMs, but that could already be extracted by the random forests.

We found stronger improvements from using synthetic data in our second experiment. The synthesis methods made it possible to combine samples with different missing sequences in one training set. Using this larger training set increased the accuracy of both linear SVMs and random forests. We found similar results by replacing the missing values with zeros, the mean intensity after normalization. This suggests that at least part of the in accuracy improvement might be the result of having more training data.

In these applications the RBMs have a practical advantage over neural networks, because RBMs learn a joint probability distribution that can be used to predict any missing sequence. In contrast, neural networks are explicitly trained to predict one sequence given the others, so they need a separate network for each sequence. In our experiments the neural networks had a slightly lower reconstruction error, because the RBMs optimize a different learning objective.

Both neural networks and RBMs are trained with unlabeled data, a useful property that makes it easier to train them on large datasets. This can be an elegant way to use unlabeled data to improve a supervised classifier.

In conclusion: synthetic data might help classification because it allows better use of available training data, and because it offers new transformations of the data. This second contribution depends on the difference in complexity of the synthesis model and the classifier. A simpler classifier is more likely to benefit from the additional features that the synthesis model can extract from the data, even though the synthetic data does not contain extra information. In contrast, more complex classifiers can extract more information from the original data and are less likely to benefit from synthetic data. Whether it is better to include the extra complexity in the classifier or in a synthesis model is up for discussion.

Acknowledgements. This research is financed by the Netherlands Organization for Scientific Research (NWO). Brain tumor image data were obtained from the NCI-MICCAI 2013 Challenge on Multimodal Brain Tumor Segmentation (`http://martinos.org/qtim/miccai2013/`).

References

1. Little, R.J.A., Rubin, D.B.: Statistical analysis with missing data, 2nd edn. Wiley, New York (2002)
2. Fischl, B., Salat, D.H., van der Kouwe, A.J.W., Makris, N., Ségonne, F., Quinn, B.T., Dale, A.M.: Sequence-independent segmentation of magnetic resonance images. NeuroImage 23, S69–S84 (2004)
3. Johansson, A., Karlsson, M., Nyholm, T.: CT substitute derived from MRI sequences with ultrashort echo time. Medical Physics 38(5) (2011)
4. Johansson, A., Garpebring, A., Asklund, T., Nyholm, T.: CT substituties derived from MR images reconstructed with parallel imaging. Medical Physics 41 (2014)
5. Eilertsen, K., Vestad, L.N.T.A., Geier, O., Skretting, A.: A simulation of MRI based dose calculations on the basis of radiotherapy planning CT images. Acta Oncologica 47(7), 1294–1302 (2008)
6. Kapanen, M., Tenhunen, M.: T1/T2*-weighted MRI provides clinically relevant pseudo-CT density data for the pelvic bones in MRI-only based radiotherapy treatment planning. Acta Oncologica (Stockholm, Sweden) 52(3), 612–618 (2013)
7. Larsson, A., Johansson, A., Axelsson, J., Nyholm, T., Asklund, T., Riklund, K., Karlsson, M.: Evaluation of an attenuation correction method for PET/MR imaging of the head based on substitute CT images. Magnetic Resonance Materials in Physics, Biology and Medicine 26(1), 127–136 (2013)
8. Hofmann, M., Steinke, F., Scheel, V., Charpiat, G., Farquhar, J., Aschoff, P., Brady, M., Schölkopf, B., Pichler, B.J.: MRI-based attenuation correction for PET/MRI: a novel approach combining pattern recognition and atlas registration. Journal of Nuclear Medicine 49(11), 1875–1883 (2008)
9. Hofmann, M., Pichler, B., Schölkopf, B., Beyer, T.: Towards quantitative PET/MRI: a review of MR-based attenuation correction techniques. European Journal of Nuclear Medicine and Molecular Imaging 36(suppl. 1), March 2009
10. Iglesias, J.E., Konukoglu, E., Zikic, D., Glocker, B., Van Leemput, K., Fischl, B.: Is synthesizing MRI contrast useful for inter-modality analysis? In: Mori, K., Sakuma, I., Sato, Y., Barillot, C., Navab, N. (eds.) MICCAI 2013, Part I. LNCS, vol. 8149, pp. 631–638. Springer, Heidelberg (2013)
11. Roy, S., Carass, A., Prince, J.: A compressed sensing approach for MR tissue contrast synthesis. In: Székely, G., Hahn, H.K. (eds.) IPMI 2011. LNCS, vol. 6801, pp. 371–383. Springer, Heidelberg (2011)
12. Li, R., Zhang, W., Suk, H.-I., Wang, L., Li, J., Shen, D., Ji, S.: Deep learning based imaging data completion for improved brain disease diagnosis. In: Golland, P., Hata, N., Barillot, C., Hornegger, J., Howe, R. (eds.) MICCAI 2014, Part III. LNCS, vol. 8675, pp. 305–312. Springer, Heidelberg (2014)
13. Menze, B.H., Jakab, A., Bauer, S., et al.: The Multimodal Brain Tumor Image Segmentation Benchmark (BRATS). IEEE Transactions on Medical Imaging (2014)
14. Bengio, Y., Courville, A., Vincent, P.: Representation Learning: A Review and New Perspectives. Technical report, Université de Montréal (2012)
15. Hinton, G.E.: A Practical Guide to Training Restricted Boltzmann Machines. Technical report, University of Toronto (2010)
16. Tieleman, T.: Training restricted Boltzmann machines using approximations to the likelihood gradient. In: ICML (2008)
17. Bergstra, J., et al.: Theano: A CPU and GPU Math Compiler in Python. In: Proceedings of the Python for Scientific Computing Conference, SciPy (2010)
18. Pedregosa, F., et al.: Scikit-learn: Machine Learning in Python. Journal of Machine Learning Research 12, 2825–2830 (2011)

Label Stability in Multiple Instance Learning

Veronika Cheplygina[1,3], Lauge Sørensen[2], David M.J. Tax[1], Marleen de Bruijne[2,3], and Marco Loog[1,2]

[1] Pattern Recognition Laboratory, Delft University of Technology, The Netherlands
[2] The Image Section, University of Copenhagen, Copenhagen, Denmark
[3] Biomedical Imaging Group Rotterdam, Erasmus MC, Rotterdam, The Netherlands

Abstract. We address the problem of *instance label stability* in multiple instance learning (MIL) classifiers. These classifiers are trained only on globally annotated images (bags), but often can provide fine-grained annotations for image pixels or patches (instances). This is interesting for computer aided diagnosis (CAD) and other medical image analysis tasks for which only a coarse labeling is provided. Unfortunately, the instance labels may be unstable. This means that a slight change in training data could potentially lead to abnormalities being detected in different parts of the image, which is undesirable from a CAD point of view. Despite MIL gaining popularity in the CAD literature, this issue has not yet been addressed. We investigate the stability of instance labels provided by several MIL classifiers on 5 different datasets, of which 3 are medical image datasets (breast histopathology, diabetic retinopathy and computed tomography lung images). We propose an unsupervised measure to evaluate instance stability, and demonstrate that a performance-stability trade-off can be made when comparing MIL classifiers.

1 Introduction

Obtaining ground-truth annotations for patches, which can be used to train supervised classifiers for localization of abnormalities in medical images can be very costly and time-consuming. This hinders the use of supervised classifiers for this task. Fortunately, global labels for whole images, such as the overall condition of the patient, are available more readily. Multiple instance learning (MIL) is an extension of supervised learning which can train classifiers using such weakly labeled data. For example, a classifier trained on images (*bags*), where each bag is labeled as healthy or abnormal and consists of unlabeled image patches (*instances*), would be able to label patches of a novel image as healthy or abnormal.

MIL is becoming more and more popular in CAD [9,13,6,20,16,3,21,18,12]. In many of these applications, it is desirable to obtain instance labels, and to inspect the instances which are deemed positive. For example, in [13], weakly labeled x-ray images of healthy subjects and patients affected by tuberculosis are used to train a MIL classifier which can provide local abnormality scores, which can be visualized across the lungs. Furthermore, the MIL classifier *outperforms*

N. Navab et al. (Eds.): MICCAI 2015, Part I, LNCS 9349, pp. 539–546, 2015.
DOI: 10.1007/978-3-319-24553-9_66

its supervised counterpart which has access to fine-grained labels, showing the potential of MIL for CAD applications.

A pitfall in using MIL classifiers to obtain instance labels is that these labels might be unstable, for example, if a different subset of the data is used for training. This is clearly undesirable in a diagnostic setting, because abnormalities would be highlighted in different parts of the image. For example, in [12] a MIL classifier is used to identify which of the 8 regions (instances) of the tibial trabecular bone (bag) are most related to cartilage loss. The "most positive" region labeled positive by only 20% of the classifiers, trained on different subsets of the data. We have not been able to identify other research where this phenomenon is investigated, which emphasizes the importance of the present work.

In rare cases where instance-level annotations are available, such as in [9], instance labels can be evaluated using AUC. The results here show that the best bag classifier does not correspond to the best instance classifier, emphasizing that bag-level results are not reliable if instance labels are needed. Another approach is to evaluate the instances qualitatively. However, this is typically done for a single run of the classifier, which raises the question whether the same abnormalities would be found if the training set would change slightly.

We propose to evaluate the *stability* of instance-labeling MIL classifiers as an additional measure for classifier comparison. We evaluate two stability measures on three CAD datasets: computed tomography lung images with chronic obstructive pulmonary disease (COPD), histopathology images with breast cancer and diabetic retinopathy images. We demonstrate how stability varies in popular MIL classifiers, and show that choosing the classifier with the best bag-level performance may not lead to reliable instance labels.

2 Multiple Instance Learning

In multiple instance learning, a sample is a bag or set $B_i = \{\mathbf{x}_k^i | k = 1, ..., n_i\} \subset \mathbb{R}^d$ of n_i instances, each instance is thus a d-dimensional feature vector. We are given labeled training bags $\{(B_i, y_i) | i = 1, ...N_{tr}\}$ where $y_i \in \{0, 1\}$. The standard assumption is that there exist hidden instance labels $z_k^i \in \{0, 1\}$ which relate to the bag labels as follows: a bag is positive if and only if it contains at least one positive instance.

Originally, the goal in MIL is to train a bag classifier f_B to label previously unseen bags. Several MIL classifiers do this by inferring an instance classifier f_I, and combining the outputs of the bag's instances, for example by the noisy-or rule, $f_B(B_i) = \max_k\{f_I(\mathbf{x}_k^i)\}$. An example of such an *instance-level* classifier is SimpleMIL, which propagates the bag label to its instances and simply trains a supervised classifier on the, possibly noisy, instance labels. Classifiers which explicitly use the MIL assumption are miSVM [1] and milBoost [19], which are MIL adaptations of popular learning algorithms. For example, miSVM extends the SVM by not only searching for the optimal hyperplane $\mathbf{w}$ which defines f_I, but also for the instance labels $\{z_i^k\}$ which are consistent with the bag label assumptions:

$$\min_{\{z_i^k\}} \min_{\mathbf{w},\xi} \frac{1}{2}||\mathbf{w}||^2 + C\sum_{i,k}\xi_i^k \qquad \text{s.t.} \tag{1}$$
$$\forall i,k: z_i^k(\langle \mathbf{w}, \mathbf{x}_i^k\rangle) \geq 1-\xi_i^k, \xi_i^k \geq 0, z_i^k \in \{-1,1\}, \max\{z_i^k\} = y_i.$$

Another group, *bag-level* classifiers, typically represent each bag as a single feature vector and use supervised classifiers for training f_B directly [4,5]. Such classifiers are often robust, but usually can not provide instance labels. A notable exception is MILES [4], which represents each bag by its similarities to a set of prototype instances, $\mathbf{s}_i = [s(B_i, \mathbf{x}_1^1), \ldots, s(B_i, \mathbf{x}_{n_1}^1), \ldots s(B_i, \mathbf{x}_{n_{N_{tr}}}^{N_{tr}})]$ where $s(B_i, \mathbf{x}) = \exp(-\min_k ||\mathbf{x} - \mathbf{x}_k^i||)$ or any other kernel. A sparse classifier then selects the most discriminative features, which correspond to instance prototypes. It is assumed that discriminative prototypes from positive bags are positive, instances can therefore be classified based on their similarity to these prototypes.

The interest in **MIL for computer aided diagnosis** has grown over the past decade, as illustrated by Table 1. Supervised evaluation of instances is only performed in a few studies – where (a part) of the data has been annotated at the instance level. Otherwise, papers examine the instances qualitatively, such as displaying the most abnormal instances [13], or not at all, although instance labels would be interesting from a diagnostic point of view [6,9]. As our proposed evaluation is unsupervised, it can easily be adopted in all these studies.

Table 1. Evaluation of MIL in CAD tasks. Columns show bag (B) and instance (I) evaluation: supervised (+), qualitative (∘) or none (–).

Task	B	I	Task	B	I
Cancer histology [9]	+	+	Diabetic retinopathy [9]	+	–
COPD in CT [6]	+	–	Tuberculosis in XR [13]	+	∘
Cancer histopathology [22]	+	+	Osteoarthritis in MRI [12]	+	∘
Diabetic retinopathy [16]	+	+	Pulmonary embolism in CT [11]	+	–
Myocardial infarction in ECG [18]	+	–	COPD in CT [17]	+	–
Colorectal cancer in CT [8]	+	–			

3 Instance Stability

We are interested in evaluating the similarity of a labeling, or vector of outputs of two classifiers $\mathbf{z} = f_I(X)$ and $\mathbf{z}' = f_I'(X)$, trained on slightly different subsets of the training data, for the test set $X = [\mathbf{x}_1^1, \ldots, \mathbf{x}_{n_N}^N]^\intercal$. The stability measure should be **monotonically increasing** with the number of instances the classifiers agree on, have **limits**, and most importantly, be **unsupervised**, i.e. not dependent on the hidden instance labels z_i.

The general concept of stability is important in machine learning, and different aspects of it have been addressed in the literature. Leave-one-out stability [15] measures to what extent a decision boundary changes when a sample is removed from the training data, but is not appropriate because it is supervised. An unsupervised version where bags are left out, and true labels are substituted by classifier outputs, is related to the measures we propose. The kappa statistic is unsupervised, but does not follow the monotonicity property in class imbalance settings which could occur in MIL. Clustering stability [2] compares the outputs of two clustering procedures and is unsupervised. It is appropriate for our goal and is in fact related to the measures proposed in what follows.

Let $n_{00} = |\{i|z_i = 0 \wedge z'_i = 0\}|$, $n_{01} = |\{i|z_i = 0 \wedge z'_i = 1\}|$, $n_{10} = |\{i|z_i = 1 \wedge z'_i = 0\}|$ and $n_{11} = |\{i|z_i = 1 \wedge z'_i = 1\}|$. An intuitive measure that satisfies the properties above is the agreement fraction:

$$S(\mathbf{z}, \mathbf{z}') = (n_{00} + n_{11})/(n_{01} + n_{10} + n_{11} + n_{00}). \tag{2}$$

In a situation with many true negative instances, the value of S would be inflated due to the negative instances that the classifiers agree on. As a result, the classifier can still be unstable with respect to the positive instances. Due to the nature of CAD tasks, we might consider it more important for the classifiers to agree on the positive instances. Therefore we also consider the agreement on positive labels only, or Jaccard distance:

$$S_+(\mathbf{z}, \mathbf{z}') = n_{11}/(n_{01} + n_{10} + n_{11}). \tag{3}$$

We emphasize that the novelty does not lie in the measures themselves, well-known as they are. The novelty resides in what they measure in this context: we derive these measures as the appropriate ones for the stability that we want to quantify.

Classifier Selection. If instance classification stability is a crucial issue, one can study our measure in combination with bag-level AUC (or any other accuracy measure) and select a MIL classifier with a good trade-off of AUC and instance stability. We can see each classifier as a possible solution, parametrized by these two values. Intermediate solutions between classifiers f_I and f'_I can in theory be obtained by designing a randomized classifier, which trains classifier f_I with probability p and classifier f'_I with probability $1-p$. In the AUC-stability plane, the Pareto frontier is the set of classifiers which are Pareto efficient, i.e. no improvement can be made in AUC without decreasing instance stability and vice versa. Optimal classifiers can therefore be selected from this Pareto frontier. While the classifier with the highest AUC is in this set, it is not necessarily the only desirable solution, if the instance labels are of importance.

4 Experiments and Results

Datasets. The datasets are shown in Table 2. The Musk datasets are benchmark problems of molecule activity prediction. In Breast, an instance is a 7×7 patch from a 896×768 tissue microarray analysis image from a patient with a malignant (+) or benign (–) tumor. In Messidor, an instance is a 135×135 patch from a 700×700 fundus image of a diabetes (+) or healthy (–) subject. In COPD, a bag is a CT image of a lung of a subject with COPD (+) or a healthy subject (–). An instance is a region of interest (ROI) of 41 × 41 × 41 voxels, with the center inside the segmentation of the lung field.

Table 2. Datasets and their properties. Musk, Breast and Messidor can be downloaded from a MIL data repository [5] (`http://www.miproblems.org`).

Dataset	Bags	Instances	Inst per bag	Features
Musk 1	47+, 45–	476	2 to 40	166
Musk 2	39+, 63–	6598	1 to 1024	166
Breast [10]	26+, 32–	2002	21 to 40	657 (intensity, LBP, SIFT)
Messidor [9,7]	654+, 546–	12352	8 to 12	687 (intensity, LBP, SIFT)
COPD [17,14]	231+, 231–	26200	50	287 (Gaussian filter bank)

Illustrative Example. Fig. 1 shows the pairwise stability measures for the COPD validation data, for 10 MILES classifiers, each trained on random 80% of the training data. There is considerable disagreement for both measures, which is surprising because of the large overlap of the training sets. The measures are quite correlated ($\rho = 0.76$), but S has higher values because it is inflated by agreement on negative instances.

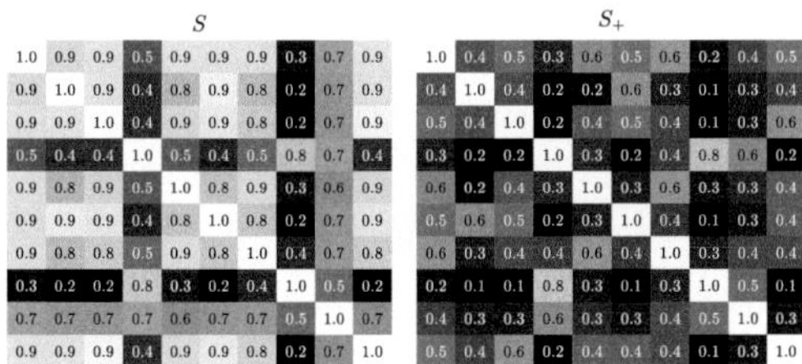

Fig. 1. Pairwise stability for 10 MILES classifiers for agreement (left) and positive agreement (right) for the COPD dataset

Fig. 2 shows how the instance classifications change in a true positive bag, i.e., CT image from a COPD patient. This bag is always classified as positive, but the instance labels are unstable. A perfectly stable classifier would have a bimodal distribution, classifying instances as positive either 0 or 10 times. We also show a number of ROIs with stable and unstable labels. Several ROIs containing emphysema have unstable classifications, and one emphysemous patch is even consistently classified as negative. This shows that while the bag is always classified correctly, the instance labels may not be very reliable.

Evaluation. We evaluate a number of classifiers (please see Sec. 2 for descriptions) from the MIL toolbox[1], which we modified to output instance labels:

- simpleMIL with SVM, nearest mean (NM) and 1-nearest neighbor (1NN)
- miSVM and its variants miNM and mi1NN (based on NM and 1NN)
- MILBoost

[1] `http://prlab.tudelft.nl/david-tax/mil.html`

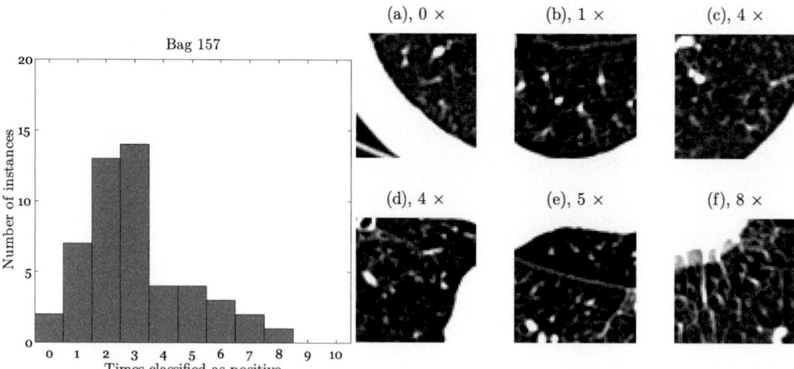

Fig. 2. "Positiveness" of 50 instances (ROIs) from a positive bag. **Left:** How often an ROI is classified positive, and for how many ROIs this holds. **Right**: Examples of 6 ROIs, for which the axial slice with most lung voxels below -910 hounsfield units is shown. ROIs (b,d,e,f) contain emphysema (low intensity areas within the lung tissue), but only (f) is often classified as positive. ROIs (a,c) are largely unaffected, but only (a) is consistently classified as negative.

– MILES

We use a linear kernel and regularization parameter $C = 1$ for SVM, miSVM and MILES. For each train/test split, we do the following 10 times: randomly sample 80% of the training bags (bag = subject), train the classifier, and evaluate on the test dataset. The splits are done randomly for Musk, Breast and Messidor and based on predefined sets for COPD.

The average bag AUCs, average pairwise instance stabilities, and the corresponding Pareto frontiers for $S+$ (S provided similar plots, but with inflated values) are shown in Fig. 3. Note that the (1, 0.5) point can be achieved by a classifier which labels all instances as positive. The main observation is that the most accurate classifier is often not the most stable one. This trade-off is especially well-illustrated in the COPD datasets. Here we see similar behavior between the two sets, which shows that if we were to use the validation set results for classifier selection, we would obtain a classifier with similar performance and stability on the test set.

With regard to the classifiers, miSVM and its variants seem to be relatively good choices. MILES, which is a popular classifier due to its good performance, can indeed be quite accurate, but at the same time unstable. The difference between the mi- classifiers and MILES is probably due to the fact that MILES trains a bag classifier f_B first, and infers f_I from f_B, while the mi- classifiers train f_I directly. MILBoost is both inaccurate and unstable, especially for COPD there is high disagreement on which instances to label as positive.

Note that the goal of these experiments is to demonstrate the trade-off between AUC and stability, not to maximize the AUC. Nevertheless, the best performances achieved by classifiers tested here are [0.91, 0.80, 0.72, 0.72] for

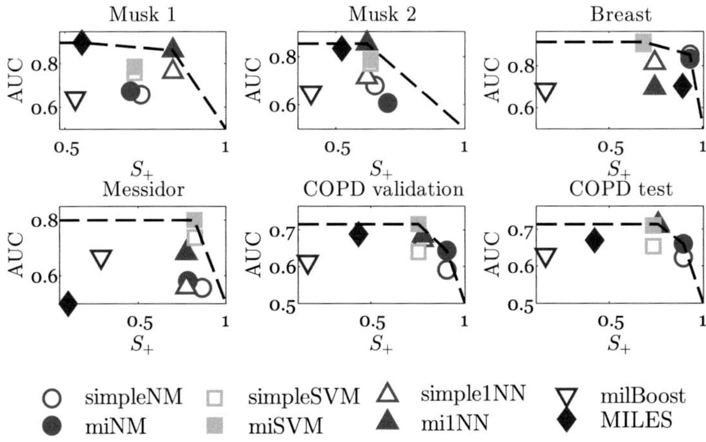

Fig. 3. Bag AUC vs positive instance stability and the corresponding Pareto frontiers

Breast, Messidor, and the COPD datasets. In previous works, the highest[2] performances for the same datasets were [0.90, 0.81, 0.74, 0.74]. This shows that our result are on par with state of the art, despite using less data and optimization.

5 Conclusions

We addressed the issue of stability of instance labels provided by MIL classifiers. We examined two unsupervised measures of agreement: S based on all labels, and S_+ based on positive (abnormal) labels, which might be more interesting from a CAD point of view. Our experiments demonstrate a trade-off between bag performance and instance label stability, and miSVM is a classifier which provides a good trade-off. In general, we propose to use instance label stability as an additional evaluation measure when applying MIL classifiers in CAD.

Acknowledgements. This research is partially financed by The Netherlands Organization for Scientific Research (NWO). We thank Dr. Melih Kandemir for kindly providing the Breast and Messidor datasets.

References

1. Andrews, S., Tsochantaridis, I., Hofmann, T.: Support vector machines for multiple-instance learning. In: NIPS, pp. 561–568 (2002)

[2] Note that [6] reports several higher AUCs for COPD, but these correspond to a larger version of the dataset, which was not used in our study.

2. Ben-Hur, A., Elisseeff, A., Guyon, I.: A stability based method for discovering structure in clustered data. In: Pac. Symp. Biocomput., pp. 6–17 (2001)
3. Bi, J., Liang, J.: Multiple instance learning of pulmonary embolism detection with geodesic distance along vascular structure. In: CVPR, pp. 1–8 (2007)
4. Chen, Y., Bi, J., Wang, J.: MILES: Multiple-instance learning via embedded instance selection. IEEE T. Pattern. Anal. Mach. Intel. 28(12), 1931–1947 (2006)
5. Cheplygina, V., Tax, D.M.J., Loog, M.: Multiple instance learning with bag dissimilarities. Pattern Recognition 48(1), 264–275 (2015)
6. Cheplygina, V., et al.: Classification of COPD with multiple instance learning. In: ICPR, pp. 1508–1513 (2014)
7. Decencière, E., et al.: Feedback on a publicly distributed image database: the Messidor database. Image Anal. Stereol., 231–234 (2014)
8. Dundar, M.M., Fung, G., et al.: Multiple-instance learning algorithms for computer-aided detection. IEEE T. Biomed. Eng. 55(3), 1015–1021 (2008)
9. Kandemir, M., Hamprecht, F.A.: Computer-aided diagnosis from weak supervision: A benchmarking study. Comput. Med. Imag. Grap. (2014) (in press)
10. Kandemir, M., Zhang, C., Hamprecht, F.A.: Empowering multiple instance histopathology cancer diagnosis by cell graphs. In: Golland, P., Hata, N., Barillot, C., Hornegger, J., Howe, R. (eds.) MICCAI 2014, Part II. LNCS, vol. 8674, pp. 228–235. Springer, Heidelberg (2014)
11. Liang, J., Bi, J.: Computer aided detection of pulmonary embolism with tobogganing and mutiple instance classification in CT pulmonary angiography. In: Karssemeijer, N., Lelieveldt, B. (eds.) IPMI 2007. LNCS, vol. 4584, pp. 630–641. Springer, Heidelberg (2007)
12. Marques, J.: Osteoarthritis imaging by quantification of tibial trabecular bone. Ph.D. thesis, Københavns Universitet (2013)
13. Melendez, J., et al.: A novel multiple-instance learning-based approach to computer-aided detection of tuberculosis on chest x-rays. TMI 31(1), 179–192 (2014)
14. Pedersen, J.H., et al.: The Danish randomized lung cancer CT screening trial-overall design and results of the prevalence round. J. Thorac. Oncol. 4(5), 608–614 (2009)
15. Poggio, T., Rifkin, R., Mukherjee, S., Niyogi, P.: General conditions for predictivity in learning theory. Nature 428(6981), 419–422 (2004)
16. Quellec, G., et al.: A multiple-instance learning framework for diabetic retinopathy screening. MedIA 16(6), 1228–1240 (2012)
17. Sørensen, L., Nielsen, M., Lo, P., Ashraf, H., Pedersen, J.H., de Bruijne, M.: Texture-based analysis of COPD: a data-driven approach. TMI 31(1), 70–78 (2012)
18. Sun, L., Lu, Y., Yang, K., Li, S.: ECG analysis using multiple instance learning for myocardial infarction detection. IEEE T. Biomed. Eng. 59(12), 3348–3356 (2012)
19. Viola, P., Platt, J., Zhang, C.: Multiple instance boosting for object detection. In: NIPS, pp. 1417–1424 (2005)
20. Wang, S., et al.: Seeing is believing: Video classification for computed tomographic colonography using multiple-instance learning. TMI 31(5), 1141–1153 (2012)
21. Wu, D., Bi, J., Boyer, K.: A min-max framework of cascaded classifier with multiple instance learning for computer aided diagnosis. In: CVPR, pp. 1359–1366 (2009)
22. Xu, Y., et al.: Weakly supervised histopathology cancer image segmentation and classification. MedIA 18(3), 591–604 (2014)

Spectral Forests: Learning of Surface Data, Application to Cortical Parcellation

Herve Lombaert[1,2], Antonio Criminisi[2], and Nicholas Ayache[1]

[1] INRIA Sophia-Antipolis, Asclepios Team, France
[2] Microsoft Research, Cambridge, UK

Abstract. This paper presents a new method for classifying surface data via spectral representations of shapes. Our approach benefits classification problems that involve data living on surfaces, such as in cortical parcellation. For instance, current methods for labeling cortical points into surface parcels often involve a slow mesh deformation toward pre-labeled atlases, requiring as much as 4 hours with the established FreeSurfer. This may burden neuroscience studies involving region-specific measurements. Learning techniques offer an attractive computational advantage, however, their representation of spatial information, typically defined in a Euclidean domain, may be inadequate for cortical parcellation. Indeed, cortical data resides on surfaces that are highly variable in space and shape. Consequently, Euclidean representations of surface data may be inconsistent across individuals. We propose to fundamentally change the spatial representation of surface data, by exploiting spectral coordinates derived from the Laplacian eigenfunctions of shapes. They have the advantage over Euclidean coordinates, to be geometry aware and to parameterize surfaces explicitly. This change of paradigm, from Euclidean to spectral representations, enables a classifier to be applied *directly* on surface data via spectral coordinates. In this paper, we decide to build upon the successful Random Decision Forests algorithm and improve its spatial representation with spectral features. Our method, Spectral Forests, is shown to significantly improve the accuracy of cortical parcellations over standard Random Decision Forests (74% versus 28% Dice overlaps), and produce accuracy equivalent to FreeSurfer in a fraction of its time (23 seconds versus 3 to 4 hours).

1 Introduction

The cerebral cortex is the center of major brain activities, including vision and perception. Its study remains, however, challenging due to its highly complex geometry, a densely convoluted surface with varying folds and fissures. In such context, efficient algorithms for surface processing and analysis are often sought. In particular, the accurate segmentation of cortical surfaces into major folds, or sulcal areas, is fundamental to many applications involving region-specific measurements. Two strategies exist for cortical parcellation and are either template based [1–7], via iterative deformations of a pre-labeled atlas, or subject based, via costly processing of sulcal data [8–10] or extracted sulcal lines [11–13]. Present methods often suffer from a heavy computational burden. For instance, FreeSurfer [6, 7], a leading software for cortical parcellation, requires 3 to

N. Navab et al. (Eds.): MICCAI 2015, Part I, LNCS 9349, pp. 547–555, 2015.
DOI: 10.1007/978-3-319-24553-9_67

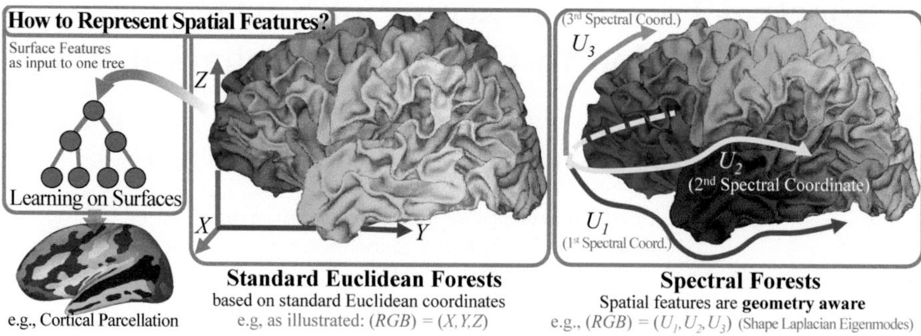

Fig. 1. Algorithm Overview – Whereas Standard Forests (RF) rely on spatial features derived from Euclidean coordinates (x,y,z), Spectral Forests (SF) build geometry-aware features using spectral coordinates ($U_{1..k}$). This change of paradigm from *extrinsic* to *intrinsic* shape representation enables learning to be performed directly on surfaces. Coloring indicates how spatial information is represented over the surface.

4 hours of computation to inflate cortices into spherical models and warp them toward a pre-labeled atlas. Machine learning techniques now carry high expectations due to their promise in classifying various types of data in a fast manner. Unfortunately, their use in cortical analysis [14] has been limited due to the high geometrical variability of the folding pattern across individuals. Classifying cortical data on larger training sets may capture additional shape variability, however, one may wonder how to better exploit existing data, and how to capture maximal information on such complex surfaces. This raises the fundamental question on how to learn data *directly* on surfaces. We propose to use a different paradigm for representing spatial features in learning techniques.

Currently, a cortical point can be represented with pointwise data information, such as its depth on the cortex or its MRI pixel intensity. Feature representations are typically augmented with spatial information to uniquely characterize points in space, for instance, with its location in the Euclidean domain [15]. This, however, poses a problem since cortical surfaces highly vary in space and shape. Moreover, neighborhood structures, often exploited in image segmentation [16], may be ambiguous on surfaces, and more challenging to interpret on highly convoluted cortical surfaces. Neighboring positions in 3D space may in fact not necessarily lie on a surface, and be even several folds away on the cortex. Consequently, standard learning approaches that use features defined in the Euclidean domain, may not be adequate for cortical parcellation. We propose to represent instead spatial information with geometry-aware features. The spectral decomposition of shapes provides means to efficiently parameterize cortical surfaces with few spectral coordinates. More specifically, surface points are uniquely characterized with the eigenfunctions of an associated graph Laplacian. Whereas its eigenvalues capture subject-wise properties, and can be used to identify subjects [17, 18], the eigenfunctions capture pointwise information directly on surfaces, and can be used, for instance, to match points between cortical surfaces [19, 20]. Such named spectral coordinates constitute, in fact, an explicit parameterization of surfaces. A learning technique could thus exploit such spectral coordinates to learn data directly on surfaces. In this paper, we improve, for instance, the Random Decision Forests (RF) [21, 22], to process surface data via spectral representations of shapes, and name our method **Spectral Forests (SF)**. The next section details the fundamentals of Spectral Forests, followed by experiments evaluating the impact of using our spectral strategy over standard Euclidean approaches. We find a substantial improvement in accuracy in terms of Dice metric (from RF: 28%, to SF: 74%) and boundary distance error (RF/SF: 6.88/2.11mm).

2 Method

We begin by briefly reminding the fundamentals of Random Forests, and extend them for classifying data directly on surfaces.

Random Forests (RF) – A standard RF consists of an ensemble of decision trees, each making probabilistic decisions from input data, for instance, classifying cortical points into cortical parcels. During training, trees are grown by finding for each node, the binary test that best splits an input training data such that *information gain* among the class distributions is maximized. Each tree t learns a class predictor $p_t(c|f)$ for a feature representation f, for instance, the sulcal depth and spatial coordinates of a cortical point, $f_i = (\texttt{depth}(i), (x, y, z)_i)$ at point i. During testing, unknown points are classified by passing down their feature representations in n_{tree} trees. The resulting class predictions are eventually averaged and a point is finally classified with the maximal prediction $\hat{c} = \arg\max_c \sum_{i=1}^{n_T} p_{t_i}(c|f)$. More details could be found in [21, 22]. In standard RF, learning shape characteristics and locating their boundaries typically rely on spatial features that are derived from Euclidean coordinates, and neighborhoods are often implemented using random rectangles on a Cartesian grid [16]. Such features are not geometry aware, and rely on *extrinsic* shape information.

Spectral Forests (SF) – We extend RF beyond the Euclidean domain, to classify surface data. To do so, spatial features are represented using spectral coordinates rather than Euclidean coordinates. They uniquely characterize surface points using the Laplacian eigenfunctions of a spectral shape decomposition [23]. These surface basis functions are *geometry aware* and have the property to be invariant to shape isometry. This is, for instance, exploited in cortical surface matching [19, 20], where, conveniently, corresponding points have similar spectral coordinates, even if they may not share the same location in space. Spectral representations effectively capture *intrinsic* shape information. Location and neighborhoods are defined explicitly on surfaces, which contrasts with the implicit representation of surfaces with Euclidean coordinates.

Spectral Coordinates – Let us build the graph $\mathscr{G} = \{\mathscr{V}, \mathscr{E}\}$ from the set of vertices with position x, and edges of a surface model S. We may define the $|V| \times |V|$

weighted adjacency matrix W in terms of node affinities, e.g., $W_{ij} = \parallel x_i - x_j \parallel^{-1}$ if $\exists e_{ij} \in \mathscr{E}$ (inverse distance between neighboring points), 0 otherwise. The diagonal node degree matrix D is the sum of all point affinities $D_i = \sum_j W_{ij}$. The graph Laplacian operator is defined [24] as a $|V| \times |V|$ matrix $\mathcal{L} = D^{-1}(D - W)$. Its spectral decomposition, $\mathcal{L} = U\Lambda U^{-1}$, provides the sorted eigenvalues $\Lambda = \mathrm{diag}(\lambda_0, ...\lambda_{|V|})$ and associated eigenfunctions $U = (u^{(0)}, ..., u^{(|V|)})$, where $u^{(\cdot)}$ is a column of U and depicts in fact a vibration mode of shape S [25]. The spectral coordinates of points $p \in \mathscr{V}$ are defined as the eigenfunction values normalized by their eigenvalues [23], $\texttt{spectral}(p) = \{\lambda_0^{-\frac{1}{2}} u^{(0)}(p), ..., \lambda_{|V|}^{-\frac{1}{2}} u^{(|V|)}(p)\}$, which is a row of matrix $\Lambda^{-\frac{1}{2}}U$. Since these coordinates are defined on surfaces, navigating with them would move us over the surface, whereas an increase in Euclidean coordinates may bring us away from the surface. For additional coherence, we further correct for slight perturbations in shape isometry, often observed as misalignment of spectral representations between subjects [26]. All representations are, therefore, realigned to an arbitrary reference, $\Lambda^{-\frac{1}{2}}UT_{i \mapsto \mathrm{ref}}$, where the transformation T is found, for instance, with Iterative Closest Points (ICP) between spectral representations [26, 27]. In practice [19, 27], only the first $k = 5$ spectral coordinates are sufficient to capture the main geometrical properties. This keeps the computational expenses low, in the order of 2 seconds for a spectral decomposition and 1.5 seconds for an ICP refinement on a standard laptop computer. The spectral coordinates $\texttt{spectral}(p)$ for a point p of subject i, are therefore the first k elements of the pth row of matrix $\Lambda^{-\frac{1}{2}}UT_{i \mapsto \mathrm{ref}}$.

Cortical Parcellation – The labeling of cortical points into major sulci and gyri, is an application where learning should be performed on surfaces. Our Spectral Forests algorithm represents spatial information with spectral coordinates, which naturally parameterize surfaces in an *intrinsic* spectral domain rather than in an *extrinsic* Euclidean space, as shown in Fig. 1. The simplest form of feature representation could be, for instance, $f_p = (\texttt{depth}(p), \texttt{spectral}(p))$, which includes data information, such as the sulcal depth at each point, and spatial information, where standard (x, y, z) point values are replaced with k spectral coordinates. This change of paradigm enables a standard RF classifier to be applied on the spectral representation f_p for learning and infering the major parcels over the brain surface.

3 Results

We now evaluate the performance of Spectral Forests (SF), with respect to standard Forests (RF) and FreeSurfer (FS), a leading software in cortical parcellation. Our dataset consists of 16 surfaces of white-grey matter interfaces generated from MRI, ranging from 109k to 174k vertices, each labeled into 77 cortical parcels obtained from a manual segmentation.

3.1 Euclidean versus Spectral Coordinates

The calcarine sulcus is of interest to studies in vision, however, its localization on the cortex remains difficult as it is deeply buried in a highly convoluted area of

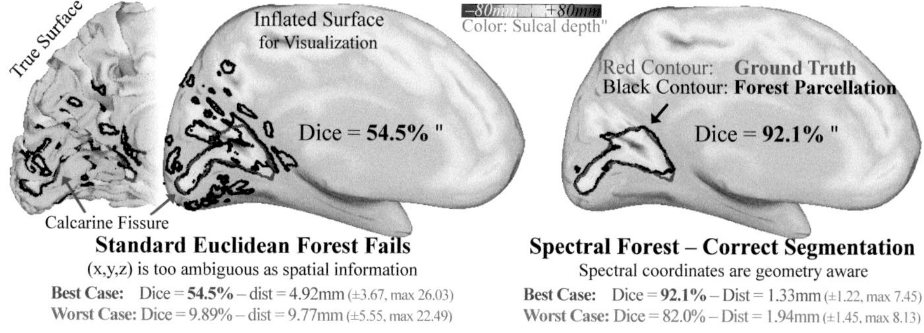

Fig. 2. Segmentation of the Calcarine Fissure – which is deeply buried in a highly convoluted area. (*Left*) Learning surface data with forests on standard Euclidean features produces low Dice scores, and a segmentation that is spatially inconsistent. (*Right*) Spectral Forests directly learn surface data via spatial features that are geometry aware. Surfaces are inflated only for visualization.

the visual cortex. Current methods, such as FS, typically involve a costly mesh deformation toward a labeled atlas. Learning approaches could be an alternative, however, their use of spatial features derived from spatial coordinates may pose problems in representing location and neighborhoods. One could augment the representation of cortical points with extra information such as their sulcal depth on the cortex. This is the strategy adopted by FS.

Standard RF – To illustrate the benefits of using spectral coordinates over Euclidean coordinates, we choose to segment the calcarine sulcus in a binary classification, i.e., calcarine or not-calcarine. We first use standard RF with a simple feature representation, $f_i = (\texttt{depth}(i), (x, y, z)_i)$, with the sulcal depth of a point i and its location in an Euclidean space. We use 50 trees, with 50k data points represented with the feature set f, and keep our parameters constant in all further experiments. We perform a leave-one-out evaluation, where 15 surfaces are used for each training, and test on the remaining surface. The average Dice overlap $(2|A \cap B|/(|A| + |B|))$ for all 16 calcarine segmentations is **36.1%** ($\pm$ 10.5, min/max = 11.3/51.3). The average distance error between boundaries is on average **7.39mm** ($\pm$ 1.92, max (Hausdorff) 53.0). As seen on Fig. 2, the best case shows, in fact, mitigated results with an overlap of 51.3%, and boundary errors of 5.63mm ($\pm$ 3.85, max 26.8). The consistent location of the predicted sulcus in deeper areas suggests that sulcal depth is a prominent feature during learning, however, spatial coherency of the resulting segmentation appears to be ambiguous. Despite a correct coarse positioning of the calcarine sulcus in the vision cortex, its precise location and delineation is imprecise. Euclidean features may not be adequate for learning on such convoluted surface. Indeed, two neighboring points in space, may not necessarily be close in term of geodesic distance on the surface, and may, in fact, even be several sulci apart.

Spectral Forests – We now only modify the spatial features in order to fully appreciate the impact of this fundamental change in Spectral Forests. We use

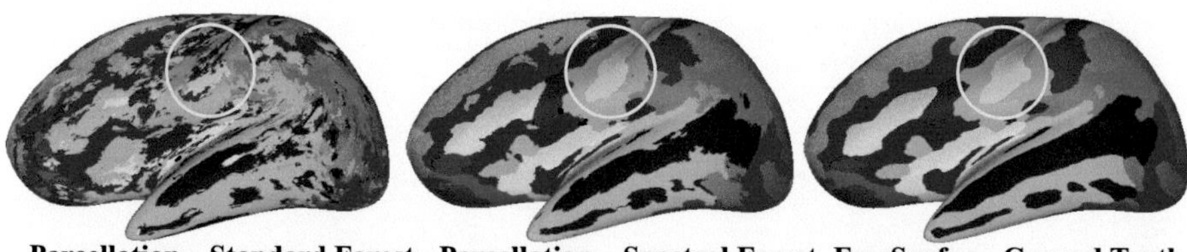
Parcellation – Standard Forest
Inconsistent Spatial Representation in Euclidean Space
Avg. Dice = 31.0% (±15.5) (One case, 77 parcels)
Avg. Boundary Dist. = 5.80mm (±4.24, max 38.02)
Parcellation – Spectral Forest
Learning directly on a Surface Space
Avg. Dice = 77.6% (±11.41)
Avg. Dist = 2.02mm (±1.67, max 17.56)
FreeSurfer – Ground Truth
Variability of 16 parcellations (FreeSurfer)
Dataset Avg. Dice = 76.1% (±8.02)
Dataset Avg. Dist = 1.91mm (±1.57, max 13.01)

Fig. 3. Cortical Parcellation – (*Left*) Best cortical parcellation using RF (31.0%), which reveals the limitation of using spatial features based on Euclidean coordinates, (*Middle*) Parcellation on same subject using SF (77.6%, our method), which shows an improved learning on cortical surfaces, (*Right*) using FS, considered here as gold standard. Inflated surfaces show 77 color-coded parcels. Central sulcus circled for visualization.

$f_i = (\mathtt{depth}(i), \mathtt{spectral}(i))$, with sulcal depth and $k = 5$ spectral coordinates. With this simple change, surface data is now represented using geometry-aware features. The average overlap of the 16 calcarine segmentations is now improved to **89.4%** (± 3.9%, min/max = 81.0/92.1), and the average boundary distance error is decreased to **1.56mm** (± 0.39, max (Hausdorff) 11.25). This is a 147% improvement in overlap, and 78% decrease in boundary error. A closer look on Fig. 2 shows indeed that this simple change of paradigm from Euclidean to spectral features produces a spatially coherent segmentation over the cortical surface. The computation time for RF and SF in this binary segmentation is 2.7 seconds for training, and 1.1 seconds for testing. Timing is measured on a 2.6GHz Core i7 with 16GB of RAM.

3.2 Full Cortical Parcellation

We now segment all 77 cortical parcels, and validate using the same leave-one-out approach with the same parameter set. **Running standard RF** produces an average overlap, for all 77 parcels on 16 surfaces, of **27.9%** (± 17.0, min/max parcels = 4.9/65.9), and an average boundary error of **6.88mm** (± 2.30, max (Hausdorff) 60.8). The required computation time is 21 seconds for training and 66 seconds for testing. **Running Spectral Forests (SF)** produces an average overlap of **74.3%** (± 8.32, min/max parcels = 38.9/94.9), and a boundary error of **2.21mm** (± 0.55, max (Hausdorff) 28.9). The computation time is 17 seconds for training and 23 seconds for testing. Fig. 3 shows the best scoring parcellation of RF, with an average overlap of 31.0% (± 15.5), which contrasts with the SF parcellation on the same subject of 77.6% (± 11.41). One can observe the improvement in spatial consistency of the surface segmentation between RF and SF, where, for instance, the central sulcus (circled in yellow) is barely distinguishable using RF. **In comparison, FreeSurfer (FS)**, which is considered here as a gold standard, performs with an average overlap of **74.4%** (± 9.7, min/max parcels = 41.2/96.6) among all possible transfers of parcellation

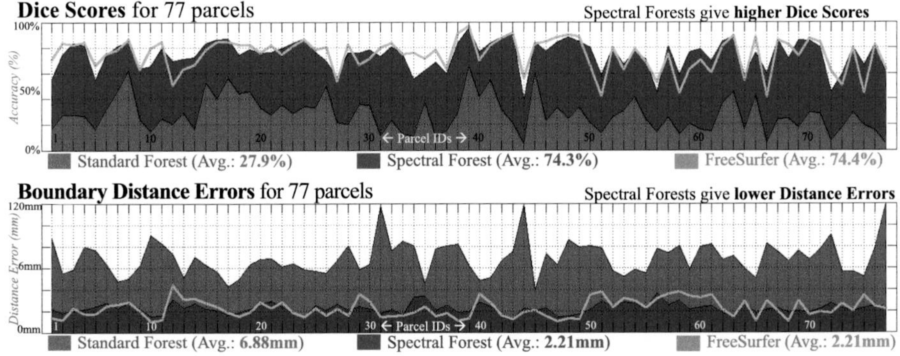

Fig. 4. Evaluation per parcel – (*Top*) Dice Metric and (*Bottom*) Boundary Distance Error for all 77 cortical parcels, using RF (*Red*), SF (*Blue*, our method), and FS (*Green* curve, given for comparison). SF provide consistently higher Dice scores than RF (74.3% vs. 27.9%), and has an equivalent accuracy than FS, but only at a fraction of its cost (23 seconds vs. 3 to 4 hours for FS).

maps from all subjects onto all possible reference subjects. The average boundary distance error between all possible transfers of cortical maps is **2.21mm** (± 0.75, max (Hausdorff) 37.5). This evaluates the variability of FS in mapping cortical parcellations. The performances of SF (74.3%, 2.21mm) and FS (74.4%, 2.21mm) are arguably similar, however SF have a clear **speed advantage** over FreeSurfer. Full cortical parcellation in SF takes on average **23 seconds** at test time, whereas FS requires 3 to 4 hours of computation due to its slow mesh inflation process. We also observed that trees have roughly 9k nodes with SF, and 23k nodes with RF. This may explain the computational advantage of SF over RF (17+23secs over 21+66secs, for training+testing time), and perhaps indicate that information may be better structured with spectral features, producing less tree nodes than with Euclidean features. Fig. 4 summarizes the overlap and boundary errors for all 77 parcels in our leave-one-out validation. It is interesting to observe that with the unique change of spatial features, from Euclidean to spectral coordinates, the average parcel overlap is consistently higher in SF than RF (74.3% vs. 27.9%). Similarly, the boundary error is consistently lower in SF than RF (2.21mm vs. 6.88mm). In addition, SF shows equivalent performance than the state-of-the-art (FreeSurfer in green) but at a significant fraction of its costs (23 seconds for SF vs. 3 to 4 hours for FS).

4 Conclusion

In this paper, we tackled the difficult problem of learning data on complex surfaces, such as the cerebral cortex. Whereas conventional approaches would represent spatial information with extrinsic, or implicit, representations, we proposed to use geometry-aware features that are based on the spectral decomposition of shapes. This change of paradigm from *extrinsic* to *intrinsic* shape representations, or from *implicit* to *explicit* surface parameterization, enables learning techniques to process data directly on surfaces. We implemented this new strategy using the Random Decision Forests model, and named our method Spectral Forests. We illustrated its impact with an application to cortical parcellation, which involves complex surfaces with highly varying folding patterns across individuals. We found that revisiting the fundamentals of spatial representations, from Euclidean to spectral-based features, improves the parcellation accuracy from 27.9% to 74.3%, which is comparable to the present state-of-the-art, but with a clear speed advantage (23 seconds vs. hours). Our experiments showed that simple spatial representations with pure spectral coordinates, on a relatively small dataset, can already track the accuracy of FreeSurfer. We may possibly expect further improvements with more advanced spectral features, for instance, by exploiting neighborhoods on surfaces. Nonetheless, our approach highlights the pertinence of using geometry-aware features in learning techniques. The use of Spectral Forests may also be relevant beyond the analysis of cortices, for instance, in studying surfaces of other organs, or more generally, in applications where data lives on surfaces.

Acknowledgment. This research is partially funded by the ERC Advanced Grant MedYMA and the Research Council of Canada (NSERC).

References

1. Behnke, K.J., Rettmann, M.E., Pham, D.L., Shen, D., Resnick, S.M., Davatzikos, C., Prince, J.L.: Automatic classification of sulcal regions of the human brain cortex using pattern recognition. TMI (2003)
2. Li, G., Shen, D.: Consistent sulcal parcellation of longitudinal cortical surfaces. NeuroImage (2011)
3. Le Goualher, G., Procyk, E., Collins, D.L., Venugopal, R., Barillot, C., Evans, A.C.: Automated extraction and variability analysis of sulcal neuroanatomy. TMI (1999)
4. Lohmann, G., von Cramon, D.Y.: Automatic labelling of the human cortical surface using sulcal basins. Med. Image. Anal. (2000)
5. Rivière, D., Mangin, J.F., Papadopoulos-Orfanos, D., Martinez, J.M., Frouin, V., Régis, J.: Automatic recognition of cortical sulci of the human brain using a congregation of neural networks. Med. Image. Anal. (2002)
6. Fischl, B., Sereno, M.I., Tootell, R.B., Dale, A.M.: High-resolution intersubject averaging and a coordinate system for cortical surface. HBM (1999)
7. Fischl, B., van der Kouwe, A., Destrieux, C., Halgren, E., Segonne, F., Salat, D.H., Busa, E., Seidman, L.J., Goldstein, J., Kennedy, D., Caviness, V., Makris, N., Rosen, B., Dale, A.M.: Automatically parcellating the human cerebral cortex. Cereb. Cortex (2004)
8. Rettmann, M.E., Han, X., Xu, C., Prince, J.L.: Automated sulcal segmentation using watersheds on the cortical surface. NeuroImage (2002)
9. Yang, F., Kruggel, F.: Automatic segmentation of human brain sulci. Med. Image. Anal. (2008)
10. Li, G., Guo, L., Nie, J., Liu, T.: Automatic cortical sulcal parcellation based on surface principal direction flow field tracking. NeuroImage (2009)
11. Shi, Y., Tu, Z., Reiss, A.L., Dutton, R.A., Lee, A.D., Galaburda, A.M., Dinov, I., Thompson, P.M., Toga, A.W.: Joint sulcal detection on cortical surfaces with graphical models and boosted priors. TMI, 361–73 (2009)

12. Shattuck, D.W., Joshi, A.A., Pantazis, D., Kan, E., Dutton, R.A., Sowell, E.R., Thompson, P.M., Toga, A.W., Leahy, R.M.: Semi-automated method for delineation of landmarks on models of the cerebral cortex. Neuroscience (2009)
13. Cachia, A., Mangin, J.F., Rivière, D., Papadopoulos-Orfanos, D., Kherif, F., Bloch, I., Régis, J.: A generic framework for the parcellation of the cortical surface into gyri using geodesic Voronoï diagrams. Med. Image Anal. (2003)
14. Tu, Z., Zheng, S., Yuille, A.L., Reiss, A.L., Dutton, R.A., Lee, A.D., Galaburda, A.M., Dinov, I., Thompson, P.M., Toga, A.W.: Automated extraction of the cortical sulci based on a supervised learning approach. TMI (2007)
15. Stough, J.V., Ye, C., Ying, S.H., Prince, J.L.: Thalamic Parcellation from Multimodal Data using Random Forests. ISBI (2013)
16. Lempitsky, V., Verhoek, M., Noble, J.A., Blake, A.: Random forest classification for automatic delineation of myocardium in real-time 3D echocardiography. In: Ayache, N., Delingette, H., Sermesant, M. (eds.) FIMH 2009. LNCS, vol. 5528, pp. 447–456. Springer, Heidelberg (2009)
17. Konukoglu, E., Glocker, B., Criminisi, A., Pohl, K.: WESD - Weighted Spectral Distance for Measuring Shape Dissimilarity. PAMI (2012)
18. Wachinger, C., Golland, P., Kremen, W., Fischl, B., Reuter, M.: BrainPrint: A Discriminative Characterization of Brain Morphology. NeuroImage (2015)
19. Lombaert, H., Grady, L., Polimeni, J., Cheriet, F.: FOCUSR: Feature Oriented Correspondence using Spectral Regularization - A Method for Accurate Surface Matching. PAMI (2012)
20. Shi, Y., Lai, R., Wang, D.J.J., Pelletier, D., Mohr, D., Sicotte, N., Toga, A.W.: Metric optimization for surface analysis in the Laplace-Beltrami embedding space. TMI (2014)
21. Breiman, L.: Random forests. Mach. Learn. 45 (2001)
22. Criminisi, A., Shotton, J.: Decision Forests for Computer Vision and Medical Image Analysis. Springer (2013)
23. Rustamov, R.M.: Laplace-Beltrami eigenfunctions for deformation invariant shape representation. In: Eurographics (2007)
24. Grady, L., Polimeni, J.R.: Discrete Calculus. Springer (2010)
25. Chung, F.: Spectral Graph Theory. AMS (1996)
26. Mateus, D., Horaud, R., Knossow, D., Cuzzolin, F., Boyer, E.: Articulated shape matching using Laplacian eigenfunctions and unsupervised point registration. In: CVPR (2008)
27. Lombaert, H., Arcaro, M., Ayache, N.: Brain transfer: Spectral analysis of cortical surfaces and functional maps. In: Ourselin, S., Alexander, D.C., Westin, C.-F., Cardoso, M.J. (eds.) IPMI 2015. LNCS, vol. 9123, pp. 474–487. Springer, Heidelberg (2015)

DeepOrgan: Multi-level Deep Convolutional Networks for Automated Pancreas Segmentation

Holger R. Roth, Le Lu, Amal Farag, Hoo-Chang Shin, Jiamin Liu, Evrim B. Turkbey, and Ronald M. Summers

Imaging Biomarkers and Computer-Aided Diagnosis Laboratory, Radiology and Imaging Sciences, National Institutes of Health Clinical Center, Bethesda, MD 20892-1182, USA

Abstract. Automatic organ segmentation is an important yet challenging problem for medical image analysis. The pancreas is an abdominal organ with very high anatomical variability. This inhibits previous segmentation methods from achieving high accuracies, especially compared to other organs such as the liver, heart or kidneys. In this paper, we present a probabilistic bottom-up approach for pancreas segmentation in abdominal computed tomography (CT) scans, using multi-level deep convolutional networks (ConvNets). We propose and evaluate several variations of deep ConvNets in the context of hierarchical, coarse-to-fine classification on image patches and regions, i.e. superpixels. We first present a dense labeling of local image patches via P-ConvNet and nearest neighbor fusion. Then we describe a regional ConvNet (R_1-ConvNet) that samples a set of bounding boxes around each image superpixel at different scales of contexts in a "zoom-out" fashion. Our ConvNets learn to assign class probabilities for each superpixel region of being pancreas. Last, we study a stacked R_2-ConvNet leveraging the joint space of CT intensities and the $P-$ConvNet dense probability maps. Both 3D Gaussian smoothing and 2D conditional random fields are exploited as structured predictions for post-processing. We evaluate on CT images of 82 patients in 4-fold cross-validation. We achieve a Dice Similarity Coefficient of 83.6±6.3% in training and 71.8±10.7% in testing.

1 Introduction

Segmentation of the pancreas can be a prerequisite for computer aided diagnosis (CADx) systems that provide quantitative organ volume analysis, e.g. for diabetic patients. Accurate segmentation could also necessary for computer aided detection (CADe) methods to detect pancreatic cancer. Automatic segmentation of numerous organs in computed tomography (CT) scans is well studied with good performance for organs such as liver, heart or kidneys, where Dice Similarity Coefficients (DSC) of >90% are typically achieved [1,2,3,4]. However, achieving high accuracies in automatic pancreas segmentation is still a challenging task. The pancreas' shape, size and location in the abdomen can vary drastically between patients. Visceral fat around the pancreas can cause large variations in contrast along its boundaries in CT (see Fig. 3). Previous methods

N. Navab et al. (Eds.): MICCAI 2015, Part I, LNCS 9349, pp. 556–564, 2015.
DOI: 10.1007/978-3-319-24553-9_68

report only 46.6% to 69.1% DSCs [1,2,3,5]. Recently, the availability of large annotated datasets and the accessibility of affordable parallel computing resources via GPUs have made it feasible to train deep convolutional networks (ConvNets) for image classification. Great advances in natural image classification have been achieved [6]. However, deep ConvNets for semantic image segmentation have not been well studied [7]. Studies that applied ConvNets to medical imaging applications also show good promise on detection tasks [8,9]. In this paper, we extend and exploit ConvNets for a challenging organ segmentation problem.

2 Methods

We present a coarse-to-fine classification scheme with progressive pruning for pancreas segmentation. Compared with previous top-down multi-atlas registration and label fusion methods, our models approach the problem in a bottom-up fashion: from dense labeling of image patches, to regions, and the entire organ. Given an input abdomen CT, an initial set of superpixel regions is generated by a coarse cascade process of random forests based pancreas segmentation as proposed by [5]. These pre-segmented superpixels serve as regional candidates with high sensitivity (>97%) but low precision. The resulting initial DSC is ~27% on average. Next, we propose and evaluate several variations of ConvNets for segmentation refinement (or pruning). A dense local image patch labeling using an axial-coronal-sagittal viewed patch ($P-$ConvNet) is employed in a sliding window manner. This generates a per-location probability response map P. A regional ConvNet (R_1-ConvNet) samples a set of bounding boxes covering each image superpixel at multiple spatial scales in a "zoom-out" fashion [7,10] and assigns probabilities of being pancreatic tissue. This means that we not only look at the close-up view of superpixels, but gradually add more contexts to each candidate region. R_1-ConvNet operates directly on the CT intensity. Finally, a stacked regional R_2-ConvNet is learned to leverage the joint convolutional features of CT intensities and probability maps P. Both 3D Gaussian smoothing and 2D conditional random fields for structured prediction are exploited as post-processing. Our methods are evaluated on CT scans of 82 patients in 4-fold cross-validation (rather than "leave-one-out" evaluation [1,2,3]). We propose several new ConvNet models and advance the current state-of-the-art performance to a DSC of 71.8 in testing. To the best of our knowledge, this is the highest DSC reported in the literature to date.

2.1 Candidate Region Generation

We describe a coarse-to-fine pancreas segmentation method employing multi-level deep ConvNet models. Our hierarchical segmentation method decomposes any input CT into a set of local image superpixels $S = \{S_1, \ldots, S_N\}$. After evaluation of several image region generation methods [11], we chose *entropy rate* [12] to extract N superpixels on axial slices. This process is based on the criterion of DSCs given optimal superpixel labels, in part inspired by the PASCAL semantic segmentation challenge [13]. The optimal superpixel labels achieve a DSC upper-bound and are used for supervised learning below. Next, we use a two-level cascade of random forest (RF) classifiers as in [5]. We only operate the RF labeling at a low class-probability cut >0.5 which is sufficient to reject the vast amount of non-pancreas superpixels. This retains a set of superpixels $\{S_{\mathrm{RF}}\}$ with high recall (>97%) but low precision. After initial candidate generation, over-segmentation is expected and observed with low DSCs of ~27%. The optimal superpixel labeling is limited by the ability of superpixels to capture the true pancreas boundaries at the per-pixel level with $DSC_{\max} = 80.5\%$, but is still much above previous state-of-the-art [1,2,3,5]. These superpixel labels are used for assessing 'positive' and 'negative' superpixel examples for training. Assigning image regions drastically reduces the amount of ConvNet observations needed per CT volume compared to a purely patch-based approach and leads to more balanced training data sets. Our multi-level deep ConvNets will effectively prune the coarse pancreas over-segmentation to increase the final DSC measurements.

2.2 Convolutional Neural Network (ConvNet) Setup

We use ConvNets with an architecture for binary image classification. Five layers of *convolutional* filters compute and aggregate image features. Other layers of the ConvNets perform *max-pooling* operations or consist of fully-connected neural networks. Our ConvNet ends with a final two-way layer with *softmax* probability for 'pancreas' and 'non-pancreas' classification (see Fig. 1). The *fully-connected* layers are constrained using "DropOut" in order to avoid over-fitting by acting as a regularizer in training [14]. GPU acceleration allows efficient training (we use *cuda-convnet2*[1]).

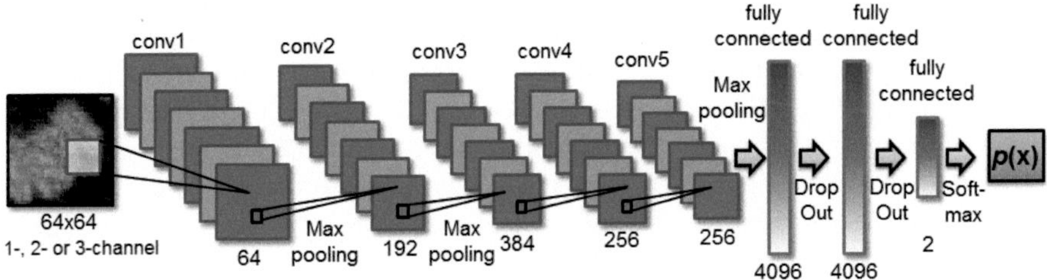

Fig. 1. The proposed ConvNet architecture. The number of convolutional filters and neural network connections for each layer are as shown. This architecture is constant for all ConvNet variations presented in this paper (apart from the number of input channels): P–ConvNet, R_1–ConvNet, and R_2–ConvNet.

[1] https://code.google.com/p/cuda-convnet2

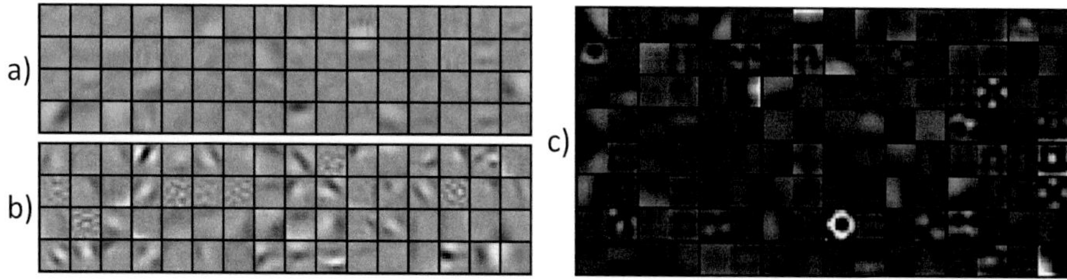

Fig. 2. The first layer of learned convolutional kernels using three representations: a) 2.5D sliding-window patches ($P-$ConvNet), b) CT intensity superpixel regions (R_1-ConvNet), and c) CT intensity + P_0 map over superpixel regions (R_2-ConvNet).

2.3 $P-$ConvNet: Deep Patch Classification

We use a sliding window approach that extracts 2.5D image patches composed of axial, coronal and sagittal planes within all voxels of the initial set of superpixel regions $\{S_{\mathrm{RF}}\}$ (see Fig. 3). The resulting ConvNet probabilities are denoted as P_0 hereafter. For efficiency reasons, we extract patches every n voxels and then apply nearest neighbor interpolation. This seems sufficient due to the already high quality of P_0 and the use of overlapping patches to estimate the values at skipped voxels.

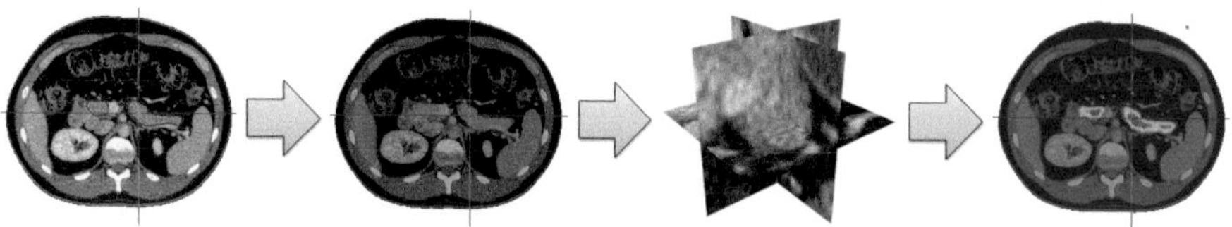

Fig. 3. Axial CT slice of a manual (gold standard) segmentation of the pancreas. From *left* to *right*, there are the ground-truth segmentation contours (in red), RF based coarse segmentation $\{S_{\mathrm{RF}}\}$, and the deep patch labeling result using $P-$ConvNet.

2.4 $R-$ConvNet: Deep Region Classification

We employ the region candidates as inputs. Each superpixel $\in \{S_{\mathrm{RF}}\}$ will be observed at several scales N_s with an increasing amount of surrounding contexts (see Fig. 4). Multi-scale contexts are important to disambiguate the complex anatomy in the abdomen. We explore two approaches: R_1-ConvNet only looks at the CT intensity images extracted from multi-scale superpixel regions, and a stacked R_2-ConvNet integrates an additional channel of patch-level response maps P_0 for each region as input. As a superpixel can have irregular shapes, we warp each region into a regular square (similar to RCNN [10]) as is required by most ConvNet implementations to date. The ConvNets automatically train their convolutional filter kernels from the available training data. Examples of trained

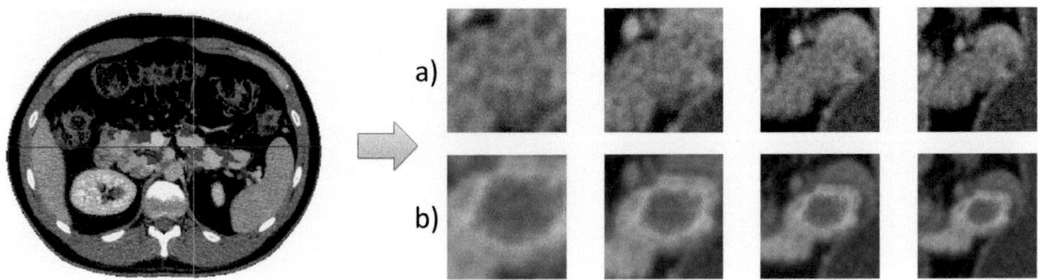

Fig. 4. Region classification using $R-$ConvNet at different scales: a) one-channel input based on the intensity image only, and b) two-channel input with additional patch-based $P-$ConvNet response.

first-layer convolutional filters for $P-$ConvNet, R_1-ConvNet, R_2-ConvNet are shown in Fig. 2. Deep ConvNets behave as effective image feature extractors that summarize multi-scale image regions for classification.

2.5 Data Augmentation

Our ConvNet models (R_1-ConvNet, R_2-ConvNet) sample the bounding boxes of each superpixel $\in \{S_{\text{RF}}\}$ at different scales s. During training, we randomly apply non-rigid deformations t to generate more data instances. The degree of deformation is chosen so that the resulting warped images resemble plausible physical variations of the medical images. This approach is commonly referred to as data augmentation and can help avoid over-fitting [6,8]. Each non-rigid training deformation t is computed by fitting a thin-plate-spline (TPS) to a regular grid of 2D control points $\{\omega_i; i = 1, 2, \dots, k\}$. These control points are randomly transformed within the sampling window and a deformed image is generated using a radial basic function $\phi(r)$, where $t(x) = \sum_{i=1}^{k} c_i \phi\left(\|x - \omega_i\|\right)$ is the transformed location of x and $\{c_i\}$ is a set of mapping coefficients.

2.6 Cross-Scale and 3D Probability Aggregation

At testing, we evaluate each superpixel at N_s different scales. The probability scores for each superpixel being pancreas are averaged across scales: $p(x) = \frac{1}{N_s}\sum_{i=1}^{N_s} p_i(x)$. Then the resulting per-superpixel ConvNet classification values $\{p_1(x)\}$ and $\{p_2(x)\}$ (according to R_1-ConvNet and R_2-ConvNet, respectively), are directly assigned to every pixel or voxel residing within any superpixel $\in \{S_{\text{RF}}\}$. This process forms two per-voxel probability maps $P_1(x)$ and $P_2(x)$. Subsequently, we perform 3D Gaussian filtering in order to average and smooth the ConvNet probability scores across CT slices and within-slice neighboring regions. 3D isotropic Gaussian filtering can be applied to any $P_k(x)$ with $k = 0, 1, 2$ to form smoothed $G(P_k(x))$. This is a simple way to propagate the 2D slice-based probabilities to 3D by taking local 3D neighborhoods into account. In this paper, we do not work on 3D supervoxels due to computational efficiency[2]

[2] Supervoxel based regional ConvNets need at least one-order-of-magnitude wider input layers and thus have significantly more parameters to train.

and generality issues. We also explore conditional random fields (CRF) using an additional ConvNet trained between pairs of neighboring superpixels in order to detect the pancreas edge (defined by pairs of superpixels having the same or different object labels). This acts as the *boundary term* together with the *regional term* given by R_2−ConvNet in order to perform a min-cut/max-flow segmentation [15]. Here, the CRF is implemented as a 2D graph with connections between directly neighboring superpixels. The CRF weighting coefficient between the boundary and the unary regional term is calibrated by grid-search.

3 Results and Discussion

Data: Manual tracings of the pancreas for 82 contrast-enhanced abdominal CT volumes were provided by an experienced radiologist. Our experiments are conducted using 4-fold cross-validation in a random hard-split of 82 patients for training and testing folds with 21, 21, 20, and 20 patients for each testing fold. We report both training and testing segmentation accuracy results. Most previous work [1,2,3] uses leave-one-patient-out cross-validation protocols which are computationally expensive (e.g., $\sim$ 15 hours to process one case using a powerful workstation [1]) and may not scale up efficiently towards larger patient populations. More patients (i.e. 20) per testing fold make the results more representative for larger population groups.

Evaluation: The ground truth superpixel labels are derived as described in Sec. 2.1. The optimally achievable DSC for superpixel classification (if classified perfectly) is 80.5%. Furthermore, the training data is artificially increased by a factor $N_s \times N_t$ using the data augmentation approach with both scale and random TPS deformations at the R−ConvNet level (Sec. 2.5). Here, we train on augmented data using $N_s = 4$, $N_t = 8$. In testing we use $N_s = 4$ (without deformation based data augmentation) and $\sigma = 3$ voxels (as 3D Gaussian filtering kernel width) to compute smoothed probability maps $G(P(x))$. By tuning our implementation of [5] at a low operating point, the initial superpixel candidate labeling achieves the average DSCs of only 26.1% in testing; but has a 97% sensitivity covering all pancreas voxels. Fig. 5 shows the plots of average DSCs using the proposed ConvNet approaches, as a function of $P_k(x)$ and $G(P_k(x))$ in both training and testing for one fold of cross-validation. Simple Gaussian 3D smoothing (Sec. 2.6) markedly improved the average DSCs in all cases. Maximum average DSCs can be observed at $p_0 = 0.2$, $p_1 = 0.5$, and $p_2 = 0.6$ in our training evaluation after 3D Gaussian smoothing for this fold. These calibrated operation points are then fixed and used in testing cross-validation to obtain the results in Table 1. Utilizing R_2−ConvNet (stacked on P−ConvNet) and Gaussian smoothing ($G(P_2(x))$), we achieve a final average DSC of 71.8% in testing, an improvement of 45.7% compared to the candidate region generation stage at 26.1%. $G(P_0(x))$ also performs well wiht 69.5% mean DSC and is more efficient since only dense deep patch labeling is needed. Even though the absolute difference in DSC between $G(P_0(x))$ and $G(P_2(x))$ is small, the surface-to-surface distance improves significantly from 1.46±1.5mm to 0.94±0.6mm, (p<0.01). An example of pancreas segmentation at this operation point is shown in Fig. 6. Training of a typical R–ConvNet with $N \times N_s \times N_t = \sim 850k$ superpixel examples of size 64 × 64 pixels (after warping) takes ~55 hours for 100 epochs on a modern GPU (Nvidia GTX Titan-Z). However, execution run-time in testing is in the order of only 1 to 3 minutes per CT volume, depending on the number of scales N_s. Candidate region generation in Sec. 2.1 consumes another 5 minutes per case.

To the best of our knowledge, this work reports the highest average DSC with 71.8% in testing. Note that a direct comparison to previous methods is not possible due to lack of publicly available benchmark datasets. We will share our data and code implementation for future comparisons[3,4]. Previous state-of-the-art results are at ~68% to ~69% [1,2,3,5]. In particular, DSC drops from 68% (150 patients) to 58% (50 patients) under the leave-one-out protocol [3]. Our results are based on a 4-fold cross-validation. The performance degrades gracefully from training (83.6±6.3%) to testing (71.8±10.7%) which demonstrates the good generality of learned deep ConvNets on unseen data. This difference is expected to diminish with more annotated datasets. Our methods also perform with better stability (i.e., comparing 10.7% versus 18.6% [1], 15.3% [2] in the standard deviation of DSCs). Our maximum test performance is 86.9% DSC with 10%, 30%, 50%, 70%, 80%, and 90% of cases being above 81.4%, 77.6%, 74.2%, 69.4%, 65.2% and 58.9%, respectively. Only 2 outlier cases lie below 40% DSC (mainly caused by over-segmentation into other organs). The remaining 80 testing cases are all above 50%. The minimal DSC value of these outliers is 25.0% for $G(P_2(x))$. However [1,2,3,5] all report gross segmentation failure cases with DSC even below 10%. Lastly, the variation $CRF(P_2(x))$ of enforcing $P_2(x)$ within a structured prediction CRF model achieves only 68.2% ±4.1%. This is probably due to the already high quality of $G(P_0)$ and $G(P_2)$ in comparison.

Table 1. 4-fold cross-validation: optimally achievable DSCs, our initial candidate region labeling using S_{RF}, DSCs on $P(x)$ and using smoothed $G(P(x))$, and a CRF model for structured prediction (best performance in bold).

DSC (%)	**Opt.**	$S_{RF(x)}$	$P_0(x)$	$G(P_0(x))$	$P_1(x)$	$G(P_1(x))$	$P_2(x)$	$G(P_2(x))$	$CRF(P_2(x))$
Mean	80.5	26.1	60.9	69.5	56.8	62.9	64.9	**71.8**	68.2
Std	3.6	7.1	10.4	9.3	11.4	16.1	8.1	**10.7**	4.1
Min	70.9	14.2	22.9	35.3	1.3	0.0	33.1	**25.0**	59.6
Max	85.9	45.8	80.1	84.4	77.4	87.3	77.9	**86.9**	74.2

[3] http://www.cc.nih.gov/about/SeniorStaff/ronald_summers.html

[4] http://www.holgerroth.com/

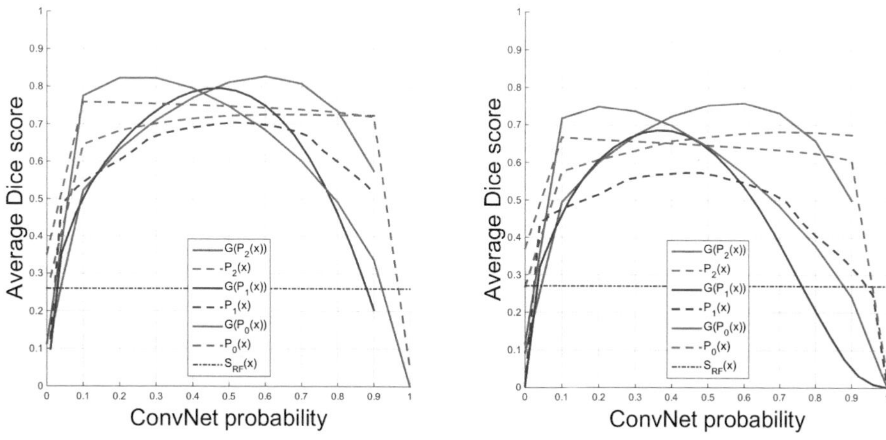

Fig. 5. Average DSCs as a function of un-smoothed $P_k(x), k = 0, 1, 2$, and 3D smoothed $G(P_k(x)), k = 0, 1, 2$, ConvNet probability maps in training (left) and testing (right) in one cross-validation fold.

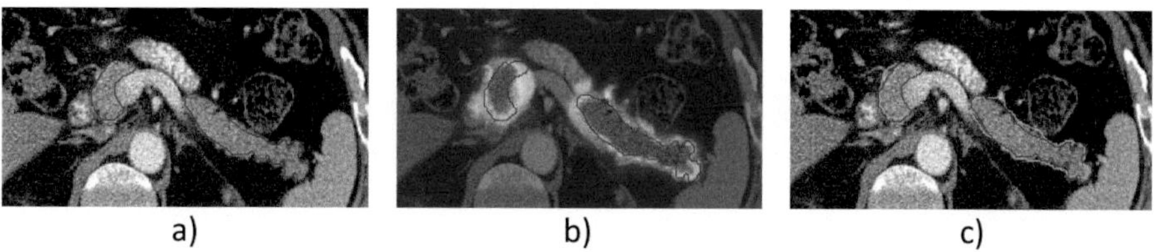

Fig. 6. Example of pancreas segmentation using the proposed R_2–ConvNet approach in testing. a) The manual ground truth annotation (in red outline); b) the $G(P_2(x))$ probability map; c) the final segmentation (in green outline) at $p_2 = 0.6$ (DSC=82.7%).

4 Conclusion

We present a bottom-up, coarse-to-fine approach for pancreas segmentation in abdominal CT scans. Multi-level deep ConvNets are employed on both image patches and regions. We achieve the highest reported DSCs of 71.8±10.7% in testing and 83.6±6.3% in training, at the computational cost of a few minutes, not hours as in [1,2,3]. The proposed approach can be incorporated into multi-organ segmentation frameworks by specifying more tissue types since ConvNet naturally supports multi-class classifications [6]. Our deep learning based organ segmentation approach could be generalizable to other segmentation problems with large variations and pathologies, e.g. tumors.

Acknowledgments. This work was supported by the Intramural Research Program of the NIH Clinical Center.

References

1. Wang, Z., Bhatia, K.K., Glocker, B., Marvao, A., Dawes, T., Misawa, K., Mori, K., Rueckert, D.: Geodesic patch-based segmentation. In: Golland, P., Hata, N., Barillot, C., Hornegger, J., Howe, R. (eds.) MICCAI 2014, Part I. LNCS, vol. MICCAI, pp. 666–673. Springer, Heidelberg (2014)
2. Chu, C., et al.: Multi-organ segmentation based on spatially-divided probabilistic atlas from 3D abdominal CT images. In: Mori, K., Sakuma, I., Sato, Y., Barillot, C., Navab, N. (eds.) MICCAI 2013, Part II. LNCS, vol. 8150, pp. 165–172. Springer, Heidelberg (2013)
3. Wolz, R., Chu, C., Misawa, K., Fujiwara, M., Mori, K., Rueckert, D.: Automated abdominal multi-organ segmentation with subject-specific atlas generation. TMI 32(9), 1723–1730 (2013)
4. Ling, H., Zhou, S.K., Zheng, Y., Georgescu, B., Suehling, M., Comaniciu, D.: Hierarchical, learning-based automatic liver segmentation. In: IEEE CVPR, pp. 1–8 (2008)
5. Farag, A., Lu, L., Turkbey, E., Liu, J., Summers, R.M.: A bottom-up approach for automatic pancreas segmentation in abdominal CT scans. MICCAI Abdominal Imaging workshop, arXiv preprint arXiv:1407.8497 (2014)
6. Krizhevsky, A., Sutskever, I., Hinton, G.E.: Imagenet classification with deep convolutional neural networks. In: NIPS, pp. 1097–1105 (2012)
7. Mostajabi, M., Yadollahpour, P., Shakhnarovich, G.: Feedforward semantic segmentation with zoom-out features. arXiv preprint arXiv:1412.0774 (2014)
8. Cireşan, D.C., Giusti, A., Gambardella, L.M., Schmidhuber, J.: Mitosis detection in breast cancer histology images with deep neural networks. In: Mori, K., Sakuma, I., Sato, Y., Barillot, C., Navab, N. (eds.) MICCAI 2013, Part II. LNCS, vol. 8150, pp. 411–418. Springer, Heidelberg (2013)
9. Roth, H.R., et al.: A new 2.5D representation for lymph node detection using random sets of deep convolutional neural network observations. In: Golland, P., Hata, N., Barillot, C., Hornegger, J., Howe, R. (eds.) MICCAI 2014, Part I. LNCS, vol. MICCAI, pp. 520–527. Springer, Heidelberg (2014)
10. Girshick, R., Donahue, J., Darrell, T., Malik, J.: Rich feature hierarchies for accurate object detection and semantic segmentation. In: IEEE CVPR, pp. 580–587 (2014)
11. Achanta, R., Shaji, A., Smith, K., Lucchi, A., Fua, P., Susstrunk, S.: Slic superpixels compared to state-of-the-art superpixel methods. PAMI 34(11) (2012)
12. Liu, M.Y., Tuzel, O., Ramalingam, S., Chellappa, R.: Entropy rate superpixel segmentation. In: IEEE CVPR, pp. 2097–2104 (2011)
13. Everingham, M., Eslami, S.A., Gool, L.V., Williams, C.K., Winn, J., Zisserman, A.: The PASCAL visual object classes challenge: A retrospective. IJCV 111(1), 98–136 (2014)
14. Srivastava, N., Hinton, G., Krizhevsky, A., Sutskever, I., Salakhutdinov, R.: Dropout: A simple way to prevent neural networks from overfitting. JMLR 15(1), 1929–1958 (2014)
15. Boykov, Y., Funka-Lea, G.: Graph cuts and efficient ND image segmentation. IJCV 70(2), 109–131 (2006)

3D Deep Learning for Efficient and Robust Landmark Detection in Volumetric Data

Yefeng Zheng, David Liu, Bogdan Georgescu, Hien Nguyen, and Dorin Comaniciu

Imaging and Computer Vision, Siemens Corporate Technology, Princeton, NJ, USA
yefeng.zheng@siemens.com

Abstract. Recently, deep learning has demonstrated great success in computer vision with the capability to learn powerful image features from a large training set. However, most of the published work has been confined to solving 2D problems, with a few limited exceptions that treated the 3D space as a composition of 2D orthogonal planes. The challenge of 3D deep learning is due to a much larger input vector, compared to 2D, which dramatically increases the computation time and the chance of over-fitting, especially when combined with limited training samples (hundreds to thousands), typical for medical imaging applications. To address this challenge, we propose an efficient and robust deep learning algorithm capable of full 3D detection in volumetric data. A two-step approach is exploited for efficient detection. A shallow network (with one hidden layer) is used for the initial testing of all voxels to obtain a small number of promising candidates, followed by more accurate classification with a deep network. In addition, we propose two approaches, i.e., separable filter decomposition and network sparsification, to speed up the evaluation of a network. To mitigate the over-fitting issue, thereby increasing detection robustness, we extract small 3D patches from a multi-resolution image pyramid. The deeply learned image features are further combined with Haar wavelet features to increase the detection accuracy. The proposed method has been quantitatively evaluated for carotid artery bifurcation detection on a head-neck CT dataset from 455 patients. Compared to the state-of-the-art, the mean error is reduced by more than half, from 5.97 mm to 2.64 mm, with a detection speed of less than 1 s/volume.

1 Introduction

There are many applications of automatic anatomical landmark detection in medical image analysis. For example, they can be used to align an input volume to a canonical plane on which physicians routinely perform diagnosis and quantification [1, 2]; A detected vascular landmark provides a seed point for automatic vessel centerline extraction and lumen segmentation [3]. Various landmark detection methods have been proposed in the literature. Most of the state-of-the-art algorithms [1–3] apply machine learning on a set of handcrafted image features. However, in practice, we found some landmark detection problems (e.g., carotid artery bifurcation landmarks in this work) are still too challenging to be solved with the current technology.

Recently, deep learning [4] has demonstrated great success in computer vision with the capability to learn powerful image features from a large training set. However, several

N. Navab et al. (Eds.): MICCAI 2015, Part I, LNCS 9349, pp. 565–572, 2015.
DOI: 10.1007/978-3-319-24553-9_69

challenges are present in applying deep learning to 3D landmark detection. Normally, the input to a neural network classifier is an image patch, which increases dramatically in size from 2D to 3D. For example, a patch of 32×32 pixels generates an input of 1024 dimensions to the classifier. However, a $32 \times 32 \times 32$ 3D patch contains 32,768 voxels. Such a big input feature vector creates several challenges. First, the computation time of a deep neural network is often too slow for a real clinical application. The most widely used and robust approach for object detection is the *sliding-window* based approach, in which the trained classifier is tested on each voxel in the volume. Evaluating a deep network on a large volume may take several minutes. Second, a network with a bigger input vector requires more training data. With enough training samples (e.g., over 10 million in ImageNet), deep learning has demonstrated impressive performance gain over other methods. However, the medical imaging community is often struggling with limited training samples (often in hundreds or thousands) due to the difficulty to generate and share images. Several approaches can tackle or at least mitigate the issue of limited training samples. One approach is to reduce the patch size. However, a small patch may not contain enough information for classification. Alternatively, instead of sampling a 3D patch, we can sample on three orthogonal planes [5] or even a 2D patch with a random orientation [6]. Although they can effectively reduce the input dimension, there is a concern on how much 3D information is contained in 2D planes.

In this work we tackle the above challenges in the application of deep learning for 3D anatomical structure detection (focusing on landmarks). Our approach significantly accelerates the detection speed by about 20 times, resulting in an efficient method that can detect a landmark in less than one second. We apply a two-stage classification strategy (as shown in Fig. 1). In the first stage, we train a shallow network with only one small hidden layer. This network is applied to test all voxels in the volume in a sliding-window process to generate 2000 candidates for the second stage classification. The second network is much bigger with three hidden layers (each has 2000 nodes) to obtain more discriminative power. The weights of a node in the first hidden layer are often treated as a filter (3D in this case). The response of the first hidden layer over the volume can be calculated as a convolution with the filter. Here, a neighboring patch is shifted by only one voxel; however, the response needs to be re-calculated from scratch. In this work we approximate the weights as separable filters using tensor decomposition. Therefore, a direct 3D convolution is decomposed as three one-dimensional convolutions along the x, y, and z axis, respectively. Previously, such approximation has been exploited for 2D classification problems [7, 8]. However, in 3D, the trained filters are more difficult to be approximated as separable filters. We propose a new training cost function to enforce smoothness of the filters so that they can be approximated with high accuracy. The second big network only applies on a small number of candidates that have little correlation. Separable filter approximation does not help to accelerate classification. However, many weights in a big network are close to zero. We propose to add L1-norm regularization to the cost function to drive majority of the weights (e.g., 90%) to zero, resulting in a sparse network with increased classification efficiency.

The power of deep learning is on the automatic learning of a hierarchical image representation (i.e., image features). Instead of using the trained network as a classifier, we can use the responses at each layer (including the input layer, all hidden layers, and the

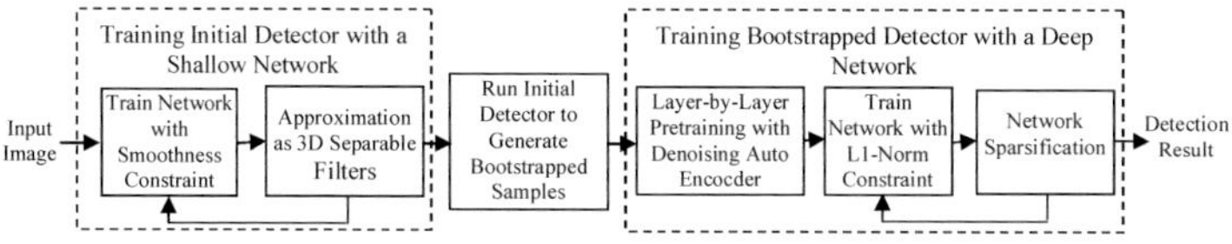

Fig. 1. Training procedure of the proposed deep network based 3D landmark detection method

output layer) as features and feed them into other state-of-the-art classifiers (e.g., boosting). After years of feature engineering, some handcrafted features have considerable discriminative power for some applications and they may be complimentary to deeply learned features. In this work we demonstrate that combining deeply learned features and Haar wavelet features, we can reduce the detection failures.

2 Efficient Detection with Neural Networks

Training Shallow Network with Separable Filters. A fully connected multilayer perceptron (MLP) neural network is a layered architecture. Suppose the input is a n_0-dimensional vector $[X_1^0, X_2^0, \ldots, X_{n_0}^0]$. The response of a node X_j^1 of the first hidden layer is

$$X_j^1 = g\left(\sum_{i=1}^{n_0} W_{i,j}^0 X_i^0 + b_j^0\right), \tag{1}$$

for $j = 1, 2, \ldots, n_1$ (n_1 is the number of nodes in the first hidden layer). Here, $g(.)$ is a nonlinear function, e.g., the sigmoid function in this work. $W_{i,j}^0$ is a weight and b_j^0 is a bias term. If we denote $\mathbf{X}^0 = [X_1^0, \ldots, X_{n_0}^0]^T$ and $\mathbf{W}_j^0 = [W_{1,j}^0, \ldots, W_{n_0,j}^0]^T$, Eq. (1) can be re-written as $X_j^1 = g\left((\mathbf{W}_j^0)^T \mathbf{X}^0 + b_j^0\right)$. Multiple layers can be stacked together using Eq. (1) as a building block. For a binary classification problem as this work, the output of the network can be a single node $\hat{X}$. Suppose there are L hidden layers, the output of the neural network is $\hat{X} = g\left((\mathbf{W}^L)^T \mathbf{X}^L + b^L\right)$. During network training, we require the output to match the class label Y (with 1 for the positive class and 0 for negative) by minimizing the squared error $E = ||Y - \hat{X}||^2$.

In object detection using a sliding window based approach, for each position hypothesis, we crop an image patch (with a pre-defined size) centered at the position hypothesis. We then serialize the patch intensities into a vector as the input to calculate response $\hat{X}$. After testing a patch, we shift the patch by one voxel (e.g., to the right) and repeat the above process again. Such a naive implementation is time consuming. Coming back to Eq. (1), we can treat the weights of a node in the first hidden layer as a filter. The first term of the response is a dot-product of the filter and the image patch intensities. Shifting the patch over the whole volume is equivalent to convolution using the filter. Therefore, alternatively, we can perform convolution using each filter $\mathbf{W}_j^0$ for $j = 1, 2, \ldots, n_1$ and cache the response maps. During object detection, we can use the cached maps to retrieve the response of the first hidden layer.

Although such an alternative approach does not save computation time, it gives us a hint for speed-up. With a bit abuse of symbols, suppose $\mathbf{W}_{x,y,z}$ is a 3D filter with size $n_x \times n_y \times n_z$. Let's further assume that $\mathbf{W}_{x,y,z}$ is separable, which means we can find three one-dimensional vectors, $\mathbf{W}_x, \mathbf{W}_y, \mathbf{W}_z$, such that

$$\mathbf{W}_{x,y,z}(i,j,k) = \mathbf{W}_x(i).\mathbf{W}_y(j).\mathbf{W}_z(k) \tag{2}$$

for any $i \in [1, n_x]$, $j \in [1, n_y]$, and $k \in [1, n_z]$. The convolution of the volume with $\mathbf{W}_{x,y,z}$ is equivalent to three sequential convolutions with $\mathbf{W}_x$, $\mathbf{W}_y$, and $\mathbf{W}_z$ along its corresponding axis. Sequential convolution with one-dimensional filters is much more efficient than direct convolution with a 3D filter, especially for a large filter. However, in reality, Eq. (2) is just an approximation of filters learned by a neural network and such a rank-1 approximation is poor in general. In this work we search for S sets of separable filters to approximate the original filter as

$$\mathbf{W}_{x,y,z} \approx \sum_{s=1}^{S} \mathbf{W}_x^s.\mathbf{W}_y^s.\mathbf{W}_z^s. \tag{3}$$

Please note, with a sufficient number of separable filters (e.g., $S \geq min\{n_x, n_y, n_z\}$), we can reconstruct the original filter perfectly.

To achieve detection efficiency, we need to cache $n_1 \times S$ filtered response maps. If the input volume is big (the size of a typical CT scan in our dataset is about 300 MB) and n_1 is relatively large (e.g., 64 or more), the cached response maps consume a lot of memory. Fortunately, the learned filters $\mathbf{W}_1^0, \ldots, \mathbf{W}_{n_1}^0$ often have strong correlation (i.e., a filter can be reconstructed by a linear combination of other filters). We do not need to maintain different filter banks for each $\mathbf{W}_i^0$. The separable filters in reconstruction can be drawn from the same bank,

$$\mathbf{W}_i^0 \approx \sum_{s=1}^{S} c_{i,s}.\mathbf{W}_x^s.\mathbf{W}_y^s.\mathbf{W}_z^s. \tag{4}$$

Here, $c_{i,s}$ is the combination coefficient, which is specific for each filter $\mathbf{W}_i^0$. However, $\mathbf{W}_x^s$, $\mathbf{W}_y^s$, and $\mathbf{W}_z^s$ are shared by all filters. Eq. (4) is a rank-S decomposition of a 4D tensor $[\mathbf{W}_1^0, \mathbf{W}_2^0, \ldots, \mathbf{W}_{n_1}^0]$, which can be solved using [9].

Using 4D tensor decomposition, we only need to convolve the volume S times (instead of $n_1.S$ times using 3D tensor decomposition) and cache S response maps. Suppose the input volume has $N_x \times N_y \times N_z$ voxels. For each voxel, we need to do $n_x n_y n_z$ multiplications using the original sliding window based approach. To calculate the response of a hidden layer with n_1 nodes, the total number of multiplications is $n_1 n_x n_y n_z N_x N_y N_z$. Using the proposed approach, to perform convolution with S set of separable filters, we need do $S(n_x + n_y + n_z)N_x N_y N_z$ multiplications. To calculate the response of n_1 hidden layer nodes, we need to combine the S responses using Eq. (4), resulting in $n_1 S N_x N_y N_z$ multiplications. The total number of multiplications is $S(n_x + n_y + n_z + n_1)N_x N_y N_z$. Suppose $S = 32$, $n_1 = 64$, the speed-up is 103 times for a $15 \times 15 \times 15$ patch.

To achieve significant speed-up and save memory footprint, we need to reduce S as much as possible. However, we found, with a small S (e.g., 32), it was more difficult to approximate 3D filters than 2D filters [7, 8]. Non-linear functions $g(.)$ are exploited in neural networks to bound the response to a certain range (e.g., [0, 1] using the sigmoid function). Many nodes are saturated (with an output close to 0 or 1) and once a node is saturated, its response is not sensitive to the change of the weights. Therefore, a weight can take an extremely large value, resulting in a non-smooth filter. Here, we propose to modify the objective function to encourage the network to generate smooth filters

$$E = ||Y - \hat{X}||^2 + \alpha \sum_{i=1}^{n_1} ||\mathbf{W}_i^0 - \overline{\mathbf{W}_i^0}||^2. \tag{5}$$

Here, $\overline{\mathbf{W}_i^0}$ is the mean value of the weights of filter $\mathbf{W}_i^0$. So, the second term measures the variance of the filter weights. Parameter α (often takes a small value, e.g., 0.001) keeps a balance between two terms in the objective function.

The training of the initial shallow network detector is as follows (as shown in the left dashed box of Fig. 1). 1) Train a network using Eq. (5). 2) Approximate the learned filters using a filter bank with S ($S = 32$ in our experiments) sets of separable filters to minimize the error of Eq. (4). The above process may be iterated a few times (e.g., three times). In the first iteration, the network weights and filter bank are initialized with random values. However, in the following iterations, they are both initialized with the optimal values from the previous iteration.

Training Sparse Deep Network. Using a shallow network, we can efficiently test all voxels in the volume and assign a detection score to each voxel. After that, we preserve 2000 candidates with the largest detection scores. The number of preserved candidates is tuned to have a high probability to include the correct detection (e.g., hypotheses within one-voxel distance to the ground truth). However, most of the preserved candidates are still false positives. In the next step, we train a deep network to further reduce the false positives. The classification problem is now much tougher and a shallow network does not work well. In this work we use a big network with three hidden layers, each with 2000 nodes. Even though we only need to classify a small number of candidates, the computation may still take some time since the network is now much bigger. Since the preserved candidates are often scattered over the whole volume, separable filter decomposition as used in the initial detection does not help to accelerate the classification. After checking the values of the learned weights of this deep network, we found most of weights were very small, close to zero. That means many connections in the network can be removed without sacrificing classification accuracy. Here, we apply L1-norm regularization to enforce sparse connection

$$E = ||Y - \hat{X}||^2 + \beta \sum_{j=1}^{L} \sum_{i=1}^{n_j} ||\mathbf{W}_i^j||. \tag{6}$$

Parameter β can be used to tune the number of zero weights. The higher β is, the more weights converge to zero. With a sufficient number of training epochs, part of weights converges exactly to zero. In practice, to speed up the training, we periodically check the magnitude of weights. The weights with a magnitude smaller than a threshold are set to zero and the network is refined again. In our experiments, we find that 90% of the weigths can be set to zero after training, without deteriorating the classification accuracy. Thus, we can speed up the classification by roughly ten times.

The proposed acceleration technologies can be applied to different neural network architectures, e.g., a multilayer perceptron (MLP) and a convolutional neural network (CNN). In this work we use the MLP. (We also tried the CNN and achieved similar,

Table 1. Quantitative evaluation of carotid artery bifurcation detection accuracy on 455 CT scans based on a four-fold cross validation. The errors are reported in millimeters.

	Mean	Std	Median	80th Percentile
Haar + PBT	5.97	6.99	3.64	7.84
Neural Network (Single Resolution)	4.13	9.39	1.24	2.35
Neural Network (Multi-Resolution)	3.69	6.71	1.62	3.25
Network Features + PBT	3.54	8.40	1.25	**2.31**
Haar + Network + PBT	**2.64**	**4.98**	**1.21**	2.39

but not superior, detection accuracy.) The shallow network is trained directly with back-propagation and the deep network is trained using the denoising auto-encoder criterion [4]. The right dashed box of Fig. 1 shows the training procedure of the sparse deep network.

3 Robust Detection by Combining Multiple Features

To train a robust neural network based landmark detector on a limited training samples, we have to control the patch size. The optimal patch size was searched and we found a size of $15 \times 15 \times 15$ achieved a good trade-off between detection speed and accuracy. However, a small patch has a limited field-of-view, thereby may not capture enough information for classification. In this work we extract patches on an image pyramid with multiple resolutions. A small patch in a low-resolution volume has a much larger field-of-view at the original resolution. To be specific, we build an image pyramid with three resolutions (1-mm, 2-mm, and 4-mm resolution, respectively). The intensities of patches from multiple resolutions are concatenated into a long vector to feed the network. As demonstrated in Section 4, a multi-resolution patch can improve the landmark detection accuracy.

Deep learning automatically learns a hierarchical representation of the input data. Representation at different hierarchical levels may provide complementary information for classification. Furthermore, through years' of feature engineering, some hand-crafted image features can achieve quite reasonable performance on a certain task. Combining effective hand-crafted image features with deeply learned hierarchical features may achieve even better performance than using them separately.

In this work we propose to use probabilistic boosting-tree (PBT) [10] to combine all features. A PBT is a combination of a decision tree and AdaBoost, by replacing a weak classification node in the decision tree with a strong AdaBoost classifier. Our feature pool is composed of two types of features: Haar wavelet features $(h_1, h_2, \ldots, h_m)$ and neural network features r_i^j (where r_i^j is the response of node i at layer j). If $j = 0$, r_i^0 is an input node, representing the image intensity of a voxel in the patch. The last neural network feature is actually the response of the output node, which is the classification score by the network. This feature is the strongest feature and it is always the first selected feature by the AdaBoost algorithm.

4 Experiments

The carotid artery is the main vessel supplying oxygenated blood to the head and neck. The common carotid artery originates from the aortic arch and runs up toward the head

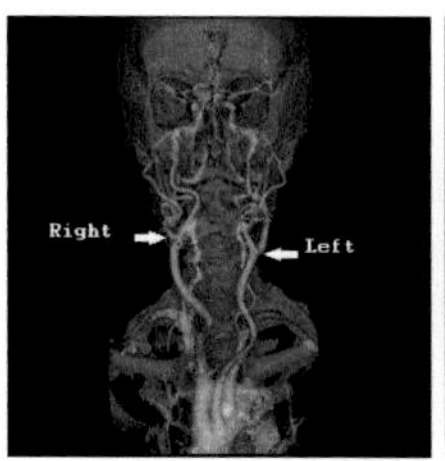

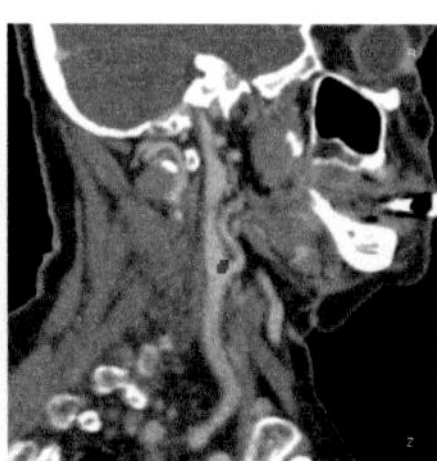
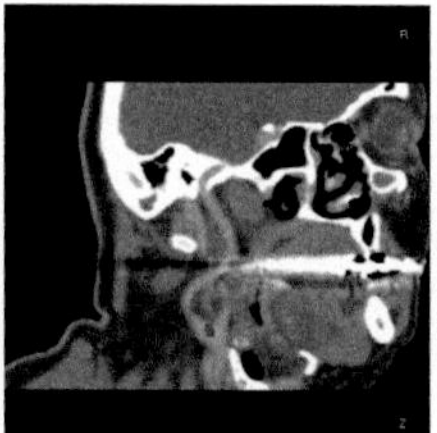
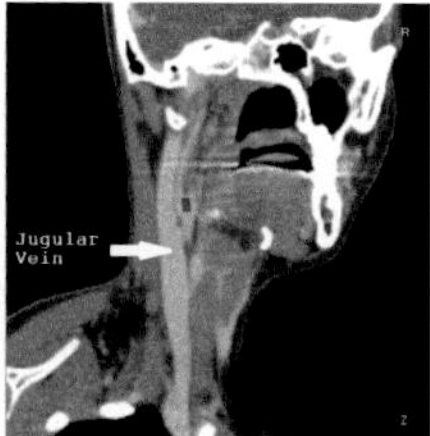

Fig. 2. Carotid artery bifurcation landmark detection in head-neck CT scans. The first column shows a 3D visualization of carotid arteries with white arrows pointing to the left and right bifurcations (image courtesy of http://blog.remakehealth.com/). The right columns show a few examples of the right carotid artery bifurcation detection results with the ground truth labeled as blue dots and detected landmarks in red.

before bifurcating to the external carotid artery (supplying blood to face) and internal carotid artery (supplying blood to brain). Examination of the carotid artery helps to assess the stroke risk of a patient. Automatic detection of this bifurcation landmark provides a seed point for centerline tracing and lumen segmentation, thereby making automatic examination possible. However, as shown in the left image of Fig. 2, the internal/external carotid arteries further bifurcate to many branches and there are other vessels (e.g., vertebral arteries and jugular veins) present nearby, which may cause confusion to an automatic detection algorithm.

We collected a head-neck CT dataset from 455 patients. Each image slice has 512×512 pixels and a volume contains a variable number of slices (from 46 to 1181 slices). The volume resolution varies too, with a typical voxel size of $0.46 \times 0.46 \times 0.50\,mm^3$. A four-fold cross validation is performed to evaluate the detection accuracy and determine the hyper parameters, e.g., the network size, smoothness constraint α in Eq. (5), sparsity constraint β in Eq. (6). There are two carotid arteries (left vs. right) as shown in Fig. 2. Due to the space limit, we only report the bifurcation detection accuracy of the right carotid artery (as shown in Table 1) with different approaches. The detection accuracy of the left carotid artery bifurcation is similar.

For each approach reported in Table 1, we follow a two-step process by applying the first detector to reduce the number of candidates to 2000, followed by a bootstrapped detection to further reduce the number of candidates to 250. The final detection is picked as the candidate with the largest vote from other candidates. Previously, Liu et al. [3] used Haar wavelet features + boosting to detect vascular landmarks and achieved promising results. Applying this approach on our dataset, we achieve a mean error of 5.97 mm and the large mean error is caused by too many detection outliers. The neural network based approach can significantly improve the detection accuracy with a mean error of 4.13 mm using a $15 \times 15 \times 15$ patch extracted from a single resolution (1 mm). Using patches extracted from an image pyramid with three resolutions, we can further reduce the mean detection error to 3.69 mm. If we combine features from all layers of the network using the PBT, we achieve slightly better mean accuracy of 3.54 mm. Combining the deeply learned features and Haar wavelet features, we achieve the best detection accuracy with a mean error of 2.64 mm. We suspect that the improvement comes from the complementary information of the Haar wavelet features and neural network features. Fig. 2 shows the detection results on a few typical datasets.

The proposed method is computationally efficient. Using the speed-up technologies presented in Section 2, it takes 0.92 s to detect a landmark on a computer with a six-core 2.6 GHz CPU (without using GPU). For comparison, the computation time increases to 18.0 s if we turn off the proposed acceleration technologies. The whole training procedure takes about 6 hours and the sparse deep network consumes majority of the training time.

5 Conclusions

In this work we proposed 3D deep learning for efficient and robust landmark detection in volumetric data. We proposed two technologies to speed up the detection using neural networks, namely, separable filter decomposition and network sparsification. To improve the detection robustness, we exploit deeply learned image features trained on a multi-resolution image pyramid. Furthermore, we use the boosting technology to incorporate deeply learned hierarchical features and Haar wavelet features to further improve the detection accuracy. The proposed method is generic and can be re-trained to detect other 3D landmarks.

References

1. Zhan, Y., Dewan, M., Harder, M., Krishnan, A., Zhou, X.S.: Robust automatic knee MR slice positioning through redundant and hierarchical anatomy detection. IEEE Trans. Medical Imaging 30(12), 2087–2100 (2010)
2. Schwing, A.G., Zheng, Y.: Reliable extraction of the mid-sagittal plane in 3D brain MRI via hierarchical landmark detection. In: Proc. Int'l Sym. Biomedical Imaging, pp. 213–216 (2014)
3. Liu, D., Zhou, S., Bernhardt, D., Comaniciu, D.: Vascular landmark detection in 3D CT data. In: Proc. of SPIE Medical Imaging, pp. 1–7 (2011)
4. Vincent, P., Larochelle, H., Lajoie, I., Bengio, Y., Manzagol, P.A.: Stacked denoising autoencoders: Learning useful representations in a deep network with a local denoising criterion. The Journal of Machine Learning Research 11, 3371–3408 (2010)
5. Prasoon, A., Petersen, K., Igel, C., Lauze, F., Dam, E., Nielsen, M.: Deep feature learning for knee cartilage segmentation using a triplanar convolutional neural network. In: Mori, K., Sakuma, I., Sato, Y., Barillot, C., Navab, N. (eds.) MICCAI 2013, Part II. LNCS, vol. 8150, pp. 246–253. Springer, Heidelberg (2013)
6. Roth, H.R., et al.: A new 2.5D representation for lymph node detection using random sets of deep convolutional neural network observations. In: Golland, P., Hata, N., Barillot, C., Hornegger, J., Howe, R. (eds.) MICCAI 2014, Part I. LNCS, vol. 8673, pp. 520–527. Springer, Heidelberg (2014)
7. Rigamonti, R., Sironi, A., Lepetit, V., Fua, P.: Learning separable filters. In: Proc. IEEE Conf. Computer Vision and Pattern Recognition, pp. 2754–2761 (2013)
8. Denton, E., Zaremba, W., Bruna, J., LeCun, Y., Fergus, R.: Exploiting linear structure within convolutional networks for efficient evaluation. In: Advances in Neural Information Processing Systems, pp. 1–11 (2014)
9. Acar, E., Dunlavy, D.M., Kolda, T.G.: A scalable optimization approach for fitting canonical tensor decompositions. Journal of Chemometrics 25(2), 67–86 (2011)
10. Tu, Z.: Probabilistic boosting-tree: Learning discriminative methods for classification, recognition, and clustering. In: Proc. Int'l Conf. Computer Vision, pp. 1589–1596 (2005)

A Hybrid of Deep Network and Hidden Markov Model for MCI Identification with Resting-State fMRI

Heung-Il Suk[1,⋆], Seong-Whan Lee[1], and Dinggang Shen[1,2]

[1] Department of Brain and Cognitive Engineering, Korea University, Republic of Korea
[2] Biomedical Research Imaging Center, University of North Carolina at Chapel Hill, USA
hisuk@korea.ac.kr

Abstract. In this paper, we propose a novel method for modelling functional dynamics in resting-state fMRI (rs-fMRI) for Mild Cognitive Impairment (MCI) identification. Specifically, we devise a hybrid architecture by combining Deep Auto-Encoder (DAE) and Hidden Markov Model (HMM). The roles of DAE and HMM are, respectively, to discover hierarchical non-linear relations among features, by which we transform the original features into a lower dimension space, and to model dynamic characteristics inherent in rs-fMRI, *i.e.*, internal state changes. By building a generative model with HMMs for each class individually, we estimate the data likelihood of a test subject as MCI or normal healthy control, based on which we identify the clinical label. In our experiments, we achieved the maximal accuracy of 81.08% with the proposed method, outperforming state-of-the-art methods in the literature.

1 Introduction

Motivated by Biswal *et al.*'s study [1] that discovered different brain regions still actively interact while a subject lies at rest, *i.e.*, not performing any cognitive task, resting-state fMRI (rs-fMRI) has been widely used as one of the major tools for investigation of brain networks. It provides insights to explore the brain's functional organization and examine the altered functional networks possibly due to brain disorders such as Mild Cognitive Impairment (MCI). In this regard, functional connectivity analysis has played core roles for brain disease diagnosis or prognosis [4, 7, 11, 12, 15, 16].

While many existing methods for MCI diagnosis with rs-fMRI typically assumed stationarity on the functional networks over time [12, 16], recent studies in neuroscience have shown that the functional organization of a brain is dynamic rather than static, changing spontaneously over time [9]. Eavani *et al.* proposed to jointly model sparse dictionary learning within a state-space model framework [2]. Leonardi *et al.* devised a method to reveal hidden patterns of coherent functional connectivity dynamics based on principal component analysis [11]. In this paper, we propose a novel method that discovers non-linear relations among brain regions in a hierarchical manner and explicitly models the dynamic characteristics inherent in rs-fMRI. It is noteworthy that rather than computing correlation matrices and extracting graph-theoretic features [14] such as small-worldness and clustering coefficients as commonly performed in the literature,

⋆ Corresponding author.

N. Navab et al. (Eds.): MICCAI 2015, Part I, LNCS 9349, pp. 573–580, 2015.
DOI: 10.1007/978-3-319-24553-9_70

we directly model functional dynamics from regional mean time series of rs-fMRI. In a testing phase, our model estimates the data likelihood of a test subject as MCI and Normal healthy Control (NC), based on which we make a clinical decision. Although different groups independently devised different types of state-space models to analyze event-related fMRI data [3, 8, 10], due to their use of variables related to external stimulus, *i.e.*, event, those models cannot be applied to rs-fMRI based disease diagnosis.

2 Materials and Preprocessing

We used a cohort[1] of 37 subjects (12 MCI patients and 25 socio-demographically matched NCs) [15]. The subjects were asked to keep their eyes open and to fixate on a crosshair during scanning. The T1-weighted anatomical MRI images were also acquired from the same scanner.

We discarded the first 10 fMRI volume images of each subject for magnetization equilibrium. In order to remove extraneous sources of variation and to isolate the fMRI signals, the remaining 140 fMRI volume images were processed by applying the procedures of slice timing, motion correction, and spatial normalization using SPM8. The images were realigned with TR/2 as a reference time point to minimize the relative errors across TRs. In the motion correction step, we realigned images to the first volume across the subjects. We considered only the signals of gray matter for further processing. The fMRI brain space was then parcellated into 116 Regions-Of-interest (ROIs) based on the Automated Anatomical Labeling (AAL) template.

By following studies in the literature, we utilized the low frequency fluctuation features in rs-fMRI with a frequency band of 0.025$\sim$0.1Hz. The representative mean time series of each ROI was computed by averaging the intensity of all voxels in an ROI. Lastly, we had a set of mean time series $\mathbf{F} \in \left\{ F^{(n)} = \left[\mathbf{f}_1^{(n)}, \ldots, \mathbf{f}_T^{(n)} \right] \in \mathbb{R}^{R \times T} \right\}_{n=1}^{N}$ of the number N(=37) of subjects, the number R(=116) of ROIs, and the number T(=140) of volumes.

3 Proposed Method

Unlike many existing methods that mostly assumed stationarity of a rs-fMRI time series and explicitly constructed a functional connectivity map, in this paper, we propose a novel probabilistic method that models functional dynamics inherent in rs-fMRI and estimates the data likelihood of a test subject as NC and MCI to make a clinical decision. Specifically, we devise a hybrid architecture by combining Deep Auto-Encoder (DAE) and Hidden Markov Model (HMM) as illustrated in Fig. 1. The roles of DAE and HMM are, respectively, to identify intrinsic networks in a hierarchical manner, from which we extract low-dimensional feature representations, and to model dynamic functional characteristics, *i.e.*, internal functional state changes. It should be noted that HMMs are trained for the classes of NC and MCI separately, while the DAE is shared between classes, and thus it is guaranteed for features of the two classes to lie in the same space.

[1] 150 volumes, TR=2,000ms; TE=32ms; flip angle=77°; acquisition matrix size=64×64; field of view=256×256mm^2; 34 axial slices parallel to the anterior commissure-posterior commissure plane; voxel size=$4 \times 4 \times 4$mm^3.

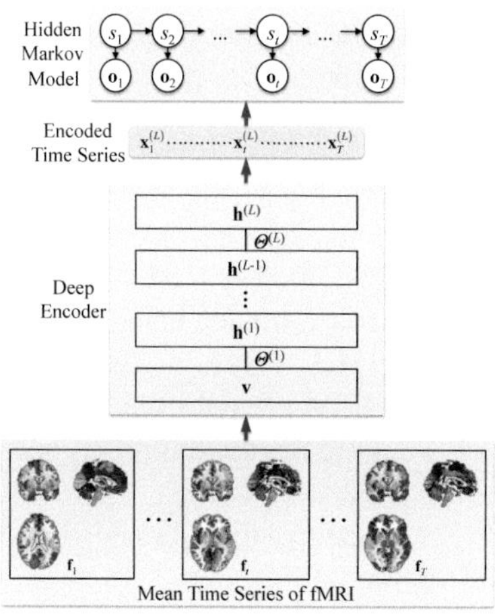

(a) A hybrid architecture of the proposed method

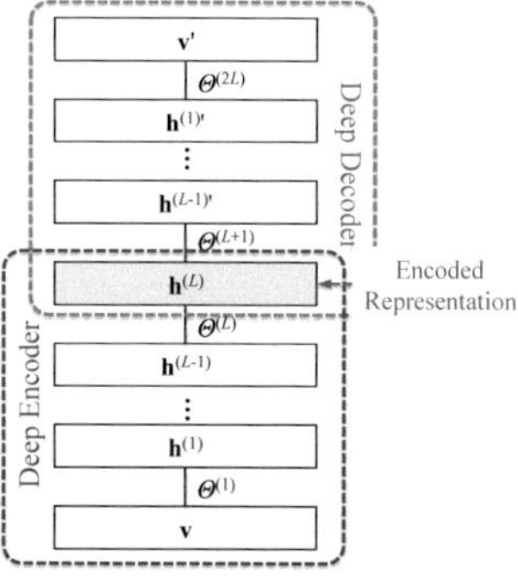

(b) Deep auto-encoder

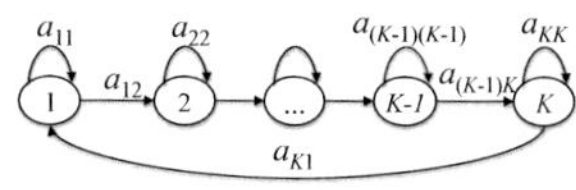

(c) Circular topology in HMM

Fig. 1. Illustration of (a) the proposed method for modelling dynamics in rs-fMRI, (b) graphical representation of a deep auto-encoder used to find internal networks and to reduce dimensionality, and (c) the state topology in HMM, where the hidden state variables $[s_1, \ldots, s_t, \ldots, s_T]$ change over time.

3.1 Deep Auto-Encoder

Recently, Hjelm *et al.* [7] demonstrated that Restricted Boltzmann Machines (RBMs) can be used to identify functional networks from fMRI and supported its use as a building block for deeper network models in neuroimaging research. Justified by their work, we design a DAE, structured by stacking multiple RBMs, to discover an embedded representation of functional patterns in a volume of rs-fMRI.

An RBM is a two-layer undirected graphical model with a number D of units in a visible layer and a number F of units in a hidden layer. It assumes symmetric inter-layer connections, but no intra-layer connections. An RBM can be specified with a parameter set Θ of inter-layer connections $\mathbf{W} = [W_{ij}] \in \mathbb{R}^{D \times F}$, a visible layer's bias $\mathbf{z} = [z_i] \in \mathbb{R}^D$, and a hidden layer's bias $\mathbf{q} = [q_j] \in \mathbb{R}^F$, *i.e.*, $\Theta = \{\mathbf{W}, \mathbf{z}, \mathbf{q}\}$, which are learned by minimizing an energy function. In this work, we consider two different energy functions, according to the value types of the visible units $\mathbf{v}$, while using a binary hidden units $\mathbf{h}$. Specifically, when the visible layer has real continuous values, we use a Gaussian-Bernoulli energy function defined as $E(\mathbf{v}, \mathbf{h}; \Theta) = \sum_{i=1}^{D} \frac{(v_i - z_i)^2}{2\sigma_i^2} - \sum_{i=1}^{D} \sum_{j=1}^{F} \frac{v_i}{\sigma_i} W_{ij} h_j - \sum_{j=1}^{F} q_j h_j$, where σ_i denotes a standard deviation of the i-th visible variable that should be learned from data. Meanwhile, for an RBM of binary visible units, it is simplified to a Bernoulli-Bernoulli energy function as $E(\mathbf{v}, \mathbf{h}; \Theta) = -\sum_{i=1}^{D} \sum_{j=1}^{F} v_i W_{ij} h_j - \sum_{i=1}^{D} z_i v_i - \sum_{j=1}^{F} q_j h_j$.

We construct a DAE by using RBMs as building blocks and taking the probability of the lower layer as the inputs to the neighbouring upper layer. The conditional probability of units in the l-th layer given the values of units in the $(l-1)$-th layer is computed as $P\left(\mathbf{h}^{(l)}|\mathbf{h}^{(l-1)},\Theta^{(l)}\right) = sigm\left(q_j^{(l)} + \sum_i W_{ij}^{(l)} h_i^{(l-1)}/\sigma_i^{(l-1)}\right)$, where $sigm(\cdot)$ denotes a sigmoid function, $\mathbf{h}^{(0)} = \mathbf{v}$, and $\sigma_i^{(l-1)} = 1$ for a binary random vector $\mathbf{h}^{(l-1)}$. Our DAE structurally consists of two parts, namely, 'encoder' and 'decoder' as shown in Fig. 1(b), similar to Hinton and Salakhutdinov's work [6]. Let L denote the number of hidden layers in the encoder, thus the decoder also has L hidden layers. It should be noted that, in our work, the units of bottom input layer, *i.e.*, $\mathbf{v}$ in Fig. 1(b), is modelled with a Gaussian function, while the units of hidden layers remain binary except for those of the middle hidden layer $\mathbf{h}^{(L)}$, for which we use a linear continuous units with Gaussian noises[2].

To learn the parameter sets $\{\Theta^{(1)},\ldots,\Theta^{(2L)}\}$, we perform the following three steps sequentially with a set of mean time series $\mathbf{F}$ as training samples:

1. Pretrain the parameters $\{\Theta^{(l)}\}_{l=1}^{L}$ of a deep encoder, *i.e.*, network in a blue box in Fig. 1(b), in a greedy layer-wise manner via contrastive divergence algorithm [5]. Note that the mean ROI intensities of the t-th fMRI volume of a subject n, *i.e.*, $\mathbf{f}_t^{(n)}$, becomes the input to $\mathbf{v}$.
2. Unfold the pretrained deep encoder to build a deeper network of encoder and decoder, which we call 'DAE', as shown in Fig. 1(b). For the decoder, *i.e.*, network in the green box in Fig. 1(b), we initially use the same weights of the encoder, pretrained in the first step, *i.e.*, $\Theta^{(L+k)} \leftarrow \Theta^{(L-k+1)}$, $k=1,\ldots,L$.
3. Fine-tune the parameter sets $\{\Theta^{(1)},\ldots,\Theta^{(2L)}\}$ of the whole deep neural network, *i.e.*, DAE, jointly by using a back-propagation algorithm [6] with the inputs $\mathbf{v}$ and target outputs $\mathbf{v}'$ kept identical.

Hereafter, we omit the subject index $^{(n)}$ for uncluttered. After completing our DAE training, we use the lower half of our DAE, *i.e.*, deep encoder, to transform the rs-fMRI feature vectors $F = [\mathbf{f}_1,\cdots,\mathbf{f}_t,\cdots,\mathbf{f}_T]$ into encoded representations $X = [\mathbf{x}_1,\cdots,\mathbf{x}_t,\cdots,\mathbf{x}_T]$, which are further fed into HMMs to identify clinical status between NC and MCI. It is remarkable that by setting the number of hidden units in the top hidden layer $\mathbf{h}^{(L)}$ of a deep encoder smaller than the dimension of the input, *i.e.*, R, it naturally has the effect of reducing dimensionality of the input vector $\mathbf{f}_t$ but still has the rich information necessary to reproduce the input in a non-linear way.

However, note that a DAE is utilized to find the highly non-linear relations among different regions at one time without considering the temporal information, which is important to discriminate MCI from NC. We handle such temporal or dynamic information with an HMM described below.

3.2 Hidden Markov Models

Based on recent studies in [4, 11], it is reasonable to assume that the groups of NC and MCI exhibit different functional characteristics, depending on the unobservable

[2] The rationale of using linear units with Gaussian noises is to obtain continuous values for better representational power of the coded representations [6].

functional states that spontaneously change over time. In this paper, we model such dynamics inherent in rs-fMRI by the first-order Markov chain in HMMs [13] for NC and MCI, separately.

An HMM is a doubly stochastic process of 1) hidden process $\{s_1, \cdots, s_t, \cdots, s_T\}$ that is latent but can be estimated by 2) observable process $\{\mathbf{o}_1, \cdots, \mathbf{o}_t, \cdots, \mathbf{o}_T\}$, which produces a sequence of observations, where s_t and $\mathbf{o}_t$ denote random variables of hidden state and observation at time t, respectively. A hidden process is represented by two probability distributions, namely, state transition probability $A = [a_{ij}]_{i,j=\{1,\ldots,K\}}$ and initial state probability $\Pi = [\pi_i]_{i=\{1,\ldots,K\}}$, where K denotes the number of hidden states, $a_{ij} = P(s_t = j | s_{t-1} = i)$, and $\pi_i = P(s_1 = i)$. Meanwhile, the observable process is depicted by emission probability density function (*pdf*) $B = \{b_i\}_{i=\{1,\ldots,K\}}$, where $b_i = p(\mathbf{o}_t = \mathbf{x}_t | s_t = i)$. In this work, we use a mixture of Gaussians for an emission *pdf* b_i. Thus, an HMM is completely defined by the parameter set of $\lambda = (A, B, \Pi)$. For simplicity, we denote, hereafter, HMMs for NC and MCI with λ_{NC} and λ_{MCI}, respectively.

Note that a functional pattern of rs-fMRI at a time-point belongs to one of a finite number K of states, which is represented by an observation probability B. Meanwhile, the changes of the unobservable states in rs-fMRI are denoted by the state transition probability A along with the initial state probability Π. By training HMMs with a Baum-Welch algorithm [13] for NC and MCI individually, they can be used as a way to represent the functional dynamic characteristics of the respective groups in a probabilistic manner. In other words, given a sequence of functional features, *i.e.*, encoded representations $X = [\mathbf{x}_1, \cdots, \mathbf{x}_t, \cdots, \mathbf{x}_T]$ in our work, we infer that how likely the sequence of functional features X is generated from HMMs of NC (λ_{NC}) and MCI (λ_{MCI}), respectively, as follows:

$$p(X|\lambda_c) = \sum_S p(X|S, \lambda_c) P(S|\lambda_c) \tag{1}$$

where $c \in \{\text{NC}, \text{MCI}\}$, $S = [s_1, \cdots, s_t, \cdots, s_T]$, and $s_t \in \{1, \ldots, K\}$. Eq. (1) can be efficiently computed by the forward algorithm [13]. We identify the clinical label of the rs-fMRI of a test subject to the class of the higher data likelihood.

4 Experiments and Discussion

4.1 Experimental Settings

With regard to the structure of our DAE, we considered four hidden layers, *i.e.*, $L = 4$, to encode the input functional features by setting the number of hidden units as 200($\mathbf{h}^{(1)}$)-100($\mathbf{h}^{(2)}$)-50($\mathbf{h}^{(3)}$)-2($\mathbf{h}^{(4)}$). Thus, the decoder was structured as 50($\mathbf{h}^{(5)}$)-100($\mathbf{h}^{(6)}$)-200($\mathbf{h}^{(7)}$)[3]. A Gaussian-Bernoulli energy function was used for the input visible units, *i.e.*, $\mathbf{v}$ in Fig. 1, while a Bernoulli-Bernoulli energy function was exploited for the hidden layers by taking the outputs of the lower layer as inputs. But the units of the top hidden layer in the encoder, *i.e.*, $\mathbf{h}^{(4)}$ in Fig. 1, had stochastic real-values, allowing the low-dimensional codes to distribute in a continuous feature space [6].

[3] Therefore, the complete structure of our DAE was 116-200-100-50-2-50-100-200-116.

For the HMMs of NC and MCI classes, we varied the number of hidden states K from 2 to 6 with different number of Gaussians for emission *pdfs*, varying between 1 and 4. Due to a small data set, a circular state topology in Fig. 1(c) was used for both classes. In order to learn the parameters (A, B, Π), we used a BNT toolbox[4].

To validate the effectiveness of the proposed method, we compared with four competing methods in the literature, namely, group Independent Component Analysis (gICA) [12], group Sparse Representation (gSR) [16], Principal Component of Functional Connectivity (PCFC) [11], and a joint framework of HMM and Sparse Dictionary Learning (HMM+SDL) [2]. We also compared with a method of combining kernel Principal Component Analysis (kPCA) with HMM to validate the effectiveness of DAE-based dimension reduction.

- gICA: We applied a fastICA algorithm using a GIFT toolbox[5]. The number of independent components was set to 30 by following Li *et al.*'s work [12]. After performing group ICA, for each subject, we computed the correlation coefficients of every pair of time courses and used them as features.
- gSR: For the regularization control parameter, we applied a grid search technique in the space of $\{0.01, 0.05, 0.1, 0.15, 0.2, 0.5\}$. We used clustering coefficients obtained from a functional connectivity map as features.
- PCFC[6]: We used a sliding window-based Functional Network (FN) modeling with a window size of 30 time points and a stride of 5 time points between consecutive windows. The estimated FNs were then projected into eigen-networks, the number of which was determined based on eigenvalues such that the transformed features hold more than 85% of the total variance. The features from each FN were then concatenated into a long vector.
- HMM+SDL[7]: We set the weighting parameters to the priors of the covariance matrices to 1 by following the original work.
- kPCA+HMM: We used a Gaussian kernel. The dimensionality of a new space was determined based on the eigenvalues so as to reflect more than 85% of the total variance.

For the competing methods of gICA, gSR, and PCFC, we further applied feature selection based on the paired t-test and used a linear support vector machine as classifier. For both HMM+SBL and kPCA+HMM, the number of hidden states was varied between 2 and 6 with a circular topology as the proposed method. To evaluate the performance, we conducted a leave-one-subject-out cross-valuation technique due to small sample sizes.

4.2 Performance Comparison

We considered five different metrics to compare performance among the competing methods and showed the results in Table 1. In a nutshell, the proposed method achieved the best accuracy of 81.08% with a sensitivity of 85.71% and a specificity of 80%.

[4] Available at '`https://github.com/bayesnet/bnt`'

[5] Available at '`http://www.nitrc.org/projects/gift`'

[6] The codes are available at '`http://miplab.epfl.ch/leonardi/`'

[7] The source codes were provided by the author of the original paper [2].

Table 1. A summary of the performances of the competing methods. The boldface denotes the best performance in each metric. (PPV: Positive Predictive Value; NPV: Negative Predictive Value)

Methods	Accuracy (%)	Sensitivity (%)	Specificity (%)	PPV (%)	NPV (%)
gICA [12]	72.97	62.51	88.00	41.67	75.85
gSR [16]	75.68	80.00	75.00	33.33	96.00
PCFC [11]	75.68	71.43	**92.00**	41.67	76.67
HMM+SDL [2]	70.27	**100.0**	69.44	8.33	**100.0**
kPCA+HMM	70.27	60.00	**92.00**	25.00	71.88
Proposed method	**81.08**	85.71	80.00	**50.00**	96.00

Note that compared to HMM+SDL and kPCA+HMM, our method enhanced the classification accuracy by 10.81%. From a clinical perspective, since it is important to consider the prevalence of the disease, we also presented Positive Predictive Values (PPVs) and Negative Predictive Values (NPVs). Statistically, PPV and NPV measure, respectively, the proportion of subjects with MCI who are correctly diagnosed as patients and the proportion of subjects without MCI who are correctly diagnosed as cognitive normal. Our method achieved the PPV of 50% and the NPV of 96%, outperforming gICA by 8.33% (PPV) and 20.15% (NPV), gSR by 16.67% (PPV), PCFC by 8.33% (PPV) and 19.33% (NPV), and kPCA+HMM by 25% (PPV) and 24.12% (NPV). While HMM+SDL achieved a high NPV of 100%, its PPV was significantly lower than that of our method.

5 Conclusion

In this paper, we proposed a novel method to model functional dynamics in rs-fMRI for MCI identification. Specifically, we designed a deep network, by which we could discover the non-linear relationships among ROIs in a hierarchical manner and effectively reduce feature dimensionality. Meanwhile, by building generative models with HMMs for each class individually, we could estimate the feature likelihood of a test subject as MCI and NC, based on which we identified the clinical label. In our experiments, we achieved the highest performance with the proposed method, outperforming state-of-the-art methods in the literature. It is noteworthy that although it is not performed in this paper because of the limited space, by decoding the state sequence for the rs-fMRI data of a testing subject via Viterbi algorithm [13], we can construct functional connectivities, one for each hidden state, based on which further neurophysiological investigation can be conducted.

Acknowledgement. This work was supported by ICT R&D program of MSIP/IITP. [B0101-15-0307, Basic Software Research in Human-level Lifelong Machine Learning (Machine Learning Center)].

References

1. Biswal, B., Yetkin, F.Z., Haughton, V.M., Hyde, J.S.: Functional connectivity in the motor cortex of resting human brain using echo-planar MRI. Magnetic Resonance in Medicine 34(4), 537–541 (1995)
2. Eavani, H., Satterthwaite, T.D., Gur, R.E., Gur, R.C., Davatzikos, C.: Unsupervised learning of functional network dynamics in resting state fMRI. In: Gee, J.C., Joshi, S., Pohl, K.M., Wells, W.M., Zöllei, L. (eds.) IPMI 2013. LNCS, vol. 7917, pp. 426–437. Springer, Heidelberg (2013)
3. Faisan, S., Thoraval, L., Armspach, J.P., Heitz, F.: Hidden Markov multiple event sequence models: A paradigm for the spatio-temporal analysis of fMRI data. Medical Image Analysis 11(1), 1–20 (2007)
4. Handwerker, D.A., Roopchansingh, V., Gonzalez-Castillo, J., Bandettini, P.A.: Periodic changes in fMRI connectivity. NeuroImage 63(3), 1712–1719 (2012)
5. Hinton, G.E., Osindero, S., Teh, Y.W.: A fast learning algorithm for deep belief nets. Neural Computation 18(7), 1527–1554 (2006)
6. Hinton, G.E., Salakhutdinov, R.R.: Reducing the dimensionality of data with neural networks. Science 313(5786), 504–507 (2006)
7. Hjelm, R.D., Calhoun, V.D., Salakhutdinov, R., Allen, E.A., Adali, T., Plis, S.M.: Restricted Boltzmann machines for neuroimaging: An application in identifying intrinsic networks. NeuroImage 96, 245–260 (2014)
8. Hutchinson, R.A., Niculescu, R.S., Keller, T.A., Rustandi, I., Mitchell, T.M.: Modeling fMRI data generated by overlapping cognitive processes with unknown onsets using hidden process models. NeuroImage 46(1), 87–104 (2009)
9. Hutchison, R.M., Womelsdorf, T., Allen, E.A., Bandettini, P.A., Calhoun, V.D., Corbetta, M., Penna, S.D., Duyn, J.H., Glover, G.H., Gonzalez-Castillo, J., Handwerker, D.A., Keilholz, S., Kiviniemi, V., Leopold, D.A., de Pasquale, F., Sporns, O., Walter, M., Chang, C.: Dynamic functional connectivity: Promise, issues, and interpretations. NeuroImage 80, 360–378 (2013)
10. Janoos, F., Machiraju, R., Singh, S., Morocz, I.: Spatio-temporal models of mental processes from fMRI. NeuroImage 57(2), 362–377 (2011)
11. Leonardi, N., Richiardi, J., Gschwind, M., Simioni, S., Annoni, J.M., Schluep, M., Vuilleumier, P., Ville, D.V.D.: Principal components of functional connectivity: A new approach to study dynamic brain connectivity during rest. NeuroImage 83, 937–950 (2013)
12. Li, S., Eloyan, A., Joel, S., Mostofsky, S., Pekar, J., Bassett, S.S., Caffo, B.: Analysis of group ICA-based connectivity measures from fMRI: Application to Alzheimer's disease. PLoS One 7(11), e49340 (2012)
13. Rabiner, L.: A tutorial on hidden Markov models and selected applications in speech recognition. Proceedings of the IEEE 77(2), 257–286 (1989)
14. Rubinov, M., Sporns, O.: Complex networks measures of brain connectivity: Uses and interpretations. NeuroImage 52(3), 1059–1069 (2010)
15. Suk, H.I., Wee, C.Y., Lee, S.W., Shen, D.: Supervised discriminative group sparse representation for mild cognitive impairment diagnosis. Neuroinformatics, 1–19 (2014)
16. Wee, C.Y., Yap, P.T., Zhang, D., Wang, L., Shen, D.: Group-constrained sparse fMRI connectivity modeling for mild cognitive impairment identification. Brain Structure and Function 219(2), 641–656 (2014)

Combining Unsupervised Feature Learning and Riesz Wavelets for Histopathology Image Representation: Application to Identifying Anaplastic Medulloblastoma

Sebastian Otálora[1], Angel Cruz-Roa[1], John Arevalo[1], Manfredo Atzori[2], Anant Madabhushi[3], Alexander R. Judkins[4], Fabio González[1], Henning Müller[2], and Adrien Depeursinge[2,5]

[1] Universidad Nacional de Colombia, Bogotá, Colombia
[2] University of Applied Sciences Western Switzerland (HES-SO)
[3] Case Western Reserve University, Cleveland, OH, USA
[4] St. Jude Childrens Research Hospital from Memphis, TN, USA
[5] Ecole Polytechnique Fédérale de Lausanne (EPFL), Switzerland

Abstract. Medulloblastoma (MB) is a type of brain cancer that represent roughly 25% of all brain tumors in children. In the anaplastic medulloblastoma subtype, it is important to identify the degree of irregularity and lack of organizations of cells as this correlates to disease aggressiveness and is of clinical value when evaluating patient prognosis. This paper presents an image representation to distinguish these subtypes in histopathology slides. The approach combines learned features from (i) an unsupervised feature learning method using topographic independent component analysis that captures scale, color and translation invariances, and (ii) learned linear combinations of Riesz wavelets calculated at several orders and scales capturing the granularity of multiscale rotation-covariant information. The contribution of this work is to show that the combination of two complementary approaches for feature learning (unsupervised and supervised) improves the classification performance. Our approach outperforms the best methods in literature with statistical significance, achieving 99% accuracy over region-based data comprising 7,500 square regions from 10 patient studies diagnosed with medulloblastoma (5 anaplastic and 5 non-anaplastic).

1 Introduction

Medulloblastoma (MB) is a type of brain cancer that represent roughly 25% of all brain tumours in children, it grows in the cerebellum on the lower, rear portion of the brain. Classifying MB is useful to determine aggressive phenotypes that require intense and early treatments [5, 7]. There are subtypes of MB based on histological appearance. These include classical, anaplastic, and desmoplastic. In anaplastic MB, the degree of anaplasia correlates to disease aggressiveness and is of clinical value when evaluating patient prognosis [7]. The problem of

N. Navab et al. (Eds.): MICCAI 2015, Part I, LNCS 9349, pp. 581–588, 2015.
DOI: 10.1007/978-3-319-24553-9_71

distinguishing between anaplastic and non anaplastic MB is difficult mainly due to the complexity of the patterns found in the histopathology images and is due to cell organization, size, shape and orientation variability towards the different malignant grades of the tumor. Examples of several tissue patterns from cases of MB whole slide images (WSI) are shown in Fig. 1. Common approaches for

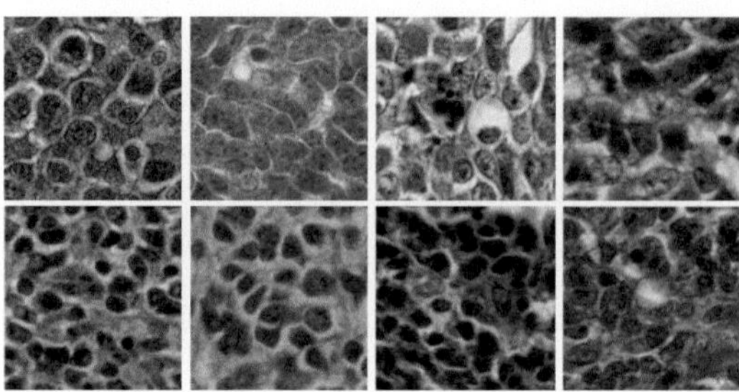

Fig. 1. Inter and intra class variability from MB tumor tiles of WSI at 40× magnification: anaplastic (Top), non-anaplastic (Bottom)

automatic tumor grading and phenotype differentiation rely on the identification of informative and discriminative features of the visual morphological patterns found in WSI. Unfortunately, they usually fail at capturing the variety of complex patterns present in the WSI, for example, considering only the subtle patterns captured by texture descriptors. This highlights the need for more powerful techniques or combinations of techniques to overcome the challenging tasks of automatical analysis of WSI [12].

Learning appropriate representations directly from data is a powerful machine learning strategy that has recently been applied with great success to pattern recognition problems, including image understanding and speech recognition [11, 10]. The representative techniques are mainly based on neural networks and can be grouped into two types: deep learning algorithms and unsupervised feature learning (UFL). An important assumption of these methods is that data patterns can be represented by the interaction of several factors at several hierarchically organized levels with semantically increasing content. Convolutional Neural Networks (CNN) are a representative technique where the features are hierarchically learned through several layers that combine convolution and pooling with non-linear functions [10].

For MB tumor differentiation, previous work [1] showed that the use of deep learning and UFL techniques outperforms classical texture descriptors. In [2], the authors made a comparative evaluation of several representation learning techniques including CNNs, Topographic Independent Component Analysis (TICA) and sparse Autoencoders (sAE), against MR8 and Haar texture descriptors. The results demonstrated the superior performance of the features learned by TICA, which builds a rotation and translation invariant representation of cell organizations in the anaplastic MB subtype.

Neural networks are the dominant approach for representation learning. However there are other representation learning strategies that are able to adapt conventional image descriptors to the needs of a particular image analysis task. In [3], the authors propose a multiscale texture signature learning approach using rotation-covariant Riesz wavelets, where most relevant combinations of orientations and scales are learned directly from the data. This approach outperformed state-of-the-art representations based on local binary patterns and grey level cooccurrence matrices for lung tissue classification [4]. Drawbacks of the data driven representations approaches are the amount of parameters involved that have to be manually tuned, which requires more time in model training. Some texture based representations fail to describe the feature patterns present in training samples that the data-driven approach is able to find [1].

In this work, we propose a joint framework for classification of MB WSI, where the invariant properties of TICA features and the multiscale rotation-covariant properties of Riesz wavelet features complement each other. We hypothesize that this fusion can lead to a better classification performance. This work join efforts of [3] and [1] in a simple manner to achieve the best accuracy reported for this histopathology WSI database.

2 Methodological Description

2.1 Topographic Independent Component Analysis

TICA is an unsupervised feature learning model, inspired by findings of the visual cortex behaviour. It groups activations of units in order to discover features that are rotation and translation invariant [1]. These are appropriate features for histopathology image characterization since shapes and cell organizations can be present regardless of the position or orientation of cells. Particularly, TICA organizes feature detectors in a square matrix for l groups such that adjacent feature detectors activate in a similar proportion to the same stimulus. To learn such groups, we need to optimize the cost function:

$$J_{\text{TICA}}(\mathbf{W}) = \frac{\lambda}{2}\sum_{i=1}^{T}\left\|\mathbf{W}^{\text{T}}\mathbf{W}x^{(i)} - x^{(i)}\right\|_2^2 + \sum_{i=1}^{m}\sum_{k=1}^{l}\sqrt{\mathbf{H}_k(\mathbf{W}x^{(i)})^2 + \epsilon} \qquad (1)$$

where $x^{(i)} \in \mathbb{R}^m$ is the *i-th* sample, T is the number of samples, $\mathbf{W} \in \mathbb{R}^{n\times m}$ is the matrix that encodes the features in each row, and $\mathbf{H} \in \{0,1\}^{l\times n}$ is the binary topographic organization where $\mathbf{H}_k^{(j)} = 1$, if the j-th feature detector, j-th row of $\mathbf{W}$, belongs to the k-th group, and 0 otherwise. This model sets $\mathbf{H}$ fixed while learning $\mathbf{W}$. In addition, TICA has two main computational advantages. First, the only parameters to be tuned are the regularization hyperparameter λ and the sparsity controller ϵ. Second, it is an unconstrained optimization problem, which can be solved efficiently by optimization techniques such as Limited memory-Broyden-Fletcher-Goldfarb-Shanno (L-BFGS).

2.2 Image Representation via Rotation-Covariant Riesz Wavelets

A fine to coarse wavelet image representation is obtained using Riesz wavelets. Class-wise texture signatures are learned for each scale as follows. First, image tiles are expressed in a feature space spanned by the energies of the responses of Riesz components. Then, an optimal linear combination of the Riesz components is learned using support vector machines (SVM) to maximize the margin between two classes. This linear combination yields class-wise texture signatures, that are locally aligned to maximize its response at the smallest scale, yielding rotation-covariant texture representations [3]. The wealth of the filterbank is controlled by the order N of the Riesz transform $\boldsymbol{\mathcal{R}}$, defined in the Fourier domain as:

$$\widehat{\mathcal{R}^{(n_1,n_2)}f}(\boldsymbol{\omega}) = \sqrt{\frac{n_1+n_2}{n_1!n_2!}}\frac{(-j\omega_1)^{n_1}(-j\omega_2)^{n_2}}{||\boldsymbol{\omega}||^{n_1+n_2}}\hat{f}(\boldsymbol{\omega}),$$

for all the combinations of (n_1, n_2) with $n_{1,2} \in \mathbb{N}$ such that $n_1 + n_2 = N$. The vector $\boldsymbol{\omega}$ is composed of $\omega_{1,2}$ corresponding to the frequencies along the two image axes and $\hat{f}(\boldsymbol{\omega})$ is the Fourier transform of $f(\boldsymbol{x})$. The Riesz transform yields $N{+}1$ distinct components behaving as N-th order directional differential operators when coupled with a multi-resolution framework based on isotropic band-limited wavelets ψ_s, with $s = 1, \cdots, S$ the number of iterations of the wavelet transform. An interesting property of Riesz wavelets is that the response of each component $\mathcal{R}^{(n_1,n_2)}$, rotated by an arbitrary angle θ, can be derived from a linear combination of the responses from all components of the filterbank. This steerability property is leveraged to obtain rotation covariant-texture features [3]. For a class c, the multiscale texture signature Γ_c^N is defined as:

$$\Gamma_c^N = w_1\left(\mathcal{R}^{(N,0)}\right)_{s=1} + w_2\left(G * \mathcal{R}^{(N-1,1)}\right)_{s=1} + \cdots + w_{SN+S}\left(G * \mathcal{R}^{(0,N+1)}\right)_{s=S}.$$

SVMs are used to find the optimal weights $\boldsymbol{w}^{\mathrm{T}} = (w_1 \ldots w_{SN+S})$[3]. Finally, the local orientations of each signature are optimized to maximize their local magnitude at the first scale $\Gamma_{c,1}^N$. The final representation is a vector of dimensionality $(N+1) \times J \times k$, where k is the number of classes.

2.3 Fusing UFL and Riesz Features

Once we have the features for each tissue tile, the features are concatenated. The latter is used as input to feed a standard softmax classifier with weight decay regularization. Two outputs of the classifier represent the probability for a tissue tile being considered as anaplastic or not, respectively. To train the models weights Θ that map the fused features into the anaplastic probability, the following cost function is minimized with an L-BFGS procedure:

$$J(\Theta) = -\frac{1}{m}\left[\sum_{i=1}^{m}\sum_{j=1}^{k}\mathbb{I}\{y^{(i)} = j\}\log\left(\frac{\exp\Theta_j x^{(i)}}{\sum_{l=1}^{k}\exp\Theta_l x^{(i)}}\right)\right] + \frac{\rho}{2}\sum_{i=1}^{k}\sum_{j=1}^{n}\Theta_{ij}^2,$$

where m stands for the number of samples, and k is the number of classes, and ρ is the weight decay parameter that penalizes large values for parameters. The fused representation of an unseen test tissue tile $x^{(p)} \in \mathbb{R}^{(N+1)Jk+l}$ is classified as anaplastic (or non-anaplastic) by calculating a probability:

$$p(y^p = 1|x^p; \Theta) = \frac{\exp(\Theta_1 x^{(p)})}{\sum_{l=1}^{2} \exp(\Theta_l x^{(p)})}.$$

A tile belongs to the anaplastic class if $p(y^p|x^p; \Theta) > 0.5$ and non-anaplastic otherwise.

3 Experimental Results and Discussion

The workflow of the proposed approach is summarized in Fig. 2. As first step, we compute the UFL features learned by TICA and the supervised features learned with Riesz wavelets for each image as described in Sections 2.1 and 2.2. Once TICA and Riesz wavelets are computed a final step of supervised classification is made using the combination of the computed features in a concatenated vector as input for a standard softmax classifier as described in Section 2.3. Parameter tuning is presented in Section 3.2.

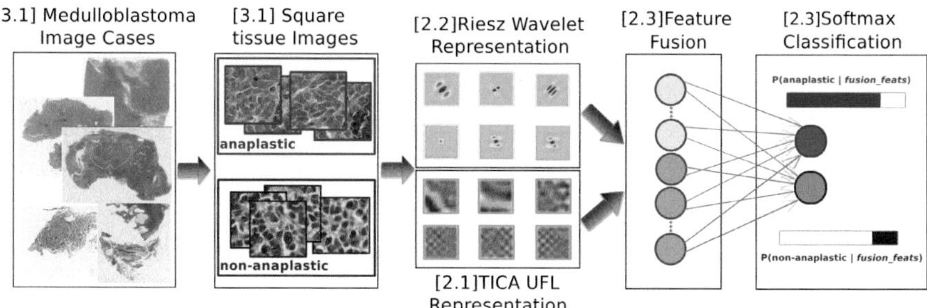

Fig. 2. Flowchart for MB feature extraction and classification for both learned representations: Riesz and TICA, the details of each stage are described in subsections.

3.1 Medulloblastoma Dataset

Our MB database is from St. Jude Childrens Research Hospital in Memphis where a neuropathologist manually annotated the cancerous regions of 10 pathology slides, 5 diagnosed as anaplastic and 5 as non-anaplastic MB. Slides were stained with hematoxylin and eosin (H&E) and digitization was done on an Aperio Scanner obtaining WSI with a resolution of 80,000×80,000 pixels. Each image can have several cancerous regions, which were manually annotated. For training, we randomly extracted a total of 7,500 square regions (750 per case) of 200×200 pixels of the tumor regions (3,750 anaplastic and 3,750 non-anaplastic).

3.2 Experimental Setup

In order to evaluate the advantages of the presented approach we compare the performance of the state-of-the art work on this database [1, 7]. In [7], the authors used a bag-of-visual-words approach using texton-based features obtained from Haar wavelets and MR8 filterbanks. In [1], the authors perform an extensive comparison between UFL techniques (sAE and TICA) and CNN, showing that the TICA outperforms by a considerable margin the previous approaches in [7]. Our evaluations follow the same leave-two-patients-out cross-validation scheme that consist of 20 trials where for each 4 of the non-anaplastic and 4 of the anaplastic cases are randomly selected for training whereas the remaining 2 slides (i.e., 1 non-anaplastic and 1 anaplastic) are used for validation. The architectures and setup for the approaches are summarized as:

- 2-Layer CNN: The best CNN model reported in baseline [1] was reproduced, consisting of a 2-layer architecture with 225 features in the first layer, and 225 units on the fully-connected layer. The feature kernel was of 8×8 pixels and a pool size of 2×2.
- TICA: The best of the three different TICA models reported in baseline [1] were reproduced: $\text{TICA}^{225}_{F:8,P:1}$ using a pool size of 1 and using 225 features with a feature kernel size of 8×8.
- Riesz wavelets: For the presented Riesz wavelet representation we explore the order N of the wavelet as well as the number of scales J as $N \in [1, 2, 3, 4, 5]$ and $J \in [1, 2, 3, 4]$. We also tried concatenations of orders and scales.
- TICA + Riesz fusion: For the combination of the best approaches we propose to build a joint vector 240 features for each of the tiles composed of the 225 best features found by TICA and the 15 features of the concatenation of the Riesz wavelets of orders 1,2,3 and scales 2,2,1 respectively.

For softmax the weight decay parameter was explored logarithmically in the range [1e-10, 100]. The performance measures are accuracy, sensitivity and specificity.

3.3 Results

Table 1 presents the results of the approaches. The best results were obtained by combining TICA and Riesz wavelets. We show some qualitative digital annotation results on 2 sample test cases in Fig. 3. We compare the statistical significance of the results of the combined representation and the TICA results with the Kruskal-Wallis test that calculates the average rank of the accuracy results of two approaches on the 20 trials, and compute the p-value for the null hypothesis that the two set of results comes from the same distribution. The test gives us a p-value of 2.5394^{-7} at a 1% significance level, hence we reject the null hypothesis.

Table 1. MB classification performance (baseline, Riesz, fusion). The measures are averaged over the 20 test runs with standard deviation where available.

Method	Accuracy	Sensitivity	Specificity
TICA + Riesz$[N_3^1, N_2^2, N_1^2]$	**0.997 ± 0.002**	**0.995 ± 0.004**	**1 ± 0**
TICA [1]	0.972 ± 0.018	0.977 ± 0.021	0.967 ± 0.031
Riesz $[N_3^1, N_2^2, N_1^2]$ [3]	0.964 ± 0.038	0.999 ± 0.001	0.932 ± 0.07
Riesz $[N_3^1]$ [3]	0.958 ± 0.062	0.963 ± 0.05	0.916 ± 0.125
Riesz $[N_2^2]$ [3]	0.94 ± 0.02	0.94 ± 0.02	0.3 ± 0.04
2-Layer *CNN* [1]	0.90 ± 0.1	0.89 ± 0.18	0.9 ± 0.0.3
sAE [1]	0.90	0.87	0.93
BOF + *A2NMF* (Haar) [2]	0.87	0.86	0.87
Riesz $[N_1^2]$ [3]	0.85 ± 0.23	0.9 ± 0.15	0.7 ± 0.47
BOF + K - NN (Haar) [7]	0.80	-	-
BOF + K - NN (MR8) [7]	0.62	-	-

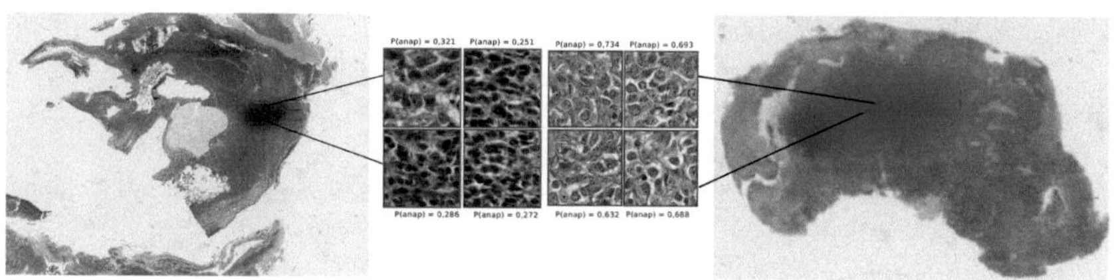

Fig. 3. Predictions over two WSIs, non-anaplastic MB (left) and anaplastic (right).

4 Concluding Remarks

We present a feature fusion between unsupervised feature learning and supervised Riesz wavelet representation that captures subtle pattern of textures as well as high level features, allowing to create a more separable feature space where the differentiation of medulloblastoma into anaplastic and non-anaplastic can be made with high classification accuracy outperforming any other result previously described in the literature. To our knowledge this is the first time that a feature fusion method is presented between UFL and the Riesz wavelets in the context of histopathology image analysis showing the complementarity between these learned features for the challenging task of tumour differentiation, we are currently working on extending the method to other patch-based histopathology image analysis problems with larger cohorts of patients.

Acknowledgments. This work was supported by the SNSF (PZ00P2_154891), by the Administrative Department of Science, Technology and Innovation of Colombia (Colciencias) (1225-569-34920) and by Microsoft Research LACCIR (R1212LAC006). Otlora and Cruz-Roa thank for the Young Researcher and Doctoral Fellowship grants (645/2014, 528/2011). The authors thank for K40 Tesla GPU donated by NVIDIA used for the training process.

References

[1] Cruz-Roa, A., Arevalo, J., Basavanhally, A., et al.: A comparative evaluation of supervised and unsupervised representation learning approaches for anaplastic medulloblastoma differentiation. In: Proc. SPIE 9287, pp. 92870G–92870G–6 (2015)

[2] Cruz-Roa, A., González, F., Galaro, J., Judkins, A.R., Ellison, D., Baccon, J., Madabhushi, A., Romero, E.: A visual latent semantic approach for automatic analysis and interpretation of anaplastic medulloblastoma virtual slides. In: Ayache, N., Delingette, H., Golland, P., Mori, K. (eds.) MICCAI 2012, Part I. LNCS, vol. MICCAI 2012, pp. 157–164. Springer, Heidelberg (2012)

[3] Depeursinge, A., Foncubierta-Rodriguez, A., Van De Ville, D., Müller, H.: Rotation–covariant texture learning using steerable Riesz wavelets. IEEE Transactions on Image Processing 23(2), 898–908 (2014)

[4] Depeursinge, A., Foncubierta–Rodriguez, A., Van de Ville, D., Müller, H.: Multiscale lung texture signature learning using the riesz transform. In: Ayache, N., Delingette, H., Golland, P., Mori, K. (eds.) MICCAI 2012, Part III. LNCS, vol. 7512, pp. 517–524. Springer, Heidelberg (2012)

[5] Ellison, D.W.: Childhood medulloblastoma: novel approaches to the classification of a heterogeneous disease. Acta Neuropathologica 120(3), 305–316 (2010)

[6] Fuchs, T.J., Buhmann, J.M.: Computational pathology: Challenges and promises for tissue analysis. Computerized Medical Imaging and Graphics 35(7–8), 515–530 (2011)

[7] Galaro, J., Judkins, A., Ellison, D., Baccon, J., Madabhushi, A.: An integrated texton and bag of words classifier for identifying anaplastic medulloblastomas. In: EMBC, 2011 Annual International Conference of the IEEE, pp. 3443–3446 (2011)

[8] Gurcan, M.N., Boucheron, L.E., Can, A., et al.: Histopathological image analysis: A review. IEEE Reviews in Biomedical Engineering 2, 147–171 (2009)

[9] Kothari, S., Phan, J.H., Stokes, T.H., Wang, M.D.: Pathology imaging informatics for quantitative analysis of whole-slide images. Journal of the American Medical Informatics Association 20(6), 1099 (2013)

[10] Krizhevsky, A., Sutskever, I., Hinton, G.E.: Imagenet classification with deep convolutional neural networks. In: Advances in Neural Information Processing Systems, vol. 25, pp. 1097–1105 (2012)

[11] Ranzato, M., Huang, F.J., Boureau, Y.L., LeCun, Y.: Unsupervised learning of invariant feature hierarchies with applications to object recognition. In: IEEE Conference on Computer Vision and Pattern Recognition, pp. 1–8 (2007)

[12] Wang, H., Cruz-Roa, A., Basavanhally, A., et al.: Mitosis detection in breast cancer pathology images by combining handcrafted and convolutional neural network features. Journal of Medical Imaging 1(3), 34003 (2014)

Automatic Coronary Calcium Scoring in Cardiac CT Angiography Using Convolutional Neural Networks

Jelmer M. Wolterink[1,⋆], Tim Leiner[2], Max A. Viergever[1], and Ivana Išgum[1]

[1] Image Sciences Institute, UMC Utrecht, Utrecht, The Netherlands
[2] Department of Radiology, UMC Utrecht, Utrecht, The Netherlands

Abstract. The amount of coronary artery calcification (CAC) is a strong and independent predictor of cardiovascular events. Non-contrast enhanced cardiac CT is considered a reference for quantification of CAC. Recently, it has been shown that CAC may be quantified in cardiac CT angiography (CCTA). We present a pattern recognition method that automatically identifies and quantifies CAC in CCTA. The study included CCTA scans of 50 patients equally distributed over five cardiovascular risk categories. CAC in CCTA was identified in two stages. In the first stage, potential CAC voxels were identified using a convolutional neural network (CNN). In the second stage, candidate CAC lesions were extracted based on the CNN output for analyzed voxels and thereafter described with a set of features and classified using a Random Forest. Ten-fold stratified cross-validation experiments were performed. CAC volume was quantified per patient and compared with manual reference annotations in the CCTA scan. Bland-Altman bias and limits of agreement between reference and automatic annotations were -15 (-198–168) after the first stage and -3 (-86 – 79) after the second stage. The results show that CAC can be automatically identified and quantified in CCTA using the proposed method. This might obviate the need for a dedicated non-contrast-enhanced CT scan for CAC scoring, which is regularly acquired prior to a CCTA scan, and thus reduce the CT radiation dose received by patients.

Keywords: Automatic coronary artery calcium scoring, Cardiac CTA, Convolutional neural network, Random Forest.

1 Introduction

Cardiovascular disease (CVD) is the global leading cause of death. The amount of coronary artery calcification (CAC) is a strong and independent predictor of CVD events, which can be identified and quantified in cardiac CT [1]. In clinical practice, CAC is routinely quantified using non-contrast enhanced, calcium scoring CT (CSCT) [2]. Recently, it has been shown that CAC may also be quantified in contrast-enhanced cardiac CT angiography (CCTA). Consequently,

⋆ This work has been financially supported by PIE Medical Imaging.

N. Navab et al. (Eds.): MICCAI 2015, Part I, LNCS 9349, pp. 589–596, 2015.
DOI: 10.1007/978-3-319-24553-9_72

a dedicated CSCT scan, which is often routinely acquired prior to CCTA, might potentially be omitted. This could reduce the radiation dose of a typical cardiac CT examination by 40-50% [3]. CAC in CSCT can be identified manually by an expert or automatically [4,5]. In both situations, a threshold of 130 HU is used to identify connected voxels representing CAC. This method is not generalizable to CCTA. The coronary artery lumen is typically enhanced beyond 130 HU, which makes differentiation of CAC and lumen challenging. Other global attenuation thresholds for manual CAC scoring in CCTA have therefore been proposed [6,7]. However, a global threshold might limit the applicability of the method to scans acquired with different protocols, scanners or contrast agents. Alternatively, patient-specific attenuation thresholds were proposed, based on HU values taken from an ROI in the ascending aorta [8] or the proximal coronary arteries [9]. A drawback of these thresholds is the limited repeatability of user-defined ROIs. Furthermore, the large number of image slices in CCTA (> 200) makes routine manual scoring of CAC in CCTA time-consuming.

To overcome these limitations, automatic methods have been proposed. Previously published automatic methods were based on a (semi)-automatically extracted segmentation of the coronary arteries. This segmentation was used to identify CAC as deviations from a trend line through the lumen intensity [10,11], deviations from a model of non-calcified artery segments [12], or as voxels in the extracted arteries with intensities above a patient-specific HU threshold [13]. These methods have shown good performance, but depend on successful coronary artery extraction. This might fail in patients with complex anatomy, in the distal segments of the coronary arteries or in scans with motion or noise artifacts. In addition, severe CAC deposits affect the performance of artery extraction algorithms, restricting their applicability in CAC identification [14]. Failure of the extraction step would result in failure of the automatic CAC scoring method.

Therefore, we propose a novel pattern recognition based method, which identifies CAC in CCTA without artery extraction. The method uses a convolutional neural network (CNN) for the identification of potential CAC voxels and subsequently a Random Forest for the identification of CAC lesions. Previous work has demonstrated that CNNs can provide insights via automatically derived feature hierarchies leading to highly accurate results [15,16]. In this paper, we combine texture features that the CNN automatically derives from image patches with basic location features that are extracted from the input image. Automatically derived CAC scores are compared with manual annotations in CCTA and CSCT.

2 Material and Methods

2.1 Data

We retrospectively inspected 116 CT examinations of consecutively scanned patients for whom both a CCTA and a CSCT scan were available. CAC scores (Agatston scores) had previously been manually determined in the CSCT scans by experts. Based on these scores, ten consecutively scanned patients from each of five CVD risk categories (I:0, II:1-10, III: 11-100, IV:101-400, V:>400) [1] were included in the data set. The CCTA of one additional patient with CAC score zero was included as an atlas. All CCTA scans were acquired on a 256-detector row scanner (Philips Brilliance iCT, Philips Medical, Best, The Netherlands) using 120 kVp and 210-300 mAs, with ECG-triggering and contrast enhancement. Reconstructed sections had 0.45 mm spacing, 0.90 mm thickness and 0.4-0.5 $\times$ 0.4-0.5 mm in-plane resolution.

To train and evaluate the method, manual reference annotations in the CCTA scans were obtained as follows. A region of interest in the ascending aorta was manually defined. The mean HU_{aorta} and standard deviation SD of the intensities in this region were used to compute a patient-specific threshold HU_{aorta} + 2 SD [8]. This threshold was locally adjusted to correct for erroneous inclusion of contrast-enhanced lumen. CAC lesions were manually annotated with region growing in the thresholded image.

2.2 Automatic CAC Scoring

The proposed method for automatic CAC scoring consisted of two stages: a voxel classification stage and a lesion classification stage. In the voxel classification stage, potential CAC locations were identified using a CNN. Based on the output of the CNN, 3D-connected voxels with a high probability of being CAC (p_{CAC}) were extracted as lesions. These lesions were described by a set of features and classified as CAC or non-CAC using a Random Forest classifier. Identified CAC volume and Agatston score were quantified per patient.

Candidates in the voxel classification stage were voxels with intensity above a patient-specific threshold θ_{PS}, the 98th percentile of the CCTA HU intensity histogram. This is a conservative threshold which correlated well (Spearman's ρ 0.89) with that proposed in [8]. Determination of this threshold required no user interaction. Each voxel was represented by three 24 $\times$ 24 patches from orthogonal planes centered at the voxel [15,16]. The patch size was chosen to be large enough to contain CAC lesions of moderate size or the surrounding coronary artery lumen, while remaining within the computational limitations of our hardware. Figure 1 shows an example candidate with orthogonal patches (bottom left). Because patches were small, they did not convey much anatomical information. Therefore, images were registered to the atlas CCTA using affine and elastic registration with *elastiX* [17] and parameters as in [5], and voxel x, y and z-coordinates in the atlas image were computed as location features.

A CNN with two convolutional and max-pooling layers, two fully connected hidden layers and a softmax output layer was used (Figure 1). Features were derived from the orthogonal input patches in the convolutional layers and combined with the three location features as input to the first hidden layer. All units used the rectifier activation function [18]. The network was trained with mini-batch learning and RMSprop, which uses a moving average of recent gradients to normalize the gradient in each iteration [19]. We sought to obtain translation invariant features by max-pooling after each convolutional layer. To prevent overfitting, Dropout was used to simulate the training of a large number

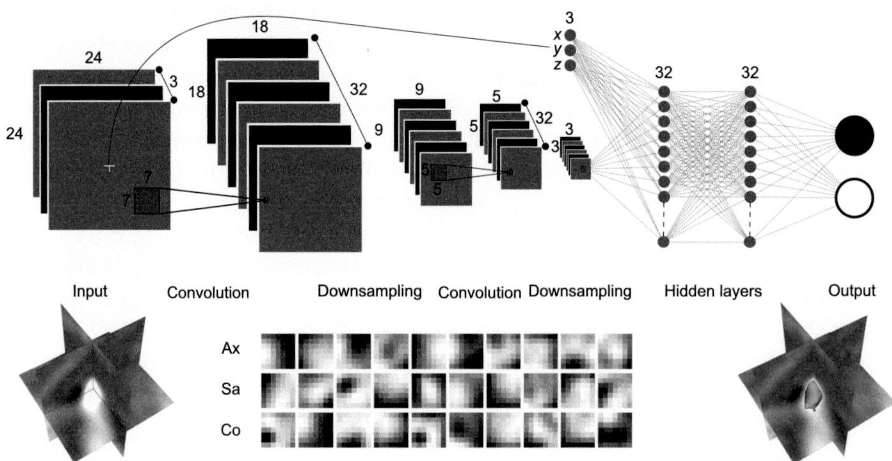

Fig. 1. *Top* CNN architecture. The CNN had two convolutional layers with max-pooling, two fully connected hidden layers and one softmax output layer. Location features (x, y, z) were additional input to the first hidden layer. *Bottom* Example input CAC voxel representation: three orthogonal input patches of size 24×24. Convolutional filters for axial (Ax), sagittal (Sa) and coronal (Co) input patches. Rendering of thresholded output for candidate and neighboring voxels.

of thinned networks [20]. The softmax output layer of the CNN returned p_{CAC}: the probability of a candidate voxel to belong to a CAC lesion.

In the lesion classification stage, p_{CAC} was first thresholded to consider only voxels that were likely CAC. The threshold value ($p_{CAC} \geq 0.75$) was set based on precision-recall analysis of the voxel classification, so that most CAC voxels were retained and individual lesions could be extracted by 3D-connected component labeling. Each extracted lesion was described by 14 features. The following statistics of the p_{CAC} values of the voxels in the candidate lesion were features: minimum, maximum, range, average and standard deviation. These features were supplemented with features that have been shown to benefit CAC detection in CSCT [4,5]: lesion volume and the minimum, maximum, range, average and standard deviation of intensity values of voxels in the lesion. Furthermore, x, y and z-coordinates of lesions in the atlas image were used as location features. All features were used as input to a Random Forest classifier [21].

3 Experiments and Results

For both CNN and Random Forest classification, experiments were performed using stratified ten-fold cross validation. Each fold contained one patient in each of five CVD risk categories.

To train and test the CNNs, approximately $800,000$ candidate voxels were extracted per patient. From these, 15,000 candidates were selected for training,

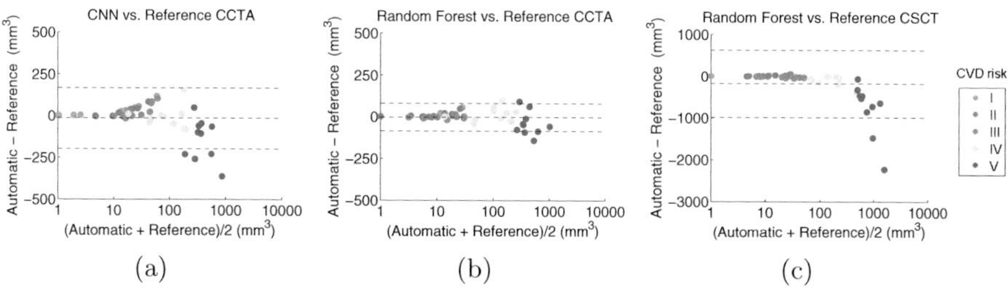

Fig. 2. Bland-Altman plots comparing reference and automatic per patient CAC volume in CCTA. Automatic results after (a) CNN output thresholding and (b) Random Forest lesion classification. In (c), Random Forest lesion classification is compared with reference CAC volume in CSCT. Patients are color-coded according to their CSCT-based CVD risk category.

including all positives (CAC) and a random selection of negatives. Hence, for each fold a CNN was trained with $45 \times 15,000 = 675,000$ candidates using mini-batch training with batches of 512 samples. The Dropout retention probability was 0.5 for all units. CNNs were implemented in Theano [22] and run on single Nvidia GRID K520 GPUs. For each fold, a separate CNN was trained for 30 epochs with a training time of 4,5 hours. Voxel classification for a single scan took approximately ten minutes. Figure 1 shows convolution filters trained in the first layer of one of the trained CNNs.

To train and test the Random Forest a total of 2268 candidate lesions were extracted by thresholding at $p_{CAC} \geq 0.75$ and 3D-connected component labeling of the thresholded image. Among candidates, 253 were positives, constituting 30% of candidate volume. All extracted candidates were used for training. Hence, for each fold a Random Forest was trained with approximately 2041 candidates. The four most important features in the Random Forest classification were the mean, maximum and standard deviation of voxel intensities and the minimum CNN output value p_{CAC} in a candidate.

The output of the CNN (p_{CAC}) may be directly thresholded for voxel classification and CAC quantification. Thresholding at $p_{CAC} \geq 0.95$ resulted in Bland-Altman mean and limits of agreement of -15 (-198–168) (Figure 2a). Lesion extraction and Random Forest classification improved these values to -2 (-86 –79) (Figure 2b). However, CAC volume was overestimated for several patients in the lower two CVD risk categories, including one patient with a calcified mediastinal lymph node and one patient with a CAC-like lesion near the sternum.

Figure 2c shows a comparison of automatically determined CAC volumes in CCTA and reference CAC volumes in CSCT. CAC volume and Agatston scores were substantially lower in CCTA than in CSCT, which agrees with previously published studies on manual CAC scoring in CCTA [8,23]. Nevertheless, CAC quantification in CCTA can differentiate between patients with zero

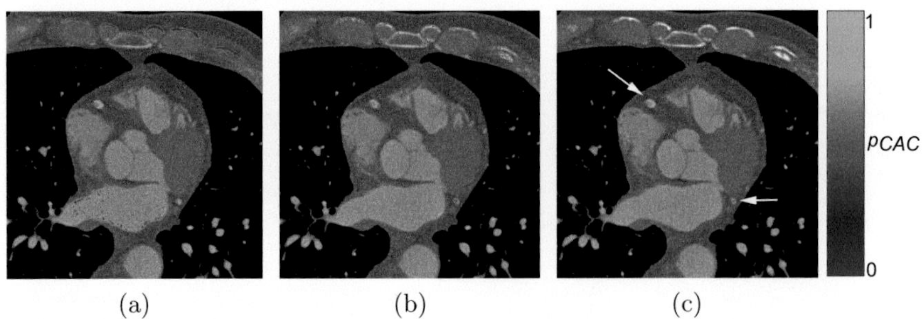

Fig. 3. Output of three CNNs on example image slice. (a) Using only location information, candidates near the center of the scan were favored. (b) Using only patch values, ribs were erroneously identified as CAC. (c) Using both patch values and location information, only true CAC in the right and left circumflex coronary artery (arrows) was detected.

CAC and non-zero CAC. Namely, the method correctly identified 8/10 patients with zero CAC according to CSCT and 36/40 patients with non-zero CAC as determined with CSCT. In addition, the method correctly identified 9/10 patients at very high risk of a CVD event (Agatston score $>$ 400) according to CSCT and 40/40 patients at low or intermediate risk of a CVD event (Agatston score $\leq$ 400).

The CNNs used features derived from the input patches, as well as information about the location of candidates. To evaluate the effect of these location features on CAC identification, we trained two additional CNNs for one fold. One CNN was trained with patch values set to zero, but location features preserved. A second CNN was trained with location features set to zero, but patch values preserved. Figure 3 shows that the CNN that only used location features (Figure 3a) favored candidates in the heart, but made no distinction between true CAC and attenuated blood. The CNN that only used patch input (Figure 3b) identified calcific objects, but made no distinction between CAC and ribs. The full CNN (Figure 3c) used both location and texture information to correctly identify two CAC lesions in the right and left circumflex coronary arteries.

4 Discussion and Conclusion

A pattern recognition method for the automatic identification of CAC in CCTA has been described. The method uses CNNs to locate likely CAC voxels and Random Forests to classify extracted CAC lesions. To our knowledge, this is the first application of CNNs to CAC scoring in CT. In contrast to other automatic CAC scoring methods, it does not rely on automatic coronary artery extraction.

The results showed that CNNs were able to identify voxels likely to be CAC. Combining automatically derived patch-based texture features and candidate location features proved advantageous. However, the use of a single atlas for location determination might introduce bias towards a single image. In future work, we will investigate a multi-atlas based coordinate space, which could also aid candidate voxel extraction. Extraction was now based on HU thresholds, similar but not equal to those for manual reference scoring. Hence, this could cause discrepancies between reference and automatic volumes. Furthermore, in the current study, candidate voxels were represented by three orthogonal patches instead of a full 3D representation. A comparable full 3D representation with 24 voxels along each dimension might contain more information, but also increases the input size eight-fold. The size of the model increases accordingly, posing memory requirements which we found could not be met by our hardware. In addition, the larger number of weights might require more training samples than provided in the current study. It has previously been shown that smaller 3D representations can be outperformed by larger sparse orthogonal patches [15]. The voxel classification output of the CNNs was enhanced by Random Forest classification of extracted lesions. This resulted in good agreement between reference and automatic per patient CAC volumes.

In conclusion, CAC can be automatically identified and quantified in CCTA using the proposed pattern recognition method. This might obviate the need for a dedicated CSCT for CAC scoring, which is regularly acquired prior to a CCTA, and thus reduce the CT radiation dose received by patients.

References

1. Rumberger, J.A., Brundage, B.H., Rader, D.J., Kondos, G.: Electron beam computed tomographic coronary calcium scanning: a review and guidelines for use in asymptomatic persons. Mayo Clin. Proc. 74(3), 243–252 (1999)
2. Hecht, H.S.: Coronary artery calcium scanning: Past, present, and future. JACC: Cardiovasc. Imag. 8(5), 579–596 (2015)
3. Voros, S., Qian, Z.: Agatston score tried and true: by contrast, can we quantify calcium on CTA? J. Cardiovasc. Comput. Tomogr. 6(1), 45–47 (2012)
4. Shahzad, R., van Walsum, T., Schaap, M., Rossi, A., Klein, S., Weustink, A.C., de Feyter, P.J., van Vliet, L.J., Niessen, W.J.: Vessel specific coronary artery calcium scoring: An automatic system. Acad. Radiol. 20(1), 1–9 (2013)
5. Wolterink, J.M., Leiner, T., Takx, R.A.P., Viergever, M.A., Išgum, I.: Automatic coronary calcium scoring in non-contrast-enhanced ECG-triggered cardiac CT with ambiguity detection. IEEE Trans. Med. Imag. 34(9), 1867–1878
6. Otton, J.M., Lønborg, J.T., Boshell, D., Feneley, M., Hayen, A., Sammel, N., Sesel, K., Bester, L., McCrohon, J.: A method for coronary artery calcium scoring using contrast-enhanced computed tomography. J. Cardiovasc. Comput. Tomogr. 6(1), 37–44 (2012)
7. Glodny, B., Helmel, B., Trieb, T., Schenk, C., Taferner, B., Unterholzner, V., Strasak, A., Petersen, J.: A method for calcium quantification by means of CT coronary angiography using 64-multidetector CT: very high correlation with Agatston and volume scores. Eur. Radiol. 19(7), 1661–1668 (2009)
8. Mylonas, I., Alam, M., Amily, N., Small, G., Chen, L., Yam, Y., Hibbert, B., Chow, B.J.: Quantifying coronary artery calcification from a contrast-enhanced cardiac computed tomography angiography study. Eur. Heart J. Cardiovasc. Imaging 15(2), 210–215 (2014)

9. Pavitt, C.W., Harron, K., Lindsay, A.C., Ray, R., Zielke, S., Gordon, D., Rubens, M.B., Padley, S.P., Nicol, E.D.: Deriving coronary artery calcium scores from CT coronary angiography: a proposed algorithm for evaluating stable chest pain. Int. J. Card. Imaging 30(6), 1135–1143 (2014)
10. Wesarg, S., Khan, M.F., Firle, E.A.: Localizing calcifications in cardiac CT data sets using a new vessel segmentation approach. J. Digit. Imaging 19(3), 249–257 (2006)
11. Ahmed, W., de Graaf, M.A., Broersen, A., Kitslaar, P.H., Oost, E., Dijkstra, J., Bax, J.J., Reiber, J.H., Scholte, A.J.: Automatic detection and quantification of the Agatston coronary artery calcium score on contrast computed tomography angiography. Int. J. Cardiovasc. Imaging 31(1), 151–161 (2014)
12. Eilot, D., Goldenberg, R.: Fully automatic model-based calcium segmentation and scoring in coronary CT angiography. IJCARS 9(4), 595–608 (2014)
13. Teßmann, M., Vega-Higuera, F., Bischoff, B., Hausleiter, J., Greiner, G.: Automatic detection and quantification of coronary calcium on 3D CT angiography data. CSRDC 26(1), 117–124 (2011)
14. Schaap, M., Metz, C.T., van Walsum, T., van der Giessen, A.G., Weustink, A.C., Mollet, N.R., Bauer, C., Bogunović, H., Castro, C., Deng, X., et al.: Standardized evaluation methodology and reference database for evaluating coronary artery centerline extraction algorithms. Medical Image Analysis 13(5), 701–714 (2009)
15. Prasoon, A., Petersen, K., Igel, C., Lauze, F., Dam, E., Nielsen, M.: Deep feature learning for knee cartilage segmentation using a triplanar convolutional neural network. In: Mori, K., Sakuma, I., Sato, Y., Barillot, C., Navab, N. (eds.) MICCAI 2013, Part II. LNCS, vol. 8150, pp. 246–253. Springer, Heidelberg (2013)
16. Roth, H.R., Lu, L., Seff, A., Cherry, K.M., Hoffman, J., Wang, S., Liu, J., Turkbey, E., Summers, R.M.: A new 2.5D representation for lymph node detection using random sets of deep convolutional neural network observations. In: Golland, P., Hata, N., Barillot, C., Hornegger, J., Howe, R. (eds.) MICCAI 2014, Part I. LNCS, vol. 8673, pp. 520–527. Springer, Heidelberg (2014)
17. Klein, S., Staring, M., Murphy, K., Viergever, M.A., Pluim, J.P.W.: elastix: a toolbox for intensity-based medical image registration. IEEE Trans. Med. Imag. 29(1), 196–205 (2010)
18. Glorot, X., Bordes, A., Bengio, Y.: Deep sparse rectifier networks. In: Proceedings of the 14th International Conference on Artificial Intelligence and Statistics, vol. 15, pp. 315–323 (2011)
19. Tieleman, T., Hinton, G.: Lecture 6.5-rmsprop: Divide the gradient by a running average of its recent magnitude. COURSERA: Neural Networks for Machine Learning 4 (2012)
20. Srivastava, N., Hinton, G., Krizhevsky, A., Sutskever, I., Salakhutdinov, R.: Dropout: A simple way to prevent neural networks from overfitting. The Journal of Machine Learning Research 15(1), 1929–1958 (2014)
21. Breiman, L.: Random forests. Machine Learning 45(1), 5–32 (2001)
22. Bastien, F., Lamblin, P., Pascanu, R., Bergstra, J., Goodfellow, I.J., Bergeron, A., Bouchard, N., Bengio, Y.: Theano: new features and speed improvements. In: Deep Learning and Unsupervised Feature Learning NIPS 2012 Workshop (2012)
23. van der Bijl, N., Joemai, R.M., Geleijns, J., Bax, J.J., Schuijf, J.D., de Roos, A., Kroft, L.J.: Assessment of Agatston coronary artery calcium score using contrast-enhanced CT coronary angiography. Am. J. Roentgenol. 195(6), 1299–1305 (2010)

A Random Riemannian Metric for Probabilistic Shortest-Path Tractography

Søren Hauberg[1], Michael Schober[2], Matthew Liptrot[1,3], Philipp Hennig[2], and Aasa Feragen[3]

[1] Cognitive Systems, Technical University of Denmark, Denmark
[2] Max Planck Institute for Intelligent Systems, Tübingen, Germany
[3] Department of Computer Science, University of Copenhagen, Denmark

Abstract. Shortest-path tractography (SPT) algorithms solve global optimization problems defined from local distance functions. As diffusion MRI data is inherently noisy, so are the voxelwise tensors from which local distances are derived. We extend Riemannian SPT by modeling the stochasticity of the diffusion tensor as a "random Riemannian metric", where a geodesic is a distribution over tracts. We approximate this distribution with a Gaussian process and present a probabilistic numerics algorithm for computing the geodesic distribution. We demonstrate SPT improvements on data from the Human Connectome Project.

1 Introduction

Diffusion weighted imaging enables inference of structural brain connectivity, assuming that water diffuses *along* brain fibers, not across. At any brain location, a local brain fiber orientation distribution function (ODF) is estimated from measured diffusion along a fixed set of directions. Integration of the field of local ODFs yields a heuristic estimate of the most likely path for a brain fiber.

We study the stochasticity of the ODF estimate and its effect on the distribution of estimated tracts through Riemannian shortest-path tractography (SPT) in diffusion tensor imaging (DTI), where the ODF is a second order tensor describing a Gaussian diffusion process at any given location. In Riemannian SPT, tracts are estimated as geodesics on a Riemannian manifold, where the Riemannian metric is constructed from the diffusion tensor [9, 14, 15]. As the diffusion tensor is estimated from data, it is subject to noise. The tensor, and the induced Riemannian metric, should therefore be treated as stochastic variables, not exact representatives of the true underlying diffusion process. This is not possible in current Riemannian tractography models, which assume a deterministic metric.

We present a solution to *probabilistic SPT* for DTI which treats diffusion tensors as stochastic variables, and returns a distribution over the tracts connecting two given points in the brain, approximated by a Gaussian process (GP). Algorithmically, we extend recent probabilistic solutions for ordinary differential equations (ODEs) [12, 18] by allowing "noisy" evaluations of the ODE due to the noisy metric. The resulting ODE solver is extendable to other problems. The combined model yields both quantitative and qualitative improvements over standard SPT algorithms.

N. Navab et al. (Eds.): MICCAI 2015, Part I, LNCS 9349, pp. 597–604, 2015.
DOI: 10.1007/978-3-319-24553-9_73

2 Shortest-Path Tractography and Random Geometries

In *shortest-path tractography* (SPT) the ODFs induce a local Riemannian metric [9, 11, 14, 15], where the most probable fiber connecting two points $\mathbf{x}$ and $\mathbf{y}$ is re-interpreted as the *geodesic*, or shortest path, connecting $\mathbf{x}$ and $\mathbf{y}$.

Why SPT? Walk-based streamline methods searching for the most likely paths from a seed point to anywhere in the brain [3, 16] suffer from path-length dependency, i.e. long paths are harder to estimate than short ones. When two endpoints are known, SPT avoids this by looking for the shortest connecting path. This ensures that long and short tracts are estimated with the same sample size. As endpoints are not always known, these are complementary methods.

Solving Riemannian SPT. In Riemannian SPT, the diffusion tensor $\mathbf{D_p}$ at $\mathbf{p}$ is commonly interpreted as the *inverse* of a Riemannian metric $\mathbf{M_p}$ [14, 15]. Geodesics returned by this *ad hoc* interpretation are typically "too straight" or are attracted to high diffusivity cortical spinal fluid (CSF) regions. Hao et al. [11] suggest a per-voxel scaling $\mathbf{M_p} = \alpha_\mathbf{p}\mathbf{D}_\mathbf{p}^{-1}$ that avoids this issue, while Fuster et al. [9] show that the *adjugate metric* $\mathbf{M_p} = \det(\mathbf{D_p})\mathbf{D}_\mathbf{p}^{-1}$ gives a metric under which free Brownian motion matches the diffusion implied by $\mathbf{D_p}$. This reduces attraction to CSF regions [9, 19], so we use the adjugate metric.

Given a Riemannian metric $\mathbf{M_p}$, the Riemannian geodesic $\mathbf{c}\colon [0,1] \to \mathbb{R}^3$ connecting two points $\mathbf{x}$ and $\mathbf{y}$ is found by solving the geodesic ODE

$$\ddot{c}_d(t) = f_d(t, \mathbf{c}, \dot{\mathbf{c}}) = -\boldsymbol{\Gamma}_d^\intercal \cdot (\dot{\mathbf{c}}(t) \otimes \dot{\mathbf{c}}(t)), \quad d = 1, \ldots, D = 3, \tag{1}$$

$$\boldsymbol{\Gamma}_d = \frac{1}{2}\sum_{k=1}^{D}\left[\mathbf{M}_{\mathbf{c}(t)}^{-1}\right]_{d,k}\left(\frac{\partial \operatorname{vec} \mathbf{M_p}}{\partial p_k}\right)_{\mathbf{p}=\mathbf{c}(t)} \in \mathbb{R}^{D^2\times 1}, \tag{2}$$

subject to the boundary conditions $\mathbf{c}(0) = \mathbf{x}$ and $\mathbf{c}(1) = \mathbf{y}$. Here $\otimes$ is the Kronecker product, $\mathbf{c}(t) = [c_1(t); c_2(t); c_3(t)]$ is a point on the shortest path $\mathbf{c}$, and $\dot{\mathbf{c}}$ and $\ddot{\mathbf{c}}$ denote the first and second derivative along the path, respectively.

Estimating a Random Geometry. The Riemannian adjugate metric $\mathbf{M_p}$ is estimated from finite noisy data and should be considered a stochastic variable. This, however, complicates the geometric interpretation as the resulting object is now a *random Riemannian metric* [13], and not a deterministic metric. Given two endpoints $\mathbf{x}$ and $\mathbf{y}$, our interest is in finding a connecting geodesic. Since the metric is stochastic, there is a distribution of geodesics connecting $\mathbf{x}$ and $\mathbf{y}$.

We approximately solve the geodesic ODE (1) using a probabilistic description of the uncertainty over $f(t, \mathbf{c}, \dot{\mathbf{c}})$, the stochastic variable arising from Eq. 1 with a stochastic metric. We approximate f with a Gaussian distribution (using the shorthand notation $f_{t,\mathbf{c},\dot{\mathbf{c}}} \equiv f(t, \mathbf{c}, \dot{\mathbf{c}})$)

$$p(f_{t,\mathbf{c},\dot{\mathbf{c}}}) = \mathcal{N}\left(f_{t,\mathbf{c},\dot{\mathbf{c}}}; m_{t,\mathbf{c},\dot{\mathbf{c}}}, \mathbf{C}_{t,\mathbf{c},\dot{\mathbf{c}}}\right). \tag{3}$$

The mean and covariance that form this approximation are computed from

$$m_d = -\mathbb{E}(\boldsymbol{\Gamma}_d)^\intercal (\dot{\mathbf{c}} \otimes \dot{\mathbf{c}}) \qquad \text{and} \qquad C_d^2 = (\dot{\mathbf{c}} \otimes \dot{\mathbf{c}})^\intercal \operatorname{cov}(\boldsymbol{\Gamma}_d)\,(\dot{\mathbf{c}} \otimes \dot{\mathbf{c}}), \tag{4}$$

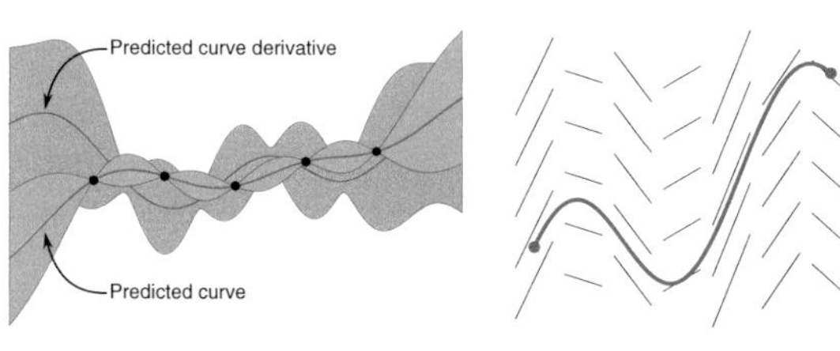

Fig. 1. *Left:* A GP regressor (blue) and its derivative (orange). *Right:* A numerical solver seeks the smooth function (blue) that best fits observed derivatives (black) while meeting the boundary constraints (red).

where $\mathbf{m}_{t,\mathbf{c},\dot{\mathbf{c}}} = [m_1; m_2; m_3]$ and $\mathbf{C}_{t,\mathbf{c},\dot{\mathbf{c}}} = \text{diag}\left(C_1^2, C_2^2, C_3^2\right)$.

We estimate the mean and covariance of $\mathbf{\Gamma}_d$ empirically, subsampling the gradient directions used to generate the local diffusion tensors into $S = 20$ batches each containing 80% of the directions. For each subsample we fit a diffusion tensor field and compute $\mathbf{\Gamma}_d$ (2). Finally, we estimate the moments $\mathbb{E}(\mathbf{\Gamma}_d) \approx \frac{1}{S}\sum_{s=1}^{S} \mathbf{\Gamma}_d^{(s)}$ and $\text{cov}(\mathbf{\Gamma}_d) \approx \frac{1}{S-1}\sum_{s=1}^{S}\left(\mathbf{\Gamma}_d^{(s)} - \mathbb{E}(\mathbf{\Gamma}_d)\right)\left(\mathbf{\Gamma}_d^{(s)} - \mathbb{E}(\mathbf{\Gamma}_d)\right)^{\intercal}$.

3 Regressing an ODE

In the Riemannian setting, geodesics are found as the solution to the geodesic ODE (1). This is a smooth curve $\mathbf{c}(t) : [0,1] \to \mathbb{R}^3$, which must be estimated numerically. We use *probabilistic numerics* that solves the ODE using Gaussian process (GP) regression [12,18,20] We extend previous work [19] to handle uncertainty in the ODE due to a noisy metric.

GP Regression. A GP $c(t) \sim \mathcal{GP}(\mu(t), k(t,u))$ [17] is a probability measure over real-valued functions $c : \mathbb{R} \to \mathbb{R}$ such that any finite restriction to function *values* $\{c(t_n)\}_{n=1}^{N}$ has a Gaussian distribution. GPs are parameterized by a mean function $\mu : \mathbb{R} \to \mathbb{R}$ and a covariance function $k : \mathbb{R} \times \mathbb{R} \to \mathbb{R}$ that determines the regularity of the paths. GPs are closed under linear transformations

$$p(c) = \mathcal{GP}(c; \mu, k) \quad \Rightarrow \quad p(\mathbf{A}c) = \mathcal{GP}(\mathbf{A}c; \mathbf{A}\mu, \mathbf{A}k\mathbf{A}^{\intercal}), \tag{5}$$

where $\mathbf{A}^{\intercal}$ denotes application of operator $\mathbf{A}$ to the left. Given observations $\{\mathbf{t}, \mathbf{Y}\} = \{(t_1, y_1), \ldots, (t_N, y_N)\}$ of likelihood $p(y_i \mid t_i) = \mathcal{N}(y_i; \mathbf{A}c(t_i), \sigma^2\mathbf{I})$, the posterior over c is a Gaussian process $\mathcal{GP}(\tilde{c}; \tilde{\mu}, \tilde{k})$ with

$$\begin{aligned} \tilde{\mu}(t) &= \mu(t) + k(t,\mathbf{t})\mathbf{A}^{\intercal}(\mathbf{A}k_{\mathbf{tt}}\mathbf{A}^{\intercal} + \sigma^2\mathbf{I})^{-1}(\mathbf{Y} - \mathbf{A}\mu(\mathbf{t})) \\ \tilde{k}(t,u) &= k(t,u) - k(t,\mathbf{t})\mathbf{A}^{\intercal}(\mathbf{A}k_{\mathbf{tt}}\mathbf{A}^{\intercal} + \sigma^2\mathbf{I})^{-1}\mathbf{A}k(\mathbf{t},u), \end{aligned} \tag{6}$$

where $(k_{\mathbf{tt}})_{ij} = k(t_i, t_j)$ is the $N \times N$ covariance of input locations [17, §2.2], and similarly for $k(t, \mathbf{t})$. Differentiation is a linear operation so (by Eq. 5) a GP belief over c implies a GP belief over $\partial c = \dot{c}$ as well (see left panel of Fig. 1).

Beliefs over multi-output functions $\mathbf{c}(t) = [c_1(t); c_2(t); c_3(t)]$ can be constructed through vectorization. If the covariance structure is assumed to factorize between inputs and outputs, $\text{cov}(c_i(t), c_j(u)) = [\mathbf{V}]_{ij}\, k(t,u)$, for covariance $\mathbf{V}$, then the belief over $\mathbf{c}$ can be written as $p(\mathbf{c}) = \mathcal{GP}(\mathbf{c}; \boldsymbol{\mu}_{\mathbf{c}}, \mathbf{V} \otimes k)$.

GP ODE Solvers. Numerical ODE solvers evalute the ODE at finitely many points and estimate a smooth curve that *fits these observations* along with either initial or boundary values (see right panel of Fig. 1). *This is statistical regression.* This view gives rise to probabilistic ODE solvers [5,12,18–20] implemented using GP regression. In these solvers, uncertainty represents the approximation of not evaluating the ODE at the true solution, but at the current approximation.

At runtime, the solver repeatedly uses the current posterior mean estimate $\tilde{\mathbf{c}}(t_i)$ for the true solution $\mathbf{c}(t_i)$ to construct approximate noisy "observations"

$$\mathbf{y}_i = f(t_i, \tilde{\mathbf{c}}(t_i), \partial\tilde{\mathbf{c}}(t_i)) = \ddot{\mathbf{c}}(t_i) + \eta_i. \tag{7}$$

This describes that $\tilde{\mathbf{c}}(t_i)$ is only an approximation to the true solution $\mathbf{c}(t_i)$ as the observation $\mathbf{y}_i$ is corrupted by an error η_i. Here, η_i is assumed to be Gaussian, and the current uncertainty over $\mathbf{c}$ is propagated through the algorithm:

At step i, assume a posterior $p(\mathbf{c}) = \mathcal{GP}(\mathbf{c}; \tilde{\boldsymbol{\mu}}^i, \tilde{k}^i)$. We construct the estimates $\tilde{\mathbf{c}}^i$ and $\partial\tilde{\mathbf{c}}^i$ as the current "best guess", the mean $[\tilde{\mathbf{c}}^i; \partial\tilde{\mathbf{c}}^i] = [\tilde{\boldsymbol{\mu}}^i(t_i); \partial\tilde{\boldsymbol{\mu}}^i(t_i)]$. An estimate for the error of this approximation is provided by the local variance

$$\operatorname{cov}\begin{pmatrix} \tilde{\mathbf{c}}^i(t_i) \\ \partial\tilde{\mathbf{c}}^i(t_i) \end{pmatrix} = \begin{pmatrix} \tilde{k}^i(t_i, t_i) & \left.\frac{\partial \tilde{k}^i(t_i,t)}{\partial t}\right|_{t=t_i} \\ \left.\frac{\partial \tilde{k}^i(t,t_i)}{\partial t}\right|_{t=t_i} & \left.\frac{\partial^2 \tilde{k}^i(t,u)}{\partial t \partial u}\right|_{t,u=t_i} \end{pmatrix} =: \boldsymbol{\Sigma}^i. \tag{8}$$

Assuming we have upper bounds $\mathbf{U} > {}^{\partial f}/_{\partial \mathbf{c}}$ and $\dot{\mathbf{U}} > {}^{\partial f}/_{\partial \dot{\mathbf{c}}}$ on the gradients of f, $\boldsymbol{\Sigma}^i$ can be used to estimate the error on y_i as $(\mathbf{U}, \dot{\mathbf{U}})^\intercal \boldsymbol{\Sigma}^i (\mathbf{U}, \dot{\mathbf{U}}) =: \boldsymbol{\Lambda}^i$, i.e. $\eta_i \sim \mathcal{N}(0, \boldsymbol{\Lambda}_i)$. This gives an observation likelihood function

$$p(\mathbf{y}_i \mid \ddot{\mathbf{c}}(t_i)) = \mathcal{N}(\mathbf{y}_i; \ddot{\mathbf{c}}(t_i), \boldsymbol{\Lambda}^i). \tag{9}$$

The belief is updated with Eq. 6 to obtain $\tilde{\mu}^{i+1}, \tilde{k}^{i+1}$, and the process repeats.

The repeated extrapolation to construct $\tilde{\mathbf{c}}(t_i)$ in the GP solver is similar to explicit Runge-Kutta methods as it defines a Butcher tableau. For some GP priors, the posterior mean even coincide with results from such methods [18].

Regressing a Noisy ODE. When the metric is *uncertain*, the geodesic ODE can only be evaluated probabilistically as $p(f)$. To handle this situation, we extend the probabilistic ODE solver to cope with Gaussian uncertain observations.

Due to noise, the curvature $\mathbf{y}_i = f(t_i, \tilde{\mathbf{c}}_i, \partial\tilde{\mathbf{c}}(t_i))$ can only be estimated up to Gaussian noise $p(\mathbf{y}_i \mid \mathbf{m}_{t,\tilde{\mathbf{c}},\partial\tilde{\mathbf{c}}}, \mathbf{C}_{t,\tilde{\mathbf{c}},\partial\tilde{\mathbf{c}}}) = \mathcal{N}(\mathbf{y}_i; \mathbf{m}_{t,\tilde{\mathbf{c}},\partial\tilde{\mathbf{c}}}, \mathbf{C}_{t,\tilde{\mathbf{c}},\partial\tilde{\mathbf{c}}})$. As the normal distribution is symmetric around the mean, this is a likelihood for y_i,

$$p(\mathbf{m}_{t,\tilde{\mathbf{c}},\partial\tilde{\mathbf{c}}} \mid \mathbf{y}_i, \mathbf{C}_{t,\tilde{\mathbf{c}},\partial\tilde{\mathbf{c}}}) = \mathcal{N}(\mathbf{m}_{t,\tilde{\mathbf{c}},\partial\tilde{\mathbf{c}}}; \mathbf{y}_i, \mathbf{C}_{t,\tilde{\mathbf{c}},\partial\tilde{\mathbf{c}}}). \tag{10}$$

Since both likelihoods (9, 10) are Gaussian, the latent $\mathbf{y}_i$ can be marginalized analytically, giving the complete observation likelihood for $\mathbf{m}_{t,\tilde{\mathbf{c}},\partial\tilde{\mathbf{c}}}$

$$p(\mathbf{m}_{t,\tilde{\mathbf{c}},\partial\tilde{\mathbf{c}}} \mid \ddot{\mathbf{c}}(t_i)) = \mathcal{N}\left(\mathbf{m}_{t,\tilde{\mathbf{c}},\partial\tilde{\mathbf{c}}}; \ddot{\mathbf{c}}_i, \mathbf{C}_{t_i,\tilde{\mathbf{c}}_i,\partial\tilde{\mathbf{c}}_i} + \boldsymbol{\Lambda}_i\right). \tag{11}$$

Solutions to noisy ODEs are then inferred by replacing Eq. 9 with Eq. 11, using $\mathbf{m}_{t,\tilde{\mathbf{c}},\partial\tilde{\mathbf{c}}} = \mathbb{E}[f_{t,\mathbf{c},\dot{\mathbf{c}}}]$ in place of the (inaccessible) function evaluations $\mathbf{y}_i = f_{t,\tilde{\mathbf{c}},\partial\tilde{\mathbf{c}}}$, such that the approximation error is modeled by the additive uncertainty $\mathbf{C}_{t,\tilde{\mathbf{c}},\partial\tilde{\mathbf{c}}}$.

The ODE solver rely on two noise terms: η_i in Eq. 7 captures the numerical error, while $\mathbf{C}$ in Eq. 10 describes the uncertainty arising from the data. While the terms are structurally similar they capture different error sources; e.g. changes in the number of grid points imply a change in η, while $\mathbf{C}$ is unaffected. Both noise terms are approximated as Gaussian to ensure efficient inference.

Adaptation to Tractography. To compute geodesics in DTI we subsample the diffusion gradients, estimate the mean and covariance of $\mathbf{\Gamma}_d$, and finally solve the noisy geodesic ODE (1) numerically. For the prior covariance we use a Gaussian kernel $k(t_i, t_j) = \exp\left[-(t_i - t_j)^2/(2\lambda^2)\right]$ with length scale λ. To estimate $\mathbf{V}$ and λ we maximize their likelihood with gradient descent on the positive definite cone. We initialize the prior mean with the Dijkstra path under the deterministic metric, which we pre-process with a GP smoother.

4 Experimental Results

Tractography was performed on pre-processed diffusion data of 20 subjects from the Q3 release of the Human Connectome Project (HCP) [7, 8, 10, 21]. The pre-processed HCP diffusion data contains 270 diffusion directions distributed equally over 3 shells with b-values $=$ 1000, 2000 and 3000 $^{\mathrm{s}}/_{\mathrm{mm}^2}$ [21]. Diffusion directions were uniformly subsampled into 20 batches each containing 80% of the directions, where DTI tensors were computed with `dtifit` [2]. Segmentation was performed with `FAST` [23]. The cortico-spinal tract (CST) and inferior longitudinal fasiculus (ILF) used for experiments were obtained from the probabilistic expert-annotated Catani tract atlas [4]. ROI atlases were constructed in MNI152 "template space" by overlapping the tract atlas with regions from the Harvard-Oxford atlas [6]. The CST ROIs are the overlap with the brainstem, the hippocampus and the amygdala for one region, and the overlap with the superior frontal gyrus, the precentral gyrus and the postcentral gyrus for the second region. The ILF ROIs are the overlap with the temporal pole for one region, and the overlap with the superior occipital cortex, the inferior occipital cortex and the occipital pole for the second region. The constructed ROIs were warped from "template space" to "subject space" using warps provided by HCP.

As a first illustration, Fig. 2 shows the density of a *single* geodesic within the CST projected onto a slice. The center column shows that the geodesic density roughly consists of two certain vertical line segments with an uncertain connection between them (green box). The bottom row shows the standard deviation of $\mathbf{\Gamma}_d$. The geodesic uncertainty appears related to data noise. This is not attained with other GP ODE solvers [19] as they model constant observation noise.

Next we sample 250 endpoint pairs and compute the corresponding geodesics. Fig. 3 shows the resulting heatmaps. The GP solution provides a more coherent picture of the tract compared to the picture generated with Dijkstra's algorithm.

To compare solution qualities we compute the set of voxels each geodesic passes through. Taking the Catani atlas as a reference we measure the percentage of voxels which are classified as part of the tract by at least one expert. Figure 4 shows the results for 20 subjects. In ILF the median accuracy is comparable

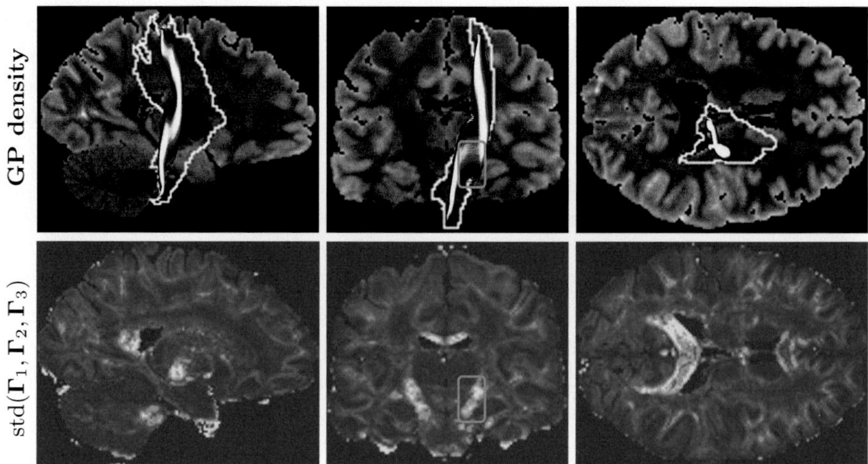

Fig. 2. *Top row:* The density of a *single* GP geodesic under the random metric. The density heatmap is projected into axis-aligned slices; the background image is the expected metric trace; and the outline is where at least one expert annotated the CST. *Bottom row:* Standard deviation of $\mathbf{\Gamma}_d$ at the same slices as the top row.

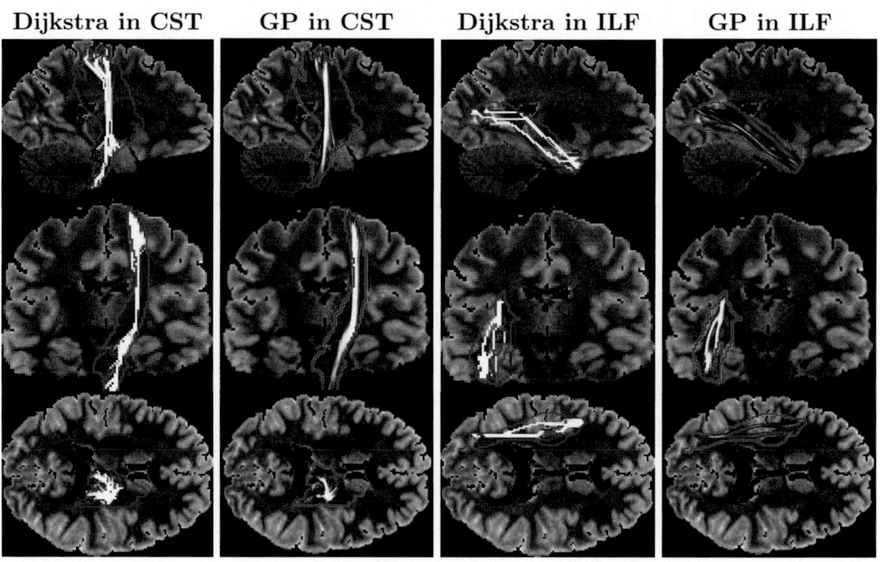

Fig. 3. Example shortest paths in the CST and ILF using both Dijkstra's algorithm on a deterministic metric, and a GP solver with a random Riemannian metric.

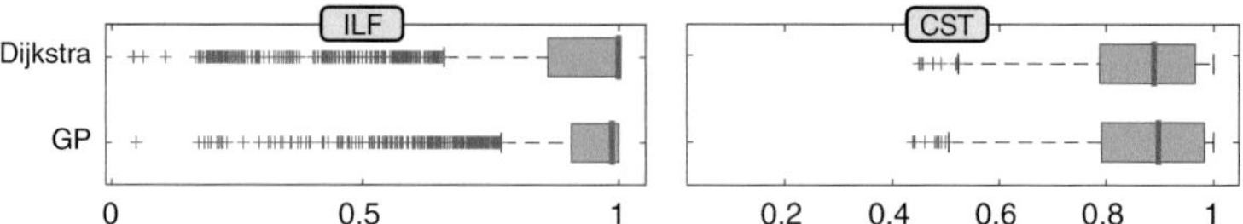

Fig. 4. Agreement with at least one expert in the Catani atlas as estimated by Dijkstras algorithm and the GP solver.

for Dijkstra and GP paths, but the GP error bars are significantly smaller. For the CST, we observe similar quality results for Dijkstra and GP paths. This is expected, as the ILF is generally considered the harder tract to estimate.

5 Discussion and Conclusion

SPT methods are advantageous for tracts that connect two brain regions, e.g. for structural brain networks. However, a long-standing problem is that SPT only finds a single connection with no insight to its uncertainty. This is in contrast to walk-based methods, which are often probabilistic in nature. In this paper, we provide a first fully probabilistic SPT algorithm that models stochastic diffusion tensors and returns a distribution over the shortest path. While uncertainty propagates in probabilistic walk-based methods, the uncertainty of probabilistic SPT only depends on local data uncertainty, not the seed point distance.

Through experiments we visualize the estimated geodesic densities between brain regions, and validate that the estimated geodesic densities are less certain in areas where the estimated diffusion tensor is uncertain. We see that the visualized geodesic densities from the probabilistic SPT yield smoother and more coherent tracts than the corresponding Dijkstra solutions.

While Riemannian SPT only applies to second order tensor models, a Finsler geometry framework has emerged enabling continuous SPT with higher order tensors for HARDI data [1]. Our proposed numerical tools also extend to these models, and can provide a probabilistic interpretation of Finsler models. Further future work includes shape analysis on the resulting estimated geodesic densities, which are suitable for GP-based tract shape analysis [22].

Acknowledgements. Data were provided [in part] by the Human Connectome Project, WU-Minn Consortium (Principal Investigators: David Van Essen and Kamil Ugurbil; 1U54MH091657) funded by the 16 NIH Institutes and Centers that support the NIH Blueprint for Neuroscience Research; and by the McDonnell Center for Systems Neuroscience at Washington University. S.H. is funded in part by the Danish Council for Independent Research (DFF), Natural Sciences. A.F. is funded in part by the DFF, Technology and Production Sciences.

References

1. Astola, L., Jalba, A., Balmashnova, E., Florack, L.: Finsler streamline tracking with single tensor orientation distribution function for high angular resolution diffusion imaging. Journal of Mathematical Imaging and Vision 41(3), 170–181 (2011)
2. Basser, P.J., Mattiello, J., LeBihan, D.: Estimation of the effective self-diffusion tensor from the NMR spin echo. J. Magn. Reson B 103(3), 247–254 (1994)
3. Basser, P.J., Pajevic, S., Pierpaoli, C., Duda, J., Aldroubi, A.: In vivo fiber tractography using DT-MRI data. Magnetic Resonance in Medicine 44(4), 625–632 (2000)
4. Catani, M., de Schotten, M.T.: A diffusion tensor imaging tractography atlas for virtual in vivo dissections. Cortex 44(8), 1105–1132 (2008)

5. Chkrebtii, O., Campbell, D., Girolami, M., Calderhead, B.: Bayesian uncertainty quantification for differential equations. arXiv stat.ME 1306.2365 (June 2013)
6. Desikan, R.S., others: An automated labeling system for subdividing the human cerebral cortex on MRI scans into gyral based regions of interest. NeuroImage 31(3), 968–980 (2006)
7. van Essen, D., et al.: The Human Connectome Project: a data acquisition perspective. NeuroImage 62(4), 2222–2231 (2012)
8. van Essen, D., et al.: The WU-Minn Human Connectome Project: an overview. NeuroImage 80, 62–79 (2013)
9. Fuster, A., Tristan-Vega, A., Haije, T., Westin, C.-F., Florack, L.: A novel Riemannian metric for geodesic tractography in DTI. In: Computational Diffusion MRI and Brain Connectivity. Math. and Visualization, pp. 97–104. Springer (2014)
10. Glasser, M., et al.: The minimal preprocessing pipelines for the human connectome project. NeuroImage 80, 105–124 (2013)
11. Hao, X., Zygmunt, K., Whitaker, R.T., Fletcher, P.T.: Improved segmentation of white matter tracts with adaptive Riemannian metrics. Medical Image Analysis 18(1), 161–175 (2014)
12. Hennig, P., Hauberg, S.: Probabilistic solutions to differential equations and their application to Riemannian statistics. In: AISTATS, vol. 33, JMLR, W&CP (2014)
13. LaGatta, T., Wehr, J.: Geodesics of random riemannian metrics. Communications in Mathematical Physics 327(1), 181–241 (2014)
14. Lenglet, C., Deriche, R., Faugeras, O.: Inferring white matter geometry from diffusion tensor MRI: Application to connectivity mapping. In: Pajdla, T., Matas, J(G.) (eds.) ECCV 2004. LNCS, vol. 3024, pp. 127–140. Springer, Heidelberg (2004)
15. O'Donnell, L., Haker, S., Westin, C.-F.: New approaches to estimation of white matter connectivity in diffusion tensor MRI: Elliptic PDEs and geodesics in a tensor-warped space. In: Dohi, T., Kikinis, R. (eds.) MICCAI 2002. LNCS, vol. 2488, pp. 459–466. Springer, Heidelberg (2002)
16. Parker, G., Haroon, H., Wheeler-Kingshott, C.: A framework for a streamline-based probabilistic index of connectivity (PICo) using a structural interpretation of MRI diffusion measurements. J. Magn. Reson. Imaging 18(2), 242–254 (2003)
17. Rasmussen, C.E., Williams, C.K.I.: GPs for Machine Learning. MIT Press (2006)
18. Schober, M., Duvenaud, D., Hennig, P.: Probabilistic ODE solvers with Runge-Kutta means. In: NIPS (2014)
19. Schober, M., Kasenburg, N., Feragen, A., Hennig, P., Hauberg, S.: Probabilistic shortest path tractography in DTI using gaussian process ODE solvers. In: Golland, P., Hata, N., Barillot, C., Hornegger, J., Howe, R. (eds.) MICCAI 2014, Part III. LNCS, vol. 8675, pp. 265–272. Springer, Heidelberg (2014)
20. Skilling, J.: Bayesian solution of ordinary differential equations. Maximum Entropy and Bayesian Methods, Seattle (1991)
21. Sotiropoulos, S.N., et al.: Effects of image reconstruction on fiber orientation mapping from multichannel diffusion MRI: reducing the noise floor using SENSE. Magn. Reson. Med. 70(6), 1682–1689 (2013)
22. Wassermann, D., Rathi, Y., Bouix, S., Kubicki, M., Kikinis, R., Shenton, M., Westin, C.-F.: White matter bundle registration and population analysis based on gaussian processes. In: Székely, G., Hahn, H.K. (eds.) IPMI 2011. LNCS, vol. 6801, pp. 320–332. Springer, Heidelberg (2011)
23. Zhang, Y., Brady, M., Smith, S.: Segmentation of brain MR images through a hidden Markov random field model and the expectation-maximization algorithm. IEEE Trans. Med. Imaging 20(1), 45–57 (2001)

Deep Learning and Structured Prediction for the Segmentation of Mass in Mammograms*

Neeraj Dhungel[1], Gustavo Carneiro[1], and Andrew P. Bradley[2]

[1] ACVT, School of Computer Science, The University of Adelaide
[2] School of ITEE, The University of Queensland

Abstract. In this paper, we explore the use of deep convolution and deep belief networks as potential functions in structured prediction models for the segmentation of breast masses from mammograms. In particular, the structured prediction models are estimated with loss minimization parameter learning algorithms, representing: a) conditional random field (CRF), and b) structured support vector machine (SSVM). For the CRF model, we use the inference algorithm based on tree re-weighted belief propagation with truncated fitting training, and for the SSVM model the inference is based on graph cuts with maximum margin training. We show empirically the importance of deep learning methods in producing state-of-the-art results for both structured prediction models. In addition, we show that our methods produce results that can be considered the best results to date on DDSM-BCRP and INbreast databases. Finally, we show that the CRF model is significantly faster than SSVM, both in terms of inference and training time, which suggests an advantage of CRF models when combined with deep learning potential functions.

Keywords: Deep learning, Structured output learning, Mammogram segmentation.

1 Introduction

Screening mammogram is one of the most effective imaging modalitites to detect breast cancer, and it is used for the segmentation of breast masses (among other tasks), which is a challenging task due to the variable shape/size of masses [1] and their low signal-to-noise ratio (see Fig. 1). In clinical practice, lesion segmentation is usually a manual process, and so its efficacy is associated with the radiologist's expertise and workload [2], where a clear trade-off can be noted between sensitivity (Se) and specificity (Sp) in manual interpretation, with a median Se of 83.8% and Sp of 91.1% [2].

The main goal of this paper is to introduce and evaluate a new methodology for segmenting masses from mammograms based on structured prediction models

* This work was partially supported by the Australian Research Council's Discovery Projects funding scheme (project DP140102794). Prof. Bradley is the recipient of an Australian Research Council Future Fellowship(FT110100623).

N. Navab et al. (Eds.): MICCAI 2015, Part I, LNCS 9349, pp. 605–612, 2015.
DOI: 10.1007/978-3-319-24553-9_74

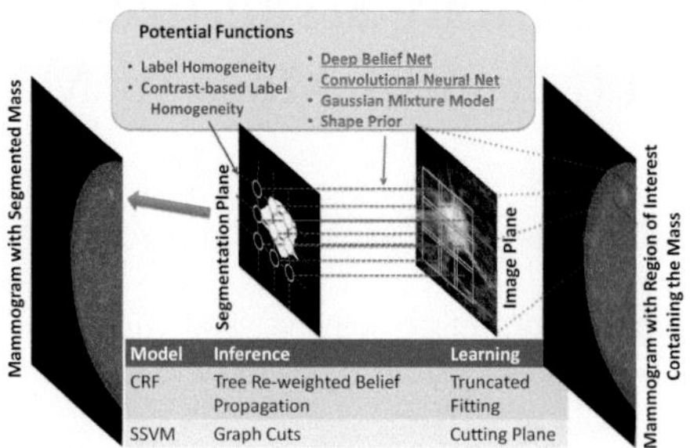

Fig. 1. Structured prediction model with a list of potential functions that include two deep learning methods and two structured prediction models

that use deep learning as their potential functions (Fig. 1). Our main contribution is the introduction of powerful deep learning appearance models, based on CNN [3,4] and DBN [5], into the following recently proposed structured output models: a) a conditional random field (CRF), and b) structured support vector machines (SSVM). The CRF model performs inference with tree re-weighted belief propagation [6] and learning with truncated fitting [7], while the SSVM model uses graph cuts [8] for inference and cutting plane [9,10] for training. We show that both structured output models produce comparable segmentation results, which are marginally superior to other recently proposed methods in the field in public datasets, and we also show that the use of both deep learning models is essential to reach such accurate results. Finally, we also demonstrate that the CRF model is significantly faster in terms of training and inference time, which suggests its use as the most efficient method in the field.

2 Methodology

Let us assume that the model parameter is denoted by $\mathbf{w}$, the image of the region of interest (ROI) containing the mass is denoted by $\mathbf{x} : \Omega \rightarrow \mathbb{R}$ ($\Omega \in \mathbb{R}^2$ denotes the image lattice of size $M \times M$) , the labeling is represented by $\mathbf{y} : \Omega \rightarrow \{-1, +1\}$, the training set is referred to as $\{(\mathbf{x}_n, \mathbf{y}_n)\}_{n=1}^{N}$, and the graph that links the image and labels is defined with $\mathcal{V}$ nodes and $\mathcal{E}$ edges between nodes. The learning process is based on the minimization of the empirical loss [11]:

$$\mathbf{w}^* = \arg\min_{\mathbf{w}} \frac{1}{N} \sum_{n=1}^{N} \ell(\mathbf{x}_n, \mathbf{y}_n, \mathbf{w}), \tag{1}$$

where $\ell(\mathbf{x}, \mathbf{y}, \mathbf{w})$ is a continuous and convex loss function that defines the structured model. We explore CRF and SSVM formulations for solving Eq.(1), described in Sections 2.1 and 2.2. In particular, CRF uses the loss

$$\ell(\mathbf{x}_n, \mathbf{y}_n, \mathbf{w}) = A(\mathbf{x}_n, \mathbf{w}) - E(\mathbf{y}_n, \mathbf{x}_n; \mathbf{w}), \tag{2}$$

where $A(\mathbf{x};\mathbf{w}) = \log \sum_{\mathbf{y}\in\{-1,+1\}^{M\times M}} \exp\{E(\mathbf{y},\mathbf{x};\mathbf{w})\}$ is the log-partition function that ensures normalization, and

$$E(\mathbf{y},\mathbf{x};\mathbf{w}) = \sum_{k=1}^{K}\sum_{i\in\mathcal{V}} w_{1,k}\phi^{(1,k)}(\mathbf{y}(i),\mathbf{x}) + \sum_{l=1}^{L}\sum_{i,j\in\mathcal{E}} w_{2,l}\phi^{(2,l)}(\mathbf{y}(i),\mathbf{y}(j),\mathbf{x}), \quad (3)$$

with $\phi^{(1,k)}(.,.)$ representing one of the K potential functions between label (segmentation plane in Fig. 1) and pixel (image plane in Fig. 1) nodes, $\phi^{(2,l)}(.,.,.)$ denoting one of the L potential functions on the edges between label nodes, and $\mathbf{w} = [w_{1,1}, ..., w_{1,K}, w_{2,1}, ..., w_{2,L}]^\top \in \mathbb{R}^{K+L}$ with $\mathbf{y}(i)$ being the ith component of vector $\mathbf{y}$. Alternatively, the SSVM minimizes the loss function

$$\ell(\mathbf{x}_n,\mathbf{y}_n,\mathbf{w}) = \max_{\mathbf{y}\in\mathcal{Y}} \left(\Delta(\mathbf{y}_n,\mathbf{y}) + E(\mathbf{y},\mathbf{x}_n;\mathbf{w}) - E(\mathbf{y}_n,\mathbf{x}_n;\mathbf{w})\right), \quad (4)$$

where $\Delta(\mathbf{y}_n,\mathbf{y})$ returns the dissimilarity between $\mathbf{y}_n$ and $\mathbf{y}$, satistfying the conditions $\Delta(\mathbf{y}_n,\mathbf{y}) \geq 0$ and $\Delta(\mathbf{y}_n,\mathbf{y}_n) = 0$.

2.1 Conditional Random Field (CRF)

The solution of Eq.(1) using the CRF loss function in Eq.(2) involves the computation of the log-partition function $A(\mathbf{x};\mathbf{w})$. Tree re-weighted (TRW) belief propagation provides an upper bound to this log-partition function [6]:

$$A(\mathbf{x};\mathbf{w}) = \max_{\mu\in\mathcal{M}} \mathbf{w}^T\mu + H(\mu), \quad (5)$$

where $\mathcal{M} = \{\mu' : \exists\mathbf{w}, \mu' = \mu\}$ denotes the marginal polytope, $\mu = \sum_{\mathbf{y}\in\{-1,+1\}^{M\times M}} P(\mathbf{y}|\mathbf{x},\mathbf{w})f(\mathbf{y})$, with $f(\mathbf{y})$ denoting the set of indicator functions of possible configurations of each clique and variable in the graph [12] (as denoted in Eq.(3), $P(\mathbf{y}|\mathbf{x},\mathbf{w}) = \exp\{E(\mathbf{y},\mathbf{x};\mathbf{w}) - A(\mathbf{x};\mathbf{w})\}$ indicating the conditional probability of the annotation $\mathbf{y}$ given the image $\mathbf{x}$ and parameters $\mathbf{w}$ (where we assume that this conditional probability function belongs to the exponential family), and $H(\mu) = -\sum_{\mathbf{y}\in\{-1,+1\}^{M\times M}} P(\mathbf{y}|\mathbf{x};\mathbf{w})\log P(\mathbf{y}|\mathbf{x},\mathbf{w})$ is the entropy. Note that for general graphs with cycles, the marginal polytope $\mathcal{M}$ is difficult to characterize and the entropy $\mathbf{H}(\mu)$ is not tractable [7]. TRW solves these issues by first replacing the marginal polytope with a superset $\mathcal{L} \supset \mathcal{M}$ that only accounts for the local constraints of the marginals, and then approximating the entropy calculation with an upper bound [7]. The learning of $\mathbf{w}$ in (2) is achieved via gradient descent in a process called truncated fitting [7], and the inference to find the label $\mathbf{y}^*$ for an image $\mathbf{x}^*$ is based on TRW.

2.2 Structured Support Vector Machine (SSVM)

The SSVM optimization to estimate $\mathbf{w}$ consists of a regularized loss minimization problem formulated as $\mathbf{w}^* = \min_{\mathbf{w}} \|\mathbf{w}\|^2 + \lambda\sum_n \ell(\mathbf{x}_n,\mathbf{y}_n,\mathbf{w})$, with $\ell(.)$ defined in Eq.(4), where the introduction of slack variable leads to [9,10]:

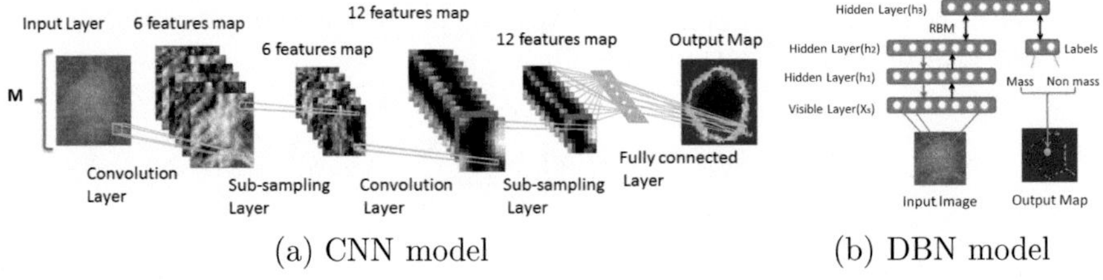

(a) CNN model (b) DBN model

Fig. 2. (a) CNN and (b) DBN models with the given mass patch as input

$$\begin{array}{ll} \text{minimize}_{\mathbf{w}} & \frac{1}{2}\|\mathbf{w}\|^2 + \frac{C}{N}\sum_n \xi_n \\ \text{subject to} & E(\mathbf{y}_n, \mathbf{x}_n; \mathbf{w}) - E(\hat{\mathbf{y}}_n, \mathbf{x}_n; \mathbf{w}) \geq \Delta(\mathbf{y}_n, \hat{\mathbf{y}}_n) - \xi_n, \forall \hat{\mathbf{y}}_n \neq \mathbf{y}_n \\ & \xi_n \geq 0. \end{array} \tag{6}$$

In order to keep the number of constraints manageable in Eq.(6), we use the cutting plane for solving the maximization problem:

$$\hat{\mathbf{y}}_n = \arg\max_{\mathbf{y}} \Delta(\mathbf{y}_n, \mathbf{y}) + E(\mathbf{y}, \mathbf{x}_n; \mathbf{w}) - E(\mathbf{y}_n, \mathbf{x}_n; \mathbf{w}) - \xi_n, \tag{7}$$

which finds the most violated constraint for the nth training sample given the parameter $\mathbf{w}$,

where $\Delta(.)$ denotes the Hamming distance [13]. The label inference for a test mammogram $\mathbf{x}$, given the learned parameters $\mathbf{w}$ from Eq.(6), is based on $\mathbf{y}^* = \arg\max_{\mathbf{y}} E(\mathbf{y}, \mathbf{x}; \mathbf{w})$, which can be optimally solved with graph cuts [8].

2.3 Potential Functions

The model in Eq.(3) can incorporate a large number of unary and binary potential functions. We propose the use of CNN and DBN in addition to the more common Gaussian mixture model (GMM) and shape prior between the nodes of image and segmentation planes (Fig. 1).

The **CNN potential function** is defined by [4] (Fig. 2-(a)):

$$\phi^{(1,1)}(\mathbf{y}(i), \mathbf{x}) = -\log P_c(\mathbf{y}(i)|\mathbf{x}, \theta_c), \tag{8}$$

where $P_c(\mathbf{y}(i)|\mathbf{x}, \theta)$ denotes the probability of labeling the pixel $i \in M \times M$ with mass or background (given the input image $\mathbf{x}$ for the ROI of the mass) and θ_c denotes the CNN parameters. A CNN model consists of multiple processing stages, each containing a convolutional layer (where the learned filters are applied to the image) and a non-linear subsampling layer that reduces the input image size for the next stage (Fig. 2), and a final stage consisting of few fully connected layers. The convolution stages compute the output at location j from input at i using the learned filter (at q^{th} stage) $\mathbf{k}^q$ and bias b^q with $\mathbf{x}(j)^q = \sigma(\sum_{i \in M_j} \mathbf{x}(i)^{q-1} * \mathbf{k}^q_{ij} + b^q_j)$, where $\sigma(.)$ is the logistic function and

M_j is the input region location; while the non-linear subsampling layers calculate subsampled data with $\mathbf{x}(j)^q = \downarrow(\mathbf{x}_j^{q-1})$, where $\downarrow(.)$ denotes a subsampling function that pools (using either the mean or max functions) the values from a region from the input data. The final stage consists of the convolution equation above using a separate filter for each output location, using the whole input from the previous layer. Inference is simply the application of this process in a feed-forward manner, and training is carried out with backpropagation to minimize the segmentation error over the training set [3,4].

The **DBN potential function** is defined as [5] (Fig. 2-(b)):

$$\phi^{(1,2)}(\mathbf{y}(i), \mathbf{x}) = -\log P_d(\mathbf{y}(i)|\mathbf{x}_S(i), \theta_{d,S}), \tag{9}$$

where $\mathbf{x}_S(i)$ is a patch extracted around image lattice position i of size $S \times S$ pixels ($S < M$, with M being the original patch size), $\theta_{d,S}$ represents the DBN parameters. The inference is based on the mean field approximation of the values in all DBN layers, followed by the computation of free energy on the top layer [5]. The learning of the DBN parameters $\theta_{d,S}$ in Eq.(9) is achieved with an iterative layer by layer training of auto-encoders using contrastive divergence, followed by a discriminative learning using backpropagation [5]. In addition to the CNN and DBN patch-based potential functions, we also use a pixel-wise **GMM model** [13] defined by $\phi^{(1,3)}(\mathbf{y}(i), \mathbf{x}) = -\log P_g(\mathbf{y}(i)|\mathbf{x}(i), \theta_g)$, where $P(.)$ is computed from the GMM class dependent probability model, learned from the training set; and the shape prior model [13] represented by $\phi^{(1,4)}(\mathbf{y}(i), \mathbf{x}) = -\log P(\mathbf{y}(i)|\theta_p)$, which computes the probability of belonging to the mass based only on the patch position (this prior is taken from the training annotations). Finally, the **pairwise potential functions** between label nodes in Eq.(3) encode label and contrast dependent labelling homogeneity as $\phi^{(2,1)}(\mathbf{y}(i), \mathbf{y}(j), \mathbf{x})$ and $\phi^{(2,2)}(\mathbf{y}(i), \mathbf{y}(j), \mathbf{x})$ [11].

3 Experiments

3.1 Materials and Methods

The evaluation of our methodology is performed on two publicly available datasets: INbreast [14] and DDSM-BCRP [15].The INbreast dataset comprises a set of 56 cases containing 116 accurately annotated masses. We divide this dataset into mutually exclusive train and test sets, each containing 58 images. The DDSM-BCRP [15] dataset consists of 39 cases (77 annotated images) for training and 40 cases (81 annotated images) for testing. We used Dice index to assess the segmentation accuracy. Efficiency is estimated with the training and testing time of the segmentation algorithm, obtained on a standard computer (Intel(R) Core(TM) i5-2500k 3.30GHz CPU with 8GB RAM). The ROI to be segmented is obtained by a manual input of location and scale, similarly to other works in the field [13,16,17]. It is important to realize that the segmentation of masses from these manually labeled regions is an important step in mass classification, so it is still an open problem [18] because of the challenges involved,

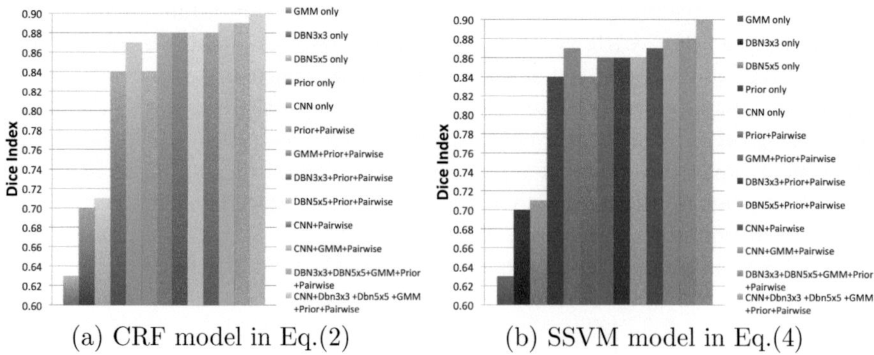

(a) CRF model in Eq.(2) (b) SSVM model in Eq.(4)

Fig. 3. Dice index over the test set of INbreast of the CRF (a) and SSVM (b) models, using various subsets of the potential functions

such as spicules segmentation, low signal-to-noise ratio, and lack of robust shape and appearance models. This ROI forms a rectangular bounding box that is resized to 40 x 40 pixels using bicubic interpolation and pre-processed with Ball and Bruce technique [1]. The model selection for the CNN/DBN structures is performed via cross validation on the training set, and for the CNN, the net structure of the first and second stages have filters of size 5×5 and a subsampling based on max pooling. The final stage of the CNN has a fully connected layer with 588 nodes and an output layer with 40×40 nodes (i.e., same size of the input layer). We use two DBN models, like the one shown in Fig. 2(b), where each of the three layers contains 50 nodes and input patches of sizes 3×3 and 5×5 (i.e., $S = 3, 5$, respectively).

3.2 Results

Fig. 3 shows the importance of adding each potential function in the model Eq.(3) to improve the Dice index using both CRF and SSVM. We show these results using several subsets of the potential functions introduced in Sec. 2.3 (i.e., the potentials $\phi^{(1,k)}$ for $k = \{1, 2, 3, 4\}$ with 3×3 and 5×5 denoting the image patch size used by the DBN). The Dice index of our methodology using all potential functions on the train set of INbreast is similar to test set at 0.93 using CRF and 0.95 using SSVM. It is also worth mentioning that the results on the INbreast test set when we do not use preprocessing [1] falls to 0.85 using all potential functions for both models (similar results are obtained on DDSM).

Tab. 1 shows the Dice index and average training (for the whole training set) and testing times (per image) of our approach with all potential functions (CNN+DBN3x3 + DBN5x5 + GMM + Prior + Pairwise) using the CRF and SSVM models on DDSM-BCRP and INbreast test sets.

Table 1. Comparison of the proposed and state-of-the-art methods on test sets

Method	#Images	Dataset	Dice Index	Test Run.Time	Train Run. time
Proposed CRF model	116	INbreast	0.90(0.06)	0.1s	360s
Proposed SSVM model	116	INbreast	0.90(0.06)	0.8s	1800s
Cardoso et al. [16]	116	INbreast	0.88	?	?
Dhungel et al. [13]	116	INbreast	0.88	0.8s	?
Proposed CRF model	158	DDSM-BCRP	0.90(0.06)	0.1s	383s
Proposed SSVM model	158	DDSM-BCRP	0.90(0.06)	0.8s	2140s
Dhungel et al. [13]	158	DDSM-BCRP	0.87	0.8s	?
Beller et al. [17]	158	DDSM-BCRP	0.70	?	?

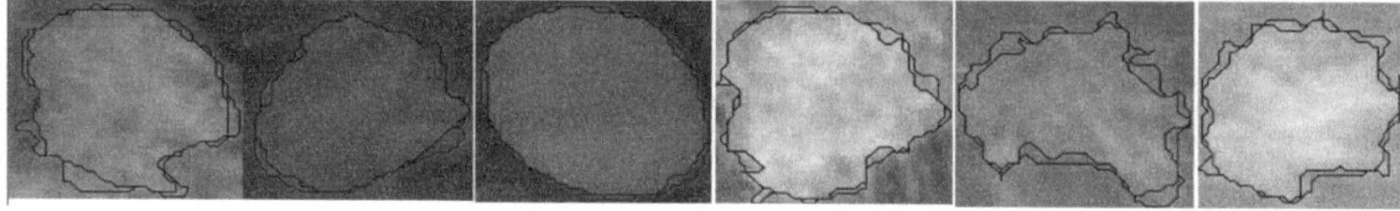

Fig. 4. Segmentation results by the CRF model on INbreast where the blue denotes the manual annotation and red denotes automatic segmentation

4 Discussion and Conclusions

From the results in Fig. 3, we notice that the use of deep learning based potential functions provide a significant improvement when compared with the shape prior alone. Also, the combination of GMM and deep learning models improve both the CRF and SSVM models. Another important observation is the fact that the image preprocessing [1] is important empirically. The comparison with other methods in Table 1 shows that our methodology produces the best results(0.90 v 0.88 and 0.90 v 0.87) for both databases. Our CRF and SSVM models demonstrate equivalent results (0.90) on both data sets. However, assuming a standard deviation of 0.06, a t-test indicates that our methods perform significantly ($p<0.01$) better than the previous methods [13,16,17]. The comparison in terms of train and test times shows a significant advantage to the CRF model over SSVM model. There are some important notes to make about the training and testing processes in these results: 1) we tried different CNN structures and the combination of more than one CNN model as additional potential functions, but the single CNN model detailed in Sec. 3.1 produced the best cross validation results; 2) for the DBN models, we tried different input sizes (3×3 and 7×7 patches), but the combinations of the ones detailed in Sec. 3.1 provided the best cross-validation results; and 3) both CRF and SSVM models estimate a much larger weight to the CNN potential function compared to others in Sec. 2.3, indicating that this is the most important potential function, but the CNN model alone overfits the training data (with a Dice of 0.87 on test and 0.95 on training), so the structural prediction models (CRF and SSVM) serve as a regularizer to the CNN model. Finally, from the visual results in Fig. 4, our CRF model produces quite accurate segmentation results even in the presence of moderately sharp corners and cusps.

References

1. Ball, J., Bruce, L.: Digital mammographic computer aided diagnosis (cad) using adaptive level set segmentation. In: 29th Annual International Conference of the IEEE EMBS 2007, pp. 4973–4978. IEEE (2007)
2. Elmore, J.G., Jackson, S.L., Abraham, L., et al.: Variability in interpretive performance at screening mammography and radiologists characteristics associated with accuracy1. Radiology 253(3), 641–651 (2009)
3. Krizhevsky, A., Sutskever, I., Hinton, G.E.: Imagenet classification with deep convolutional neural networks. In: NIPS, vol. 1, p. 4 (2012)
4. LeCun, Y., Bengio, Y.: Convolutional networks for images, speech, and time series. In: The Handbook of Brain Theory and Neural Networks, vol. 3361 (1995)
5. Hinton, G.E., Salakhutdinov, R.R.: Reducing the dimensionality of data with neural networks. Science 313(5786), 504–507 (2006)
6. Wainwright, M.J., Jaakkola, T.S., Willsky, A.S.: Tree-reweighted belief propagation algorithms and approximate ml estimation by pseudo-moment matching. In: Workshop on Artificial Intelligence and Statistics, vol. 21, p. 97. Society for Artificial Intelligence and Statistics Np (2003)
7. Domke, J.: Learning graphical model parameters with approximate marginal inference. arXiv preprint arXiv:1301.3193 (2013)
8. Boykov, Y., Veksler, O., Zabih, R.: Fast approximate energy minimization via graph cuts. PAMI 23(11), 1222–1239 (2001)
9. Szummer, M., Kohli, P., Hoiem, D.: Learning cRFs using graph cuts. In: Forsyth, D., Torr, P., Zisserman, A. (eds.) ECCV 2008, Part II. LNCS, vol. 5303, pp. 582–595. Springer, Heidelberg (2008)
10. Tsochantaridis, I., Joachims, T., Hofmann, T., Altun, Y.: Large margin methods for structured and interdependent output variables. In: JMLR, pp. 1453–1484 (2005)
11. Nowozin, S., Lampert, C.: Structured learning and prediction in computer vision. Foundations and Trends in Computer Graphics and Vision 6(3–4), 185–365 (2011)
12. Meltzer, T., Globerson, A., Weiss, Y.: Convergent message passing algorithms: a unifying view. In: Proceedings of the Twenty-Fifth Conference on Uncertainty in Artificial Intelligence, pp. 393–401. AUAI Press (2009)
13. Dhungel, N., Carneiro, G., Bradley, A.P.: Deep structured learning for mass segmentation from mammograms. arXiv preprint arXiv:1410.7454 (2014)
14. Moreira, I.C., Amaral, I., Domingues, I., Cardoso, A., Cardoso, M.J., Cardoso, J.S.: Inbreast: toward a full-field digital mammographic database. Academic Radiology 19(2), 236–248 (2012)
15. Heath, M., Bowyer, K., Kopans, D., Moore, R., Kegelmeyer, P.: The digital database for screening mammography. In: Proceedings of the 5th International Workshop on Digital Mammography, pp. 212–218 (2000)
16. Cardoso, J.S., Domingues, I., Oliveira, H.P.: Closed shortest path in the original coordinates with an application to breast cancer. International Journal of Pattern Recognition and Artificial Intelligence (2014)
17. Beller, M., Stotzka, R., Müller, T.O., Gemmeke, H.: An example-based system to support the segmentation of stellate lesions. In: Bildverarbeitung für die Medizin 2005, pp. 475–479. Springer, Heidelberg (2005)
18. Rahmati, P., Adler, A., Hamarneh, G.: Mammography segmentation with maximum likelihood active contours. Medical Image Analysis 16(6), 1167–1186 (2012)

Learning Tensor-Based Features for Whole-Brain fMRI Classification

Xiaonan Song, Lingnan Meng, Qiquan Shi, and Haiping Lu*

Department of Computer Science, Hong Kong Baptist University, Hong Kong
haiping@hkbu.edu.hk

Abstract. This paper presents a novel tensor-based feature learning approach for whole-brain fMRI classification. Whole-brain fMRI data have high exploratory power, but they are challenging to deal with due to large numbers of voxels. A critical step for fMRI classification is dimensionality reduction, via *feature selection* or *feature extraction*. Most current approaches perform voxel selection based on *feature selection* methods. In contrast, *feature extraction* methods, such as principal component analysis (PCA), have limited usage on whole brain due to the small sample size problem and limited interpretability. To address these issues, we propose to directly extract features from natural tensor (rather than vector) representations of whole-brain fMRI using multilinear PCA (MPCA), and map MPCA bases to voxels for interpretability. Specifically, we extract low-dimensional tensors by MPCA, and then select a number of MPCA features according to the captured variance or mutual information as the input to SVM. To provide interpretability, we construct a mapping from the selected MPCA bases to raw voxels for localizing discriminating regions. Quantitative evaluations on challenging multiclass tasks demonstrate the superior performance of our proposed methods against the state-of-the-art, while qualitative analysis on localized discriminating regions shows the spatial coherence and interpretability of our mapping.

1 Introduction

Over the past decades, functional Magnetic Resonance Imaging (fMRI) has emerged as a powerful instrument to collect vast quantities of data for measuring brain activities. It becomes a popular tool in applications such as brain state encoding/decoding and brain disease detection, including Alzheimer's disease, Mild Cognitive Impairment, and Autism Spectrum Disorder [2,14]. Most existing studies on fMRI classification restrict the analysis to specific brain *regions of interest* (ROIs). However, ROI analysis is labor-intensive, subject to human error, and requires the assumption that a functionally active brain region will be within an anatomically standardized index [10]. In contrast, *whole-brain* fMRI data have higher exploratory power and lower bias (with no prior user-dependent hypothesis/selection of spatial voxels) [5,17], and recent works reported promising results on whole-brain-based classification [1,16,17]. Inspired by these works, this paper focuses on whole-brain fMRI classification.

* Corresponding author.

N. Navab et al. (Eds.): MICCAI 2015, Part I, LNCS 9349, pp. 613–620, 2015.
DOI: 10.1007/978-3-319-24553-9_75

It is challenging to analyze all voxels in the whole brain. The number of whole-brain voxels usually far exceeds the number of observations available in practice, leading to *overfitting* [17]. We need to perform dimensionality reduction first, through either *feature selection* or *feature extraction* [12].

Feature selection methods are more popular for fMRI classification, partly due to their good interpretability. There are two main approaches: univariate and multivariate feature selection [14]. For the *univariate* approach, mutual information (MI) is a popular choice [3,15], e.g., Chou et al. [3] select informative fMRI voxels with high MI values individually for brain state decoding and report good improvement in classification accuracy. In contrast, the *multivariate* methods consider interactions between multiple features, e.g., Ryali et al. [17] and Kampa et al. [7] present sparse optimization frameworks for whole-brain fMRI feature selection and demonstrate the effectiveness of logistic regression (LR) with the elastic net penalty, which outperforms LR with ℓ_1-norm regularization and recursive feature elimination [16], and serves as the *state-of-the-art.*

The other dimensionality reduction approach is feature extraction. Principal component analysis (PCA) is arguably the most popular *linear* feature extraction method. To apply PCA to whole-brain fMRI, we need to concatenate all voxels into a very high-dimensional vector, making the small sample size problem more severe. Moreover, though individual PCA bases can be well interpreted [6], a group of PCA bases are seldom interpreted together effectively [12,13]. On the other hand, *multilinear* feature extraction methods, such as the multilinear PCA (MPCA) [9], are getting popular recently. They represent *multidimensional data* as tensors rather than vectors, with *three key benefits*: preserved multidimensional structure, lower computational demand, and less parameters to estimate. For example, for 3D $128 \times 128 \times 64$ volumes, a PCA basis needs $128 \times 128 \times 64 = 1,048,576$ parameters, while an MPCA basis needs only $128 + 128 + 64 = 320$ parameters [8]. fMRI data are *multidimensional* so it is more intuitive to analyze them using tensor representations [1,8].

In this paper, we propose a novel tensor-based feature learning approach via MPCA for whole-brain fMRI classification and a new mapping scheme to localize discriminating regions based on MPCA features. We perform evaluations on a challenging multiclass fMRI dataset [11]. Our contributions are twofold:

- Our methods directly extract features from tensor representations of fMRI using MPCA for the three key benefits mentioned above. The extracted MPCA features are then selected according to variance or mutual information to be fed into the Support Vector Machine (SVM). Superior performance on both binary and multiclass tasks is achieved without requiring vectorization or a priori identification of localized ROIs.
- Our mapping scheme localizes discriminating regions in the voxel space via MPCA bases for interpretability. It is different from the scheme in [12] of mapping the coefficients of the optimal hyperplane in linear SVM, which tends to be noisy and fragmented, as pointed out in [4]. We can obtain spatial maps with good spatial coherence and good interpretability for neuroscience.

2 Methods

Our proposed methods use the fMRI data represented by the mean percent signal change (PSC) over the time dimension [11] as input features and model them directly as third-order tensors (3D data). We use MPCA to learn multilinear bases from these tensorial input to obtain low-dimensional tensorial MPCA features. We then select the most informative MPCA features to form feature vectors for the SVM classifier. We present the key steps of our methods in detail below.

Notations and Basic Operations. Following [8], we denote vectors by lowercase boldface letters, e.g., $\mathbf{x}$; matrices by uppercase boldface, e.g., $\mathbf{X}$; and tensors by calligraphic letters, e.g., $\mathcal{X}$. An index is denoted with a lowercase letter, spanning the range from 1 to the uppercase letter of the index, e.g., $i = 1, \ldots, I$. We denote an Nth-order tensor as $\mathcal{A} \in \mathbb{R}^{I_1 \times \cdots \times I_N}$ and their elements with indices in parentheses $\mathcal{A}(i_1, \ldots, i_N)$. The n-mode index is denoted with i_n, $n = 1, \ldots, N$. The n-mode product of a tensor $\mathcal{A}$ by a matrix $\mathbf{U} \in \mathbb{R}^{J_n \times I_n}$, is written as $\mathcal{B} = \mathcal{A} \times_n \mathbf{U}$, with its entries obtained as [8]:

$$\mathcal{B}(i_1, \ldots, i_{n-1}, j_n, i_{n+1}, \ldots, i_N) = \sum_{i_n} \mathcal{A}(i_1, \ldots, i_N)\mathbf{U}(j_n, i_n), j_n = 1, \ldots, J_n. \tag{1}$$

The scalar product of two tensors $\langle \mathcal{A}, \mathcal{B} \rangle \in \mathbb{R}^{I_1 \times I_2 \times \cdots \times I_N}$ is defined as:

$$\langle \mathcal{A}, \mathcal{B} \rangle = \sum_{i_1} \cdots \sum_{i_N} \mathcal{A}(i_1, \ldots, i_N)\mathcal{B}(i_1, \ldots, i_N). \tag{2}$$

A rank-one tensor $\mathcal{U}$ equals to the outer product of N vectors [8]:

$$\mathcal{U} = \mathbf{u}^{(1)} \circ \cdots \circ \mathbf{u}^{(N)}, \text{ where } \mathcal{U}(i_1, \ldots, i_N) = \mathbf{u}^{(1)}(i_1) \cdots \mathbf{u}^{(N)}(i_N). \tag{3}$$

MPCA Feature Extraction. MPCA [9] is an unsupervised learning method to learn features directly from tensorial representations of multidimensional data. Thus, we represent our M training fMRI samples as third-order tensors $\{\mathcal{X}_1, \ldots, \mathcal{X}_M \in \mathbb{R}^{I_1 \times I_2 \times I_3}\}$ as input to MPCA. MPCA then extracts low-dimensional tensor features $\{\mathcal{Y}_1, \ldots, \mathcal{Y}_M \in \mathbb{R}^{P_1 \times P_2 \times P_3}\}$ through three ($N = 3$) projection matrices $\{\mathbf{U}^{(n)} \in \mathbb{R}^{I_n \times P_n}, n = 1, 2, 3\}$ as follows:

$$\mathcal{Y}_m = \mathcal{X}_m \times_1 \mathbf{U}^{(1)^T} \times_2 \mathbf{U}^{(2)^T} \times_3 \mathbf{U}^{(3)^T}, m = 1, \ldots, M, \tag{4}$$

where $P_n < I_n$. In this way, the tensor dimensions are reduced from $I_1 \times I_2 \times I_3$ to $P_1 \times P_2 \times P_3$. The solutions for the projection matrices $\{\mathbf{U}^{(n)}\}$ are obtained via maximizing the total tensor scatter $\Psi_{\mathcal{Y}} = \sum_{m=1}^{M} \| \mathcal{Y}_m - \bar{\mathcal{Y}} \|_F^2$, where $\bar{\mathcal{Y}} = \frac{1}{M} \sum_{m=1}^{M} \mathcal{Y}_m$ is the *mean tensor feature* and $\| \cdot \|_F$ is the Frobenius norm [9]. This problem is solved through an iterative alternating projection method in [9]. Each iteration involves N modewise eigendecompositions to get the n-mode eigenvalues and eigenvectors. We denote the i_nth n-mode eigenvalue as $\lambda_{i_n}^{(n)}$.

There are two parameters to set in MPCA. One is Q for determining the tensor subspace dimensions $\{P_1, P_2, P_3\}$. Specifically, the first P_n eigenvectors

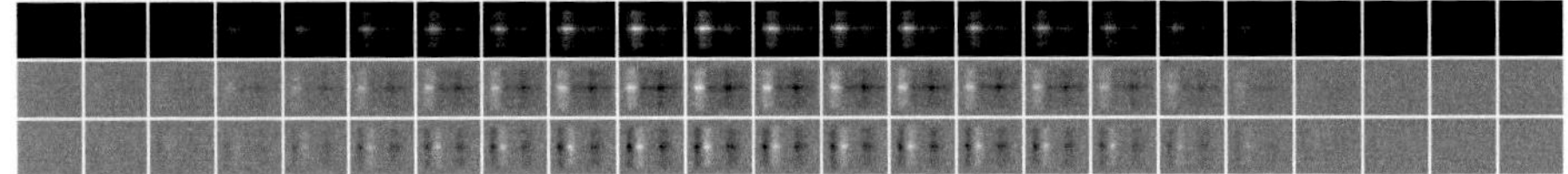

Fig. 1. Illustration of three selected eigentensors (MPCA features), where each row corresponds to an eigentensor with the third (depth) dimension concatenated

are kept in the n-mode so that the same (or similar) amount of variances is kept in each mode: $Q^{(1)} = Q^{(2)} = Q^{(3)} = Q$, where $Q^{(n)}$ is the ratio of variances kept in the n-mode defined as $Q^{(n)} = \sum_{i_n=1}^{P_n} \lambda_{i_n}^{(n)*} / \sum_{i_n=1}^{I_n} \lambda_{i_n}^{(n)*}$, and $\lambda_{i_n}^{(n)*}$ is the i_nth n-mode eigenvalue in the full projection [9]. The second parameter is the maximum number of iterations K, which can be safely set to 1 following [9].

MPCA Feature Selection. The MPCA projection matrices $\{\mathbf{U}^{(n)}, n = 1, 2, 3\}$ can be viewed as $P_1 \times P_2 \times P_3$ *eigentensors* [9] using (3):

$$\mathcal{U}_{p_1 p_2 p_3} = \mathbf{u}_{p_1}^{(1)} \circ \mathbf{u}_{p_2}^{(2)} \circ \mathbf{u}_{p_3}^{(3)} \in \mathbb{R}^{I_1 \times I_2 \times I_3}, \; p_n = 1, \ldots, P_n, \tag{5}$$

where $\mathbf{u}_{p_n}^{(n)}$ is the p_nth column of $\mathbf{U}^{(n)}$. Each eigentensor $\mathcal{U}_{p_1 p_2 p_3}$ is an MPCA feature and it can be mapped to the voxel space. Figure 1 illustrates three eigentensors capturing the most variance of the fMRI data studied in this paper. Each eigentensor is shown in a row by concatenating the third dimension. It is rich in structure because it is a rank-one tensor. Since our objective is whole-brain fMRI classification, it will be beneficial to select the P most informative (rather than all) features to be fed into a classifier such as the SVM [9].

Therefore, we further perform feature selection based on an importance score using either the variance or the MI criterion. We arrange the entries in $\{\mathcal{Y}_m\}$ into feature vectors $\{\mathbf{y}_m\}$ according to the importance score in descending order. Only the first P entries of $\{\mathbf{y}_m\}$ are selected as SVM input. We can determine the optimal value for P via cross-validation. For convenience, we denote the eigentensor corresponding to the pth selected feature as $\mathcal{U}_p$ so the pth feature y_p can be written as $y_p = \langle \mathcal{X}, \mathcal{U}_p \rangle$ using (2).

The **variance** is an *unsupervised* criterion. We obtain the variance $S_{p_1 p_2 p_3}$ captured by the eigentensor $\mathcal{U}_{p_1 p_2 p_3}$ using a scatter measure as

$$S_{p_1 p_2 p_3} = \sum_{m=1}^{M} \left[\mathcal{Y}_m(p_1, p_2, p_3) - \bar{\mathcal{Y}}(p_1, p_2, p_3) \right]^2. \tag{6}$$

The **MI** is a criterion to quantify statistical dependence between two discrete random variables A and B (for example) as [3]:

$$\mathrm{MI}(A; B) = \sum_{a \in A} \sum_{b \in B} p(a, b) \log \frac{p(a, b)}{p(a) p(b)}, \tag{7}$$

where $p(a, b)$ is the joint probability distribution, and $p(a)$ and $p(b)$ are the marginal probability distribution. In feature selection, we can use MI in a *supervised* way to measure the relevancy between a feature $\mathcal{Y}(p_1, p_2, p_3)$ and the class label c. A higher MI indicates a greater dependency or relevancy between them.

Table 1. Details of the four classification tasks for experimental evaluation

#Class	#Sample	Semantic categories (classes)
2	120	Animals (animal+insect) / tools (tool+furniture) [7]
4	120	Animal/insect/tool/vegetable [7]
6	180	Animal/insect/tool/vegetable/building/vehicle
8	240	Animal/insect/tool/vegetable/building/vehicle/buildingpart/clothing

Mapping for Interpretability. It is often useful to localize regions in the original voxel space of the brain for interpretation. Good features for classification are expected to be closely related to discriminating regions. Since $y_p = \langle \mathcal{X}, \mathcal{U}_p \rangle$, we can view y_p as a weighted summation of the voxels in $\mathcal{X}$, where the weights are contained in $\mathcal{U}_p$. Therefore, we propose a scheme to map the selected MPCA features (the eigentensors) to the voxel space. We perform a weighted aggregation of the selected eigentensors first and then determine the D most informative voxels to produce a spatial map $\mathcal{M}$ by choosing an appropriate threshold T (depending on D): $\mathcal{M} = \sum_{p=1}^{P} w_p \, |\mathcal{U}_p| > T$, where w_p is the weight for the pth eigentensor, and $|\cdot|$ denotes the absolute value (magnitude). Note that $\mathcal{M}$ is actually a low-rank tensor (rank P) since it is a summation of P rank-one tensors $\{\mathcal{U}_p\}$ [8].

3 Experiments and Discussions

Data. We choose a challenging multiclass dataset, the CMU Science 2008 fMRI data (CMU2008) [11]. It aims to predict brain activities associated with the meanings of nouns. The data acquisition experiments had 9 subjects viewing 60 different word-picture stimuli from 12 semantic categories, with 5 exemplars per category and 6 runs per stimulus. The acquisition matrix was 51×61 with 23 slices, with the numbers of brain voxels for 9 subjects ranging from 19,750 to 21,764. The mean PSC values over time are extracted as input fMRI features.[1]

Multiclass Tasks. We study four classification tasks: the binary (2-class) and 4-class tasks with the same settings as [7], and two additional, more challenging, 6-class and 8-class tasks. Table 1 summarizes the details.

Algorithms.[2] We evaluate seven feature selection/extraction algorithms in Table 2 on the four tasks above: the MI-based univariate feature selection (MI) [3], variance-based univariate feature selection (Var), LR with the elastic net penalty (LR+ENet) for multivariate feature selection [5,7]; PCA-based feature extraction followed by MI-based and variance-based feature selection (PCA-MI and PCA-Var), and the proposed methods of MPCA with MI-based and variance-based feature selection (MPCA-MI and MPCA-Var).

[1] `http://www.cs.cmu.edu/afs/cs/project/theo-73/www/science2008/data.html`

[2] We have also tested MPCA alone and MPCA with Lasso-based feature selection. They have similar accuracy as MPCA-MI/Var, but using much more features. In addition, replacing PCA with its popular extension, kernel PCA, gives only slightly better results than PCA-MI/Var.

Table 2. The classification accuracy in percentage (Acc) and average numbers of features selected (#Features) by five competing methods and the proposed two methods for the four tasks. The top two results in accuracy are highlighted in bold font.

Task	2-Class		4-Class		6-Class		8-Class	
Method	Acc	#Features	Acc	#Features	Acc	#Features	Acc	#Features
MI	72.78	2276	42.59	3472	37.65	4157	33.94	4208
Var	73.43	5120	39.26	5795	35.31	5405	33.52	5662
LR+ENet	72.13	629	42.78	3058	**40.19**	1441	34.58	3136
PCA-MI	71.30	65	36.85	59	34.14	78	30.19	102
PCA-Var	71.39	58	37.31	56	34.20	78	31.30	98
MPCA-MI	**75.83**	701	**44.35**	995	**40.86**	968	**36.06**	1088
MPCA-Var	**77.41**	910	**44.81**	973	40.06	1165	**34.68**	1034

Experimental Settings. We follow [7] to arrange testing, validation, and training sets in the format of $(1:1:4)$ for the six runs in all the experiments. Following [3], we use the SVM classifier with the linear kernel to classify selected features for all methods except LR+ENet which serves as a classifier itself [7,17]. We use the average classification accuracy as the evaluation metric.

Algorithm Settings. Parameters for LR+ENet are set following [7] and the number of selected features is determined according to the weight matrix in LR [17]. Other methods use the validation set to determine the number of selected features with the same steps as in [3]. For our MPCA-MI and MPCA-Var methods, we set the parameter $Q = 80$ in MPCA to report the results. Empirical studies to be shown in Fig. 2(a) show that the classification performance is not sensitive to Q as long as it is not too small (e.g., for $Q \geq 70$).

Classification Accuracy. As shown in Table 2, our proposed methods, MPCA-MI and MPCA-Var achieve the top two overall accuracy (highlighted in bold font), with MPCA-Var achieving the best results on 2-class and 4-class tasks and MPCA-MI achieving the best results on 6-class and 8-class tasks. MPCA-Var and MPCA-MI outperform the state-of-the-art (LR+ENet) by an average of 1.82% and 1.86%, respectively. Though inferior to our methods, LR+ENet indeed outperforms the other existing methods on the whole. In particular, LR+ENet achieves the second best result on 6-class task, slightly better than MPCA-Var. PCA gives the worst results.

Number of Selected Features. The number of features selected varies for different methods in Table 2. It fluctuates drastically (from 629 to 3,136) for LR+ENet. It is stable for the Var method but exceeds 5,000. It increases monotonically with the class number for the MI method. PCA can extract only $(M-1)$ features, e.g., $M = 150$ for the 6-class task. MPCA-Var and MPCA-MI use fewer features in general than MI, Var, and LR+ENet, and the number is relatively stable in contrast.

Parameter Sensitivity. Figure 2(a) plots the average accuracy against the Q values for each task. The four curves share a similar trend. The accuracy increases monotonically with Q till $Q = 70$ and then remains almost constant for $Q \geq 70$.

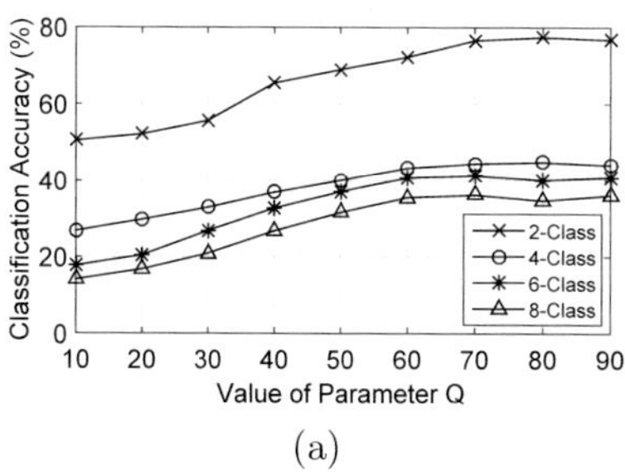

(a)

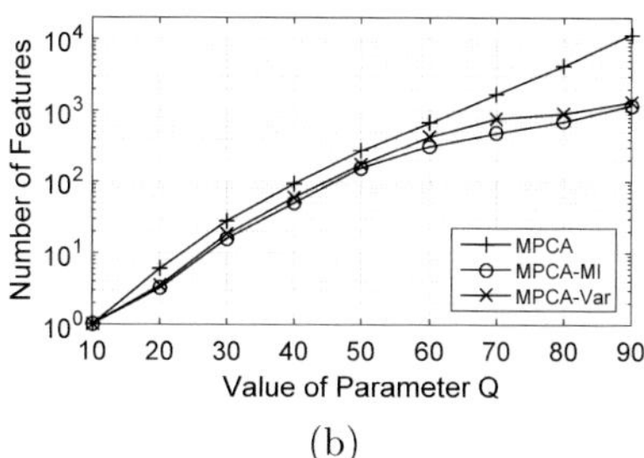

(b)

Fig. 2. Sensitivity against Q: (a) average accuracy of MPCA-Var (MPCA-MI has similar trends), and (b) average number of extracted (for MPCA) and selected (for MPCA-MI/MPCA-Var) features on the 2-class task (other tasks share similar trends).

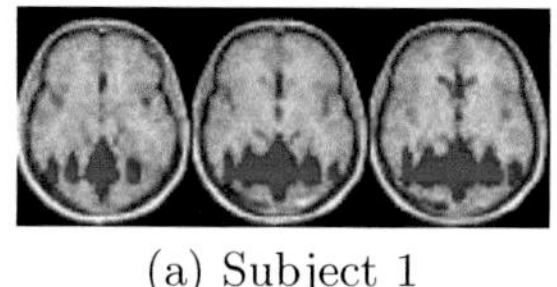

(a) Subject 1

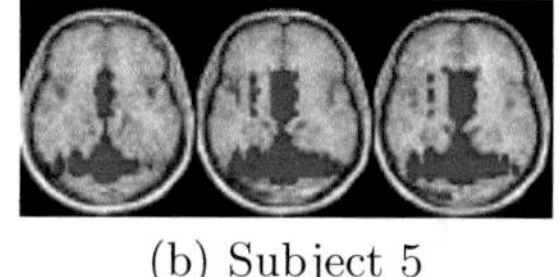

(b) Subject 5

Fig. 3. Discriminating regions localized by MPCA-MI for a 2-class task

Thus we choose $Q = 80$ to report the results. In addition, as shown in Fig. 2(b), the Q value has a greater effect on the number of features, which affects the efficiency in turn. The number of features extracted by MPCA increases almost exponentially with Q, while that by MPCA-MI or MPCA-Var increases with Q at a much slower rate for $Q > 60$.

Mapping and Interpretation. Since raw fMRI data are not provided in the CMU2008, we overlay the regions localized by our mapping scheme on a properly scaled and cropped version of the MRI template in "mri.mat" (Matlab R2013b). We set the weight $w_p = 1/p$ to give higher weights to MPCA features with higher importance scores. The regions localized with $D = 2000$ voxels are highlighted in red in Fig. 3 for the 9th-11th slices of two subjects for MPCA-MI on the 2-class task. The localized regions are spatially coherent and largely consistent between different subjects. Moreover, the localized discriminating regions of Subject 5 have significant overlap with the interpretable regions of the same subject depicted in Fig. 3(B) of [11], indicating good interpretability.

4 Conclusion

In this paper, we propose to learn features directly from tensor representations of whole-brain fMRI data via MPCA for classification. We use a variance-based or an MI-based criterion to select the most informative MPCA features for SVM classification. In addition, we propose a novel scheme to localize discriminating regions by mapping the selected MPCA features to the raw voxel space. Experimental results on challenging multiclass tasks show that our methods outperform the state-of-the-art methods. Furthermore, the proposed mapping scheme can localize discriminating regions that are spatially coherent and consistent cross subjects, with good potential for neuroscience interpretation.

Acknowledgments. We thank the support of Hong Kong Research Grants Council (under Grant 22200014 and the Hong Kong PhD Fellowship Scheme).

References

1. Batmanghelich, N., Dong, A., Taskar, B., Davatzikos, C.: Regularized tensor factorization for multi-modality medical image classification. In: Fichtinger, G., Martel, A., Peters, T. (eds.) MICCAI 2011, Part III. LNCS, vol. 6893, pp. 17–24. Springer, Heidelberg (2011)
2. Chen, M., et al.: Survey of encoding and decoding of visual stimulus via fMRI: An image analysis perspective. Brain Imaging and Behavior 8(1), 7–23 (2014)
3. Chou, C.A., et al.: Voxel selection framework in multi-voxel pattern analysis of fMRI data for prediction of neural response to visual stimuli. IEEE Transactions on Medical Imaging 33(4), 925–934 (2014)
4. Cuingnet, R., Rosso, C., Lehéricy, S., Dormont, D., Benali, H., Samson, Y., Colliot, O.: Spatially regularized SVM for the detection of brain areas associated with stroke outcome. In: Jiang, T., Navab, N., Pluim, J.P.W., Viergever, M.A. (eds.) MICCAI 2010, Part I. LNCS, vol. 6361, pp. 316–323. Springer, Heidelberg (2010)
5. Ecker, C., et al.: Investigating the predictive value of whole-brain structural MR scans in autism: A pattern classification approach. NeuroImage 49(1), 44–56 (2010)
6. Irimia, A., Van Horn, J.D.: Systematic network lesioning reveals the core white matter scaffold of the human brain. Frontiers in Human Neuroscience 8, 1–14 (2014)
7. Kampa, K., Mehta, S., et al.: Sparse optimization in feature selection: application in neuroimaging. Journal of Global Optimization 59(2-3), 439–457 (2014)
8. Lu, H., Plataniotis, K.N., Venetsanopoulos, A.: Multilinear Subspace Learning: Dimensionality Reduction of Multidimensional Data. CRC Press (2013)
9. Lu, H., Plataniotis, K.N., et al.: MPCA: Multilinear principal component analysis of tensor objects. IEEE Trans. Neural Networks 19(1), 18–39 (2008)
10. McKeown, M.J., et al.: Local linear discriminant analysis (LLDA) for group and region of interest (ROI)-based fMRI analysis. NeuroImage 37(3), 855–865 (2007)
11. Mitchell, T.M., Shinkareva, S.V., et al.: Predicting human brain activity associated with the meanings of nouns. Science 320(5880), 1191–1195 (2008)
12. Mourão-Miranda, J., et al.: Classifying brain states and determining the discriminating activation patterns: Support vector machine on functional MRI data. NeuroImage 28(4), 980–995 (2005)
13. Mourão-Miranda, J., et al.: The impact of temporal compression and space selection on SVM analysis of single-subject and multi-subject fMRI data. NeuroImage 33(4), 1055–1065 (2006)
14. Mwangi, B., Tian, T.S., Soares, J.C.: A review of feature reduction techniques in neuroimaging. Neuroinformatics 12(2), 229–244 (2013)
15. Rasmussen, P.M., et al.: Model sparsity and brain pattern interpretation of classification models in neuroimaging. Pattern Recognition 45(6), 2085–2100 (2012)
16. Retico, A., Bosco, P., et al.: Predictive models based on support vector machines: Whole-brain versus regional analysis of structural MRI in the alzheimer's disease. Journal of Neuroimaging, 1–12 (2014)
17. Ryali, S., Supekar, K., Abrams, D.A., Menon, V.: Sparse logistic regression for whole-brain classification of fMRI data. NeuroImage 51(2), 752–764 (2010)

Prediction of Trabecular Bone Anisotropy from Quantitative Computed Tomography Using Supervised Learning and a Novel Morphometric Feature Descriptor

Vimal Chandran, Philippe Zysset, and Mauricio Reyes

Institute for Surgical Technology and Biomechanics, University of Bern, Swizerland
{vimal.chandran,philippe.zysset,mauricio.reyes}@istb.unibe.ch

Abstract. Patient-specific biomechanical models including local bone mineral density and anisotropy have gained importance for assessing musculoskeletal disorders. However the trabecular bone anisotropy captured by high-resolution imaging is only available at the peripheral skeleton in clinical practice. In this work, we propose a supervised learning approach to predict trabecular bone anisotropy that builds on a novel set of pose invariant feature descriptors. The statistical relationship between trabecular bone anisotropy and feature descriptors were learned from a database of pairs of high resolution QCT and clinical QCT reconstructions. On a set of leave-one-out experiments, we compared the accuracy of the proposed approach to previous ones, and report a mean prediction error of 6% for the tensor norm, 6% for the degree of anisotropy and 19° for the principal tensor direction. These findings show the potential of the proposed approach to predict trabecular bone anisotropy from clinically available QCT images.

Keywords: Trabecular anisotropy, QCT, HRpQCT, Implicit coordinate system, Tensor, Multi-output regression.

1 Introduction

Musculoskeletal diseases, such as osteoporosis, are characterized by low bone mass and impaired trabecular structure, leading to bone fragility and an increased risk for fractures. An improved fracture risk assessment is provided by evaluating the patient's bone strength at an anatomical site at risk (spine, hip) via clinical quantitative computer tomography (QCT)-based finite element analyses [1]. These models can be improved. Indeed, trabecular bone anisotropy, the most important determinant of the mechanical behaviour of trabecular bone after bone volume fraction [2], can be accounted for in numerical simulations to better predict bone strength [3,4]. Unfortunately, such information is derived from high resolution peripheral QCT (HRpQCT) and is not directly available for the axial skeleton from clinical CT.

Predicting trabecular bone anisotropy using prior knowledge from QCT images has been of interest and two types of strategies have been proposed in

N. Navab et al. (Eds.): MICCAI 2015, Part I, LNCS 9349, pp. 621–628, 2015.
DOI: 10.1007/978-3-319-24553-9_76

the literature. Firstly, Hazrati-Marangalou et al. [4], proposed a registration driven prediction mechanism. From a database of HRpQCT images, the closest to the patient's image was chosen by minimizing the root-mean-square error and trabecular bone anisotropy was mapped by a mesh morphing technique. Taghizadeh et al. [5], used a template based morphing mechanism where the patient's QCT image was rigidly and non-rigidly registered with a QCT template image. The computed registration transformation was then applied to the corresponding HRpQCT template image to map trabecular bone anisotropy. Although the registration-based approaches have shown good performance, in practice they are computationally expensive and careful registration parameter tuning is required.

A second group of approaches are based on supervised learning. Lekadir et al. [6] used a statistical predictive model, constructed from a database of HRpQCT images. A partial least square (PLS) regression model was built from training data to predict trabecular bone anisotropy. Their approach involves a linear regression and a non-rigid registration step that requires manual landmark annotations.

Given the inherent difficulty involved in deriving trabecular bone anisotropy from clinical scans, and to circumvent the need for time-consuming registration procedures or manual landmark annotations, we proposed a supervised learning approach to predict trabecular bone anisotropy in the human proximal femur. Differently from previous approaches, we used a multi-output decision tree regressor that relies on a novel set of pose invariant feature descriptors. An implicit coordinate system of the proximal femur was constructed that enables computation of pose invariant features. Trabecular bone anisotropy was described as a tensor and its statistical relationship with the feature descriptors was learned from a database of aligned HRpQCT and clinical QCT pairs of images. We compared our approach to a registration based and PLS based approaches, and demonstrated on a set of leave-one-out experiments the ability of the approach to predict trabecular bone anisotropy from clinical QCT images.

2 Methods

Our aim is to establish a mapping from the pose invariant features $\boldsymbol{x} = (x_1, ...x_d) \in \mathbb{R}^d$ computed on clinical QCT to the corresponding tensor $\boldsymbol{y} \in \mathbb{R}^6$ computed on HRpQCT. Consequently the construction of the mapping is cast as a regression problem. Given a training set $\{\langle \boldsymbol{X_i}, \boldsymbol{Y_i} \rangle | i = 1, ..., N\}$ of N QCT and HRpQCT aligned pairs of images, we extract from each i_{th} image, $\boldsymbol{X_i} = (\boldsymbol{x}_1, ...\boldsymbol{x}_C) \in \mathbb{X}$ with an output response $\boldsymbol{Y_i} = (\boldsymbol{y}_1, ...\boldsymbol{y}_C) \in \mathbb{Y}$ over a grid of C nodes. We construct a function $\hat{\boldsymbol{y}} : \mathbb{X} \mapsto \mathbb{Y}$ from a space of images $\mathbb{X}$ to the space of responses $\mathbb{Y}$ that predicts the response for any new test image $\boldsymbol{X_{test}} \in \mathbb{X}$.

2.1 Feature Extraction

Implicit Coordinate System. For feature extraction, an implicit coordinate system of the proximal femur bone was constructed, and shown in Figure 1.

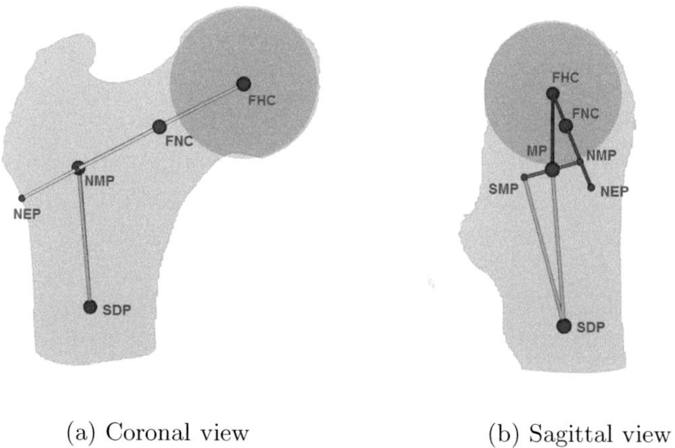

(a) Coronal view (b) Sagittal view

Fig. 1. Implicit coordinate system of the human proximal femur. It was used to extract a total of 10 morphometric pose invariant feature descriptors (see Table.1).

First, the center of the femoral head (FHC) was defined by a mass center of a spherical region with minimal cross-section area. The neck axis was constructed by following the procedure reported by Kang et al. [7,8]. In short, the radius of the spherical region of the femoral head was enlarged by 25% and an initial neck center was defined. Using Powell's optimization, the center of the femoral neck (FNC) was computed and the neck axis was defined. The intersection point between the neck axis and the lateral surface of the proximal femur was defined as neck-axis-end-point (NEP). Then, the mass center of each slice distal to NEP was computed. The shaft axis was constructed by RANSAC fitting. The most distal point of the shaft axis was chosen as shaft-axis-distal-point (SDP). Since the neck and shaft axes does not intersect, a midpoint (MP) was defined as the shortest distance between the neck and shaft axes. By connecting SDP, MP and FHC, the implicit coordinate system was defined. The caput-collum-diaphyseal (CCD) angle was represented as $\angle(SDP)(MP)(FHC)$. All the images are re-positioned to the common coordinate system with origin at neck-midpoint (NMP), $+x$ axis as the neck axis and $+y$ axis towards the distal surface of the femur. From experiments, the procedure has shown to be robust, fast, and thus clinically applicable.

Input Features. A uniform sampling grid with isotropic grid spacing of $5.3mm$ [5] was defined over the QCT and HRpQCT images. At each node c_j of the grid $j = \{1, ...C\}$ lying inside the trabecular region, a volume of interest (VOI) was extracted on which feature descriptors and tensors (responses) were computed.

We propose to use two family of pose invariant features, morphometric- and texture-based. The morphometric features are computed with respect to the femoral implicit coordinate system [section 2.1]. We remark that in contrast to

Table 1. List of features computed at each grid node

Morphometric Features		Texture Features	
Scalar	**Angle**	**1st Order Statistics**	**GLCM**
Distance b/w FHC-FNC	CCD	Mean	Energy
Distance b/w FHC-MP		Std.Dev	Entropy
Distance b/w FNC-MP		Skewness	Correlation
Distance b/w FHC-c_j		Kurtosis	Inertia
Distance b/w FNC-c_j		Minimum	Cluster Shade
Distance b/w MP-c_j		Maximum	Cluster Prominance
Femoral Head Diameter			Inverse Difference Moment
Femoral Neck Min.Cross.Area			Haralick Correlation

previous approaches, this property results in a registration-free approach. The texture based features includes first order statistical features and GLCM [9,10]. The list of features is presented in Table 1. The input feature set $\boldsymbol{x} = (x_1, ...x_d)$ includes all the morphometric features, mean and variance of all the texture features. For texture based features, a feature pooling was performed, followed by principal component analysis (PCA) to reduce dimensionality and redundancy of feature sets. This leads to a reduced feature space of $\mathbb{R}^{214}$ to $\mathbb{R}^{58}$.

Output Response. Tensors were computed on the corresponding VOI at each grid node c_j using the Mean Intercept Length technique (MIL) [11]. As tensors lie on a Riemannian manifold, we used the Log-Euclidean framework to perform Euclidean operations as follows [12]. The MIL tensor is a 3×3 positive semi-definite matrix $\boldsymbol{M}$ with associated eigenvectors $\boldsymbol{e_1}$, $\boldsymbol{e_2}$, $\boldsymbol{e_3}$ and eigenvalues λ_1,λ_2,λ_3. The matrix logarithm of $\boldsymbol{M}$ is calculated as

$$\boldsymbol{L} = \log(\boldsymbol{M}) = \sum_{k=1}^{3} \log(\lambda_k)(\boldsymbol{e_k} \otimes \boldsymbol{e_k}), \tag{1}$$

where $\otimes$ represents the dyadic product. The response variable is then defined as

$$\boldsymbol{y} = (L_{11}, L_{22}, L_{33}, \sqrt{2}L_{12}, \sqrt{2}L_{13}, \sqrt{2}L_{23}) \tag{2}$$

The tensor $\boldsymbol{M}$ can be obtained from the Log-Euclidean vector $\boldsymbol{y}$ by performing matrix exponential [12].

2.2 Multi-output Regression Model

Decision forests are a group of learning methods widely used for classification and regression tasks in machine learning and computer vision. An extension of decision forest with extra trees algorithm has been proposed to handle multi-output image classification [13,14]. We adopted this technique as a regression approach as it promotes preservation of tensor structure ($trace(\boldsymbol{M}) = 3$). During supervised learning, the algorithm randomly selects without replacement K

input variables $\{x_1, ...x_k\}$ from the training data $\boldsymbol{D} := \{\langle \boldsymbol{X_i}, \boldsymbol{Y_i} \rangle | i = 1, ..., N\}$. For each selected input variable, within the interval $[x_i^{min}, x_i^{max}]$ a cutpoint s_i was randomly defined and splitting $[x_i < s_i]$ was performed. Among the K candidate splits, the best split was chosen via optimizing the L2 mean square error [14]. This was a reasonable choice due to the Log-Euclidean transform being applied to the tensor.

3 Results and Discussion

3.1 Datasource

The study was performed on a database of QCT and HRpQCT images of human proximal femora. The training data comprises 30 femurs (15 males, 15 females with age 76±11 years, range 46-96) and were obtained from a previous study [15]. In summary, the clinical QCT images (Brillance64, Phillips, Germany, intensity: 100 mA, voltage: 120 kV, voxel size: 0.33 0.33 1.00 mm^3) and HRpQCT images (Xtreme CT, Scanco, Switzerland, intensity: 900 A, voltage: 60 kVp, voxel size: 0.082 0.082 0.082 mm^3). The clinical QCT images were resampled to have isotropic voxel spacing, and the cortical bone in the HRpQCT images was masked out according to the procedure reported in [16].

3.2 Evaluation Metric

For numerical evaluation of the proposed approach, a leave-one-out strategy was followed for the available 30 femurs. The MIL tensor $\boldsymbol{M}$ was measured from the HRpQCT images. The predicted tensor was represented as $\widehat{\boldsymbol{M}}$ with eigenvectors $\widehat{\boldsymbol{e_1}}$, $\widehat{\boldsymbol{e_2}}$, $\widehat{\boldsymbol{e_3}}$ and eigenvalues $\widehat{\lambda_1}$, $\widehat{\lambda_2}$, $\widehat{\lambda_3}$. We adopted the same evaluation metric described in [6]. The tensor norm error $TN_{error} = \|\boldsymbol{M} - \widehat{\boldsymbol{M}}\| / \|\boldsymbol{M}\|$, degree of anisotropy error $DA_{error} = |DA - \widehat{DA}|/DA$ and angular error of the principal tensor direction $PTD = \arccos(\boldsymbol{e_1}, \widehat{\boldsymbol{e_1}})$.

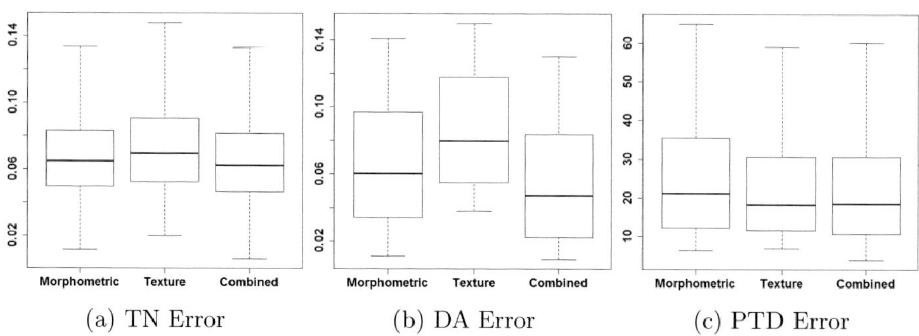

(a) TN Error (b) DA Error (c) PTD Error

Fig. 2. Prediction error of morphometric, texture and combined features for different evaluation metrics

3.3 Experiment

Experiment 1: Feature Importance. On a first experiment, we evaluated the individual and combined predictive power of our feature descriptors. The number of trees used for the experiment was empirically found as 80. In comparison to the texture features, morphometric features offered a better tensor prediction and preservation of degree of anisotropy (Figure 2a, 2b). This supports the fact that trabecular bone anisotropy was related to the bone morphology. In contrast, texture features better predicted the principal tensor direction (Figure 2c). Trabecular bone anisotropy is characterized by specific orientations to support the stresses acting on the femur and they form an internal texture pattern. This motivated us to combine the features and perform the analysis. It resulted in a higher predictive power for the combined feature set (Figure 2).

Experiment 2: Comparative Study with Previous Approaches. On the second experiment, we compared the proposed approach to registration based- and PLS based approaches. For registration based, the image closest to the test image was taken and mapping was performed using rigid and non-rigid registration [17]. In the case of PLS based, the regression model was built using the proposed combined set of features. The number of trees used for the experiment was empirically found as 80. The prediction accuracy of our approach yielded comparable results to the registration based method and outperformed PLS based method (Figure 3a). In addition, a similar trend was observed for the degree of anisotropy (Figure 3b). Furthermore, our approach better predicted the principal tensor direction, which is of primary interest for finite element simulations (Figure 3c). The prediction accuracy in different regions of femur revealed that our approach offered a better prediction with lower tensor norm error (Figure 4). Further, it was able to track the main loading direction of the femur with higher accuracy.

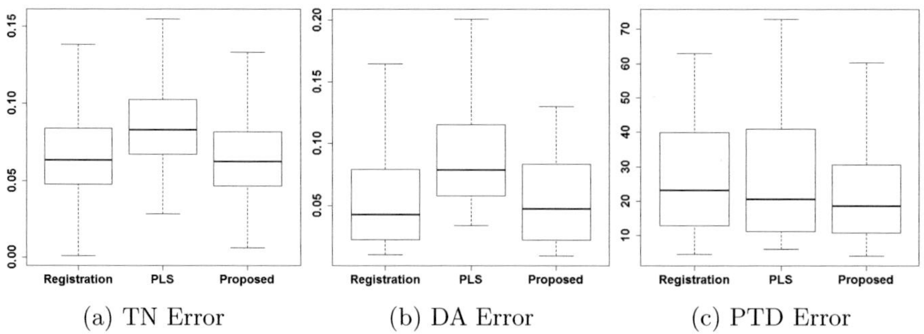

(a) TN Error (b) DA Error (c) PTD Error

Fig. 3. Prediction error of Registration-based, PLS-based and proposed approach for different evaluation metrics

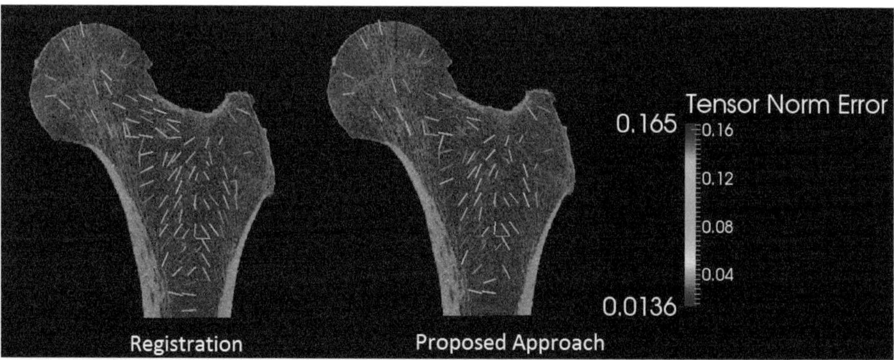

Fig. 4. Illustration of trabecular bone anisotropy prediction accuracy achieved on a test case. The lines indicate the principal orientation of the tensors computed on the HRpQCT image and displayed on an image slice. The colors correspond to the tensor norm error at each grid node. Left: tensor prediction accuracy by registration based approach, Right: tensor prediction accuracy by the proposed approach.

In comparison to the other approaches, the preference of the proposed approach can be explained by its ability of preserving tensor structure ($trace(\boldsymbol{M}) = 3$) and a prior knowledge of trabecular bone anisotropy over the entire population. This was supported by (Figure 4) that illustrates the possible problem of registration approach in handling highly homogenized bone areas.

4 Conclusion and Future Work

In finite element analysis, trabecular bone anisotropy contributes significantly to the assessment of the bone strength and improves diagnosis of musculoskeletal diseases [3,4]. In comparison to previous approaches in predicting trabecular bone anisotropy, we propose a multi-output nonlinear supervised learning technique that uses pose invariant feature descriptors, which makes the approach registration-free. The nature of multi-output regression promotes preservation of tensor structure ($trace(\boldsymbol{M}) = 3$). According to our knowledge this is the first study predicting trabecular bone anisotropy from clinical QCT. The study also shows the potential of statistical approaches in predicting trabecular bone anisotropy. The approach can be extended to other anatomical sites where trabecular bone anisotropy plays an important role.

Future work includes a thorough comparison to other approaches on a larger dataset, incorporation of cortical information and evaluation through finite element analysis.

Acknowledgements. This work is supported by the Swiss National Science Foundation, Project number - 143769. The authors thank Dr. Ghislain Maquer for his comments on mechanical aspects and proof reading.

References

1. Kopperdahl, D.L., Aspelund, T., Hoffmann, P.F., Sigurdsson, S., Siggeirsdottir, K., Harris, T.B., Gudnason, V., Keaveny, T.M.: Assessment of incident spine and hip fractures in women and men using finite element analysis of CT scans. Journal of Bone and Mineral Research 29(3) (2014)
2. Maquer, G., Musy, S.N., Wandel, J., Gross, T., Zysset, P.K.: Bone Volume Fraction and Fabric Anisotropy Are Better Determinants of Trabecular Bone Stiffness than Other Morphological Variables. Journal of Bone and Mineral Research (2014)
3. Enns-Bray, W.S., Owoc, J.S., Nishiyama, K.K., Boyd, S.K.: Mapping anisotropy of the proximal femur for enhanced image based finite element analysis. Journal of Biomechanics 47(13) (2014)
4. Hazrati Marangalou, J., Ito, K., Cataldi, M., Taddei, F., van Rietbergen, B.: A novel approach to estimate trabecular bone anisotropy using a database approach. Journal of Biomechanics 46(14) (2013)
5. Taghizadeh, E., Maquer, G., Reyes, M., Büchler, P.: Including the trabecular anisotropy from registered microCT data in homogenized FE model improves the bones mechanical predictions. In: CMBBE (2014)
6. Lekadir, K., Hazrati-Marangalou, J., Hoogendoorn, C., Taylor, Z., van Rietbergen, B., Frangi, A.F.: Statistical estimation of femur micro-architecture using optimal shape and density predictors. Journal of Biomechanics 48(4) (2015)
7. Kang, Y., Engelke, K., Fuchs, C., Kalender, W.A.: An anatomic coordinate system of the femoral neck for highly reproducible BMD measurements using 3D QCT. Computerized Medical Imaging and Graphics 29(7) (2005)
8. Kang, Y., Engelke, K., Kalender, W.A.: A New Accurate and Precise 3-D Segmentation Method for Skeletal Structures in Volumetric CT Data. IEEE TMI 22(5) (2003)
9. Haralick, R.M., Shanmugam, K.: Textural Features for Image Classification. IEEE TSMC 3(6) (1973)
10. Ortiz, A., Palacio, A.A., Górriz, J.M., Ramírez, J., Salas-González, D.: Segmentation of brain MRI using SOM-FCM-based method and 3D statistical descriptors. Computational and Mathematical Methods in Medicine (2013)
11. Harrigan, T., Mann, R.: Characterization of microstructural anisotropy in orthotropic materials using a second rank tensor. Journal of Materials Science 19(3) (1984)
12. Pennec, X., Fillard, P., Ayache, N.: A Riemannian Framework for Tensor Computing. International Journal of Computer Vision 66(1) (2006)
13. Dumont, M., Marée, R.: Fast multi-class image annotation with random windows and multiple output randomized trees. In: Proc. of VISAPP, vol. 2 (2009)
14. Marée, R., Wehenkel, L., Geurts, P.: Extremely randomized trees and random subwindows for image classification, annotation, and retrieval. In: Decision Forests for Computer Vision and Medical Image Analysis (2013)
15. Dall'Ara, E., Luisier, B., Schmidt, R., Kainberger, F., Zysset, P., Pahr, D.: A nonlinear QCT-based finite element model validation study for the human femur tested in two configurations in vitro. Bone 52(1) (2013)
16. Pahr, D.H., Zysset, P.K.: From high-resolution CT data to finite element models: development of an integrated modular framework. CMBBE Journal 12(1) (2009)
17. Klein, S., Staring, M., Murphy, K., Viergever, M.A., Pluim, J.P.W.: elastix: A toolbox for intensity-based medical image registration. IEEE Trans. Med. Imaging 29(1) (2010)

Automatic Diagnosis of Ovarian Carcinomas via Sparse Multiresolution Tissue Representation

Aïcha BenTaieb[1], Hector Li-Chang[2], David Huntsman[2], and Ghassan Hamarneh[1]

[1] Medical Image Analysis Lab, Simon Fraser University, Burnaby, BC, Canada
[2] Departments of Pathology and Laboratory Medicine and Obstetrics and Gynaecology, University of British Columbia, Vancouver, Canada

Abstract. It has now been convincingly demonstrated that ovarian carcinoma subtypes are not a single disease but comprise a heterogeneous group of neoplasms. Whole slide images of tissue sections are used clinically for diagnosing biologically distinct subtypes, as opposed to different grades of the same disease. This new grading scheme for ovarian carcinomas results in a low to moderate interobserver agreement among pathologists. In practice, the majority of cases are diagnosed at advanced stages and the overall prognosis is typically poor. In this work, we propose an automatic system for the diagnosis of ovarian carcinoma subtypes from large-scale histopathology images. Our novel approach uses an unsupervised feature learning framework composed of a sparse tissue representation and a discriminative feature encoding scheme. We validate our model on a challenging clinical dataset of 80 patients and demonstrate its ability to diagnose whole slide images with an average accuracy of 91% using a linear support vector machine classifier.

Keywords: Histopathology, ovarian carcinomas, machine learning.

1 Introduction

Recent advances in epithelial ovarian cancer diagnosis have shown that morphologic subtypes of ovarian carcinomas (OC) are associated with distinct pathologic and molecular characteristics. This resulted in the introduction of a new grading system for OC diagnosis [12,15]. The World Health Organization recommends characterizing OC as five distinct tumour types: High Grade Serous Carcinoma, Low Grade Serous Carcinoma, Endometrioid Carcinoma, Mucinous Carcinoma and Clear Cell Carcinoma (HGSC, LGSC, EN, MC and CC). At present, targeted therapies are being introduced for each subtype and successful treatments are highly correlated with the accurate classification of these subtypes [13].

Pathologists diagnose OC from tumour biopsies (Fig. 1). Samples of the tumorous tissue are collected and examined using Hematoxylin & Eosin (H&E) stained tissue sections at different microscope magnifications [10]. However, diagnosis from histopathology images is impaired by technical factors (e.g. lighting, staining variability, operator acquisition procedure) and by pathologists'

N. Navab et al. (Eds.): MICCAI 2015, Part I, LNCS 9349, pp. 629–636, 2015.
DOI: 10.1007/978-3-319-24553-9_77

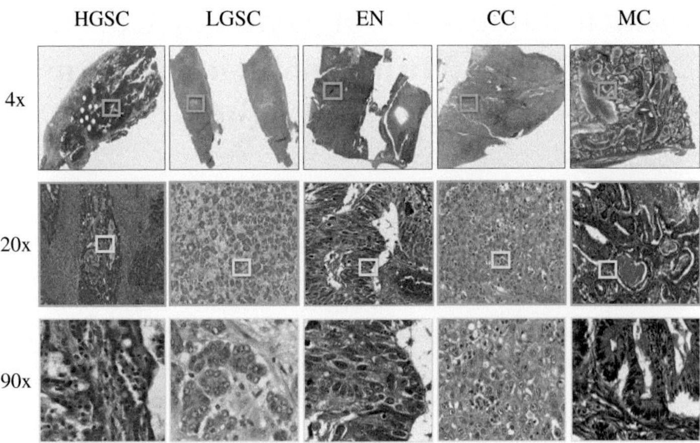

Fig. 1. Ovarian carcinoma subtypes at different microscope resolutions. HGSC: High Grade Serous Carcinoma, LGSC: Low Grade Serous Carcinoma, EN: Endometrioid carcinoma, CC: Clear cell Carcinoma and MC: Mucinous Carcinoma. Each carcinoma subtype is shown at 4x, 20x and 90x microscope zoom.

experience. Non-expert pathologists often end up performing additional costly tests (e.g. immunohistochemistry) or asking for second opinions. The variability among tissues coupled with the limited knowledge of ovarian carcinomas subtypes translates into a moderate agreement among pathologists [11] and a high mortality rate among patients [1].

A system capable of automatically classifying OC subtypes from whole slide histopathology images would be valuable for several reasons. First, an automatic system provides computational abilities enabling rapid screening and learning from large scale multiresolution images (i.e. too large/detailed for a human observer to examine thoroughly). Second, such an automated system may act as a second reader while mimicking expert pathologists. Finally, it can benefit the diagnostic procedure by minimizing the inter-observer variability among pathologists while adding robustness to the diagnosis.

There is a vast literature on classification and grading of cancer from histopathology images [7,8]. One widely used approach is to design a set of features, usually based on texture (e.g. SIFT, Gabor filters) or segmentation [14,4]. More recent studies have applied unsupervised feature learning techniques to classify cancerous from non-cancerous regions of tissues [9,3]. For cancer typing from a tissue section (i.e. classification of subtypes of ovarian cancer), the task has been shown to be more challenging [16]. Xu et al. [16] proposed to classify subtypes of colon cancer using multiple instance learning. This weakly-supervised framework uses hand-designed features and annotated data to first classify a tissue section as cancerous (or not). Then, a patch-based clustering is applied on cancerous tissue slides to identify different subtypes of colon cancer at different spatial locations. In OC diagnosis, this clustering framework is not fully suitable. In fact, different regions of OC tissues do not correspond to a different type but to different grades of the same subtype, which increases the intra-class variability. Thus, OC diagnosis is a multiclass classification rather than a patch-based clustering problem.

To the best of our knowledge, no existing work has addressed the automatic typing of OC subtypes. The question we raise in this paper is whether it is possible to automate the analysis of OC subtypes despite the limited existing pathogenetic understanding of the disease, the high variability among patients and within tissues (in terms of staining and grades) and the low agreement between pathologists. To this end we make the following contributions: (i) we design an unsupervised feature learning technique based on a hybrid model combining a sparse multiresolution representation of tissue sections with a discriminative feature encoding scheme; (ii) we demonstrate that our technique achieves a better performance on OC than state-of-the-art unsupervised feature learning methods proposed in histopathology image classification; (iii) we show that our unified framework captures more complex and discriminative patterns of textures and shapes that are more suitable for a multiclass typing of tissues. Ultimately, we validate the proposed approach on real clinical data and show that our pipeline provides marked improvements over existing techniques.

2 Approach

At a high level, our approach proceeds as follows. We represent a tissue slide X with a set of unlabeled multiresolution patches $[x_1, ...x_P]$ extracted at different spatial locations. For each patch x_i we learn a new sparse image representation using a multi-layer deconvolution network (DN) [17]. This representation is then used to encode a high-dimensional set of discriminative features $\psi(x_i)$ via Fisher Vector Encoding (FVE) [5]. Finally, using a linear SVM, we predict a carcinoma subtype $y_i \in \mathcal{Y}$ where $\mathcal{Y} = \{HGSC, CC, EN, MC, LGSC\}$ for each multi-resolution patch of a tissue section. To infer a final carcinoma for the whole slide, we aggregate the classifiers' prediction probabilities, $P(y_i|\psi(x_i))$, for all patches. Next, we provide the details of these methodological components.

Feature Learning: To begin, our goal is to find a new image representation more suitable for classification. This representation can then be used to extract robust local image descriptors. This is specifically challenging for OC as the appearance of the tissue widely differs at different locations and among patients. To overcome these challenges, we adopt an unsupervised feature learning approach which has shown to produce more robust features in presence of wide technical and biological variations [4]. Using a DN, we learn a set of filters that allow us to reconstruct the original image from convolutions with feature maps (Fig. 2-a). A feature map can be considered as an activation map where the values are filters' responses. These filters and feature maps are estimated using a unified optimization technique based on the convolutional decomposition of an image under a sparsity constraint [17]. Feature maps are inferred in a hierarchical fashion (Fig. 2-b) by stacking layers of sparse convolutions to form a multi-layer DN. More concretely, a single layer DN decompose an RGB patch x_i into a linear sum of

K_1 latent feature maps $z^i_{k,1}$ convolved with filters $f_{k,1}$ where $k = [1, \ldots, K_1]$. This reconstruction relies on optimizing the following energy with respect to z and f:

$$E(x_i) = \lambda || \sum_{k=1}^{K_1} z^i_{k,1} \circledast f_{k,1} - x_i||_2^2 - ||z^i_{k,1}||_1, \tag{1}$$

where the first term is the reconstruction error and the second term encourages sparsity in the latent feature maps. λ controls the balance between the contributions of the reconstruction and sparsity. The sign $\circledast$ corresponds to the convolution operation. For a $N \times M$ image and filters f_k of size $H \times H$, the resulting feature maps are of size $(N + H - 1) \times (M + H - 1)$. To better capture multiresolution patterns, we use a set of filters with adaptive sizes.

In practice, first layer filters of a DN $f_{k,1}$ (learnt from minimizing E over all training set) are Gabor-like filters and represent low-level visual information from the image (Fig. 2-a). To capture more complex patterns, we learn a hierarchy of filters by stacking multiple layers of deconvolutions. The hierarchy is formed by treating the feature maps of layer $l - 1$ as input to layer l. Each of these layers attempts to directly minimize the reconstruction error of the input patch while inferring sparse feature maps. During learning, we use the entire set of patches to seek for latent feature maps for each image and learnt filters. At layer l, we minimize the following energy function:

$$E_l(x) = \lambda \sum_{i=1}^{P} \sum_{j=1}^{K_{l-1}} || \sum_{k=1}^{K_l} (z^i_{k,l} \circledast f_{k,l}) - z^i_{j,l-1}||_2^2 + \sum_{i=1}^{P} \sum_{k=1}^{K_l} ||z^i_{k,l}||_1 \tag{2}$$

where P is the total number of images, K_{l-1} and K_l are the total number of feature maps at layer $l-1$ and l respectively, $z_{k,l}$ are the inferred feature maps at layer l, and $f_{k,l}$ are the learnt filters. Feature maps $z^i_{j,l-1}$ are inferred at layer $l-1$. A max-pooling operation is applied on feature maps between layers. The energy function $E_l(x; z, f)$ is biconvex with respect to z and f thus the optimization is solved using an iterative procedure [17]. At inference, we set the optimal z given a set of filters f and input images x. This corresponds to solving a convex energy function with a sparsity constraint. This step is optimized via stochastic gradient descent which showed to be efficient for large-scale problems [17].

Each patch is now represented by a hierarchical set of feature maps. We densely construct local image descriptors by splitting each feature map into overlapping quadrants of fixed size and pooling over the absolute value of activations in each quadrant. This pooling procedure adds translation invariance to the local descriptors [17]. We obtain a final set of local descriptors $\phi(x_i)$ by concatenation of the pooled activations from each feature map (Fig. 2-c).

Fisher Vector Encoding: Encoding features from the local descriptors $\phi(x_i)$ is a critical step for designing discriminative features [6]. We use FVE to define a mapping or "encoding" of the descriptors ϕ into a higher dimensional feature space. Here, our assumption is that higher dimensional features facilitate class-separation and enable us to use simple linear classifiers. To do this, we first

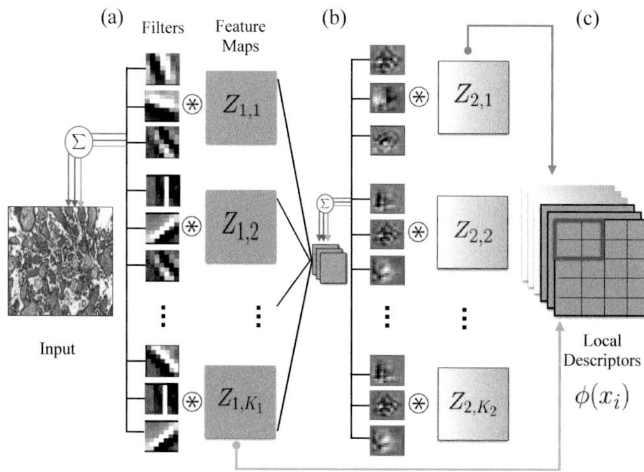

Fig. 2. Representation of a 2-layer DN. Feature maps $Z_{j,k}$, convolved with learnt low and mid-level filters, form a sparse representation of an image. K_1 and K_2 refer to the number of feature maps in each layer. Aggregation of the feature maps is used to construct dense local descriptors ϕ. In our implementation, we use a 3-layer DN.

learn a codebook of Gaussian Mixture Models (GMM) from the total set of local descriptors. Each Gaussian models the probability $P(\phi|\theta)$, where $\theta = (\mu_g, \sigma_g, \pi_g : g = 1, \ldots, G)$ are the parameters representing the mean, covariance and prior probabilities of the Gaussian distribution. The GMM can be thought of as a soft dictionary of words in a bag-of-words (BoW) scheme. To encode features from dense local descriptors, we used FVE to compute the average first and second order differences between descriptors and GMM centers. For each GMM g and descriptor $d \in \phi$, we compute the following vectors:

$$\begin{aligned}
\mathcal{G}_{\mu,g} &= \frac{1}{\mathcal{D}\sqrt{\pi_g}} \sum_{k=1}^{\mathcal{D}} \gamma_d(g) \frac{(d - \mu_g)}{\sigma_g}, \\
\mathcal{G}_{\sigma,g} &= \frac{1}{\mathcal{D}\sqrt{2\pi_g}} \sum_{k=1}^{\mathcal{D}} \gamma_d(g) \left[\frac{(d - \mu_g)^2}{\sigma_g^2} - 1 \right], \\
\gamma_d(g) &= \frac{\pi_g \mathcal{N}(d; \mu_g, \sigma_g)}{\sum_{i=1}^{G} \pi_i \mathcal{N}(d; \mu_i, \sigma_i)},
\end{aligned} \tag{3}$$

$\mathcal{D}$ is the total number of local descriptors per patch and d represents one local descriptor for patch x_i. $\gamma_d(g)$ is a weight for the gth Gaussian distribution. We note $\psi(x_i) = [\mathcal{G}_{\mu,1}, \ldots, \mathcal{G}_{\mu,G}, \mathcal{G}_{\sigma,1}, \ldots, \mathcal{G}_{\sigma,G}]$ the final feature vector for a given patch in each training image. The dimensionality of the feature vector is $2 \times \mathcal{D} \times G$ where G is the codebook size (number of Gaussians).

Classification: Given the final feature representation for each patch in all training images, we train a linear multiclass SVM classifier. When used with high-dimensional feature vectors, linear SVM is more suitable than other non-linear classifiers (e.g. Random Forests or Kernel SVM) as it has faster training time and is less likely to overfit to the data. To predict a carcinoma subtype for a novel tissue slide X, we extract the local descriptors ϕ for all patches x_i of this new tissue. Then, we encode features ψ via FVE and classify these features using the trained SVM. The classifier's output probabilities $P(y_i|\psi(x_i))$ are aggregated using geometric mean to infer a final tissue label $P(y_i|X)$.

3 Experiments and Discussion

We evaluated our approach on a dataset composed of 80 patients (29 HGSC, 21 CC, 11 EN, 10 MC and 9 LGSC). Each tissue was labeled by two expert pathologists [10]. We extracted 50 patches at 20x and 90x resolution on every whole slide image. Using these colour patches, we trained a 3-layer DN with filter sizes 7×7 for 20x patches and 10×10 for 90x patches, at each layer. In all our experiments, the SVM classifier was trained on 40 patients (selected randomly) and tested on the rest. We compared the different components of our method to existing approaches used in histopathology image classification. All parameters inherent to each technique were determined via cross-validation on the training set. Table 1 reports our results for the following experiments.

Sparse Tissue Representation: We tested the discriminative ability of our features. A sparse representation was obtained from the feature maps of a multi-layer DN from which we densely constructed local descriptors. These descriptors were then vector-quantized using a BoW representation [2] and used to classify each patch. We used the traditional SIFT local descriptors and Sparse Coding (SC) [3] as comparison. We extracted 16×16 multiresolution samples from each image on a grid with step size 8 pixels to generate dense SIFT descriptors and SC dictionary. The same BoW quantization was applied on top of both descriptors. We observe in Table 1 that our representation allows for better discrimination between OC subtypes even when used with a simple quantization technique (BoW). Additionally, we see that higher layers of the DN induce a discrimination gain. This is linked to the convolutional property of the DN, which enables the model to learn more complex representations at higher layers (Fig. 3).

Feature Encoding: We also tested the performance of FVE compared to the traditional BoW with Spatial Pyramid Matching (SPM) pooling technique [4]. Table 1 shows the significant gain achieved using FVE instead of BoW encodings. Using a relatively small number of GMMs, FVE gives an accuracy of 92.1% . In contrast, similar accuracy could not be achieved using BoW even with a larger number of visual words (e.g. 1024).

Classification: We report the final multiclass accuracy after using the geometric mean to aggregate the classifiers probabilities and predict a tissue label from multiresolution patches. We note how this fairly simple aggregation technique results in performance gain in all experiments. We also report the mean Area Under ROC Curve (AUC) after one-against-all classification to better appreciate the differences between methods.

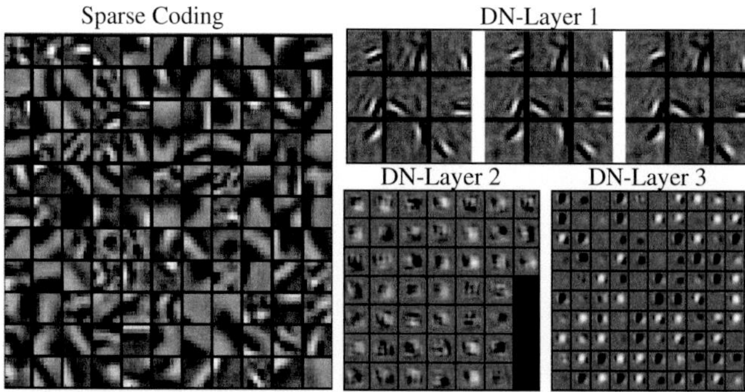

Fig. 3. Filters learnt using SC and multi-layer DN. We note how filters obtained with DN are more diverse at higher layers and span different orientations more uniformly.

Table 1. Performance of different methods on ovarian carcinomas dataset. We report the average accuracy of prediction on patches and tissue sections. Experiments were repeated 3 times on shuffled training and test sets of 40 patients each. The best dictionary size is shown for each experiment. Mean AUC is shown using one-against-all.

Features	Encoding	Pooling	Dictionary Size	Accuracy (Patches)	Accuracy (Tissues)	Mean AUC (Tissues)
SIFT	BoW	–	1024	32.5%±0.8	37.5%±0.6	–
SIFT	BoW	SPM	512	57.5%±0.5	61.5%±0.8	–
SIFT	**FVE**	**SPM**	**64**	66.7%±0.5	**68.5%**±0.5	0.67
SC	BoW	–	1024	57.5%±0.4	59.5%±0.5	–
SC	**BoW**	**SPM**	**1024**	68.0±2.0	**71.5%**±1.5	0.71
DN-1	BoW	–	256	35%±0.1	37.5%±0.8	–
DN-2	BoW	–	256	42.8±0.2	45.5%±0.8	–
DN-3	BoW	–	1024	48.0±0.8	51.5%±0.9	–
DN(1-2)	FVE	SPM	64	67.9±1.5	69.5%±1.2	–
DN(2-3)	FVE	SPM	64	83.7±1.2	85.0%±0.9	–
DN(1-3)	**FVE**	**SPM**	**128**	89.4%±1.7	**91.0%**±1.0	**0.86**

4 Conclusion

This paper is the first work to automate ovarian carcinomas subtypes classification from histopathology images. We proposed a method that learns robust features by capturing complex tissue patterns. The unsupervised nature of our feature learning framework enabled us to discover discriminative patterns from limited data. Our approach proved more suitable for the classification of OC and outperformed existing methods. Future work will focus on combining this hybrid feature representation with latent classification models to discover discriminative regions on tissues. We are also interested in experimenting with larger datasets, as new problems arises when more data becomes available, which together motivate new solutions to be developed.

Acknowledgment. We would like to thank NSERC for their financial support and our collaborators at the British Columbia Cancer Agency for providing insight and expertise that greatly assisted the research.

References

1. Baak, J.P., et al.: Interpathologist and intrapathologist disagreement in ovarian tumor grading and typing. In: Analytical and Quantitative Cytology and Histology (1986)
2. Caicedo, J.C., et al.: Histopathology image classification using bag of features and kernel functions. In: AI in Medicine, pp. 126–135 (2009)
3. Chang, H., Nayak, N., Spellman, P.T., Parvin, B.: Characterization of tissue histopathology via predictive sparse decomposition and spatial pyramid matching. In: Mori, K., Sakuma, I., Sato, Y., Barillot, C., Navab, N. (eds.) MICCAI 2013, Part II. LNCS, vol. 8150, pp. 91–98. Springer, Heidelberg (2013)
4. Chang, H., et al.: Classification of tumor histology via morphometric context. In: CVPR, pp. 2203–2210 (2013)
5. Chatfield, et al.: The devil is in the details: an evaluation of recent feature encoding methods (2011)
6. Coates, A., Ng, A.Y.: The importance of encoding versus training with sparse coding and vector quantization. In: ICML, pp. 921–928 (2011)
7. Demir, C., Yener, B.: Automated cancer diagnosis based on histopathological images: a systematic survey. Rensselaer Polytechnic Institute, Tech. Rep. (2005)
8. Gurcan, M.N., et al.: Histopathological image analysis: A review. Reviews in Biomedical Engineering, 147–171 (2009)
9. Han, J., et al.: Comparison of sparse coding and kernel methods for histopathological classification of gliobastoma multiforme. In: ISBI, pp. 711–714 (2011)
10. Köbel, M., et al.: Diagnosis of ovarian carcinoma cell type is highly reproducible: a transcanadian study. The American Journal of Surgical Pathology 34(7), 984–993 (2010)
11. Malpica, A., et al.: Interobserver and intraobserver variability of a two-tier system for grading ovarian serous carcinoma. The American Journal of Surgical Pathology, 354–357 (2007)
12. McCluggage, W.G.: Morphological subtypes of ovarian carcinoma: a review with emphasis on new developments and pathogenesis. Pathology Journal of the RCPA, 420–432 (2011)
13. McCluggage, W.G.: Ten problematical issues identified by pathology review for multidisciplinary gynaecological oncology meetings. Journal of Clinical Pathology, 420–432 (2011)
14. Naik, S., et al.: Automated gland and nuclei segmentation for grading of prostate and breast cancer histopathology. In: ISBI, pp. 284–287 (2008)
15. Soslow, R.A.: Histologic subtypes of ovarian carcinoma: an overview. International Journal of Gynecologic Pathology, 161–174 (2008)
16. Xu, Y., et al.: Multiple clustered instance learning for histopathology cancer image classification, segmentation and clustering. In: CVPR, pp. 964–971 (2012)
17. Zeiler, M.D., et al.: Deconvolutional networks. In: ICCV, pp. 2528–2535 (2010)

Scale-Adaptive Forest Training via an Efficient Feature Sampling Scheme

Loïc Peter[1], Olivier Pauly[1,2,⋆], Pierre Chatelain[1,3], Diana Mateus[1,2], and Nassir Navab[1,4]

[1] Computer Aided Medical Procedures, Technische Universität München, Germany
[2] Institute of Computational Biology, Helmholtz Zentrum München, Germany
[3] Université de Rennes 1, IRISA, France
[4] Computer Aided Medical Procedures, Johns Hopkins University, USA

Abstract. In the context of forest-based segmentation of medical data, modeling the visual appearance around a voxel requires the choice of the scale at which contextual information is extracted, which is of crucial importance for the final segmentation performance. Building on Haar-like visual features, we introduce a simple yet effective modification of the forest training which automatically infers the most informative scale at each stage of the procedure. Instead of the standard uniform sampling during node split optimization, our approach draws candidate features sequentially in a fine-to-coarse fashion. While being very easy to implement, this alternative is free of additional parameters, has the same computational cost as a standard training and shows consistent improvements on three medical segmentation datasets with very different properties.

1 Introduction

Among the existing statistical learning techniques, randomized forests [1] became one of the most popular methods for the analysis of medical images [2], as they are suitable for both classification and regression tasks and scale well with large data like 3D volumes. Recent applications of the forest framework to the medical field include multi-organ segmentation within computed tomography (CT) volumes [3], segmentation of the midbrain in transcranial ultrasound volumes [4], multi-organ localization in magnetic resonance (MR) [5] and CT [6] data, semantic labeling of brain structures in MR scans [7], depth video classification to quantify the progression of multiple sclerosis [8], and localization of anatomical landmarks within hand MR scans [9].

In the case of voxelwise tasks such as segmentation, the visual information around each voxel is quantified by a set of features, on which the forest decision rule is built. However, the choice of the most relevant scale at which these features must be extracted is a crucial problem whose impact on the final performance can be enormous (Fig. 1). In general, medical images contain useful information

⋆ Olivier Pauly's new affiliation is: Siemens Healthcare GmbH, Medical Imaging Technology, Erlangen, Germany.

N. Navab et al. (Eds.): MICCAI 2015, Part I, LNCS 9349, pp. 637–644, 2015.
DOI: 10.1007/978-3-319-24553-9_78

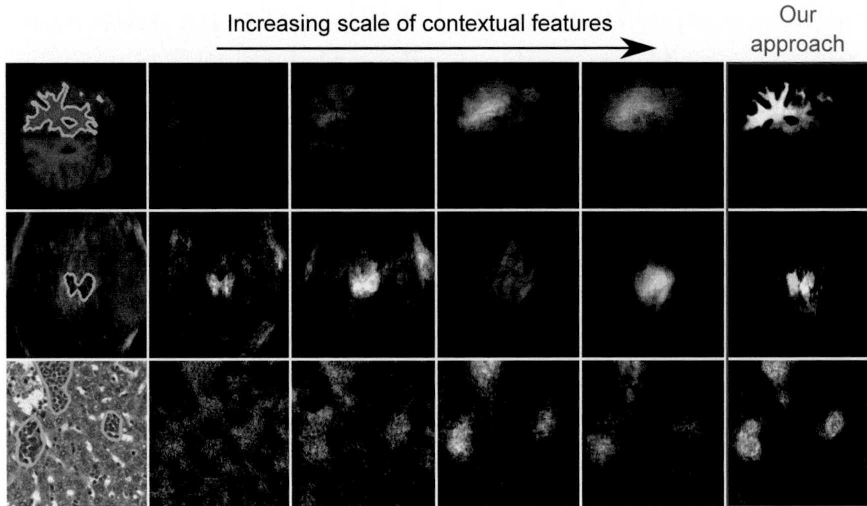

Fig. 1. How to choose the right scale when extracting visual context? This figure illustrates the motivation of this work. For an example label (outlined in green), the maximum range δ at which the visual features are extracted impacts the forest probabilistic output (from left to right: $\delta = 10, 20, 50, 100$). At small scales, fine structures like edges are captured but the lack of long-range information leads to unrealistic predictions. At larger scales, the opposite effect occurs: the approximate position of the structure of interest is correctly inferred, but the level of detail is strongly reduced. Our approach achieves an effective trade-off without computational overhead.

at several complementary scales, going from the local texture around a voxel of interest to the more global anatomical arrangement between organs. For this reason, incorporating multi-scale information during training is of great interest, and several approaches have been proposed to achieve this objective. A common but computationally costly strategy is to perform several independent learning stages at various scales and combine their outputs at prediction time [6,9,10]. Geremia et al. [11] explicitly create a hierarchy of supervoxels and refine the representation when necessary during the forest training. Zikic et al. [7] incorporate the global information via a label prior which is registered to the data at hand and used as an additional image modality. Montillo et al. [3] learn the distribution of the features selected by a preliminary forest, and sample according to this distribution during the final training. In spite of their advantages, these approaches present a computational overhead at training or testing time and raise other issues in terms of design, such as having to choose explicitly the different scales to combine.

In this work, we introduce a simple yet effective modification of the forest training which captures automatically the visual context at the appropriate scales. Our approach builds on the generic Haar-like features [12] which demonstrated lately high performance for a variety of medical objectives and imaging modalities [3,4,5,6,7,8,9]. Instead of sampling Haar-like features uniformly at each node, we sample them sequentially in a fine-to-coarse fashion. This preserves the simplicity of the original training as it (i) does not prompt any additional parameter tuning, (ii) leaves by construction the computational training and testing times unchanged, and (iii) does not require any preliminary step such as feature or scale selection. Our method shows consistent improvements with respect to standard approaches on three very different segmentation datasets.

2 Methods

Consider segmentation as a voxelwise[1] classification problem, where the goal is to assign to each voxel p a label $y(p)$. The decision rule predicting $y(p)$ is inferred from a set of labeled examples via a random forest classifier. To do so, the visual content around a voxel has to be quantitatively described by visual features (Sec. 2.1). After recalling the standard framework of classification forests in Sec. 2.2, we introduce in Sec. 2.3 our contribution, i.e. an alternative feature sampling strategy during training which enables an automatic extraction of the visual appearance at the relevant scales.

2.1 Haar-Like Features for Segmentation

Like most supervised learning techniques, random forests require a description of training and testing instances (voxels, in our case) through visual features encoding quantitatively the information available for the prediction task. While they can be specifically designed for an application if some domain knowledge is available, a popular and effective approach [3,4,5,6,7,8,9] consists in extracting a large number of low-level Haar-like features corresponding to visual cues at offset locations. Each Haar-like feature is characterized by a parameter vector $\boldsymbol{\lambda} \in \Lambda$ which defines, for each pixel p, a certain type of contextual information $x_{\boldsymbol{\lambda}}(p) \in \mathbb{R}$ as follows. Every parameter vector $\boldsymbol{\lambda}$ is expressed as

$$\boldsymbol{\lambda} = (\underbrace{\boldsymbol{v_1}, \boldsymbol{v_2}, \mathbf{s}_1, \mathbf{s}_2,}_{scale-related}\ \underbrace{c_1, c_2, \omega}_{categorical}\ ), \tag{1}$$

where $\boldsymbol{v_1}, \boldsymbol{v_2} \in \mathbb{R}^3$ are two offset vectors, $\mathbf{s}_1, \mathbf{s}_2 \in \mathbb{R}^3_+$ the dimensions of two boxes respectively attached to each offset, and c_1 and c_2 two color channels (or modalities). In each box of size $\mathbf{s}_i$ located at $p + \boldsymbol{v_i}$ ($i \in \{1, 2\}$), the mean intensity $\bar{I}_i$ over the color channel c_i is computed. The two quantities $\bar{I}_1$ and $\bar{I}_2$ are combined in a way determined by a last parameter $\omega \in \{\texttt{diff}, \texttt{binary\_diff}, \texttt{abs\_diff}, \texttt{sum}\}$, respectively corresponding to $x_{\boldsymbol{\lambda}}(p) = \bar{I}_1 - \bar{I}_2$, $\mathcal{H}(\bar{I}_1 - \bar{I}_2)$, $|\bar{I}_1 - \bar{I}_2|$, and $\bar{I}_1 + \bar{I}_2$. $\mathcal{H}$ denotes the Heaviside function so that $\mathcal{H}(\bar{I}_1 - \bar{I}_2)$ is the binarized difference between the two mean intensities, which has the useful property of being invariant to changes of illumination and contrast. The use of integral volumes [12] allows a fast access to any of these features during training.

[1] We expose our method for 3D volumes. The 2D case is obtained *mutatis mutandis.*

2.2 Classification Forests

A random forest is an ensemble of T decorrelated binary decision trees. A decision tree is a hierarchically organized set of nodes such that, starting from a root node, each node has exactly 0 or 2 child nodes. A node without children is called a leaf (or terminal node) and contains a posterior probability, whereas each non-terminal node contains a binary decision called splitting function designed to route instances towards the left or right child node. At prediction time, a testing instance is sent initially to the root and recursively passed through the tree until it reaches a leaf providing a treewise belief on the instance label. The forest prediction is the average of the T treewise posteriors.

The forest training step consists in the automatic design of the structure and content of each tree from a set of labeled training instances. The T trees are trained in parallel and independently as follows. For a given tree, a set of labeled training samples S is sent to the root node. In the present work, a splitting function is defined as a couple $(\boldsymbol{\lambda}, \theta) \in \Lambda \times \mathbb{R}$ composed of a visual feature and a threshold. We define the subsets $S_L^{\boldsymbol{\lambda},\theta} = \{p \in S | x_{\boldsymbol{\lambda}}(p) \leq \theta\}$ and $S_R^{\boldsymbol{\lambda},\theta} = \{p \in S | x_{\boldsymbol{\lambda}}(p) > \theta\}$ and the information gain generated by this split as

$$IG(S, \boldsymbol{\lambda}, \theta) = G(S) - \frac{\left|S_L^{\boldsymbol{\lambda},\theta}\right|}{|S|} G(S_L^{\boldsymbol{\lambda},\theta}) - \frac{\left|S_R^{\boldsymbol{\lambda},\theta}\right|}{|S|} G(S_R^{\boldsymbol{\lambda},\theta}), \tag{2}$$

where $G(S)$ is a purity measure of the set S (the Gini index in our case). In practice, to create a split given a feature $\boldsymbol{\lambda}$ and a set of samples S, we consider t thresholds $\theta_1, \ldots, \theta_t$ regularly distributed between the extreme values of $x_{\boldsymbol{\lambda}}(p)$ observed over all $p \in S$. The threshold providing the highest information gain is retained and defines the information gain $IG(S, \boldsymbol{\lambda})$ of the feature $\boldsymbol{\lambda}$ given S. This greedy threshold optimization is a popular choice due to its computational efficiency [2]. More sophisticated but costlier alternatives have been proposed, e.g. using a differentiable version of the information gain [13].

At each node, the retained splitting function $(\hat{\boldsymbol{\lambda}}, \hat{\theta})$ is determined by drawing randomly N features $\boldsymbol{\lambda}^{(1)}, \ldots, \boldsymbol{\lambda}^{(N)}$ and keeping the feature $\hat{\boldsymbol{\lambda}}$ providing the highest information gain, together with its corresponding best threshold $\hat{\theta}$. After splitting, $S_L^{\hat{\boldsymbol{\lambda}},\hat{\theta}}$ and $S_R^{\hat{\boldsymbol{\lambda}},\hat{\theta}}$ are respectively sent to the left and right child nodes. The process is recursively repeated until a maximum depth is reached or until the number of samples sent to child nodes is too low, in which case a leaf is created. The posterior probability stored at a leaf is defined as the class distribution over the arriving subset of labeled samples.

2.3 Fine-to-Coarse Sequential Feature Sampling

In the standard forest training framework, N candidate features $\boldsymbol{\lambda}^{(1)}, \ldots, \boldsymbol{\lambda}^{(N)}$ are drawn uniformly and independently at each node. Since each $\boldsymbol{\lambda}^{(i)}$ is a vector, this is practically achieved by sampling each coordinate $\lambda_d^{(i)}$ of $\boldsymbol{\lambda}^{(i)}$ uniformly over a predefined set of possible values Λ_d. In particular, since scale-related parameters (see Eq.1) are unbounded by definition, an upper limit δ must be set so that offset coordinates take their values in $\{-\delta, \ldots, \delta\}$ and box dimensions in $\{1, 3, \ldots, \delta + 1\}$. δ encodes the maximum scale at which the visual context is extracted. Deciding on an appropriate value of δ is usually problematic as it strongly impacts the forest prediction (see Fig. 1 for qualitative insights and Table 1 for quantitative results). In this section, we expose our alternative sampling scheme which alleviates this difficulty at no additional cost.

Instead of sampling the $\boldsymbol{\lambda}^{(i)}$ independently, we proceed sequentially by letting each candidate feature depend on the previous one. At each node, given an arriving set of training samples S, the feature sampling is conducted as follows:

- Sample a first feature $\boldsymbol{\lambda}^{(1)}$ by setting the scale-related parameters to values corresponding to the finest scale, i.e. 0 for offset coordinates and 1 for box dimensions. The categorical parameters are set randomly.
- At each iteration (for $1 \leq i \leq N-1$) :
  - Given the current feature $\boldsymbol{\lambda}^{(i)}$, suggest a slight modification $\tilde{\boldsymbol{\lambda}}$ of $\boldsymbol{\lambda}^{(i)}$ by picking at random one of the dimensions $\lambda_d^{(i)}$ (with $d \in \{1, \ldots, D\}$ uniformly drawn) and redraw it uniformly among its possible values Λ_d. The other components of $\boldsymbol{\lambda}^{(i)}$ are left unchanged.
  - Accept this modification if it does not decrease the information gain. Formally, define $\boldsymbol{\lambda}^{(i+1)} = \tilde{\boldsymbol{\lambda}}$ if $IG(S, \tilde{\boldsymbol{\lambda}}) \geq IG(S, \boldsymbol{\lambda}^{(i)})$, else $\boldsymbol{\lambda}^{(i+1)} = \boldsymbol{\lambda}^{(i)}$.

This procedure generates N features $\boldsymbol{\lambda}^{(1)}, \ldots, \boldsymbol{\lambda}^{(N)}$, exactly like the standard uniform sampling technique, and requires the same amount of information gain evaluations so that the computational time is identical by construction. Intuitively, the chosen initialization of the scale-related parameters corresponds to the finest possible scale which only provides information contained at the voxel of interest. Through the creation of candidate moves $\tilde{\boldsymbol{\lambda}}$, changes towards larger scales are then progressively suggested, but only accepted if they convey more information than the current one, in a hill climbing fashion. Hence, the maximum scale δ can be set as high as necessary in practice.

Our approach can also be seen as the design of a Markov chain at each node, where each feature corresponds to a state of the Markov chain and where moves are sequentially suggested from a proposal distribution and accepted if they do not decrease the information gain. This shares some similarities with the Metropolis-Hastings algorithm. The difference lies in the fact that the acceptance criterion is here deterministic, and that the application of the Metropolis-Hastings algorithm usually requires more iterations than the desired number N of samples to ensure decorrelation between consecutive samples.

3 Experiments

For each experiment, we train $T = 10$ trees of maximal depth 20 and so that each leaf contains at least 10 training samples. At each node, $N = 500$ candidate features are sampled and, for each of them, $t = 10$ thresholds are tested. Following a bagging strategy, we send to each tree a randomly-chosen fraction of the training data, at a rate of 5% which was experimentally found as a good compromise between accuracy and training time. Our approach is evaluated on three segmentation datasets consisting of MR, 3D ultrasound and histological data. For each of them, we train 5 standard forests with uniform sampling at the scales $\delta = 10$, 20, 50, 100, and 200 pixels respectively. Fig. 1 provides a qualitative intuition on the scale influence as well as an example image from each dataset. Our method using fine-to-coarse feature sampling is trained at the largest scale $\delta = 200$, which includes all the relevant visual information for the segmentation task. As additional baseline, we perform multi-scale prediction by multiplying the posterior probabilities obtained by the 5 standard forests [10]. Since absolute intensity values are unreliable for MR and ultrasound modalities, we also investigate a variant of the feature space which only allows binarized differences ('*Binary*' in Table 1, whereas '*All*' denotes the case where the 4 operation types are allowed) to guarantee invariance to changes of illumination and contrast. The approximate training times per tree are respectively 10 min (MR), 40 min (ultrasound) and 4 h (histology). The total testing time is 1 min per volume (or large 2D slice). Table 1 shows the mean Dice scores over patients.

Table 1. Mean Dice scores. To assess the statistical significance of the mean Dice scores, we compared our approach with each baseline by performing a paired sample t-test over the individual Dice scores obtained for each volume (or large slice). All p-values were lower than 0.05, and almost all of them were below 0.001 with only four exceptions. These are marked with a letter (from a to d) in the table below. The corresponding p-values were respectively 0.0024, 0.033, 0.010 and 0.0077. Finally, we also report the state-of-the-art performance among forest-based methods (when available) and the extension of our method to 40 trees to assess its asymptotical performance.

Dataset	IBSR2-18		Midbrain		Histology
Feature Space	Binary	All	Binary	All	All
Uniform Sampling ($\delta = 10$)	17.7	23.4	31.3	36.7	11.8[a]
Uniform Sampling ($\delta = 20$)	38.1	39.2	40.0	39.6	12.1
Uniform Sampling ($\delta = 50$)	62.8	61.5	42.1	31.8	17.3
Uniform Sampling ($\delta = 100$)	64.7	64.1	56.5	49.9	11.8
Uniform Sampling ($\delta = 200$)	64.2	63.9	57.4[b]	53.7	3.0
Multi-Scale Product [10]	75.1	73.7	62.3[c]	53.9[d]	9.3
Fine-to-Coarse Sampling	**83.1**	**82.5**	**73.1**	**63.1**	**22.3**
State of the art	83.5 [7]		33.0 [4]		-
Fine-to-Coarse Sampling (40 trees)	85.5	85.1	76.1	65.8	24.5

We conclude this section with a short description of the three datasets together with some specific discussions of the results in each case.

1. **IBSR2-18 Brain Dataset.** This is a publicly available[2] set of 18 brain MR scans with up to 32 labeled regions. Since the spacing varies between volumes, we rescale them to obtain an anisotropic spacing of 1 mm. Training

[2] http://www.nitrc.org/projects/ibsr

voxels are densely collected every 5 mm. A leave-one-out cross-validation is performed. Interestingly, when training a standard forest at the largest scale $\delta = 200$, we recover the performance of an affinely registered label prior which was reported by Zikic et al. [7] (64.2 vs 65.8). This confirms the idea that forests trained at large scales capture the general organization of labels.

2. **Midbrain Segmentation in Ultrasound.** This dataset made available by Ahmadi et al. [14] aims at segmenting the midbrain in 3D transcranial ultrasound. We downsample the volumes by a factor 2, resulting in a spacing of 0.9 mm in all directions. A 7-fold cross-validation is conducted over the 21 volumes. Our method outperforms the state-of-the-art forest-based result [4]. Due to the unreliability of raw intensities in ultrasound data, considering only binary differences is clearly beneficial here (73.1 vs 63.1).
3. **Hematopoiesis Quantification in High-Resolution Liver Slices.** This dataset is a set of high-resolution 2D liver slices extracted from 16 mice, extending the one used by Peter et al. [15]. Here, the objective is to segment hematopoietic cell clusters within the tissue. The image spacing is 1 μm after resizing the images by 2. We perform 4-fold cross-validation. It is a very challenging dataset which is subject to high variability of visual interpretation between experts. While the two other datasets were structured by the skull, hematopoietic cells can be located everywhere so that no label prior can be designed. In spite of these difficulties, a relative improvement of our method in comparison to the baselines can still be observed.

4 Conclusion

In the context of medical image segmentation, we introduced a novel and easy-to-implement alternative for sampling Haar-like features within the random forest framework. Our method is able to infer automatically the most informative scale at each stage of the training, resulting in an effective combination of local and global context at no additional cost. The experimental validation on three datasets showed the generality and the benefit of the approach.

Acknowledgments. This work was partially supported by the Collaborative Research Center 824: "Imaging for Selection, Monitoring and Individualization of Cancer Therapies", and by the EU 7th Framework Program project EndoTOFPET-US (GA-FP7/2007-2013-256984). We are very grateful to Kai Bötzel, Annika Plate and Seyed-Ahmad Ahmadi for kindly providing the midbrain data through the Lüneburg Heritage and Deutsche Forschungsgesellschaft (DFG) Grant BO 1895/4-1. We also would like to acknowledge Gabriele Multhoff, Stefan Stangl and Noemi Schworm for making the histological dataset available.

References

1. Breiman, L.: Random forests. Machine Learning (2001)
2. Criminisi, A., Shotton, J.: Decision Forests for Computer Vision and Medical Image Analysis (2013)

3. Montillo, A., Shotton, J., Winn, J., Iglesias, J.E., Metaxas, D., Criminisi, A.: Entangled decision forests and their application for semantic segmentation of CT images. In: Székely, G., Hahn, H.K. (eds.) IPMI 2011. LNCS, vol. 6801, pp. 184–196. Springer, Heidelberg (2011)
4. Chatelain, P., et al.: Learning from multiple experts with random forests: application to the segmentation of the midbrain in 3D ultrasound. In: Mori, K., Sakuma, I., Sato, Y., Barillot, C., Navab, N. (eds.) MICCAI 2013, Part II. LNCS, vol. 8150, pp. 230–237. Springer, Heidelberg (2013)
5. Pauly, O., Glocker, B., Criminisi, A., Mateus, D., Möller, A.M., Nekolla, S., Navab, N.: Fast multiple organ detection and localization in whole-body MR dixon sequences. In: Fichtinger, G., Martel, A., Peters, T. (eds.) MICCAI 2011, Part III. LNCS, vol. 6893, pp. 239–247. Springer, Heidelberg (2011)
6. Gauriau, R., Cuingnet, R., Lesage, D., Bloch, I.: Multi-organ localization combining global-to-local regression and confidence maps. In: Golland, P., Hata, N., Barillot, C., Hornegger, J., Howe, R. (eds.) MICCAI 2014, Part III. LNCS, vol. 8675, pp. 337–344. Springer, Heidelberg (2014)
7. Zikic, D., Glocker, B., Criminisi, A.: Encoding atlases by randomized classification forests for efficient multi-atlas label propagation. Medical Image Analysis 18(8), 1262–1273 (2014)
8. Kontschieder, P., et al.: Quantifying progression of multiple sclerosis via classification of depth videos. In: Golland, P., Hata, N., Barillot, C., Hornegger, J., Howe, R. (eds.) MICCAI 2014, Part II. LNCS, vol. 8674, pp. 429–437. Springer, Heidelberg (2014)
9. Ebner, T., Stern, D., Donner, R., Bischof, H., Urschler, M.: Towards automatic bone age estimation from MRI: Localization of 3D anatomical landmarks. In: Golland, P., Hata, N., Barillot, C., Hornegger, J., Howe, R. (eds.) MICCAI 2014, Part II. LNCS, vol. 8674, pp. 421–428. Springer, Heidelberg (2014)
10. Lay, N., Birkbeck, N., Zhang, J., Zhou, S.K.: Rapid multi-organ segmentation using context integration and discriminative models. In: Gee, J.C., Joshi, S., Pohl, K.M., Wells, W.M., Zöllei, L. (eds.) IPMI 2013. LNCS, vol. 7917, pp. 450–462. Springer, Heidelberg (2013)
11. Geremia, E., Menze, B.H., Ayache, N.: Spatially adaptive random forests. In: IEEE 10th International Symposium on Biomedical Imaging (ISBI), pp. 1344–1347 (2013)
12. Viola, P., Jones, M.: Robust real-time face detection. IJCV (2004)
13. Montillo, A., Tu, J., Shotton, J., Winn, J., Iglesias, J., Metaxas, D., Criminisi, A.: Entanglement and differentiable information gain maximization. In: Decision Forests for Computer Vision and Medical Image Analysis, pp. 273–293. Springer (2013)
14. Ahmadi, S.-A., Baust, M., Karamalis, A., Plate, A., Boetzel, K., Klein, T., Navab, N.: Midbrain segmentation in transcranial 3D ultrasound for parkinson diagnosis. In: Fichtinger, G., Martel, A., Peters, T. (eds.) MICCAI 2011, Part III. LNCS, vol. 6893, pp. 362–369. Springer, Heidelberg (2011)
15. Peter, L., Mateus, D., Chatelain, P., Schworm, N., Stangl, S., Multhoff, G., Navab, N.: Leveraging random forests for interactive exploration of large histological images. In: Golland, P., Hata, N., Barillot, C., Hornegger, J., Howe, R. (eds.) MICCAI 2014, Part I. LNCS, vol. 8673, pp. 1–8. Springer, Heidelberg (2014)

Multiple Instance Cancer Detection by Boosting Regularised Trees

Wenqi Li, Jianguo Zhang, and Stephen J. McKenna

CVIP, School of Computing, University of Dundee, Dundee, UK

Abstract. We propose a novel multiple instance learning algorithm for cancer detection in histopathology images. With images labelled at image-level, we first search a set of region-level prototypes by solving a submodular set cover problem. Regularised regression trees are then constructed and combined on the set of prototypes using a multiple instance boosting framework. The method compared favourably with competing methods in experiments on breast cancer tissue microarray images and optical tomographic images of colorectal polyps.

1 Introduction

Multiple instance learning (MIL) has recently been applied to histopathology image analysis for both segmentation and classification tasks [10,16]. While training a tumour detector usually requires a large amount of high quality manual annotation [1], MIL methods can potentially infer tumour regions with image-level annotation, i.e., binary labels indicating whether tumour is present in the image. The MIL formulation is attractive as it does not require the effort of manually delineating image regions.

The general MIL inference rules are defined in the context of binary classification: a bag of instances is positive if at least one instance in the bag is positive, negative if all of the instances in the bag are negative. A common implementation of the rules in image classification treats each image as a bag, and regions in an image as instances. In terms of histopathology image analysis, an example application is to label an image as *cancer* if cancer is present in at least one region of the image, and as *non-cancer* otherwise.

In this paper, following the MIL setting, we propose a novel tree boosting algorithm for training a cancer detector. Our algorithm extends Multiple Instance Boosting (MILBoosting) [17] by boosting regularised trees with instance-to-prototype distances as features. The discriminative prototypes in our algorithm are searched by solving a submodular set cover problem. Our approach is validated on two types of histopathology images, namely, breast cancer tissue microarray (TMA) images and optical projection tomographic (OPT) images of colorectal polyps.

2 Related Work

Although MIL has been extensively studied since [12] and there exists a large literature (for a general review of MIL, see [2]), it was only recently applied to

N. Navab et al. (Eds.): MICCAI 2015, Part I, LNCS 9349, pp. 645–652, 2015.
DOI: 10.1007/978-3-319-24553-9_79

histopathology image analysis. Here we give a brief review of some of the most relevant work.

Zhao et al. [19] applied MILES [4] for 10 category histopathology image classification. Xu et al. [16] extended MILBoosting [17] to simultaneously detect and cluster multiple types of tissue region in TMA images. Kandemir et al. [9] evaluated MIL formulations on diagnosis of Barrett's cancer with H&E images. Xu et al. [15] used MIL to classify colon cancer histopathology images with features extracted from convolutional neural networks.

Selecting instances as prototypes for bag classification was used previously with bags represented in terms of distances to prototypes [4,7]. Our work extends MILBoosting to select prototypes with instance-to-prototype distances. We search a set of positive instance prototypes that is both discriminative and covers multiple modes of the appearance distribution. Instance-to-prototype distances are considered as features. A regularised regression tree boosting method is proposed to further select and combine the features.

Prototypes should satisfy three criteria; they should be 1) relevant: present in many positive images, 2) discriminative: dissimilar to negative instances, and 3) complementary: covering multiple types of positive instances. Song et al. [13] formalised these intuitions as a submodular set cover problem solved by a greedy algorithm. The set of prototypes was used as an initial training set for latent SVM. In this paper we adopt the 'discriminativeness' of each prototype as a regularisation strength in a MILBoosting framework.

3 Method

3.1 Notation

Here we introduce notation adopted throughout the paper. We denote $\mathbf{x}_{ij} \in R^d$ as a d-dimensional feature representation of an instance (patch). Index ij represents the jth instance in the ith bag (image). $y_i \in \{0, 1\}$ represents the label of the bag, where 0 denotes non-cancer and 1 denotes cancer. The kth prototype $\mathbf{p}_k \in R^d$ is an instance selected from the training instance set. In the following sections we introduce the two steps of our proposed method: searching for a set of discriminative prototypes and learning cancer detectors.

3.2 Discriminative Prototypes

The discriminativeness of a prototype $g(\mathbf{p}_k)$ can be estimated as follows [13]: first find the m nearest neighbours of $\mathbf{p}_k$ from the set of training instances $\{\mathbf{x}_{ij}\}$; then, counting the number of neighbours from the positive bags (denoted as m_{pos}), the ratio m_{pos}/m can be a measurement of discriminativeness. Greedy search for a set of prototypes starts with an empty set of prototypes and a candidate set comprising all training instances. The most discriminative instance from the candidate set is then added to the prototype set, at the same time removing the prototype's m nearest neighbours from the candidate set. This is repeated until the candidate set is small enough (e.g., only 10% of initial candidates remain).

Song et al. [13] used the prototypes as an initialisation set for training latent SVM. We propose to combine the set of prototypes in a boosting framework. We further select prototype subsets and simultaneously learn an instance classifier by boosting regularised trees where we utilise $g(\mathbf{p}_k)$ as the regularisation strength.

3.3 Boosting with Regularised Regression Trees

To learn detectors we adopt multiple instance boosting (MILBoosting) [17]. In MILBoosting, the instance classifier $F(\mathbf{x}_{ij})$ is formulated as a linear combination of T weak learners, i.e., $F(\mathbf{x}_{ij}) = \sum_{t=1}^{T} \alpha_t f_t(\mathbf{x}_{ij})$, where $f_t(\mathbf{x}_{ij})$ gives a score to each instance $\mathbf{x}_{ij}$; α_t is the weight of f_t. The probabilities that cancer presents in an instance P_{ij} and in a bag P_i are respectively modelled as

$$P_{ij} = \frac{1}{1 + \exp(-F(\mathbf{x}_{ij}))} \qquad \text{and} \qquad P_i = 1 - \prod_j (1 - P_{ij}). \tag{1}$$

The instance classifier can be estimated by minimising the negative log-likelihood L of the bag labels:

$$L(y_i, F(\mathbf{x}_{ij})) = -\log \prod_i P_i^{y_i} (1 - P_i)^{(1-y_i)}. \tag{2}$$

Using the gradient boosting framework [6], L can be optimised by iteratively fitting weak learners f_t and optimising coefficients α_t. We adopt J-terminal regression trees as weak learners with a boosting shrinkage parameter ν [8]. However, instead of fitting regression trees to the feature set $\{\mathbf{x}_{ij}\}$, we first represent each instance in terms of distances to prototypes, i.e.,

$$\hat{\mathbf{x}}_{ij} = [d(\mathbf{x}_{ij}, \mathbf{p}_1), \ldots, d(\mathbf{x}_{ij}, \mathbf{p}_k)], \tag{3}$$

where $d(.,.)$ is a distance measure, e.g., ℓ_2-distance. Regression trees are then constructed on the new feature set $\{\hat{\mathbf{x}}_{ij}\}$. Each of the regression trees partitions the feature space into disjoint regions. The best variables to split and the optimal thresholds of the tree are searched by maximising information gain. In $\{\hat{\mathbf{x}}_{ij}\}$ each variable is associated with a prototype $\mathbf{p}_k$. Our method encourages trees constructed on $\{\hat{\mathbf{x}}_{ij}\}$ to split at those variables that are associated with large $g(\mathbf{p}_k)$. The motivation is to further select prototypes so that regression trees split at a few very discriminative prototypes, instead of splitting at many non-informative prototypes which could result in poor generalisation.

We introduce regularisation to properly control the variable to split in the tree construction process. The method we adopted is guided regularisation for tree construction [5]. It was first proposed as a feature selection technique integrated in a random forest classifier; the selection of variables was guided by pre-computing variable importance from a preliminary random forest training. Here we combine the regularisation method with boosting trees. We utilise the discriminativeness $g(\mathbf{p}_k)$ as the regularisation strength instead of a preliminary random forest training.

Algorithm 1. Summary of the proposed algorithm

```
procedure BOOSTING PROTOTYPES({x_ij}, {y_i}, ν, J, T)
    {p_k} ← Greedy search for prototypes (Section 3.2)
    {x̂_ij} ← Transform {x_ij} with {p_k} (Formula (3))
    for t ← 1 ··· T do
        for all i,j do
            Compute r^t_ij ← −∂L/∂f |_{f=f_{t−1}}
        end for
        Fit a J-terminal regression tree f_t to r^t_ij (regularised by Formula (4))
        Line search: α_t ← arg min_α L(y_i, F_{t−1}(x̂_ij) + α f_t)
        Update classifier: F_t ← F_{t−1} + ν α_t f_t (shrinkage ν is a fixed parameter)
    end for
    return instance classifier F_T
end procedure
```

Specifically given a set of K prototypes, we normalise $g(\mathbf{p}_k)$ as $\hat{g}(\mathbf{p}_k) = \frac{g(\mathbf{p}_k)}{\max_{k=1}^{K} g(\mathbf{p}_k)}$; when the tree chooses to split on the kth feature of $\{\hat{\mathbf{x}}_{ij}\}$, the information gain is regularised by a function of $\hat{g}(\mathbf{p}_k)$:

$$\text{Gain}_{\text{R}}(k) = ((1 - \lambda) \cdot \gamma + \lambda \cdot \hat{g}(\mathbf{p}_k)) \cdot \text{Gain}(k), \tag{4}$$

where $\lambda \in [0, 1]$ is a free parameter to control the overall regularisation; $\gamma \in [0, 1]$ is a base regularisation coefficient. We calculate Gain(k) as the reduction of variance at all leaf nodes when splitting at the kth feature. The regularised regression tree can directly utilise discriminativeness to control the regularisation strength via Formula (4). The tree-based feature selection can capture non-linear variable interactions if $J > 2$. We set $J = 4$, $\gamma = 1$, and grid search for λ in our experiments. Algorithm 1 summarises the proposed procedure.

4 Evaluations

We evaluated the proposed method on cancer detection at 1) image level (predicting the presence of cancer in an unseen image) and 2) region level (localising the cancer region in an image). Two datasets were used in the experiments: a breast cancer TMA dataset and a colorectal polyp OPT dataset.

4.1 Breast Cancer TMA Images

The first dataset consists of 58 TMA breast cancer images stained with hematoxylin and eosin (H&E). 26 images are diagnosed as malignant, 32 as benign. For a fair comparison we used the feature sets made publicly available[1] by Kandemir et al. [10]. Each image was divided into 49 equally-sized instances. Each instance was further encoded with a 708-dimensional feature vector. This feature vector

[1] Link: `http://www.miproblems.org/datasets/ucsb-breast/`

Table 1. Cancer detection performance at image-level measured with AUC

Method	GPMIL [10]	RGPMIL [10]	Proposed
AUC	0.86	0.90	0.93

was comprised of SIFT descriptors, local binary patterns, colour histograms, and cell-level morphological features. Since instance location information is not available in the feature set, we focus on image-level performance evaluation.

We follow the 4-fold cross validation protocol used in [10]. For the proposed method we first applied the set cover search with $m = 20$. This usually selects 100 to 200 positive prototypes from a total of $1,500$ instances. We set shrinkage parameter ν to 0.05, and the maximum number of iterations T to 300. The regularisation parameter λ was searched in the value set $\{0.1, 0.2, 0.3, \ldots, 1.0\}$ with a 10-fold cross validation on the training folds. Averaged area under the ROC curve (AUC) was computed as the image classification performance measure (Table 1). The standard error of our method was 0.04. Equal Error Rate was 0.16 ± 0.03. Note that Relational Gaussian Process MIL (RGPMIL) was designed for TMA images by explicitly modelling cells with a graph. Both GPMIL and RGPMIL outperformed widely-used MIL methods including EMDD [18], MILBoosting [17] and MI-SVM [3]. As shown in Table 1 our method achieved better image-level performance than the top-ranked methods.

4.2 OPT Images of Colorectal Polyps

Dataset. We evaluated both image- and instance-level cancer detection performance on 60 OPT images of colorectal polyps acquired using ultraviolet light and Cy3 dye [11]. Each 3-D image was of one colorectal polyp and consisted of 1024^3 voxels. 30 of the polyps were diagnosed as invasive cancer (ICA), and the other 30 as low-grade dysplasia (LGD). 3-D regions of cancer were annotated as sequences of 2-D slices by a trained pathologist. Our dataset for MIL evaluations consists of 200 2-D slices, with 100 slices randomly selected from ICA polyps and 100 from LGD. Fig. 2 shows some of the cancer slices and their annotations.

The pathologist was only asked to delineate major cancer regions with relatively high confidence rather than exhaustively trace all the cancer locations. Part of our motivation for applying MIL is that complete region-level annotations are difficult to obtain and validate. As a result, in ICA images, instance labels outside annotated regions were unknown. Since the instance annotations are not used in training MIL classifiers, quality of region annotation is not a concern in the training stage. We report instance-level test results based on the classifier output over all instances in LGD images, and all instances that have at least 50% overlap with ICA annotations.

Experiment Protocol. We treated each slice as a bag and densely extracted patches as instances. The size of each instance was 48×48 pixels. The sampling step size was 24 pixels in the training stage, and 12 in the test stage in both

Table 2. Cancer detection at image-level and instance-level (with standard errors).

Method	MILBoosting [17]	Proposed	Inst-SVMs
AUC (image-level)	0.74 ± 0.04	0.79 ± 0.01	0.85 ± 0.03
F-measure (instance-level)	0.41 ± 0.01	0.45 ± 0.03	0.53 ± 0.05

horizontal and vertical directions. We combined local binary patterns, SIFT features, and intensity histograms as instance features. The set cover search parameter was $m = 10$. Three-fold cross validation was conducted with the proposed method using the same grid search of parameters described in Section 4.1. Fig. 1(a) shows the image-level AUC of the proposed method plotted against the parameters T and ν on a validation set. The performance in terms of AUC is not very sensitive to T and ν. Choosing a large T and a small ν tends to give a high AUC. We set ν to 0.05, and T to 300.

We also implemented MILBoosting [17] as a baseline. Differences between the proposed method and MILBoosting are that the latter fits regression trees directly to $\{\mathbf{x}_{ij}\}$ without transformation and regularisation. In addition to the MIL methods we trained instance-level support vector machines (Inst-SVM) in a *fully supervised* setting as a comparison. In training Inst-SVM, instances with at least 50% overlap with the annotations were treated as cancer; the instances from LGD images were treated as non-cancer.

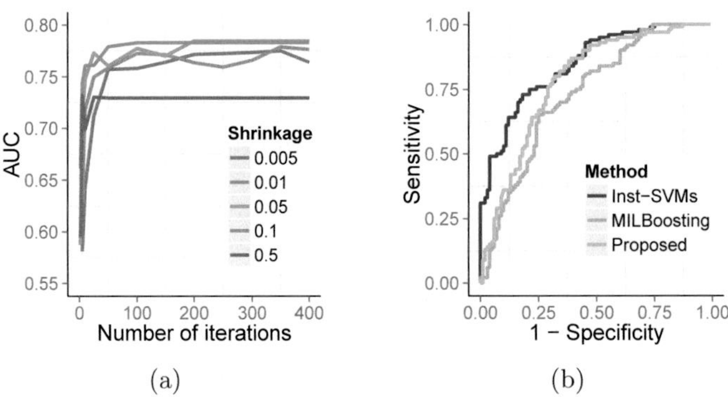

(a) (b)

Fig. 1. Cancer detection at image-level (best viewed in color). (a) AUC of the proposed method against number of iterations T and shrinkage parameter ν. (b) ROC curves.

Results. Table 2 compares image- and instance-level performance in terms of AUC and F-measure respectively. At image-level, Inst-SVM score was calculated as the maximum of instance scores in the image. At instance-level, score thresholds of each method were searched on the training set by maximising training F-measures. Our method outperformed MILBoosting in both image- and instance-level classification. However it was worse than fully supervised classification, as would be expected. Fig. 1(b) shows ROC curves at image-level. Fig. 2 shows a few cancer detection examples.

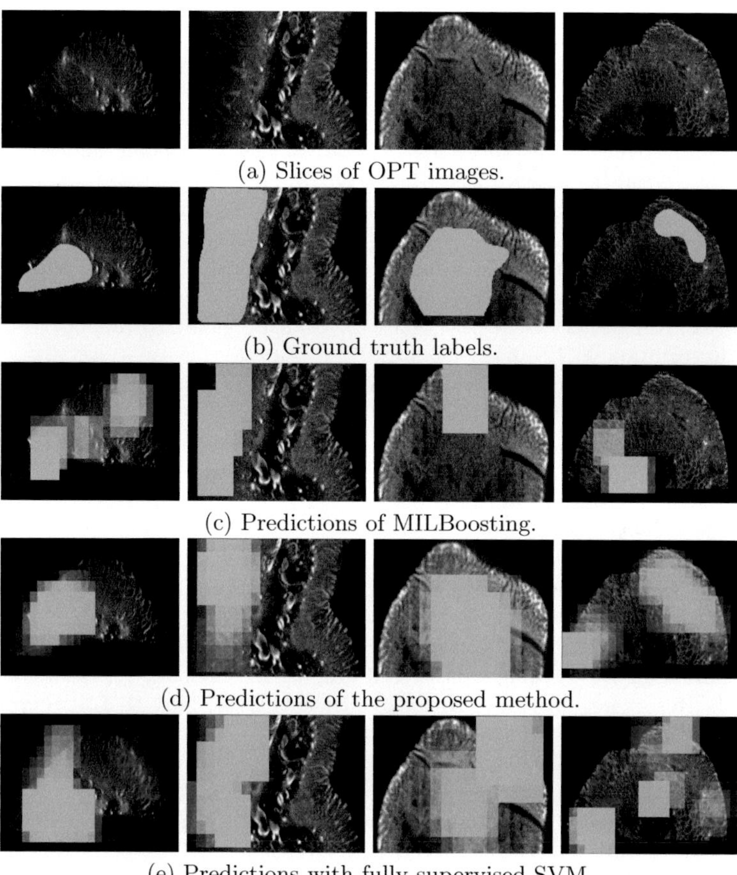

(a) Slices of OPT images.

(b) Ground truth labels.

(c) Predictions of MILBoosting.

(d) Predictions of the proposed method.

(e) Predictions with fully supervised SVM.

Fig. 2. Instance-level annotations and predictions. Green patches in third to fifth rows indicate scores of the instances are greater than the learned threshold. Instances with higher scores were mapped to higher opacity values (best viewed in colour).

5 Conclusions

This paper introduced a novel multiple instance learning algorithm by combining discriminative prototype search with boosting of regularised regression trees. Empirical studies on two histopathology datasets showed that the method can achieve more accurate results than competing methods for both image- and instance-level classification. This work is based on an implementation of MIL inference rules in which instances are rectangular patches. In future we would consider generating instance regions using visual information [14].

Acknowledgement. The authors would like to thank Ruixuan Wang and Siyamalan Manivannan for fruitful discussions.

References

1. Akbar, S., Jordan, L., Thompson, A.M., McKenna, S.J.: Tumor localization in tissue microarrays using rotation invariant superpixel pyramids. In: ISBI (2015)
2. Amores, J.: Multiple instance classification: Review, taxonomy and comparative study. Artificial Intelligence 201, 81–105 (2013)
3. Andrews, S., Tsochantaridis, I., Hofmann, T.: Support vector machines for multiple-instance learning. In: NIPS, pp. 561–568 (2002)
4. Chen, Y., Bi, J., Wang, J.Z.: Miles: Multiple-instance learning via embedded instance selection. TPAMI 28(12), 1931–1947 (2006)
5. Deng, H., Runger, G.: Gene selection with guided regularized random forest. Pattern Recognition 46(12), 3483–3489 (2013)
6. Friedman, J.H.: Greedy function approximation: a gradient boosting machine. Annals of Statistics, 1189–1232 (2001)
7. Fu, Z., Robles-Kelly, A., Zhou, J.: Milis: Multiple instance learning with instance selection. TPAMI 33(5), 958–977 (2011)
8. Hastie, T., Tibshirani, R., Friedman, J.: The elements of statistical learning. Springer (2009)
9. Kandemir, M., Feuchtinger, A., Walch, A., Hamprecht, F.A.: Digital pathology: Multiple instance learning can detect barrett's cancer. In: ISBI, pp. 1348–1351 (2014)
10. Kandemir, M., Zhang, C., Hamprecht, F.A.: Empowering multiple instance histopathology cancer diagnosis by cell graphs. In: Golland, P., Hata, N., Barillot, C., Hornegger, J., Howe, R. (eds.) MICCAI 2014, Part II. LNCS, vol. 8674, pp. 228–235. Springer, Heidelberg (2014)
11. Li, W., Zhang, J., McKenna, S.J., Coats, M., Carey, F.A.: Classification of colorectal polyp regions in optical projection tomography. In: ISBI, pp. 736–739 (2013)
12. Maron, O., Lozano-Pérez, T.: A framework for multiple-instance learning. In: Advances in Neural Information Processing Systems, pp. 570–576 (1998)
13. Song, H.O., Girshick, R., Jegelka, S., Mairal, J., Harchaoui, Z., Darrell, T., et al.: On learning to localize objects with minimal supervision. In: ICML, vol. 32 (2014)
14. Uijlings, J.R.R., van de Sande, K.E.A., Gevers, T., Smeulders, A.W.M.: Selective search for object recognition. IJCV 104(2), 154–171 (2013)
15. Xu, Y., Mo, T., Feng, Q., Zhong, P., Lai, M., Chang, E.I., et al.: Deep learning of feature representation with multiple instance learning for medical image analysis. In: ICASSP, pp. 1626–1630. IEEE (2014)
16. Xu, Y., Zhu, J.Y., Eric, I., Chang, C., Lai, M., Tu, Z.: Weakly supervised histopathology cancer image segmentation and classification. Medical Image Analysis 18(3), 591–604 (2014)
17. Zhang, C., Platt, J.C., Viola, P.A.: Multiple instance boosting for object detection. In: NIPS, pp. 1417–1424 (2005)
18. Zhang, Q., Goldman, S.A.: Em-dd: An improved multiple-instance learning technique. In: NIPS, pp. 1073–1080 (2001)
19. Zhao, D., Chen, Y., Correa, N.: Automated classification of human histological images, a multiple-instance learning approach. In: Life Science Systems and Applications Workshop, IEEE/NLM, pp. 1–2. IEEE (2006)

Uncertainty-Driven Forest Predictors for Vertebra Localization and Segmentation

David Richmond[1,⋆], Dagmar Kainmueller[1,⋆], Ben Glocker[2], Carsten Rother[3,⋆⋆], and Gene Myers[1,⋆⋆]

[1] Max Planck Institute of Molecular Cell Biology and Genetics, Germany
[2] Biomedical Image Analysis Group, Imperial College London, UK
[3] Computer Vision Lab Dresden, Technical University Dresden, Germany
{richmond,kainmueller}@mpi-cbg.de

Abstract. Accurate localization, identification and segmentation of vertebrae is an important task in medical and biological image analysis. The prevailing approach to solve such a task is to first generate pixel-independent features for each vertebra, e.g. via a random forest predictor, which are then fed into an MRF-based objective to infer the optimal MAP solution of a constellation model. We abandon this static, two-stage approach and mix feature generation with model-based inference in a new, more flexible, way. We evaluate our method on two data sets with different objectives. The first is semantic segmentation of a 21-part body plan of zebrafish embryos in microscopy images, and the second is localization and identification of vertebrae in benchmark human CT.

1 Introduction

State-of-the-art approaches for object localization or semantic segmentation typically employ pixel-wise forest predictors combined with MAP inference on a graphical constellation model [1,2,3] or a (super-)pixel graph [4,5], respectively. A recent trend in computer vision replaces single-level forest predictors by deep, *cascaded* models for feature generation, such as CNNs [6] and Auto-Context Models [7]. These models play the role of learning a complex non-linear mapping from images to features that are relevant for the task at hand.

This modeling framework is however static, as it separates feature generation from inference (i.e., "model fitting"). It has been shown that better features can be generated by *interleaving* feature generation with MAP inference [8,9,10].[1] In this work we take this idea a step further: Instead of interleaving feature generation with a pixel-level structured model or model-agnostic smoothing, we

⋆ Shared first authors.

⋆⋆ Shared last authors.

[1] Note that this is conceptually different from the classical "hierarchical" approach that, purely for the sake of pruning the search space to reduce run-time, performs feature generation and inference/model fitting multiple times on different scales.

N. Navab et al. (Eds.): MICCAI 2015, Part I, LNCS 9349, pp. 653–660, 2015.
DOI: 10.1007/978-3-319-24553-9_80

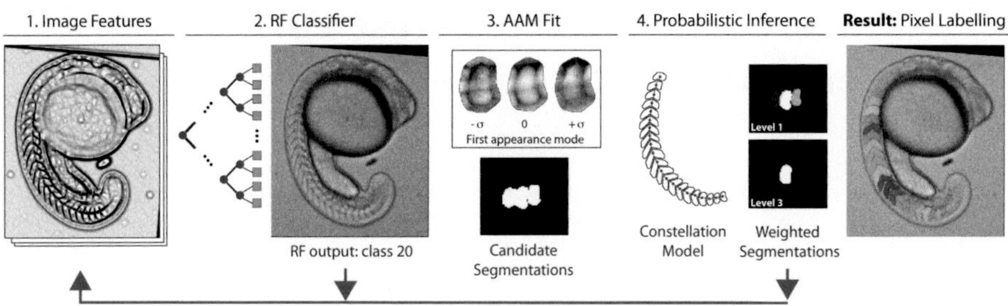

Fig. 1. Our proposed pipeline for multi-class, semantic segmentation. A stack of feature images is created by a standard filter bank, and used to train a random forest classifier. The random forest output is then used in combination with the original image to generate candidate segmentations for each class, by fitting multiple instances of appearance models. These candidate segmentations are weighted by means of probabilistic inference in a constellation model that captures relative locations of classes. The weighted and fused candidate segmentations are then fed back as additional "smoothed" features into a new random forest classifier, forming a cascade.

interleave with a global, generative constellation model. We suggest a cascaded pipeline, as illustrated in Figure 1.

We explore two applications: (1) Segmentation of *somites*, the self-similar units that give rise to muscle and bone, including vertebrae, in microscopy images of zebrafish embryos. (2) Localization and identification of vertebrae in benchmark human spine CTs [1]. Figures 1 (right) and 2 (left) show exemplary zebrafish images with and without overlaid segmentation of somites, respectively.

The most important aspect of our cascaded pipeline is the question of what to infer from a constellation model at intermediate stages of the cascade. Options are the MAP solution or the marginal distributions. Interestingly, marginal distributions are a winner for the zebrafish application. The reason that *uncertainty is beneficial* here is that individual somites are highly ambiguous with respect to shape, appearance, and importantly also the appearance of surrounding tissue. Hence only the relative spatial arrangement can disambiguate them. We show that as opposed to MAP inference, the soft marginals do not commit to a certain – potentially wrong – solution "at first sight".

Closely related to our work are (1) Auto Context [7], but they do not perform any smoothing between levels of the cascade. (2) Geodesic Forests [10], but they do not use a structured model for smoothing. (3) Cascaded classifiers interleaved with MAP inference [8,9], but they do not use a (global generative) constellation model and do not explore marginals for inference. (4) Constellation models for the widely studied application of human vertebrae localization (see e.g. [11]) but none of the respective methods runs a Random Forest cascade.

To summarize, our work makes the following main **contributions**: (1) We show, for the first time, that probabilistic inference can give a boost in performance in cascaded MRF-Forest-based models. This is compared to standard MAP inference (as in e.g. [1,3]) and model-agnostic geodesic smoothing [10]. (2) We outperform a state-of-the-art method [2] on benchmark human spine CTs of challenging pathological cases. (3) We are the first to tackle somite detection in zebrafish, where we achieve an overall average Dice score of 0.82.

2 Method

Background: Random Forests classifiers (RF) [12] are widely used in medical image analysis for organ localization, particularly for vertebrae [13,1,2]. We use RFs in a cascaded fashion [7], where the probability maps yielded by an RF are treated as features that are fed into subsequent RFs, forming a cascade. In variants of this approach, inference or smoothing operations on these probability maps are interleaved with the RF prediction, and the "smoothed" probability maps are then used as features [8,9,10]. For comparison to our proposed model-based smoothing we explore model-agnostic geodesic smoothing [10]. The rationale behind geodesic smoothing is that pixels within a small geodesic distance of each other likely belong to the same class. See [10] for details.

Generating Candidate Segmentations: We train an n-class RF, where n is the number of object parts (e.g. the number of vertebrae in the human spine), plus one background class. At test time, an RF generates one probability map per class. Given an RF-generated probability map for some foreground class, we first compute its mode via the mean shift algorithm. Second, we fit a learned, static constellation of landmarks to these centroids, yielding an optimal affine transformation w.r.t. the sum of squared landmark distances. Third, we sample a number of candidate locations around these points to get sets of initializations for the respective classes. Fourth, we fit a class specific appearance model to the image, multiple times, starting at the initial locations computed in the previous step. Depending on the application, we either use active appearance models (AAM) [14], or static average and variance images [2]. Each appearance model fit results in a binary segmentation, together with a cost for the fit. We denote the cost for the l-th fit for class v as $a(v, l)$. The cost is the sum of squared differences between the target and the template image generated by the (active) appearance model. In case of static appearance models, we weigh the squared differences by the respective pixel-wise variances stored in the variance image.

Weighting and Fusing Candidate Segmentations: The above method generates a number of candidate segmentations per class. We assign weights to these by means of a constellation model in the form of a pairwise CRF. The nodes $v \in V$ of the respective graph $G = (V, E)$ correspond to the classes. The labels $l \in L$ that each node can take correspond to the respective candidate segmentations. The edges $E \subseteq V \times V$ encode the pairs of classes for which we model relative locations. We employ either a chain model that only connects spatially neighboring classes, or a fully connected model, depending on the application.

Let Ω denote the image domain. We define unary terms $\phi(v, l)$ of the CRF as a linear combination of the cost of the respective appearance model fit $a(v, l)$ and the negative logarithm of the RF probability map $RF_v : \Omega \to [0, 1]$ accumulated over the foreground of the respective binary segmentation $S_{v,l} : \Omega \to \{0, 1\}$,

$$\phi(v,l) := a(v,l) + \frac{\lambda}{|S_{v,l}^{-1}(1)|} \sum_{i \in \Omega} -log(RF_v(i)) \cdot S_{v,l}(i). \tag{1}$$

A parameter λ weighs the relative influence of the two terms. We set this parameter heuristically. We define pairwise terms to reflect the probability of relative locations of neighboring proposals. We learn the average distances $d(v,w)$ between the centroids of any two vertebrae v,w, as well as respective standard deviations $\sigma(v,w)$, and assume an according Gaussian distribution. Let $c(v,l)$ denote the centroid of the l-th candidate segmentation of class v. Our pairwise terms read

$$\psi(v,w,k,l) := \frac{(|c(v,k) - c(w,l)| - d(v,w))^2}{\sigma(v,w)^2}. \tag{2}$$

We compute weights for each proposal and each class by means of inference in this CRF. We explore two well-known variants of inference, namely MAP inference and probabilistic inference. MAP inference finds a label l_v for each node such that the energy of the CRF,

$$E(\{l_v\}_{v \in V}) = \sum_{v \in V} \phi(v,l_v) + \sum_{(v,w) \in E} \psi(v,w,l_v,l_w), \tag{3}$$

is minimized, thus yielding binary weights $w(v,l) \in \{0,1\}$ for each proposal. Probabilistic inference computes the marginal probabilities $p_v(l)$ of the respective Gibbs distribution $p(\{l_v\}_{v \in V}) = \frac{1}{Z} \exp(-E(\{l_v\}_{v \in V}))$, yielding continuous weights $w(v,l) \in [0,1]$ for each proposal. $W_v := \sum_{l \in L} p_v(l) \cdot S_{v,l}$. We call W_v a *smoothed probability map* or *smoothed RF output* for class v.

For a chain model, both MAP and probabilistic inference can be solved optimally by means of dynamic programming. For a fully connected model, the respective optimization problem is NP hard. However, probabilistic inference by Loopy Belief Propagation, and approximate MAP inference by TRWS [15] followed by Iterated Conditional Modes (ICM) [16], yields good results in practice.

3 Experiments

Zebrafish: We applied our approach to semantic segmentation of 21 somites in a data set of 32 images of developing zebrafish. All images were automatically pre-aligned to a reference image by rigid registration. Experts in biology manually created ground truth segmentations of these images. This data set poses multiple challenges for automated segmentation, due to (1) the similar appearance of neighboring segments, and (2) the small amount of training data. We train three-level cascades. We compare our approach with Auto-context [7] and GeoF [10], as well as with state-of-the-art RF-predict-and-MAP. Figure 2 gives an overview of the different types of inference/smoothing that we evaluate, and an idea of how the smoothed features look. For all algorithms, we evaluate the Dice score averaged over all 21 foreground classes, employing two-fold cross-validation to obtain scores for all 32 images. Forest parameters are as follows:

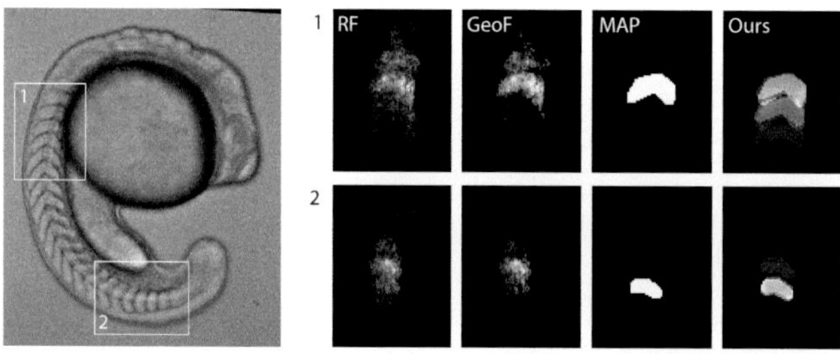

Fig. 2. Different types of inference/smoothing. Left: Zebrafish embryo. Right: Probability maps of two exemplary classes. RF probability map; geodesic smoothing (GeoF); MAP inference in our constellation model; probabilistic inference, *i.e.* marginals (Ours).

16 trees, maximum depth 12, features from a standard filter bank and local contextual features. We use a chain model as respective MRF.

Spine CT: The data used for experimental evaluation is the publicly available database of pathological spine CT[2]. For vertebrae localization in spine CT images, we use a static appearance model constructed from a mean and variance image pair as described in [1]. We use a fully connected MRF. Forest parameters are as follows: 25 trees, maximum depth 24, features from local and contextual average intensity, as described in [2].

4 Results and Discussion

Zebrafish: Figure 3 shows box plots of the Dice scores obtained from the smoothed RF output at all three levels of the cascade, for all four methods. Figure 3a lists the average Dice scores and standard deviations of the RF output as well as the smoothed RF output for all four methods after the final level of the cascade. Auto-context returns a final average Dice score of 0.60. Compared to Auto-context, GeoF generates considerably smoother posteriors, and performs better at every level of the cascade (green vs. cyan box plots in Figure 3). The best average score obtained by GeoF is 0.66 after three levels. This increase of 6% w.r.t. Auto-context is comparable to the gains reported in [10] when applying geodesic smoothing without changing the training objective.

After the first level of the cascade MAP inference performs best among all approaches (red box plots in Figure 3), with a mean Dice Score of 0.66. This approach also improves over the cascade, reaching a final Dice score of 0.76 after three levels. However, probabilistic instead of MAP inference yields the highest overall average Dice Score of 0.82, outperforming MAP by 6%. Also, the accuracy increases considerably from level to level (blue box plots in Figure 3).

Observe that the accuracy of every approach increases over the levels of the cascade. Furthermore, approaches that employ any kind of smoothing between levels perform better than auto-context, confirming the power of cascading with

[2] `http://research.microsoft.com/spine/`

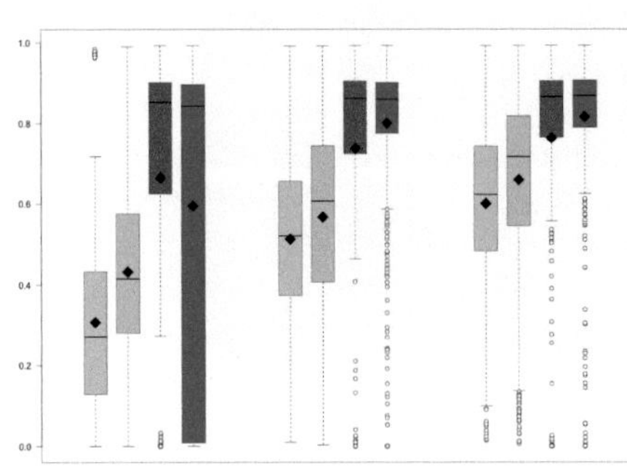

	RF	SRF
Auto Context	0.60 (0.20)	-
Geodesic	0.63 (0.21)	0.66 (0.22)
MAP	0.71 (0.27)	0.76 (0.27)
Ours	**0.82 (0.16)**	**0.82** (0.18)

(a)

	MAP			Ours		
Level	FF	RF	SRF	FF	RF	SRF
1	1	0	0	1	0	0
2	0.16	**0.60**	0.24	0.11	0.34	**0.55**
3	0.15	**0.60**	0.25	0.10	0.43	**0.47**

(b)

Fig. 3. Evaluation of four methods on 32 zebrafish datasets. Left: Segmentation accuracy as Dice scores after each level of a three-level cascade. RF (green), GeoF (cyan), MAP (red), our proposed marginals (blue). Right: (a) Average Dice Score (over 32x21 values), and standard deviation (in brackets), for segmentations obtained directly from RF-generated probability maps (RF), and from respective "smoothed" RF probability maps (SRF). (b) Variable importance of features, normalized over the three classes: Filter bank features (FF), RF output (RF) and smoothed RF output (SRF).

interleaved smoothing. Model-based smoothing performs considerably better than model-agnostic geodesic smoothing, likely due to the more specific prior knowledge induced by the constellation model.

Interestingly, while MAP inference yields the best results after the first level of our cascade, probabilistic inference undergoes a much more dramatic increase in the mean Dice score and concurrent reduction in the standard deviation over the 3 levels of the cascade. We observe that this is due to failure cases that are "rescued" by our approach, but not by MAP, as shown in Figure 4.

We quantify the relative strength of features generated by probabilistic inference vs. MAP inference by means of their variable importance [12]. Figure 3b reveals that the features generated by probabilistic inference are significantly more important for forest performance than the respective MAP features.

Human Spine CT: We evaluate the results of a single-level RF and a two-level cascade on publicly available data (cf. [2]) in terms of True Positive Rates (TPR) as listed in Table 1. Note that [2] reports Precision as opposed to TPR on this data for the sake of comparability to another dataset that is guaranteed to contain all vertebrae of the spine. This measure neglects false negative detections. However, the data we evaluate shows arbitrary subsets of vertebrae. This poses an additional challenge to an automated localisation method, because it has to decide which vertebrae are present at all. Hence we decided for an error measure that accounts for false negative detections, namely TPR.

We calculated the TPR for the results of [2] obtained exactly with their method, which is 63%. Our one-level cascade without inference is a re-implementation of [2], with the slight modifications of training deeper trees and limiting image thresholds to a HU window of $[0, 1000]$. These modifications improve the

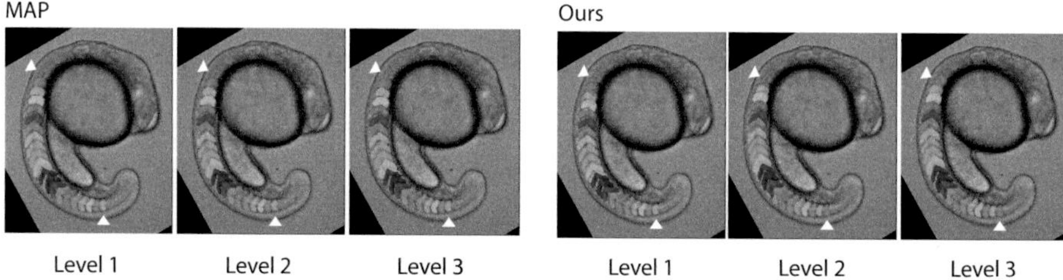

Fig. 4. Exemplary failure case that is "rescued" by our approach, but not by MAP inference. Arrows point to true locations of first and last somites in the sequence. After the first level, segmentations are off by one somite. This stays constant for MAP; however, our approach gradually recovers a correct segmentation.

Table 1. Evaluation of spine localization on pathological CTs. Median / mean distance, standard deviation (in brackets), True Positive Rate [in square brackets]. Distances are in mm. Rows: RF output without inference (None), MAP inference, and probabilistic inference (Ours). First column: One-level RF. Second column: Two level cascade.

	One Level	Cascade	
		Level 1	Level 2
None	8.7 / 12.7 (15.7) [0.67]	9.0 / 14.1 (17.7) [0.66]	9.0 / 12.7 (12.0) [0.68]
MAP	**7.8** / **10.1** (**8.0**) [0.73]	8.0 / 10.7 (8.6) [0.69]	**7.8** / 10.3 (8.3) [**0.74**]
Ours	-	8.0 / 10.6 (8.6) [0.70]	7.9 / 10.7 (8.5) [**0.74**]

TPR to 67%. Our best result, obtained by cascading and inference, has a TPR of 74%. Hence we outperform [2] by 11% in terms of TPR. For our best result we also computed the Precision, which is 79%. The Precision reported by [2] is 70%. Hence, we outperform [2] by 9% in terms of Precision.

Cascading is less powerful for the human spine CT than for the zebrafish, and MAP and marginals are en par. Potentially this is due to the extreme pathologies present in many if not most cases in this data set.

5 Conclusion

We have presented cascaded forest predictors interleaved with inference in MRF constellation models for the task of semantic segmentation and localization of vertebrae in biomedical applications. In a 21-class semantic segmentation task on biological data, probabilistic inference in the constellation model yields considerably better segmentation accuracy than the common MAP inference. Here, marginals of the constellation model allow for maintaining uncertainty in the predictions and hence help avoid sticking to a (MAP) solution too early in a cascade. These findings are of impact not only for the many types of constellation models employed in related work, but also for the recent trend of learning deep models combined with physically motivated structured models. For vertebrae localization, MAP and marginal inference are en par on a challenging pathological spine CT dataset, potentially due to the strong pathologies present in the data. However, our proposed approach of cascading interleaved with inference does improve considerably on state of the art.

Acknowledgments. The authors would like to acknowledge Daniele Soroldoni and Andrew Oates for kindly supplying the zebrafish images.

References

1. Glocker, B., Feulner, J., Criminisi, A., Haynor, D.R., Konukoglu, E.: Automatic localization and identification of vertebrae in arbitrary field-of-view CT scans. In: Ayache, N., Delingette, H., Golland, P., Mori, K. (eds.) MICCAI 2012, Part III. LNCS, vol. 7512, pp. 590–598. Springer, Heidelberg (2012)
2. Glocker, B., Zikic, D., Konukoglu, E., Haynor, D.R., Criminisi, A.: Vertebrae localization in pathological spine CT via dense classification from sparse annotations. In: Mori, K., Sakuma, I., Sato, Y., Barillot, C., Navab, N. (eds.) MICCAI 2013, Part II. LNCS, vol. 8150, pp. 262–270. Springer, Heidelberg (2013)
3. Seifert, S., Barbu, A., Zhou, S.K., Liu, D., Feulner, J., Huber, M., Suehling, M., Cavallaro, A., Comaniciu, D.: Hierarchical parsing and semantic navigation of full body CT data. In: SPIE Medical Imaging 2009: Image Processing, vol. 7259, pp. 725902–725902–8 (2009)
4. Shotton, J., Winn, J.M., Rother, C., Criminisi, A.: *textonBoost*: Joint appearance, shape and context modeling for multi-class object recognition and segmentation. In: Leonardis, A., Bischof, H., Pinz, A. (eds.) ECCV 2006, Part I. LNCS, vol. 3951, pp. 1–15. Springer, Heidelberg (2006)
5. Schroff, F., Criminisi, A., Zisserman, A.: Object class segmentation using random forests. In: BMVC (2008)
6. Krizhevsky, A., Sutskever, I., Hinton, G.E.: Imagenet classification with deep convolutional neural networks. In: Pereira, F., Burges, C., Bottou, L., Weinberger, K. (eds.) NIPS, pp. 1097–1105. Curran Associates, Inc. (2012)
7. Tu, Z.: Auto-context and its application to high-level vision tasks. In: CVPR 2008, pp. 1–8 (June 2008)
8. Nowozin, S., Rother, C., Bagon, S., Sharp, T., Yao, B., Kohli, P.: Decision tree fields. In: ICCV, pp. 1668–1675 (2011)
9. Schmidt, U., Rother, C., Nowozin, S., Jancsary, J., Roth, S.: Discriminative non-blind deblurring. In: CVPR, pp. 604–611 (2013)
10. Kontschieder, P., Kohli, P., Shotton, J., Criminisi, A.: Geof: Geodesic forests for learning coupled predictors. In: CVPR, pp. 65–72 (2013)
11. Yao, J., Glocker, B., Klinder, T., Li, S.: Recent advances in computational methods and clinical applications for spine imaging (2015)
12. Breiman, L.: Random forests. Machine Learning 45(1), 5–32 (2001)
13. Roberts, M.G., Cootes, T.F., Adams, J.E.: Automatic location of vertebrae on dxa images using random forest regression. In: Ayache, N., Delingette, H., Golland, P., Mori, K. (eds.) MICCAI 2012, Part III. LNCS, vol. 7512, pp. 361–368. Springer, Heidelberg (2012)
14. Cootes, T.F., Edwards, G.J., Taylor, C.J.: Active appearance models. IEEE Transactions on Pattern Analysis and Machine Intelligence 23(6), 681–685 (2001)
15. Kolmogorov, V.: Convergent tree-reweighted message passing for energy minimization. IEEE TPAMI 28(10), 1568–1583 (2006)
16. Besag, J.: On the statistical analysis of dirty pictures. Journal of the Royal Statistical Society. Series B (Methodological), 259–302 (1986)

Who Is Talking to Whom: Synaptic Partner Detection in Anisotropic Volumes of Insect Brain

Anna Kreshuk[1,3], Jan Funke[2], Albert Cardona[3], and Fred A. Hamprecht[1]

HCI/IWR, University of Heidelberg
Institute of Neuroinformatics, UZH/ETH Zurich
HHMI Janelia Research Campus

Abstract. Automated reconstruction of neural connectivity graphs from electron microscopy image stacks is an essential step towards large-scale neural circuit mapping. While significant progress has recently been made in automated segmentation of neurons and detection of synapses, the problem of synaptic partner assignment for polyadic (one-to-many) synapses, prevalent in the *Drosophila* brain, remains unsolved. In this contribution, we propose a method which automatically assigns pre- and postsynaptic roles to neurites adjacent to a synaptic site. The method constructs a probabilistic graphical model over potential synaptic partner pairs which includes factors to account for a high rate of one-to-many connections, as well as the possibility of the same neuron to be pre-synaptic in one synapse and post-synaptic in another. The algorithm has been validated on a publicly available stack of ssTEM images of *Drosophila* neural tissue and has been shown to reconstruct most of the synaptic relations correctly.

Keywords: Circuit reconstruction, graphical model, electron microscopy.

1 Introduction

Recent advances in electron microscopy instrumentation and sample preparation allow neuroscientists to acquire unprecedented volumes of data. Automating the analysis of the acquired images, however, still poses unsolved challenges to the computer vision community [7,14]. In order to reconstruct the connectivity in a block of neural tissue, neuroscientists have to trace all the neurons in the image stack and establish which of them are connected by synapses and in which direction. In the mammalian cortex, most synapses connect a single presynaptic neuron (sender) to a single postsynaptic neuron (receiver). Moreover, within the relatively small fields of view accessible to electron microscopy, mammalian cortex neurons mostly play an unambiguous sending or receiving role. Matters get more complicated in fruitfly neural tissue, where most synapses are polyadic (one-to-many, Fig. 1, Fig. 3), and, due to higher overall density of connections, more neurites are populated by both pre- and postsynaptic sites [3]. For such

N. Navab et al. (Eds.): MICCAI 2015, Part I, LNCS 9349, pp. 661–668, 2015.
DOI: 10.1007/978-3-319-24553-9_81

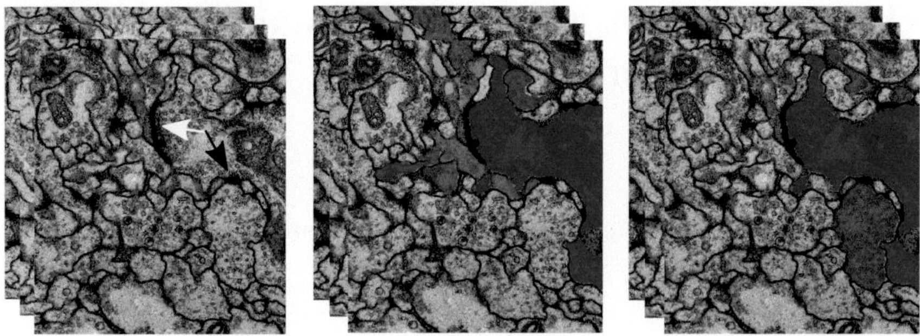

Fig. 1. A small substack of the data, showing the synaptic partners involved in two synapses. Left: raw data; black arrow points to a one-to-one synapse, white arrow to a one-to-many synapse from inside the presynaptic neuron. Center: pre- and postsynaptic neurons, participating in the larger one-to-many synapse (not all connections happen in the top section). Right: pre- and postsynaptic partners of the one-to-one synapse.

data, it becomes necessary to both find all the partners in a synaptic connection and to establish the direction of signal flow.

Until recently, all image analysis for neural circuit mapping has been performed manually. While manual processing continues to play a major role, latest advances in neuron segmentation and synapse detection algorithms allow neuroscientists to switch to a semi-automated mode with automated processing followed by targeted proofreading [10,17]. For FIB/SEM data with isotropic resolution [11], performance of automated synapse detection methods [2,13,18] is already comparable to that of human annotators. While anisotropic ssTEM data is more difficult, several methods have very recently been suggested to tackle this problem ([9,12,19]). The significantly more challenging problem of automated neuron segmentation has been the subject of even more active research. While human performance is not yet reached, substantial progress has been made in recent years [1,5,8,15,16,21]. Overshadowed by the challenges of neuron segmentation and synapse detection, the problem of synaptic partner assignment has so far been left to fully manual annotation. Automating this painstakingly laborious and error prone analysis step is the target of our contribution.

We propose to build a probabilistic graphical model, where synaptic roles of pairs of spatially adjacent neurites are modeled by random variables. Morphological properties of the neurons are incorporated into unary factors; general synapse properties, such as the prevalence of one-to-many connections, are modeled by pairwise factors. Our motivation for choosing this method is the simplicity of modeling rules of different strengths, from slight preference of certain neuron/synapse configurations to rules with almost no exceptions, such as neurons not synapsing on themselves. Pairwise factors allow us to model much more prior biological knowledge and substantially improve the results.

A detailed description of the model can be found in the next section. In section 3 we apply the method to a stack of *Drosophila* larva neural images with anisotropic resolution and demonstrate that this model is superior to neuron pair classification. Finally, in section 4 we discuss how this model could be extended to isotropic data or used jointly with a neural segmentation procedure.

2 Methods

Our method starts from a segmentation of the stack into neurons and detection of its synapses. In the following we refer to individual images of the stack as sections and to cross sections of neurons in the image as neuron slices. Similar to neuron segmentation methods for anisotropic data, we consider the stack section by section and then introduce inter-section links.

In each section of the stack, we group adjacent neuron slices into pairs of neighbors. For a pair of neighbor neuron slices i and j we then introduce a random variable P_{ij} with three possible states: 1) no synaptic connection, 2) the first neuron of the pair is presynaptic, the second is postsynaptic, 3) the first neuron is postsynaptic, the second is presynaptic. Note that pre- and postsynaptic roles of the neuron slices are defined individually for each potential synaptic connection rather than globally. Thus, a neuron slice can be presynaptic to one and postsynaptic to another one of its neighbors.

2.1 Unary Factors

The unary factors for each pair represent the prediction we can make on the state of the pair, when considering each pair individually. These are computed as predictions of a Random Forest classifier. The features for prediction are inspired by rules typically employed by human annotators, namely: 1) neurotransmitter vesicles are found on the presynaptic side of the connection; 2) presynaptic neuron slices are usually larger than postsynaptic ones; 3) there is a synaptic density (electron dense region, showing as a darker spot in the images) very near to the boundary between the slices. These cues are shown in Fig. 3(left). To compute the first feature, we train another Random Forest classifier to detect vesicles on the pixel level. The ilastik toolkit [20] has been used to train the classifier interactively on very sparse user labels. A similar classifier was used by [9] to detect vesicles in the retina, while [2] employ similar features to implicitly encode the presence of vesicles on one and absence on the other side of the synapse. The number of segmented vesicles is used as a feature for the unary Random Forest. To obtain an estimate of the synapse presence between the neurons of the pair, we either use smoothed precomputed synapse detections or, if these are not available, train another pixelwise classifier on synaptic densities. The summed predictions of this classifier in the vicinity of neuron-neuron boundary are also taken as a feature for the unary Random Forest. The remaining features are areas of the two neuron slices. The prediction of the Random Forest for the neuron slices i and j is then taken as the unary factor ψ_{ij} associated with the random variable P_{ij}.

2.2 Pairwise Factors

The unary factors predict the synaptic relation for each pair of neuron slices individually. To reflect dependencies between pairs of neuron pairs, we augment our model by pairwise factors. In particular, we strive to encode the following biological knowledge: i) a single synapse should have only one presynaptic neuron (there are no convergent synapses in our test data); ii) one-to-many connections are more likely than one-to-one; iii) in cases when a neuron slice is both pre- and postsynaptic through different synapses, these synapses are usually not located immediately next to each other.

A pairwise factor is introduced for two random variables whenever their constituent pairs share one of the slices. For example, if P_{ij} represents the pair of slices i and j, and P_{ik} the pair of slices i and k, then we introduce a pairwise factor $\psi_{ij,ik}$ between them. The values of this factor depend not only on the states of P_{ij} and P_{ik}, but also on the conditions of them belonging to the same synapse and j and k being neighbors. Consequently, we introduce four variants of the $\psi_{ij,ik}$ factor with different value tables (see also Fig. 2):

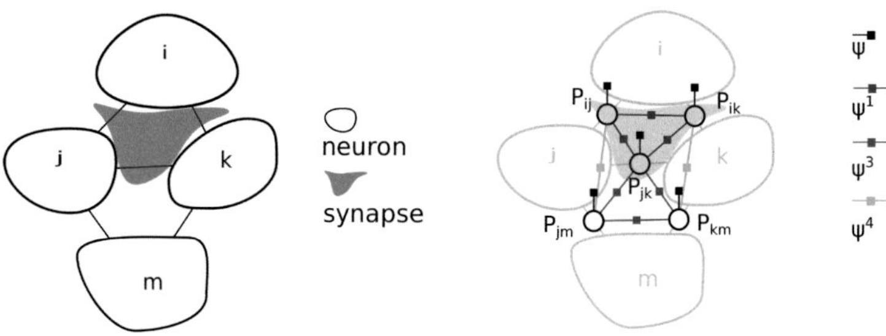

Fig. 2. An example of a region adjacency graph of neurons and synapses and the corresponding factor graph model. Left: a region adjacency graph for four neuron slices i, j, k, m and one synapse. Note that i and m are not neighbors, and the j to m and k to m boundaries are not covered by the synapse. Right: the corresponding factor graph for variables P_{ij}, P_{ik}, P_{jk}, P_{jm}, P_{km}. Connections across different sections of the stack are omitted. See main text in Section 2.2 for the factor legend.

1. $\psi^1_{ij,ik}$: j and k are neighbors, i, j and k touch the same synapse. In this case, we penalize the variable states which give rise to the configurations with two presynaptic neurons in the same synapse (cost c_0), neuron being pre- and postsynaptic through the same synapse (cost c_1) and one-to-one rather than one-to-many connection (cost c_2). This potential, along with the corresponding variable states, is shown in Fig. 3(right).
2. $\psi^2_{ij,ik}$: j and k are *not* neighbors, i, j and k touch the same synapse. In this case we again penalize variable states which lead to two presynaptic neurons in the same synapse and a neuron being both pre- and postsynaptic through the same synapse.

3. $\psi^3_{ij,ik}$: j and k are neighbors, i, j and k do *not* touch the same synapse. Here we penalize the state with a many-to-one connection, as well as the state with one neuron being both pre- and post-synaptic, but with a lower cost than for neurons touching the same synapse.
4. $\psi^4_{ij,ik}$ (j and k are *not* neighbors, i, j and k do *not* touch the same synapse. In this case we slightly penalize the state, where one neuron is both pre- and postsynaptic.

Fig. 3 shows the values of $\psi^1_{ij,ik}$ as a function of the state of P_{ij} and P_{ik}.

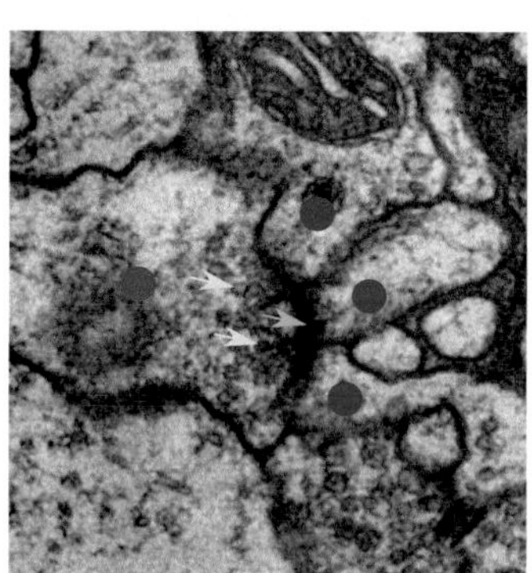

$\psi_{ij,ik}$	$P_{ij}=0$	$P_{ij}=1$	$P_{ij}=2$
$P_{ik}=0$	$\psi_{ij,ik}=0$	$\psi_{ij,ik}=c_2$	$\psi_{ij,ik}=0$
$P_{ik}=1$	$\psi_{ij,ik}=c_2$	$\psi_{ij,ik}=0$	$\psi_{ij,ik}=c_1$
$P_{ik}=2$	$\psi_{ij,ik}=0$	$\psi_{ij,ik}=c_1$	$\psi_{ij,ik}=c_0$

Fig. 3. Left: a typical one-to-many synapse. Red dot marks the pre-synaptic neuron, blue dots its post-synaptic partners. Yellow arrows point to vesicles and the green arrow to the electron-dense area of the membrane. Right: the value table for the $\psi^1_{ij,ik}$ factor for different values of P_{ij} and P_{ik}. Random variable states are denoted by arrows showing synapse direction: $P_{ij} = 0$ – no synaptic connection, $P_{ij} = 1$ – i is presynaptic, j is postsynaptic, $P_{ij} = 2$ – vice versa.

To link the variables between consecutive sections, we additionally introduce pairwise factors between pairs of slices of the same neurons which encourage consistency of the synaptic role assignment between sections. For illustration, let neuron n_i be represented by slice i_s in section s and by slice i_{s+1} in section $s+1$, while neuron n_j is represented by j_s and j_{s+1} respectively. If both i_s, j_s and i_{s+1}, j_{s+1} form neighor pairs, touching the same synapse in both sections, we add a pairwise factor between variables $P_{i_s,j_s}, P_{i_{s+1},j_{s+1}}$.

The MAP estimation problem for this factor graph can be reformulated as an energy minimization problem, with the usual transition from potentials to energies ($\mathcal{N}$ stands for the set of all pairs of neighbors):

$$\psi_{ij}(P_{ij}) = \exp(-E_{ij}(P_{ij})), \qquad \psi_{ij,ik}(P_{ij}, P_{ik}) = \exp(-E_{ij,ik}(P_{ij}, P_{ik}))$$

$$\operatorname*{argmin}_{P_{ij},(i,j)\in\mathcal{N}} E(P) = \operatorname*{argmin}_{P_{ij},(i,j)\in\mathcal{N}} \sum_{(i,j)\in\mathcal{N}} E_{ij} + \sum_{(i,j),(i,k)\in\mathcal{N}} E_{ij,ik}$$

We solve this problem to global optimality by an ILP solver.

3 Results

The proposed algorithm has been validated on a publicly available dataset from *Drosophila* larval neuropil volume [6]. Two 1024×1024×20 image stacks are provided along with manual neuron segmentation and synapse detections for the first stack. We annotated the synapses in the second stack and the pre- and post-synaptic neuron slices in both stacks. The first stack has been used for training the unary Random Forest and the first 9 sections of the second stack have been used for the grid search of the best values for the costs in the pairwise potentials.

Table 1. Algorithm results. First and second column show recall and precision of the synaptic partner detection. The third column shows the total number of synaptic partner pairs in the groundtruth annotation. Fourth column shows the number of synapses, for which all partners have been detected automatically (with possible false positive pairs besides true detections). Fifth and sixth columns show the number of synapses, where not all or no partners at all have been found. See main text for evaluation details.

Method	Recall	Precision	Total pairs	Fully recovered synapse groups	Partially recovered synapse groups	Not recovered synapse groups
Unary only	90%	64%	163	36	6	5
Full model	90%	78%	163	38	2	7

The evaluation procedure ran as follows: groundtruth neuron segmentation and synapse detection were provided as input to the algorithm. Each synaptic partner pair, detected by the algorithm, was assigned to its closest synapse, if it was within a 10 pixel distance from it on any section. Pairs with no synapse at such distance were discarded. Recall was computed as the number of groundtruth pairs found by the algorithm, divided by the total number of groundtruth pairs; precision as the number of algorithm pairs found in the groundtruth, divided by the total number of algorithm pairs. A synapse group is "fully recovered"/"partially recovered", if all/at least one of its pairs are found. The groundtruth contained 47 synapses, connecting 163 neuron pairs. For 7 such synapses, the algorithm did not find any of the pairs. We analyzed these synapses in more detail and found that 4 out of 7 were small synapses, only visible in the first or last slice. Another missed synapse was located very close to the image border. A difficult missed connection of a partially recovered synapse group is shown in Fig. 4(A, B, C, D). Other connections of this synapse, found in consecutive sections, were reconstructed correctly. A typical false positive, caused by the preference for the same label for neighboring pairs, is shown in Fig. 4(E,F). The same preference explains the reduced number of partially recovered synapse groups for the full model in Table 1.

4 Discussion

We have introduced an algorithm for synaptic partner detection, which, by constructing a probabilistic graphical model to couple synaptic partner pairs,

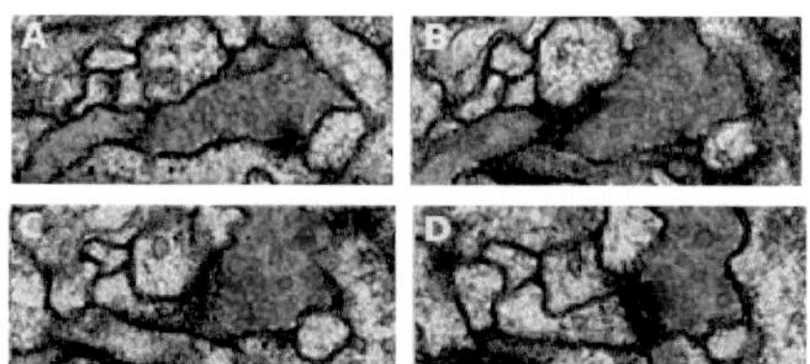

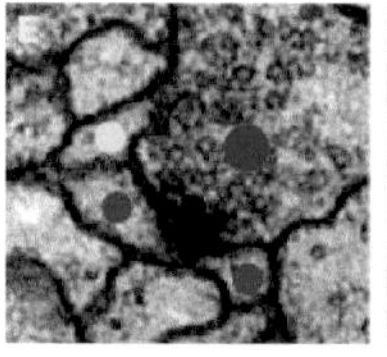

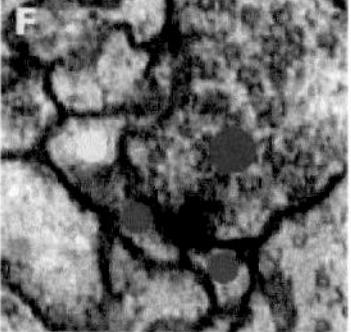

Fig. 4. A, B, C, D: serial sections of a missed connection. Presynaptic slice is colored blue, postsynaptic red. E, F: a typical false positive error over two sections. Blue dot: presynaptic neuron, red dots: correct postsynaptic neurons, yellow dot: false positive.

can benefit from more biological prior knowledge than an estimator considering each pair individually. On a test dataset, our evaluation shows a significant improvement of precision without a loss in recall.

In its current form, our algorithm explicitly uses 2D neuron slices and links them together across the lower resolution z-axis. It could, however, also be extended to isotropic 3D data, such as data produced by FIB/SEM microscopes. For a fully 3D approach, we would consider neuron pairs within a spherical neighborhood of each synapse detection and replace the features by their 3D counterparts.

Assignment of synaptic partners could also be incorporated directly into the neuron segmentation procedure and perhaps improve both the segmentation and the partner assignment steps. For methods operating on neuron hypotheses [4,15,21], this could be achieved by explicitly introducing synaptic relations between neuron slice candidates. Segmentation could then make use not only of the general prior knowledge of neuron appearance, but also more specific local pre- and postsynaptic features.

We believe that the proposed algorithm can substantially reduce human annotation effort for insect brain circuit reconstruction by shifting the synaptic partner detection task from fully manual to at least semi-automated domain, as well as pointing out the human attention errors.

References

1. Andres, B., Kroeger, T., Briggman, K.L., Denk, W., Korogod, N., Knott, G., Koethe, U., Hamprecht, F.A.: Globally Optimal Closed-surface Segmentation for Connectomics. In: Fitzgibbon, A., Lazebnik, S., Perona, P., Sato, Y., Schmid, C. (eds.) ECCV 2012, Part III. LNCS, vol. 7574, pp. 778–791. Springer, Heidelberg (2012)
2. Becker, C., Ali, K., Knott, G., Fua, P.: Learning Context Cues for Synapse Segmentation in EM Volumes. In: Ayache, N., Delingette, H., Golland, P., Mori, K. (eds.) MICCAI 2012, Part I. LNCS, vol. 7510, pp. 585–592. Springer, Heidelberg (2012)
3. Cardona, A., Saalfeld, S., Preibisch, S., Schmid, B., Cheng, A., Pulokas, J., Tomancak, P., Hartenstein, V.: An integrated micro- and macroarchitectural analysis of the Drosophila brain by computer-assisted serial section electron microscopy. PLoS Biology 8(10) (January 2010)

4. Funke, J., Andres, B., Hamprecht, F.A., Cardona, A., Cook, M.: Efficient automatic 3D-reconstruction of branching neurons from EM data. In: Proceedings of CVPR (2012)
5. Funke, J., et al.: Candidate Sampling for Neuron Reconstruction from Anisotropic Electron Microscopy Volumes. In: Golland, P., Hata, N., Barillot, C., Hornegger, J., Howe, R. (eds.) MICCAI 2014, Part I. LNCS, vol. 8673, pp. 17–24. Springer, Heidelberg (2014)
6. Gerhard, S., Funke, J., Julien, M., Cardona, A., Fetter, R.: Segmented anisotropic ssTEM dataset of neural tissue, `http://dx.doi.org/10.6084/m9.figshare.856713`
7. Helmstaedter, M., Mitra, P.P.: Computational methods and challenges for large-scale circuit mapping. Current Opinion in Neurobiology 22(1), 162–169 (2012)
8. Huang, G.B., Jain, V.: Deep and Wide Multiscale Recursive Networks for Robust Image Labeling. In: Proceedings of ICLR (2014)
9. Jagadeesh, V., Anderson, J., Jones, B., Marc, R., Fisher, S., Manjunath, B.S.: Synapse Classification and Localization in Electron Micrographs. Pattern Recognition Letters (2013)
10. Kaynig, V., Knowles-barley, S., Jones, T.R.: Large-Scale Automatic Reconstruction of Neuronal Processes from Electron Microscopy Images. arxiv:1303.7186v1 (2013)
11. Knott, G., Marchman, H., Wall, D., Lich, B.: Serial section scanning electron microscopy of adult brain tissue using focused ion beam milling. The Journal of Neuroscience 28(12), 2959–2964 (2008)
12. Kreshuk, A., Köthe, U., Pax, E., Bock, D.D., Hamprecht, F.A.: Automated Detection of Synapses in Serial Section Transmission Electron Microscopy Image Stacks. PLoS One 9, 2 (2014)
13. Kreshuk, A., Straehle, C.N., Sommer, C., Koethe, U., Cantoni, M., Knott, G., Hamprecht, F.A.: Automated detection and segmentation of synaptic contacts in nearly isotropic serial electron microscopy images. PloS One 6(10), e24899 (2011)
14. Lichtman, J.W., Pfister, H., Shavit, N.: The big data challenges of connectomics. Nature Neuroscience 17(11), 1448–1454 (2014)
15. Liu, T., Jones, C., Seyedhosseini, M., Tasdizen, T.: A modular hierarchical approach to 3D electron microscopy image segmentation. Journal of Neuroscience Methods 226, 88–102 (2014)
16. Nunez-Iglesias, J., Kennedy, R., Parag, T., Shi, J., Chklovskii, D.B.: Machine Learning of Hierarchical Clustering to Segment 2D and 3D Images. PloS One 8(8), e71715 (2013)
17. Plaza, S.M.: Focused Proofreading: Efficiently Extracting Connectomes from Segmented EM Images. arXiv:1409.1199v1 (2014)
18. Plaza, S.M., Parag, T., Huang, G.B., Olbris, D.J., Saunders, M.A., Rivlin, P.K.: Annotating Synapses in Large EM Datasets. arXiv:1409.1801v2 (2014)
19. Roncal, W.G., Kaynig-Fittkau, V., Kasthuri, N., Berger, D., Vogelstein, J.T., Fernandez, L.R., Lichtman, J.W., Vogelstein, R.J., Pfister, H., Hager, G.D.: Volumetric Exploitation of Synaptic Information using Context Localization and Evaluation. arXiv:1403.3724 (2014)
20. Sommer, C., Straehle, C., Kothe, U., Hamprecht, F.A.: Ilastik: Interactive learning and segmentation toolkit. In: Proceedings of ISBI (2011)
21. Vazquez-Reina, A., Gelbart, M., Huang, D., Lichtman, J., Miller, E., Pfister, H.: Segmentation fusion for connectomics. In: Proceedings of ICCV (2011)

Direct and Simultaneous Four-Chamber Volume Estimation by Multi-Output Regression

Xiantong Zhen[1], Ali Islam[3], Mousumi Bhaduri[4], Ian Chan[4], and Shuo Li[1,2]

[1] The University of Western Ontario, London, ON, Canada
[2] GE Healthcare, London, ON, Canada
[3] St. Joseph's Health Care, London, ON, Canada
[4] London Health Sciences Centre, ON, Canada

Abstract. Cardiac four-chamber volumes provide crucial information for quantitative analysis of whole heart functions. Conventional cardiac volume estimation relies on a segmentation step; recently emerging direct estimation without segmentation has shown better performance than than segmentation-based methods. However, due to the high complexity, four-chamber volume estimation poses great challenges to these existing methods: four-chamber segmentation is not feasible due to intensity homogeneity of ventricle and atrium without implicit boundaries between them; existing direct methods which can only handle single or bi-ventricles are not directly applicable due to great combinatorial variability of four chambers. In this paper, by leveraging the full strength of direct estimation, we propose a new method for direct and simultaneous four-chamber volume estimation using multi-output regression that can disentangle complex relationship of image appearance and four-chamber volumes via statistical learning. To accomplish accurate and efficient estimation, we propose using a supervised descriptor learning (SDL) algorithm to generate a compact and discriminative feature representation. By casting into generalized low-rank approximations of matrices with a supervised manifold regularization, the SDL jointly removes irrelevant and redundant information by feature reduction and extracts discriminative features directly related to four chambers via supervised learning, which overcomes the high complexity of four chambers. We evaluate the proposed method on a cardiac four-chamber MR dataset from 125 subjects including both healthy and diseased cases. The experimental results show that our method achieves a high correlation coefficient of up to 91.5% with manual segmentation obtained by human experts. Our method for the first time achieves simultaneous and direct four-chamber volume estimation, which enables more efficient and accurate functional assessment of the whole heart.

1 Introduction

Cardiac four-chamber volumes offer comprehensive measurement for heart functional assessment by capturing the dynamic pattern of the whole heart [1]. The left/right ventricles (LV/RV), which have been extensively studied, play a critical role in heart disease diagnosis, while the left/right atrium (LA/RA) volumes

N. Navab et al. (Eds.): MICCAI 2015, Part I, LNCS 9349, pp. 669–676, 2015.
DOI: 10.1007/978-3-319-24553-9_82

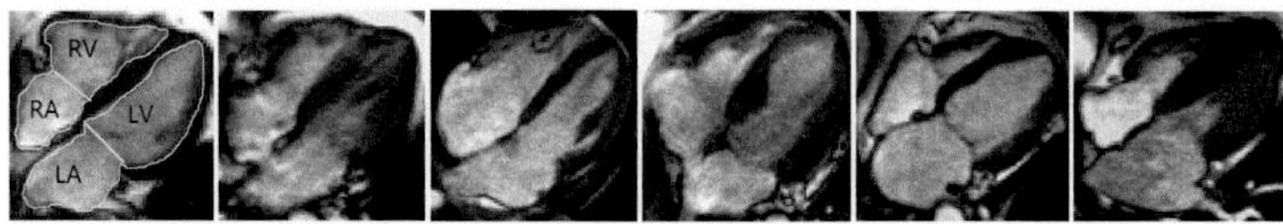

Fig. 1. Cardiac four-chamber MR images from different subjects with different temporal frames

are strongly associated with heart functions and indicate severity of diastolic dysfunctions and cardiovascular disease burden; together, four chambers provide crucial information for quantitative functional analysis of the whole heart. However, the LA and RA have long been overlooked due to the difficulty in measuring their volumes. Efficient simultaneous four-chamber volume estimation would enable more accurate and comprehensive cardiac functional analysis.

Four-chamber volume estimation poses great challenges to existing methods due to the huge complexity of four chambers stemming from highly complex contours, temporal deformations, anatomical interdependency of chambers, low tissue contrast and large patient variability as shown in Fig. 1. Conventional segmentation-based methods for cardiac volume estimation mainly focus on the LV with few on the RV. LA and RA volume estimation has not yet been addressed, not to mention simultaneous four-chamber volume estimation. Although automatic segmentation becomes more reliable, accurate and less time-consuming, four-chamber segmentation is still a challenging task and far from being used in clinical practice. Whole heart segmentation [1] potentially offers a solution to simultaneous four-chamber volume estimation; however, it is currently unable to segment four chambers separately to obtain their individual volumes due to the fact that ventricle and atrium are of intensity homogeneity with vague boundary between them, and two atriums are mostly connected with a very thin wall as shown in Fig. 1.

Recently, direct estimation [2–4] without segmentation has emerged as an effective tool for cardiac ventricular volume estimation [5, 6] which outperforms segmentation-based estimation in terms of both accuracy and efficiency [6]. More importantly, direct estimation allows us to leverage fast evolving state-of-the-art machine learning techniques which makes automatic detection and diagnosis comparable to a well-trained and experienced radiologist [7]. Although direct estimation has gained great success in single and bi-ventricular volume estimation [2–4], existing direct methods are not directly applicable to simultaneous four-chamber volume estimation due to the great combinatorial variability of four chambers and even more complicated relationship between image appearance and four-chamber volumes compared to single or bi-ventricles.

In this paper, we formulate four-chamber volume estimation as a multi-output regression problem. This formulation naturally models four-chamber volumes simultaneously, successfully handles the great challenge of four chambers, and provides clinical more meaningful volume estimation of four chambers. By removing unreliable segmentation, our method enables accurate and convenient functional analysis of the whole heart. To establish compact and discriminative feature representation for accurate and efficient volume estimation, we propose using a supervised descriptor learning (SDL) algorithm [8] formulated as generalized low-rank approximations of matrices with a supervised manifold regularization (SMR). The SDL jointly removes irrelevant and redundant information by feature reduction, i.e., generalized low-rank approximation and extracts discriminative features directly related to four-chamber volumes via supervised learning, i.e., supervised manifold regularization. The obtained cardiac four-chamber image representations by SDL are compact and discriminative, which enables efficient and accurate four-chamber volume estimation.

This work contributes in three folds: **1)** Our method is the first to achieve direct and simultaneous cardiac four-chamber volume estimation, which removes unreliable segmentation and enables more accurate and convenient whole heart functional analysis. The method can be conveniently extended to other clinical direct organ volume estimation; **2)** We formulate four-chamber volume estimation as a multi-output regression problem, which leverages the strength of statistical learning to achieve simultaneous four-chamber volume estimation. Other similar clinical data prediction from medical images can be modeled and solved in the same way; **3)** We propose using a supervised descriptor learning (SDL) algorithm [8] to generate compact and discriminative cardiac image representations, which overcomes the huge complexity of four chambers. The SDL provides a general supervised descriptor learning framework that can be widely used in other clinical multivariate estimation tasks.

2 Cardiac Four-Chamber Volume Estimation via Multi-Output Regression

2.1 Cardiac Image Representations

We are given a set of annotated data $\{X_1, \ldots, X_L\}$ and the corresponding multivariate targets $\{Y_1, \ldots, Y_L\}$, where L is the number of training samples and $Y_i \in \mathbb{R}^d$ denote four-chamber volumes. We start with matrix representations of four chamber cardiac images, *i.e.*, $X_i \in \mathbb{R}^{M \times N}$, which could be any matrix representations, *e.g.*, raw pixel intensities. We use the gradient orientation matrix (GOM) which is constructed from pyramid histogram of gradients (PHOG) of images by stacking spatial cells in rows and orientation bins in columns. The GOM takes advantages of prior knowledge to capture characteristic spatial layout and local shape which are the key characteristics of four chambers. The GOM is fed into the proposed SDL to learn a compact and discriminative representation of four chambers.

Generalized Low-Rank Approximation. We propose using the generalized low-rank approximation of matrices due to its efficient computation of dimension reduction of matrices [9]. This is to find two transformations: $W \in \mathbb{R}^{M \times m}$ and $V \in \mathbb{R}^{N \times n}$ with $m \ll M$ and $n \ll N$, and L matrices $D_i \in \mathbb{R}^{m \times n}$ such that

WD_iV^{T} is an appropriate approximation of each X_i, $i = 1, \ldots, L$. We solve the following optimization problem of minimizing the reconstruction errors:

$$\underset{\substack{W,V,D_1,\ldots,D_L \\ W^{\mathrm{T}}W=I_m, V^{\mathrm{T}}V=I_n}}{\arg\min} \quad \frac{1}{L}\sum_{i=1}^{L} \|X_i - WD_iV^{\mathrm{T}}\|_F^2 \tag{1}$$

where $\|\cdot\|_F$ is the Frobenius norm of a matrix, I_m is an identity matrix of size $m \times m$ and the constraints $W^{\mathrm{T}}W = I_m$ and $V^{\mathrm{T}}V = I_n$ ensure that W and V have orthogonal columns to avoid redundancy in the approximations.

From (1), we know that D_i is the low-rank approximation of X_i in terms of the transformations of W and V, and it is worth to mention that the matrices $D_1, \ldots, D_L$ are not required to be diagonal. It is also proven in [9] that given the W and V, for any i, D_i is uniquely determined by $D_i = W^{\mathrm{T}}X_iV$ which is the compact representation of X_i that will reduce regression complexity for efficient multivariate estimation. (1) only minimize the reconstruction error in the low-rank space leading to indiscriminate representations $\{D\}_{i=1}^L$.

Supervised Manifold Regularization (SMR). We impose discrimination on the low-rank representation $\{D_i\}_{i=1}^L$ by integrating the proposed SMR into (1). To this end, we first construct a weighted graph $G = (V, E)$ using the ϵ-neighborhood method [10], where V and E respectively represent L vertices and edges between vertices. The graph is built on the multivariate targets $(Y_1, \ldots, Y_L)$, *i.e.*, the four-chamber volume values, rather than on inputs in conventional manifold regularization [11], which naturally induces the supervision. We denote $S \in \mathbb{R}^{L\times L}$ as the symmetric similarity matrix with non-negative elements corresponding to the edge weight of the graph G, where each element S_{ij} is computed by a heat kernel with parameter σ: $S_{ij} = \exp\left(\frac{-\|Y_i - Y_j\|^2}{2\sigma^2}\right), i, j = 1, \ldots, L$. We set the diagonal elements of S to be zeros, *i.e.*, $S_{ii} = 0$. In the low-rank space, we would like to minimize the following term

$$\sum_{i,j} \|D_i - D_j\|_F^2 S_{ij}. \tag{2}$$

Since the similarity matrix S characterizes the manifold structure of the multivariate target space, low-rank approximations $\{D_i\}_{i=1}^L$ preserve the intrinsic local geometrical structure of the target space and are therefore automatically aligned to their regression targets. The discrimination is then naturally injected into the low-rank representations $\{D_i\}_{i=1}^L$.

Feature Learning with SMR. By integrating the SMR term in (2) into (1), we obtain the compact objective function of generalized low-rank approximation of matrices with the supervised manifold regularization (SMR) as follows:

$$\underset{\substack{W,V,D_1,\ldots,D_L \\ W^{\mathrm{T}}W=I_m, V^{\mathrm{T}}V=I_n}}{\arg\min} \quad \frac{1}{L}\sum_{i=1}^{L} \|X_i - WD_iV^{\mathrm{T}}\|_F^2 + \beta\sum_{i,j} \|D_i - D_j\|_F^2 S_{ij} \tag{3}$$

where $\beta \in (0, \infty)$ is a tuning parameter to balance the tradeoff between reconstruction errors and discrimination of the low-rank approximations, which also serves to keep the flexibility of the model.

In the objective function of (3), the first term guarantees the reconstruction fidelity in the low-rank approximation while the second SMR term introduces the discrimination to learned new representations. The objective function is solved by an iterative algorithm via alternate optimization: fixing W, solve V and fixing V, solve W.

2.2 Multi-Output Regression with Random Forests

Regression forests, an efficient way of mapping a complex input space to continuous output, started to attract interest in medical image analysis [4,12]. Due to the strong capability of naturally handling multivariate estimation, regression forests offer a best-suited tool for simultaneous cardiac four-chamber volume estimation. They can **1)** effectively handle the non-linear relationship between the cardiac image appearance and four-chamber volumes; **2)** naturally deal with multiple outputs, i.e., four-chamber volumes, by capturing the interdependency among them; and **3)** provide accurate and clinically more meaningful volume estimation without overfitting due to the nature of ensemble learning.

We adopt the adaptive K-cluster regression forests (AKRF) recently proposed in [13] for multivariate estimation. In the AKRF, a novel node splitting method formulated as a classification problem is proposed to replace simple thresholding in conventional regression forests [14], which allows each node to have more than two child nodes. This enhances the ability to handle the complex distributions of four-chamber volumes. It has been shown in [13] that the AKRF significantly outperforms other regressors, *e.g.*, support vector regression (SVR), conventional random forests and kernel partial least squares [13].

3 Experiments

3.1 Dataset and Implementation Details

The dataset contains four-chamber cardiac MR images from 125 subjects each of which has 25 frames across a temporal cardiac cycle. Images were acquired on a 1.5T scanner with fast imaging employing steady-state acquisition (FIESTA) image sequence mode, using these acquisition parameters: TR=35.5 ms, TE=1.2 ms and slice thickness=6mm. The performance of the proposed method is quantitatively evaluated by comparing with ground truth by manual segmentation. The correlation coefficient between the ground truth and the estimation is used as measurement to evaluate estimation performance as in [4,5], and higher correlation coefficient indicates better performance. The leave-one-subject-out cross validation is used for evaluation.

We estimate cavity areas of four chambers in MR images, and the volumes are computed by integrating cavity areas in the sagittal direction. Note that we use the normalized areas as the targets, *i.e.*, the number of pixels in a chamber divided by the total number of pixels of the images. A region of interest (ROI) is placed to enclose four chambers in an MR image according to the method in [3]. We use a three-level pyramid HOG (PHOG) obtaining a matrix of size 84×31 from an image of 64×64 pixels. To show the advantage of our SDL algorithm, we have also compared with popular descriptors, *e.g.*, GIST and histogram of LBP both of which are implemented with a similar spatial pyramid to the PHOG descriptor, and dimensionality reduction methods, *e.g.*, generalized principal component analysis (GPCA) [15] and principal component analysis (PCA). In the implementation of adaptive K-clustering random forests (AKRF) [13], we use 20 trees to construct the regression forests, which can keep low computational cost with satisfactory performance.

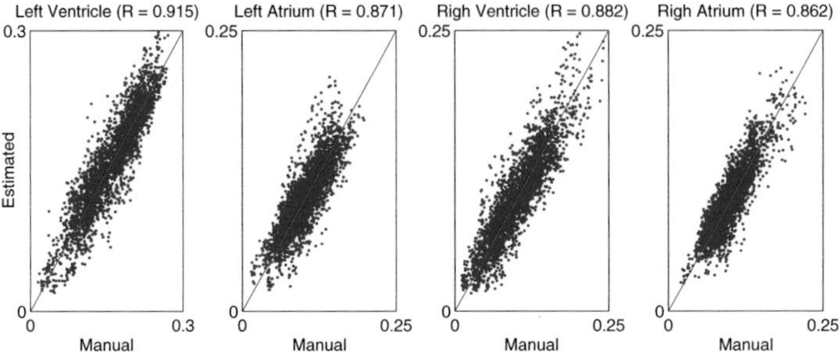

Fig. 2. The correlation coefficients between estimated and manually obtained volumes for four chambers. R is the correlation coefficient.

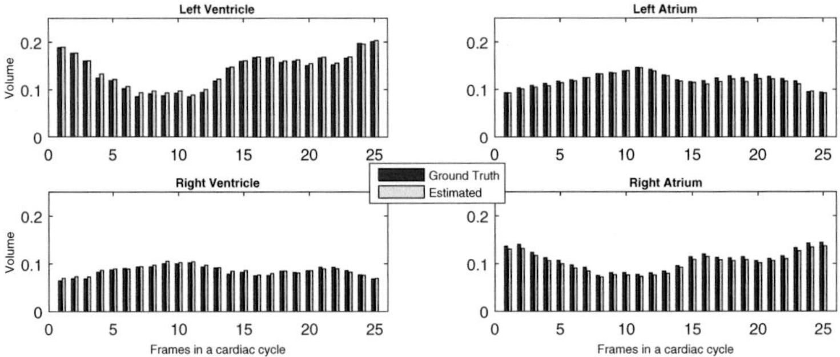

Fig. 3. The illustration of ground truth against estimation by the proposed method for 25 frames in cardiac cycle averaged over subjects

Table 1. The comparison results for cardiac four-chamber volume estimation

Methods	Left Ventricle	Left Atrium	Right Ventricle	Right Atrium
SDL	**0.915**	**0.871**	**0.882**	**0.862**
PHOG	0.869	0.819	0.832	0.811
GPCA	0.885	0.838	0.843	0.822
PCA	0.871	0.812	0.825	0.807
LBP	0.868	0.799	0.827	0.794
GIST	0.864	0.828	0.815	0.843

3.2 Simultaneous Four-Chamber Volume Estimation

The proposed method for the first time achieves simultaneous four-chamber volume estimation and produces high estimation accuracy for all the four chambers despite of the great challenge of four chambers, especially for the LV with a high correlation coefficient of 91.5% as illustrated in Fig. 2. Although the boundary between ventricle and atrium is mostly invisible and not supported by edge and region homogeneity, the proposed method can successfully predict four-chamber volumes due to the use of multi-output regression via statistically learning. Moreover, LA and RA volumes not measured previously due to their complex anatomical geometry are successfully predicted by our method with high accuracy. The results are clinically significant showing the great potential in clinical use [4,6].

The average estimation results by our method against ground truth is shown in Fig. 3 for 25 frames (aligned across a cardiac cycle) over subjects. Our method can produce very close estimations with low errors for frames of all the four chambers to the ground truth manually obtained by human experts. The volume change pattern in a cardiac cycle is successfully captured by our method providing further information for cardiac pathologies, e.g., diastolic dysfunction, which indicates its practical use in clinical cardiac functional assessment and enables much wider clinical applications.

The strength of the proposed SDL algorithm for cardiac four-chamber image representation is also demonstrated by comparing with other methods as shown in Table 1. The SDL substantially outperforms both state-of-the-art descriptors, *e.g.*, LBP and GIST and dimensionality reduction techniques, *e.g.*, GPCA and PCA by up to 7.2% showing the effectiveness of the SDL for continuous multivariate estimation. The generalized low-rank approximation removes redundant information while the supervised manifold regularization extracts most discriminative features that are directly related to four-chamber volumes. By integrating them, we obtain compact and discriminative image representations for efficient and accurate cardiac four-chamber volume estimation.

4 Conclusion

In this paper, we proposed a new method for direct and simultaneous cardiac four-chamber volume estimation. Without depending on an intractable four-chamber segmentation step, we formulate four-chamber volume estimation as a multi-output regression problem. To achieve accurate and efficient estimation, we proposed using a supervised descriptor learning (SDL) algorithm to generate compact and discriminative cardiac image representation. Experimental results show that our method can produce highly accurate four-chamber volume estimation close to that obtained by human experts.

References

1. Zheng, Y., Barbu, A., Georgescu, B., Scheuering, M., Comaniciu, D.: Four-chamber heart modeling and automatic segmentation for 3-d cardiac ct volumes using marginal space learning and steerable features. IEEE TMI 27(11), 1668–1681 (2008)
2. Afshin, M., Ayed, I.B., Islam, A., Goela, A., Peters, T.M., Li, S.: Global assessment of cardiac function using image statistics in MRI. In: Ayache, N., Delingette, H., Golland, P., Mori, K. (eds.) MICCAI 2012, Part II. LNCS, vol. 7511, pp. 535–543. Springer, Heidelberg (2012)
3. Wang, Z., Ben Salah, M., Gu, B., Islam, A., Goela, A., Li, S.: Direct estimation of cardiac bi-ventricular volumes with an adapted bayesian formulation. IEEE TBME, 1251–1260 (2014)
4. Zhen, X., Wang, Z., Islam, A., Bhaduri, M., Chan, I., Li, S.: Direct estimation of cardiac bi-ventricular volumes with regression forests. In: Golland, P., Hata, N., Barillot, C., Hornegger, J., Howe, R. (eds.) MICCAI 2014, Part II. LNCS, vol. 8674, pp. 586–593. Springer, Heidelberg (2014)
5. Wang, Z., Salah, M., Ayed, I., Islam, A., Goela, A., Li, S.: Bi-ventricular volume estimation for cardiac functional assessment. In: RSNA (2013)
6. Zhen, X., Wang, Z., Islam, A., Chan, I., Li, S.: A comparative study of methods for cardiac ventricular volume estimation. In: RSNA (2014)
7. Wang, S., Summers, R.M.: Machine learning and radiology. Medical Image Analysis 16(5), 933–951 (2012)
8. Zhen, X., Wang, Z., Yu, M., Li, S.: Supervised descriptor learning for multi-output regression. In: CVPR (2015)
9. Ye, J.: Generalized low rank approximations of matrices. Machine Learning 61(1-3), 167–191 (2005)
10. He, X., Niyogi, P.: Locality preserving projections. In: NIPS, vol. 16, p. 153 (2004)
11. Belkin, M., Niyogi, P., Sindhwani, V.: Manifold regularization: A geometric framework for learning from labeled and unlabeled examples. JMLR 7, 2399–2434 (2006)
12. Criminisi, A., Robertson, D., Konukoglu, E., Shotton, J., Pathak, S., White, S., Siddiqui, K.: Regression forests for efficient anatomy detection and localization in computed tomography scans. Medical Image Analysis 17(8), 1293–1303 (2013)
13. Hara, K., Chellappa, R.: Growing regression forests by classification: Applications to object pose estimation. In: Fleet, D., Pajdla, T., Schiele, B., Tuytelaars, T. (eds.) ECCV 2014, Part II. LNCS, vol. 8690, pp. 552–567. Springer, Heidelberg (2014)
14. Breiman, L.: Random forests. Machine Learning 45(1), 5–32 (2001)
15. Ye, J., Janardan, R., Li, Q.: GPCA: an efficient dimension reduction scheme for image compression and retrieval. In: ACM SIGKDD, pp. 354–363 (2004)

Cross-Domain Synthesis of Medical Images Using Efficient Location-Sensitive Deep Network

Hien Van Nguyen, Kevin Zhou, and Raviteja Vemulapalli

Imaging and Computer Vision, Siemens Corporate Technology

Abstract. Cross-modality image synthesis has recently gained significant interest in the medical imaging community. In this paper, we propose a novel architecture called location-sensitive deep network (LSDN) for synthesizing images across domains. Our network integrates intensity feature from image voxels and spatial information in a principled manner. Specifically, LSDN models hidden nodes as products of features and spatial responses. We then propose a novel method, called ShrinkConnect, for reducing the computations of LSDN without sacrificing synthesis accuracy. ShrinkConnect enforces simultaneous sparsity to find a compact set of functions that accurately approximates the responses of all hidden nodes. Experimental results demonstrate that LSDN+ShrinkConnect outperforms the state of the art in cross-domain synthesis of MRI brain scans by a significant margin. Our approach is also computationally efficient, e.g. 26× faster than other sparse representation based methods.

1 Introduction

Recently, cross-modality synthesis has gained significant interest in the medical imaging community. Existing approaches do not have a systematic way to incorporate the spatial information which is important for accurate synthesis. As an illustration, we plot the intensity correspondences of registered MRI-T1 and MRI-T2 of the same subject in Fig. 1a. We can notice that the intensity transformation is not only non-linear but also far from unique, i.e. there are multiple feasible intensity values in MRI-T2 domain for one intensity value in MRI-T1 domain. The non-uniqueness comes from a well-known fact that intensity values depend on the regions in which voxels reside. By restricting to a local neighborhood of, say $10 \times 10 \times 10$ voxels, the intensity transformation is much simpler as shown in Fig. 1b. In particular, it could be reasonably well described as a union of two linear subspaces represented by the two red lines. That is to say, the spatial information helps simplify the relations between modalites which in turn could enable more accurate prediction.

In this paper, we propose a novel architecture called location-sensitive deep network (LSDN) to integrate image intensity features and spatial information in a principled manner. Our network models the responses of hidden nodes as the product of feature responses and spatial responses. In LSDN formulation, spatial information is used as soft constraints whose parameters are learned.

N. Navab et al. (Eds.): MICCAI 2015, Part I, LNCS 9349, pp. 677–684, 2015.
DOI: 10.1007/978-3-319-24553-9_83

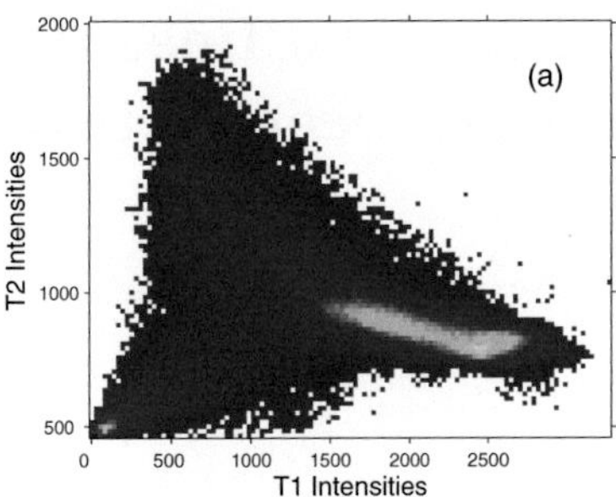

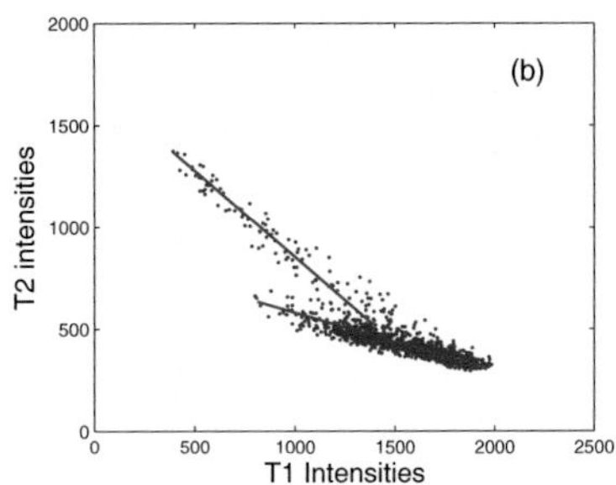

Fig. 1. a) 2D histogram of intensity correspondences between T1 and T2 scans over an entire image. Brighter color indicates higher density regions. b) Intensity correspondences of a restricted region of $10 \times 10 \times 10$ voxels. Red lines indicate the main directions of variation. All images are registered using rigid transformations.

As a result, LSDN is able to capture the joint distribution of feature and spatial information. We also propose a network simplification method for speeding up LSDN prediction. Experimental results demonstrate that our approach achieves better synthesis quality compared to the state-of-the-art. It is also more computationally efficient because the algorithm only uses feed-forward operations instead of expensive sparse coding or nearest neighbor search.

Contributions: 1) We incorporate spatial location and image intensity feature for cross-domain image synthesis in a principled manner. To perform such an integration, we propose a novel deep network architecture called location-sensitive deep network. We derive the gradients necessary for training LSDN. 2) We propose a network simplification technique for speeding up LSDN. 3) We provide experiments to demonstrate that LSDN outperforms state-of-art methods on brain MRI synthesis.

2 Location-Sensitive Deep Network

Our goal is to learn a deep network that uses an image of one domain (e.g., MRI-T1) to predict the corresponding image from another domain (e.g., MRI-T2). It is ineffective to train a network that operates on the entire image since the number of variables becomes too large for the learning algorithm to generalize well. Instead, our network operates on small voxels. Let $\mathbf{s}$ and $\mathbf{x}$ denote the voxel's intensity feature and spatial coordinates from the input domain, respectively. Let $\psi(.)$ represent a mapping that is carried out by a multi-layer network. This function operates on $(\mathbf{s}, \mathbf{x})$ and gives out a scalar value approximating the corresponding intensity t in the output domain. The error function that we want to minimize can be written as:

$$E = \frac{1}{2N} \sum_{n=1}^{N} \|\psi(\mathbf{s}_n, \mathbf{x}_n) - t_n\|^2 \tag{1}$$

where N is the total number of voxels sampled from all training images. The minimization is with respect to network variables which will be explained in detail shortly. As E is just a sum over the individual error on each training sample, it is sufficient to study the optimization with respect to a single sample. For the simplicity of notation, the subscript "n" would be omitted in our derivations of gradients. Motivated by the observation in Fig. 1, which shows that output intensity depends on voxel's location, we make our mapping dependent on both local feature and spatial coordinates.

We introduce a location-sensitive deep network for effectively fusing image feature and spatial information in a principled manner. Fig. 2a shows the architecture of a LSDN, where $(\mathbf{F}^{(k)}, \mathbf{h}^{(k)}, \mathbf{b}^{(k)})$ are the set of filters, hidden nodes, and biases at k-th layer, respectively. LSDN has multiple feed-forward layers. Moreover, the hidden nodes in the second layer of LSDN is modeled as products of feature and spatial functions:

$$\mathbf{h}^{(2)} = \kappa(\mathbf{s}) \odot \varsigma(\mathbf{x}), \quad \kappa(\mathbf{s}) = \gamma(\mathbf{u}^{(2)}), \quad \mathbf{u}^{(2)} = \mathbf{F}^{(2)}\mathbf{s} + \mathbf{b}^{(2)} \tag{2}$$

$$\varsigma(\mathbf{x}) = 2\gamma\left(-\left[\frac{\|\mathbf{x} - \hat{\mathbf{x}}_1\|^2}{\sigma^2}, \ldots, \frac{\|\mathbf{x} - \hat{\mathbf{x}}_{p_2}\|^2}{\sigma^2}\right]^T\right) \tag{3}$$

Here, $\kappa(\mathbf{s})$ is a feature response computed by a linear filtering followed by a sigmoid function denoted as $\gamma(.)$. The spatial response function $\varsigma(\mathbf{x})$ is parameterized by $\hat{\mathbf{X}} = [\hat{\mathbf{x}}_1, \ldots, \hat{\mathbf{x}}_{p_2}]$, which are learned, and a constant σ. We use "$\odot$" to indicate the Hadamard product. The reason we choose ς as in (3) is because we want to enforce locality property within the network. Specifically, we associate each hidden node in the second layer with a latent coordinates $\hat{\mathbf{x}}_i$. As can be seen from (3), i-th hidden node of the second layer only turns on when the voxel is close enough to location $\hat{\mathbf{x}}_i$. The combination of on/off hidden nodes effectively creates multiple sub-networks, each tuned to a small spatial region in the image. This novel property is an important advantage of our network compared to other approaches. We recall from the observation in Fig. 1b that the input-output mapping becomes much simpler when restricted to a smaller spatial region. Therefore, LSDN has the potential to yield more accurate prediction. Our experimental results in section 4 confirm this intuition.

For spatial coordinates $\mathbf{x}$ to convey useful information, training and test images are registered to a reference image using rigid transformations, as done in [6,2]. This makes the same location in different images corresponding to roughly the same anatomical region. Alternatively, one could eliminate the need for registration by using relative coordinates with respect to some landmarks. This direction is open for future research. We note that in [4], three-way multiplicative interactions were used with Restricted Boltzmann Machine to model the transformation between two images. Their hidden nodes are products of learned weights and pixel intensities from two different images. In contrast, our network uses multiplicative interactions between a spatial function and an intensity function computed from a single image. LSDN is similar to the convolutional neural network (CNN) [3] in the sense that it is applied on every voxel during the synthesis phase. However, the two networks differ in how they incorporate the

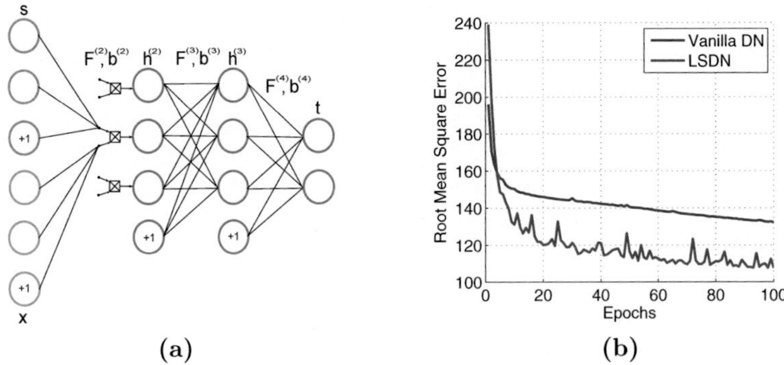

Fig. 2. a) Location-sensitive deep network. Green color and cyan color indicate feature **s** and spatial location **x**, respectively. For better clarity, we only draw connections between input layer and one product node. b) Comparison of training errors.

spatial information. CNN uses spatial pooling while LSDN uses multiplicative interactions.

2.1 Training LSDN

We use stochastic gradient descent [1] to optimize the loss function in (1). The optimization is with respect to the network's parameters such as filters' coefficients, biases, and latent coordinates. As mentioned earlier, all derivations in this section are for based on one training sample $(\mathbf{s}, \mathbf{x}, t)$. Recall that the second-layer hidden nodes' responses are given in (2). We can write the responses of hidden nodes in higher layers as:

$$\mathbf{h}^{(k)} = \gamma(\mathbf{u}^{(k)}), \text{ where } \mathbf{u}^{(k)} = \mathbf{F}^{(k)}\, \mathbf{h}^{(k-1)} + \mathbf{b}^{(k)}, \ \forall k \in [3, K] \tag{4}$$

where K is the number of layers. First, the gradients of the bias terms $\mathbf{b}^{(k)}$, denoted as $\mathbf{d}^{(k)}$, can be computed recursively as in (5), where $\gamma'(.)$ denotes the derivative of the sigmoid function. This recursive relationship can be verified easily using the chain rule.

$$\mathbf{d}^{(k)} = (\mathbf{F}^{(k+1)})^T \mathbf{d}^{(k+1)} \odot \gamma'(\mathbf{u}^{(k)}), \text{ where } \mathbf{d}^{(k)} = \frac{\partial E}{\partial \mathbf{b}^{(k)}}, \ \forall k \in [3, K-1]. \tag{5}$$

The above expression only applies to the intermediate layers. The gradients of biases in the second layer and the last layer take slightly different forms:

$$\mathbf{d}^{(2)} = {\mathbf{F}^{(3)}}^T \mathbf{d}^{(3)} \odot \gamma'(\mathbf{u}^{(2)}) \odot \varsigma(\mathbf{x}), \text{ and } \mathbf{d}^{(K)} = (\psi(\mathbf{s}, \mathbf{x}) - t) \odot \gamma'(\mathbf{u}^{(K)}) \tag{6}$$

Once all $\mathbf{d}^{(k)}$ and $\mathbf{h}^{(k)}$ are computed, the other gradients could be easily derived from using the chain rule. For completion, the gradients of filters coefficients and latent coordinates are provided below. We use $[.]_i$ to denote the i-th element of a vector.

$$\frac{\partial E}{\partial \mathbf{F}^{(k)}} = \mathbf{d}^{(k)}\, \mathbf{h}^{(k-1)^T}, \ \forall k \in [2, K] \tag{7}$$

$$\frac{\partial E}{\partial \hat{\mathbf{x}}_i} = \left[\mathbf{F}^{(3)^T}\, \mathbf{d}^{(3)} \odot \gamma(\mathbf{u}^{(2)}) \odot \varsigma(\mathbf{x}) \odot (2 - \varsigma(\mathbf{x})) \right]_i \times \frac{(\mathbf{x} - \hat{\mathbf{x}}_i)}{\sigma^2}, \ \forall i \in [1, p_2] \tag{8}$$

The learning rate is one of the most important tuning parameters. We empirically found that 0.25 is a good learning rate for our experiments. We also slowly decrease the learning rate after each iteration by multiplying it by 0.99. Fig. 2b shows the evolution of training error over 100 epochs which we obtained when training a LSDN to predict MRI-T2 intensity values from MRI-T1 intensity values. More details of this experiment will be explained in section 4. We can see that LSDN error goes significantly lower than that of the vanilla network despite they have the same parameter setting such as learning rate and number of hidden nodes. Similar patterns were observed for different learning rates and network sizes.

3 Network Simplification

Applying LSDN on every voxel during the synthesis process can be computationally expensive because medical images usually contains hundreds of thousands of voxels. In what follows, we propose a post-processing approach for simplifying the network in order to improve the speed of LSDN without losing much in its prediction accuracy. Our method is based on a central observation that, at each hidden layer of a network, there exists a smaller subset of functions that approximately span the same functional space of the entire layer. Let $\mathcal{I}^{(k)}$ denote the index set of such subset, we have:

$$h_{i,n}^{(k)} \approx \sum_{j \in \mathcal{I}^{(k)}} \alpha_{ij}^{(k)} h_{j,n}^{(k)}, \ \forall i \in [1, p_k], \ \forall n \in [1, N] \tag{9}$$

where p_k is the number of hidden nodes at k-th layer, $h_{i,n}^{(k)}$ is the response of i-th hidden node at k-layer for n-th training sample, and $\alpha_{ij}^{(k)}$ is an unknown coefficient of the linear approximation. We propose the following optimization to find $\mathcal{I}^{(k)}$ and $\alpha_{ij}^{(k)}$:

$$\operatorname*{argmin}_{\mathbf{A}^{(k)}} \|\mathbf{H}^{(k)} - \mathbf{A}^{(k)}\mathbf{H}^{(k)}\|_F^2, \ \text{subject to } \|\mathbf{A}^{(k)}\|_{col-0} \leq T^{(k)} \tag{10}$$

$$\mathbf{A}_{ij}^{(k)} = \begin{cases} \alpha_{ij}^{(k)}, & \text{if } j \in \mathcal{I}^{(k)} \\ 0, & \text{otherwise} \end{cases}, \qquad \mathbf{H}^{(k)} = \begin{pmatrix} h_{1,1}^{(k)} & \dots & h_{1,N}^{(k)} \\ \vdots & \ddots & \vdots \\ h_{p_k,1}^{(k)} & \dots & h_{p_k,N}^{(k)} \end{pmatrix} \tag{11}$$

The optimization in (10) enforces a small number of hidden nodes to linearly represent well all hidden nodes for all training samples. This is achieved by constraining the quasi-norm $\|\mathbf{A}^{(k)}\|_{col-0}$, which is the number of nonzero columns, to be less than $T^{(k)}$. Since the formulation in (10) is a special case of the simultaneous sparsity, we use simultaneous orthogonal matching pursuit [5] to efficiently minimize the loss function. It takes less than 2 seconds for each network in our experiments. Finally, the subset $\mathcal{I}^{(k)}$ is obtained from the indices of non-zero columns in $\mathbf{A}^{(k)}$.

Once we find $\mathcal{I}^{(k)}$ and all the coefficients, the computation can be reduced by shrinking the connection at each layer (in short, ShrinkConnect). This is done by discarding the hidden nodes at k-layer and their associated rows in $\mathbf{F}^{(k)}$ whose indices are not in $\mathcal{I}^{(k)}$. In addition, the latent coordinates $\hat{\mathbf{x}}_i$ is removed if $i \notin \mathcal{I}^{(2)}$. Since the hidden nodes of k-layer connect to $(k+1)$-layer, we also need to update $\mathbf{F}^{(k+1)}$. Intuitively, the update should preserve $\mathbf{F}^{(k+1)}\mathbf{h}^{(k)}$ as much as possible so that the output at $(k+1)$-layer is similar to that of the original network. From (9), we can derive the update rule for $\mathbf{F}^{(k+1)}$ whose details are given in the appendix. The update step can be summarized as follows:

$$\mathbf{F}^{(k)} \leftarrow \mathbf{F}^{(k)}_{\mathrm{row}\in\mathcal{I}^{(k)}} \text{ and } \mathbf{F}^{(k+1)} \leftarrow \mathbf{F}^{(k+1)}\mathbf{A}^{(k)}_{\mathrm{column}\in\mathcal{I}^{(k)}} \tag{12}$$

where $\mathbf{F}^{(k)}_{\mathrm{row}\in\mathcal{I}^{(k)}}$ and $\mathbf{A}^{(k)}_{\mathrm{column}\in\mathcal{I}^{(k)}}$ are the matrices formed by the rows of $\mathbf{F}^{(k)}$ and columns of $\mathbf{A}^{(k)}$ whose indices are in $\mathcal{I}^{(k)}$, respectively. In practice, we set the sparsity level $T^{(k)}$ of all layers to a certain percentage of the original layer's size (e.g. from 10% to 90%) and pick the smallest network that does not degrade the prediction accuracy on training data by more than 2%. We retrain LSDN with 10 epochs after performing ShrinkConnect to refine the whole network. In most cases, the network could be reduced $4\times$ without losing much in prediction accuracy. We note that training a LSDN of the same size from scratch or randomly removing hidden nodes yield worse results.

4 Experiments

We perform experiments on NAMIC brain dataset with leave-one-out cross validation. All images are registered, within domain and across domain, to a reference image using rigid transformations, as done in [6,2].

Training Phase: We are given a set of training pairs of images. Each pair has one image from a source domain (e.g. MRI-T1) and another image from a target domain (e.g. MRI-T2) of the same subject. We assume that our data are 3-dimensional volumes. Source images are cropped into small voxels of size $3\times3\times3$. The source voxels's intensities and their corresponding center's coordinates, denoted as $(\mathbf{s}, \mathbf{x})$, are used as input for training a LSDN network. The intensities at centers of target voxels are treated as the desirable outputs. We investigate two network configurations denoted LSDN-1 and LSDN-2 whose layers sizes are [30-200-20-1] and [30-400-40-1], respectively. In the first layer, 27 dimensions are from the intensity feature and 3 dimensions are from the spatial coordinates. The learning rate λ is set to 0.25, and the constant σ to 0.5.

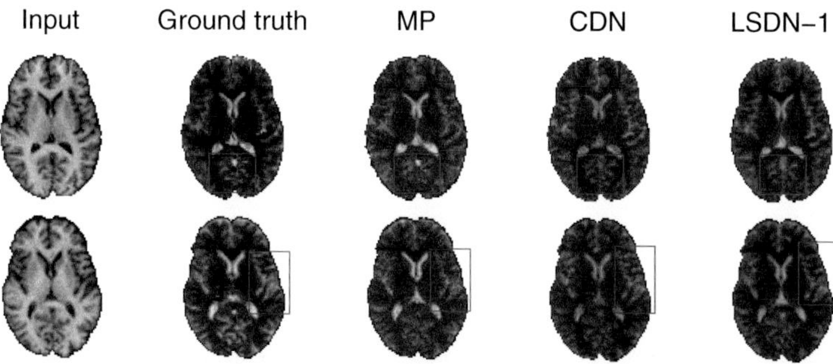

Fig. 3. Visual comparison of synthesized MRI-T1 volumes using different approaches. Red boxes indicates regions where there are significant differences among approaches.

Test Phase: We apply LSDN over all voxels of a given source image in a sliding-window fashion. The predicted intensity values of all source-domain voxels are arranged according to the voxel centers' coordinates to create a synthesized target image. We note that computational complexity for applying LSDN to one voxel is $\mathcal{O}(p_s p_2 + p_x p_2 + \sum_{k=3}^{K} p_{k-1} p_k)$, where p_s and p_x are the dimensions of the intensity feature and the spatial coordinates, respectively. This is slightly more expensive than that of a vanilla network, which is $\mathcal{O}(p_s p_2 + \sum_{k=3}^{K} p_{k-1} p_k)$. However, we will see that ShrinkConnect further reduces the computation of LSDN, making our network significantly faster than the vanilla deep network.

Results and Discussion: We use signal-to-noise ratio (SNR) as the measure to evaluate different methods. Table 1 compares average SNR for different methods. One of the methods trains a vanilla deep network (VDN) of size [27-400-40-1] on only intensity features. Another approach, denoted as concatenation deep network (CDN), trains a vanilla deep network of size [30-400-40-1] on the concatenation of intensity features and spatial coordinates. We also compare with recent methods in literature such as modality propagation (MP) [6] and coupled sparse representation [2]. The improvements in SNR is quite significant for LSDN compared to other approaches, especially for the case of T2→T1 synthesis. It is interesting to see that the synthesis results from T2→T1 is much better than from T1→T2. We conjecture that more details of the brain are visible under T2 than under T1. From CDN results, we observe that the concatenation of intensity feature and spatial feature is not as effective as LSDN. ShrinkConnect reduces the LSDN-1 and LSDN-2 sizes respectively to [30-50-5-1] and [30-100-10-1] without losing much in prediction accuracy, as shown in the last two rows of Table 1. To validate if we could obtain the same accuracy without ShrinkConnect, we train a LSDN network of size [30-50-5-1] from scratch, denoted as LSDN-Small. We can easily notice the accuracy of LSDN-Small is significantly lower than that of LSDN+ShrinkConnect. This demonstrates the effectiveness of our network simplification technique.

The results also indicate that increasing network size improves the accuracy, at the cost of higher run-time computation. Table 1 provides training time of

Table 1. Comparison of signal to noise ratios and speeds on NAMIC brain dataset

Method	**SNR (T1→T2)** (dB)	**SNR (T2→T1)** (dB)	**Training** (hour)	**Synthesis** (second)
MP [6]	13.64 ± 0.67	15.13 ± 0.88	n/a	928
Coupled Sparse [2]	13.72 ± 0.64	15.24 ± 0.85	2.8	245
VDN	12.67 ± 0.6	14.19 ± 0.82	1.2	23.5
CDN	13.79 ± 0.68	15.36 ± 0.88	1.2	23.6
LSDN-Small	12.53 ± 0.75	13.85 ± 0.86	0.6	9.2
LSDN-1	**14.82 ± 0.72**	**17.09 ± 0.94**	**1.4**	**29.5**
LSDN-2	**14.93 ± 0.73**	**17.39 ± 0.91**	**2.5**	**68.0**
LSDN-1+ShrinkConnect	**14.79 ± 0.72**	**17.05 ± 0.91**	**1.4**	**9.2**
LSDN-2+ShrinkConnect	**14.80 ± 0.74**	**17.1 ± 0.86**	**2.5**	**21.5**

LSDN with 300 epochs. The average time it takes LSDN-1 to synthesize an image is 29.5 seconds compared to 23.5 seconds of VDN. With ShrinkConnect, the run time is reduced to 9.2 seconds per image, which is 26× faster than the coupled sparse method and 100× faster than modality propagation. Fig 3 provides visual comparisons for different methods.

5 Conclusions

We proposed LSDN as a way to incorporate both image intensity feature and spatial information into a deep network. We also proposed a novel network simplification technique for reducing computation of LSDN. Our approach outperforms the state of the art in both accuracy and computation on MR brain image synthesis. In the future, we plan to investigate the use of LSDN for other applications such as segmentation.

References

1. Bottou, L.: Large-scale machine learning with stochastic gradient descent. In: Proceedings of COMPSTAT 2010, pp. 177–186. Springer (2010)
2. Cao, T., Zach, C., Modla, S., Powell, D., Czymmek, K., Niethammer, M.: Multimodal Registration for Correlative Microscopy Using Image Analogies. MIA 18(6), 914–926 (2014)
3. LeCun, Y., Bottou, L., Bengio, Y., Haffner, P.: Gradient-based learning applied to document recognition. Proceedings of the IEEE 86(11), 2278–2324 (1998)
4. Memisevic, R.: Learning to relate images. IEEE Transactions on Pattern Analysis and Machine Intelligence 35(8), 1829–1846 (2013)
5. Tropp, J.A., Gilbert, A.C., Strauss, M.J.: Simultaneous sparse approximation via greedy pursuit. In: IEEE ICASSP. vol. 5, p. v–721 (2005)
6. Ye, D.H., Zikic, D., Glocker, B., Criminisi, A., Konukoglu, E.: Modality Propagation: Coherent Synthesis of Subject-Specific Scans with Data-Driven Regularization. In: Mori, K., Sakuma, I., Sato, Y., Barillot, C., Navab, N. (eds.) MICCAI 2013, Part I. LNCS, vol. 8149, pp. 606–613. Springer, Heidelberg (2013)

Grouping Total Variation and Sparsity: Statistical Learning with Segmenting Penalties

Michael Eickenberg, Elvis Dohmatob, Bertrand Thirion, and Gaël Varoquaux

Inria Parietal, Neurospin, CEA Saclay, 91191 Gif-sur-Yvette
michael.eickenberg@nsup.org

Abstract. Prediction from medical images is a valuable aid to diagnosis. For instance, anatomical MR images can reveal certain disease conditions, while their functional counterparts can predict neuropsychiatric phenotypes. However, a physician will not rely on predictions by black-box models: understanding the anatomical or functional features that underpin decision is critical. Generally, the weight vectors of classifiers are not easily amenable to such an examination: Often there is no apparent structure. Indeed, this is not only a prediction task, but also an inverse problem that calls for adequate regularization. We address this challenge by introducing a convex region-selecting penalty. Our penalty combines total-variation regularization, enforcing spatial contiguity, and ℓ_1 regularization, enforcing sparsity, into one group: Voxels are either active with non-zero spatial derivative or zero with inactive spatial derivative. This leads to segmenting contiguous spatial regions (inside which the signal can vary freely) against a background of zeros. Such segmentation of medical images in a target-informed manner is an important analysis tool. On several prediction problems from brain MRI, the penalty shows good segmentation. Given the size of medical images, computational efficiency is key. Keeping this in mind, we contribute an efficient optimization scheme that brings significant computational gains.

1 Introduction

For certain pathologies, medical images carry weak indicators of external phenotype. For instance, in Magnetic Resonance images, a pattern of brain atrophy centered on the thalamus predicts the evolution in Alzheimer's disease [19]. Functional Magnetic Resonance Imaging (fMRI) can be used to infer subjects' behavioral state from their brain activity [11]. Machine learning methods can identify these biomarkers. With linear predictors, the weight vectors form spatial maps in the image domain. However, minimizing a prediction error gives little control on the corresponding maps. Indeed, the prediction problem is often an ill-posed inverse problem in the sense that there are less samples than features available: many different weight maps can generate exactly the same predictions. A choice among these candidates is implicitly taken by the estimator employed. In the empirical risk minimization framework, this choice is imposed via a penalty which favors maps according to certain criteria, interpretable as a "prior". Sparsity for

N. Navab et al. (Eds.): MICCAI 2015, Part I, LNCS 9349, pp. 685–693, 2015.
DOI: 10.1007/978-3-319-24553-9_84

instance, imposable in convex optimization via the ℓ_1 norm, is very useful as it selects a small number of voxels for the prediction. It has been widely used in medical imaging, from fMRI [21] to regularizing diffeomorphic registration [8].

However, imposing sparsity can often lead to less stable weight maps. Indeed, for images with high spatial correlations, adjacent voxels contain similar information and only one of them is needed for prediction. To counter this behavior, several estimators incorporate the notion of spatial contiguity in weight maps. For instance *GraphNet* [15,10,12] uses an ℓ_2 penalty on image gradients, to force adjacent voxels to have similar weights. An improvement upon this method is to impose sparsity on the spatial derivative [14], or to combine sparsity of the derivative with sparsity of the weights [1,9]. These penalties come with the mathematical property of positive homogeneity, which makes model selection easier. A drawback for these methods is that they favor flat or staircased weight maps, while one would tend to expect smooth variation within an active region.

Our goal is to detect spatially-contiguous patches in statistically estimated images and to inform their estimation of the image with these detections. Thus, our work bridges two fields: sparsity and segmentation.

Specifically, we are interested in a foreground segmentation problem: recovering small, non-zero predictive regions from a noisy background. However, in many applications, such as CT or medical imaging, the measurement process leads to strong correlations in columns of the design matrix corresponding to neighboring pixels, rendering recovery theorems non-applicable and sparse support estimation highly unstable.

The other body of literature that we draw from is that of segmentation, specifically convex variational approaches, as they can be expressed as penalties in a risk minimizer. A central aspect is the Chan-Vese functional [5] for segmentation that computes piecewise constant approximations. This variational formulation is not convex, but [16] have shown that good solutions can be achieved with a similar but convex functional, based on total variation (TV), *i.e.* the ℓ_1 norm of the image gradient. For our purposes, this approach is appealing, as the use TV as a regularizing penalty shows good properties for image denoising [17] or estimation in a linear model [4]. However, all these segmentation approaches model an object as a homogeneous constant-valued domain, thus washing out internal structure. Here, for foreground-background segmentation, we want to impose a constant structure on the background, but not in the selected image domain.

Our contribution is twofold: 1) We introduce a new penalty, *Sparse Variation*, which forces zeros on coordinates and spatial derivative jointly and smooth variations in spatially-contiguous active zones. 2) We present *FAASTA*, a novel optimization scheme for fast estimation up to a very high precision. Importantly, control on spatial maps requires solving the optimization to a tight tolerance [7]. We empirically evaluate *Sparse Variation* in regression and classification on fMRI and structural MRI data, comparing it to TV-ℓ_1 and GraphNet.

2 Sparse Variation: A New Spatially Regularizing Penalty

2.1 Penalized Regression: Problem Formulation and Prior Art

Penalized Generalized Linear Models. Let $X \in \mathbb{R}^{n \times p}$ be the design matrix and $y \in \mathbb{R}^n$ the prediction target, where $n, p \in \mathbb{N}$ are the number of samples and features. The weight vector w and the offset c are obtained by solving the optimization problem: $\arg\min_{w,c} \ell(Xw + c, y) + \Omega(w)$. Ω is the regularizer and ℓ the loss, typically a logistic loss for classification or a squared loss for regression.

Existing Regularizers. Two regularizers successfully applied to medical volume data are the GraphNet and TV-ℓ_1. In the following, ∇ will denote a finite differences spatial gradient operator acting upon an image. Generally, for a 3D grid of size $p = p_x p_y p_z$, we have $\nabla \in \mathbb{R}^{3p \times p}$. To write a function gradient, we will indicate the variable with respect to which it is calculated in subscript, e.g. "∇_w". $\| \cdot \|_2$ is the euclidean norm. For a partition $\mathcal{G}$ of coordinates the $\ell_{2,1}$ group norm is written $\|v\|_{2,1} = \sum_{g \in \mathcal{G}} \|v_g\|_2$. For all penalties, $\lambda > 0$ regulates the strength and $\rho \in [0, 1]$ is a parameter controlling the trade-off between coordinate sparsity and spatial regularity. GraphNet consists of the sum of an ℓ_1 penalty on all coordinates and a squared ℓ_2 penalty on the spatial gradient, whereas TV-ℓ_1 is the sum of an ℓ_1 penalty and an $\ell_{2,1}$ group penalty on the spatial derivative:

$$\Omega_{\mathrm{GN}}(w) = \lambda((1 - \rho)\|\nabla w\|_2^2 + \rho\|w\|_1)$$
$$\Omega_{\mathrm{TV}-\ell_1}(w) = \lambda((1 - \rho)\|\nabla w\|_{2,1} + \rho\|w\|_1),$$

2.2 A New Penalty for Segmentation Purposes: Sparse Variation

We propose a new penalty, *Sparse Variation*, which enforces contiguous zones of smooth activation against a background of zeros. Indeed, in TV-ℓ_1, the penalties for sparsity of the signal and sparsity of the gradient are separable: they can be active and inactive independently. A non-zero constant block, for example, is active for the ℓ_1 penalty, but inactive for the gradient, except at the borders. This property induces step functions and blockiness where one would expect smoothness. We address this issue in *Sparse Variation* by grouping coordinate activation with spatial derivative activation: Either a coordinate is active (nonzero) and its derivative is active as well - allowing for smooth variation in active zones - or both are inactive (zero). We define the *Sparse Variation* penalty as

$$\Omega_{\mathrm{SV}}(w) = \lambda\|Kw\|_{2,1}, \qquad \text{where} \quad K = \begin{pmatrix} (1 - \rho)\nabla \\ \rho\,\mathrm{Id}_p \end{pmatrix}, \tag{1}$$

with Id_p the $p \times p$ identity matrix. For 3D grids, $K \in \mathbb{R}^{4p \times p}$. The $\ell_{2,1}$ norm consists of groups containing the coordinate and all derivatives at each coordinate.

2.3 Optimization Strategy

All optimization problems mentioned in this manuscript - GraphNet, TV-ℓ_1 and *Sparse Variation*, with either the logistic loss or the squared loss - have a similar global structure: a sum of two convex functions, one being smooth, that we write F, the other nonsmooth, G. This structure can be exploited in proximal splitting algorithms [6], of which we contribute a new optimized variant. These algorithms rely on an implicit subgradient step in the non-smooth function called the *proximal operator* $\text{prox}_{tG}(y) := \arg\min_x \frac{1}{2t}\|y - x\|_2^2 + G(x)$.

The simplest method is the Iterative Shrinkage-Thresholding Algorithm (ISTA) [6]. It amounts to iterations of $w_{k+1} = \text{prox}_{\frac{1}{L}G}\left(w_k - \frac{1}{L}\nabla_w F(w_k)\right)$, where L is the Lipschitz constant of $\nabla_w F$. To accelerate convergence, the *fast iterative shrinkage-thresholding algorithm* (fISTA) [3] adds a momentum term: the gradient steps are applied to a combination of w_k and w_{k-1}. The acceleration brought by this method comes at the cost that there is no guarantee that each step of fISTA decreases the objective function and large rebounds are common. This non-monotone behaviour can be remedied by switching to ISTA iterations whenever an increase in cost is detected, as in *monotone fISTA* (mfISTA) [2].

There is no closed-form expression for proximal operators for TV-ℓ_1 and *Sparse-Variation*: they must be solved with a second, "inner" optimization problem. Both penalties can be written as $\lambda\|K\cdot\|$ for an appropriate norm $\|\cdot\|$. The projected-gradient algorithm used in [2] for TV denoising can then be adapted to iteratively solve the proximal operator with control of the dual gap.

Fast Adaptively Accurate Shrinkage Thresholding Algorithm. Importantly, solving $\text{prox}_{G/L}$ numerically is an inexact operation, which can easily prevent convergence of the outer loop. However, proximal algorithms converge if the error on $\text{prox}_{G/L}$ decreases sufficiently with the iteration number k of the outer loop [18]. Accuracy can be captured by the dual gap value. Instead of using a fixed dual gap refinement strategy, we devise an adaptive method, increasing accuracy (*dgtol*) as needed, if the energy $\mathcal{L}$ increases during an $ISTA$ step (Alg. 1).

3 Empirical Results

3.1 A Simple 1D Signal Recovery Problem

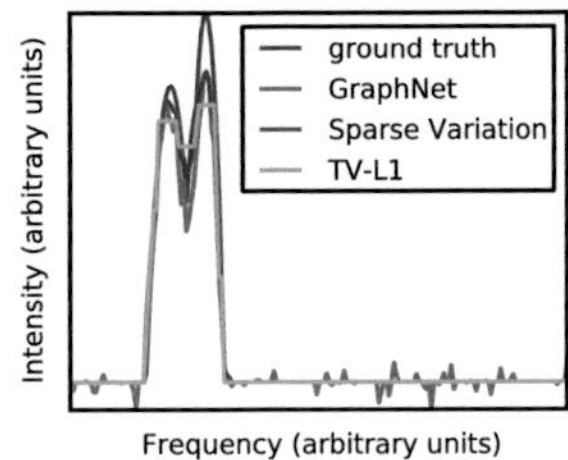

Fig. 1. Recovery for 1D spectroscopy. Note the blocky nature of the TV-ℓ_1 solution, and the noise in the GraphNet estimation.

To develop intuitions, we study a 1D recovery problem with simulated data. We mimic spectroscopy settings: a signal with a spectrum on a small spatially-contiguous support is measured with additive noise. The spectrum is recovered via an inverse problem with a discrete cosine transform operator. Measurements are given by $y = X_{\text{DCT}}^{-1}w + \varepsilon$, where X_{DCT} is the DCT operator, w the spectrum and ε Gaussian noise of 40% signal norm. We use w of size 200, with 80% zeros and an activated region resembling that of a chemical

Algorithm 1. fAASTA

```
Data: w_0
ISTA ← False,   v_1 ← w_0,   k ← 0,   t_1 ← 1,   dgtol ← 0.1;
while not converged do
    k ← k + 1,   w_k ← prox_{G/L}(v_k − (1/L)∇F(v_k), dgtol);
    if L(w_k) > L(w_{k−1}) then
        w_k ← w_{k−1},   v_k ← w_{k−1};
        if ISTA then
            dgtol ← dgtol/2;
            while L(prox_{G/L}(v_k − (1/L)∇_w F(v_k), dgtol)) > L(w_{k−1}) do
                dgtol ← dgtol/2
        ISTA ← True;
    else
        if ISTA then
            v_k ← w_k,   ISTA ← False
        else
            t_k ← (1+sqrt(1+4t_{k−1}^2))/2,   v_k ← w_k + ((t_{k−1}−1)/t_k)(w_k − w_{k−1});
```

compound signature: two overlapping smooth peaks. Fig. 1 shows the ground truth and the best recovery results: We selected the λ, ρ parameters minimizing ℓ_2 error with the ground truth. By construction, TV-ℓ_1 promotes flat signals, whereas *Sparse Variation* recovers better the smooth nature of the signal.

3.2 Segmenting Regions from MRI Data

We run experiments in both fMRI and structural MRI as well as both regression and classification settings. We compute prediction for the target variable from brain images over a full parameter grid λ, ρ. For each regularizer, weight maps of the best performing parameters in cross-validation are shown.

Classification: Intra-subject Object Recognition Study. The human ventral temporal cortex exhibits specialization to recurrent concepts such as faces, but also other object categories. We revisit the data from a seminal publication on this topic [11]: responses to visual stimuli of different categories. We test two classic contrasts, *faces versus houses* and *objects versus scramble*, with the logistic loss. Maps for optimal parameters overall detect similar regions. The top row of Fig. 2 shows the segmented right Fusiform Face Area. TV-ℓ_1 and *Sparse Variation* detect similar region size, whereas GraphNet selects a stronger sparsity. On the right, an F-statistic indicates extents of regions correlated to the stimuli. The bottom row shows the mapping of the Lateral Occipital Complex (LOC). *Sparse Variation* selects larger regions than the other two penalties. The focality of the maps is due to the single subject nature of the experiment.

Regression: Inter-subject Gain Prediction in Gambling Task. For linear regression in a multi-subject setting, we examine an fMRI experiment with gambles with varying gains [20]. Here we predict the gain of a given gamble from

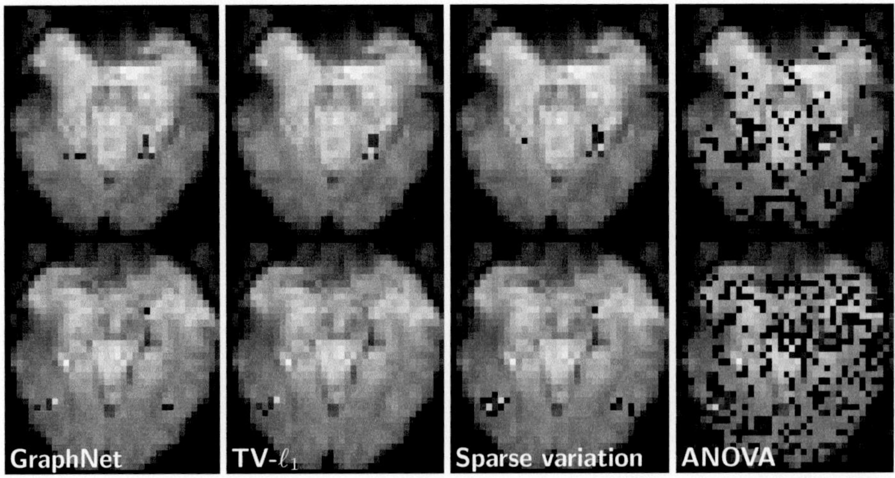

Fig. 2. Weight maps obtained from discrimination tasks between two visual concepts on data from [11]. **Top**: **FFA** (Fusiform Face Area) segmented in a face vs house discrimination. Cut at $z = -20$mm. Accuracies on held-out data: GN: 95.5%, TV-ℓ_1: 96.6%, SV: 97.7% **Bottom**: **LOC** (Lateral Occipital Complex) segmented in an object vs scramble discrimination. In this intra-subject analysis the maps are very well localized. Cut at $z = -16$mm. Accuracies: GN: 78.8%, TV-ℓ_1: 80.0%, SV: 80.0%

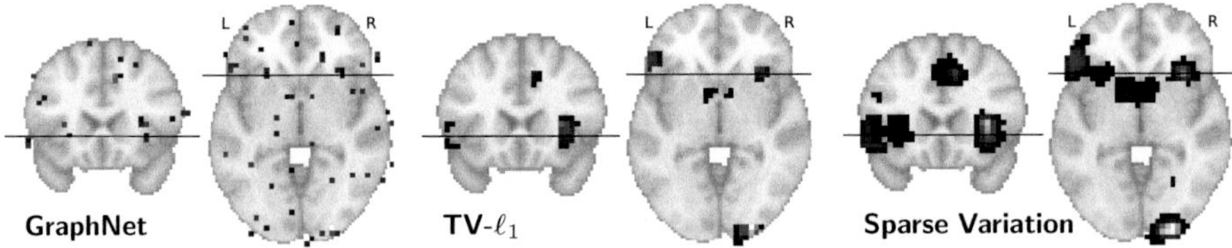

Fig. 3. Weight vectors from estimating gain on the mixed gambles task [20]. This inter-subject analysis shows broader regions of activation. Mean correlation scores on held out data: GN: 0.128, TV-ℓ_1: 0.147, SV: 0.149

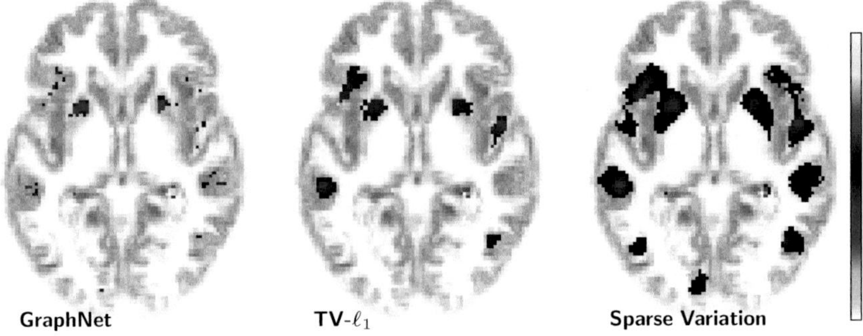

Fig. 4. Weight vectors for age prediction from VBM maps from the Oasis dataset. *Sparse Variation* selects clearly defined regions which are easily amenable to further analysis. Mean correlation scores on held-out data: GN:0.805, TV-ℓ_1:0.793, SV:0.794

the fMRI activation. At fixed $\rho = 0.5$, we evaluated the regularizers on a grid of λ. The weight maps of the best predicting parameters are shown in Fig. 3. At optimal predictive power the weight maps of TV-ℓ_1 and *Sparse Variation* show spatial contiguity and activation in expected regions, whereas GraphNet weights are scattered. The main distinction between TV-ℓ_1 and *Sparse Variation* is the "smoothness or zero" enforced by the latter in comparison to more blocky activations for the former. Larger activated regions do justice to the multi-subject setting. Note the segmentation of the Insulae, mentioned in the original study.

Regression: Estimating Age from Voxel-Based Morphometry (VBM) The Oasis database contains anatomical MRI for 400 subjects [13]. We extracted VBM images and used the different regularizers in a regression to estimate subjects' age. Fig. 4 shows the resulting weight maps. All identify the putamen, insula and para-hippocampal regions. TV-ℓ_1 selects contiguous regions where GraphNet finds sparse clouds of voxels. *Sparse Variation* segments smoother versions of regions selected by TV-ℓ_1, as well as several additional regions.

3.3 Optimization Speed of FASTAA

In data analysis optimization speed is important, practitioners may often decide to use less accurate but faster methods. We compare the adaptive refinement of the tolerance in FAASTA to others approaches: setting the dual gap tolerance to a constant, one strict (10^{-10}), one lax (0.1), and the refinement strategy of [18] (decrease dual gap as k^{-4}). We also compare to using ISTA in the outer loop in a constant dual gap (0.1) or an adaptive refinement setting.

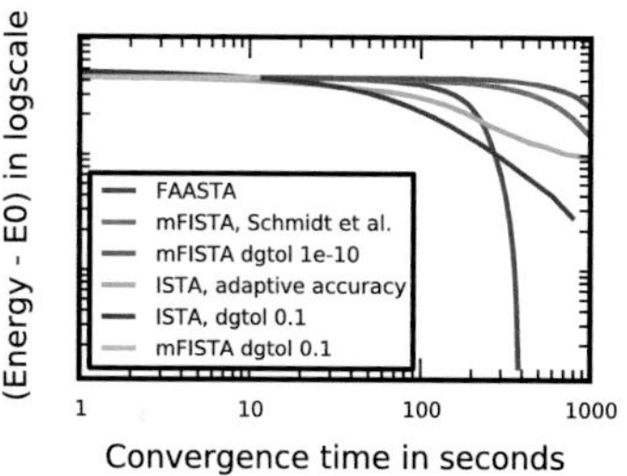

Fig. 5. Convergence on *object vs scramble*. FAASTA converges in 7mn, whereas other methods take more than 15mn

The results on Fig. 5 are striking. While the adaptive strategy always provides enough dual gap accuracy to ensure energy descent, the technique from [18] quickly becomes too strict, slowing convergence. Using a lax dual gap or the adaptive method with ISTA stalls at insufficient accuracy rates. The proposed adaptive method provides by far the fastest convergence.

Conclusion. We introduced a new region-selecting sparse convex penalty, *Sparse Variation*. It forces large regions of an image to zero, but, unlike prior art, allows smooth variation within spatially-contiguous active zones. On three brain imaging problems, this penalty shows best region segmenting properties with respect to prior art. Good convergence of the associated optimization problem is crucial to obtain reliable spatial maps. As with TV regularization, the optimization procedure necessitates an inner optimization to evaluate the proximal operator. A line-search strategy on dual gap tolerance is employed to refine the tolerance only as much as needed for fast convergence. Compared to other schemes, our method converges fastest. In conclusion, *Sparse Variation* with $fAASTA$ is the optimal choice for segmentation of medical images in a target-informed manner.

Acknowledgements. This work was funded by the European Union Seventh Framework Programme (FP7/2007-2013) under grant agreement no. 604102 ("Human Brain Project").

References

1. Baldassarre, L., Mourao-Miranda, J., Pontil, M.: Structured sparsity models for brain decoding from fMRI data. In: PRNI, p. 5 (2012)
2. Beck, A., Teboulle, M.: Fast gradient-based algorithms for constrained total variation image denoising and deblurring problems. IEEE Trans. Image Proc. (2009)
3. Beck, A., Teboulle, M.: A fast iterative shrinkage-thresholding algorithm with application to linear inverse problems. SIAM 2, 183–202 (2009)
4. Candes, E., Romberg, J.: Signal recovery from random projections. In: Wavelet Applications in Signal and Image Processing XI, SPIE. vol. 5674, p. 76 (2005)
5. Chan, T.F., Vese, L.A.: Active contours without edges. IEEE Transactions on Image Processing 10, 266 (2001)
6. Combettes, P.L., Pesquet, J.C.: Proximal splitting methods in signal processing. In: Fixed-Point Algorithms for Inverse Problems in Science and Engineering (2011)
7. Dohmatob, E., Gramfort, A., Thirion, B., Varoquaux, G.: Benchmarking solvers for TV-l1 least-squares and logistic regression in brain imaging. PRNI (2014)
8. Durrleman, S., Prastawa, M., Gerig, G., Joshi, S.: Optimal data-driven sparse parameterization of diffeomorphisms for population analysis. In: IPMI, p. 123 (2011)
9. Gramfort, A., Thirion, B., Varoquaux, G.: Identifying predictive regions from fMRI with TV-L1 prior. In: PRNI, pp. 17–20 (2013)
10. Grosenick, L., Klingenberg, B., Katovich, K., et al.: Interpretable whole-brain prediction analysis with graphnet. NeuroImage 72, 304 (2013)
11. Haxby, J., Gobbini, I., Furey, M., et al.: Distributed and overlapping representations of faces and objects in ventral temporal cortex. Science 293, 2425 (2001)
12. Kandel, B.M., Wolk, D.A., Gee, J.C., Avants, B.: Predicting cognitive data from medical images using sparse linear regression. In: IPMI, p. 86 (2013)
13. Marcus, D.S., Wang, T.H., Parker, J., et al.: Open access series of imaging studies (OASIS): cross-sectional MRI data in young, middle aged, nondemented, and demented older adults. J. Cogn. Neurosci. 19, 1498 (2007)
14. Michel, V., Gramfort, A., Varoquaux, G.: other: Total variation regularization for fMRI-based prediction of behavior. IEEE Trans. Med. Im. 30, 1328 (2011)
15. Ng, B., Vahdat, A., Hamarneh, G., et al.: Generalized sparse classifiers for decoding cognitive states in fMRI. Machine Learning in Medical Imaging, p. 108 (2010)
16. Pock, T., Chambolle, A., Cremers, D., Bischof, H.: A convex relaxation approach for computing minimal partitions. In: CVPR, p. 810 (2009)

17. Rudin, L.I., Osher, S., Fatemi, E.: Nonlinear total variation based noise removal algorithms. Physica D: Nonlinear Phenomena 60, 259 (1992)
18. Schmidt, M., Roux, N.L., Bach, F.R.: Convergence rates of inexact proximal-gradient methods for convex optimization. In: NIPS, p. 1458 (2011)
19. Stonnington, C., Chu, C., Klöppel, S., et al.: Predicting clinical scores from magnetic resonance scans in alzheimer's disease. Neuroimage 51, 1405 (2010)
20. Tom, S.M., Fox, C.R., Trepel, C., Poldrack, R.A.: The neural basis of loss aversion in decision-making under risk. Science 315(5811), 515–518 (2007)
21. Yamashita, O., Sato, M.A., Yoshioka, T., et al.: Sparse estimation automatically selects voxels relevant for the decoding of fMRI activity patterns. NeuroImage 42, 1414 (2008)

Scandent Tree: A Random Forest Learning Method for Incomplete Multimodal Datasets

Soheil Hor[1] and Mehdi Moradi[2,⋆]

[1] University of British Columbia, Vancouver, British Columbia, Canada
[2] IBM Almaden Research Center, San Jose, CA, USA
mmoradi@us.ibm.com

Abstract. We propose a solution for training random forests on incomplete multimodal datasets where many of the samples are non-randomly missing a large portion of the most discriminative features. For this goal, we present the novel concept of scandent trees. These are trees trained on the features common to all samples that mimic the feature space division structure of a support decision tree trained on all features. We use the forest resulting from ensembling these trees as a classification model. We evaluate the performance of our method for different multimodal sample sizes and single modal feature set sizes using a publicly available clinical dataset of heart disease patients and a prostate cancer dataset with MRI and gene expression modalities. The results show that the area under ROC curve of the proposed method is less sensitive to the multimodal dataset sample size, and that it outperforms the imputation methods especially when the ratio of multimodal data to all available data is small.

1 Introduction

In recent years there has been an interest in multimodality data analysis for disease detection. Ideally, multimodality methods should leverage the strengths of each modality and compensate for weaknesses. Another advantage of multimodality data analysis is discovering novel relations between different modalities. One example is finding the connection between genes related to Alzheimer's disease and related areas in functional MRI [1]. Acquiring multimodal data is, in general, more costly and time consuming than a single modality. As a result, multimodal datasets usually have valuable features, but small sample sizes. This makes it difficult to build classifiers, with large training data, for highly multimodal protocols. Multomodal data is also often high dimensional and pose difficulties in feature selection and classifier building. Ensemble classifiers such as random forest provide a solution for the large feature space in small datasets using feature bagging.

To tackle the issue of incomplete datasets, a variety of data imputation techniques exist. Some of these are non-parametric methods like hot deck imputation, KNN imputation or mean substitution. These methods ignore the possible correlations in data and could add bias. Model-based methods, on the other hand,

⋆ Corresponding author.

N. Navab et al. (Eds.): MICCAI 2015, Part I, LNCS 9349, pp. 694–701, 2015.
DOI: 10.1007/978-3-319-24553-9_85

assume a certain structure to the missing samples, like missing completely at random (MCAR) or missing not at random (MNAR). Examples of these methods include multiple imputation [2], maximum likelihood, stochastic regression [3], expectation maximization [3] and Bayesian methods [4]. While these methods could result in reduced bias, the assumption of specific pattern in the missing components may not be justified, especially in the case of small datasets with complex features. Therefore, a third approach to treating missing data has emerged that maximizes the performance of a classifier. An example is the imputation method proposed by Breiman in [5,6]. This method uses the proximity matrix of the random forest to iteratively predict the missing values in a way that maximizes the overall performance of the random forest and is designed to perform well even in MNAR conditions.

Our motivation in this area stems from the work on combining genomic biomarkers of prostate cancer with imaging biomarkers from multiparametric MRI (mpMRI) to enhance risk stratification. While imaging data is routinely acquired and archived from prostate cancer patients, there are very few patients with imaging data and spatially registered tissue specimens for genomic analysis. As a result, we have a relatively large number of data samples with only mpMRI data (which we call the single modality dataset in this work), and a small set of samples with both mpMRI and gene expression analysis from the same regions of interest (which we call multimodality data). While most of the imputation methods assume a small number of missing values (typically 10%-30% of the whole data), we are dealing with a situation where the multimodal samples only constitute around 10% of the data. While the patients recently recruited into the study provide multimodal data, we intend to find a solution to include the archival data with imaging only samples. In this work, we develop a solution to leverage a large single modality dataset to enhance the training of a classifier based on multimodal data. The proposed method is based on decision trees. However, we describe an entirely novel technique to link different feature sets and predict the class label using information from all of the datasets, multimodal and single modal. We use a large clinical benchmark dataset to show that our method outperforms the current state of the art in random forest imputation methods, particularly in the case of dataset with large missing ratio. We also report very promising preliminary results on our prostate cancer dataset.

2 Method

Let us assume that the training data consists of at least one single modality dataset defined as $S = (s_1, s_2, \ldots, s_{N_s})$ and at least one multimodality dataset defined as $M = (m_1, m_2, \ldots, m_{N_m})$ which is described by the multimodality feature set $F_m = (f_1, f_2, \ldots, f_{km})$. The aim is to train a classifier using both S and M that can predict the outcome class C, for any test data described by F_m. While we do not set conditions on feature or sample sizes, in practical scenarios, the multimodality dataset has fewer samples ($N_m < N_s$). In practice F_s is often a subset of F_m and is missing some of the more discriminative features.

As an advantage of having all the important features, trees formed by the multimodal dataset are expected to partition the feature space very effectively. But because of the low multimodal sample size, the estimation of outcome probability at each leaf may not be accurate. The idea of our method is to reduce prediction error at each leaf of the multimodal tree by using single modality samples that are likely to belong to the same leaf. In order to find these single modality samples, a feature space partitioning algorithm is needed that can simulate the feature space division of the target multimodal tree on the single modality dataset. The proposed method is to grow single modality trees that mimic the feature space division structure of the multimodal decision tree. Growing a tree that follows the structure of another tree from the root to the top brings analogy to the behaviour of "scandent" trees in nature that climb a stronger "support" tree. Considering this analogy, the proposed method can be divided into three basic steps: First, division of the sample space by a multimodal decision tree, called "the support tree". Second, forming the single modality trees that mimic the structure of the support tree, called "scandent trees". And third, leaf level inference of outcome label C, using the multimodal samples in each leaf and the single modal samples that are most likely to belong to the selected leaf.

Support Tree: The first step in the proposed method is growing a decision tree to predict the outcome class based on the multimodal dataset.

Scandent Trees: The second step is to form the scandent trees which enable the assignment of single modality samples to the leaves of the support tree. The process of feature space division in the support tree can be considered as grouping the multimodal data set (M) to different multimodal subsets at each node. Let us define the subset of the samples of the multimodal dataset (M) in the i_{th} node as M_i. The algorithm to form a scandent tree is as follows:

for each node i in the support tree starting from the root node,
{
    for each sample n in M_i and each child node j of node i
    {
        if $n \in M_j$, $C^{'}_{i,n} = j$
    }
    Grow T_i, as optimum tree that for each sample n in M_i,
    predicts $C^{'}_{i,n}$ using only F_s.
}

The above algorithm forms sub-trees T_i for each node i that divide M_i to the child datasets M_j using only the single modality features F_s. Let us assume that the sample space division at node i of the support tree is based on feature f. If $f \in F_s$, then T_i is expected to divide M_i to the child subsets (M_j) using only a single division node and with perfect accuracy. But if $f \notin F_s$, then T_i will be optimized to form the smallest tree that can divide the sample space in a similar manner to the support tree. Using T_i's for feature space division at each node, we can form a new tree that consists of the same division nodes as the support tree but only uses features of a single modality (F_s) for feature space division, we name this single modality tree, a scandent tree. Since the scandent tree is a single modality tree, it can be used to predict the probability that each single modality sample s belongs to each node j calculated by:

$$p(s \in Node_j) = p(s \in Node_j | s \in Node_i) p(s \in Node_i)$$

In which $Node_i$ is the parent node of $Node_j$. The term $p(s \in Node_j | s \in Node_i)$ in the above equation can be estimated by the corresponding sub-tree T_i and $p(s \in Node_i)$ is calculated by recursion. This method is expected to be generally more accurate than direct estimation of the leaves by any other single modality classifier. Because the scandent tree only has to predict the feature division for features that do not belong in F_s and other divisions will be perfectly accurate. Moreover, if two features are dependent over the whole sample space (unconditional dependence), they will also be predictable by each other over a sub-space of the sample space. But if the dependence is conditional, they cannot be universally predicted by each other. The scandent tree locally estimates each division and does not require a global dependence. As a result, it can predict the set of single modality samples that belong to each leaf of the support tree which may not be possible by any other single modality classifier.

Leaf Level Inference: The standard method for leaf-level inference is majority voting. However, if there are single modality samples misplaced by the scandent tree, they may flood the true observations. The proposed method for weighted majority voting is to re-sample from each leaf i and calculate the probability of outcome C by non-uniform bootstrapping. The bootstrap probability of each sample x in leaf i is defined by:

$$p(x)_{bootstrap,leaf_i} = \begin{cases} 1/\mathrm{N}, & x \in M_i \\ p(x \in Leaf_i)/N, & x \notin M_i \quad \& \quad p(x \in Leaf_i) > q \\ 0, & x \notin M_i \quad \& \quad p(x \in Leaf_i) < q \end{cases}$$

In which q is the selected minimum threshold for the probability that a single modality sample belongs to the selected leaf i, and N is the total number of samples in leaf i (single modal and multimodal). As q value increases, the probability that a misplaced sample is used in the leaf-level inference is reduced. This may increase the accuracy of the majority voting but increasing q will also reduce the number of single modality samples at each leaf which decreases the accuracy of the probability estimation. This tradeoff is more evident at the two ends of the spectrum, for $q = 1$ the tree will be the same as the support tree which suffers from low sample size at the leaves. For $q = 0$ all the single modality samples will be used for inference at each leaf and the feature space division of the support tree will have no direct effect on the inference. The optimization of the q parameter for each leaf is essential for optimal performance of the resulting tree. This can be done by cross validation over the multimodal dataset. Because M_i is smaller at deeper nodes, as the support tree gets deeper and develops more division points, it gets harder for the scandent tree to accurately follow the tree structure. Moreover, a higher number of consequent divisions by T_i's leads to accumulative errors. So forming smaller trees and ensembling those in form of a random forest may lead to a more accurate classifier.

Implementation: In building the support trees, we bagged 2/3 of bootstrapped samples and the square root of the dimension of the multimodal feature set. The out of bag samples are used for optimization of the q parameter at each leaf. After growing and optimizing each of the trees, the probability of outcome class C is calculated by averaging the corresponding probabilities of all trees in the forest. We use the R package "rpart" [7] to grow the support tree. This package uses internal cross validation to form the optimal tree. But for the purpose of controlling the bias-variance of the resulting forest, the depth of support tree is limited by controlling the minimum of samples needed for each division. The depth of T_i's in each scandent tree is optimized by cross validation.

Evaluation: We evaluate the performance of the proposed method using a dataset available from University of California at Irvine (UCI) Machine Learning Repository [8]. We also report preliminary results on a prostate cancer multimodal dataset. The datasets are summarized in Table 1.

Heart disease data: This set consists of data from two different studies reported in [9]. One set (data from the Hungarian Institute of Cardiology) is missing two out of 14 features. We use this as the single modal dataset in our experiments. In real world problems, such as our prostate cancer study, the single modal dataset is missing some of the most discriminative features. To simulate this condition we used a classical random forest feature ranking approach. We study the effect of decreasing the number of features in the single modality dataset on the overall performance by sweeping from 12 to two features, always removing the most top-ranking ones. The multimodal dataset in this experiment was the Cleveland dataset consisting of 303 samples. 100 samples were randomly separated and used as test data. The remaining samples were used as the multimodal data for training the support trees. We experimented with scenarios that included 10% to 90% of this data in training of the support trees.

Table 1. Evaluation Datasets

Datasets	Heart Disease		Prostate Cancer	
	Cleveland	Hungarian	MRI and Genetic	MRI only
Sample Size	303	294	27	400
Feature size	14	12	43	4

Prostate cancer data: We also test our method on a dataset that is a perfect example of the target scenario, a small multimodal prostate cancer dataset ($N_m = 27$) accompanied by a relatively large single modal dataset ($N_s = 400$). The single modality dataset consists of four multiparametric MRI features from dynamic contrast enhanced (DCE) MRI and diffusion MRI on a 3 Tesla scanner.

We used the apparent diffusion coefficient (ADC) from diffusion MRI, and three pharmacokinetic parameters from DCE MRI: volume transfer constant, k^{trans}, fractional volume of extravascular extracellular space, v_e, and fractional plasma volume v_p [10,11].

For the 27 multimodal samples, besides the four described imaging features, biopsy tissue samples with known pathologic state (cancer or normal determined by a histopathologist) were also available. RNA was extracted and purified [12]. The expression level of 39 genes that form the most recent consensus on the genetic signature of prostate cancer for patients with European ancestry were used as features. This signature is reported and maintained by National Institute of Health [13]. We have 27 samples with genomic analysis and registered imaging data (14 normal, 13 cancer) from 19 patients. The evaluation of the proposed method on this small dataset was carried out in a leave-one-out scheme. Each time, the support trees were trained using 26 multimodal samples, with all the 400 single modality data samples used for forming the scandent trees.

3 Results and Discussion

Heart Disease Dataset: Figure 1 shows the AUC of the proposed method and the rfImpute method for different multimodal sample sizes. Each box in this figure shows AUC values for different single modal feature set sizes and a fixed multimodal dataset sample size. The expected upward trend in AUC *vs.* multimodal sample size is evident and it can be seen that the proposed method outperforms the rfImpute method especially in smaller samples sizes. For example, when only 14 multimodal samples are available, the rfImpute method results in a mean AUC of 0.90 whereas the proposed method delivers an AUC of 0.94. As the number of multimodal samples increases to 112, the performances increase for rfImpute and scandent tree to 0.96 and 0.97, respectively. In other words, the scandent tree approach has a clear advantage when the dataset with multimodal data is significantly smaller.

Figure 2 shows the AUC of the proposed method and the rfImpute method for different single modality feature set sizes. Each box shows changes of AUC for different sample sizes at a fixed feature set in the single modality data. Smaller variances of the boxes for the proposed method, especially in smaller feature set sizes, show that the proposed method is on average less sensitive to the multimodal sample size especially when the single modality dataset has a large number of missing features. For example, at feature vector size of 2 for the single modality dataset, the performance of rfImpute varies from 0.88-0.98, whereas scandent tree shows a performance range of 0.93-0.98. This stable behavior is due to the unique ability of the scandent trees to predict division points for missing features that only conditionally depend on the available features.

Prostate Cancer Dataset: In leave one out validation, the proposed method resulted in an AUC of 0.95 for the prostate cancer data. The rfImpute approach resulted in an AUC of 0.8. The difference was statistically significant (p <0.02). This dataset is an example of the worst case scenario of missing data: a large

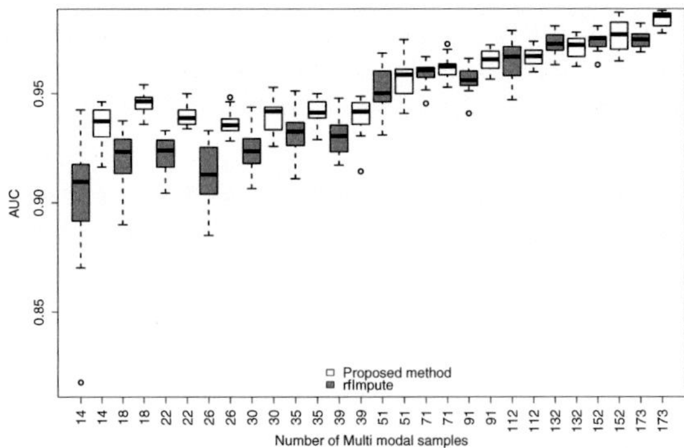

Fig. 1. AUC vs multimodal sample size for heart disease dataset (each box shows AUC values for different single modal feature sets)

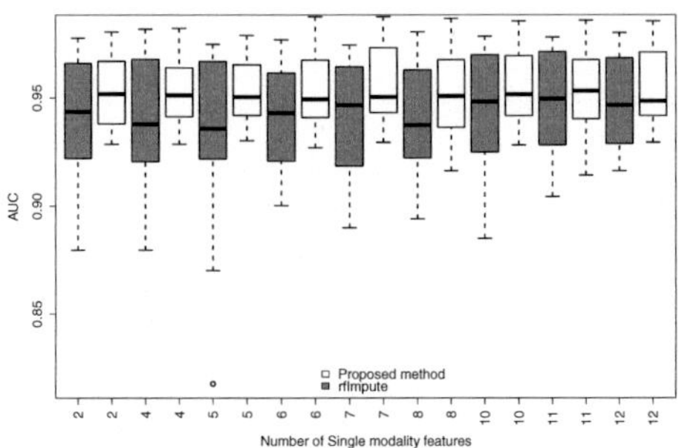

Fig. 2. AUC vs single modal feature set size for heart disease dataset (each box shows AUC values for different multimodal sample sizes)

non-random portion of the data is missing the potentially more powerful genomic features resulting in a very small multimodal dataset. At the same time, the number of features on the single modality (imaging) side is small. As a result, the power of the proposed method in comparison with rfImpute is on full display. It is also important to understand that the scandent tree is providing a platform to incorporate the genomic data, despite the very limited number of samples. In the absence of such methodology, if one uses only the imaging features with an optimized random forest, the AUC is 0.74.

4 Conclusion

In this paper we addressed the problem of incomplete multimodal datasets in random forest learning algorithms in a scenario where many of the samples are non-randomly missing a large portion of the most discriminative features. We introduce the novel concept of scandent trees. The results show that the proposed method outperforms the embedded missing value imputation method of random forests introduced in [5], particularly in smaller samples sizes. The method is in general less sensitive to the number of missing features and the multimodal sample size. We showed that the proposed method enables the integration of a small genomic plus imaging dataset, with a relatively large imaging dataset.

In this paper we used a single modal dataset to improve the accuracy of leaf-level inference in multimodal trees. Future work will address the possibility of using single modality data at the test stage.

Acknowledgment. Funding from Canadian Institutes of Health Research (CIHR). Prostate imaging and genomic data were obtained at Vancouver General Hospital and UBC Hospital with approval from Clinical Research Ethics Board and informed patient consent. The authors would like to acknowledge Drs. Peter Black, Larry Goldenberg, Piotr Kozlowski, Jennifer Locke, Silvia Chang, Edward C. Jones, Ladan Fazli, all from UBC; Dr. Elai Davicioni, Christine Buerki, Heesun Shin, and Zaid Haddad from GenomeDx Biosciences Inc.

References

1. Liu, J., Calhoun, V.D.: A review of multivariate analyses in imaging genetics. Frontiers in Neuroinformatics 8, 29 (2014)
2. Rubin, D.B.: Multiple imputation for nonresponse in surveys, vol. 81. John Wiley & Sons (2004)
3. Gold, M.S., Bentler, P.M.: Treatments of missing data: A Monte Carlo comparison of RBHDI, iterative stochastic regression imputation, and expectation-maximization. Structural Equation Modeling 7(3), 319–355 (2000)
4. Kong, A., Liu, J.S., Wong, W.H.: Sequential imputations and bayesian missing data problems. Journal of the American Statistical Association 89(425), 278–288 (1994)
5. Breiman, L.: Random forests. Machine Learning 45(1), 5–32 (2001)
6. Liaw, A., Wiener, M.: Classification and regression by randomforest. R News 2(3), 18–22 (2002)
7. Therneau, T.M., Atkinson, B., Ripley, B.: rpart: Recursive partitioning. R package version 3.1-46. Ported to R by Brian Ripley 3 (2010)
8. Lichman, M.: UCI machine learning repository (2013)
9. Detrano, R., Janosi, A., Steinbrunn, W., Pfisterer, M., Schmid, J.J., Sandhu, S., Guppy, K.H., Lee, S., Froelicher, V.: International application of a new probability algorithm for the diagnosis of coronary artery disease. The American Journal of Cardiology 64(5), 304–310 (1989)
10. Haq, N.F., Kozlowski, P., Jones, E.C., Chang, S.D., Goldenberg, S.L., Moradi, M.: A data-driven approach to prostate cancer detection from dynamic contrast enhanced MRI. Computerized Medical Imaging and Graphics 41, 37–45 (2015)
11. Moradi, M., Salcudean, S.E., Chang, S.D., Jones, E.C., Buchan, N., Casey, R.G., Goldenberg, S.L., Kozlowski, P.: Multiparametric MRI maps for detection and grading of dominant prostate tumors. Journal of Magnetic Resonance Imaging 35(6), 1403–1413 (2012)
12. Erho, N., et al.: Discovery and validation of a prostate cancer genomic classifier that predicts early metastasis following radical prostatectomy. PloS One 8(6), e66855 (2013)
13. National Institutes of Health: National cancer institute: PDQ genetics of prostate cancer (Date last modified February 20, 2015)

Disentangling Disease Heterogeneity with Max-Margin Multiple Hyperplane Classifier

Erdem Varol, Aristeidis Sotiras, and Christos Davatzikos

Center for Biomedical Image Computing and
Analytics University of Pennsylvania Philadelphia, PA 19104, USA
{erdem.varol,aristeidis.sotiras,christos.davatzikos}@uphs.upenn.edu

Abstract. There is ample evidence for the heterogeneous nature of diseases. For example, Alzheimer's Disease, Schizophrenia and Autism Spectrum Disorder are typical disease examples that are characterized by high clinical heterogeneity, and likely by heterogeneity in the underlying brain phenotypes. Parsing this heterogeneity as captured by neuroimaging studies is important both for better understanding of disease mechanisms, and for building subtype-specific classifiers. However, few existing methodologies tackle this problem in a principled machine learning framework. In this work, we developed a novel non-linear learning algorithm for integrated binary classification and subpopulation clustering. Non-linearity is introduced through the use of multiple linear hyperplanes that form a convex polytope that separates healthy controls from pathologic samples. Disease heterogeneity is disentangled by implicitly clustering pathologic samples through their association to single linear sub-classifiers. We show results of the proposed approach from an imaging study of Alzheimer's Disease, which highlight the potential of the proposed approach to map disease heterogeneity in neuroimaging studies.

1 Introduction

Brain disorders often assume a heterogeneous clinical presentation: Autism Spectrum Disorder (ASD) encompasses neurodevelopmental disorders characterized by deficits in social communication and repetitive behaviors [5]; Schizophrenia can be subdivided into distinct groups by separating its symptomatology to discrete symptom domains [2]; Alzheimer's Disease (AD) can be separated into three subtypes on the basis of the distribution of neurofibrillary tangles [8]; and Mild Cognitive Impairment (MCI) may be further classified based on the type of specific cognitive impairment [11].

Disentangling disease heterogeneity may greatly contribute to our understanding and lead to more accurate diagnosis, prognosis and targeted treatment. However, most commonly used neuroimaging analysis approaches assume a single unifying pathophysiological process and perform a monistic analysis to identify it. These approaches aim to either identify voxels that characterize group differences through mass-univariate statistical techniques [1], or reveal patterns of

N. Navab et al. (Eds.): MICCAI 2015, Part I, LNCS 9349, pp. 702–709, 2015.
DOI: 10.1007/978-3-319-24553-9_86

variability through high-dimensional pattern classification analysis, towards categorizing population with respect to the underlying pathology [10]. Thus, the heterogeneity of the disease is completely ignored.

Contrarily, few research efforts have been focused on revealing the inherent disease heterogeneity. These methods can mainly be classified into two groups. The first class assumes an a priori subdivision of the diseased samples into coherent groups, based on independent criteria, and opts to identify group-level anatomical differences using univariate statistical methods [7, 12]. Thus, multivariate effects are ignored, while the a priori definition of disease subtypes is either difficult to obtain (*e.g.*, from autopsy near the date of imaging), or noisy and non-specific (*e.g.*, cognitive or clinical evaluations). The second class focuses on the diseased population and maps it to distinct anatomical subtypes by applying multivariate clustering driven by considering all image elements [11, 9]. Thus, disease heterogeneity may be confounded due to considering the whole brain anatomy instead of the disease-specific information, and disentangling it may not be possible.

In order to tackle the aforementioned limitations, it is necessary to develop a principled machine learning approach that will allow for the simultaneous identification of a class of images with pathological changes and its separation to coherent subgroups. To the best of our knowledge, only one approach has been proposed in this direction [3], which makes strong assumptions regarding the number of the existing disease subgroups (that there are exactly 2 subgroups). Here, we propose a novel non-linear machine learning algorithm for integrated binary classification and subpopulation clustering. The proposed approach is motivated by recent machine learning approaches that derive non-linear classifiers through the use of multiple-hyperplanes [4, 6]. Multiple max-margin classifiers are combined to form a convex polytope that separates healthy controls from pathological samples, while heterogeneity is disentangled by implicitly clustering pathologic samples through their association to single linear sub-classifiers. By varying the number of estimated hyperplanes (faces of polytope), it is possible to capture multiple modes of heterogeneity.

2 Method

In high dimensional spaces, linear Support Vector Machines (SVMs) are able to separate by a large margin two classes. However, in the case that the one class is drawn from a multimodal distribution (as in the presence of heterogeneity), the classes may be still linearly separated, albeit with a smaller margin. This may be remedied by the use of a non-linear classifier, allowing for larger margins and thus, better generalization. However, while kernel methods, such as Gaussian kernel SVM, provide non-linearity, they lack interpretability when aiming to characterize heterogeneity. Instead, we introduce non-linearity by means of using multiple linear classifiers that form a locally linear hyperplane whose linear segments separate the clusters of negative samples from the positive class (Fig 1). In this way, subjects are explicitly clustered, giving rise to interpretable directions of variability that may be useful in discovering heterogeneity.

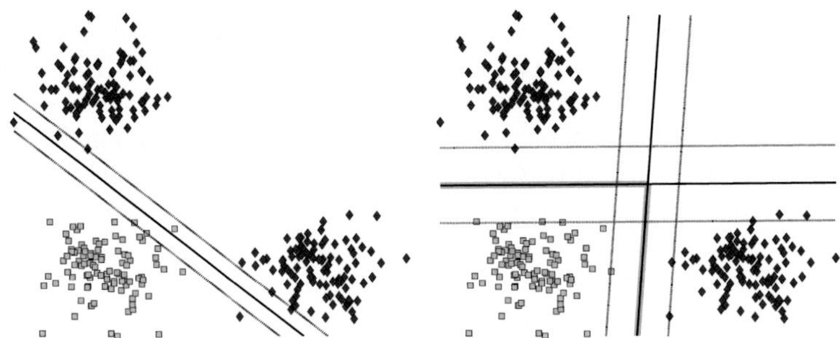

Fig. 1. Heterogeneity due to the presence of two clusters. **Left:** Result obtained by linear SVM (small margin). **Right:** Result obtained by separately classifying each cluster (large margin). Solid lines correspond to the classifier, dashed lines indicate margin, while highlighted linear segments define the separating convex polytope.

Suppose that our dataset consists of n binary labeled d-dimensional data points ($\mathcal{D} = (\mathbf{x}_i, y_i)_{i=1}^n, \mathbf{x}_i \in \mathbb{R}^d$ and $y_i \in \{-1, 1\}$). Without loss of generality, we assign the negative class to be pathologic whose heterogeneity we seek to reveal.[1] Our aim is twofold. First, we aim to estimate k hyperplanes that form a convex polytope that separates the two classes with a large margin. Second, we aim to assign each pathologic sample to the hyperplane that best separates it from the normal controls. Towards fulfilling these aims, we introduce the proposed approach by extending standard linear maximum margin classifiers.

2.1 Margin for Multiple Hyperplanes — Polytope

The hypothesis class of standard linear maximum margin classifiers comprises the set of all linear classifiers $\mathbf{w}$ that separate the two classes by a halfspace. Here, we extend the hypothesis class by considering the set of sets of K hyperplanes, generalizing the geometry of the classifier to that of a convex polytope. Due to the interior/exterior asymmetry of the polytope, it is necessary to confine one class to its interior, while restricting the other class to its exterior. Without loss of generality, we confine the positive class to the interior of the polytope. Thus, the search space $\mathcal{F}_K$ is defined as:

$$\mathcal{F}_K \triangleq \{\{\mathbf{w}_j, b_j\}_{j=1}^K \mid \text{if } y_i = +1 \; \forall j, \mathbf{w}_j^T \mathbf{x}_i + b_j \geq 1, \; \text{if } y_i = -1, \; \exists j : \mathbf{w}_j^T \mathbf{x}_i + b_j \leq -1\}$$

In other words, $\mathcal{F}_K$ comprises all sets of k classifiers such that all classifiers correctly classify all members of the positive class, while for every member of the negative class, there is at least one classifier that correctly classifies it. The latter gives rise to an assignment problem, which can also be seen as a clustering task. Thus, if $\mathbf{S}^- = [s_{i,j}] \in \{0, 1\}^{n^- \times K}$ denotes the binary matrix that describes the assignment of the negative class samples to the jth face of the polytope, then the search space becomes:

$$\mathcal{F}_K(\mathbf{S}^-) \triangleq$$
$$\{\{\mathbf{w}_j, b_j\}_{j=1}^K \mid \text{if } y_i = +1 \; \forall j, \mathbf{w}_j^T \mathbf{x}_i + b_j \geq 1, \; \text{if } y_i = -1, s_{i,j} = 1 : \mathbf{w}_j^T \mathbf{x}_i + b_j \leq -1\}$$

[1] Label reversal would enable us to seek heterogeneity in the control samples.

Given the assignment $\mathbf{S}^-$, there are K margins; each one corresponding to one face of the polytope. Analogous to the SVM formulation, the margin for the jth face of the polytope is $\frac{2}{\|\mathbf{w}_j\|_2}$. However, due to the piecewise nature of the convex polytope, there are multiple notions of margin for the surface of the polytope. In this work, we aim to maximize the average margin across all the faces of the polytope: $\bar{m} = \frac{1}{K}\sum_{j=1}^{K}\frac{2}{\|\mathbf{w}_j\|_2}$ in order to keep the problem tractable. Thus, for a given dataset $\mathcal{D}$ and assignment $\mathbf{S}^-$ for the negative class, the objective of maximizing polytope margin becomes:

$$\begin{aligned} &\underset{\{\mathbf{w}_j, b_j\}_{j=1}^K}{\text{maximize}} \ \frac{1}{K}\sum_{j=1}^{K}\frac{2}{\|\mathbf{w}_j\|_2} && (1)\\ &\text{subject to } \mathbf{w}_j^T\mathbf{x}_i + b_j \geq 1 && \text{if } y_i = +1\\ &\qquad\qquad \mathbf{w}_j^T\mathbf{x}_i + b_j \leq -1 && \text{if } y_i = -1, s_{i,j} = 1 \end{aligned}$$

Note that given the assignments, the objective and the constraints are separable into K independent subproblems. Each subproblem is analogous to the SVM formulation after adding the slack terms $\xi_{i,j}$, or:

$$\begin{aligned} &\underset{\mathbf{w}_j, b_j, \xi}{\text{minimize}} \ \frac{\|\mathbf{w}_j\|_2^2}{2} + C\sum_{i=1}^{n}\xi_{i,j} &&\\ &\text{subject to } \mathbf{w}_j^T\mathbf{x}_i + b_j \geq 1 - \xi_{i,j} && \text{if } y_i = +1\\ &\qquad\qquad \mathbf{w}_j^T\mathbf{x}_i + b_j \leq -1 + \xi_{i,j} && \text{if } y_i = -1, s_{i,j} = 1\\ &\qquad\qquad \xi_{i,j} \geq 0 && \end{aligned}$$

where C is a penalty parameter on the training error. If we now use the definition of the slack terms as $\xi_{i,j} = \max\{0, 1 - y_i(\mathbf{w}_j^T\mathbf{x}_i + b_j)\}$, and consider all hyperplanes ($\{\mathbf{w}_j, b_j\}_{j=1}^K$) at the same time, we get the objective function:

$$\underset{\{\mathbf{w}_j, b_j\}_{j=1}^K}{\text{minimize}} \ \sum_{j=1}^{K}\frac{\|\mathbf{w}_j\|_2^2}{2K} \qquad (2)$$

$$+ C\sum_{\substack{i|y_i=+1\\ j}}\frac{1}{K}\max\{0, 1 - \mathbf{w}_j^T\mathbf{x}_i - b_j\} + C\sum_{\substack{i|y_i=-1\\ j}} s_{i,j}\max\{0, 1 + \mathbf{w}_j^T\mathbf{x}_i + b_j\}$$

So far, we have assumed that the assignment matrix $\mathbf{S}^-$ is known. However, this is not the case in practice and $\mathbf{S}^-$ has to be estimated too. We relax the 0-1 assignment to a soft assignment; $s_{i,j}$ is allowed to be in the interval $[0, 1]$, satisfying the constraint that $\sum_{j=1}^{K} s_{i,j} = 1$ for all i. Given this relaxation the problem becomes convex with respect to the blocks $\{\mathbf{W}, \mathbf{b}\}$ and $\{\mathbf{S}^-\}$.

For $\mathbf{S}^-$ fixed, the solution to $\mathbf{W}$ can be obtained using K calls to a modified version of LIBSVM[2] that allows for adaptive sample weightings, where the weights are given by

$$c_{i,j} = \begin{cases} Cs_{i,j} & \text{if } y_i = -1\\ \frac{C}{K} & \text{if } y_i = +1 \end{cases} \qquad (3)$$

[2] http://www.csie.ntu.edu.tw/~cjlin/libsvmtools/weights/

Algorithm 1. — Max-Margin Multiple Hyperplane

Input: $\mathbf{X} \in \mathbb{R}^{n \times d}$, $\mathbf{y} \in \{-1, +1\}^n$ (training signals), C, K (parameters)
Output: $\mathbf{W} \in \mathbb{R}^{d \times K}$ (Classifier); $\mathbf{S}^- \in \mathbb{R}^{n^- \times K}$ (Soft Clustering Assignment)
Initialization: Set rows of $\mathbf{S}^-$ with probability $\text{Dir}(\mathbf{1}_K)$ (Dirichlet Assignment)
Loop: Repeat until convergence (or a fixed number of iterations)
• Fix $\mathbf{S}^-$ — Solve for $\mathbf{W}$ by LIBSVM[1] (sample weights set by equation (Eq. 3)
• Fix $\mathbf{W}$ — Solve for $\mathbf{S}^-$ by equation (Eq. 4)

For $\mathbf{W}$ fixed, the problem of estimating $\mathbf{S}^-$ is a linear program (LP) of assignment which has infinite solutions when the loss function $\max\{0, 1 + \mathbf{w}_j^T \mathbf{x}_i + b_j\}$ is equal to 0 for multiple classifiers j and for the same sample i. In this case, we choose the solution that is proportional to the margin:

$$s_{i,j} = \begin{cases} 0 & \text{if } \max\{0, 1 + \mathbf{w}_j^T \mathbf{x}_i + b_j\} > 0 \\ \frac{1 + \mathbf{w}_j^T \mathbf{x}_i + b_j}{\sum_j (1 + \mathbf{w}_j^T \mathbf{x}_i + b_j) \mathbf{1}(\max\{0, 1 + \mathbf{w}_j^T \mathbf{x}_i + b_j\} \le 0)} & \text{otherwise} \end{cases} \tag{4}$$

where $\mathbf{1}(\cdot)$ is the indicator function. The previous steps are summarized in Algorithm (1). Note that we don't explicitly give solution for the bias terms b_j. This is because all data points $\mathbf{x}_i$ can include a constant unitary component that corresponds to the bias term. In this case, last element of $\mathbf{w}_j$ contains the solution for the bias term.

Once the polytope classifier $[\mathbf{W}, \mathbf{b}]$ is trained, predicting the class y^* of a new instance $\mathbf{x}^*$ is straightforward:

$$y^* = \text{sign}(\min_j \mathbf{w}_j^T \mathbf{x}^* + b_j) \tag{5}$$

In other words, if $\mathbf{x}^*$ is in the interior of the polytope defined by $\mathbf{W}, \mathbf{b}$, then $\mathbf{w}_j^T \mathbf{x}^* + b_j > 0$ for all faces of the polytope resulting in the prediction $y^* = +1$. Otherwise, if $\mathbf{x}^*$ is in the exterior of the polytope defined by $\mathbf{W}, \mathbf{b}$, then $\mathbf{w}_j^T \mathbf{x}^* + b_j < 0$ for at least one face of the polytope, resulting in the prediction $y^* = -1$. Analogously, the prediction score is simply $\min_j \mathbf{w}_j^T \mathbf{x}^* + b_j$. Also, the clustering assignment $s_{*,j}$ is done in the same manner as Eq. (4).

3 Experimental Validation

We validated our approach on both low dimensional synthetic data and clinical data. For all of our experiments, the features were z-normalized and the default parameter setting ($C = 1$) was used for the LIBSVM subroutine of the proposed method. Thus, the only free parameter to be tuned was the number of polytope faces K (note that $K = 1$ corresponds to linear SVM). Increasing K has two effects on the performance of the algorithm: 1) the model complexity increases; and 2) the number of subject clusters increases. To assess the performance of the method, it is important to check for overfitting and clustering stability. These two effects were examined by examining the out-of-sample classification accuracy and the adjusted Rand clustering overlap index.

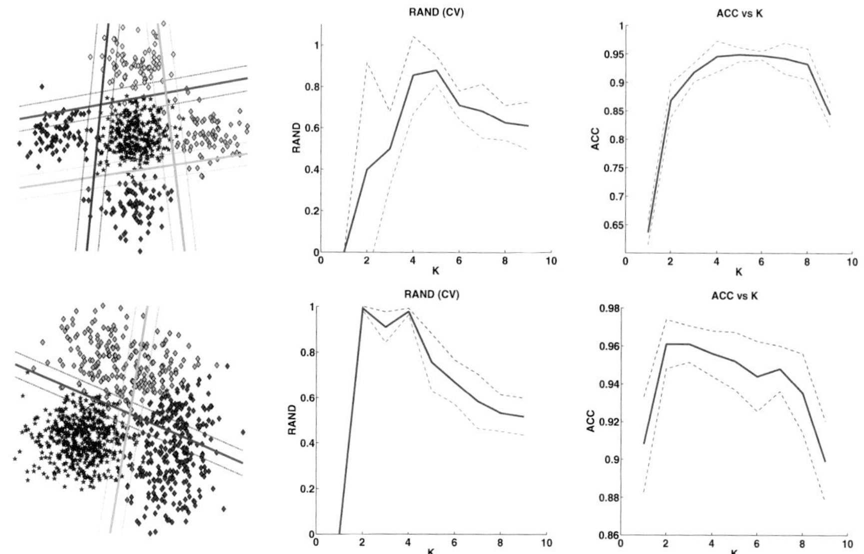

Fig. 2. Sythetic data experiments: **Left:** Data, optimal polytope classifier and the cluster assignments, **Middle:** Cross-validated adjusted Rand index across folds. **Right:** Cross-validated classification accuracy. **Note:** $K = 1$ corresponds to linear SVM.

The first set of experiments consisted of classification of 2 dimensional synthetic data with known ground truth about the underlying clusters. We simulated two cases: 1) a single (+) group with 4 disjoint (−) groups, (Fig. 2 (Top)); and 2) a single (+) group with heterogeneous (−) group distributed along a semicircle (Fig. 2 (Bottom)). The out-of-sample accuracy was computed using 10-fold cross-validation. The cross-validated Rand index was computed using the cluster assignments of the common subjects between folds and taking the average Rand index across all folds. Since only the (−) group was clustered, the (+) samples were ignored in the Rand index calculation.

The synthetic data experiments revealed two key insights. First, it demonstrated that our method is able to separate the two classes, while meaningfully clustering the negative group when K equals the number of underlying subgroups (Fig. 2 (Left)). Second, its performance - as quantified by the Rand index (Fig. 2 (Middle)) and the classification accuracy (Fig. 2 (Right)) - varied smoothly for increasing K, reaching a maximum for the ideal number and thus, allowing us to perform model selection. We note that our method is able to capture heterogeneity in the presence of distinct patterns of variability (case #1), while it provides reasonable estimates in more complex cases (case #2).

Having established a model selection strategy, we evaluate our method using data from the Alzheimer's disease neuroimaging initiative (ADNI[3]). The ADNI dataset comprises the baseline scans of 190 controls (CN), and 133 AD patients. The images were 1.5 Tesla T1-weighted MRI volumetric scans that were processed using an in-house pipeline of 1) bias correction, 2) skull stripping, 3)

[3] `http://adni.loni.usc.edu/`

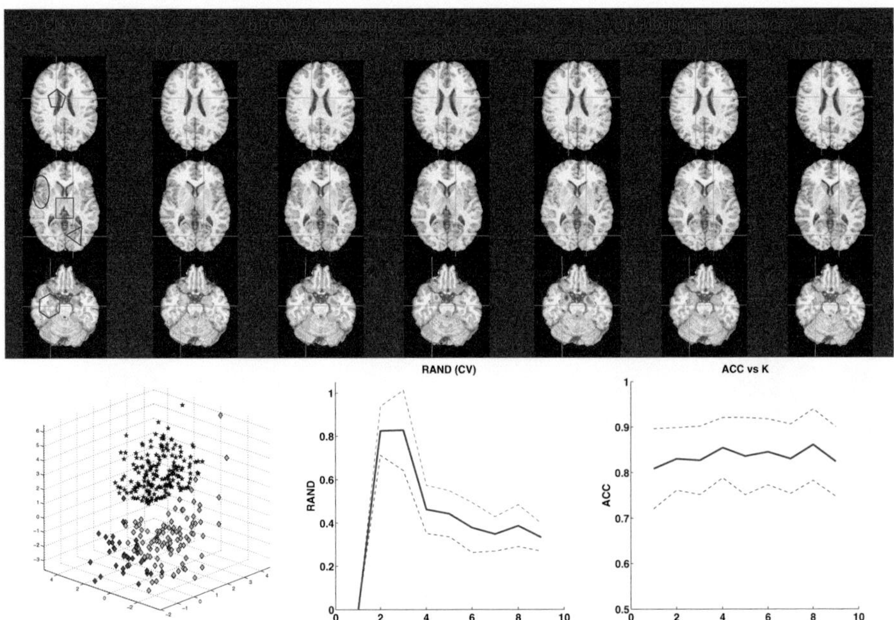

Fig. 3. Top: a) Gray Matter Group Differences (p<0.05) between CN and AD. Shape glossary: pentagon=caudate, ellipse=insula, square=thalamus, triangle=left cuneus, hexagon=right hippocampus **b)** Group differences (p<0.05) between CN vs. 3 subtypes of AD **c)**. Group differences (p<0.05) between 3 different AD subtypes. **Color-map:** Right group compared to left group [Red: loses volume] / [Cyan: gains volume] — **Bottom: Left:** Imaging features projected along the 3 faces of the polytope classifier, CN, AD group 1, AD group 2, AD group 3. **Middle:** Cross-validated adjusted Rand index across folds. **Right:** Cross-validated classification acccuracy.

tissue segmentation and 4) deformable registration that resulted in 151 cortical and sub-cortical anatomical volumes for each subject.

For the ADNI dataset, setting $2 \leq K \leq 9$ resulted in comparable out-of-sample accuracies with statistically insignificant differences (Fig 3 (Bottom right)). The fact that the cross-validation accuracy at $K = 1$ is > 0.80 suggests that the data is already separable and introducing non-linearity will only marginally improve separability. However, the clustering reproducibility analysis revealed that setting $K = 2, 3$ results in stable clusterings (Fig 3 (Bottom middle)) despite the shuffling of samples across folds. This suggests that there may be distinct patterns of variability between controls and these K AD subgroups. The drop of the Rand index for $K > 4$ further strengthens this observation.

In order to investigate the previous observation, we fixed $K = 3$ and found AD subgroups that differed in age composition. Subgroup 1 (G1) comprised younger patients, while subgroups 2 and 3 (G2 and G3) comprised older patients. Then, we performed Voxel-Based Morphometry (VBM) analysis between the CN group and the whole AD population (Fig. 3a); between the CN group and each AD subgroup (Fig. 3b) and between pairs of AD subgroups (Fig. 3c). The VBM analysis allows us to study the structural differences between the respective groups.

Typical CN vs AD VBM analysis reveals a common AD pattern with reduced gray matter in cortical and subcortical regions. However, when examining the AD subgroups separately, we observe a heterogeneous behavior: G1 does not exhibit thalamus or insula atrophy as it is observed for the other two groups; G2 differs from the typical AD pattern in caudate, cuneus and hippocampal regions; and G3 shows a typical AD profile. The differences between the AD subgroups are highlighted by the VBM results shown in Fig. 3c. To further illustrate the heterogeneity of the disease patterns, we projected the imaging features for both the CN and AD subgroups along the $K = 3$ polytope faces. The result is shown in Fig 3 (Bottom left) and emphasizes the segregation of the three subgroups.

4 Conclusion

In this paper, we proposed a novel machine learning method for simultaneous binary classification and subgroup clustering. The proposed method mapped disease heterogeneity in a data-driven way, revealing distinct imaging subtypes in a robust and generalizable fashion.

References

[1] Ashburner, J., Friston, K.J.: Voxel-Based Morphometry–The Methods. NeuroImage 11(6), 805–821 (2000)

[2] Buchanan, R.W., Carpenter, W.T.: Domains of psychopathology: an approach to the reduction of heterogeneity in schizophrenia. The Journal of Nervous and Mental Disease 182(4), 193–204 (1994)

[3] Filipovych, R., Resnick, S.M., Davatzikos, C.: Jointmmcc: Joint maximum-margin classification and clustering of imaging data. IEEE Transactions on Medical Imaging 31(5), 1124–1140 (2012)

[4] Fu, Z., Robles-Kelly, A., Zhou, J.: Mixing linear svms for nonlinear classification. IEEE Transactions on Neural Networks 21(12), 1963–1975 (2010)

[5] Geschwind, D.H., Levitt, P.: Autism spectrum disorders: developmental disconnection syndromes. Current Opinion in Neurobiology 17(1), 103–111 (2007)

[6] Gu, Q., Han, J.: Clustered support vector machines. In: Proceedings of the Sixteenth International Conference on Artificial Intelligence and Statistics, pp. 307–315 (2013)

[7] Koutsouleris, N., et al.: Structural correlates of psychopathological symptom dimensions in schizophrenia: a voxel-based morphometric study. NeuroImage 39(4), 1600–1612 (2008)

[8] Murray, M.E., et al.: Neuropathologically defined subtypes of Alzheimer's disease with distinct clinical characteristics: a retrospective study. The Lancet. Neurology 10(9), 785–796 (2011)

[9] Noh, Y., et al.: Anatomical heterogeneity of alzheimer disease based on cortical thickness on mris. Neurology 83(21), 1936–1944 (2014)

[10] Vemuri, P., et al.: Alzheimer's disease diagnosis in individual subjects using structural MR images: validation studies. NeuroImage 39(3), 1186–1197 (2008)

[11] Whitwell, J.L., et al.: Patterns of atrophy differ among specific subtypes of mild cognitive impairment. Archives of Neurology 64(8), 1130–1138 (2007)

[12] Whitwell, J.L., et al.: Neuroimaging correlates of pathologically defined subtypes of Alzheimer's disease: a case-control study. The Lancet. Neurology 11(10), 868–877 (2012)

Marginal Space Deep Learning: Efficient Architecture for Detection in Volumetric Image Data

Florin C. Ghesu[1,2], Bogdan Georgescu[1], Yefeng Zheng[1], Joachim Hornegger[2], and Dorin Comaniciu[1]

[1] Imaging and Computer Vision, Siemens Corporate Technology, Princeton NJ, USA
[2] Pattern Recognition Lab, Friedrich-Alexander-Universität, Erlangen-Nürnberg

Abstract. Current state-of-the-art techniques for fast and robust parsing of volumetric medical image data exploit large annotated image databases and are typically based on machine learning methods. Two main challenges to be solved are the low efficiency in scanning large volumetric input images and the need for manual engineering of image features. This work proposes Marginal Space Deep Learning (MSDL) as an effective solution, that combines the strengths of efficient object parametrization in hierarchical marginal spaces with the automated feature design of Deep Learning (DL) network architectures. Representation learning through DL automatically identifies, disentangles and learns explanatory factors directly from low-level image data. However, the direct application of DL to volumetric data results in a very high complexity, due to the increased number of transformation parameters. For example, the number of parameters defining a similarity transformation increases to 9 in 3D (3 for location, 3 for orientation and 3 for scale). The mechanism of marginal space learning provides excellent run-time performance by learning classifiers in high probability regions in spaces of gradually increasing dimensionality, for example starting from location only (3D) to location and orientation (6D) and full parameter space (9D). In addition, for parametrized feature computation, we propose to simplify the network by replacing the standard, pre-determined feature sampling pattern with a sparse, adaptive, self-learned pattern. The MSDL framework is evaluated on detecting the aortic heart valve in 3D ultrasound data. The dataset contains 3795 volumes from 150 patients. Our method outperforms the state-of-the-art with an improvement of 36%, running in less than one second. To our knowledge this is the first successful demonstration of the DL potential to detection in full 3D data with parametrized representations.

1 Introduction

Effective data representation is essential for the performance of machine learning algorithms [1]. This motivates a large effort invested into handcrafting features, which encompass the underlying observation in a learning space easy to tackle. For this purpose, complex data preprocessing and transformation pipelines are used to design representations that can ensure an effective learning process.

N. Navab et al. (Eds.): MICCAI 2015, Part I, LNCS 9349, pp. 710–718, 2015.
DOI: 10.1007/978-3-319-24553-9_87

This type of approach is however subject to severe limitations, since it targets exclusively human ingenuity to disentangle and understand prior information hidden in the data and then use such knowledge for feature engineering [2,3].

Representation learning through Deep Learning (DL) addresses these limitations and is aimed to expand the scope and general applicability of machine learning algorithms [1]. This is achieved by applying a mechanism that supports the joint learning of the underlying phenomena and the required features. The capability of automatically identifying and disentangling data-describing attributes directly from low-level image data eliminates the need for complex, manual prerequisites. Hierarchical representations encoded by deep neural networks (NN) [1,4] are used to effectively model this learning approach. Such deep architectures outperform state-of-the-art classifiers on a variety of publicly available benchmark tests [5–8]. Nonetheless, the current applications of these architectures concentrate on 2D data, with no generic extension to any 3D image modality. Capturing the complex appearance of a 3D object and supporting the efficient scanning of high-dimensional spaces are not straightforward, given the increased number of parameters (9 to describe a rigid transformation in 3D).

In this work we propose novel *sparse deep neural networks* for learning parametrized representations from 3D medical image modalities and supporting the effective parsing of volumetric medical image data. We use the concept of network simplification through sparsity injection to replace the standard, predetermined sampling pattern used for handcrafted features, with an adaptive, sparse, self-learned pattern. This brings a considerable increase in computational performance and also serves as regularization against overfitting. Our method for imposing sparsity is based on an iterative learning process using a greedy approach. In order to address the problem of efficiently scanning large parameter spaces for detecting objects in 3D images, we propose MSDL, a novel integration of our sparse deep neural network into the Marginal Space Learning (MSL) pipeline [3]. The Probabilistic Boosting Tree (PBT) classifier [9] used in the MSL framework is replaced with our generic, sparse feature-learning engine, which we apply in marginal spaces of increasing dimensionality to estimate the rigid transformation parameters of the target object. The proposed framework combines the computational efficiency of MSL with the potential of DL architectures. We

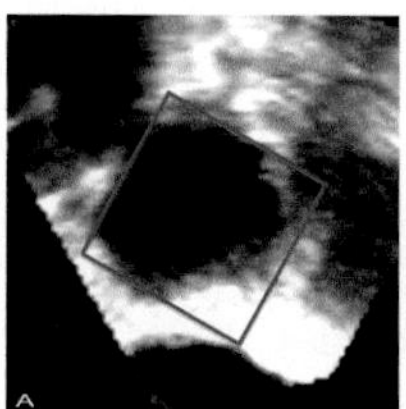

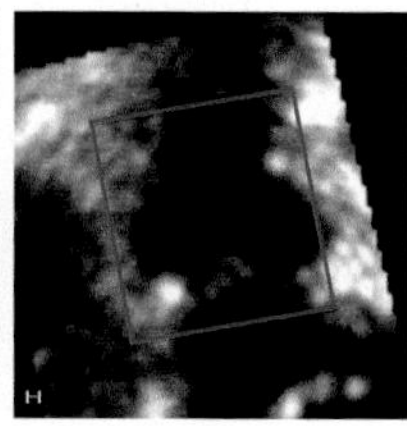

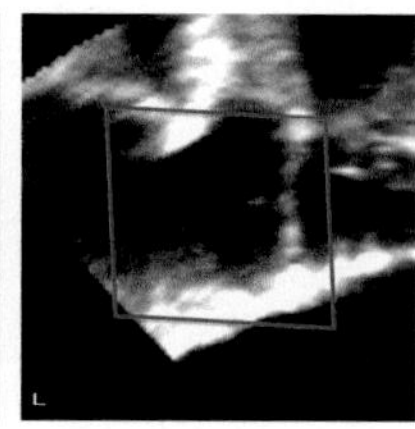

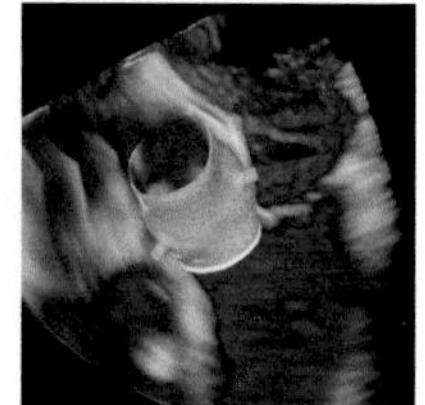

Fig. 1. Planar cuts displaying the bounding box of the aortic valve in a transesophageal ultrasound volume, as well as the 3D geometry of the valve depicted in the last image

evaluate the framework for the problem of detecting the pose of a bounding box enclosing the aortic valve in 3D ultrasound images of the heart (see Figure 1).

2 Related Work

Representation learning, also known under the header of *deep learning* or *feature learning*, is a rapidly developing field in the machine learning community. Correlated with the increase in computational power, recent publications show remarkable result improvements for tasks ranging from speech recognition, object recognition, natural language processing to transfer learning.

For the generic task of object recognition/tracking the impact of this technology started with the break of supremacy of the support vector machines on the MNIST image classification problem [5,6]. This motivated a further improvement through the introduction of multi-column deep neural networks [8] or state-of-the-art network regularization techniques based on a random dropping of units [7]. For more specific tasks within the medical imaging field, stacked sparse autoencoders are applied for multiple organ detection and classification [10]. Using the same pixel-based classification approach, deep neural architectures are also used for the segmentation of brain structures [11]. More recent publications present solutions to emulate 3D learning tasks using 2D feature fusion from predetermined planar cuts [12] or representation sets from random observations.

All investigated methods are devised for 2D or hybrid image modalities, with no extension or direct solution for parsing 3D data. The application of deep learning for object detection with high-dimensional representations is, to the best of our knowledge, not attempted yet.

3 Method

In the following we present our Marginal Space Deep Learning architecture for efficiently estimating the anisotropic similarity transformation parameters of an object in a 3D image. We model the pose of the sought object by using a bounding box, defined by 9 parameters: $\boldsymbol{T} = (t_x, t_y, t_z)$ for the translation, $\boldsymbol{R} = (\phi_x, \phi_y, \phi_z)$ for the orientation and $\boldsymbol{S} = (s_x, s_y, s_z)$ for the anisotropic scale of the object (see Figure 1 for the aortic valve examples). We tackle the object detection problem with machine learning, by training a classifier which can decide if a given parametrized volume patch contains the target object or not.

3.1 Sparse Deep Learning Architectures

A deep Neural Network (NN) is a powerful feature-learning engine, built on hierarchies of data representations [4]. Structurally, the network architecture can be divided into multiple layers, organized and connected hierarchically. In such networks, data representations are obtained by applying learned filters or kernels over representations defined in the previous layer. The same holds for fully

Algorithm 1. Learning algorithm with iterative threshold-enforced sparsity

Pre-training stage using all weights (small # epochs)
for # iterations **do**
  for all filter i with sparsity **do**
    p - proportion of absolute smallest non-zero $w_j^{(i)} \leftarrow 0$
    Re-normalize to preserve $\|\boldsymbol{w}^{(i)}\|_1$
  end for
  Train network on active coefficients (small # epochs)
end for

connected layers, where the kernel size is restricted to the size of the underlying representation map. As such, a deep NN can be defined by the parameters $(\boldsymbol{w}, \boldsymbol{b})$, where $\boldsymbol{w} = (\boldsymbol{w}^{(1)}, \boldsymbol{w}^{(2)}, \cdots, \boldsymbol{w}^{(n)})^\top$ represents the list of concatenated kernel parameters over n layers and $\boldsymbol{b}$ encodes the biases of all neurons contained in the network. The underlying learning problem is supervised, meaning that for a given set of input patches $\boldsymbol{X}$ (i.e. observations), we are given a corresponding set of class assignments $\boldsymbol{y}$, specifying if the patches contain the target object or not. Considering the independence of the input observations, using the Maximum Likelihood Estimation (MLE) method, we learn the network parameters in order to maximize the likelihood function:

$$\left(\hat{\boldsymbol{w}}, \hat{\boldsymbol{b}}\right) = \arg\max_{\boldsymbol{w},\boldsymbol{b}} \mathcal{L}(\boldsymbol{w}, \boldsymbol{b}) = \arg\max_{\boldsymbol{w},\boldsymbol{b}} \prod_{i=1}^{m} p(y^{(i)}|\boldsymbol{x}^{(i)}; \boldsymbol{w}, \boldsymbol{b}), \tag{1}$$

where m represents the number of training samples. For a linear regression model this is equivalent to minimizing the least square distance between the estimated output $\hat{\boldsymbol{y}}$ and the ground truth reference $\boldsymbol{y}$ [4]. We solve this with the Stochastic Gradient Descent (SGD) method, based on the back-propagation algorithm to update the network coefficients according to the computed gradient [13].

As presented in [4], it is conjectured that most networks are oversized for the underlying task. Starting from this observation and the need for optimal runtime performance, we propose a novel network simplification technique based on the injection of sparsity. Defining the network response function as $\mathcal{R}(\,\cdot\,; \boldsymbol{w}, \boldsymbol{b})$, we aim to find a sparsity map $\boldsymbol{s}$ over the network parameters, such that the response residual ϵ given by:

$$\epsilon = \|\mathcal{R}(X; \boldsymbol{w}, \boldsymbol{b}) - \mathcal{R}(X; \boldsymbol{w} \odot \boldsymbol{s}, \boldsymbol{b})\|, \text{ where } s_i \in \mathbb{R}^+, \forall i, \tag{2}$$

is minimal, where $\odot$ denotes the element-wise multiplication of vectors. For this, we apply an iterative learning process, enforcing sparsity in a gradual manner in the layers of the neural network by removing weights with smallest absolute value, in other words with minimal impact on the network response. Algorithm 1 presents the training method.

By using this kind of approach we learn adaptive, sparse features, more specifically in the first layer we learn an adaptive sampling pattern over the input. This is used to replace the standard uniform sampling pattern defined in hand-

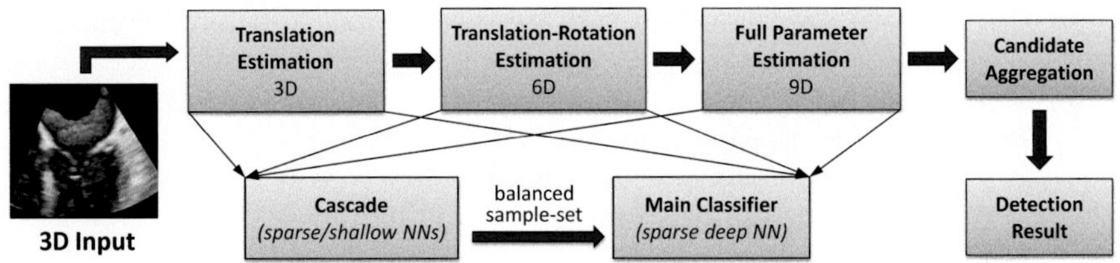

Fig. 2. Scheme depicting the Marginal Space Deep Learning pipeline.

crafted features, eliminating the need for feature engineering. The sparsity enforcement is essential for efficient feature computation under different transformations, bringing a speed-wise improvement of two orders of magnitude. Also, by simplifying the model, the network is more robust against overfitting.

3.2 Marginal Space Deep Learning

In order to perform the detection with the introduced classifier in a given volumetric image I, we aim to find the parameters $(\boldsymbol{T}, \boldsymbol{R}, \boldsymbol{S})$ such that we maximize the posterior probability $p(\boldsymbol{T}, \boldsymbol{R}, \boldsymbol{S}|I)$ over the space of all possible transformations, namely:

$$\left(\hat{\boldsymbol{T}}, \hat{\boldsymbol{R}}, \hat{\boldsymbol{S}}\right) = \arg\max_{\boldsymbol{T}, \boldsymbol{R}, \boldsymbol{S}} p(\boldsymbol{T}, \boldsymbol{R}, \boldsymbol{S}|I). \tag{3}$$

Due to the exponential increase of the number of pose hypotheses with respect to the dimensionality of the pose parameter space, an exhaustive search is impractical. To address this we propose *Marginal Space Deep Learning*, a framework combining the concept of Marginal Space Learning [3] with the presented sparse DL architecture. We split the parameter space in marginal sub-spaces of increasing dimensionality, learning the underlying classifier only in high probability regions, estimating consequently the translation, orientation and scale of the target object. This approach is expressed by the factorization of the posterior probability as:

$$p(\boldsymbol{T}, \boldsymbol{R}, \boldsymbol{S}|I) = p(\boldsymbol{T}|I)p(\boldsymbol{R}|\boldsymbol{T}, I)p(\boldsymbol{S}|\boldsymbol{T}, \boldsymbol{R}, I). \tag{4}$$

We use our sparse DL-based classifier to estimate in turn the posterior probabilities $p(\boldsymbol{T}|I)$, $p(\boldsymbol{T}, \boldsymbol{R}|I)$ and $p(\boldsymbol{T}, \boldsymbol{R}, \boldsymbol{S}|I)$ which are then used to obtain the factors contained in Eq. 4, using the relations: $p(\boldsymbol{R}|\boldsymbol{T}, I) = \frac{p(\boldsymbol{T}, \boldsymbol{R}|I)}{p(\boldsymbol{T}|I)}$ and $p(\boldsymbol{S}|\boldsymbol{T}, \boldsymbol{R}, I) = \frac{p(\boldsymbol{T}, \boldsymbol{R}, \boldsymbol{S}|I)}{p(\boldsymbol{T}, \boldsymbol{R}|I)}$. Using this kind of approach, as shown in [3], we achieve a speed-up of 6 orders of magnitude compared to the exhaustive search.

A challenge arising with the use of deep neural networks as discriminating engine in each stage of the marginal space pipeline, is the high class imbalance. This imbalance can reach ratios of $1 : 1000$ positive to negative samples. A deep architecture cannot be trained with an SGD approach on such an unbalanced set and simply re-weighting the penalties for the network cost function further worsens the vanishing gradient effect. Instead, we propose to use a *negative filtering cascade* of classifiers to hierarchically eliminate as many negatives as possible, while preserving the positive samples across cascade stages. More specifically, in each stage of the cascade we employ a simple, shallow, sparse neural network and manually tune its decision boundary to eliminate the maximum number of true negatives. The remaining samples are propagated through to the next cascade stage where the same filtering procedure is repeated, unless we achieve a balanced sample set. In order to train a network within the cascade, we iterate at epoch level over the complete positive sample set, while at each batch level, we randomly sample the negative space to obtain a balanced training batch. Figure 2 shows a schematic visualization of the complete framework.

4 Experimental Results

For a comprehensive evaluation, we refer to the problem of detecting the aortic valve in 3D Ultrasound volumes and compare the results to the reference state-of-the-art MSL approach [3]. We model the pose of the aortic valve using a bounding box defined in a 9-dimensional parameter space (see Section 3). The dataset used for evaluation stems from 150 patients. Over multiple acquisitions and time frames we extracted a set of 3795 volumes. The size of the frames present a high variation between $100 \times 100 \times 50$ and $250 \times 250 \times 150$ voxels, at an original isotropic resolution of 0.75 mm, adjusted to 3 mm for our experiments. The intensity of each volume is normalized to unit range and annotated with the ground truth box, enclosing the aortic valve at an average scale of $32 \times 32 \times 28$ mm [14]. To set up the training environment for both the proposed MSDL pipeline and the reference MSL approach, the dataset is split randomly at patient level in a $90\% - 10\%$ proportion to determine the training set and the validation examples for testing.

The meta-parameters defining the sub-space sampling and candidate propagation in the MSL pipeline, as well as the network dependent parameters for both the main classifier and the cascade used in each stage are estimated using a grid search. For the proposed MSDL approach we distinguish in our experiments

Table 1. Comparison of the performance of the state-of-the-art MSL [3] and the proposed MSDL framework. The measures used to quantify the quality of the results w.r.t to the groundtruth data are the error of the position of the box and mean corner distance (both measured in millimetres). The superior results are displayed in bold.

	Position Error [mm]				**Corner Error [mm]**			
	Training Data		**Test Data**		**Training Data**		**Test Data**	
	MSL	MSDL	MSL	MSDL	MSL	MSDL	MSL	MSDL
Mean	3.24	**1.66**	3.52	**2.26**	5.73	**3.29**	6.49	**4.57**
Median	2.91	**1.51**	3.31	**2.04**	5.21	**3.02**	6.22	**3.98**
STD	1.83	**0.99**	1.60	**1.13**	2.58	**1.44**	**2.06**	2.07

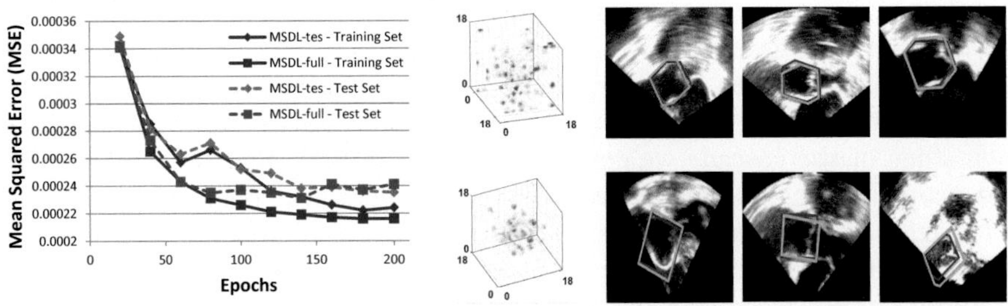

Fig. 3. Left: Plot depicting the error progression on the training set and hold-out test set in the translation stage, with the highlight on the impact of the sparsification on the accuracy. Centre: Example sparse patterns for translation (top) and full space (bottom), note more compact representation for the latter due to better data alignment. Right: Example images showing detection results for different patients from the test set. In order to capture also the underlying image information (i.e. the anatomy) we use 2D planar cuts through the volume. Please note that depending on the cutting plane, the visualized boxes can be viewed as complex polygons (ground-truth shown in red, detection shown in green).

two variants: **MSDL-tes** (using the gradual sparsity enforcement technique) and **MSDL-full** (using all weights in the network). We achieve with 0% false negative rate the sample balancing, using in each cascade less than 3 shallow networks. All used networks are composed of fully connected layers of nodes with sigmoid activation. For all 3 marginal spaces we use the same architecture for the cascade and main classifier; cascade: 2 layers = 5832 (sparse) $\times$ 60 $\times$ 1 and main classifier: 4 layers = 5832 (sparse) $\times$ 150 $\times$ 80 $\times$ 50 $\times$ 1 hidden units.

To quantify the results, we consider the position error of the center of the box and the mean corner distance error (measuring the estimation accuracy of the full transformation). The latter measure represents the average distance between the 8 corners of the detected box and the ground truth box. Table 1 shows the obtained results. The MSDL approach outperforms the state-of-the-art MSL method by improving the mean position error by 36%. Figure 3(left) shows the error measured during training for MSDL-tes and MSDL-full. The error variation on the training data is explained by the injection of sparsity. As can be seen, the enforced sparsity acts as regularization on the hold-out test set, preventing the network from overfitting the data. As such applying sparsity minimally impacts the accuracy on unseen data. In Figure 3(center) we illustrate an example of the learned sparse weights showing a more distributed pattern on the translation stage and more compact (and around the aortic root) on the full parameters estimation stage, due to better data alignment. Qualitative results are depicted in Figure 3(right). In terms of time performance, running the full MSDL pipeline requires under 0.5 seconds compared to 1.9 seconds for MSL (using only CPU). By imposing sparsity we achieve a speed-up of $\times$300 compared to MSDL-full, hence the large computational benefit of the network simplification.

5 Conclusion

This work introduces the MSDL framework for efficient and robust scanning of 3D volumetric medical image data. We proposed to tackle the parameter estimation in hierarchical sub-spaces of increasing dimension by using a deep neural architecture, simplified through sparsity injection. The training of such a classifier is based on an iterative learning process. Within the pipeline, the described learning engine is preceded by a negative sample filtering cascade of shallow sparse neural networks, which addresses the high class imbalance associated with each learning space. By using this kind of approach, the need for complex handcrafted features is eliminated. In terms of performance our method outperforms the state-of-the-art MSL for the problem of detecting the aortic valve in 3D ultrasound images. For future work, we plan on evaluating the framework on more complex problems, with the target of completing the detection pipeline with the full segmentation of the shape.

References

1. Bengio, Y., Courville, A.C., Vincent, P.: Unsupervised Feature Learning and Deep Learning: A Review and New Perspectives. CoRR abs/1206.5538 (2012)
2. Lowe, D.G.: Object recognition from local scale-invariant features. In: ICCV, vol. 2, pp. 1150–1157 (1999)
3. Zheng, Y., Barbu, A., Georgescu, B., Scheuering, M., Comaniciu, D.: Four-Chamber Heart Modeling and Automatic Segmentation for 3-D Cardiac CT Volumes Using Marginal Space Learning and Steerable Features. IEEE TMI 27(11), 1668–1681 (2008)
4. Lecun, Y., Bottou, L., Bengio, Y., Haffner, P.: Gradient-based learning applied to document recognition. Proceedings of the IEEE 86(11), 2278–2324 (1998)
5. Hinton, G.E., Osindero, S., Teh, Y.W.: A Fast Learning Algorithm for Deep Belief Nets. NIPS 18(7), 1527–1554 (2006)
6. Bengio, Y., Lamblin, P., Popovici, D., Larochelle, H., Montréal, U.D., Québec, M.: Greedy layer-wise training of deep networks. In: NIPS. MIT Press (2007)
7. Krizhevsky, A., Sutskever, I., Hinton, G.E.: ImageNet Classification with Deep Convolutional Neural Networks. In: NIPS, pp. 1097–1105. Curran Associates, Inc. (2012)
8. Ciresan, D.C., Meier, U., Schmidhuber, J.: Multi-column Deep Neural Networks for Image Classification. CoRR abs/1202.2745 (2012)
9. Tu, Z.: Probabilistic Boosting-Tree: Learning Discriminative Models for Classification, Recognition, and Clustering. In: IEEE 10th ICCV, ICCV, pp. 1589–1596 (2005)
10. Shin, H.C., Orton, M., Collins, D.J., Doran, S.J., Leach, M.O.: Stacked Autoencoders for Unsupervised Feature Learning and Multiple Organ Detection in a Pilot Study Using 4D Patient Data. IEEE PAMI 35(8), 1930–1943 (2013)
11. Ciresan, D., Giusti, A., Gambardella, L.M., Schmidhuber, J.: Deep Neural Networks Segment Neuronal Membranes in Electron Microscopy Images. In: Pereira, F., Burges, C., Bottou, L., Weinberger, K. (eds.) NIPS, pp. 2843–2851. Curran Associates, Inc. (2012)

12. Roth, H.R., et al.: A New 2.5D Representation for Lymph Node Detection Using Random Sets of Deep Convolutional Neural Network Observations. In: Golland, P., Hata, N., Barillot, C., Hornegger, J., Howe, R. (eds.) MICCAI 2014, Part I. LNCS, vol. 8673, pp. 520–527. Springer, Heidelberg (2014)
13. Rumelhart, D.E., Hinton, G.E., Williams, R.J.: Parallel Distributed Processing: Explorations in the Microstructure of Cognition, pp. 318–362. MIT Press (1986)
14. Ionasec, R.I., Voigt, I., Georgescu, B., Wang, Y., Houle, H., Vega-Higuera, F., Navab, N., Comaniciu, D.: Patient-specific modeling and quantification of the aortic and mitral valves from 4-D cardiac CT and TEE. IEEE Trans. Med. Imaging 29(9), 1636–1651 (2010)

Nonlinear Regression on Riemannian Manifolds and Its Applications to Neuro-Image Analysis*

Monami Banerjee[1], Rudrasis Chakraborty[1], Edward Ofori[2], David Vaillancourt[2], and Baba C. Vemuri[1,**]

[1] Department of CISE, University of Florida, Gainesville, Florida, USA
{monami,rudrasis,vemuri}@cise.ufl.edu
[2] Department of Applied Physiology and Kinesiology, University of Florida, Florida, USA
{eofori,vcourt}@ufl.edu

Abstract. Regression in its most common form where independent and dependent variables are in $\mathbb{R}^n$ is a ubiquitous tool in Sciences and Engineering. Recent advances in Medical Imaging has lead to a wide spread availability of manifold-valued data leading to problems where the independent variables are manifold-valued and dependent are real-valued or vice-versa. The most common method of regression on a manifold is the geodesic regression, which is the counterpart of linear regression in Euclidean space. Often, the relation between the variables is highly complex, and existing most commonly used geodesic regression can prove to be inaccurate. Thus, it is necessary to resort to a non-linear model for regression. In this work we present a novel Kernel based non-linear regression method when the mapping to be estimated is either from $M \to \mathbb{R}^n$ or $\mathbb{R}^n \to M$, where M is a Riemannian manifold. A key advantage of this approach is that there is no requirement for the manifold-valued data to necessarily inherit an ordering from the data in $\mathbb{R}^n$. We present several synthetic and real data experiments along with comparisons to the state-of-the-art geodesic regression method in literature and thus validating the effectiveness of the proposed algorithm.

1 Introduction

Regression is an essential tool for quantitative analysis to find the relation between independent and dependent variables. Here, we are given a training set of both of these variables and we seek a relation between them. When, both of these variables are in Euclidean space, and there is a linear relation between them, i.e., $y_i = ax_i + b$ for a set of $\{x_i, y_i\}$, a common way to solve for the unknowns a and b is using linear least-square estimator, i.e., minimizing the sum of square distances between the two sets of variables over the training set. But, in many real applications, the relation is seldom linear, hence a non-linear least squares estimator or any other sophisticated regression tool like Support Vector Regression [4] can be used.

Often, either of the independent or dependent variables are manifold-valued and lie on a smooth Riemannian manifold. In such instances, *embedding* the manifold valued

* This research was funded in part by the NIH grant NS066340 to BCV.
** Corresponding author.

N. Navab et al. (Eds.): MICCAI 2015, Part I, LNCS 9349, pp. 719–727, 2015.
DOI: 10.1007/978-3-319-24553-9_88

variables in Euclidean space (using the Whitney Embedding [1]) might result in a poor estimation of the underlying model. Also, as any general manifold globally lacks the vector space structure, any linear combination of points on the manifold may not lie on the manifold. For example, suppose the data points lie in a Kendall's shape space [14], then an arbitrary linear combination of the shapes will not yield a point on in the shape space. These problems motivate the development of novel regression methods for manifold-valued data. We will now briefly present earlier work that addresses this problem.

Related Work: Curve fitting on Riemannian manifolds where some notion of ordering is imposed on the manifold-valued data has been quite common lately in literature [2,18,7,13,5,16]. We will present a brief review within the limited space. Samir et al. [18] developed a gradient descent algorithm for time ordered manifold-valued data using a variational formulation, where the cost function entails a data fidelity and a regularization constraint on the curve being sought. This formulation itself is quite common to finding smooth approximation of both real-valued and manifold-valued data. What is then different between methods is the kind of metric used and at times even the data fidelity terms. Each could facilitate the solution sought from an efficiency and/or accuracy.

In the recent past, several researchers [7,13] have proposed geodesic regression on manifolds, as well as non-parametric regression models [2]. The geodesic regression models correspond to linear regression in $\mathbb{R}^n$. Most recently however, a variational spline regression for the manifold of diffeomorphisms was presented in a large deformation diffeomorphic mapping (LDDMM) setting [19]. Fletcher [7] proposed *geodesic regression* to regress manifold-valued data against the real-valued variables. Taking cues from [7], authors in [5], developed a regression technique for points that lie on unit Hilbert sphere. In [2], authors estimate the correlation between shape and age using manifold regression. The aforementioned methods dealt mostly with the independent scalar variable. A multivariate general linear model was proposed in [16] where given a dataset, authors try to model a functional relation from a $\mathbb{R}^n$ to a manifold $\mathcal{M}$. In [15], they extend Canonical Correlation Analysis (CCA) on Riemannian manifold, where both of the variables are manifold-valued. Hong et al. [12] proposed a shooting spline formulation to regress points on Grassmann manifold with reals. In [9], Hinkle et al. has proposed a polynomial regression method formulated as a variational minimization problem on the manifold using covariant derivatives. The minimization tends to covariant differential equations.

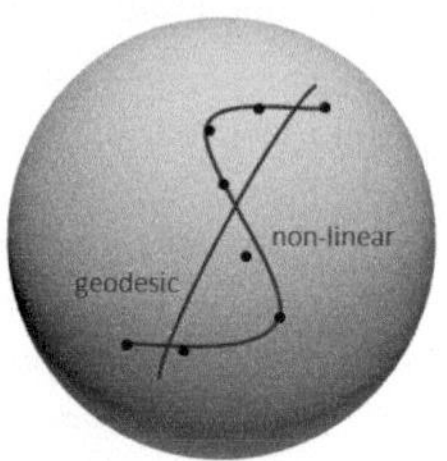

Fig. 1. Examples of nonlinear & geodesic regression.

In this paper, we present a nonlinear kernel regression technique to handle both of the following commonly encountered cases, $\mathbb{R}^n \to \mathcal{M}$ and $\mathcal{M} \to \mathbb{R}^n$. We dub our proposed kernel based regression from $\mathbb{R}^n \to \mathcal{M}$ as *Manifold-valued Kernel Regression* (MVKR). A key advantage of this approach is that there is no requirement for the manifold-valued data to necessarily inherit an ordering from the multi-variate data in $\mathbb{R}^n$, a necessary requirement in most existing methods. An example in Fig. 1 depicts the usefullness in terms of accuracy in using the nonlinear regression over the geodesic regression model.

2 Methodology

Regression is ubiquitous in scientific analysis where given a set of tuples $\{x_i, y_i\}_{i=1}^N \subset \mathcal{X} \times \mathcal{Y}$, the goal is to find a functional relation between $\{x_i\}_{i=1}^N$ and $\{y_i\}_{i=1}^N$. Here, one variable is the observed data (*independent variable*) and the other one is the response (*dependent variable*). We propose a kernel interpolation to find the relation between observed data and responses where one of them lies in the Euclidean space and the other one lies on a Riemannian manifold. Given $\{x_i\}_{i=1}^N \subset \mathbb{R}^n$ and $\{y_i\}_{i=1}^N \subset \mathcal{M}$, we pose the two cases as following interpolation problems:

- **Manifold valued independent variable:** Find a function $f : \mathcal{M} \to \mathbb{R}^n$ such that $x_i = f(y_i), \forall i$.
- **Manifold valued dependent variable:** Find a function $h : \mathbb{R}^n \to \mathcal{M}$ such that $y_i = h(x_i), \forall i$.

In both the above cases, $\mathcal{M}$ is a Riemannian manifold equipped with a Riemannian metric g. We will address these above two problems separately in the following subsections.

2.1 Manifold Valued Independent Variable

Given $\{x_i, y_i\}_{i=1}^N$ as before, we try to model the function $\hat{f} : \mathcal{M} \to \mathbb{R}^n$ by minimizing the following error function: $E = \frac{1}{N}\sum_{i=1}^N ||\hat{x}_i - x_i||^2$ where, $\hat{x}_i = \hat{f}(y_i) = \sum_{j=1}^k \mathcal{K}(c_j, y_i)t_j$. Here $\{c_j\}_{j=1}^k \subset \mathcal{M}$ and $\{t_j\}_{j=1}^k \subset \mathbb{R}^n$ are the *representatives* on $\mathcal{M}$ and $\mathbb{R}^n$ respectively. $\mathcal{K} : \mathcal{M} \times \mathcal{M} \to \mathbb{R}$ is the *kernel function*. Thus, $\hat{x}$, the approximation of x is the weighted mean of t_j's. The weights here are computed by using a suitable kernel function and representatives, $\{c_j\}_{j=1}^k$, on the manifold, $\mathcal{M}$. We learn the $\{t_j\}_{j=1}^k$ by minimizing the above error function, E, whereas, $\{c_j\}_{j=1}^k$ are taken to be the cluster representatives. Here, we used the steepest descent technique to estimate $\{t_j\}_{j=1}^k$. The gradient of the objective function with respect to t_j is given by, $\nabla_{t_j} E = \frac{2}{N}\sum_{i=1}^N (\hat{x}_i - x_i)\mathcal{K}(c_j, y_i)$.

Note that, as the objective function, E is convex in t_j, the global minimum can be achieved using a steepest descent technique. In a similar fashion, we can initialize c_j to be the cluster representatives and estimate them along the gradient direction. The gradient of the objective function with respect to c_j is given by, $\nabla_{c_j} E = \frac{2\, t_j}{N}\sum_{i=1}^N (\hat{x}_i - x_i)\nabla_{c_j}\mathcal{K}(c_j, y_i)$.

Since any kernel function depends on the underlying metric, if the underlying manifold $\mathcal{M}$ has a closed form expression for the geodesic distance, so will $\nabla_{c_j}\mathcal{K}(c_j, y_i)$. In this work, we use the kernel $\mathcal{K}(c, y) = \exp\{-\frac{b}{2\sigma^2}\, d(c, y)^2\}$, where b, σ^2 are the kernel parameters, and $d(.,.)$ is the geodesic distance on $\mathcal{M}$. Then, $\nabla_{c_j}\mathcal{K}(c_j, y_i) = \frac{b}{2\sigma^2}\mathcal{K}(c_j, y_i)Log_{c_j} y_i$ where, $Log_{c_j} y_i$ is the Riemannian inverse exponential map. Note that, the b value is tuned according to the structure of the dataset. By drawing an analogy with the Gaussian kernel on $\mathbb{R}^n$, we chose a small b value for a well clustered data, and a high b value otherwise. The parameter σ^2 is taken as the variance over the training data.

2.2 Manifold Valued Dependent Variable

Given $\{x_i, y_i\}_{i=1}^N$ as above, we now try to model the function $\hat{h} : \mathbb{R}^n \to \mathcal{M}$ such that $y_i \approx \hat{h}(x_i)$. As before, let $\mathcal{M}$ be equipped with a Riemannian metric g. Also, let $d : \mathcal{M} \times \mathcal{M} \to \mathbb{R}$ be the geodesic distance on $\mathcal{M}$ defined as follows: $d(y_i, y_j)^2 = g_{y_i}(Log_{y_i} y_j, Log_{y_i} y_j)$, where $Log_{y_i} y_j$ is the inverse-exponential map. We can now estimate h by minimizing the following error function: $E = \frac{1}{N}\sum_{i=1}^N d(\hat{y}_i, y_i)^2$ where,

$$\hat{y}_i = \hat{h}(x_i) = \arg\min_{\mu \in \mathcal{M}} \sum_{j=1}^k \mathcal{K}_{Euc}(t_j, x_i)\, d(c_j, \mu)^2 \tag{1}$$

Analogous to the manifold valued independent variable case, here $c_j \in \mathcal{M}$ and $t_j \in \mathbb{R}^n$, $\forall j$. $\mathcal{K}_{Euc} : \mathbb{R}^n \times \mathbb{R}^n \to \mathbb{R}$ is the kernel function on the Euclidean space. Thus, y_i is estimated as the weighted Fréchet mean (FM) [8] of the representatives, $\{c_j\}_{j=1}^k$, where weights are given by the kernel function, yielding the MVKR. We use $\{t_j\}_{j=1}^k$ as the cluster representatives and estimate $\{c_j\}_{j=1}^k$ using the steepest descent on the objective function. The gradient direction of E with respect to c_j is given by,

$$\nabla_{c_j} E = -\frac{2}{N}\sum_{i=1}^N Log_{\hat{y}_i} y_i \, \nabla_{c_j} \hat{y}_i. \tag{2}$$

As c_j and $\hat{y}_i$ both are on $\mathcal{M}$, we will use charts to compute $\nabla_{c_j}\hat{y}_i$. Let $\mathcal{M}$ be an m dimensional manifold. Consider two charts (U, Φ) and (V, Ψ) containing c_j and $\hat{y}_i$, respectively. By fixing x_i, we can take $\hat{y}_i$ as a function of c_j's. Let the function be F. Then, $\nabla_{c_j}\hat{y}_i$ can be defined as $\nabla_{c_j}\hat{y}_i := \nabla_{\tilde{c}_j} G$, where $\tilde{c}_j = \Phi(c_j)$ and $G = \Psi \circ F \circ \Phi^{-1} : \mathbb{R}^m \to \mathbb{R}^m$. Hence, $\nabla_{\tilde{c}_j} G$ is the Jacobian of G. Note that, $\nabla_{c_j} E \in T_{c_j}\mathcal{M}$, so in order to make the RHS of equation 2 to be in $T_{c_j}\mathcal{M}$, we use parallel transport of $Log_{\hat{y}_i} y_i$ from $\hat{y}_i$ to c_j. For a general Riemannian manifold $\mathcal{M}$, we can approximate this parallel transport, $\Lambda_{c_j} Log_{\hat{y}_i} y_i$ as $\Lambda_{c_j} Log_{\hat{y}_i} y_i \approx Log_{c_j} y_i - Log_{c_j} \hat{y}_i$.

Since there is no closed form solution for the weighted FM of more than two samples on general Riemannian manifolds, computation of $\nabla_{\tilde{c}_j} G$, or the Jacobian of G, is not straightforward. Hence, in spirit of [16,11], we approximate Equation 1 as $\hat{y}_i \approx Exp_p\big(\sum_{j=1}^k \mathcal{K}_{Euc}(t_j, x_i) Log_p c_j\big)$, where $p \in \mathcal{M}$ is any arbitrary point on M, and Exp is the Riemannian Exponential map. In the absence of such an approximation, the problem would become analytically intractable as estimating both the control points and the FM jointly is nontrivial. With this simplification, $\nabla_{c_j}\hat{y}_i = \mathcal{K}_{Euc}(t_j, x_i) \times I_m$, where I_m is the identity matrix of size m. For the case of $P(n)$, we resort to use of the efficient recursive FM estimator in [10] and a similar one for and S^n.

3 Experimental Results

We now evaluate the performance of the proposed regression method on both synthetic and real datasets. In the following two subsections, we will experimentally show effectiveness of our method to (1) regress real vector-valued dependent variables against manifold-valued independent variables and (2) regress manifold-valued dependent variables against real vector-valued independent variables. In order to quantify the performance of our $\mathbb{R}^n$ to manifold regression, we use the R^2 statistical measure and the $p-$value. The R^2 statistical measure on a manifold is defined in [7] and repeated here for convenience. Let $\{y_i\}_{i=1}^N$ be the manifold-valued data with its corresponding predicted value to be $\{\hat{y}_i\}_{i=1}^N$. Let the *unexplained variance* be defined as $\sum_{i=1}^N d(y_i, \hat{y}_i)^2$. Then, the R^2 statistic is defined as: $R^2 = 1 - \frac{\text{unexplained variance}}{\text{data variance}}$. The value of R^2 statistic lies in the interval $[0, 1]$, and a value close to one in general denotes better regression performance. We use a $t-$test over 30 independent runs to reject the null hypothesis, H_0: *mean of the unexplained variance is not less than the mean of the data variance* with a significance level of 0.001. For the manifold to $\mathbb{R}^n$ regression, we present an application to the classification on Parkinson's dataset and report the average classification accuracy over 30 runs.

3.1 Manifold Valued Independent Variable

In this section, we present results of our regression scheme applied to classification of MR T2 brain scans obtained from, (1) controls (CON), and patients with (2) essential tremor (ET), and (3) Parkinson's disease (PD). We aim to automatically discriminate between these three classes, using features derived from the data.

In [20], authors have used DTI based analysis, specifically the scalar-valued features to address the problem of movement disorder classification. In this section, we use the shape of the Substatia Nigra across the input population as our key discriminatory feature. Sample Substantia Nigra shapes for the three classes are shown in Fig. 2. The shapes of interest are first segmented and then are converted into a probability density function. Then using the square root density parameterization, this shape can be represented as a point on the unit Hilbert sphere using the Schrodinger Distance Transform (SDT) [3].

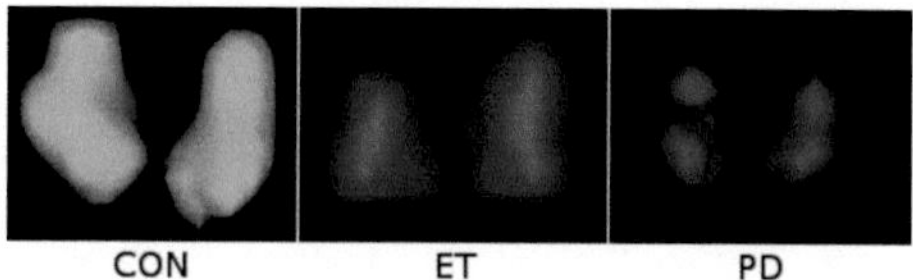

Fig. 2. Examples of Substantia Nigra

The key feature used in our classification of the aforementioned disease classes is the shape of the Substantia Nigra. The Substantia Nigra was hand-segmented from all rigidly pre-aligned datasets, consisting of 25 controls, 15 ET and 24 PD images. The T2 brain scans were acquired using a 3T Phillips MR scanner with the following parameters: $TR = 774\,ms, TE = 86\,ms$ and voxel size = $2 \times 2 \times 2\,mm^3$.

We first collected random (point) samples on the boundary of each 3-D Substantia Nigra shape, and applied the SDT to represent each shape as a point on the unit hypersphere. The size of the ROI for the 3-D shape of interest was set to $(28 \times 28 \times 15)mm^3$, resulting in a 11760-dimensional unit vectors using SDT. Therefore, the samples now live on the $\mathbb{S}^{11759}$ manifold.

We randomly selected 10 Control, 10 PD and 5 ET images as the test set, and used the rest of the data for training. The details of our classification method are described next. First, we regress the dependent variable against the independent variable on $\mathbb{S}^{11759}$. In order to make the dependent variable lie in $[0, 1]$, we apply the logistic function $\mathcal{L}$ on the dependent variable $f(y)$. Then, we classify a point y as belonging to class-1, if $\mathcal{L}(f(y)) < 0.5$, else we assign it to class-2. The classification task is repeated 30 times using various randomly chosen training sets and the average accuracy is reported. The results are shown in Table 1. We compare our method with the standard PCA and PGA (Principal Geodesic Analysis) [6], and report the accuracy of classification.

Table 1. Result based on Substantia Nigra shape

	Control vs. ET			Control vs. PD			PD vs. ET		
	Proposed	PGA	PCA	Proposed	PGA	PCA	Proposed	PGA	PCA
Accuracy	**100.00**	90.14	75.69	**95.26**	92.95	67.32	85.71	**87.58**	64.60

The results show that our proposed method performs well compared to the other two in classifying Control versus PD and ET. In case of PD vs. ET classification, our method gives slightly lower accuracy compared to PGA.

3.2 Manifold Valued Dependent Variable

In this section, we applied our MVKR method on synthetic and real datasets. In all of these experiments, we have made a comparison with the recently proposed MGLM method in [16] and MKRE (Manifold kernel regression estimator) in [2]. As MVKR and MKRE both use the same Nadaraya-Watson kernel, we have used the same choice of parameters for both of these methods.

Table 2. Synthetic data results

	MVKR	MGLM	MKRE
Train Error	**0.00**	0.60	0.07
Test Error	**0.00**	0.61	0.07
R^2 Stat.	**1.00**	0.29	0.92
$p-$value	$<$ **0.001**	$<$ **0.001**	$<$ **0.001**

Synthetic Data Experiment: For this experiment, we synthesized a dataset $\{\mathbf{x}_i, y_i\}_{i=1}^{500} \subset \mathbb{R}^2 \times S^2$ by defining a function $h : \mathbf{x}_i = [\theta_i, \phi_i] \rightarrow y_i$ as follows: $h([\theta_i, \phi_i]) := (\cos(\theta_i) \cos(\phi_i), \cos(\theta_i)\sin(\phi_i), \sin(\theta_i))$ where $\theta_i \in [0, \pi/2)$, $\phi_i \in [0, 2\pi]$, $\forall i$. Thus, all the y_is are on the northern hemisphere of the $2-$sphere, so FM is uniquely defined. We have partitioned this dataset into 90%, 10% for training and testing respectively. The $p-$value and average R^2 statistics are reported in Table 2 over 30 runs. From these figures, we can clearly see that our MVKR method performs better in comparison to MGLM [16] and gives comprative performance to MKRE [2].

OASIS Dataset [17]: We used the publicly available OASIS data [17] to regress manifold-valued data with reals. This dataset consists of T1 MR brain scans of subjects with ages from 18 to 96 including individuals with early stage Alzheimer's Disease.

We randomly chose 4 brain scans from each of the decades in the $18 - 96$ age group, totalling 36 brain images, out of which 32 were randomly chosen and used as training and the rest were used as the test set. Corpus callosum (CC) shapes of individuals of varying ages are shown in Fig. 3. We seek to model the relationship between age and shape of the CC, captured using three different features as described in the following. From each of the brain images of the 36 individuals, we construct three different data representations as follows. (1) We segmented out the CC from the brain images. Then, we take the boundary of the CC and

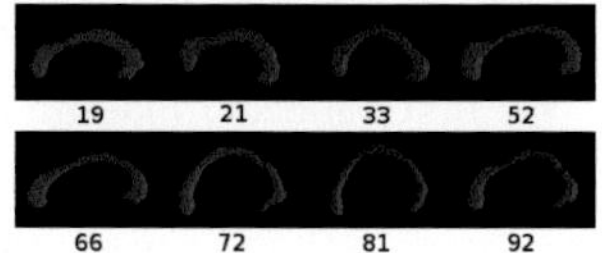

Fig. 3. Corpus callosum shapes

map it to S^{24575} using the SDT [3]. (2) After segmenting out the CC, we used a set of landmark points on the boundary and map each of these point sets into the Kendall's shape space [14], which is a *complex projective space*. (3) We took the whole brain image and computed the normalized histogram and used the square root of the normalized histogram to map each image on to S^{255}.

The average R^2 statistics of 30 runs on each of these three representations of the chosen OASIS datasets is given in Table 3. From the table, it is evident that the performance of MVKR is significantly better compared to the MGLM method. It should be noted that the R^2 statistics reported by MVKR is not very high (not close to 1). But it can be argued that, as we are only considering relation between age and the manifold-valued data, the relation is highly nonlinear.

Table 3. Results on the OASIS dataset

	Dataset using SDT			Kendall's shape space			Dataset using histogram		
	MVKR	MGLM	MKRE	MVKR	MGLM	MKRE	MVKR	MGLM	MKRE
R^2 Stat.	**0.49**	0.05	0.46	**0.35**	-0.27	0.33	**0.48**	-0.18	0.40
$p-$value	$<$ **0.001**	$<$ **0.001**	$<$ **0.001**	$<$ **0.001**	$>$ 0.001	$<$ **0.001**	$<$ **0.001**	$>$ 0.001	$<$ **0.001**

Hence, it is not possible to truly capture the "relation in full" based on age alone, of an individual. Also, the brain images are chosen randomly without considering gender, educational background or even symptoms of AD, all of which makes the relation between age and the shape of the CC very complex. So, given these confounding parameters that could influence the structure, the R^2 statistics for MVKR depicts a significantly good performance. Note that, for second and third variant of this dataset, MGLM results in a negative R^2 statistic. From the definition of R^2 statistics, we can see that a negative value indicates that the regressor performed worse than the most trivial choice, which is FM of the dataset for any given test point x (value of the independent variable).

Thus, MGLM's unsatisfactory performance on these datasets indicates that a linear regressor is inept for this problem and motivates the use of a nonlinear regression technique such as the one presented here. The $p-$values reported in Table 3 indicate the higher statistical significance and hence the superior performance of our MVKR method. In comparison to MKRE, the performance of MVKR is consistently better, though not by a significant amount.

So, in summary, as for most of the real cases, the data on the manifold do not lie close to a geodesic, the performance of MGLM is not comparable to MVKR. This is due to the fact that MGLM assumes that data lie close to a geodesic while MVKR does not require any such assumption. When the data lie or are close to a geodesic, MVKR and MGLM have comparable performance as can be seen from the following toy example. In this example, we have used the sythetic data on $P(3)$, the space of symmetric positive definite matrices, in [16]. The R^2 statistics value for MGLM and MVKR are 0.98 and 0.99 respectively. We would also like to point out that although compared to MKRE, performance of MVKR is not significantly better, MVKR is applicable for $\mathbb{R}^n$ to M regression and vice versa, whereas, the method in [2] is applicable only to regression for the case of $\mathbb{R}$ to M.

4 Conclusions

In this paper, we presented a novel nonlinear regression technique for estimating the functional relationship between manifold-valued independent variables and $\mathbb{R}^n$ valued dependent variables and vice versa. Earlier work in this area involved use of geodesic regression and is ill suited for many situations involving complex relationships between the aforementioned independent and dependent variables. Our method involved a Kernel-based technique and we presented several experiments to demonstrate the performance of our methods in comparison to the state-of-the-art (MGLM method) on a variety of data sets. Results depict that our method yields superior performance for both the applications namely, classification of movement disorders and finding a correlation between age and CC shape of patients from the OASIS database.

References

1. Adachi, M., Hudson, K.: Embeddings and immersions. American Mathematical Soc. (2012)
2. Davis, B.C., Fletcher, P.T., et al.: Population shape regression from random design data. In: IEEE ICCV, pp. 1–7 (2007)
3. Deng, Y., Rangarajan, A., et al.: A Riemannian framework for matching point clouds represented by the Schrodinger distance transform. In: IEEE CVPR, pp. 3756–3761 (2014)
4. Drucker, H., Burges, C.J., et al.: Support vector regression machines. In: NIPS, pp. 155–161 (1997)
5. Du, J., Goh, A., et al.: Geodesic regression on orientation distribution functions with its application to an aging study. Neuroimage, 416–426 (2014)
6. Fletcher, P., Lu, C., et al.: Principal geodesic analysis for the study of nonlinear statistics of shape. In: IEEE TMI, pp. 995–1005 (2004)
7. Fletcher, P.T.: Geodesic regression and the theory of least squares on Riemannian manifolds. International Journal of Computer Vision, 171–185 (2013)
8. Fréchet, M.: Les éléments aléatoires de nature quelconque dans un espace distancié. Annales de l'institut Henri Poincaré, pp. 215–310 (1948)
9. Hinkle, J., Muralidharan, P., Fletcher, P.T., Joshi, S.: Polynomial regression on Riemannian manifolds. In: Fitzgibbon, A., Lazebnik, S., Perona, P., Sato, Y., Schmid, C. (eds.) ECCV 2012, Part III. LNCS, vol. 7574, pp. 1–14. Springer, Heidelberg (2012)
10. Ho, J., Cheng, G., et al.: Recursive Karcher expectation estimators and geometric law of large numbers. In: AISTATS, pp. 325–332 (2013)
11. Ho, J., Xie, Y., et al.: On a nonlinear generalization of sparse coding and dictionary learning. In: ICML, pp. 1480–1488 (2013)
12. Hong, Y., Kwitt, R., Singh, N., Davis, B., Vasconcelos, N., Niethammer, M.: Geodesic regression on the Grassmannian. In: Fleet, D., Pajdla, T., Schiele, B., Tuytelaars, T. (eds.) ECCV 2014, Part II. LNCS, vol. 8690, pp. 632–646. Springer, Heidelberg (2014)
13. Hong, Y., Singh, N., Kwitt, R., Niethammer, M.: Time-warped geodesic regression. In: Golland, P., Hata, N., Barillot, C., Hornegger, J., Howe, R. (eds.) MICCAI 2014, Part II. LNCS, vol. 8674, pp. 105–112. Springer, Heidelberg (2014)
14. Kendall, D.: A survey of the statistical theory of shape. Stat. Science, 87–99 (1989)
15. Kim, H.J., Adluru, N., Bendlin, B.B., Johnson, S.C., Vemuri, B.C., Singh, V.: Canonical Correlation analysis on Riemannian Manifolds and its Applications. In: Fleet, D., Pajdla, T., Schiele, B., Tuytelaars, T. (eds.) ECCV 2014, Part II. LNCS, vol. 8690, pp. 251–267. Springer, Heidelberg (2014)

16. Kim, H.J., Bendlin, B.B., et al.: MGLM on Riemannian manifolds with applications to statistical analysis of diffusion weighted images. In: IEEE CVPR, pp. 2705–2712 (2014)
17. Marcus, D.S., Wang, T.H., et al.: OASIS: cross-sectional mri data in young, middle aged, nondemented, and demented older adults. Journal of Cognitive Neuroscience, 1498–1507 (2007)
18. Samir, C., Absil, P.-A., et al.: A gradient-descent method for curve fitting on Riemannian manifolds. Foundations of Comput. Mathematics, 49–73 (2012)
19. Singh, N., Niethammer, M.: Splines for diffeomorphic image regression. In: Golland, P., Hata, N., Barillot, C., Hornegger, J., Howe, R. (eds.) MICCAI 2014, Part II. LNCS, vol. 8674, pp. 121–129. Springer, Heidelberg (2014)
20. Vaillancourt, D., Spraker, M., et al.: High-resolution diffusion tensor imaging in the substantia nigra of de novo parkinson disease. Neurology, 1378–1384 (2009)

Author Index

Printed in the United States
By Bookmasters